With the Assistance of

MARGARET R. BECKLAKE, M.D. (Witwatersrand), M.D. (Hon.) (Witwatersrand), F.R.C.P, F.R.C.P. (C).

Professor, Departments of Epidemiology and Biostatistics and of Medicine, McGill University, Montreal and
Career Investigator, Medical Research Council of Canada.
(Section on Pulmonary Function Tests in Epidemiology, Chapter 5)

MOIRA CHAN-YEUNG, M.B. B.S. (Hong Kong), F.R.C.P. (Edin.), F.R.C.P. (C).

Professor of Medicine; Head of the Respiratory Division, Vancouver General Hospital, University of British Columbia, Vancouver.
(Section on Challenge Tests to the Lung, Chapter 5)

JOHN A. FLEETHAM, M.B. (London), F.R.C.P. (C).

Associate Professor of Medicine; Director, Respiratory Sleep Disorder Clinic, and Respiratory Division, UBC Health Sciences Centre Hospital, University of British Columbia, Vancouver.
(Section on Sleep Disorders, Chapter 4)

JAMES C. HOGG, M.D. (Manitoba), Ph.D. (McGill), F.R.C.P. (C).

Professor of Pathology; Director, Pulmonary Research Laboratory, St. Paul's Hospital, University of British Columbia, Vancouver.
(Chapter 1)

MALCOLM KING, Ph.D. (McGill)

Associate Research Professor, Pulmonary Defense Group, University of Alberta, Edmonton.
(Section on Mucus and Mucocilary Clearance, Chapter 3)

JOHN R. LEDSOME, M.D. (Edin.)

Head, Department of Physiology, University of British Columbia, Vancouver.
(Chapter 2)

JEREMY D. ROAD, M.D. (Saskatoon), F.R.C.P. (C).

Assistant Professor, Department of Medicine, UBC Health Sciences Centre Hospital, University of British Columbia, Vancouver.
(Chapter 22)

RESPIRATORY FUNCTION IN DISEASE

THIRD EDITION

DAVID V. BATES

M.D. (Cantab), F.R.C.P. (C), F.R.C.P. (London), F.A.C.P., F.R.S. (C).

Professor of Medicine & Physiology, and Emeritus Dean, Faculty of Medicine;
and Physician, UBC Health Sciences Centre Hospital, University of British Columbia;
Sometime Senior Physician, Royal Victoria Hospital, and Chairman, Department of Physiology,
McGill University, Montreal, Canada

1989
W. B. SAUNDERS COMPANY
Harcourt Brace Jovanovich, Inc.
Philadelphia • London • Toronto • Montreal • Sydney • Tokyo

W. B. SAUNDERS COMPANY
Harcourt Brace Jovanovich, Inc.

The Curtis Center
Independence Square West
Philadelphia, PA 19106

Library of Congress Cataloging-in-Publication Data

Bates, David V.

Respiratory function in disease/David V. Bates—3rd ed.   p.   cm.

Includes bibliographies.

1. Lungs—Diseases.   I. Title. [DNLM: 1. Lung Diseases—
   physiopathology.   2. Respiratory Tract Diseases—
   physiopathology. WF 140 B329r]

RC756.B36 1989   616.2′4–dc19   DNLM/DLC

ISBN 0–7216–1592–9   88–15844

Editor: William Lamsback
Designer: Karen O'Keefe
Production Manager: Carolyn Naylor
Manuscript Editor: Mark Crowe
Cover Design: Paul Fry
Illustration Coordinator: Walter Verbitski

Listed here are the latest translated editions of this book together with the language of the translation and the publisher.

Italian (1st Edition)—Piccin Editore, Padova, Italy

Japanese (2nd Edition)—Hirokawa Publishing Co., Tokyo, Japan

Respiratory Function in Disease   ISBN 0–7216–1592–9

Last digit is the print number: 9   8   7   6   5   4   3   2   1

This book is dedicated to the memory of
RONALD V. CHRISTIE
1902–1986

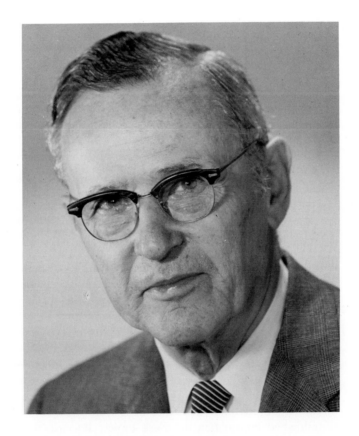

If a man will begin with certainties, he shall end in doubts; but if he will be content to begin with doubts, he shall end in certainties.

FRANCIS BACON
Advancement of Learning (1605)

PREFACE
to the Third Edition

The second edition of this book, published in 1971, was very different in content from the first edition, which had been published 7 years before. This edition is completely different from the second and is intended to serve a somewhat different purpose from its two predecessors. What the three editions have in common is a philosophy that for graduate teaching, statements should be carefully referenced to the literature, and opinion should be clearly identifiable as such. All but a handful of the bibliography refers to work published since 1970; its volume testifies to the very considerable effort that has proceeded internationally to explore the derangements of function that occur in every clinical situation. Yet the reader should be cautioned that the literature coverage is not encyclopedic; only about half of the references that I have annotated have been included, and many clinical and specialty medical journals have not been systematically searched.

The reporting of pulmonary function tests can be done at several different levels of sophistication. The simplest is to be content with noting airflow limitation, or changes in lung volume indicative of "restrictive" disease, and not to attempt to provide any further information. The second level is to be able to answer such questions as "Are these findings typical of simple silicosis?" "Is the dyspnea after a myocardial infarction likely to be due to pulmonary congestion or to airway disease?" "Are the findings typical of those found in stage 2 sarcoidosis in non-smokers?" "Are the findings typical of those found in someone 3 months after recovery from adult respiratory distress syndrome?" To give authoritative answers to these (and hundreds of similar) questions requires a detailed knowledge of the published information on these topics. Because the physician rarely has time to look up the answers by consulting original papers, all too often only a very superficial report is written. This edition is designed to be a guide to the second level of pulmonary function test reporting.

The interpretation of studies of regional lung function, of detailed exercise studies, or of lung mechanics (what might be termed "third-level" reporting) may also be assisted by the information in this volume.

This edition contains six special sections for more detailed coverage of questions of contemporary importance; in addition, such topics as the effects of cigarette smoking and of other environmental agents, exercise tests, the effects of drugs on the lungs, and occupational lung disease receive detailed attention in the main body of the text. Over the past 15 years, there have been an increasing number of longitudinal studies of pulmonary function; these have been noted in sufficient detail to allow the physician to place in context similar observations from his or her own laboratory.

No attempt has been made to present the recent very important advances made in understanding lung biochemistry, the role of oxygen radicals, or pulmonary immunology (except briefly in the first chapter), not because the physician does not need to be apprised of these but because the volume would have been far too long had any attempt been made to do so. No doubt these advances will eventually lead to major improvements in our management of lung disease; in the meantime, however, there are many sick patients to whose welfare the informed analysis of pulmonary function can contribute.

The 6-year task of preparing this edition has been facilitated by many individuals. Dr. Peter Macklem and Dr. Nick Anthonisen provided useful critiques of early drafts of the manuscripts, and the outline of this edition was planned with their assistance. During my sabbatical in Australia, Dr. Bryan Hudson of the Florey Institute and Dr. Peter Sutherland and Dr. Michael Pain of the Royal Melbourne Hospital provided a great deal of help. My sabbatical in France was made possible by Dr. Paul Sadoul and the members of his staff at INSERM U-14 in Nancy, Lorraine. Their library of pulmonary literature was invaluable, and their pulmonary conferences were of great interest (and somewhat of a challenge for the visitor). Dr. Ben Burrows, on sabbatical in Vancouver from Tucson, Arizona, read the whole of the penultimate draft of the manuscript and made many useful suggestions. I am also much indebted to my son, Andrew Bates, who introduced me to word processing in 1980 and who instructed me in the technology.

Finally, I am indebted to the many physicians of all levels of experience, and in many different places, with whom I have enjoyed exchanging ideas and prejudices over the past 40 years.

The staff of W.B. Saunders have been most patient with me, and as relieved as I have been when the manuscript was finally in their hands. Once there, they have dealt with it with their customary courtesy and efficiency.

DAVID V. BATES

PREFACE
to the Second Edition

The welcome given to the first edition of this book has encouraged us to bring the book up-to-date, in the hope that it will continue to prove useful in the training of physicians in the field of lung disease and as a reference source for those whose work necessitates an understanding of the lung.

Since the first edition was prepared in 1964, there have been many important advances in the understanding of pulmonary physiology and abnormalities of pulmonary function. In comparison with the state of knowledge at that time, the contribution of different-sized airways to the flow-resistance of the whole tracheobronchial tree is much better defined today, and we now understand that such measurements as the FEV_1 are insensitive indicators of changes occurring in small airways; measurements of regional lung function have clarified the effects of aging on the lung and emphasized the importance of small-airway closure in a wide variety of clinical circumstances; important new observations have been made of the hypoxemia that occurs in spasmodic asthma and in respiratory failure secondary to shock; and the treatment of respiratory failure has been greatly advanced by careful application of controlled oxygen therapy. This period has also seen the first attempts, so far unsuccessful, at human lung transplantation, and much new information has been contributed in other clinical and physiological areas.

To incorporate in a new edition these and other advances in our knowledge, extensive revision and redrafting have been necessary. Most of the first seven chapters have been entirely rewritten and the chapter on respiratory failure has been modified to a major extent. We have completely revised the sequence of presentation of pulmonary physiology and hope that we have achieved thereby a more satisfactory approach to the understanding of pulmonary function. This reorganization and updating necessitated a total rewriting of the chapters on physiology.

The additions have been accommodated in the present volume with little increase in length, since specialized books or monographs have now been published on such topics as pulmonary surfactant, pediatric chest disease, dyspnea, exercise physiology, and by our colleagues on the radiological and clinical basis of the diagnosis of lung disease. These contributions have led us to change the emphasis in some aspects of the original text and have permitted us to curtail or omit altogether detailed discussion of these areas.

Since many students and trainees should, in our opinion, be encouraged to begin their reading with early literature, we have decided not to eliminate from the present bibliography any of the references that were in the first edition, although many of these references are not now specifically referred to in the text. This bibliography, together with 1476 new references that have been added, summarizes the field of pulmonary function and respiratory physiology since 1945. We have provided an index to the now extensive bibliography that we hope will permit the physician and the trainee to make better use of the references contained within it.

Our colleagues, Dr. R.G. Fraser and Dr. J.A.P. Paré, have now published a text of their own. Their extensive involvement in the preparation of that work has limited their participation in the revision of this edition, but, nevertheless, they have both made valuable contributions. Heavy responsibilities have prevented Prof. Thurlbeck from a detailed involvement in the preparation of this new edition, but much of his original contribution has been retained and he has been good enough to edit many of the changes and supervise the drafting of the new chapter on the anatomy of the lung. His assistance in many other parts of the book is gratefully acknowledged. Dr. M.R. Becklake, who contributed much of the original section on occupational lung disease, was too heavily committed with other work to undertake the revision, but her contribution to the present volume is, nevertheless, gratefully acknowledged.

We are specially indebted to friends and colleagues who have allowed us to use illustrations for this edition, in particular, Dr. John West, Dr. Maurice McGregor, and the editor of the *Scientific American*. We are also very much indebted to all those who have made suggestions to us for the improvement of the first edition and hope that critical readers will continue to be of assistance to us in improving the present volume.

One of us (D.V.B.) wishes to record his gratitude to Dr. L. Donato and to Dr. C. Giuntini of the University of Pisa for making it possible for him to begin the task of preparation of the second edition of this volume in the comparative tranquillity of Tuscany.

Finally, we would like to acknowledge the assistance given us by the staff members of the W. B. Saunders Company, who, with their usual patience, have accepted explanations for our delay in completing this task and have dealt very expeditiously with the manuscript, once it was finally delivered into their hands.

DAVID V. BATES
PETER T. MACKLEM
RONALD V. CHRISTIE

PREFACE
to the First Edition

"This book is intended mainly for those engaged in the practice and teaching of Medicine. We trust that our friends and colleagues who are concerned with the more technical and purely physiological aspects of respiration will not judge too severely our presentation of the subject. We have attempted to give physicians a working knowledge of the chemical and physiological facts concerning respiration, indicating their clinical applications and as far as possible avoiding a highly technical dissertation on the subject.

"We are fully conscious of the incompleteness in our knowledge of respiratory function. As there are many points still in dispute regarding the physiology of normal respiration, it is not surprising to find that there are even more deficiencies in our understanding of the abnormal. We have attempted to point out many of these, hoping in this way to focus attention on our ignorance. At times opposing views have been given in as impartial a manner as possible. We quite acknowledge our difficulty and perhaps weakness in not always keeping ourselves from inclining towards one or other point of view. This possible bias is in all cases quite open to correction, and we trust that the near future may settle some debatable points beyond fear of contradiction."

This was written by Jonathan C. Meakins and H. Whitridge Davies in their preface to their book "Respiratory Function in Disease," which was published in 1925. We cannot improve upon it to describe our purpose in writing this volume, which we have dedicated to the memory of Jonathan Meakins. He was a pioneer in the application of physiological methods to the problems of clinical medicine. In 1923 he developed in the McGill University Clinic of the Royal Victoria Hospital what must have been one of the first respiratory function laboratories, if not the first, to be established in any hospital. It was in this laboratory that one of us received his early training; and it has been in the same laboratory that the patients referred to in this book have been studied.

During the past forty years the contribution of physiologists and biochemists to our understanding of functional impairment in disease has been remarkable. It has led, however, to a degree of specialization tending to separate disciplines which are, by their nature, interdependent. An understanding of the clinical patterns of disease and of the morphological changes that underlie disease is still necessary if the physiological and biochemical changes that occur are to be understood in proper perspective. We are hopeful that the brief reviews of clinical patterns, radiological findings, and morphology of lung disease that we have included will be valuable to those scientists whose major interest lies outside these fields. Such sections are not aimed at the experienced chest physician, radiologist, or pathologist respectively, any more than are the sections on normal physiology written for the physiologist.

The literature on respiratory function is already so vast that we have been able to include only sufficient references to provide the essential background, and from these the reader will be able to obtain a more comprehensive bibliography.

It is our hope that our many friends and colleagues, who have not hesitated to stimulate us with their criticisms in the past, will bring to our attention any deficiencies and inaccuracies they detect in the present volume.

DVB
RVC

Montreal
1964

CONTENTS

GLOSSARY OF TERMS

AIRWAY CONDUCTANCE (Gaw)—The reciprocal of airway resistance, expressed as L/sec/cm H_2O.

AIRWAY RESISTANCE (Raw)—The pressure between the airway opening (i.e., mouth or nose) and the alveoli, in relation to simultaneous air flow; expressed as cm H_2O/L/sec.

ALVEOLAR–ARTERIAL DIFFERENCES for O_2, CO_2, and N_2 [(A − a) D_{O_2}]—The difference (in mm Hg) between a measured arterial gas tension and a simultaneously measured or computed mean alveolar gas tension. The differences reflect, among other factors, abnormalities of $\dot{V}/\dot{Q}$ ratio (see Figure 2–19).

ALVEOLAR–ARTERIAL END-CAPILLARY GRADIENT—The pressure difference (in mm Hg) that exists between alveolar gas and pulmonary capillary blood as the latter leaves the alveolus (see Figure 2–18).

ALVEOLAR GAS—Expired gas that has come from alveoli. The definition of mean alveolar gas concentration is complicated by the discontinuous nature of lung ventilation and perfusion, and by the non-uniform behavior of the lung in regard to these aspects of function.

ALVEOLAR VENTILATION—If the lungs behaved as a completely uniform system, alveolar ventilation could be defined as the tidal volume minus the anatomic dead-space volume, multiplied by the respiratory frequency. In many situations, however, alveolar ventilation can be defined only in terms of the arterial P_{CO_2}, the level of which ordinarily reflects the total effective alveolar ventilation.

BLOOD-GAS TENSION—The pressure in mm Hg of a gas in the blood. Note that pressures between a liquid and a gas must always be in equilibrium, regardless of solubility, buffer systems, partition coefficients, or dissociation curves.

CLOSING VOLUME—The volume at which there is an inflection between the alveolar expiratory nitrogen slope (Phase III) and the terminal change in nitrogen percentage (Phase IV), believed to indicate the onset of airway closure. A preceding full inspiration of 100% oxygen must be taken, and expiratory flow rate must be controlled.

COEFFICIENT OF VARIATION—The ratio of a standard deviation of a distribution to its arithmetic mean. It is determined by making replicate measurements on the same individual.

COMPLIANCE, DYNAMIC (C_{dyn})—The ratio of the tidal volume to the difference in pressure at points of zero gas flow, expressed in L/cm H_2O.

COMPLIANCE, STATIC (C_{st})—The slope of a static-pressure–volume curve at a point, or the linear approximation of the nearly straight portion of such a curve, in the tidal volume range, expressed in L/cm H_2O.

DEAD SPACE, ANATOMIC (inert-gas dead space)—The volume of all non-gas-exchanging passages in the lung, normally comprising the upper airway and bronchial tree as far as the respiratory bronchioles.

DEAD SPACE, PHYSIOLOGIC—A number (not a topographic volume) that, by comparison with the anatomic or inert-gas dead space, expresses the non-uniformity of $\dot{V}/\dot{Q}$ ratios in the lung. When expressed for a particular gas, the physiologic dead space is the number that has to be used for V_D in the Bohr equation if the correct arterial tension is to be computed from inspired and mixed expired concentrations.

DIFFUSING CAPACITY (D_L)—The rate of gas transfer through a membrane in relation to a constant pressure difference across it. A simple physical concept that in biology is usually a complex measurement because of difficulty in accurate determination of the effective pressure difference.

DIFFUSING CAPACITY COMPONENTS—Components of the total diffusing capacity ($D_{L_{CO}}$) may be summed as resistances as follows:

$$\frac{1}{D_{L_{CO}}} = \frac{1}{D_M*} + \frac{1}{\theta V_C**}$$

ELASTANCE—The reciprocal of compliance, expressed in cm H_2O/L.

ELASTIC RECOIL (P_{st})—The difference between intrapleural and alveolar pressure at a given long volume under static conditions.

FORCED EXPIRATORY VOLUME (FEV)—The volume of a maximally fast expiration starting from a full inspiration. The time in fractions of a second over which the FEV has been measured is indicated by suitable subscripts (i.e., $FEV_{0.75,}$ $FEV_{1,}$ etc.).

FUNCTIONAL RESIDUAL CAPACITY (FRC)—The volume of gas contained in the lungs at the end of a normal quiet expiration.

INERT-GAS DISTRIBUTION—The distribution of a non-exchanging gas between alveoli, theoretically perfect only when each alveolus receives from the tidal volume the same quantum of inspired gas in relation to its original volume as does every other alveolus.

---

*Membrane diffusion coefficient (q.v.).
**Pulmonary capillary blood volume (q.v.).

INSPIRATORY CAPACITY (IC)—The volume of gas that can be taken into the lungs on a full inspiration, starting from the resting expiratory position.

KINETIC CONSTANT (θ)—The rate of combination of CO with red blood cells, expressed as ml CO/min/mm Hg/mL of blood. Affected by the oxygen tension simultaneously present.

MAXIMAL BREATHING CAPACITY (MBC)—The maximal volume of gas that can be breathed per minute by voluntary effort.

MAXIMAL MIDEXPIRATORY FLOW RATE (MMFR or FEF_{25-75})—The velocity (in L/sec) of a forced expiration over the middle half of the total expired volume.

MAXIMAL STATIC NEGATIVE INTRAPLEURAL PRESSURE—The difference between intrapleural and alveolar pressures at full inspiration.

MEMBRANE DIFFUSION COEFFICIENT (D_M)—A component of total diffusing capacity that sums every factor affecting CO transfer other than pulmonary capillary blood volume (V_c) and the kinetic constant (θ). It thus includes both qualitative and quantitative aspects of the alveolar surface, together with other addition factors.

MINUTE VOLUME—The volume of gas expired per minute.

MOUTH OCCLUSION PRESSURE ($P_{0.1}$)—The pressure measured at FRC in the seated subject when a normal inspiration is interrupted by occlusion of the airway for a time interval of 0.1 second. It is an index of the neural drive to ventilate.

PULMONARY CAPILLARY BLOOD VOLUME (V_C)—The volume of blood in the lung in contact with alveolar gas at any instant.

RESIDUAL VOLUME (RV)—The volume of gas in the lungs that cannot be expelled by expiratory effort; hence, the total lung capacity minus the vital capacity.

RQ—The ratio of CO_2 production to oxygen uptake, as follows:

$$\frac{\dot{V}_{CO_2}}{\dot{V}_{O_2}}$$

SINGLE-BREATH NITROGEN TEST OF VENTILATION DISTRIBU-TION—The change in nitrogen percentage expressed as $\%N_2/L$, when an expiration is made after a full inspiration of 100% oxygen, measured between 750 mL and 1250 mL of the full expiration.

TIDAL VOLUME—The volume of gas expired with each breath.

TIME CONSTANT—In pulmonary mechanics, this term is used to indicate the product of compliance and airway resistance.

TOTAL LUNG CAPACITY (TLC)—The volume of gas contained in the lungs at the end of a full inspiration.

VITAL CAPACITY (VC)—The volume of gas that can be expelled from the lungs from a position of full inspiration, with no time limit to the duration of expiration.

$\dot{V}/\dot{Q}$—The ratio between ventilation and perfusion, each being expressed in the same units.

WORK OF BREATHING—The cumulative product of instantaneous pressure developed by the respiratory muscles and volume of air moved in a breathing cycle, expressed as g · cm/mL.

AIRWAY STRUCTURE AND FUNCTION

INTRODUCTION

This chapter starts by reviewing the normal anatomy and the defense mechanisms of the airways in order to facilitate the later discussion of the pathologic processes that occur in them. These are discussed with respect to the general pathology of the inflammatory response, although gaps in our knowledge of them make firm conclusions about the nature of airway lesions difficult. At the same time there are now enough data to suggest that the common features of airway inflammation can be recognized in most situations in which airway disease exists. This general topic of the nature of airway inflammation is central to allergic lung disease, to the pathogenesis of chronic airflow obstruction, and to the airway response to inhaled irritants.

NORMAL ANATOMY

Examination of a normal bronchogram (Fig. 1–1A) shows that there is an irregularity to the branching pattern of the airways. This means that it is possible to get to the terminal airways (Fig. 1–1B) by passing relatively few branches if a pathway to the apical segment of the lower lobe is followed or by passing many branches if the longer pathways to the basal segments are taken. It also shows (Fig. 1–1C) that the number of divisions to airways 2 millimeters in diameter varies from four to 14 and that the total cross-sectional area at each division (Fig. 1–1D) increases substantially toward the periphery of the lung. Weibel's[5239, 5240] analysis of the airways is based on the assumption of a regularly dichotomous branching system in which the trachea

is given the number 0, the left and right main-stem bronchi the number 1, and so on, so that there is a ratio of "daughter" to "parent" of 2:1. He divided the airways into conducting, transitional, and respiratory zones (Fig. 1–2), which means that the transitional zone begins somewhere between the fifth and sixteenth generations, depending on the pathway that is taken.

An alternative system that tries to take the irregularity of the branching system into account has been popularized by Horsfield and his associates.[5164] Horsfield and Cumming[5163] used the Stahler system in which the numbering is started from the terminal unit (Fig. 1–3) and in which the branching ratio is approximately 1.4:1. The importance of the branching ratio is that in each generation the airway diameter is reduced by the cube root of the branching ratio:

$$d_z = d_o \cdot 2^{-z/3}$$

where z = the generation and d_o = the diameter of the initial branch.

Weibel has shown (Fig. 1–4) that the average airway diameter at each generation follows this relationship until the respiratory bronchioles are reached. He has argued[5240] that this means that the central airways are constructed for optimal mass flow, whereas the larger cross-section of the terminal airways is optimal for the diffusion of gas. Macklem and his associates partitioned resistance of the bronchial tree in animals[5184] and humans[5160] and confirmed that very little of the total resistance is present beyond bronchi 2 millimeters in size. A similar finding has been reported from several other laboratories, but there is also evidence to the contrary, suggesting that peripheral airway resistance may be higher in normal lungs.[5201, 5234]

The peripheral airway resistance of children is disproportionately high,[5161] but this gradually changes with lung growth until the ratio of peripheral to total airway resistance becomes similar to that in the adult. This is likely to be due to the fact that the actual dimensions of the intrapulmonary conducting airways change little, while the lung is growing primarily by the addition of alveoli. Later, when the alveoli begin to increase in size as well as number, the dimensions of the entire peripheral unit begin to increase. These small changes in peripheral airway dimensions are responsible for a substantial fall in intrapulmonary airways resistance because the resistance is inversely proportional to the fourth power of the radius.

When a gas is inhaled at a constant flow rate, its velocity at each location in the respiratory tract depends on the cross-sectional area of the airways at that point. This means that at the same flow rate, the gas velocity will be very high in the upper airways, larynx, and central conducting airways and very low at the level of the terminal bronchioles. If the gas contains particles and makes a sudden change in direction at a branch point (Fig. 1–1), the particles tend not to change from their path because of their momentum.[23] This means that larger particles are filtered out of the airstream in the upper airways, larynx, and major bronchi because these airways have a narrow cross section and therefore high gas velocities.[2303] Particles with a density greater than that of air are accelerated downward by the force of gravity until the retarding force caused by their motion through the air balances their weight. If the particle is spherical, then Stokes' Law can be used to predict the retarding force.[23] This states

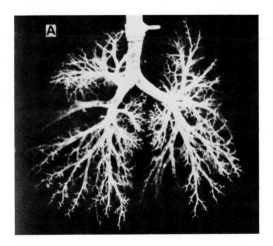

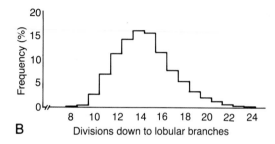

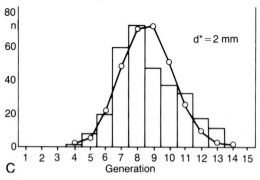

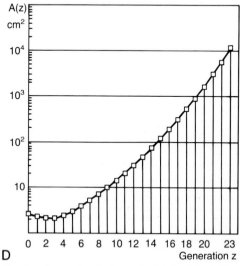

Figure 1–1. *A*, A normal human bronchogram performed on a postmortem lung using finely particulate lead dust. Note that it is possible to get to the peripheral portions of the lung by following either a relatively small number of branches to the apical segment of the lower lobe or a greater number of branches to the basal segment of the lower lobe. *B* shows frequency distribution of the number of divisions down to the gas exchanging surface. (From Horsfield and Cumming,[5163] with permission of authors and publisher.) *C* shows that it is possible to get to the 2-mm airways with as few as four branches or as many as 14 branches, depending on the pathway that is taken. (From Weibel,[5239] with permission of author and publisher.) *D* shows a cross-sectional area (cm²) at each generation of branching. Note that the cross-sectional area increases markedly beyond the 14th generation of airways. (From Weibel,[5239] with permission of author and publisher.)

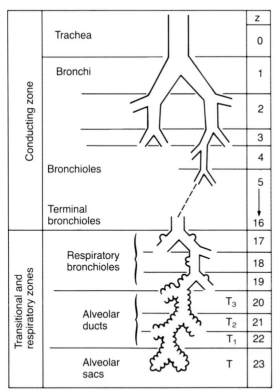

	z
Trachea	0
Bronchi	1
	2
	3
	4
Bronchioles	5
Terminal bronchioles	16
Respiratory bronchioles	17
	18
	19
Alveolar ducts	T₃ 20
	T₂ 21
	T₁ 22
Alveolar sacs	T 23

Figure 1–2. The distribution of conducting, transitional, and respiratory zones as a function of airway generation z. (From Weibel,[5239] with permission of author and publisher.)

that at low velocities the frictional force on a spherical body moving through a fluid at constant velocity is equal to six times the product of the velocity, the fluid viscosity, and the radius of the sphere.[3670]

Particles small enough not to be deposited in the central airways reach the lung parenchyma, where they settle to the surface if there is sufficient time. Those that do not reach the surface are removed by the subsequent exhalation. Even in the absence of gravity, small particles are moved around in the air by the Brownian motion of the gas molecules. This displacement increases as particle size decreases and is independent of density. In general, settling is much more important than Brownian motion for deposition of particles of about 0.5 micrometer in diameter. Below this diameter, Brownian motion becomes a more important factor than settling.[23]

The very wide cross-sectional area of the peripheral airways is of great importance to aerosol deposition. Because the central airways are relatively narrow, the velocity of flow in them is so high that inertial impaction at the branch points is maximized. Toward the periphery of the lung, deposition is governed largely by settling, so that particles deposit in relation to their settling times. From these considerations, one would predict that large particles would be deposited in the central airways and smaller particles would be retained peripherally. As noted in Chapter 3, this is what is found. Studies by Gerrity and his colleagues[5150] showed that radioactive particles between 5 and 10 micrometers in diameter were deposited largely in airway generations 0 to 12, whereas those from 1 to 3 micrometers in diameter were predominantly deposited in generations 14 to 20 (Fig. 1–5). Other aspects of particle deposition are noted in Chapter 3.

STRUCTURAL ASPECTS OF CILIARY FUNCTION

A general discussion of the physics of mucus and mucociliary clearance can be found in

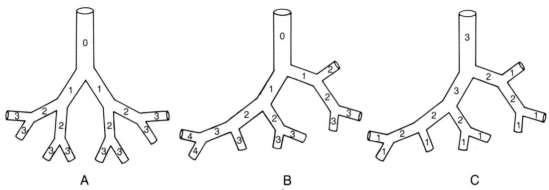

A B C

Figure 1–3. Compares a regular dichotomous branching system compared with an irregular one. Weibel used the model shown in (A), while Horsfield and his associates have used the model shown in (C). While the irregular dichotomous system is more consistent with the real anatomy (Fig. 1–1A), the arguments concerning the distribution of cross-sectional area in the airways are similar, no matter what branching system is used. (From Weibel,[5239] with permission of author and publisher.)

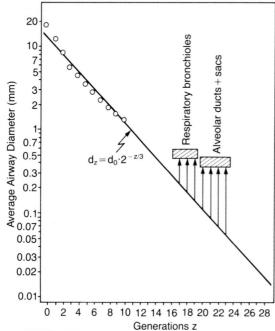

Figure 1–4. The average airway diameter at each airway generation is shown using a regularly branching dichotomous model. The data points show that the conducting airways fit this model. However, the respiratory bronchioles and alveolar ducts and sacs fall well off the line predicted by the equation. This means that the respiratory bronchioles and alveolar ducts and sacs have a wider cross-sectional area than predicted by this model and are therefore more suited to diffusion than to bulk flow. (From Weibel,[5239] with permission of author and publisher.)

Chapter 3. As noted there, the mucociliary system protects the conducting airways by trapping inhaled particles and sweeping them back up the airway and through the glottis, where they are swallowed. The system is two-layered,[2872, 5167] consisting of a non-viscid, serous fluid, which surrounds the cilia, and an upper layer of mucus, which is visco-elastic and propelled by the cilial beat (Fig. 1–6). The cilia[5220] conduct their power stroke when they are fully extended and attached to the surface layer of mucus. The recovery stroke takes place by a bending motion, which allows them to remain in the non-viscous periciliary fluid. This is analogous to swimming when the body is propelled through the water with the fully extended arm that recovers by a bending motion through the less viscous air. As noted in Chapter 3, the mean linear velocity of the mucous layer is influenced by the ciliary beat frequency, the viscosity and depth of the serous fluid, and the nature of the mucoid layer.

The cilia are made up of microtubules, which are arranged in nine doublets round a central pair. The central microtubules are surrounded by a sheath, and each of the nine doublets is connected to the sheath by a radial spoke.[5220] The individual doublets are attached to one another by arms. The cilia are capable of beating independently of the underlying cell and have been shown to continue to beat after separation from the cell by laser beams.[5220] Their beat is accomplished by a sliding motion of the microtubules over one another, with no shortening of individual microtubules. This action has been beautifully illustrated by Satir and his colleagues,[5220] who have shown crowding and spreading of the doublets as the cilia move from side to side. Recently it has been suggested that chronic infectious processes in the lung may be associated with abnormal ciliary function.[5139] This has been established for the bronchiectasis present in Kartagener's syndrome[5105] and may be important in other forms of chronic bronchiectasis.[5238] However, not all observers agree that the syndrome can be diagnosed morphologically.[5146] Pulmonary function in these conditions is discussed in Chapter 10.

Because the surface area of the peripheral airways is much greater than that of the trachea, it follows that the speed of clearance must be greater in the trachea or the mucus would collect in this airway and drown the lung. Morrow and his associates[5197] have estimated that the half-time of clearance in the trachea is 2.7 minutes, as compared with 80 to 300 minutes in the lower bronchi. Computed velocity in centimeters/minute is therefore 1.4 cm/min in the trachea, as compared with 0.06 cm/min in smaller bronchi.

Clearance from Non-ciliated Airways

Clearance from the peripheral parts of the lung that do not have ciliated cells is a slower process. The primary mechanism of clearance from the alveolar surface is the alveolar macrophage, but clearance from the intermediate zone between the alveolated surface and ciliated airways is less well understood. Movement between these regions may be accomplished by differences in the surface tension of the lining fluid, which may cause movement from areas covered by surfactant to areas covered by mucus or may cause an actual flow of fluid up the airways.

THE ALVEOLAR MACROPHAGE

The alveolar macrophage is part of the mononuclear phagocyte system. The cells of this

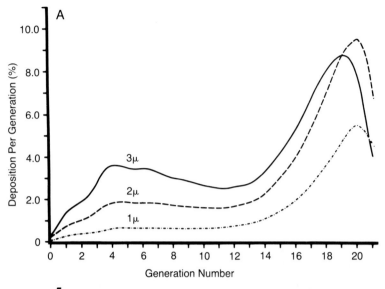

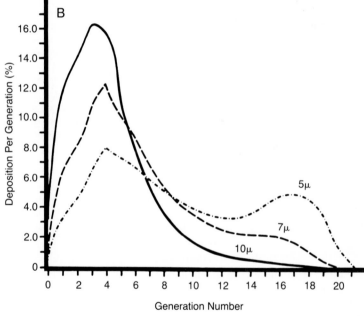

Figure 1–5. Deposition of particulates of different size as a function of airway generation. These data show that the small particles of 1 to 3 microns in diameter deposit mainly in the peripheral airways, whereas the larger particles are found largely in the central airways. (Reprinted with permission from Gerrity, T. R., Lee, T. S., Haas, F. J., et al. Calculated deposition of inhaled particles in the airway generations of normal subjects. J. Appl. Physiol. 47: 867–873, 1979.)

system originate from precursor cells in the bone marrow,[5117, 5152] are transported in the blood as monocytes, and eventually become tissue macrophages.[5116, 5214] As there are differences in morphologic, metabolic, and functional characteristics between the blood monocyte and the alveolar macrophage, several authors have suggested that a maturation process occurs in these cells before the macrophage reaches the air space. Bowden and Adamson[5115] have suggested that there is an intermediate interstitial compartment of cells between the blood monocyte and the free alveolar macrophage. In

studies using whole body radiation to suppress circulating monocytes and organ culture, they found that cell division occurred in the interstitial cells of the explant but not in the cells in the alveoli. They suggested that a normal steady state exists in which macrophage loss in the mucociliary escalator is balanced by cell production in the interstitial compartment.

The alveolar macrophages probably cover less than 5% of the total alveolar surface. Studies of the clearance of iron particles from the lung by Brain and his associates[5116] suggest that these cells are actively motile and capable of cleaning

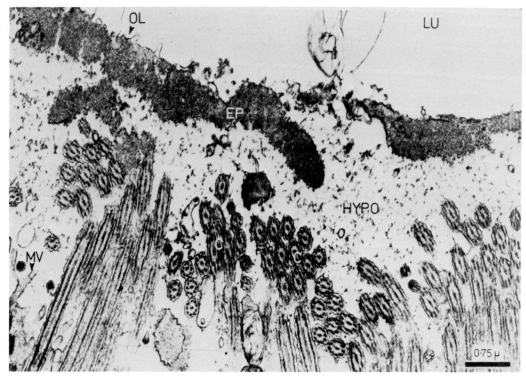

Figure 1–6. Electron micrograph of the surface lining the ciliated surface of the airways. Note the height of the epiphase (EP) is electron-dense as compared with the hypophase (HYPO). The cilia carry out their recovery stroke in the less viscous hypophase and their power stroke by attaching to the dense epiphase. Particles on the epiphase are swept toward the mouth by this movement. OL = osmiophilic layer; LU = lumen; MV = microvilli. (Reprinted with permission from Hulbert, W. C., Forster, B. B., Laird, W., et al. An improved method of fixation of the respiratory epithelial surface with mucus and surfactant layers. Lab. Invest. 47:354–363, 1982, © by US & Canadian Academy of Pathology, Inc.)

up the surface after it has been covered by foreign particles. However, it is less clear what happens to the macrophages after they have ingested the particles. The majority probably make their way to the mucociliary escalator and are cleared in the airways; but it remains controversial whether any of them migrate back through the epithelium to the interstitium. Although inhaled particulate material can be found in regional lymph nodes, and some of it is demonstrable within macrophages, Brain and colleagues have argued that this is a result of free particles penetrating the epithelium and being picked up by macrophages on the other side.[5116] However, a recent study[5129] has produced evidence that macrophages may penetrate the epithelium and make their way to the lymph nodes.

Clearance by Blood and Lymph

The epithelial surfaces of the airways are quite impermeable to large molecules.[5223] Ra-

diolabeled compounds and other tracers, such as horseradish peroxidase, are cleared from these surfaces into the blood at a rate per hour that represents less than 1% of the total deposited dose in that time.[5166, 5168] In experiments in which all the lung lymph has been collected, the relative clearance into the blood has been estimated to be five times greater than clearance into the lymph.[5195]

The lung lymphatics consist of loose collections of lymphoid cells in the peripheral portions of the lung that gradually become more organized as they approach the hilum.[5199] True intrapulmonary lymph nodes with a marginal sinus, germinal center, and an efferent lymph vessel can be found in relation to segmental and lobar airways. Miller in 1911[5196] concluded that the peripheral lymphoid tissues were related to both the bronchi and blood vessels in normal lungs and that those underlying the pleura were principally related to pulmonary veins. He believed that the intrapulmonary lymphoid tissues proliferated upon stimulation by anthracotic deposits. The bronchial-associated lymphoid tissue (designated BALT) is much more conspicuous in some species than in others but is present in humans and has been shown to increase with irritant stimuli.[5110] The layer lining the surface of these tissues is somewhat different from that covering the surrounding airway. The BALT is thought to be capable of absorbing solid particles, including bacteria, and transporting them via lymphatics to regional lymph nodes.

IMMUNOLOGIC DEFENSE

The deposition of foreign material on the surface of the respiratory tract, its entry into the tissues, and its clearance by macrophages, blood, and lymph provide ample opportunity for the body's immune system to mount a defensive response. This response is partially determined by the genetic make-up of the host. The immune response genes of experimental animals are thought to be closely located on chromosome 6, which is responsible for formation of the human leukocyte–associated, or HLA, antigens.[5178] Because of the close association between HLA antigens and the immune response genes, the relationship between HLA typing and immunologically determined lung disease has been the focus of considerable recent research.[5111, 5231] It is to be hoped that a complete understanding of how the genes control the inflammatory process will provide clearer insights into individual susceptibility to disease.

Respiratory Immunoglobulins

Local humoral immunity plays an important role in respiratory tract defense. IgG and IgM are produced from cells within the germinal follicles of the regional lymph nodes, whereas IgE is produced in the lymphoid tissue in the upper respiratory tract, particularly in the tonsils.[5233] IgA is also formed in the regional lymph nodes, but it can also be produced in plasma cells lining the respiratory mucosa, especially in the neighborhood of the bronchial glands.[5189]

The IgA found in secretions has several distinctive structural, immunologic, and biologic differences from the IgA present in serum.[5189] In the sputum it occurs mainly as dimers, condensation products consisting of two molecules linked to two types of low molecular

weight junctional pieces. The first of these to be described was the secretory T-piece, or secretory component, which is believed to link IgA molecules through their Fc portions.[5189] This component is probably formed in the mucosal glands and epithelial cells, since immunofluorescent studies have demonstrated the presence of secretory component IgA within mucosal cells. The major function of IgA appears to be preventing the adherence of organisms to the mucosal surface.[5189] This probably accounts for the experimental observations that virus infections can be more readily prevented by a vaccine intranasally instilled than parenterally injected. It has now been amply confirmed that the protective immunity following intranasal immunization is more closely related to levels of secretory IgA than to serum levels of either IgA or IgG. A reasonable conclusion would be that the IgA provides the first line of defense against surface invaders deposited on the airway mucosa. The antibodies in serum provide a back-up defense against those organisms that have penetrated the mucosal barrier into the interstitial tissue.[5233]

When an individual encounters an infecting agent for the first time, specific IgM is the first immunoglobulin to increase and is detectable within 3 to 4 days.[5233] Its production tends to be transient, and increases indicate a recent infection. It is characteristic of blood group isoagglutinins, cold agglutinins, and some bacterial antibodies. IgG increases more slowly, beginning at about 10 days after infection and rising to a peak at 3 weeks. With re-infection, the IgG response is accelerated and reaches a much higher peak at 3 weeks. IgG occurs in the greatest amount in serum and is the major specific antibody against bacteria, viruses, and other organisms.

IgE has a short half-life of 2 to 3 days in serum but survives in tissue, where it is linked to the surfaces of basophils and mast cells.[5170] It is formed in the lymphoid tissue and plasma cells of the upper respiratory tract, in the tonsils, and to a lesser extent in the trachea and main bronchi.[5233] Salvaggio and Laskowitz[5216] were able to show that the intranasal administration of a variety of antigens stimulated production of circulating skin-sensitizing antibodies in atopic individuals, whereas no such response was observed in controls. This contrasted to parenteral administration of the antigen, which produced mainly IgG antibody production. Very low levels of IgE are found in the neonate; this level begins to rise by about 6 weeks and reaches adult values at about 5 years of age.[5233] IgE increases during the pollen season in allergic subjects, and excessively high IgE values are found in the presence of parasitic infections. Antigen interaction with IgE on the surface of mast cells causes the release of mediators that modulate the inflammatory response to the inhaled antigen.[5170]

Cell-Mediated Immunity

The cell-mediated immune reaction has been best studied as the response to bacterial antigens, such as those of the tubercle bacillus, but it is now recognized that this reaction can be expressed in a variety of biologic events. In experimental studies it can be induced by proteins or other chemical determinants conjugated to proteins. In some cases the chemical may be quite simple (such as haptene), but the cell-mediated response appears to be directed against both haptene and protein. This differs from the antibody response, which can be directed against either the haptene or the protein.[5154]

Another important feature of the cell-mediated immune response is the route of antigen introduction. Large amounts of soluble antigen given intravenously often fail to induce cell-mediated immunity, whereas small amounts of particulate or adjuvant-associated antigen introduced into an area with appropriate lymphocyte drainage produce a local cellular sensitization that involves the draining lymph nodes.[5106, 5126] The T cells are recognized as the instruments of cell-mediated immunity, but there is debate as to how they interact with antigen. The general consensus[5247] is that the antigen is presented to the T cell by the macrophage. The T cell then differentiates to a "blast" form and begins to divide. The sensitized T cell thus provides the basis for immunologic memory, and an expansion of this clone of cells increases the intensity of the response.[5247] The observation by Tada[5229] that an intact thymus was required to shut off the IgE response in skin-sensitized rats after antigen challenge led to the discovery of the T suppressor cell. The control of antibody synthesis by helper and suppressor T cells is now an established concept.

The nature of the histologic changes in the cell-mediated immune response are characteristic but not specific.[5247] They depend on the tissue site, the species of animal, and the method of exposure to the antigen. The lymphocytes responsible for producing the reaction make up a small proportion of the cells present in the expression of the reaction. This appears to be possible because the sensitized T cell is able to release factors that control the inflammatory response. Some of these factors have been reasonably well characterized. They include: (1) migratory inhibitory factor (MIF), which modulates the accumulation of inflammatory cells; (2) interleukins, which induce cell proliferation; (3) cytotoxins, which damage other cells; and a rapidly growing list of other less well-characterized factors.

AIRWAYS INFLAMMATION

An inflammatory response generally follows the injury of these tissues by the inhalation of a noxious gas or aerosol. Florey and his associates[5145] were the first to show that an inflammatory process involving a mucosal surface, such as that found in the airways, had some features that were typical of all inflammatory responses and others that were characteristic for mucosal surfaces. The common features include vascular congestion, increased vascular permeability, and the formation of an exudate. The features that are specific are mucus hypersecretion and shedding of the epithelium. In the central airways, a chronic inflammatory process is associated with hypertrophy of the mucous glands and the excess formation of mucous secretory cells in the epithelium. The immune system plays a major role in this response following some injuries, but not in others. The unfortunate fact is that we have a very incomplete understanding of the relative importance of each of the factors that may contribute to this inflammatory reaction. However, it seems likely that the acute inflammatory response in these airways is similar to that in other tissues in that the injury is followed by a fluid exudative phase, which is followed in turn by a proliferative repair phase.[5246]

The exudative phase consists of a movement of fluid and then cells out of the vascular space, into the tissue, and onto the surface of the airway lumen (Fig. 1–7A). The presence of exudate on the surface of the peripheral airways causes the airways to close prematurely by replacing the surfactant that is normally found there[5185] with fluid with a much higher surface tension. The combination of excess mucus production by glands and goblet cells, together with the inflammatory exudate, results in the

Text continued on page 13

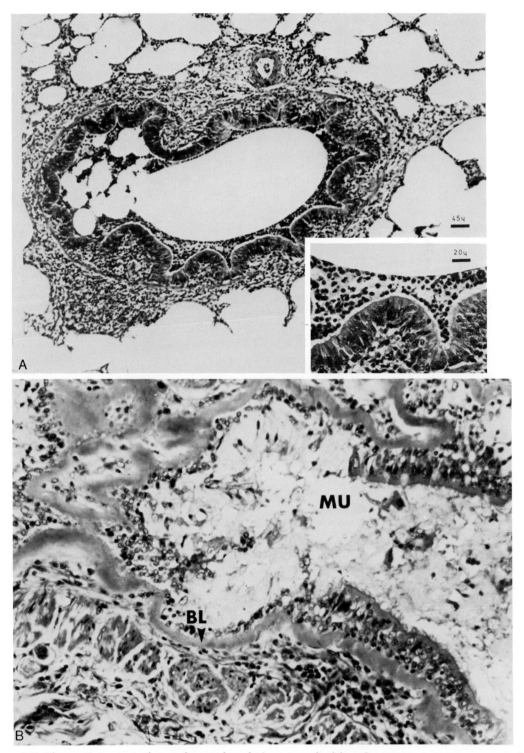

Figure 1–7. Changes that occur in the membranous bronchioles as a result of the inflammatory process are summarized. Figure 1–7A shows an acute inflammatory exudate into the airway wall and on to the airway surface. Figure 1–7B shows a chronic inflammatory mucous exudate (MU) from a case of asthma that occludes the airway lumen. Note that the epithelium is disrupted and that the epithelial basement membrane (BL) is quite thick.

Illustration continued on following page

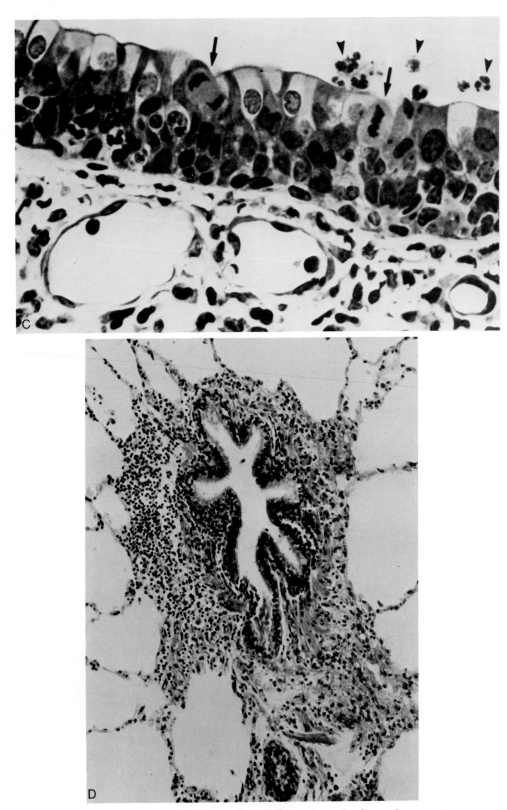

Figure 1–7 *Continued* In Figure 1–7C, the presence of mitotic figures (arrows) indicates that a repair process is present in the airway epithelium. These begin to increase 12 hours after airway injury (From Hulbert et al.,[5168] with permission from the American Lung Association). Figure 1–7D shows a bronchiole where the airway wall has been infiltrated with inflammatory cells but the lumen remains empty.

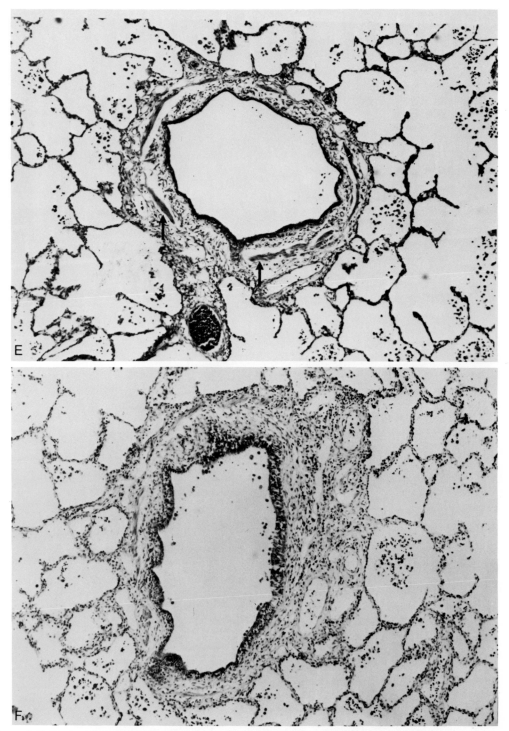

Figure 1–7 *Continued* Figure 1–7E shows a bronchiole with inflammatory cells infiltrating the wall and prominent bronchial smooth muscle (arrows). Figure 1–7F shows a bronchiole with the airway wall thickened by inflammatory cells and the deposition of connective tissue.

Illustration continued on following page

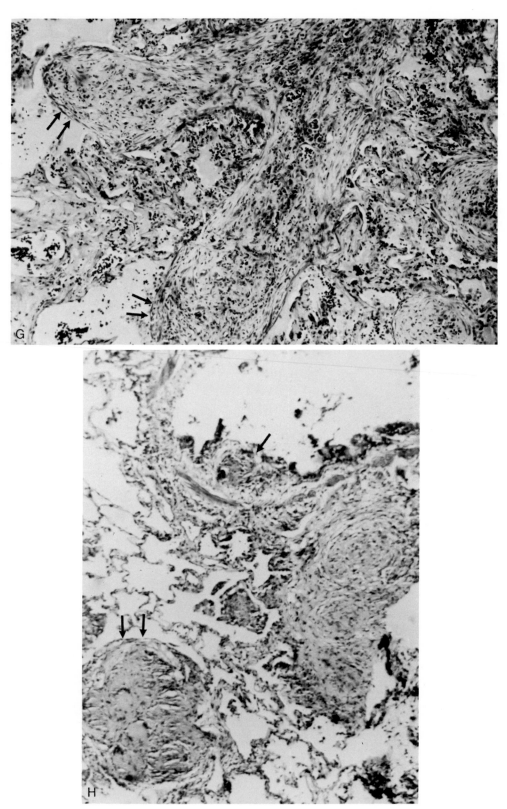

Figure 1–7 *Continued* Figure 1–7G shows a bronchiole that has been occluded by an inflammatory exudate that has been organized by fibrous connective tissue (arrows). Figure 1–7H shows a peripheral airway involved by chronic granulomatous inflammation (double arrows) with granulomas present just below the airway surface (single arrow).

sputum production associated with airway inflammation.

The source of the mediators responsible for this movement of fluid and cells in the exudate is probably the same as in other inflammatory responses, but this phenomenon has been very little studied in the peripheral airways. In some cases the mediators may come from mast cells, but they may also be generated from the injured epithelial cell membranes from the plasma, and from the inflammatory cells that migrate from the vascular space to the injured site.

Failure to clear the exudate can result in the occlusion of the airway lumen (Fig. 1–7B). This is often referred to as mucous plugging but it is more complicated than this term might imply. Although there may indeed be an excess production of mucus from both goblet cells and bronchial glands, the fluid protein and cells of the exudate make a major contribution to the airway plug. Some recent studies by Man and his associates[5187] are of interest with respect to sloughing of the epithelium. They showed that increasing the osmotic pressure on the submucosal side of the epithelium resulted in shrinkage and disruption. It seems likely that fluid exudation into the airways would have this effect; the tight epithelial junctions could restrict the movement of solute so that the osmotic pressure would rise in the submucosa, producing the same phenomenon. After the epithelium is shed, mitotic figures appear (Fig. 1–7C) and the new epithelium begins to proliferate to repair the defect in the membrane. The generation of epithelial cells can restore a normal epithelium or an epithelium in which goblet or squamous cells predominate.

The ability of the airway epithelium to repair itself completely and to reline the lumen may be an important determinant of this response. For example, an injury leading to a rapid turnover of cells in the epithelium may result in a thickened basement membrane (Fig. 1–7B) due to collagen deposition in the basal lamina, but there may be very little organization of the exudate that plugs the lumen (Fig. 1–7B). These changes are observed frequently in the lungs of patients who die in status asthmaticus.

In other cases the inflammatory response may cause relatively little change in the lumen and may be dominated by an infiltration of cells into the wall of the airway (Fig. 1–7D). This is often seen in viral infections of the peripheral airways and is a common occurrence in chronic obstructive lung disease that is thought to be related to cigarette smoking. The precise mechanisms that control this infiltration of cells are very poorly understood.

The repair phase of the inflammatory reaction is characterized by an increase in connective tissue in the peripheral airways. In some cases this is dominated by hypertrophy and/or hyperplasia of the muscle (Fig. 1–7E). In others, there is an accumulation of collagen in the wall of the airway (Fig. 1–7F), which can narrow the lumen as it contracts and form a scar. In conditions in which the airway epithelium is more completely disrupted, a necrotic ulcerated surface forms. When this occurs in the peripheral airways, an eosinophilic exudate can extend down the airway to the second or third order respiratory bronchioles. The organization of this exudate transforms it into a polypoid mass of fibroblastic granulation tissue (Fig. 1–7G) that obliterates the airway lumen.

The changes occurring in the airways that are summarized in Figure 1–7 show a response that varies from an exudate onto the surface of the lumen (Fig. 1–7A) to a complete obliteration of the airway lumen by connective tissue (Fig. 1–7G). An interesting difference between inflammatory exudate that plugs the lumen without becoming organized by connective tissue (Fig. 1–7B) and one that does (Fig. 1–7G) is that the epithelium remains intact in the former (Fig. 1–7B), but not in the latter (Fig. 1–7G). The ability of the epithelium to recover and remain more or less intact may be a critical event in preventing the organization of the exudate in the lumen of the airway and the possibility of obliteration (Fig. 1–7G).

Experimental Studies of Airways Inflammation

In a classic series of studies, Winternitz and his associates over 60 years ago[5244] introduced strong concentrations of acid into the airways to produce lesions that were associated with a proliferation of connective tissue into the air space. Five years ago in our laboratory, Baile and her colleagues,[3141] using an aerosolized dose of a much weaker concentration of acid, showed that functional abnormalities in the small airways occurred when very minimal inflammation had been induced. These experiments suggest a dose-response relationship between the severity of the injury and the nature of the response, but the details of this dose-response relationship have yet to be explored in a systematic fashion.

Castleman[5121] carried out an interesting series of studies on the inflammatory response by infecting rats with para-influenza type 1 (Sendai) virus and observing the animals for up to 90 days. He found that the virus infected the bronchiolar epithelium, and this resulted in epithelial necrosis. This was subsequently associated with an inflammatory reaction with proliferation of connective tissue polyps in the airway lumen. On the basis of studies such as these, it seems reasonable to hypothesize that minimal epithelial injury leads to exudation of fluid and cells with little deposition of connective tissue. With more severe injury, there may be deposition of connective tissue in the airway wall, but the lumen remains patent as long as the epithelium can regenerate. However, with severe injury and permanent loss of the epithelium, exudation into the airway lumen becomes organized into a polypoid mass of connective tissue.

Granulomatous Inflammation in the Peripheral Airways

Until 1959, granulomatous inflammation was thought to be a non-specific response to lipids and other foreign material that resulted primarily from non-digestible bacterial cell walls.[5237] More recently, granuloma formation has been shown to be part of the tissue response in the delayed hypersensitivity reaction to particulate antigens (Fig. 1–7H). The formation of granulomata in response to mycobacterial infection has also been shown to be suppressed in animals lacking functional T lymphocytes and by measures directed against T lymphocytes.[5113] The fact that the T cell recognized macrophage-associated antigen probably accounts for the granulomatous inflammation caused by intracellular parasites such as *Mycobacterium tuberculosis* and *Brucella*, as well as a variety of viral, chlamydial, and fungal organisms.[5112, 5113] However, not all granuloma form as part of a clearly defined immunologic response, and some that form in response to inorganic particles, such as silica, are not associated with cell-mediated immunity.

Extrinsic allergic bronchioloalveolitis is an important cause of peripheral airway inflammation in humans. These lesions occur as a result of sensitization to a wide variety of antigens and can be produced in animals by several experimental protocols. The development of the lesion appears to depend on a particulate antigen that can penetrate to the peripheral airways. In humans, acute reactions are usually reversible, but repeated attacks can result in airway narrowing due to connective tissue deposition in the wall and complete obliteration of the airway lumen by organization of the exudate. The common finding of a lowered FEF_{25-75} in these cases, noted in Chapter 11, is the functional correlate of these morphologic airway changes.

Acute Viral Bronchitis and Bronchiolitis

Acute inflammatory processes of the central airways cause cough with sputum, with the sputum containing obvious evidence of an inflammatory process. These events frequently complicate upper respiratory tract infections and are commonly attributed to viruses. The high cost of investigation of viral infections means that such episodes are rarely precisely characterized by laboratory evidence. A bronchial biopsy study by Lindsay and associates[5181] showed that patients with uncomplicated influenza had cellular infiltrates into the airway mucosa. As noted in Chapter 18, there is evidence that rhinovirus infections are capable of producing an abnormality in the diffusing capacity,[2707, 5181] and this may also be reduced in uncomplicated influenza.[2708] The authors of these studies attribute the reduced diffusing capacity to the abnormal $\dot{V}/\dot{Q}$ distribution, which in turn is a consequence of the bronchiolar component of the infection.

Peripheral Airway Inflammation Associated with Viral Infection

In 1898, Holt[5162] provided an excellent description of childhood airway disease. He divided acute catarrhal bronchitis into a mild form involving the larger tubes and a more severe form involving the small tubes, which he called "capillary" bronchitis. He recognized that the pathology was that of acute inflammation of the mucous membrane with swelling, desquamation of the epithelium, and exudation of mucus and pus cells. He noted that the lungs were more often inflated than collapsed at autopsy and that there was enlargement of the lymph nodes at the hilum. He also clearly separated this condition from bronchopneumonia in which there is an exudate into the air spaces.

Wohl and Chernick[5245] credit Engle and Newns[5140] with being the first to use the term "bronchiolitis" and also for suggesting that it could have a viral etiology that was not related to measles, influenza, or pertussis. The development of immunofluorescent techniques and bedside inoculation of secretions into susceptible cell lines have allowed this viral infection to be studied. A number of investigators have shown that this airway disease can be initiated by respiratory syncytial virus,[5188] adenovirus,[5153] para-influenza virus,[5136] rhinovirus,[5171] influenza virus,[5122] and mumps.[5147] Because small bronchi, bronchioles, and respiratory bronchioles are all involved in this condition, the term "peripheral airway inflammation" probably provides a better description than "bronchiolitis."

The importance of respiratory syncytial virus as a cause of life-threatening peripheral airway inflammation in infants and children under the age of 2 is now widely recognized. Jacobs and his associates[5171] found that respiratory syncytial virus accounted for a high percentage of the cases of bronchiolitis in this age group and estimated that the disease was fatal in 2 to 6% of these children. Population studies have shown that epidemics of respiratory syncytial virus occur every year, last for up to 5 months, and usually peak in a month between November and March. Because infected persons continue to shed virus for months, the rate of nosocomial infection is high.

The reason why the disease is life-threatening in young children and relatively mild in older children and adults is incompletely understood. One possibility is the point that has already been made, namely, peripheral airway resistance is disproportionately high in younger children[5161] so that any further airway narrowing caused by a virus-induced inflammatory reaction interferes with ventilation and gas exchange. A second possibility[5245] is that adults are protected by a previous exposure to the virus so that they are resistant to infection. A third possibility[5140] is that the virus replicates only in the upper airways of adults but in both upper and lower airways of children. Whatever the reason, the fact remains that viral disease in the peripheral airways can be severe in small children but is usually mild and self-limiting in older children and adults.

Adenovirus infection has been associated with a particularly severe form of peripheral airway disease; up to 60% of proven cases develop long-term complications in the form of obstructive airway disease.[5241] In the most severe cases,

this may take the form of unilateral hyperlucent lung, which was first described in children by Swyer and James[5227] and in adults by Mac-Leod.[5182] Reid and Simon[5209] have pointed out the probable relationship between bronchiolitis and hyperlucent lung, and this relationship has now been confirmed in several studies. In addition to the hyperlucent lung, other complications, such as obliterative bronchiolitis and bronchiectasis, are frequently reported following adenovirus infection.[5109] Details of function test abnormalities in acute infections are given in Chapter 18.

Bronchiectasis: A Complication of Childhood Airway Inflammation

This anatomic disorder was first described by Laennec[5176] and is characterized by dilatation and distortion of the central airways. He illustrated his analysis of this condition in the first edition of his book with a 3½-year-old child who developed severe bronchiectasis after whooping cough and a 62-year-old woman who had been troubled with cough and hemoptysis from early life. These instances pointed to the conclusion that this disorder was a manifestation of chronic airway disease in childhood that could produce symptoms in adult life. The fact that bronchiectasis was a disease that began in young people was clearly established more than a century later by Mallory.[5186]

Bachman and his associates[5107] showed that acute airway inflammation could cause the central airways to dilate. They performed bronchograms on 60 cases of acute pneumonia and found large airway dilatation in 25 of them. However, Mallory[5186] pointed out that the presence of inflammation by itself could not explain the ectasia, because he found severe bronchitis in only 35 of the 50 cases of bronchiectasis that he studied. Because he found far worse inflammation in the airways in cases of asthma in which no bronchiectasis was observed, he concluded that central airway inflammation was not an important cause of the bronchiectasis.

The classic studies of Reid[5208] showed that permanent bronchiectasis was associated with obliteration of the peripheral bronchial tree, as well as dilatation of the central airways. Whitwell[5243] provided a large series of cases in which he described the appearance of follicular hyperplasia of the lymphatics and introduced the term "follicular bronchiectasis." It seems likely that repeated episodes of inflammation are responsible for both the follicular hyperplasia of the lymphatics and the peripheral airway obliteration. This is illustrated by a case of bronchiectasis (Fig. 1–8) in which aspiration of a plastic toy produced severe bronchiectasis and obliteration of the peripheral airways by a process similar to that shown in Figure 1–7G, together with hyperplasia of the lymph nodes.

The early experimental studies of Lander[5177] showed that atelectasis was important in the production of bronchiectasis. By introducing mobile acacia gum plugs into the airways of cats, which were sucked down into peripheral airways, both atelectasis and dilation of the proximal bronchi were produced. As the dilated central airways could be returned to normal caliber by introducing a pneumothorax, he argued that the bronchi were dilated because of increased traction from the partially atelectatic lobe. This contrasted with the earlier work of Tannenberg and Pinner,[5230] who obstructed the main bronchus and could only produce ectasia by introducing infected material beyond the obstruction.

In the light of Mead and colleagues' recent analysis[5192] of the interdependence of airways and parenchyma, it seems likely that inflammation leads to occlusion of airways, which results in atelectasis of the parenchyma and consequent dilatation of central airways by increased traction on the peribronchial sheath.

However, an awkward fact in relation to this hypothesis is that children with bronchiolitis most often have hyperinflated rather than atelectatic lungs. It seems likely that the increase in breathing frequency, together with the prolongation of the time required to empty the lung, may combine to produce hyperinflation of the parenchyma. As hyperinflation, as well as atelectasis, would increase the traction on the central airways, either could contribute to the initial dilation of them. It seems probable that the natural course of the inflammatory reaction in the central airways would weaken their walls, leading to further dilatation; the deposition of connective tissue would cause the permanent changes of dilatation and distortion that we recognize as bronchiectasis.

Pulmonary Complications of Fibrocystic Disease

The pulmonary complications of fibrocystic disease of the pancreas provides an illustration of the relationship between repeated episodes of airway inflammation that lead to obliteration of peripheral airways and dilatation of the bronchi. The fact that bronchiectasis is a common event in the lungs of patients dying of fibrocystic disease has been well recognized by many authors.[5224] In 1968, Esterly and Oppenheimer[5142, 5143] reported 84 autopsies on infants

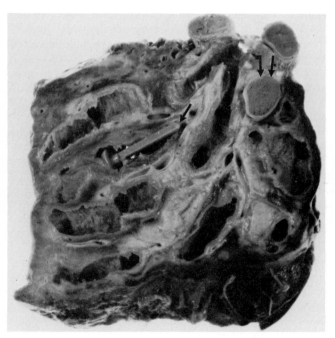

Figure 1–8. Resected bronchiectatic lobe of lung of a young adult. The bronchiectasis was produced by the aspiration of the plastic toy (single arrow) when the patient was a child. This foreign body was present in the lobe for many years and produced chronic inflammation, obliteration of the peripheral airways, bronchiectasis, and hyperplasia of the lymphatics (double arrows).

and children with cystic fibrosis and found that bronchiectasis was present in 53 of them. The airways from these patients very frequently showed hypertrophy and hyperplasia of the bronchial mucous gland layer, as well as chronic inflammation of bronchial and bronchiolar walls, where the inflammation was severe and obliterative in character.

Figure 1–9 shows the morphology of a case of fibrocystic disease. The bronchiectatic sacs are evident on the cut surface of the lung (Fig. 19A), and the bronchogram (Fig. 1–9B) shows that the peripheral airways have been obliterated and the central airways dilated. It seems likely that repeated pneumonia with abscess formation and systemic sepsis result from the chronic airway disease. Furthermore, the expansion of the bronchial circulation that occurs as a result of the chronic airway inflammation[5180] provides an opportunity for bleeding into the airway lumen and probably accounts for the occurrence of hemoptyses that can be severe enough to be life-threatening. Pulmonary function tests in adults with cystic fibrosis are discussed in Chapter 10.

ASTHMA

As noted in Chapter 9, this disorder has proved difficult to define,[5124] but it is usually thought of in terms of reversible airflow obstruction. Those who have the propensity to develop asthmatic attacks have hyperresponsive airways,

as noted in Chapter 5; such patients can be identified by challenge tests.[5127] Patients who have hyperresponsive airways are also known to develop airflow limitation upon exercise[1476] or breathing cold air.[5133] These phenomena are described in Chapter 9.

It is of interest that relatively few subjects have a clearly established allergic mechanism for their asthma. The majority seem to acquire hyperreactivity and asthma in a non-specific fashion. In those patients in whom an immune mechanism can be demonstrated, it occurs as a result of specific IgE binding to mast cells. When antigen interacts with this antibody, the mast cells release preformed mediators, such as histamine, and also generate a wide variety of other mediators, including the leukotrienes. The subject of mediator release has been comprehensively reviewed[5123, 5170, 5221] and will not be further discussed. In recent years it has become apparent that airways hyperreact when an inflammatory reaction occurs in them.[3167, 5159] This inflammatory reaction can be induced by a specific antigen reacting with IgE on mast cells[5170]; or with upper respiratory tract infections[2748]; or by non-specific irritants, such as cigarette smoke,[693] ozone,[160] and possibly NO_2,[776] as noted in Chapter 6.

In models of asthma, such as allergic bronchoconstriction in the guinea pig, Jeffries and associates[5172] in our laboratory showed that smooth muscle contraction can occur without associated airway edema or mucous plugging in the airways. This contrasts with human autopsy

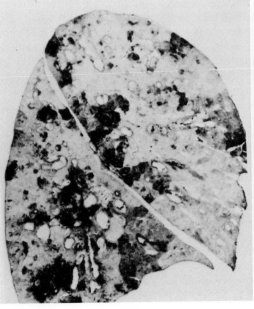
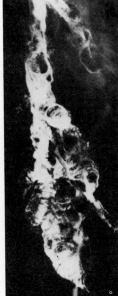

Figure 1–9. The lung from a case of fibrocystic disease of the pancreas. The bronchiectasis is apparent on the cut surface of the lung (A), and the bronchogram (B) shows that the central airways are dilated and the peripheral airways are obliterated.

findings in asthma in which small bronchi and bronchioles nearly always show edema of airway walls and mucous plugging of the lumen.[5137, 5138] This suggests that airway smooth muscle contraction plays an important role in those asthma patients in whom the airflow limitation is easily and rapidly reversed by bronchodilator therapy and that inflammation of the wall and mucous plugging of the lumen may be important anatomic features of asthma as it becomes more severe. In Chapter 9, recent studies by Laitinen and colleagues[4192] are noted; these have shown that acute inflammatory changes are often found in the airways of asthma patients at a time when their airflow limitation is only moderately severe.

The dominant control of the smooth muscle is provided by the cholinergic system, which constricts smooth muscle,[3734] and the beta-adrenergic system, which relaxes it.[5228] Alpha-adrenergic receptors are sparse in the airway muscle of most species and probably relate to the bronchial vasculature or mucus-secreting apparatus rather than to the muscle. A third system of nerves, the so-called non-adrenergic inhibitory system,[3734] has been described more recently. As its name suggests, this system is thought to relax the smooth muscle by release of an as yet unidentified mediator. Several theories of asthma have developed that relate to one or another aspect of smooth muscle airway control. One theory[5228] stresses the possibility of a partial beta blockade; a second theory details a hyperreactive cholinergic pathway[5198]; a third theory suggests that a basic abnormality is suppression of the non-adrenergic inhibitory system[5211]; and finally, another theory suggests that asthmatic airways may be associated with smooth muscle that functions as a single unit so that the whole network contracts when part of it is stimulated.[3734]

As allergic asthmatic attacks are initiated by the interaction of antigen with IgE on mast cells,[5170] the relationship of the mast cell to the airway lumina is of critical importance in the initiation of these attacks. Studies on mast cell distribution are not easy because their fixation requires alcohol- rather than water-based fixatives, and these are seldom used routinely. Salvato[5217, 5218] has demonstrated that mast cells are depleted in asthma, and those that remain are markedly degranulated. Guerzon and associates[5155] have shown that there are relatively few mast cells in the mucosa as compared with the large concentration of them in the submucosa of the airways. Although there are

a very important number of mast cells on the surface of the airway lumen, this number can be overestimated by washing and brushing techniques, which also harvest mast cells from the mucosa. For example, Guerzon[5155] estimated that there was approximately one mast cell for every million epithelial cells, whereas Patterson and his colleagues[5204] found one mast cell for every 200 epithelial cells in lung washings. It seems likely that large antigen molecules unable to penetrate the mucosa react with the relatively small number of mast cells on the epithelial surface and that chemical mediators released from these mast cells are responsible for opening the tight epithelial junctions and allowing the antigen to penetrate to the mast cells located deep in the mucosa in the airway wall.

Thickening of the epithelial basement membrane is an important histologic feature of the asthmatic lung (Fig. 1–7B). Callerame and associates[5120] showed that the mean width of the basement membrane from asthmatics was 17.5 micrometers, whereas that from normal persons was only 7.0 micrometers. They attributed this thickening to the deposition of immunoglobulins. However, recent data on airway inflammation suggest that the basement membrane begins to increase in thickness in association with the increased mitotic activity that heralds the beginning of epithelial repair. This suggests that the increased thickness of the basement membrane may be due to collagen deposition associated with increased epithelial cell turnover in much the same way that the basement membrane of the microvasculature in diabetes mellitus thickens in relation to the increased endothelial cell turnover.[5235, 5236] As early as 1882, Curschmann[5130] noted that asthmatics had a large number of epithelial cells in their sputum, and this has subsequently been confirmed by many investigators.[5128, 5200] They have also demonstrated that squamous cells, as well as compact clusters of columnar cells (known as Creola bodies), are commonly found. The loss of mucosal cells has been attributed to muscle spasm by Houston and colleagues[5165] and to submucosal edema by Dunnill,[5137, 5138] but it also seems likely that direct toxic injury to epithelial cells, perhaps by products of the eosinophil,[5151] is also important. This increased epithelial turnover is also associated with active division of the epithelial cell layer, with an increase in the number of goblet cells present in the epithelium.

At autopsy, the lungs from patients who have

died in status asthmaticus are hyperinflated and tend not to collapse after the thorax is opened because the segmental and subsegmental airways and bronchioles are filled with inflammatory mucous plugs. In addition to mucus, these plugs contain fluid, solute, and cellular elements derived from the blood.[5145, 5219] The eosinophilic leukocyte is the cell that tends to predominate in these plugs, but other inflammatory cells and a large number of epithelial cells can also be found. The submucosa shows evidence of an inflammatory reaction, which consists of a congested microvasculature, and of an edematous interstitial space containing the same inflammatory cellular infiltrate as the airway lumen. The reason for the excess mucus in airways is probably related both to increased production and to decreased clearance. Increased mucus production can result from hypertrophy of the bronchial mucous glands, as well as from goblet cell metaplasia of the mucosal lining,[5137, 5138] whereas decreased clearance would result from the disrupted epithelium. The fact that the plugs have a high protein content, with much of the protein being albumin,[5219] suggests that the inflammatory exudate contributes to their formation.

The nature and source of the fluid that normally lines the airways has proved difficult to clarify. It seems possible that the lining fluid emanates largely as a fluid secretion in the distal airways and that its final composition is influenced by water absorption in the central airways.[5114] This absorption of fluid and the more rapid movement of the lining layer in the central airways[5197] are both required to prevent the airways' relatively narrow cross sections from being occluded. An increase in the production of fluid in the form of exudate, interference with a normal fluid resorptive process, and decreased mucociliary clearance tend to increase the amount of fluid in the airways. In severe asthma, all of these factors appear to combine to produce severe airway obstruction in the form of tenacious plugs. Whether or not plugging occurs in less severe forms of asthma is not clear. Early bronchographic studies of patients with chronic asthma[5213] showed that the airways were often occluded by mucus, but this form of investigation is now known to be dangerous in these patients.

Airway Changes in Chronic Obstructive Pulmonary Disease

As noted in Chapter 7, a major problem in describing the pathology of chronic obstructive pulmonary disease is the terminology used. The definition of chronic bronchitis is based on clinical symptoms of cough and sputum production that are thought to be related to mucous hypersecretion.[5125] However, as noted in Chapters 7 and 8, chronic airflow obstruction and chronic cough and sputum may not be closely related. Because most authors[599, 5160, 5234] seem to agree that the site of airway obstruction is in the peripheral airways, it is incorrect to use the term "severe chronic bronchitis" to describe patients with more severe chronic airflow obstruction—a point noted in Chapter 7.

Several studies have established the fact that lesions in the peripheral airways in cases of chronic airflow limitation are inflammatory in nature.* The changes in the epithelium range from metaplasia to ulceration and are associated with an infiltration of inflammatory cells into the airway wall, deposition of connective tissue, and hypertrophy and perhaps hyperplasia of the airway muscle layer.

As noted in Chapter 6, several recent studies have shown that there is also an increased permeability of the airways in asymptomatic smokers,[3980, 5172] and experimental studies in animals[5168, 5223] suggest that this occurs in relation to the fluid exudation phase of the inflammatory response. While the lesions seen in the airways of smokers represent a trivial inflammatory response as compared with that seen in bronchiectasis,[5208] as already noted, experimental studies in animals[3141] have shown that minimal lesions can cause measurable airway dysfunction. It seems likely that reversible airway dysfunction is accounted for either by fluid exudation onto the airway surface or by an increased responsiveness of the peripheral airway smooth muscle, rather than by a permanent structural alteration. However, when severe fixed airflow limitation is present, connective tissue deposition in the airway wall narrows the airways.[1202]

Several authors have suggested that emphysema contributes to the peripheral airway obstruction by either decreasing the tension in the outer wall of the airway[5119] or causing it to behave as a check valve through the reduction of alveolar attachments to the outer wall of the airway.[5131, 5179] However, direct measurements[5160] have shown that the increased peripheral resistance was not reversed by lung inflation and that it was not possible to get these airways to behave as a check valve. Therefore,

---

*See references 625, 3146, 5190, 5191, 5201, 5206.

it seems more likely that the increased airway resistance is due to inflammatory disease in the wall and lumen of the peripheral airways. This fixed airway obstruction, which is the same on inspiration as on expiration, leads to dynamic compression of the larger airways during forced expiration,[5148, 5183, 5193] which in turn accounts for the so-called check valve obstruction.

The Transition from Health to Obstructive Airway Disease

If one accepts that peripheral airways account for little of the total airway resistance in normal adult lungs but are the major site of airflow obstruction in diseased lungs, it follows that pathologic changes may be advanced in these airways before their effects are apparent clinically. This concept led to a period of investigation based on the attractive hypothesis that early detection of peripheral lung disease might allow measures to be taken to reverse the process prior to the onset of severe airflow obstruction. The tests designed to detect early disease have been summarized[584] and are dealt with in other chapters. It is clear that a number of special tests of peripheral airway function become abnormal at a stage when the FEV_1 is still normal.[3160] The function tests may revert to normal with cessation of smoking even though the pathology does not appear to change.[3118]

Cigarette smoking is the most important cause of airway disease, but epidemiologic studies indicate that only some fraction of those who smoke develop chronic airflow obstruction.[5118] It may be that those who do develop severe obstructive lung disease from smoking constitute a susceptible group. Just why such a susceptible group might exist is of some interest, and there are several possibilities.[5194] De Vries and his associates[5132] have suggested that patients with the most severe bronchospastic airway obstruction components were the most likely to develop chronic airflow limitation. This has subsequently been referred to as the "Dutch" hypothesis; the major problem with it is that it is difficult to test. This difficulty is caused partially from our limited understanding of the nature of bronchial hyperresponsiveness and partially from the fact that an adequate test of the hypothesis requires long-term epidemiologic surveys. As noted above, studies both in humans and in animals have shown that acute airway inflammation induced by a variety of mechanisms can cause the airways to hyperreact to another inhaled irritant or stimulant. The Dutch hypothesis would suggest that those with the greatest reactivity for a given degree of inflammation would be the most susceptible to the development of chronic obstruction. A greater understanding of the factors responsible for airway hyperresponsiveness would obviously be of value in predicting those likely to develop chronic disease. Similarly, new knowledge concerning the genetic control of the inflammatory response would be of obvious value in throwing light on this problem.

Alternatively, the susceptibility to develop severe airflow obstruction (apart from that due to concomitant emphysema) could be acquired. Several studies have suggested that episodes of viral bronchiolitis in childhood result in airway abnormalities in adult life.[2636, 2899, 5225] It has also been suggested that viral bronchiolitis may lead to wheezing and/or bronchial hyperreactivity.[5156] If this were so, one could argue that viral infection might be important in the development of chronic peripheral airway obstruction. There have also been case reports[5135, 5202] of rapidly progressive airway obstruction in adults in whom viral infections have been implicated (see Chapter 18 and Chapter 19). This suggests the possibility that rapidly progressive chronic airflow obstruction could be a result of a viral infection superimposed on the lesions initiated by cigarette smoke. It is of interest that Homma and his associates[3343] have described an entity characterized by chronic inflammation of the bronchioles without obliteration, which they have termed "panbronchiolitis." This could well be a result of a combination of insults that might include cigarette smoking, viral bronchiolitis, and exposure to air pollutants. This type of bronchiolitis is discussed in Chapter 19.

BRONCHIOLITIS OBLITERANS

The pathologic features of severe peripheral airway inflammation in which the exudate in the peripheral airways becomes organized into a polypoid connective tissue plug extending into peripheral airways have been noted earlier in this chapter. The clinical spectrum of this pathologic abnormality was reviewed by Epler and Colby[3741] in 1983. They classified the clinical setting in which it occurs into:

1. Toxic fume bronchiolitis obliterans
2. Post-infectious bronchiolitis obliterans.

3. Bronchiolitis obliterans associated with connective tissue disease.

4. Bronchiolitis obliterans occurring with a localized lesion.

5. Idiopathic bronchiolitis obliterans.

More recently, they and their colleagues[4268] have reviewed a larger number of patients with idiopathic bronchiolitis obliterans, which they have grouped into a clinical syndrome they call "bronchiolitis obliterans with organizing pneumonia" (see Chapter 19 for function test data on their cases). The major difference between this latter syndrome and other forms of bronchiolitis obliterans is that it does not appear to be associated with irreversible airway obstruction and has a much better prognosis. It seems very likely that severe bronchiolitis obliterans with irreversible airway obstruction results from a diffuse airway injury, whereas the patchy injury described by Epler and his associates may result from an organizing bronchopneumonia.[4268] The fact that a lung biopsy would reveal bronchiolitis obliterans in both cases is not surprising in view of the fact that the pathologic process is stereotyped.

The occurrence of bronchiolitis obliterans in rheumatologic disease with or without the administration of penicillamine[1320, 3367, 5141] (noted in Chapter 13) and as an isolated event following bone marrow transplantation[4782] points strongly to a host factor in its pathogenesis. Whether this host factor is genetic or acquired remains to be determined. This condition may lead to severe chronic airflow limitation.

PERIPHERAL AIRWAY DISEASE IN HYPERSENSITIVITY PNEUMONITIS

A great many antigens have been associated with hypersensitivity pneumonitis.[5233] The majority of these are occupational in origin, but as noted in Chapter 11, cases are also caused by naturally occurring organisms.[5144, 5207, 5215] As the materials to which patients are exposed are complex and contain a wide variety of antigenic materials, it is often difficult to be sure which antigen has caused the pneumonitis.

In an experimental study on rabbits, Joubert and associates[5174] used a relatively pure antigen (horseradish peroxidase); they found that one major component of this mixture of antigenic materials caused the alveolitis, while other components were responsible for the precipitating antibody in the serum and for positive skin tests. This means that the demonstration of a positive skin test and/or a precipitating antibody to crude extracts provides evidence of exposure to the material but does not establish that a particular molecule in the crude material is responsible for the lung disease. This suggests that the most effective way of establishing a relationship between a crude mixture of antigens and lung disease is to challenge the patient with an aerosol of the crude material and to make objective measurements of the pulmonary response (see Chapter 5). Unfortunately, it is not possible to be dogmatic as to whether this sort of test is indicated in every case. In some cases, particularly when the patient's livelihood may be involved, a challenge test may be necessary to establish a firm diagnosis. However, in other cases remission of symptoms and signs of disease when the patient leaves an environment may be all that is necessary for satisfactory management of the disease.

Histologic Features of Hypersensitivity Pneumonitis

The histologic appearance of hypersensitivity pneumonitis is stereotyped, in spite of the fact that it can be caused by so many different materials. In general, hypersensitivity pneumonitis appears as a granulomatous inflammatory lesion that involves the central portion of the lobule, including the terminal and respiratory bronchioles (Fig. 1–7H).* Bronchiolitis is such an important feature of the disease that Turner-Warwick[5233] has suggested that it should be called "extrinsic allergic bronchioloalveolitis."

As noted in Chapter 11, a careful analysis of 60 patients with farmer's lung[3468] showed that common findings were an alveolar interstitial infiltrate (consisting of plasma cells, lymphocytes, and, occasionally, eosinophils) in all cases; a granulomatous interstitial reaction in 70% of the cases (with the granulomas tending to be located in the center of the lobule); and a mild form of bronchiolitis obliterans in about half the cases, with connective tissue proliferating in the respiratory bronchioles. Other histologic features, such as unresolved pneumonia, the presence of alveolar foam cells, and pleural fibrosis, seem more likely to have occurred as a result of the airway obstruction produced by

*See references 3468, 5108, 5134, 5140, 5175, 5222, 5226, 5232.

the primary disease. Foreign bodies are commonly found in extrinsic allergic alveolitis, but it is rare to be able to demonstrate the nature of the etiologic agent. However, cork dust has been identified within the lesions in suberosis,[2490] vegetable fibers in bagassosis,[5242] and fungi in maple bark disease. Although these crude materials are the source of the responsible antigens, it seems very likely that different antigens present in the crude material are responsible for different aspects of the disease.

Kawanami and his associates[5175] have reported light and electron microscopy findings in 18 patients who had biopsies for extrinsic allergic alveolitis. Their findings were similar to earlier reports but provided electron microscopic evidence that the primary cell infiltrating the alveolar wall was the lymphocyte. They also provided very good photomicrographs of the granulomas; these tended to be poorly formed and showed the deposition of interstitial connective tissue. This latter event was often associated with the formation of "alveolar buds," which represent masses of loose connective tissue located within the air space. This probably reflects the organization of an exudate that has developed in an area with extensive epithelial damage and is likely to be the preliminary event in the formation of bronchiolitis obliterans.

In recent years, several groups of investigators[4296, 5149, 5158, 5169] have claimed that this diagnosis can also be established by bronchoalveolar lavage. The value of this procedure in the diagnosis of lung disease has recently been questioned by Whitcomb and Dixon.[4387] However, this does not mean that bronchoalveolar lavage will not prove to be a useful method of investigation of the pathogenesis of hypersensitivity pneumonitis and other interstitial lung diseases.

Patients with extrinsic allergic alveolitis develop symptoms when they are challenged with crude extracts of the source of the antigens to which they have become allergic. These challenge tests may show (1) an immediate response in which the FEV_1 falls significantly within a few minutes after exposure to the aerosol; (2) a delayed response in which it falls several hours later; or (3) a combination of both immediate and delayed responses (see Chapter 5). The immediate response is known to be IgE-mediated, but the nature of the delayed response is much more controversial. The timing of the response and the indirect evidence that precipitating antibody was present caused original investigators[5203, 5205] to favor an Arthus reaction as the mechanism producing the phenomenon. However, a vasculitis consistent with this reaction has not been found in most studies, although in some[5108] it has been considered to be a cause of early pathologic changes. More recently, studies of experimental models of the disease indicate the probability of a pathogenesis induced by a delayed type of hypersensitivity,[5174, 5212] rather than by an Arthus reaction. The development of the granulomatous bronchioloalveolitis that is typical of human disease would seem to require both a particulate antigen and a delayed type of hypersensitivity reaction.

SUMMARY

This chapter has reviewed the manifestations of an inflammatory process in the conducting airways. While it is not possible to be dogmatic, there is a reasonable amount of data that suggests that certain patterns of abnormality become manifest in different situations. These changes are summarized in Figure 1–7, which shows a range of patterns including acute exudation into the lumen, plugging of the lumen with a mucous exudate, infiltration of the wall with inflammatory cells, deposition of connective tissue and hypertrophy of muscle in the wall, and obliteration of the lumen by organization of the exudate. The nature and extent of the changes in the peripheral airways determine whether or not the airway disease leads to symptoms or develops into severe airway obstruction. As the changes are all manifestations of the inflammatory response, it follows that future efforts aimed at understanding the nature of this response in the airways more fully could well prove highly relevant to a better understanding of the various forms of obstructive lung disease.

BASIC PULMONARY PHYSIOLOGY

INTRODUCTION

The principal function of the lung is to exchange gas between the blood and the atmospheric air. It follows from this that the measurement of the tension of gases in the blood leaving the lung might be regarded as the only required test of lung function. However, the "pulmonary reserve" is so large and the mechanisms that adjust the amount of ventilation and that relate the blood flow to ventilation within the lung are so efficient that these gas tensions may remain within normal limits, despite the presence of extensive lung disease. Indeed, the symptoms of lung disease, in particular the sensation of dyspnea, bear little relationship to the efficiency of gas exchange. For these reasons, measurements of the properties of the lung—such as size (or volume), expansibility (elasticity), ventilatory ability (forced expiratory volume), or efficiency of gas transfer (diffusing capacity)—often provide a much more complete picture of the state of the lung than measurements of arterial blood gases, important though these are.

This chapter is intended as an introduction to the physiologic considerations that lie behind the interpretation of derangements of function and is not concerned with details of methods and procedure. The factors that influence the choice of methods of testing pulmonary function are discussed in Chapter 5. It should be emphasized here that no single test of lung function can ever measure all the attributes that constitute the function of the whole lung and caution should be used in extrapolating conclusions from a simple test. The limits of interpretation are based on a knowledge of the physiologic principles embodied in the test, the biologic

variability of the measured quantity, and the accuracy and reproducibility of the measurement. Reference will be made to the appropriate volumes of the *Handbook of Physiology (Section 3, The Respiratory System)* recently published by the American Physiological Society, where comprehensive reviews of individual topics may be found. The third edition of *The Lung*[5402] provides an excellent summary of the field.

The terms, symbols, and abbreviations used in respiratory physiology were chosen and approved by the Commission of Respiratory Physiology of the International Union of Physiological Sciences in 1980. A full list of the symbols may be found on the inside cover of the *Handbook of Physiology* series published by the American Physiological Society (Section 3).

VENTILATION

Spirometry: Subdivisions of Lung Volume

The subdivisions of lung volume may be measured using a spirometer. The desirable characteristics of a spirometer for routine use have been defined.[2881] It is usual for volumes of air breathed to be expressed as volumes at body temperature and pressure saturated with water vapor (BTPS). Oxygen consumption and carbon dioxide output are expressed at standard temperature and pressure, dry (STPD), because equal volumes at STPD contain equal numbers of molecules (Avogadro's hypothesis). Since measurements are normally made at ambient (room) temperature and pressure (ATP), vol-

23

umes must be corrected using the gas laws and taking into account the presence of water vapor. Many current spirometers have an electrical output that allows computerized measurement of the subdivisions of lung volume; however, a printed record of the expiration data should always be available.[53][78]

The terms now commonly used to describe the subdivisions of lung volume are indicated in Figure 2–1. It may be noted that there are primary "volumes," which do not overlap each other, and there are "capacities," which are combinations of the primary volumes. It follows from a study of these that sufficient data to calculte all of the subdivisions can be provided by a selection of the measurements. For example, by giving total lung capacity (TLC), functional residual capacity (FRC), and vital capacity (VC); or residual volume (RV), expiratory reserve volume (ERV), and VC, the other subdivisions of lung volume may be calculated.

RV, FRC, and TLC cannot be measured directly using a spirometer because they include air that cannot be expelled from the lungs. FRC is the most frequently measured because the subject is in a rest position where the tendency of the chest wall to spring out is equally balanced by the tendency of the lungs to collapse inward and away from the chest wall. Thus, no effort is required by the subject to reach and maintain this position. To measure the absolute gas volume in the lung, one of four different methods may be used: closed-circuit helium equilibration, open-circuit nitrogen washout, whole body plethysmography, or radiologic techniques.

Closed-Circuit Helium Equilibration

The method in most frequent use for the measurement of FRC employs helium dilution. A closed-circuit spirometer system is used, and carbon dioxide is absorbed from the system. To the spirometer system is added a known amount of 100% helium. The helium concentration is measured and from its dilution the volume of the spirometer system can be calculated. The subject is then connected to the spirometer through a mouthpiece and breathes the helium mixture until mixing is complete (3 minutes in normal subjects but may be longer in patients with disease). Because helium is poorly soluble and little is absorbed in the lungs, the volume of the spirometer plus the volume of the lungs can be calculated from the dilution of the helium. Subtracting the volume of the spirometer system from the volume of the spirometer plus the lungs gives the volume of gas in the lungs. In practice, during the breathing from the closed-circuit, carbon dioxide is absorbed, and oxygen is added to the system to keep the volume of the spirometer system at end-expiration equal to that of the spirometer system before the patient was connected.

Single-Breath Helium Dilution

This method is frequently used during the measurement of single-breath diffusing capacity. The subject expires to residual volume and takes a full inspiration to TLC of a gas containing a known concentration of helium. The average helium concentration in the subsequent expirate is then measured. Dead space is estimated and TLC may be calculated. This method assumes the mean concentration in the expirate is close to that in the residual volume. Although this is true in normal subjects errors arise in subjects with obstructive disease.

Open-Circuit Nitrogen Washout

This method involves the displacement of the nitrogen in the lungs by breathing 100% oxygen

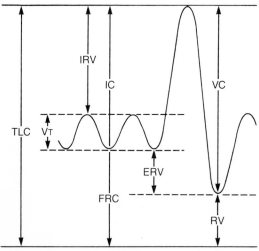

Figure 2–1. *Subdivisions of Lung Volume*

TLC = Total lung capacity
FRC = Functional residual capacity
VC = Vital capacity
ERV = Expiratory reserve volume
RV = Residual volume
IC = Inspiratory capacity
V_T = Tidal volume
IRV = Inspiratory reserve volume

and the calculation of the volume of nitrogen expired by analysis of the nitrogen concentration in the expired air. Breathing of the oxygen is usually continued for 7 minutes. Nitrogen analysis of the expired air is most conveniently performed by a nitrogen meter. The meter must be carefully calibrated because the method depends on the multiplication of a large gas volume by a value for the nitrogen concentration and small analytical errors cause considerable changes in the FRC computed. The technical details and precautions to ensure accuracy have been described.[5379]

Both the closed-circuit helium and the open-circuit nitrogen techniques give satisfactory results when normal subjects are being tested (see Chapter 5). In the presence of airways obstruction, equilibration takes longer than the standard time. It is important that with the closed-circuit technique breathing should be continued until a steady helium concentration is reached (possibly up to 18 minutes). It had been previously thought that if the helium closed-circuit or the nitrogen elimination procedure were continued for long enough, values for FRC computed from these methods would be not very different from those found by body plethysmography. However, it now appears that body plethysmography may overestimate FRC in some situations; thus, provided that the stability of the equilibrated helium concentration is carefully observed, the latter technique may provide the best estimate (see Chapter 5).

Body Plethysmography

The concept of plethysmography in the study of the lung dates from 1882, when Pfluger measured his own intrathoracic gas volume by applying Boyle's Law to relate changes in alveolar pressure to simultaneous changes in lung volume.[5380] He used a wooden chamber or plethysmograph that completely enclosed the subject and communicated with a spirometer. The principle led to the development of the pressure plethysmograph as an airtight box in which volume changes in the intrathoracic gas can be calculated from the simultaneous pressure change in the gas surrounding the subject.[5380]

The subject sits inside the chamber and breathes through an outlet in the wall of the chamber. At the end of a normal expiration, a shutter closes the mouthpiece and the subject is asked to make rapid shallow respiratory efforts. As the subject inhales, the gas in the lungs is expanded and the box pressure rises as its gas volume decreases. Using Boyle's Law and knowing the pre-inspiratory box volume (by prior calibration), the change in the volume in the box can be calculated. The gas in the lung must have changed by this same volume, and Boyle's Law is then applied to the gas in the lungs. Knowing the changes in pressure in the mouth (and also in the lung, as there is no air flow), the volume of gas in the lung (FRC) can be calculated. The volume-displacement plethysmograph was later revived using a pneumotachograph to measure volume flow in and out of the box.[5381] It has the advantage that there are less stringent requirements regarding leaks.

The body plethysmograph has the advantage that it measures the total volume of gas in the lung, including any that is trapped behind closed airways and does not communicate with the mouth. However, recent studies have suggested that under some circumstances mouth pressure may underestimate alveolar pressure and may lead to an overestimate of the calculated FRC (Chapter 5).

Radiologic Methods

Lung volume may be estimated from the anteroposterior x-ray of the chest with some estimate of the anteroposterior diameter. Various formulae have been used, and volumes are subtracted to account for heart, blood, and lung tissue. The results correlate closely with physiologic measurements but only under defined conditions and for specific volumes (see Chapter 5).

MEASUREMENTS OF VENTILATION

Resting Ventilation

Resting ventilation is defined as the quantity of air expired per minute ($\dot{V}E$). It is most frequently measured using a mouthpiece and a three-way valve, air being collected into a Neoprene bag. The volume of gas collected is then measured in a Tissot spirometer or by using a dry gas meter. More recently, the improved quality of pneumotachographs has allowed measurements of air flow to be integrated and a direct read-out of minute ventilation to be obtained. Careful calibration is required to maintain accuracy, but these instruments may be useful for bedside monitoring. Turbine flowmeters have also been designed for measurement of air flow during exercise.[5382] However, the "lag" in the system leads to unacceptable errors in the calculation of $\dot{V}_{CO_2}$ and $\dot{V}_{O_2}$ at low flow rates. The Wright Respirometer remains a practical and economic means of taking bedside measurements. If a value of dead space is assumed and the respiratory rate is known, it is possible to make an approximate estimate of alveolar ventilation from the measured resting ventilation.

The measurement of resting ventilation plays little part in routine pulmonary assessment, since patients with advanced lung disease frequently breathe with a normal tidal volume and respiratory rate. Normal values for resting ventilation are difficult to obtain. As soon as the subject knows that ventilation is being measured, breathing no longer remains an unconscious process and the pattern may alter (see Chapter 4). In addition, the presence of a mouthpiece and noseclip, even in trained normal subjects, may cause the rate and depth to change. However, the pattern of breathing may be of importance and may be recorded noninvasively using impedance or inductive plethysmography. The output of these instruments may be calibrated by taking breaths, the volume of which is measured by spirometry; both the volume and the pattern of the breaths may then be followed. Values of tidal volume with inductive plethysmography are claimed to be within ±10% of the values observed with spirometry.

In contrast to its insignificant role in routine pulmonary assessment, the measurement of resting ventilation may be important in the management of patients who are in danger of developing respiratory failure from hypoventilation, especially if facilities are not available for the measurement of blood gases. Hypoventilation may arise in postoperative states, in barbiturate intoxication, or in neuromuscular disease. There are, of course, many situations in which the minute ventilation may be normal while the alveolar ventilation is grossly deficient. Even in this case, measurement of minute ventilation (and calculation of alveolar ventilation) may reduce the need for frequent sampling of arterial blood.

Anatomic Dead Space

A part of each breath remains within the upper airway and tracheobronchial tree and does not reach the gas-exchanging surfaces of the alveoli. Therefore, it does not contribute to the exchange of O_2 and CO_2. This part of the airway is referred to as the *anatomic dead space* and is commonly designated V_D. That fraction of the total ventilation ($\dot{V}_E$) that enters the gas exchanging surface is called the *alveolar ventilation* or $\dot{V}_A$. To measure $\dot{V}_A$ it is necessary to subtract the dead space ventilation ($\dot{V}_D$) from $\dot{V}_E$. This is given by the following expression:

$$\dot{V}_A = \dot{V}_E - \dot{V}_D$$

V_D may be measured directly or estimated from body height or body weight (1 mL/0.5 kg body weight).

In 1948 Fowler described a single-breath method of measuring V_D. This method involves the simultaneous registration of expired nitrogen concentration and volume or flow, following a deep inspiration of a nitrogen free gas. The same technique is used to measure the distribution of ventilation and closing volume (see later). Details of the method of measurement of dead space are shown in Figure 2–2.

Under normal conditions, the gas volume measured by this method is the volume of those parts of the respiratory tract that, at the beginning of expiration, contain gas whose composition is unchanged from that of inspired air. This volume approximates that of the bronchial tree down to the terminal bronchioles. It has been shown that the extrathoracic fraction of the dead space, mainly comprising the pharynx and mouth, contributes about 66 milliliters of dead space to the average total of about 150 milliliters for a normal man.[5393] This value falls with depression of the jaw and flexion of the neck, and protrusion of the jaw and neck extension increases it. The dead space measured by Fowler's technique is smaller in the supine position than when sitting and is increased with advancing age.[5378] The volume of the dead space is decreased after pneumonectomy and is decreased 60% by tracheostomy.

The Bohr Equation and the Physiologic Dead Space

The anatomic dead space may be calculated by applying *Bohr's equation*. This equation is derived from the simple proposition that any gas expired must consist of two distinct portions, a volume of gas from the non-exchanging

Figure 2–2. *Calculation of Inert-Gas Dead Space After Single Breath of 100% Oxygen*

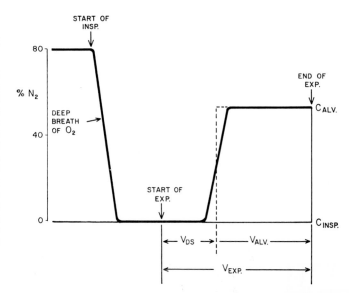

Idealized diagram illustrating the recorded nitrogen percentage at the mouth, using a fast analyzer. At the start of expiration the gas coming from the anatomic dead space contains no nitrogen. The nitrogen concentration then rises steeply until all the gas being expired is coming from the alveoli. The inert-gas dead space (V_{DS}) may be calculated from the volume of expiration from the start of expiration until the point indicated on the curve of nitrogen concentration. This point is selected by determining the point at which the two triangles (made up of the dotted line and the nitrogen curve) have equal area. This method may be used even if the alveolar nitrogen concentration is not uniform.

dead space plus a volume derived from alveolar gas. Thus

$$\dot{V}_E = \dot{V}_A + \dot{V}_D$$

and for CO_2,

$$\dot{V}_E \cdot F_{E_{CO_2}} = \dot{V}_A \cdot F_{A_{CO_2}} + \dot{V}_D \cdot F_{D_{CO_2}}$$

However, because $F_{D_{CO_2}}$ at the beginning of expiration is zero,

$$\dot{V}_E \cdot F_{E_{CO_2}} = \dot{V}_A \cdot F_{A_{CO_2}}$$

$$\dot{V}_E \cdot F_{E_{CO_2}} = (\dot{V}_E - \dot{V}_D)F_{A_{CO_2}}$$

Rearranging,

$$\dot{V}_D = \frac{(F_{A_{CO_2}} - F_{E_{CO_2}})}{F_{A_{CO_2}}} \cdot \dot{V}_E$$

(equation 1)

The fractional concentration of a gas is proportional to its partial pressure. Thus

$$\frac{\dot{V}_D}{\dot{V}_E} = \frac{P_{A_{CO_2}} - P_{E_{CO_2}}}{P_{A_{CO_2}}}$$

(equation 2)

This equation provides a value for $\dot{V}_D$ that is valid if a single number can be used to correctly define the mean alveolar gas tension ($P_{A_{CO_2}}$). If the assumption is made that arterial P_{CO_2} is equal to alveolar P_{CO_2}, equation 2 can be rewritten as follows:

$$\frac{\dot{V}_D}{\dot{V}_E} = \frac{P_{a_{CO_2}} - P_{E_{CO_2}}}{P_{a_{CO_2}}}$$

(equation 3)

The validity of this assumption is discussed later.

Since the expired volume and the arterial and mixed expired CO_2 tensions can be measured easily and accurately, a value for $\dot{V}_D$ can be readily calculated from equation 3. This number is called the *physiologic dead space*. When arterial and mixed alveolar gas tensions are the same, as they are in normal subjects, the calculated anatomic and physiologic dead spaces will be the same, and both are an approximate measure of the volume of the conducting airways. However, if areas of the lung are poorly perfused relative to their ventilation, $P_{a_{CO_2}}$ will be greater than $P_{A_{CO_2}}$ and the use of $P_{a_{CO_2}}$ in equation 3 will give a larger value for dead space. The difference in these circumstances between the anatomic dead space (equation 2) and the physiologic dead space (equation 3) has been termed the *alveolar dead space*. The physiologic dead space is increased in relation to anatomic dead space when there are significant volumes of the lung with a ventilation disproportionately high in relation to perfusion. The measurement of physiologic dead space is therefore a measure of ventilation/perfusion discrepancy.

The dead space to tidal volume ratio ($\dot{V}_D/\dot{V}_E$) is usually about 0.3 and normally decreases as tidal volume increases, as for example, in exercise. The failure of $\dot{V}_D/\dot{V}_E$ to decrease in exercise may be an early sign of pulmonary vascular disease.

Functional Distribution of Ventilation

Functionally, ventilation may be divided into the alveolar ventilation, corresponding to the ventilation of those areas of the lung where gas exchange between alveolar gas and blood takes place, and the dead space ventilation, corresponding to the ventilation of those areas where there is no gas exchange with blood. As noted earlier, the dead space ventilation may be considered to consist of two components: (1) the anatomic dead space, consisting of the air passages proximal to the respiratory bronchioles, and (2) the alveolar dead space, consisting of alveoli that have no blood flow but that are ventilated. These two components, the anatomic dead space plus the alveolar dead space, form the physiologic dead space. It should be noted that the alveolar dead space need not necessarily exist as an area of alveoli to which there is zero blood flow and in which there is no gas exchange. An area of the lung that is hyperventilated relative to its blood flow will function as if there were some normal lung plus a region that is ventilated but not perfused. Thus, there need not be an identifiable morphologic correlate of the alveolar dead space.

Alveolar Ventilation

Once the physiologic dead space is known (or in the normal lung if the anatomic dead space is known), the alveolar ventilation may be calculated by subtracting the dead space ventilation from the minute ventilation.

When the ventilation/perfusion ratios are similar throughout the lungs, as in normal subjects, an alveolar ventilation at rest of about 4 liters per minute is usually adequate. However, alveolar ventilation can be considered adequate only if it maintains within physiologic limits the tension of the respiratory gases leaving the lung. Thus, the only satisfactory measurement of effective alveolar ventilation in many clinical circumstances is by the measurement of arterial carbon dioxide tension. It is of interest that, at very low tidal volumes, alveolar ventilation is greater than would be predicted from the measured anatomic dead space, probably as a result of mixing at the interface between alveolar and dead space gases.

The arterial P_{CO_2} is inversely proportional to alveolar ventilation and if alveolar ventilation is unchanged is directly proportional to CO_2 production. This relationship is expressed in the equation

$$\dot{V}_A \text{ (BTPS)} = \frac{863 \times \dot{V}_{CO_2} \text{ (STPD)}}{Pa_{CO_2}}$$

Thus, the direct measurement of arterial P_{CO_2} is the only accurate way of assessing alveolar ventilation.

Maximal Voluntary Ventilation

Maximal voluntary ventilation (MVV) is the maximum volume of air that a subject can breathe per minute. It is measured over a limited period of hyperventilation, usually lasting 15 seconds. The test requires a high level of motivation and co-operation and is exhausting for the subject. Because the results correlate closely with the $FEV_{1.0}$, most laboratories assess ventilatory capacity by studying forced expiration.

PULMONARY MECHANICS

Air flows from a region of higher pressure to one of lower pressure. For inspiration to occur, alveolar pressure must be less than atmospheric pressure. Normal breathing in humans is accomplished by active contraction of the inspiratory muscles that enlarge the thorax. A full discussion of the function of the respiratory muscles appears in Chapter 22, and this will not be considered here. Expansion of the chest wall pulls on the lungs, enlarging the alveoli, alveolar ducts, and smaller airways. The expansion of the alveolar gas decreases its pressure below atmospheric, and air flows into the mouth, nose, and trachea and to the alveoli.

The active muscular contraction provides the force necessary to overcome (1) the elastic recoil of the lungs and chest wall, and (2) the frictional resistance to air flow through the airways.

Elastic Recoil of the Lungs

The outer surface of the lungs, which is covered by the visceral pleura, is in close contact with the inner surface of the thoracic cage, which is covered by the parietal pleura. It is characteristic of the lung that it tends to recoil inward, away from the chest wall; if the thorax is opened, the lung collapses. This property is due to the connective tissues, elastin and collagen, in the lung and is also due to the surface tension generated at the air-liquid interface in the alveoli. At the same time, at FRC the chest wall is at a volume lower than its resting volume. If the thorax is opened, the chest wall volume expands by about 600 to 1000 milliliters. The outward pull of the chest wall, whether passive or caused by inspiratory muscle activity, and the inward recoil of the lung tend to separate the visceral pleura from the parietal pleura. Under normal physiologic conditions, there is a small amount of fluid in the pleural cavity that allows the two layers of the pleurae to slide easily over each other. The mechanisms that keep the pleural space free of air and maintain only a minimal amount of liquid have been fully discussed by Agostoni.[5384] The tendency of the lung to recoil away from the chest wall may be measured as the pleural pressure (P_{pl}). This pressure can be measured directly by introducing a needle and a small amount of air into the pleural space. A safer but indirect method is to measure pressure in a thin-walled balloon introduced into the middle third of the esophagus. Changes in esophageal pressure follow changes in pleural pressure because the esophagus lies between the lungs and the chest wall and because the walls of the esophagus are thin and have little tone.

To understand any discussion of the elastic properties of the lung and chest wall it is essential to comprehend the different pressures that must be considered. These are shown in Figure 2–3.

Elasticity is the property of matter that causes it to return to its resting shape after deformation by an external force. A highly elastic material, e.g., steel, thus resists deformation. A perfectly elastic body when acted upon by one unit of force will stretch one unit of length until the elastic limit is reached, after which it will rapidly deform. The tissues of the lungs and chest wall are elastic; they must be stretched by an external force during inspiration. When the external force is removed, the tissues recoil to their resting position. In the lung the force is indicated by the pressure exerted on the lung, the transpulmonary pressure ($P_L = P_A - P_{pl}$), and the degree of stretch is indicated by the

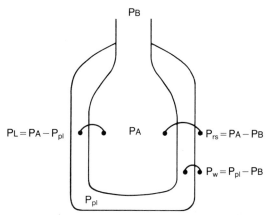

Figure 2–3. *Diagram Showing the Pressures Affecting the Respiratory System*

P_A = Alveolar pressure
P_B = Barometric pressure
P_{pl} = Pleural pressure
P_L = Transpulmonary pressure
P_{rs} = Pressure of the respiratory system
P_w = Pressure across the chest wall

change in volume. The relationship of the change in lung volume to the change in transpulmonary pressure (dV/dP) under static conditions (i.e., a few seconds are allowed to come to rest at each state) is known as the *compliance* of the lung. In the past, this measurement was usually made over the range of tidal volume. Over a small volume range, the relationship between pressure and volume could be regarded as linear. For comparison between lungs of different size, compliance may be expressed per unit of lung volume; this measurement is then known as *specific compliance*. Recoil of the lung is more usually assessed by measuring the full pressure/volume (PV) curve of the lung. The relationship between pressure and volume exhibits hysteresis; that is, the relationship is not the same during inflation and deflation, and PV curves are usually measured during deflation from TLC. The subject inhales to TLC, the airway is occluded, and transpulmonary pressure (P_L) is measured. Measurements are repeated during stepwise deflation obtained by releasing the airway occlusion (Fig. 2–4). After obtaining the PV curve, it may be described quantitatively by assuming it to be an exponent.[5385] In patients with emphysema, the curve is shifted upward and to the left, indicating a marked loss of elastic recoil. In patients with pulmonary fibrosis, the curve is shifted downward and to the right, indicating a significant increase in elastic recoil (Fig. 2–5).

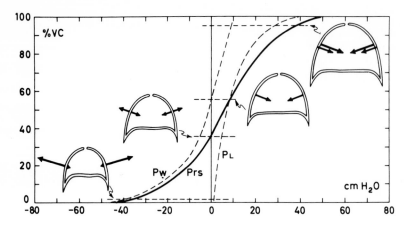

Figure 2–4. Static pressure-volume curves of the lung (PL), chest wall (Pw), and total respiratory system (Prs) during relaxation in the sitting posture. *Large arrows*, static forces of lung and chest wall (dimensions not to scale). *Horizontal broken lines*, volume for each drawing. (Reprinted with permission from Hyatt, R. E. Forced expiration. In: Handbook of Physiology, Section 3, Vol. 3, Part 1. American Physiological Society, Bethesda, Md., 1986, p. 116.)

Factors Influencing Elastic Recoil

Lung volume history is clearly an important factor in the shape of the pressure/volume curve of the lung, as shown by the difference between the inflation and deflation curves. Another important factor is age, since the elastic recoil falls with age. The recoil pressure of the lung is also influenced by the nature of the air-liquid interface and the surface tension in the lung.

Surface tension is the manifestation of the attracting forces between atoms and molecules. It has the units of force per unit length (dynes/cm). Many substances when placed in a liquid lower surface tension; such "surface active" or "surfactant" molecules exert lesser attracting forces for other molecules and thus lower surface tension. Pulmonary surfactant has been

found to be present in the lungs of all air-breathing vertebrates. It is formed in the Type II alveolar epithelial cells, which store surfactant in characteristic osmiophilic lamellar bodies and secrete their contents into the alveolar lumen.

The main constituent of surfactant is the phospholipid dipalmitoyl phosphatidylcholine. However, specific apoproteins are also important to its function. Pulmonary surfactant is able to markedly decrease the surface tension of an air-liquid interface. The relationship between the radius of a bubble, pressure inside, and tension in the wall is given by the Law of Laplace:

$$P = \frac{2T}{r}$$

where P = pressure across the wall, T =

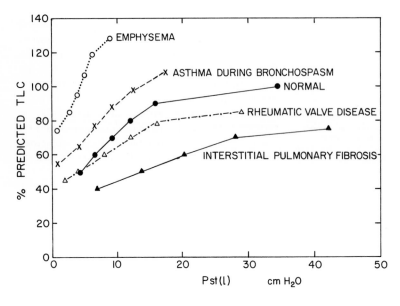

Figure 2–5. Static deflation pressure-volume curves of the lung in a variety of conditions.

tension in the wall, and r = radius of the sphere.

A reduction in wall tension reduces the pressure that must be exerted to increase the size of the sphere. This increases the compliance of the lung and reduces the work required to expand the alveolus with each breath. The influence of the surface tension of the air-liquid interface is best illustrated by comparing the PV curves for lungs inflated with air and those inflated with saline (Fig. 2–6). Peak recoil with saline, at the same volume as with air inflation to 30 cm H_2O, may be only 10 to 15 cm H_2O.[5386] The surfactant also has the important property that when the layer of surfactant (which probably exists as a monolayer) is compressed, the surface tension becomes lower. This property has been said to stabilize the lung. During expiration the alveoli become smaller; according to the Laplace relationship, the smaller alveoli would empty into the larger ones if wall tension did not also decrease. Another factor which

tends to stabilize the lung is the "interdependence" of lung units. The fact that adjacent alveoli share a common wall means that the tendency of any one alveolus or lung unit to collapse is opposed by the support of surrounding units.

Surfactant forms relatively late in gestation. The surfactant phospholipids and specific apoproteins appear simultaneously when the first lamellar bodies are observed—about the twenty-fifth week of gestation in humans. The amount of disaturated phosphatidylcholine increases first in the tissue and then in amniotic fluid, where it can be detected and its presence or absence used to predict the risk of postnatal respiratory distress. Factors controlling the biosynthesis of surfactant have been the object of numerous studies. The effects of glucocorticoids are best understood; in a complex sequence the Type II cells are stimulated to produce surfactant. However, glucocorticoids are no longer used for accelerating lung maturation because of their deleterious effects on the maturation of other organs.[5387] It is widely accepted that hyaline membrane disease, of which neonatal respiratory distress syndrome is the most frequent clinical manifestation, is the consequence of inadequate amounts of surfactant, either because of prematurity or because of a pathologic condition associated with pregnancy. Surfactant replacement can improve the status of infants suffering the syndrome, but only natural or "semisynthetic" surfactants containing both phospholipids and apoproteins are effective.

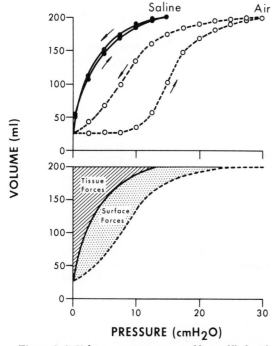

Figure 2–6. Volume-pressure curves of lungs filled with saline and with air (*upper panel*). The use of saline eliminates the effect of surface forces at the air-liquid interface and allows subdivision of the total pressure required to inflate the lung into the amounts necessary to overcome tissue forces and surface forces (*lower panel*). The arrows indicate whether the lung is being inflated or deflated; note that when using saline, hysteresis (the difference between the inflation and deflation limbs of the curve) is almost eliminated. (From Murray, J. The Normal Lung. W. B. Saunders, Philadelphia, 1976, p. 83.)

Chest Wall Recoil

The static recoil of the chest wall is assessed by measuring the pressure exerted by the relaxed respiratory system against an occluded airway over the range of the voluntarily achieved vital capacity. This assessment of the compliance of the total respiratory system is often unreliable because most subjects find it difficult to relax completely. Compliance of the chest wall can be calculated from the relationship:

$$(\text{total compliance})^{-1} = (\text{lung compliance})^{-1} + (\text{chest wall compliance})^{-1}$$

The chest wall progressively stiffens with age. Obesity decreases chest wall compliance (see Chapter 4), and chest deformities such as kyphoscoliosis and ankylosing spondylitis are associated with extreme chest wall stiffness (see Chapter 21).

Resistance to Air Flow

Most of the work of breathing is done to overcome the recoil of the lungs and thoracic cage. However, when respiration is rapid or the airways are narrowed, much work is done to overcome the frictional resistance to air flow. There is also frictional resistance of the tissues of the lung and chest wall; these comprise less than half the total pulmonary resistance.

The physical principles affecting the flow of air through tubes are similar to those for other fluids. Although there may be some turbulence in the larger airways, in most of the lung as the total cross-sectional area of the airways increases, flow is laminar. For laminar flow, Poiseuille's Law holds:

$$\dot{Q} = \frac{(P_1 - P_2) \cdot r^4 \cdot P_i}{8nl}$$

where $\dot{Q}$ = flow per unit time, $P_1 - P_2$ = driving pressure, r = radius, l = length, and n = viscosity of fluid. Because the factor $8nl/P_i r^4$ is fixed in a rigid system of tubes, this factor is referred to as resistance and

$$\text{Resistance} = \frac{P_1 - P_2}{\dot{Q}} = \frac{8nl}{P_i \cdot r^4}$$

For the lung,

$$\text{Airway resistance} = \frac{P_A - P_B}{\text{air flow}}$$

The units of airway resistance are cm $H_2O/L/$ sec.

A measurement of alveolar pressure is needed to calculate airway resistance, and this may be obtained, together with air flow, through the use of a body plethysmograph. The total resistance of the respiratory system (including the chest wall) can be estimated by imposing oscillating flow patterns upon spontaneous breaths, for example, with a loudspeaker placed in series with a mouthpiece. Normal values for airway resistance are in the range 1 to 1.5 cm $H_2O/L/sec$. For a discussion of techniques for partitioning the resistance between the chest wall, lung, and airways, see reference 5388. The upper or extrathoracic airways contribute a major share of the airway resistance, particularly when nose breathing is employed. Since the airways become narrow as they approach the alveoli, it is natural to expect that the smaller airways would be the major site of resistance to air flow. However, as noted in Chapter 1, there are so many of these small airways, each with a high resistance and parallel to each other, that the total resistance of the small airways is comparatively low and accounts for only a small proportion of the total resistance to air flow. Thus, less than 20% of the total airway resistance is created by airways of less than 2 millimeters in diameter. It follows that considerable changes can occur in the resistance to flow through smaller airways before this can be detected by a measure of total airway resistance.

Factors Influencing Airway Resistance

Lung Volume. Airway resistance decreases in a hyperbolic fashion because of the increase in the diameter of the airways as lung volume increases. The measurement of resistance may be normalized by expressing the ratio of conductance (which, as the reciprocal of resistance, is linearly related to lung volume) to the volume at which the measurement was made; the ratio is termed *specific airway conductance*. At very low lung volumes the small airways may close completely, especially in dependent lung zones.

Phase of Respiration. At any lung volume, resistance is less during inspiration than during expiration.

Vagal and Sympathetic Tone. Pharmacologic cholinergic blockade decreases pulmonary resistance in both large and small airways. Stimulation of bronchial beta$_2$-receptors produces bronchodilatation and increased airway conductance in both large and small airways. Beta blockade may be associated with an increase in airway resistance. In normal subjects there is little or no resting vagal or sympathetic tone.

Respiratory Gases. Hypocapnia is associated with bronchoconstriction and increased resistance, apparently as a result of a direct action on bronchiolar smooth muscle. Increased CO_2 does not affect airway conductance. This may provide a mechanism by which the ventilation is reduced to an area of the lung that is poorly perfused.

The density of the inspired gas affects the

Figure 2–7. *Left,* flow-volume plot for a normal subject. $\dot{V}_{max}$ values are plotted against their corresponding volume at A, B, and C and define the MEFV curve (*solid line*). *Right,* three isovolume pressure-flow curves from the same subject. Curves A, B, and C were measured at volumes of 0.8, 2.3, and 3.0 liters from total lung capacity (TLC), respectively. Transpulmonary pressure is the difference between pleural (estimated by esophageal balloon) and mouth pressures. (Reprinted with permission from Hyatt, R. E. Forced expiration. In: Handbook of Physiology. American Physiological Society, Bethesda, Md., 1986, p. 296.)

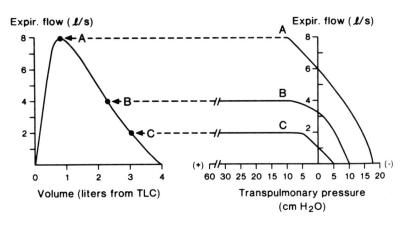

resistance to flow. Resistance is increased during a deep dive because the increased pressure raises gas density; conversely, the resistance may be reduced when a mixture of helium and oxygen is breathed.

Effects of Increased Airway Resistance

Because of increased resistance during expiration, gas may be trapped in the lungs, leading to increased FRC. This leads to a reduction in inspiratory capacity and limits the ability to increase ventilation on demand. Significant dyspnea may not become a symptom until airway resistance is increased five- to fifteenfold. An increase of threefold in airway resistance may be present without the subject's being aware of it.

Forced Expiration

Direct measurement of airway resistance with the use of a body plethysmograph is complex and requires expensive equipment. It is possible to assess the effects of increased airway resistance, by means of forced expiration into a suitable spirometer. The subject inspires maximally and then immediately exhales as rapidly and as completely as possible. This is called a forced vital capacity (FVC) maneuver. The performance of the forced expiration is evaluated by examining the change in volume over time and also by examining the relationship between volume and flow rate. It has been shown that during a forced expiration flow becomes limited at modest transpulmonary pressures (PL), and

that at any lung volume increasing effort and thereby increasing PL does not lead to an increase in flow.

It is this expiratory flow limitation that explains why the FVC maneuver has proved to be so useful. The relationships between PL, respiratory gas flow, and lung inflation are shown in Figure 2–7. The isovolume pressure/flow curves on the right of the figure demonstrate three important points:

1. The peak flow *(A)* increases as pressure increases; therefore, the peak flow ($\dot{V}_{max}$) near TLC is highly dependent on the subject's effort.

2. Curves *B* and *C* measured at lower lung volumes show increases in flow until maxima are reached, beyond which further increases in pressure produce no increases in flow. Maximum flow values decrease with decreasing lung volume.

3. During the FVC, maximum flow requires less than maximal effort, at lung volumes lower than that associated with peak flow.

In practice, it is usual to plot the flow on the y-axis of a suitable recorder and the volume signal on the x-axis (Fig. 2–7, *left*). The subject performs the FVC while flow and volume are plotted, simultaneously yielding the maximum expiratory flow volume (MEFV) curve. In the initial portion of the FVC near TLC, the respiratory muscles are unable to develop sufficient pressure to reach maximal flows. $\dot{V}_{max}$ is therefore largely dependent on patient effort and is sensitive to extrathoracic airway resistance; as a result, there is wide variability. Over the volume range below 80% of TLC, maximal flow does not require maximal effort and flow does not vary appreciably with effort. Thus, the curves are quite reproducible at these volumes.

The mechanisms of flow limitation have been discussed in detail[5389, 5390] and will be mentioned only briefly here. The equal pressure point concept postulates that during forced expiration, although the alveolar pressure is high, there is a rapid pressure drop down the airway because of the high flow rate and that at some point the intra-airway pressure will equal the intrapleural pressure (the equal pressure point or EPP). Downstream from this point, intrapleural pressure exceeds airway pressure and compression of the airway occurs. The maximum driving force for flow then becomes the difference between alveolar pressure and intrapleural pressure, which is determined not by effort but by the volume and compliance of the lung. The flow-limiting site in human airways is typically in the second and third generations of airways. The EPP hypothesis appears to be a good but approximate description of flow limitation at high lung volumes in humans. As lung volume decreases, the change in recoil pressure has a significant effect; flow decreases, and the flow-limiting site moves peripherally. However, this analysis does not explain the mechanism of the drop in airway pressure and thus the flow limitation.

It appears there are two flow-limiting mechanisms. One depends on the fact that compliant tubes like the airways cannot carry a greater flow than the flow at which the fluid velocity equals wave speed at some point in the system (wave-speed mechanism). The wave speed is the speed at which a small disturbance travels in a compliant tube filled with fluid. The wave speed in a compliant tube depends on the cross-sectional area and the density of the fluid. At high lung volumes, lateral pressure in the peripheral airways is large and the total cross-sectional area for flow is large so that velocity of flow is low. However, as the central airways are approached, the cross-sectional area decreases and flow velocity increases. This, by the Bernoulli effect, decreases lateral pressure relative to pleural pressure, further reducing cross-sectional area and contributing to the flow limitation. The second flow-limiting mechanism is more important at low lung volumes and depends on viscous flow limitation as described by the Poiseuille equation.

Measurement and Analysis

When measurements of FVC are made and analyzed, the results may be divided into three categories:

The first category measures peak flow (PEF) during the initial part of the FVC. Because of the marked volume dependence of $\dot{V}_{max}$, it is important that these tests are initiated from full inspiration.

The second category measures the volume of air exhaled per unit time. The most widely used measurement is the volume expired in 1 second (FEV_1) (Fig. 2–8). The result may be expressed either as the absolute volume exhaled or as the volume exhaled expressed as a percentage of the FVC ($FEV_1 \times 100/FVC$, FEV_1 %).

The third category relates expiratory flow to lung volume. Two types of measurements are made. First, the volume of air exhaled over a specified volume range of the FVC is divided by the time required to exhale this volume. The most common measure is the volume between 25% and 75% of the FVC divided by time (FEF_{25-75}). Second, absolute flow at a specified volume during the FVC is measured. The usual measurements are maximal flow at

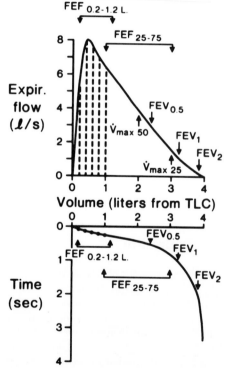

Figure 2–8. *Top,* flow-volume plot of a forced expired vital capacity maneuver from a normal subject. *Bottom,* derived volume-time trace of the same breath. $\dot{V}_{max}$, maximum expiratory flow; TLC, total lung capacity; FEF, mean forced expiratory flow between two designated volume points in FVC; FEV, forced expiratory volume in time interval. (Reprinted with permission from Hyatt, R. E. Forced expiration. In: Handbook of Physiology. American Physiological Society, Bethesda, Md., 1986, p. 301.)

75% of FVC ($\dot{V}max_{75\%}$), maximal flow at 50% of FVC ($\dot{V}max_{50\%}$), and maximal flow at 25% of FVC ($\dot{V}max_{25\%}$).

The use of these measures and their limitations in the assessment of pulmonary function are discussed in Chapter 5.

Work of Breathing

Work in a fluid system is performed when a pressure produces a volume change in the system. For the respiratory muscles, the work done on the lung during the breathing cycle is given by the area under the PV curve of the lung. The work calculated by such an analysis includes the elastic work required to inflate the lungs and the flow-resistive work required to generate flow through the airways. Such analyses underestimate the rate of the mechanical work of breathing (or power output of the respiratory muscles) because they neglect the considerable work expended on chest wall distortion. Respiratory muscle power increases in a curvilinear manner with increasing ventilation during exercise.

Mammals of different sizes naturally breathe at rates and depths that represent their own minimal rates of respiratory work. Such a relationship also appears to hold in a number of pathologic conditions. An associated concept is that it is the minimum average force of the respiratory muscles rather than the minimum work that determines the optimal frequency of breathing. Because respiratory muscle force is better related to the oxygen cost of breathing, this concept suggests there is an attempt to minimize the energy cost of breathing.

Maximum power output of the respiratory muscles is usually thought of as occurring during MVV, but this output can be maintained for only a limited time. Of more interest perhaps is the level of ventilation that can be maintained for long periods. This level (maximal sustained ventilatory capacity or MSVC) varies from 55 to 80% of MVV in normal subjects, although values approaching 90% have been demonstrated in highly fit athletes.[5391] Work rates requiring ventilations between MSVC and MVV are thought to induce ventilatory limitation due to ventilatory muscle fatigue. Two groups may be at risk of ventilatory limitation by ventilatory muscle fatigue when performing exercise: subjects with a low MVV, as in persons with airways obstruction, and highly fit subjects

with a normal MVV but high ventilatory requirements.

REGIONAL DISTRIBUTION OF VENTILATION

During normal tidal breathing in the upright position, the lower regions of the lung receive more ventilation per unit volume than do the upper regions.[5392] This vertical gradient has been clearly demonstrated during inhalation of radioactive xenon. The distribution of ventilation to different regions of the lung depends on two factors: first, a gradient in intrapleural pressure that is gravity-dependent and is related to the weight of the lung, and second, the shape of the static pressure/volume curve of the lung. In erect humans, the forces acting on the lung function as if the intrapleural pressure is less negative at the bottom of the lung than at the top; this pressure gradient amounts to about 0.25 cm H_2O/cm lung height. Thus with a lung height of 30 centimeters, the pressure difference between the top and bottom of the intrapleural space is effectively 7.5 cm H_2O. This is, of course, difficult to measure directly since if

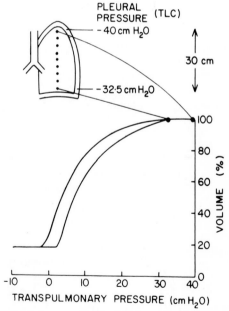

Figure 2–9. At maximally negative transpulmonary pressure (40 cm H_2O), the lungs are fully expanded (at TLC). Although there is a 7.5 cm H_2O difference between the top and the bottom of the lung, the volume of alveoli will be the same at the top and bottom of the lung, since the pressure-volume curve is nearly flat at this point. It is assumed that the pressure increases at a constant rate of 0.25 cm H_2O/cm vertical distance.

air is introduced into the intrapleural cavity to allow pressure measurement, the measured pressure would equalize throughout the introduced air. Measurements in animals, made with liquid and without introducing air into the system, have confirmed the presence of a gravity-dependent gradient of pleural pressure.[5384]

Because the intrapleural pressure is more negative at the top of the lung, it follows that the transpulmonary pressure (PL) is greatest or most positive in this region. At FRC the alveoli at the top of the lung are inflated to a greater degree than are the alveoli at the bottom of the lung. The degree of inflation of the alveoli in different regions depends on their transpulmonary pressure and their individual pressure/volume relationships; there is evidence that the latter are similar in different regions of the lung.[5392] The implications of these observations are illustrated in Figures 2–9, 2–10, and 2–11. With the lung at FRC, the alveoli at the bottom of the lung are at about 40% of their TLC and will have a large increase in volume for a given change in PL (for example, 5 cm H_2O) during inspiration. The alveoli at the top of the lung are at 70% of TLC and will have smaller increments in volume for the same change in PL. Thus, when an individual inspires from FRC, a greater proportion of the inspired gas goes to the lower alveoli.

The situation is quite different when the individual expires to RV and then inspires. At

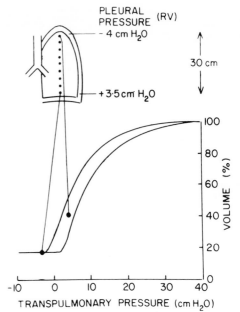

Figure 2–11. At residual volume (full expiration), airways at the bottom of the lung have closed, whereas airways at the top are still open because the upper lung regions are still at 40% of their maximal volume.

the start of the inspiration, alveoli at the lower part of the lungs may be on a horizontal portion of the PV relationship, whereas alveoli at the top of the lungs may be partially inflated and on the steep part of their PV relationship. Since P_{pl} at the base of the lungs may exceed airway pressure, the smaller airways may be closed and may not open until the adjacent pleural pressure becomes less than airway pressure. Thus, the first part of the inspiration goes almost exclusively to the apex. The lung volume at which airway closure occurs on expiration is referred to as *closing volume*. This volume is close to RV in healthy adults but becomes greater with age and may approach FRC in elderly subjects. This change with age is due to the loss of elastic recoil of the lung. Under these circumstances, the lower portions of the lung may be poorly ventilated during normal tidal breathing and gas exchange will be limited, leading to a decrease in Pa_{O_2} (see Chapter 4).

Causes of Uneven Ventilation

Ventilation is distributed as described above in relation to gravitational forces and the PV curve of the lung. This distribution will be different in the supine position as compared with the erect position, since gravity will act along the anteroposterior axis. Since the vertical

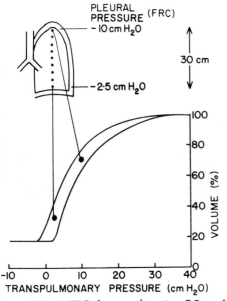

Figure 2–10. At FRC, because there is a 7.5 cm H_2O difference between the top and the bottom of the lung, alveoli in these regions are expanded to different degrees.

height of the lung will be less, the distribution of ventilation will be more uniform in this position.

In disease states in which there are regional differences in compliance and resistance of areas of the lung, ventilation will be unevenly distributed. Suppose there are two areas of the lungs with compliances of 0.1 L/cm H_2O and 0.2 L/cm H_2O, respectively. During inspiration the first area will only fill by half the volume of the second one. If there were areas with equal compliances but varying resistances, on inspiration both areas would fill to equal volume, but it would take longer to fill the area with high resistance. If expiration began before filling was complete, the two areas would have received different volumes. An area that had both a high compliance and a high resistance would take a long time to fill, whereas an area with low resistance and low compliance would fill quickly. The concept that the degree of filling of a lung unit may depend on the time available for filling has led to the concept of the *time constant* of a lung unit. The time constant of an area of the lung depends on both the compliance and on the resistance.

If compliance is measured by comparing the changes in lung volume and transpulmonary pressure (PL) during the breathing cycle rather than under static conditions, the measurement is called *dynamic compliance*. In normal subjects, the dynamic compliance is equal to static compliance, even at high breathing rates (90/min). In patients with increased airway resistance, the dynamic compliance decreases as the breathing rate increases; this is called *frequency dependence of compliance*. As the breathing rate increases, those areas of the lung with long time constants may not have time to fill completely before the next expiration starts, thus causing an apparent decrease in compliance.

In normal lungs, the resistance is sufficiently low that all lung units empty synchronously. In an abnormal lung, if there are units with long time constants, these units will fill slowly and at higher breathing frequency will be relatively poorly ventilated. On expiration, the areas with short time constants (the better ventilated areas) will empty first and the areas with the long time constants (less well ventilated) will empty later. Thus, there is sequential emptying of lung units rather than the normal synchronous emptying.

A final factor that may contribute to uneven alveolar ventilation is the delivery of inspired gas to terminal lung units. Flow of gas to the terminal bronchioles is by volume flow (bulk flow) down the airways. Beyond that region, the distribution of the gas depends on diffusion. Since the distances are very small and diffusion in gases is extremely rapid, mixing is usually complete. However, if there is dilatation of the terminal airways (as in emphysema), diffusion distances may become relatively large. This factor may play a role in determining the gas tensions in emphysema.

The factors that conspire to produce unequal ventilation of lung units are to some extent opposed by other mechanisms in the lungs. These mechanisms include the interdependence of lung units; that is, contiguous units may not move independently of each other. Also, collateral channels of ventilation between adjacent alveoli (pores of Kohn) contribute to a more even distribution of ventilation. Transfer of gas in the distal airways is also aided by the mixing effect of pulsations associated with the heart beat.

The Assessment of Uneven Ventilation

Frequency Dependence of Compliance

Transpulmonary pressure is measured from an esophageal balloon, air flow and volume are recorded, and the subject breathes at frequencies varying from 5 to 10 breaths/min to 60 to 90 breaths/min. Tidal volume is divided by the difference in transpulmonary pressure between the points of zero flow at end inspiration and at end expiration. This is a difficult test to perform, for both the subject and the investigator.

Single-Breath Oxygen Test

The subject makes a maximal expiration, then makes a full inspiration of 100% O_2, and finally breathes out slowly and steadily to residual volume. The N_2 concentration in the expired gas is continuously measured. Characteristic changes in N_2 concentration are observed (Fig. 2–12). The first portion of the expirate (Phase I) is dead space gas containing zero N_2. The second portion (Phase II) is mixed dead space and alveolar gas. The third phase (Phase III) is gas from the alveoli. In normal subjects in whom the alveoli empty synchronously, this phase shows a "plateau" during which N_2 concentration rises only slowly. The slope of Phase

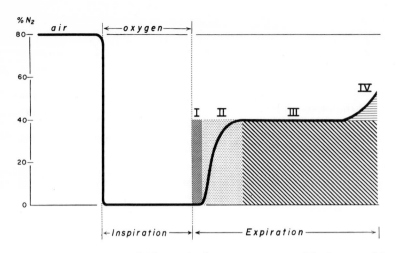

Figure 2–12. Single-breath oxygen test. The N_2 analyzer continuously samples, analyzes, and records the N_2 concentration of gas being inspired or expired. During air breathing the N_2 analyzer records 79% to 80% N_2 in inspired and expired gas. The subject is then requested to take a maximum inspiration of O_2 and breathe out slowly and evenly. During inspiration the N_2 analyzer records 0% N_2. At the beginning of expiration about 50 ml of pure O_2 (0% N_2) is expired (Phase I); this is followed by about 200 to 300 mL of gas of rapidly rising N_2 concentration (Phase II), which represents the washout of the remainder of the dead space gas by alveolar gas. Then alveolar gas is expired (Phase III). The N_2 concentration of the last part of the expiration (Phase IV) rises because of progressive closure of small airways at the bases of the lung. (Reprinted with permission from Forster, R. E., II, DuBois, A. B., Briscoe, W. A., and Fisher, A. B. The Lung. 3rd ed. Year Book Medical Publishers, Chicago, 1986, p. 34.)

III should be less than 1.5% N_2/500 mL expired. A greater slope than this indicates uneven ventilation with sequential emptying of the alveoli. Since the more poorly ventilated units empty later, there is a gradual rise in N_2 concentration. Finally, at a volume close to residual volume, there is a sharp increase in N_2 concentration (Phase IV).

The start of Phase IV is said to indicate the volume at which closure of airways occurs in the lower part of the lungs (closing volume). The increase in N_2 concentration in Phase IV is due to the fact that during inspiration of a single breath of 100% O_2 from residual volume, the first part of the inspired gas (which is dead space gas containing high N_2 concentration) goes to the upper part of the lungs. This helps to establish a gradient of N_2 concentration, with the upper alveoli having a higher N_2 concentration than the lower alveoli. During the next expiration, as residual volume is approached, airways in the lower parts of the lungs close. Air is then expelled selectively from the upper regions, which contain a higher N_2 concentration.

Similar measurements may be made using other trace gases such as xenon, argon, or helium. It was thought that this test might detect chronic airway disease before it was clinically apparent, but it has not conclusively been shown to be more sensitive than other tests. Most patients with established disease and an abnormal slope of Phase III do not produce single-breath tests from which closing volumes can be measured.

THE PULMONARY CIRCULATION

The major function of the pulmonary circulation is to provide a flow of mixed venous blood to the terminal respiratory units to allow gas exchange to take place. The pulmonary arteries accompany the bronchi down the center of the secondary lobules as far as the terminal bronchioles. There are no thick-walled muscular vessels in the pulmonary circulation that correspond to the arterioles of the systemic circulation. The pulmonary arteries with diameters of 100 to 1000 micrometers have, relatively, the most muscle in their walls and are sometimes referred to as *muscular pulmonary arteries*. The smooth muscle disappears as the capillary bed is approached. The capillaries form a complex sheet of segments—each about 10 micrometers long and 10 micrometers across—forming a complete network over the alveolar walls and making an efficient arrangement for gas exchange. The oxygenated blood is collected from the capillary bed by small pulmonary venules, which join and run between the lobules to eventually form the pulmonary veins and to drain into the left atrium.

The larger pulmonary arteries are extremely distensible, and the vascular resistance to flow is so low that the pressures developed in the pulmonary arteries are only about one-sixth of those in the systemic circulation, although the blood flows in the two systems are the same. The pulmonary arterial mean pressure, which is about 14 mm Hg at rest with a cardiac output of 5 L/min, increases to only about 20 mm Hg during exercise when cardiac output may be 25 L/min. This indicates a marked decrease in vascular resistance during exercise. The decrease in vascular resistance is achieved by the opening of vessels previously closed (recruitment) and by the passive dilatation of the very distensible vessels.

Factors Affecting Pulmonary Vascular Resistance

The major site of pulmonary vascular resistance remains controversial, but it is likely that at least 50% of the resistance to flow is in the capillary bed. Different agents may have their effects on different segments of the pulmonary vascular bed.

Because of their distensibility and low pressures, the pulmonary vessels are acted upon by a number of passive factors. Whenever pulmonary arterial pressure rises, there is an increase in distending pressure (transmural pressure) in the vessels, leading to an increase in diameter and reducing resistance to flow. An increase in left atrial pressure also increases the distending pressure in the pulmonary vascular bed and leads to a decrease in the resistance to flow. Because the pulmonary capillaries have alveolar air spaces on each side of them, the caliber of the capillaries may be influenced by the alveolar pressure. Not all the vessels in the lung are exposed to alveolar pressure, and vessels that are extra-alveolar may be acted upon by retractive forces in the connective tissue of the lung. The extra-alveolar vessels tend to be held open more effectively as lung volume increases, and therefore their resistance to flow falls. The alveolar vessels, on the other hand, tend to be compressed as transpulmonary pressure rises with lung volume. The total pulmonary vascular resistance appears to be minimal at about FRC.

In addition to the passive mechanisms that influence the pulmonary circulation, there are a number of active factors that can alter pulmonary vascular resistance. The pulmonary vessels are innervated by the sympathetic nervous system, and electrical stimulation of these nerves causes contraction of the pulmonary vascular smooth muscle. However, it has not been possible to demonstrate significant changes in pulmonary vascular resistance due to physiologic modifications of sympathetic nerve activity. Vasconstriction is produced by circulating catecholamines, as well as by histamine, angiotensin-II, and prostaglandins. Vasodilatation is produced by acetylcholine, serotonin, and other prostaglandins. The pulmonary vessels are very sensitive to alveolar oxygen tension, with alveolar hypoxia causing pulmonary vasoconstriction. The precise site of action and the mechanism by which hypoxia leads to an increase in pulmonary vascular resistance are not known. In the presence of alveolar hypoxia, there is an increase in vascular resistance, whether the lungs are perfused in the normal manner or whether the perfusion is from the veins to the arteries. The response to hypoxia is exaggerated in the presence of acidemia.

At altitude, there is a close relationship between pulmonary arterial pressure and alveolar hypoxia. The increase in pulmonary vascular resistance in chronic hypoxia leads to pulmonary hypertension and eventually to congestive heart failure. The effect of hypoxia on the pulmonary vessels is a local one: if an area is poorly ventilated and there is alveolar hypoxia, vessels to that area may be constricted, reducing blood flow to the poorly ventilated area.

Regional Distribution of Blood Flow

Because of the low pressure in the pulmonary circulation, the distribution of blood flow is significantly affected by the force of gravity. Gravity affects the hydrostatic pressure within the vessels: the transmural pressure is relatively high in the vessels at the bottom of the lung, and these vessels are therefore distended (low resistance). Conversely, the pressure within the vessels is low at the top of the lung; the vessels are therefore narrowed (high resistance). As already pointed out, the pulmonary capillaries have alveolar air spaces on each side and may be influenced by alveolar pressure, especially when capillary pressure is low.

The lung has been divided into four zones according to the relative magnitude of the three pressures that determine the flow—pulmonary arterial pressure, pulmonary venous pressure, and alveolar pressure. At the top of the lung is *Zone 1*, in which alveolar pressure (PA) is greater than the pulmonary arterial pressure (Pa). Hence, there is no flow.

Below this is *Zone 2*, in which the pulmonary arterial pressure is greater than the alveolar pressure. This pressure in turn is greater than the pulmonary venous pressure (Pv). In this situation, the driving pressure for flow is the difference between pulmonary arterial pressure and alveolar pressure (Pa − PA), and flow is independent of pulmonary venous pressure. Because PA is constant through the lung and Pa increases on moving down the lung, the driving force for flow, and therefore the blood flow, increases on moving down this zone.

In the next zone, *Zone 3*, the pulmonary arterial pressure is greater than the pulmonary venous pressure, which in turn is greater than the alveolar pressure. The driving force for flow (Pa − Pv) is constant; both pressures increase equally on moving down the lung, but the transmural pressure is greater so that resistance to flow decreases on moving down the zone.

There is a small zone, *Zone 4*, at the extreme base of the lung, where the blood flow becomes reduced. There is some uncertainty as to the cause of the reduced flow in this zone. Flow may be limited by loss of fluid from the vessels and a high interstitial pressure around the small vessels. It has been suggested that hypoxia secondary to airway closure might also contribute to a low flow in this region.

Fluid Balance in the Pulmonary Circulation

Net flow across the pulmonary capillary wall takes place according to the Starling hypothesis and depends on the hydrostatic pressures in the capillary (P_{cap}) and interstitial space (P_{int}) and also on the colloid osmotic pressures in these spaces (π_{cap}, π_{int}). The permeability of the capillary membrane, the effectiveness of the membrane in preventing the movement of plasma proteins out of the capillary (reflection coefficient = σ), and the filtration coefficient (K_r)—a function of both microvascular permeability and exchange vessel surface area—also contribute to the balance. Thus

$$J_v = K_r [(P_{cap} - P_{int}) - \sigma (\pi_{cap} - \pi_{int})]$$

where J_v is the total volume of fluid crossing the microvascular exchange barrier and entering the pulmonary tissue spaces.

The colloid osmotic pressure in the capillary is about 26 mm Hg. The colloid osmotic pressure in the interstitial space is unknown; in the lymph draining the lung it is about 20 mm Hg, and the pressure in the interstitial space must be close to this. The capillary hydrostatic pressure must lie between the pulmonary arterial pressure (14 mm Hg) and the pulmonary venous pressure (8 mm Hg) and is probably about 10 mm Hg. The interstitial hydrostatic pressure is unknown but is thought to be less than atmospheric pressure (about −3 mm Hg). It is thought that the interstitial pressure would be considerably more negative in the absence of surfactant, since the recoil of the alveoli would be greater. It is probable that there is normally a small net outward movement of fluid from the pulmonary capillaries into the interstitial space. This fluid is readily removed via the lung lymphatics.[53][93] The lung lymphatics have a considerable capacity for an increased flow, to at least 10 times the normal lymph flow. However, once the capacity of the lymphatics to remove the fluid is exceeded, the fluid collects, first in the interstitial space and then in the alveoli, leading to pulmonary edema. Since the lymphatic drainage is into the systemic venous system, the lymph flow from the lung can be influenced not only by factors in the pulmonary circulation but also by systemic venous pressure.

Metabolic Functions of the Pulmonary Circulation

The lung has important metabolic functions in addition to its function of gas exchange, and much remains to be learned about these functions. A number of vasoactive substances are metabolized in the lung, and since it receives the whole of the circulating blood, it is uniquely suited to modify blood-borne substances. The pulmonary capillary bed presents a large surface area of capillary endothelial cells, where many of the modifications take place.

Angiotensin-I is formed in the blood by the action of the enzyme renin, which acts on a peptide precursor. Angiotensin-I is converted to angiotensin-II by a converting enzyme located in small pits in the surface of the capillary endothelial cells. Angiotensin-II is a powerful vasoconstrictor.

Many vasoactive substances are partially or completely inactivated during passage through the lung. The lung is the major site of inactivation of serotonin, the inactivation being achieved mainly by uptake and storage. Bradykinin, a potent vasodilator, is about 80% inactivated on a single passage through the lung. The prostaglandins E_1, E_2, and $F_2\alpha$ are also inactivated in the lung. The significance of many of these functions remains unclear.

THE TRANSPORT OF GASES IN THE BLOOD

Oxygen absorbed in the lungs is transported to the organs and the tissues by the blood, and carbon dioxide formed there is carried by the blood to the lungs. This operation is fundamentally dependent upon the erythrocytes, which contain the red pigment hemoglobin. Hemoglobin is capable of combining with oxygen in the lung capillaries and releasing it again in the tissues. In addition, hemoglobin can bind some of the carbon dioxide produced by metabolism and is also capable of buffering some of the hydrogen ions released when CO_2 enters the blood. The chemical properties of hemoglobin will not be dealt with here.

Transport of Oxygen

Oxygen is carried in the blood in physical solution and in chemical combination with hemoglobin. The partial pressure of a gas and its solubility coefficient are the factors determining the amount of a gas that is dissolved in a liquid. Oxygen is a relatively insoluble gas, and 100 milliliters of plasma take up only approximately 0.3 milliliter of oxygen for each 100 mm Hg Po_2. Most of the oxygen in the blood is chemically bound to hemoglobin; 1 gram of hemoglobin is capable of combining with 1.34 milliliters of O_2. The average hemoglobin concentration in the blood is 15.8 g/dL for men and 14.0 g/dL for women; the blood of the newborn contains an average of 20.0 g/dL. The *oxygen capacity* of a blood sample is the maximum amount of oxygen that will combine with the available hemoglobin at high Po_2 (with a hemoglobin concentration of 15 g/dL, this gives an oxygen capacity of 20 mL/dL). The actual amount of oxygen combined with the hemoglobin at any time depends on the Po_2 and is referred to as the *oxygen content* of the sample.

The amount of oxygen combined with hemoglobin is not linearly related to the Po_2 as it is in the case of dissolved O_2. A graph on which the amount of oxygen combined with the he-

moglobin is plotted on the ordinate against Po_2 on the abscissa is an S-shaped curve. It has a steep slope between 20 and 40 mm Hg and becomes flatter at Po_2 greater than 70 mm Hg (Fig. 2–13). In plotting such a graph (*oxygen dissociation curve*), it is usual to plot the percentage saturation of hemoglobin on the ordinate rather than the actual amount of O_2, as this takes into account individual variations of hemoglobin concentration.

$$\text{Saturation (\%)} = \frac{\text{amount } O_2 \text{ combined with Hb}}{O_2 \text{ capacity of Hb}} \times 100$$

Biologic Significance of the O_2 Dissociation Curve

The characteristic shape of the O_2 dissociation curve is of great physiologic significance. At the Po_2 normally existing in the lungs and in the arterial blood (100 mm Hg), hemoglobin is 97.5% saturated with O_2. Between O_2 tensions of 75 and 100 mm Hg, there is little change in the amount of O_2 combined with hemoglobin. Thus, if arterial Po_2 decreases from 100 mm Hg to 70 mm Hg as a result of either disease or age, arterial blood will still be almost maximally saturated. At oxygen tensions greater than 100 mm Hg, hemoglobin cannot accept more oxygen, and oxygen carriage can be enhanced only by raising Po_2 greatly and increasing the amount of oxygen dissolved. When the arterial blood passes into the capillaries, oxygen leaves the blood and the oxygen tension in the capillaries falls to about 40 mm Hg. At this tension, relatively large amounts of oxygen can be given up for relatively small changes in oxygen tensions. Since the driving force for the diffusion of oxygen from the capillaries to the cells is the capillary Po_2, this aids the maintenance of the diffusion of O_2 to the cells.

Factors Affecting the O_2 Dissociation Curve

The O_2 dissociation curve is not "fixed" in position, but its position varies with a number of factors. Variations in the position of the curve are described as changes in the "affinity" of hemoglobin for O_2. The position of the curve may be described by the Po_2 at which the available hemoglobin is 50% saturated (P_{50}). The P_{50} of normal human blood is 26.6 mm Hg. When affinity decreases (P_{50} increases), the new curve is shifted to the right and more oxygen is

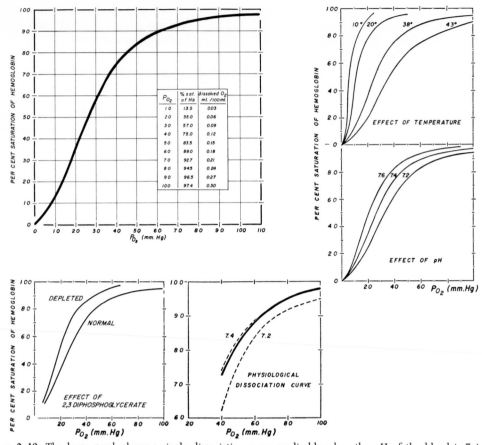

P_{O_2}	% sat. of Hb	dissolved O_2 ml. /100 ml.
10	13.5	0.03
20	35.0	0.06
30	57.0	0.09
40	75.0	0.12
50	83.5	0.15
60	89.0	0.18
70	92.7	0.21
80	94.5	0.24
90	96.5	0.27
100	97.4	0.30

Figure 2–13. The large graph shows a single dissociation curve applicable when the pH of the blood is 7.4 and the temperature 37° C. The blood oxygen tension and saturation in patients with CO_2 retention, acidosis, alkalosis, fever, or hypothermia or 2,3-diphosphoglycerate changes will not fit this curve because the curve "shifts" to the right or left.

Effects on the O_2 hemoglobin dissociation curve of changes in temperature (*upper right*), pH (*lower right*), and 2,3-DPG concentration (*bottom left*) are shown in the smaller graphs. (Reprinted with permission from Forster, R. E., II, DuBois, A. B., Briscoe, W. A., and Fisher, A. B. The Lung. 3rd ed. Year Book Medical Publishers, Chicago, 1986, p. 224.)

released into the tissues at low P_{O_2}. Since the upper portions of the curve are flat, and eventually reach 100% saturation, there is little effect on the amount of O_2 picked up in the lungs at 100 mm Hg.

A single molecule of adult hemoglobin consists of four polypeptide (globin) chains, each associated with an iron atom. The iron atom is contained within an iron-porphyrin compound (heme), which is joined to the polypeptide chain. The four chains are twisted into a kind of basket within which fit the iron-containing heme groups. In adult hemoglobin, two of the polypeptide chains contain 141 amino acid residues (alpha-chains) and two contain 146 amino acid residues (beta-chains). The hemoglobin molecule undergoes a conformational change when it reacts with O_2, this change probably occurring when the third of the possible four O_2 molecules combines with the hemoglobin.

The readiness with which such conformational changes occur is influenced by reactions with hydrogen ions, CO_2, and organic phosphates (particularly 2,3-diphosphoglycerate or 2,3-DPG) found within the red cells.

Increases in hydrogen ion concentration (decreased pH) cause a shift of the O_2 dissociation curve to the right (decreased affinity). This effect of the hydrogen ion is known as the *Bohr effect*. In active tissues, pH may be low because of the products of metabolism, and the increased production of CO_2 in active tissues also directly increases the hydrogen ion concentration. This effect means that more O_2 is unloaded from the blood at any given P_{O_2}. An increase in P_{CO_2} also shifts the curve to the right, and this effect cannot be ascribed entirely to the associated pH change. An increase in temperature shifts the O_2 dissociation curve to the right. Changes in body temperature are usually small, but this effect may be of significance in fever and in hypothermia. Also, there may be an increase of temperature in the working muscles during exercise. The O_2 dissociation curve is also shifted to the right by an increase in the concentration of organic phosphates in the red blood cells.

The red blood cells contain a large amount of 2,3-DPG relative to other cells, and it appears that 2,3-DPG is synthesized in the red cells, with the synthesis increasing during hypoxia. The normal position of the O_2 dissociation curve is dependent upon the presence of 2,3-DPG, which has been shown to bind to the deoxygenated form of hemoglobin, decreasing its oxygen affinity. It has been documented that patients with cardiac or respiratory disease associated with hypoxia have higher than normal levels of 2,3-DPG in their red cells, with a corresponding increase in the P_{50}.

Abnormal Hemoglobins

A large number of genetic variants of the hemoglobin molecule have been described. In only a small number of cases is the difference in the molecule associated with a change in oxygen affinity, although a number of the variants are of clinical importance, e.g., sickle cell disease. Fetal hemoglobin differs from adult hemoglobin in that in the fetus the two beta-chains are replaced by two gamma-chains. 2,3-DPG is unable to bind to the gamma-chains and thus does not exert its usual effect of decreasing O_2 affinity. Thus, the oxygen dissociation curve of fetal blood is to the left of the adult curve. This is advantageous to the fetus, since fetal arterial P_{O_2} is low (40 mm Hg) as is fetal pH. The increased affinity means that more O_2 can be picked up in the placenta.

Oxidizing agents may promote the conversion of the iron in the hemoglobin molecule from the ferrous to the ferric state. As this occurs, the oxygen affinity of the remaining ferrous atoms increases, shifting the O_2 dissociation curve to the left.

Hemoglobin and Carbon Monoxide

Carbon monoxide appears to bind with hemoglobin at the same sites as does oxygen, but the affinity of hemoglobin for CO is about 240 times that for O_2. CO is released from combination with hemoglobin much more slowly than O_2. Exposure to CO lowers the O_2 capacity of the blood by reducing the amount of O_2 that

can combine with hemoglobin. Even in very low concentrations, CO can displace O_2 from hemoglobin and make the latter unavailable for the transport of O_2. When part of the hemoglobin has been converted to CO-hemoglobin, the hemoglobin that remains unblocked has an O_2 dissociation curve that is shifted to the left. Together, these factors lead to severe tissue hypoxia and explain why the formation of 50% CO-hemoglobin has more serious consequences and leads to a lower P_{O_2} in working tissues than when hemoglobin concentration is reduced by 50% in anemia.

Transport of Carbon Dioxide

Carbon dioxide is continuously produced in all metabolizing cells and must diffuse from regions of high P_{CO_2} within the cells to regions with lower P_{CO_2} in the capillaries. Once the CO_2 has diffused from the cells into the blood, it may be transported in one of several forms. Some of the CO_2 molecules dissolve in the plasma, some diffuse into the red blood cells, and some dissolve in the water in the cells. Most of the CO_2 undergoes chemical conversion by hydration to form carbonic acid, which then dissociates to form bicarbonate and hydrogen ions.

$$CO_2 + H_2O \rightleftharpoons H_2CO_3 \rightleftharpoons HCO_3^- + H^+$$

The hydration of CO_2 is a slow reaction, but in the red cells it proceeds about 10,000 times faster than in plasma because of the presence of an enzyme, *carbonic anhydrase*, that catalyzes the reaction. This means that the bicarbonate concentration rises much faster in the red cells, and bicarbonate diffuses out of the red cells into the plasma. Since cations do not easily cross the cell membrane, to maintain electrical neutrality, chloride ions diffuse into the cell from the plasma. This exchange is called the *chloride shift*. The hydrogen ions that are formed in the cells by the dissociation of carbonic acid are buffered by the hemoglobin molecule. This process is aided by the fact that non-oxygenated hemoglobin is a weaker acid than oxygenated hemoglobin, and at the same time that CO_2 is entering the blood, oxygen is leaving the hemoglobin. The reverse effect occurs in the lungs, where the oxygenation of the hemoglobin helps with the unloading of CO_2. Some of the CO_2 combines with terminal amine groups in the blood proteins, especially the globin of hemoglobin, to form carbaminohemoglobin.

$$Hb \cdot NH_2 + CO_2 \rightleftharpoons Hb \cdot NH \cdot COO^- + H^+$$

This reaction occurs rapidly and non-oxygenated hemoglobin can bind more CO_2 in this form than oxygenated hemoglobin. Although only a small proportion of the total CO_2 carried is in the carbamino form (5%), the carbamino-bound CO_2 may provide a more significant proportion (20 to 30%) of the CO_2 exchanged.

Most of the CO_2 in the blood (90%) is in the form of bicarbonate, with approximately two-thirds being in the plasma and one-third in the red cells. The proportions are different if the amount of CO_2 exchanged in the lungs or given up by the tissues is examined. Then, about 10% of the exchanged CO_2 comes from dissolved CO_2, 30% from carbamino compounds, and 60% from bicarbonate.

The Carbon Dioxide Dissociation Curve

The relationship between the P_{CO_2} and the total CO_2 concentration in the blood is known as the carbon dioxide dissociation curve. The CO_2 dissociation curve is more linear than the O_2 dissociation curve, and Figure 2–14 shows that the position of the curve is influenced by the state of oxygenation of the hemoglobin. The differential binding of CO_2 is called the *Haldane effect* and can be explained by the better ability of non-oxygenated hemoglobin to take up hydrogen ions and the greater facility with which it forms carbaminohemoglobin. The extent to which the Haldane effect assists the exchange of CO_2 is illustrated by examining the *physiologic CO_2 dissociation curve*, which is thought of as occurring between the mixed venous blood and the arterial blood (Fig. 2–14). Both the uptake of CO_2 in the tissues and the release of CO_2 in the lungs are aided by the simultaneous change in the oxygenation of the hemoglobin.

RESPIRATORY REGULATION OF ACID-BASE BALANCE

Definitions

For biomedical purposes an acid is a compound that can serve as a proton donor in the living organism. Similarly, bases are defined as compounds that function as proton acceptors in the body. Two classes of acids can be defined on the basis of certain chemical and physical properties and on the way the acid is processed in the body. The first class is composed of a single acid, *carbonic acid* (H_2CO_3), which can dissociate into hydrogen ion and HCO_3^-. It is also in equilibrium with CO_2 and H_2O.

$$CO_2 + H_2O \rightleftharpoons H_2CO_3 \rightleftharpoons H^+ + HCO_3^-$$

Carbonic acid differs from other acids in that (1) CO_2 readily permeates cell membranes and thus rapidly influences intracellular pH; (2) large amounts of CO_2 are continuously being produced by metabolic processes; and (3) CO_2 is continuously eliminated from the lungs, and its concentration is regulated by the ventilatory system. The second class of physiologic acids is composed of all the acids in the body other than carbonic acid; these are known as *fixed acids*.

Hydrogen Ion Concentration

Under normal circumstances, the hydrogen ion concentration of the arterial blood is maintained close to pH 7.4, with a maximum range of 6.7 to 7.8. This control is achieved by both physicochemical buffers and physiologic factors. The major buffer system in the blood is the carbonic acid/bicarbonate system. It is of importance not because it is an efficient chemical buffer at normal body pH but because of the ability to lose or gain CO_2 if pulmonary ventilation is changed. The next most important buffers are the proteins; the imidazole groups of the histidine residues provide most of the protein buffering at body pH. Because hemoglobin is present in much higher concentration than any other protein, it is of particular importance. Also, as noted previously, the conversion of hemoglobin from the oxygenated to the non-oxygenated form allows the uptake of additional hydrogen ions. Phosphate buffer systems provide a small contribution (<5%) to the non-bicarbonate buffering in the blood and extracellular fluid. The buffer properties of the blood are determined by the combined effects of all the anionic groups of weak acids, the most important of which are bicarbonate and proteinate. All of these anions with buffer effects are called *buffer bases*. The concentration of buffer bases in arterial blood is about 48 mmol/L and does not change when P_{CO_2} changes. Because the total buffer base is independent of P_{CO_2}, it

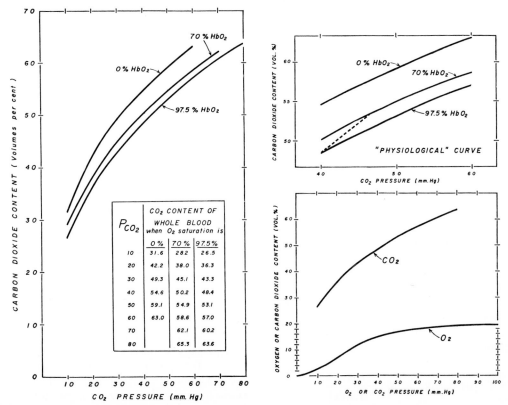

Figure 2–14. The large graph shows the relationship between P_{CO_2} and CO_2 content of whole blood; this varies with changes in the saturation of hemoglobin with oxygen. *Above right*, greatly magnified portion of the large graph to show the change that occurs as mixed venous blood (70% HbO_2, P_{CO_2} = 46 mm Hg) passes through the pulmonary capillaries and becomes arterial blood (97.5% HbO_2, P_{CO_2} = 40 mm Hg). The dashed line is a hypothetical transition between the two curves. *Below right*, O_2 and CO_2 dissociation curves plotted on the same scale to show that the O_2 curve has a steep and a flat portion and the CO_2 curve does not. (Reprinted with permission from Forster, R. E., II, DuBois, A. B., Briscoe, W. A., and Fisher, A. B. The Lung. 3rd ed. Year Book Medical Publishers, Chicago, 1986, p. 238.)

is a suitable measure of the non-respiratory component of acid-base balance. Departures from the normal buffer-base concentration are called *base excess*, the normal base excess being zero.

The major physiologic factor that influences hydrogen ion concentration is the elimination of CO_2 by changes in pulmonary ventilation. In addition, changes in the intake or excretion of fixed acids or bases and changes in their metabolic production may change hydrogen ion concentration. For instance, tissue hypoxia leads to the production of lactic acid, and in diabetes changes in carbohydrate metabolism may lead to the production of keto acids. The kidneys, together with the lungs, are involved in the regulation of acid-base balance. They excrete about 40 to 60 millimoles of fixed acid per day. The kidneys are capable of considerably increasing the rate of excretion of acid and returning a falling pH to normal. Similarly, an increase

in pH reduces the rate of renal excretion (Fig. 2–15).

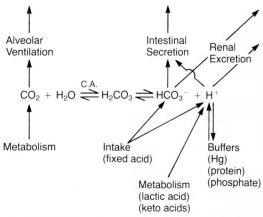

Figure 2–15. Diagram of factors affecting the hydrogen ion concentration in the plasma. (C.A. is carbonic anhydrase.)

Measurement of Hydrogen Ion Activity

Hydrogen ion activity in arterial blood is measured by means of sensitive glass electrodes. Automated systems allow the measurement to be made at body temperature and without the sample being exposed to the air. It is customary to express hydrogen ion activity in terms of pH units (the negative logarithm of the hydrogen ion concentration).

The Carbonic Acid/Bicarbonate Buffer System

The amount of hydrogen ion activity in the blood is governed by the interrelationships of all the blood acids, bases, and buffer systems. It is this same hydrogen ion activity that determines the dissociation of carbonic acid. The hydrogen ion concentration in the bicarbonate buffer system may be expressed in the form of the *Henderson-Hasselbalch* equation:

$$pH = pK' + \log \frac{[HCO_3^-]}{[H_2CO_3]}$$

where pK' is the first dissociation constant for H_2CO_3. The carbonic acid concentration is difficult to measure. It is in equilibrium with the amount of CO_2 dissolved in the solution. The concentration of the dissolved CO_2 is about 1000 times greater than that of H_2CO_3. Dissolved CO_2 concentration may be calculated as the product of the P_{CO_2} and the solubility constant for CO_2 in plasma (0.03 at 37° C). Thus

$$pH = pK'' + \frac{\log [HCO_3^-]}{0.03 \times P_{CO_2}}$$

pK'' then has a value of 6.1.

Terminology of Disturbances in Acid-Base Balance

Normal Values

pH = 7.4 units	Range:	7.36–7.44
P_{CO_2} = 40 mm Hg		36–44
$[HCO_3^-]$ = 25 mmol/L		23–27

Acidemia denotes an increase in the hydrogen ion concentration in the arterial blood. Alkalemia denotes a decrease in the hydrogen ion concentration in the arterial blood. Acidosis and alkalosis are terms used to describe increases or decreases in acid in the body as a whole (usually based on measurements in the blood). There are two main types of disorder, those in which the primary cause is a change in alveolar ventilation (respiratory) and those in which the primary cause is non-respiratory. During hypoventilation there is an increase in Pa_{CO_2}, which leads to an increase in $[H^+]$ and also to an increase in $[HCO_3^-]$. There is therefore a decrease in pH and a respiratory acidosis. Hyperventilation causes an increase in pH and a respiratory alkalosis. The difference in Pa_{CO_2} from its normal value of 40 mm Hg is directly proportional to the magnitude of the respiratory disturbance.

Non-respiratory acid-base disorders occur when there is excessive retention or elimination of fixed acid or base by the body. Acidosis due to loss of alkaline intestinal secretions may be caused by diarrhea. Alkalosis may be due to persistent vomiting with loss of secretions high in acid or by absorption of alkalinizing salts.

A primary acidosis or alkalosis, regardless of cause, elicts physiologic responses that oppose the deviation of pH from normal. Thus, a non-respiratory acidosis causes stimulation of breathing and a secondary or compensatory respiratory alkalosis. Conversely, respiratory alkalosis leads to increased excretion of base by the kidney and thus a secondary non-respiratory acidosis. Respiratory compensation for non-respiratory alkalosis is usually poor because depression of ventilation causes not only retention of CO_2 but also hypoxemia; this limits the degree of compensation. Thus, neither the magnitude of the pH change nor the change in $[HCO_3^-]$ alone is a reliable indicator of the magnitude of the acid-base disturbance because compensatory mechanisms will have been stimulated.

Assessment of Acid-Base Balance

An adequate portrayal of the type and severity of a disturbance of acid-base balance requires information about at least three factors: hydrogen ion concentration, Pa_{CO_2}, and HCO_3^- concentration. Clinically, practicable methods have made use of measurements of two of these variables, the third being predicted from the Henderson-Hasselbalch equation. The accuracy of such predictions in the presence of rapid or severe changes in acid-base balance has been questioned, but the accuracy is usually adequate for clinical purposes. The choice of the two variables to be measured and the presentation of data have been governed by the ease and availability of the methods of measurement. At present, pH and Pa_{CO_2} are the normally measured variables, $[HCO_3^-]$ being calculated or read from a nomogram.

The following steps are taken to interpret acid-base balance in terms of acidosis versus alkalosis and respiratory versus non-respiratory disturbances:

1. The pH of the arterial blood indicates the overall degree of acidemia or alkalemia. A normal pH does not necessarily mean that the acid-base balance is undisturbed.

2. The presence of an elevated or a lowered Pa_{CO_2} indicates a primary or secondary respiratory disturbance, the severity of which is indicated by the deviation of the Pa_{CO_2} from normal.

3. The plasma bicarbonate concentration is calculated from the Henderson-Hasselbalch equation or read from a nomogram. In general, primary respiratory acid-base disturbances produce relatively small changes in plasma $[HCO_3^-]$ as compared with the change in plasma $[HCO_3^-]$ when a similar change in pH is caused by a non-respiratory disturbance. Because both respiratory and non-respiratory disturbances influence plasma $[HCO_3^-]$, interpretation of the acid-base balance on the basis of a change in plasma $[HCO_3^-]$ alone is sometimes difficult.

4. The base excess (BE) reveals whether or not there is a non-respiratory disturbance and the magnitude of the disturbance. (The normal range of BE is from -2.5 to $+2.5$ mmol/L).

Earlier methods of quantification of non-respiratory disturbances utilized data obtained from the equilibration of whole blood *in vitro* at different P_{CO_2} values and with different amounts of fixed acid or base added. Under these circumstances, hemoglobin is the major buffer in blood, and variations in hemoglobin concentration produce significant changes in the buffering power of the blood. More recently, it has become obvious that when acute changes in acid-base balance occur *in vivo*, there is rapid equilibration of CO_2 throughout both the blood and extracellular fluid. Hemoglobin remains the major buffer, but the system has a buffering capacity similar to that of blood, with a hemo-globin concentration of only 60 g/L. The effects of changes in hemoglobin concentration are then small, and under clinical circumstances may be ignored if the buffer capacity of the system is taken to be equal to that of blood *in vitro* with a hemoglobin concentration of 60 g/L. The base excess for the extracellular fluid (ECF) has been determined in experimental animals and humans for acute acid-base disturbances. The BE represents the amount of acid or base that would have to be added or removed per liter of ECF to return the plasma pH to 7.4 at a P_{CO_2} of 40 mm Hg. The BE may be derived from the measurements of pH and Pa_{CO_2} by means of either the Siggaard-Andersen chart[5400] (Fig. 2–16) or a nomogram. The use of BE has been criticized on the basis that it may give a false sense of precision, particularly when used in chronic acid-base disturbances accompanied by significant changes in the intracellular acid-base state. However, provided it is realized that BE is not always a precise index, it is a useful tool.

Correction of Acid-Base Disturbances

Treatment of ventilatory failure or hyperventilation must be directed to reversing the respiratory defect and will depend on the primary cause of the respiratory abnormality. In some cases, this may mean instituting mechanical ventilation.

In subjects with severe non-respiratory acidosis, especially if cardiac arrhythmias are present, it may be desirable to correct the abnormality in a short period of time. This is most easily accomplished by the infusion of sodium bicarbonate. The amount needed for correction is indicated by the BE. It is usual to give about half the calculated amount and then to remeasure pH and P_{CO_2}. Further treatment is based on these measurements.

GAS EXCHANGE

A simplified approach to the problem of O_2 transport has been described by Otis,[5403] who visualized the gas exchange-transport system as consisting of five major compartments: (1) inspired gas, (2) alveolar gas, (3) pulmonary capillary blood, (4) tissue capillary blood, and (5) tissue.

These compartments are viewed as being

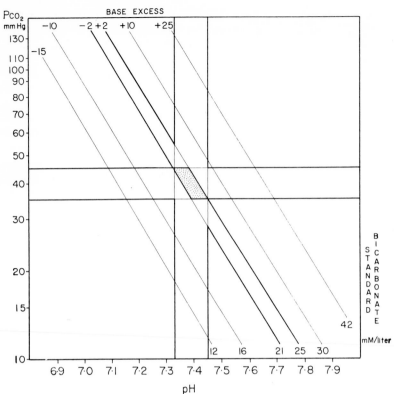

Figure 2–16. *Acid-Base Diagram*

The diagram illustrates in convenient form the interrelationship between pH, P_{CO_2}, and base excess. Standard bicarbonate is the bicarbonate concentration the plasma of the sample would have if P_{CO_2} were 40 mm Hg. The shaded area in the center of the diagram indicates the normal range. (Adapted from Sigaard-Andersen, O., and Engel, K. A new acid-base nomogram. Scand. J. Clin. Lab. Invest. 12:177, 1960.)

connected in series, to form a continuous pathway along which there is net flow of O_2 from compartment 1 to compartment 5. This hypothesis allows one to consider the flow of O_2 as being opposed by a series of resistances between compartments or as a "cascade," with a loss of partial pressure as oxygen flows down the cascade and loses energy in proportion to the conductance at each step (Fig. 2–17).

The gradient between inspired gas and alveolar gas depends on the alveolar ventilation:

$$\dot{V}_{O_2} = (F_{I_{O_2}} - F_{A_{O_2}})\dot{V}_A$$

The conductance (G_1 or the reciprocal of resistance) between the two compartments depends on the alveolar ventilation and is determined by breathing frequency, tidal volume, and dead-space volume.

The conductance (G_2) between the alveolar gas and the pulmonary capillary blood is what is more usually called the diffusing capacity of the lungs:

$$D_L = \frac{\dot{V}_{O_2}}{(P_{A_{O_2}} - P_{c,L_{O_2}})}$$

where $P_{c,L_{O_2}}$ is the partial pressure of O_2 in the

lung capillaries. The reciprocal conductance between the alveolar gas and blood can be subdivided into two compartments: a true diffusion barrier of the membrane, $1/D_M$, and a virtual barrier that depends on the reaction rate (θ) of O_2 with hemoglobin and on the volume of blood in the pulmonary capillaries:

$$\frac{1}{D_L} = \frac{1}{D_M} + \frac{1}{\theta V_c}$$

The conductance of the flow of O_2 from the pulmonary capillary blood to the tissue capillary blood is given by:

$$\text{Conductance } (G_3) = \frac{\dot{V}_{O_2}}{(P_{c,L_{O_2}} - P_{c,ti_{O_2}})}$$

where $P_{c,ti_{O_2}}$ is tissue capillary oxygen tension and

$$\dot{V}_{O_2} = (C_{a_{O_2}} - C_{v_{O_2}})\dot{Q} = (P_{a_{O_2}} - P_{v_{O_2}})Bb \cdot \dot{Q}$$

where Bb is the slope of the oxygen dissociation curve between Pa and Pv. Thus, the conductance is

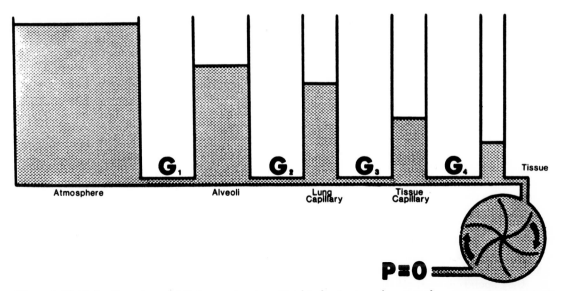

Figure 2–17. Hydraulic analogue of O_2 transport system. Height of water in each rectangular compartment represents the partial pressure of O_2 (Po_2) in that compartment. The last circular compartment represents the participation of O_2 in metabolic energy generation, a process in which Po_2 is reduced to zero. In any given situation atmospheric Po_2 is considered constant; the height in the succeeding four compartments is determined by O_2 flow and the four conductances (G_{1-4}). The volume of a compartment is immaterial in a steady state but is of great importance in transient events. (Reprinted with permission of Otis, A. B. An overview of gas exchange. In: Handbook of Physiology, Section 3, Vol. 4. American Physiological Society, Bethesda, Md., 1986, p. 3.)

$$G_3 = (Pa_{O_2} - Pv_{O_2})Bb \cdot \frac{\dot{Q}}{(Pc,L_{O_2} - Pc,ti_{O_2})}$$

and the variables determining the conductance are the blood flow and the slope of the oxygen dissociation curve.

The conductance of the oxygen flow from the tissue capillary blood to the tissue is the mean oxygen flow divided by the mean difference in partial pressure of oxygen between the capillaries and the tissue (Pti_{O_2}).

$$G_4 = \frac{\dot{V}o_2}{(Pc,ti_{O_2} - Pti_{O_2})}$$

The principal physiologic variables determining G_4 are the kinetics of oxyhemoglobin dissociation and the geometry of the capillaries perfusing the metabolizing tissues.

Diffusion of Gases in the Lung

The exchange of O_2 and CO_2 in the lung depends upon the process of diffusion. Diffusion is a process that depends on the random movement of molecules and is an efficient means of transfer of molecules over very short distances. The rate of diffusion of gases through tissues is governed by Fick's Law. This states that the rate of transfer of a gas is proportional to the area (A) through which diffusion occurs and the pressure difference. It is inversely proportional to the distance for diffusion (or thickness of the tissue, T). In addition, the rate of transfer is proportional to a diffusivity constant (D), which depends on the properties of the tissue and the gas. This constant is proportional to the solubility of the gas and is inversely proportional to the square root of the molecular weight of the gas.

$$\dot{V}gas = \frac{A \cdot D}{T}(P_1 - P_2)$$

$$D = \frac{solubility}{\sqrt{molecular\ weight}}$$

Carbon dioxide diffuses about 20 times more rapidly than O_2 because it has a higher solubility and a relatively similar molecular weight.

The transfer of oxygen from the alveoli to the red blood cells may be thought of as occurring in stages. The final mixing of the inspired gas with the alveolar gas depends on diffusion. Because diffusion in gases is rapid, this is not normally a limiting step. However, if the terminal air spaces are very large (as in emphysema), diffusion may become significant. Oxygen must diffuse from the air spaces through the surface film containing surfactant, through the epithelium of the alveolus, through the basement membranes, and through the endothelium of the pulmonary capillary. The total thickness of this barrier is about 0.4 micrometer over most of the alveolocapillary area. The oxygen must also diffuse within the blood and combine with hemoglobin. The reaction time with hemoglobin was originally thought to be instantaneous, but it is now known to require a finite time and to impose a measurable delay on the diffusion process. This knowledge is made use of in measuring separately the two components of the diffusion process.

As the red blood cells move through the lung, they spend, at rest, about 0.75 second in the capillaries. Equilibration between the oxygen in the alveoli and the partial pressure of oxygen in the capillary blood is achieved in about 0.25 second. Thus, normally the transfer of oxygen is not limited by diffusion, and the amount of oxygen transferred is said to be "perfusion limited." If the time for diffusion is reduced, for instance as it is during exercise, and if the transfer of oxygen is reduced (decreased surface area; increased distance for diffusion), equilibration may not be achieved in the time available. In this case the transfer of oxygen would be "diffusion limited." If $P_{A_{O_2}}$ is low, the rate of transfer of oxygen to the pulmonary capillary blood is slower and full equilibration may not be reached even though the diffusing properties of the lung are normal (Fig. 2–18).

Measurement of Diffusing Capacity

The diffusing capacity of the lung for any gas ($D_{L}g$) is the quantity of gas transferred from the alveoli to the blood in unit time, per unit of pressure difference between the alveoli and the blood.

$$D_{L}g = \frac{\dot{V}g}{P_{A}g - P_{c}g} \text{ (mL/min/mm Hg)}$$

Carbon monoxide is the gas usually chosen to measure diffusing capacity in the lung. Because the affinity of hemoglobin for carbon monoxide is very high, equilibrium is not reached and the transfer of carbon monoxide is primarily diffusion limited. When carbon monoxide is inhaled in low concentration, all the molecules that diffuse across the alveolocapillary membrane enter the red cells and are bound to the hemoglobin, so that the the mean capillary P_{CO} remains zero. Then

$$D_{L_{CO}} = \frac{\dot{V}_{CO}}{P_{A_{CO}}}$$

This conveniently avoids the problem of having to measure the mean capillary P_{CO}. Many different techniques have been used to measure $P_{A_{CO}}$ (see Chapter 5). The major differences are between techniques that employ a "single breath" of CO and those techniques in which a CO mixture is breathed in a "steady state," usually over 3 minutes.[5404] The practical consequence of the use of the different techniques is that the single-breath method gives higher values for $D_{L_{CO}}$ than does the steady-state method.

Diffusing capacity is related to the size of the lung, as indicated by the height of the individual, and also increases with the state of inflation of the lung. The index $D_{L_{CO}}/V_{A}$ is sometimes calculated since it compensates to some extent for changes in V_{A} within an individual patient. Diffusing capacity increases during growth and development and then decreases with age. There is an increase in diffusing capacity during exercise probably associated with improved perfusion of the lung, and the diffusing capacity decreases with decreasing hemoglobin concentration (see Chapter 19).

As noted earlier the reciprocal conductance, or the resistance to CO flow between the alveolar gas and blood ($1/D_{L_{CO}}$), can be partitioned into two compartments: the resistance to diffusion through the pulmonary membrane ($1/D_{M}$) and the resistance to CO uptake by the red blood cells in the capillary bed ($1/\theta CO \cdot V_{c}$). Thus

$$\frac{1}{D_{L_{CO}}} = \frac{1}{D_{M}} + \frac{1}{\theta CO \cdot V_{c}}$$

Values for D_{M} and V_{c} can be obtained because $D_{L_{CO}}$ depends on the inspired O_2 concentration. Oxygen and CO compete for binding with hemoglobin. The higher the $P_{A_{O_2}}$, the less is the rate of uptake of CO per milliliter of blood (θCO) and the lower is the $D_{L_{CO}}$. If $D_{L_{CO}}$ is determined at normal and at high $P_{A_{O_2}}$, two values for $D_{L_{CO}}$ will be obtained. If θCO, which can be measured *in vitro*, is also known at the same $P_{A_{O_2}}$ values, D_{M} and V_{c} can be calculated.

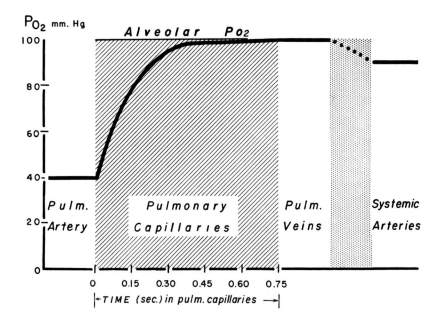

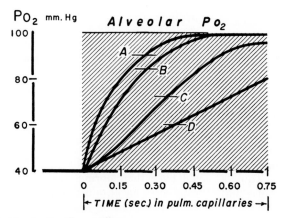

Figure 2–18. *Alveolar-Capillary Diffusion*

Above, mixed venous blood enters pulmonary capillaries with a P_{O_2} of 40 mm Hg. Blood normally requires about 0.75 second to pass through the capillaries. At the end of this time, its P_{O_2} has risen to 100 mm Hg. The P_{O_2} of the arterial blood is lower because of venous to arterial shunts.

Below, illustration of different rates at which venous blood may be oxygenated in pulmonary capillaries, depending on the diffusing capacity of the lung. End-pulmonary capillary blood in *A, B,* and *C* would all have normal O_2 saturation, although diffusing capacity is different in each case. If the time in the capillary were shortened, as during exercise, from 0.75 to 0.30 second, O_2 saturation in the end-capillary blood would be low in *B, C,* and *D*. (Reprinted with permission from Forster, R. E., II, DuBois, A. B., Briscoe, W. A., and Fisher, A. B. The Lung. 3rd ed. Year Book Medical Publishers, Chicago, 1986, p. 208.)

Normal values for D_M average about 57 mL/min/mm Hg; V_c is about 90 to 110 milliliters.

Normal Gas Exchange

For gas exchange to be efficient, each terminal lung unit must receive an appropriate amount of ventilation and blood flow. This "matching" of ventilation and perfusion in each terminal unit is critical to efficient gas exchange. As the gas exchange in individual units cannot be examined, the average gas exchange in the lungs is assessed. In the resting state, when $\dot{V}_A$, $\dot{V}_{O_2}$, and $\dot{V}_{CO_2}$ are constant, the partial pressures of O_2 and CO_2 in the alveolar gas and in the arterial and venous blood may be regarded as constant (Table 2–1). Because equilibration between the alveolar gas and the pulmonary capillary blood is virtually complete, the tensions of the gases in these compartments are almost identical. The small alveolar-arterial difference for oxygen, $(A - a) D_{O_2}$, that is normally found is due to the anatomic shunt and to variations in the distribution of ventilation and perfusion (see later). The $(A - a) D_{O_2}$ is usually 8 mm Hg and the upper limit of normal is 15 mm Hg. Because CO_2 equilibrates so readily, there is rarely an $A - a$ difference for CO_2. The $(A - a) D_{O_2}$ can be calculated only if the average PA_{O_2} is known, and this has been difficult to measure directly. However, "ideal" PA_{O_2} can be calculated from the alveolar air equation:

$$PA_{O_2} = PI_{O_2} - PA_{CO_2} \left[FI_{O_2} + \frac{1 - FI_{O_2}}{R} \right]$$

or in its simpler form:

$$PA_{O_2} = PI_{O_2} - \frac{PA_{CO_2}}{R}$$

where R = respiratory exchange ratio = $\dot{V}CO_2/\dot{V}O_2$.

R varies between 0.7 and 1, depending on the particular substrate being metabolized, but it is usually 0.8. Since PA_{CO_2} can usually be considered equal to Pa_{CO_2}, the arterial PCO_2, measured at the same time as Pa_{O_2}, can be used for the calculation of the average PA_{O_2}. Thus, a value for the difference between alveolar and arterial PO_2 can be calculated as $(A - a) D_{O_2}$.

Abnormal Gas Exchange

The best guide to the adequacy of gas exchange is the measurement of Pa_{O_2} and Pa_{CO_2}.

Table 2–1. PARTIAL PRESSURES OF GASES (mm Hg)*

	Dry Air	Alveolar Gas	Arterial Blood	Venous Blood
PO_2	159.1	104	100	40
PCO_2	0.3	40	40	46
PH_2O	0	47	47	47
PN_2	600.6	569	573	573
TOTAL	760	760	760	706

*Average values of partial pressures of the respiratory gases at sea level. The values of PO_2, PCO_2, and PN_2 fluctuate from breath to breath and during a single breath.

Calculation of the $(A - a) D_{O_2}$ sometimes gives additional insight into the mechanisms involved. If abnormalities are present, further studies may be necessary to determine which processes are at fault. The major causes of abnormalities of gas exchange and their effects on $(A - a) D_{O_2}$ are presented in Figure 2–19.

Hypoventilation

The simplest derangement of gas exchange occurs when alveolar ventilation is inadequate. When this happens, the PA_{O_2} falls and the Pa_{CO_2} rises. Since PA_{CO_2} is inversely proportional to alveolar ventilation, when alveolar ventilation is halved Pa_{CO_2} is doubled. The effect of hypoventilation on PA_{O_2} is less dramatic and can be calculated from the alveolar air equation.

Decreased Inspired Oxygen Concentration

PI_{O_2} may be decreased because of a decrease in the percentage of O_2 in the inspired air or, more commonly, because of a reduction in barometric pressure at high altitude. The decrease in PA_{O_2} may be calculated from the alveolar air equation. The hypoxemia stimulates breathing, so that there is usually hyperventilation and a decrease in Pa_{CO_2}.

Diffusion Abnormality

When there is a diffusion defect, it may take a longer than normal time in the pulmonary capillaries for equilibrium to be reached. However, it should be realized that a pure "alveolocapillary block" is rare. Reduction in the pulmonary capillary bed with a consequent decrease in transit time in the remaining capillaries is a more common cause of reduced gas transfer. In either case, the effect will be enhanced during exercise or in the presence of a low PA_{O_2}. The only occasion on which gas transfer is diffusion limited in healthy individuals is during heavy exercise in the presence of a low PI_{O_2}. Under these circumstances, PA_{O_2} will be low and there will be an increased $(A - a) D_{O_2}$.

Right to Left Shunt

In the normal lung, some blood from the bronchial venous drainage reaches the pulmonary veins, and there is also a small portion of the coronary venous blood flow that enters the

Figure 2–19. Effects of various disturbances on alveolar-arterial differences. The various disturbances are listed in the first column, and the effects on (A − a) D appear at the proper boxes. The effects are graded from ○ (no effect), through ◌ (theoretically present, but too small to be measured), to + + + +. (A − a) D or (a − A) D values, which are specific for a given disturbance, are indicated by shaded background. (Reprinted with permission from Farhi, L. E. Recent Advances in Respiratory Physiology. Ventilation–perfusion relationship and its role in alveolar gas exchange. W. H. Arnold, London, 1965.)

		$(A-a)Do_2$ on air	$(A-a)Do_2$ on 100% O_2	$(A-a)Do_2$ on low O_2	$(a-A)Dco_2$	$(a-A)Dn_2$
Venous admixture		+ +	+ + / + +	+	◌	O
Diffusion limitation		+	◌	+ +	◌	O
Uneven $\dot{V}A/\dot{Q}$	High $\dot{V}A/\dot{Q}$	+ +	+	+	+ + / + +	+
	Low $\dot{V}A/\dot{Q}$	+ +	+	+	+	+ + / + +

cavity of the left ventricle through the thebesian veins. The effect of this addition of venous blood is to decrease Pa_{O_2}. Thus, in the ideal lung, even though there is complete equilibration in the alveolus and PA_{O_2} equals Pc_{O_2}, there will always be a small A − a difference. The amount of the blood in the shunt (i.e., the blood that has not been oxygenated in the lungs) can be calculated if it assumed that the blood in the shunt has the same O_2 content as the mixed venous blood. The shunt is referred to as *venous admixture*, which is defined as the amount of mixed venous blood that would have to be added to the pulmonary end-capillary blood to give the observed Pa_{O_2}. This can be calculated from the shunt equation:

$$\dot{Q}_t \times Ca_{O_2} = (\dot{Q}_s \times Cv_{O_2}) + ((\dot{Q}_t - \dot{Q}_s) \times Cc'_{O_2})$$

or

$$\frac{\dot{Q}_s}{\dot{Q}_t} = \frac{Cc'_{O_2} - Ca_{O_2}}{Cc'_{O_2} - Cv_{O_2}}$$

where $\dot{Q}_s$ is the shunt flow and $\dot{Q}_t$ is the cardiac output. PA_{O_2} is calculated from the alveolar air equation and used to give Cc'_{O_2} from an oxygen dissociation curve.

A true shunt is by definition composed of blood that does not take part in gas exchange. It is therefore unaffected by breathing 100% oxygen. The arterial PCO_2 is not significantly affected by the shunt because Pv_{CO_2} is not very different from Pa_{CO_2}, so that a large shunt would be needed to raise Pa_{CO_2}. In addition to the shunt through the bronchial veins and thebesian veins, shunts may occur through intracardiac channels and pulmonary arteriovenous fistulas and in conditions leading to complete closure of lung units. The last may be associated with pneumonia, pulmonary edema, atelectasis, or drowning.

Ventilation/Perfusion Imbalance

In the normal lung the ratio of alveolar ventilation ($\dot{V}A$ = 4 L/min) to blood flow ($\dot{Q}$ = 5 L/min) averages 0.8. Because of inequalities in the distribution of both ventilation and blood flow and because the gravitational effects are somewhat greater on blood flow than they are on ventilation in the upright position, the $\dot{V}A/\dot{Q}$ ratio is about 3.0 at the apex of the lung and about 0.6 at the base.

Variations in the $\dot{V}A/\dot{Q}$ ratio in different lung regions affect gas exchange in specific ways. Decreasing the $\dot{V}A/\dot{Q}$ causes the area to become hypoventilated, so that the PA_{O_2} falls and PA_{CO_2} increases. However, the increase in PA_{CO_2} is limited by the fact that Pv_{CO_2} is only 46 mm Hg (Fig. 2–20). Any such lung unit will effectively act as if there were a shunt acting together with some normal lung. The virtual shunt will differ from a true shunt by the fact that giving 100% oxygen to breathe will eventually wash the N_2 out of all lung units, leading to high PA_{O_2} and full saturation of blood leaving that region (Pa_{O_2} > 560 mm Hg). Thus, if the magnitude of the shunt were measured, the calculated venous admixture would be reduced by giving 100% oxygen to breathe. Alternatively, if a lung region has a high $\dot{V}A/\dot{Q}$, it will be hyperventilated and the PA_{O_2} will rise and the PA_{CO_2} will fall. Under these circumstances, the PA_{CO_2} will fall in proportion to the increase in ventilation, but

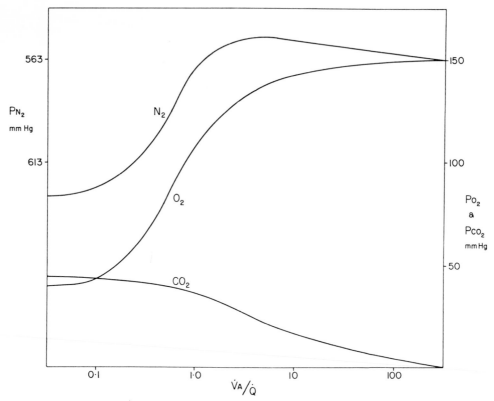

Figure 2–20. *Effects of Variations of Ventilation and Perfusion Ratio on the Oxygen, Carbon Dioxide, and Nitrogen Tensions in Alveoli*

The left-hand ordinate refers to nitrogen tension and the right-hand to tensions of oxygen and carbon dioxide. Note that the nitrogen tension varies most in regions of low $\dot{V}_A/\dot{Q}$ ratio, whereas changes in CO_2 tension are more affected by high $\dot{V}_A/\dot{Q}$ regions. (Diagram from Dr. Leon Farhi.)

the increase in $P_{A_{O_2}}$ will not significantly increase pulmonary capillary blood oxygen content because this blood is normally nearly fully saturated. Such a unit can be considered to function as if there were a region of normally ventilated lung plus a portion of lung that was ventilated but not perfused (dead space). The magnitude of the defect may be quantitatively assessed by the measurement of physiologic dead space.

These concepts have been incorporated into a "three compartment model" to quantitate the degree of $\dot{V}_A/\dot{Q}$ inhomogeneity.[5405] This model consists of (1) an ideal compartment having the same $\dot{V}_A/\dot{Q}$ throughout; (2) a dead space compartment consisting of an anatomic dead space and an alveolar dead space, the latter derived from ventilation of a virtually unperfused compartment; and (3) a shunt compartment consisting of a true anatomic shunt plus blood flow through a virtual compartment that is perfused but not ventilated.

Another approach has been to use the presence of alveolar-arterial N_2 differences to assess inhomogeneity.[5405] It may be noted from Figure 2–20 that the different effects of variations of $\dot{V}_A/\dot{Q}$ on $P_{A_{O_2}}$ and $P_{A_{CO_2}}$ lead to variations in $P_{A_{N_2}}$. These, in turn, give rise to an alveolar-arterial N_2 difference in the presence of ventilation/perfusion inhomogeneity.

In most instances, changes in resistance and compliance in different lung units lead to the formation of areas of both high and low $\dot{V}_A/\dot{Q}$. The effect of this is that there is an increased "scatter" of $\dot{V}_A/\dot{Q}$ ratios in the lung. There is then an increase in venous admixture and an increase in physiologic dead space. The primary effect is to produce a decrease in Pa_{O_2}. The $P_{A_{CO_2}}$ is less affected because the hypoxia leads to an overall stimulus to breathe that lowers $P_{A_{CO_2}}$. It has been shown that with increasing age the loss of lung elasticity is associated with an increased scatter of $\dot{V}_A/\dot{Q}$ ratios. This contributes to the decrease in Pa_{O_2} with age (see

Chapter 4). Changes in ventilation/perfusion relationships are by far the most common cause of hypoxemia in human subjects.

THE CONTROL OF BREATHING

Minute ventilation is controlled with respect to metabolic demands so that under normal circumstances arterial Po_2 and Pco_2 remain constant. The regulation of the alveolar ventilation and the rate and depth of breathing by which this is achieved must depend upon information provided to the central nervous system regarding both metabolic requirements and ventilation. This information is provided by several sensory systems.

Peripheral Chemoreceptors

Chemoreceptors are sensitive to changes in the chemical composition of the blood. They are contained in groups of cells found close to the bifurcation of the carotid arteries and close to the arch of the aorta, between the aorta and the pulmonary artery. These groups of cells are difficult to find on dissection, as they usually measure only 1 to 2 millimeters in diameter. The *carotid bodies* are usually found lying between the internal and external carotid arteries. They receive their blood supply from a small branch of the occipital artery, and their venous drainage joins the internal jugular vein. The afferent nerve fibers from the carotid bodies join the carotid sinus nerve, a branch of the glossopharyngeal nerve. The *aortic bodies* are groups of cells scattered between the arch of the aorta and the pulmonary artery. They receive their blood supply from small vessels leaving the arch of the aorta and from branches of the coronary arteries. The afferent fibers from the aortic bodies join the vagus nerves.

The structure and function of the carotid and aortic bodies are believed to be similar, although most physiologic investigations have been carried out on the carotid bodies because of their greater accessibility. It is generally believed, although the evidence is not entirely convincing, that stimulation of the carotid bodies has more influence on ventilation than does stimulation of the aortic bodies. Chemoreceptor tissue has an extremely high blood flow per gram of tissue, so that although it also has a very high oxygen usage there is only a small fall in saturation between the arterial and ve-

nous blood. Thus, tissue Po_2 and Pco_2 are close to arterial values.

Histologically, chemoreceptor tissue is complex; the following discussion outlines only the main features. The structure and function of the chemoreceptors have recently been reviewed in detail.[5394] The glomus cells (Type I cells) are believed to be the cells that are sensitive to chemical change. They are cells with prominent granules and mitochondria and contain a high concentration of pseudocholinesterase and dopamine. There are afferent nerve fibers closely associated with the glomus cells, and they are both myelinated and nonmyelinated. There appears to be some sort of close synaptic connection between the glomus cells and the afferent nerve fibers. One theory suggests that release of acetylcholine stimulates the nerve endings; another theory suggests that dopamine is released and inhibits the activity of the nerve endings, which are spontaneously active. In addition to the glomus cells, there are interstitial cells (Type II or sustentacular cells), which appear to wrap around the nerve fibers and the glomus cells. Their function is unknown, and they do not contain transmitter granules. There are also efferent nerve fibers in the glossopharyngeal nerve; their function is not established, but stimulation appears to inhibit activity in afferent fibers. There are efferent sympathetic nerve fibers which are preganglionic to ganglion cells and postganglionic to blood vessels. Stimulation of the postganglionic fibers causes constriction of the blood vessels. There are ganglion cells within the carotid and aortic bodies. These are few in number but may release transmitters that affect blood vessels.

The impulse activity in the afferent nerve fibers from the peripheral chemoreceptors is of low frequency (0 to 15 Hz) and has a random pattern.[5395] The major stimulus for increased activity is a decrease in arterial Po_2. The relationship between impulse discharge and Pa_{O_2} is shown in Figure 2–21. It may be noted that there is little, but not zero, activity at very high Pa_{O_2} (>500 mm Hg). There is a slight increase in impulse activity as Pa_{O_2} is decreased to between 500 and 100 mm Hg. There is a marked increase in impulse activity only when Pa_{O_2} falls below 60 mm Hg, and maximum activity is reached at about 30 mm Hg. The chemoreceptors are sensitive to Pa_{O_2} rather than to the oxygen content of the blood (Ca_{O_2}), and the response to a change in Pa_{O_2} is almost immediate. Thus, they are not normally stim-

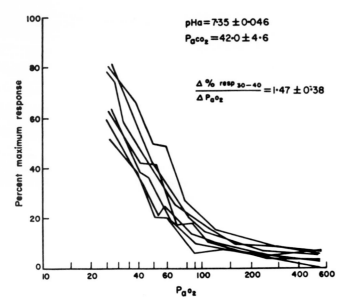

$pHa = 7.35 \pm 0.046$

$P_aco_2 = 42.0 \pm 4.6$

$$\frac{\Delta\% \; resp_{30-40}}{\Delta P_aO_2} = 1.47 \pm 0.38$$

Figure 2–21. Average neural discharge (expressed as a percentage of maximum asphyxial activity) from carotid bodies of seven cats anesthetized with pentobarbital and paralyzed with gallamine in response to changing arterial O_2 tension (Pa_{O_2}) plotted semi-logarithmically. Mean values $\pm$ 1 SD are shown for arterial pH (pHA) and arterial CO_2 tension (Pa_{CO_2}) and slope of the response curve between PaO_2 of 30 and 40 mm Hg. (Reprinted with permission from Fidone, S. J., and Gonzalez, C. Initiation and control of chemoreceptor activity in the carotid body. In: Handbook of Physiology, Section 3, Vol. 2, Part 1. American Physiological Society, Bethesda, Md., 1986, p. 258.)

ulated in anemia or in carbon monoxide poisoning except when Ca_{O_2} decreases to such low values that the oxygen usage by the chemoreceptor cells leads to a decrease in PO_2 in the chemoreceptor tissue. Recent work has suggested that the aortic chemoreceptors may be more sensitive to changes in Ca_{O_2} than are the carotid chemoreceptors.

The activity of the chemoreceptors is also influenced by Pa_{CO_2} and by pH. Increasing Pa_{CO_2}, at constant Pa_{O_2} and pH, causes an almost linear increase in nerve activity. The increase in nerve activity for a given increase in Pa_{CO_2} is much greater when the Pa_{O_2} is low ($<$ 60 mm Hg); hypoxia is said to potentiate the effects of CO_2. A decrease in arterial pH at constant Pa_{O_2} and constant Pa_{CO_2} causes stimulation of the chemoreceptors. Under circumstances in which the blood flow through the chemoreceptors is reduced to about 25% of normal, there is impaired O_2 delivery and the chemoreceptors are stimulated. This may occur with hemorrhaging when there is hypotension and increased sympathetic nerve activity.

Stimulation of the peripheral chemoreceptors causes an increase in the rate and depth of breathing and plays a major role in the defense against hypoxia. In experimental animals, after removal of the peripheral chemoreceptors, hypoxia causes depression of ventilation. Stimulation of chemoreceptors also causes reflex vasoconstriction and a decrease in heart rate. These reflex responses contribute to the cardiovascular changes associated with the diving reflex. There is some evidence that stimulation of the aortic chemoreceptors may cause an increase in heart rate.

Central Chemoreceptors

The central chemoreceptors are located close to (within 2 millimeters) the ventral surface of the medulla oblongata. They are situated laterally and rostrally, close to the area of entry of the eighth through eleventh cranial nerve roots. This area can be stimulated in experimental animals by applying solutions of low pH or a low PCO_2 to the surface of the brain. Stimulation in this way causes an increase in the rate and depth of breathing. Application of local anesthetics or cold substances to this area depresses breathing. The precise neural elements responsible for the response have not been identified histologically.

It is believed that the cells close to the surface of the medulla are sensitive to changes in the pH of their ECF. The composition of the ECF in this area can be affected by changes in either the cerebrospinal fluid (CSF) or the blood. When blood Pa_{CO_2} rises, CO_2 diffuses rapidly into the ECF and CSF. Because there is relatively little buffering in the CSF or ECF, there is greater change in pH in these fluids than in the blood for a given change in Pa_{CO_2}. Changes in blood pH have less of an effect than changes in CO_2 because H^+ diffuses less readily across the blood-brain barrier. Because the response depends on the equilibration between PCO_2 in the blood and that in the ECF, it may take several minutes before equilibrium and a steady-state response are achieved. Changes in ECF pH may be assessed by measuring changes in CSF pH. Normally, the CSF pH is constant at 7.32 units. If there is a long-term change in Pa_{CO_2}, such as might occur in a patient who is chronically hypoventilating, the CSF pH, which is initially decreased, returns to normal in about 8 to 48 hours. This change is accompanied by an increase in CSF HCO_3^- concentration. Thus, initially the increase in Pa_{CO_2} tends to stimulate an increase in breathing, but as the CSF pH is restored to normal, this stimulus disappears. The effect is to stabilize Pa_{CO_2} at the new level, since an increase in ventilation now increases CSF pH and has a depressant effect on breathing.

Most of the increased stimulus to breathe provided by increased P_{CO_2} is dependent on stimulation of the central chemoreceptors. In experimental animals, when the peripheral chemoreceptors are denervated, it can be demonstrated that less than 20% of the response to CO_2 is mediated by the peripheral chemoreceptors.

Sensory Nerve Endings in the Airways, Lung, and Chest

Nasal Receptors. Nerve endings in the nasal mucosa are stimulated by inhaled irritants. Stimulation causes sneezing but may also cause apnea. The apnea is a part of the "diving response," which also includes intense bradycardia and vasoconstriction in the skin, muscle, and splanchnic and renal vascular beds but not in the cerebral and coronary circulation.[5396]

Pharyngeal and Laryngeal Receptors. These nerve endings are stimulated by irritants or by the presence of foreign bodies. Stimulation causes coughing but may also cause laryngeal spasm.

Receptors in the Lungs. There are three major groups of receptors in the lungs.

The *bronchopulmonary stretch receptors* are sensory nerve endings that lie within the smooth muscle surrounding the trachea and larger bronchi. The afferent fibers from these receptors are carried in myelinated fibers in the vagus nerves. The receptors are activated by lung distension. If the distension is maintained, they are found to be only slowly adapting. When activated these receptors shorten inspiration and prolong expiration. It has been postulated that the bronchopulmonary stretch re-

ceptors, by providing information regarding the degree of inflation of the lung, may regulate the rate and depth of breathing to achieve the optimal combination of mechanical work and/or inspiratory force. In experimental animals, these receptors can be demonstrated to function over the normal tidal volume range. If the trachea is clamped at end-inspiration (high lung volume), breathing movements are inhibited. If the trachea is clamped at end-expiration (low lung volume), there are rapid and forceful respiratory movements. When the vagus nerves are cut, breathing is slow and deep and is unaffected by clamping the trachea. These effects are referred to as the *Hering-Breuer reflex*, otherwise known as the inspiratory-inhibitory reflex. The reflex appears to be weak in adult humans, in whom lung volume must be raised to about 1 liter greater than FRC before inspiratory inhibition can be demonstrated. Stimulation of these receptors also causes a reflex increase in heart rate and peripheral dilatation.

The pulmonary stretch receptors are also stimulated by a decrease in airway P_{CO_2}. In experimental animals, a large decrease in P_{CO_2} to less than 20 mm Hg is needed to demonstrate this effect. The physiologic significance of the sensitivity to CO_2 is at present unknown.

The *tracheobronchial irritant receptors* are nonspecialized nerve endings that are thought to terminate between the epithelial cells close to the mucosal surface of the airways. The afferent fibers are myelinated fibers in the vagus nerves. They have an irregular spontaneous discharge and are stimulated by large inflations or deflations of the lungs and by a large number of inhaled irritants, such as cigarette smoke, sulfur dioxide, and ammonia. They are also stimulated in the presence of histamine. The receptors adapt rapidly to maintained stimuli.

Stimulation of the irritant receptors causes cough, bronchoconstriction, laryngeal constriction, and hyperpnea and is usually associated with increased mucus secretion.

The *pulmonary and bronchial C-fibers* arise from a wide area of the lung and bronchial tree. They are said to be stimulated by harmful stimuli, such as pulmonary edema and congestion, and by embolization of the pulmonary vascular bed. Stimulation causes rapid shallow breathing, bronchoconstriction, and increased airway secretion and may often be associated with cardiovascular depressor effects.[5397]

Chest Wall Receptors. The intercostal muscles have a rich innervation of muscle spindles.[5398] Opinion is divided on the importance of this innervation in the control of breathing in humans. One view is that they are mainly concerned with stabilizing the chest wall during postural movements and movements of the upper limbs and head. The other view is that the muscle spindles provide information related to lung volume. This information is used in the brain stem control of tidal volume, especially in the presence of added respiratory loads. If this is so, it is not the only mechanism, since patients with high spinal cord lesions respond normally to both resistive and elastic loading.

Central Control of Breathing

The characteristic rhythm of respiration may be recorded from "respiratory rhythm" (RR) neurons in the brain stem, in the neural output to the respiratory muscles in the phrenic and intercostal nerves, and in the electromyogram of the respiratory muscles. The most frequent RR consists of three phases: an abrupt onset of inspiratory activity on a background of silence in late expiration, a gradual augmentation of activity during inspiration, and an abrupt decline to silence during the expiratory phase. Other neurons may become active during expiration or may be "phase-spanning" neurons active during both inspiration and expiration. The major timing event in the cycle is thought to be the transition between inspiration and expiration (the "inspiratory off-switch"). The source of the RR is thought to be in the medulla, but it has not been localized to a single identifiable group of neurons. However, it is clear that the respiratory control mechanisms and their output pathways are represented on both sides of the brain stem as two bilaterally symmetric systems.[5399]

Localization of Respiratory Control

Areas of the brain stem concerned with respiratory control have been localized by means of three techniques: ablation (local destruction), electrical stimulation, and electrophysiologic recording of action potentials. In addition to groups of neurons in the ventrolateral medulla that serve the laryngeal, pharyngeal, tongue, and alae nasi muscles, there are two groups of RR neurons in the medulla. One aggregate forms a longitudinal column in the ventrolateral part of the medulla in the general region of the nucleus ambiguus (NA). It extends caudally, almost to the bulbospinal border, and rostrally to the bulbopontine border; it is known as the ventral respiratory group (VRG). The other aggregate is located dorsally and more medially, close to the nucleus tractus solitarius (NTS). This aggregate is more circumscribed, with only a limited extension caudally and rostrally. It is referred to as the dorsal respiratory group (DRG) (Fig. 2–22).

The cells of the DRG lie close to the NTS, which is the site of termination of afferents from arterial baroreceptors, peripheral chemoreceptors, and lung receptors. The majority of the cells of the DRG are active during inspiration (IR cells) and show the typical RR. They are classified as either IR-alpha (inhibited by lung inflation) or IR-beta cells (excited by lung inflation) on the basis of their responses to lung inflation. It has been proposed that the IR-beta cells are excited directly by the pulmonary stretch receptor afferents and then act as interneurons inhibiting the IR-alpha cells. However, this appears to be an oversimplification. In addition to the input from the pulmonary stretch receptors, both types of DRG cells receive a similar driving input of a central inspiratory activity (CIA). The source of the CIA is unknown, but it is mainly dependent on chemical drive inputs for its activity. The majority of the IR-alpha neurons project, after crossing the midline close to the obex, to the phrenic motor neurons in the spinal cord. There are also projections from the DRG to the VRG.

The cells of the VRG form a long chain of cells that correspond closely to the nucleus ambiguus (NA, rostral) and nucleus retroambigualis (NRA, caudal). The NA contains the somatic motor neurons for the laryngeal muscles and also the pharyngeal and facial muscles involved in the respiratory control of the upper airways. The VRG can be divided into three functional parts. The most caudal region consists almost entirely of neurons active in expiration (ER) that project to the expiratory intercostal and abdominal muscles. The intermediate region contains mainly IR neurons that project to the contralateral spinal cord and terminate on the phrenic (25%) and intercostal (75%) motorneurons. There is a distinct group of neurons in this region that is active early in inspiration (early burst neurons), and this group does not project to the spinal cord. Their projections probably cross the midline and inhibit the expiratory premotor neurons during inspiration, thereby contributing to the pattern-

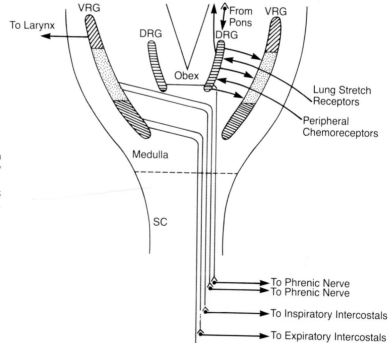

Figure 2–22. Simplified diagram of the connections of the respiratory control centers in the medulla. DRG, dorsal respiratory group; VRG, ventral respiratory group; SC, spinal cord.

generating system. The most rostral group of neurons is mainly expiratory and is thought to play a complex role in the control of the breathing pattern.

There is also a group of respiratory neurons in the dorsolateral pons in the area of the nucleus parabrachialis medialis (NPBM). These cells have been described by the term *pneumotaxic center*. The cells have activity in inspiration, expiration, or both inspiration and expiration. Electrical stimulation of this area causes respiratory phase switching (inspiration terminates and becomes expiration). It is believed these cells influence the pattern generator to determine the operation of the inspiratory off-switch. This may be of particular importance in humans in whom there is a high threshold for the inhibitory effects of lung inflation. There appears to be a monosynaptic connection from the DRG to the NPBM that becomes active during inspiration, exciting the cells of the NPBM. There is a polysynaptic connection from the NPBM to the region of the DRG that forms a negative feedback, leading to the termination of inspiration. Lesions of the NPBM in humans are associated with apneusis.

Voluntary control of breathing probably originates from a rather circumscribed area of the cerebral cortex. The descending pathways from the cortex providing voluntary control of the respiratory muscles are separate from those of the involuntary system from the medulla. The voluntary pathways run in the dorsolateral columns of the spinal cord (corticospinal tract), whereas the involuntary pathways are in the ventrolateral columns (bulbospinal tract). It is likely that the integration of voluntary and involuntary controls occurs at the spinal motor neurons.

Respiratory Responses to Hypercapnia and Hypoxia

Hypercapnia

Under normal conditions, respiration is regulated to maintain Pa_{CO_2} at or close to 40 mm Hg. An increase in Pa_{CO_2} causes an increase in minute ventilation with an increase in both tidal volume and minute ventilation. When inspired CO_2 concentration is suddenly increased, it takes 3 to 7 minutes before a steady state of ventilation is reached. Over the range of 40 to 70 mm Hg there is a nearly linear relationship between ventilation and Pa_{CO_2}. Although variation in the magnitude of the response between individuals is high (1 to 6 L/min/mm Hg), there is good reproducibility in any one subject. The maximum ventilatory response induced by CO_2 is about 70 to 80 L/min, significantly less than that seen at maximum exercise. When Pa_{CO_2} exceeds 70 mm Hg in a normal subject, there may be depression of ventilation and eventually coma and death. Low concentrations of inspired CO_2 can be tolerated for many days. But as the inspired concentration increases above 7% there may be headache, irritability, and spontaneous muscular movements, as well as respiratory stimulation.

The ventilatory response to CO_2 may be tested by having the subject re-breathe from a bag filled with 7% CO_2 and 93% O_2. If the bag has an initial volume of about 2 to 4 liters, the P_{CO_2} of the bag increases at a rate of about 4 mm Hg/min. The relationship between ventilation and alveolar (end-tidal) P_{CO_2}, when plotted, provides a *CO_2 response curve* (Fig. 2–23). The ventilatory response curve may be used to determine the effects of other agents influencing ventilation. For instance, lowering the P_{O_2} produces two effects: there is a higher ventilation for a given P_{CO_2}, and the slope of the line becomes steeper. Drugs that depress the respiratory center (such as morphine and barbiturates) reduce the slope of the CO_2 response curve.

Acidemia

A rise in P_{CO_2} is usually accompanied by a decrease in pH of the arterial blood, and it is sometimes difficult to separate the ventilatory effects of the CO_2 from those of pH. However, in experimental animals, it is possible to demonstrate a ventilatory response to a change in pH when P_{CO_2} is held constant and also a ventilatory response to CO_2 when pH is held constant. The major site of action of pH is on the peripheral chemoreceptors, although some hydrogen ions may cross the blood-brain barrier.

Hypoxia

The ventilatory response to hypoxia may be studied by having the subject breathe gas mixtures containing a lower than normal percentage of O_2. Because stimulation of ventilation by the hypoxia decreases P_{CO_2}, the ventilatory response to hypoxia is small and is limited by the fall in P_{CO_2}. If the inspired gas mixture is adjusted to keep P_{CO_2} constant, the response to hypoxia can be examined. The relationship between minute ventilation and PA_{O_2} is hyperbolic. At a P_{CO_2} of 40 mm Hg there is little change in ventilation until PA_{O_2} falls below 50 mm Hg (Fig. 2–24). If arterial O_2 saturation is measured by means of an ear oximeter and if Sa_{O_2} is plotted against minute ventilation, the relationship is nearly linear. The ventilatory response to hypoxia is very variable between individuals and is about 0.6 L/min/1% desaturation. Although hypoxia does not play a significant role in the day-to-day control of ventilation at sea level, the hypoxic drive to ventilation becomes very important in patients with chronic hypercapnia. In these patients, the pH of the brain ECF has returned to normal in spite of the raised Pa_{CO_2}. Plasma pH may also be nearly normal because of renal compensation. Under conditions in which the CSF bicarbonate concentration is high, further changes in CSF P_{CO_2} produce relatively smaller changes in CSF pH, and the major stimulus to ventilation becomes hypoxia. If such a patient is given a high O_2 mixture to breathe to relieve the

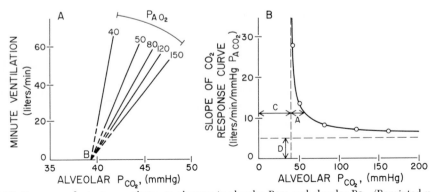

Figure 2–23. Response of minute ventilation to changes in alveolar P_{CO_2} and alveolar P_{O_2}. (Reprinted with permission from Forster, R. E., II, DuBois, A. B., Briscoe, W. A., and Fisher, A. B. The Lung. 3rd ed. Year Book Medical Publishers, Chicago, 1986, p. 278.)

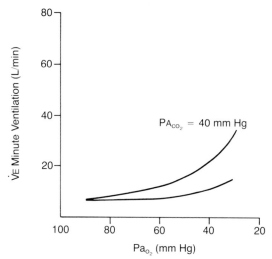

Figure 2–24. *Upper curve,* minute ventilation as a function of the arterial oxygen tension (PaO_2) at constant alveolar P_{CO_2} (PA_{CO_2} = 40 mm Hg). *Lower curve,* ventilatory response ordinarily observed when PA_{CO_2} is not controlled.

hypoxia, ventilation may become severely depressed.

VENTILATION DURING EXERCISE

Oxygen Delivery to the Tissues

During physical exercise there is an increase in the oxygen requirements of the tissues from about 250 mL/min at rest to between 3 and 6 L/min at maximal exercise. To provide for the increased oxygen requirements, there are profound changes in the cardiovascular and respiratory systems. Since the cardiac output increases by only about a factor of five (from 5 L/min to 25 L/min), there must be an increased extraction of oxygen from the blood in its passage through the working muscles. Mixed venous oxygen content may fall from 14 mL/100 mL to 6 mL/100 mL. The increased oxygen extraction is aided by the low PO_2 in the working muscles and by the effects of pH, PCO_2, and temperature on the oxygen dissociation curve, as noted earlier in this chapter.

The Ventilatory Response to Exercise

At the beginning of exercise there is an immediate increase in ventilation that begins with the first breath after the start of the exercise. Following this, there is a hyperbolic increase in ventilation that, if work rate remains constant, reaches a steady state in about 4 minutes. When exercise terminates, there is an equally rapid decrease in ventilation and then a gradual return to the former resting ventilation (Fig. 2–25). During exercise in the steady state, the respiratory minute volume is directly related to the rate of working and oxygen consumption. The relationship is linear up to an oxygen consumption of about 2 to 3 L/min, after which the respiratory minute volume increases more steeply for a given increment in work done (Fig. 2–26). During mild and moderate exercise, Pa_{CO_2}, Pa_{O_2}, and pH of the arterial blood remain constant. At higher work rates there is a lactic acidosis as a result of anaerobic metabolism. Pa_{CO_2} decreases and Pa_{O_2} increases since there is a relative hyperventilation secondary to the decrease in pH. The work rate at which the anaerobic metabolism causes a decrease in pH and the ventilation increases above its linear relationship with work rate is called the *anaerobic threshold.* Surprisingly, the precise mechanisms that regulate the minute ventilation to achieve a linear relationship between ventilation and the rate of working remain unknown. A number of neural, humoral, and hemodynamic factors probably contribute to the response.[5401, 5402]

Neurogenic Factors

It has been proposed that impulses originating in the motor cortex and destined for the skeletal muscles are accompanied by an "irradiation" of impulses to the respiratory centers, leading to a stimulation of breathing. There is no direct experimental evidence in support of this hypothesis. During movements of the limbs, both in experimental animals and in humans, there is a proprioceptive stimulus to respiration. Evidence suggests that stimulation of muscle spindle afferents is not a major component of the proprioceptive stimulus, which probably arises from receptors in the tendons and joints.

Humoral Factors

During mild to moderate exercise, ventilation is more closely related to $\dot{V}CO_2$ than it is to $\dot{V}O_2$. However, it is unlikely that changes in Pa_{CO_2} provide the stimulus for hyperpnea, as Pa_{CO_2} does not change, and with more severe exercise Pa_{CO_2} decreases. The Pa_{O_2} does not alter appreciably during mild to moderate exercise, and

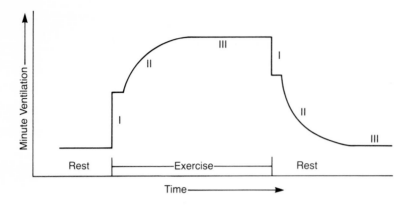

Figure 2–25. Scheme of ventilation before, during, and after a period of exercise at a moderate work rate. Phase I identifies a period of abrupt change in ventilation during the transition between rest and exercise. The second phase (Phase II) occurs after about 15 seconds, and there is a gradual (exponential) change in ventilation to reach a new steady state (Phase III). Phase II has a time constant of 60 to 70 seconds, so that Phase III is reached in about 4 minutes.

at high work loads it may increase. Thus, hypoxia cannot be the stimulus for the hyperpnea. But there is a good correlation between ventilation and $\dot{V}O_2$. During severe exercise, breathing 100% O_2 causes a small decrease (10%) in ventilation, suggesting there is a hypoxic stimulus. The role of the peripheral chemoreceptors in human subjects during exercise has been examined by observing the ventilatory response to exercise in patients who have had both carotid bodies removed. The steady-state ventilatory responses were unaffected by this procedure during mild to moderate exercise (there was a reduction in ventilation during severe exercise), but there was a slight time-lag in reaching the steady-state ventilation. There is

no change in pH of the arterial blood during mild to moderate exercise, and during severe exercise there is a decrease in pH. The hyperventilation during severe exercise can be accounted for by the decrease in pH. Because mixed venous PO_2 and PCO_2 show large changes in exercise, it has been suggested that there may be chemoreceptors sensitive to chemical changes in venous blood. Despite vigorous efforts, no convincing evidence has been presented for the existence of venous chemoreceptors.

Cardiodynamic Factors

A strong correlation has been noted between ventilation and the CO_2 flux to the lung. The

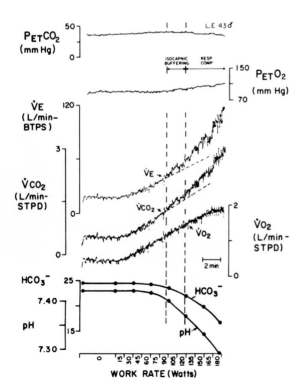

Figure 2–26. Breath-by-breath measurement of end-tidal partial pressure of CO_2 and O_2 (PET_{CO_2} and PET_{O_2}), minute expiratory ventilation ($\dot{V}E$), CO_2 output ($\dot{V}CO_2$), O_2 uptake ($\dot{V}O_2$), and, at the times indicated by points, arterial HCO_3 and pH measurements for a 1 minute incremental work test on a cycle ergometer in a normal subject. During the isocapnic buffering period $\dot{V}E$ and $\dot{V}CO_2$ increase curvilinearly at the same rate, keeping PET_{CO_2} constant by increasing PET_{O_2}. During the respiratory compensation (Resp Comp) period PET_{CO_2} starts to decrease. (Reprinted with permission from Wasserman, K., Whipp, B. J., and Casaburi, R. Respiratory control during exercise. In: Handbook of Physiology, Section 3, Vol. 2, Part 2. American Physiological Society, Bethesda, Md., 1986, p. 598.)

amount of CO_2 returning to the lungs is the product of the mixed venous CO_2 content and the venous return. A number of investigators have shown that manipulation of either the mixed venous CO_2 content or cardiac output leads to immediate changes in ventilation that maintain constant arterial P_{CO_2}.[5391] It has also been shown that cardiac output and venous return increase immediately at the start of exercise and could therefore contribute to the immediate increase in ventilation at the start of exercise. It has not, however, been possible to identify the receptors that would be stimulated by an increase in cardiac output or venous return.

It should be remembered that if the ventilatory response did not match the CO_2 load reaching the lung there would be changes in Pa_{CO2} that would stimulate chemoreceptor responses. For the present, it must be assumed that the overall ventilatory level is determined by the simultaneous action of neurogenic, humoral, and cardiodynamic stimuli.

BREATHING AT ALTITUDE

As one progressively rises from sea level to higher and higher altitudes, the barometric pressure decreases, so that although oxygen concentration remains constant the partial pressure falls. As a rule of thumb, the barometric pressure halves for each 6000 meters of ascent. The PI_{O_2} at altitude can be calculated, and the PA_{O_2} can be estimated from the alveolar air equation. At 6000 meters:

$$\text{Barometric pressure} = \frac{760}{2} = 380$$

$$PI_{O_2} = (380 - 47) \times \frac{21}{100} = 70 \text{ mm Hg}$$

$$PA_{O_2} = 70 - \frac{Pa_{CO_2}}{0.8} = 70 - \frac{40}{0.8}$$
$$= 20 \text{ mm Hg}$$

Thus, unless ventilation is increased to lower PA_{CO_2}, PA_{O_2}, will be too low to be compatible with life. However, a doubling of ventilation would decrease PA_{CO_2} to 20 mm Hg, and PA_{O_2} becomes 45 mm Hg.

Effects of Hypoxia

Those symptoms that appear on acute exposure to hypoxia may be discussed by imagining the subject being exposed to different altitudes.

Sensory Function. The earliest effect of hypoxia is a decreased efficiency of night vision. This loss becomes apparent at altitudes above 2000 meters, and at 3000 meters a 60% increase in illumination is needed to restore visual acuity. There is no loss of visual acuity in bright light, and the loss of night vision appears to be the only sensory loss.

Mental Function. The first hypoxic symptoms appear at about 3000 meters and are said to be somewhat similar to alcoholic intoxication, varying widely between individuals and perhaps reflecting the underlying personality. There may be lightheadedness and euphoria with unwarranted self-confidence, sometimes changing to resentment and surliness if challenged. Simultaneously, critical judgment and insight are impaired and fixed ideas prevail. Short-term memory is affected, and later there may be impairment of fine motor movements. The most common complaint of subjects voluntarily subjected to hypoxia is of headache and dizziness. There are also difficulty in concentrating and lassitude. It should be emphasized that more usually the subject is completely unaware of any functional changes. The effects of hypoxia become marked at 4000 to 5000 meters.

When there is a *sudden onset* of oxygen deficiency at altitudes above 7000 meters (e.g., loss of pressure in an airplane), there is a brief period of grace during which normal function continues. At the end of this period, consciousness becomes impaired; this is followed by coma and death. This "time of useful consciousness" is 5 minutes at 7000 meters, but only 1 minute at 10,000 meters.

Acute Mountain Sickness. When lowlanders ascend rapidly to altitudes of 3000 to 4000 meters, they commonly experience a series of symptoms that are termed acute mountain sickness. These symptoms include lassitude, loss of appetite, and sometimes vomiting and insomnia. If the subject is able to remain at altitude, the symptoms frequently disappear after 2 to 3 days. It has been suggested that the symptoms may be secondary to hypoxia and to respiratory alkalosis. Over the next 3 to 6 weeks, a series of adaptations (acclimatization) take place that improve the individual's ability to cope with the hypoxia.

Chronic Mountain Sickness. Long-term residents at high altitude may develop gradually increasing fatigue and somnolence and decreasing mental activity. They become cyanotic and develop a very high hematocrit. There appears to be an insufficient ventilatory response to the hypoxia, and at least some patients have been shown to be almost totally without a ventilatory response.

High Altitude Pulmonary Edema. Unacclimatized individuals at altitudes above 3000 meters are prone to a very rapid onset of pulmonary edema. The cause of the pulmonary edema is not completely known, but it may be associated with hypoxic pulmonary vasoconstriction and/or hypoxic damage to the pulmonary capillaries, which alter their permeability. Prompt treatment with rest, oxygen, and diuretics is required.

Adaptation to Altitude (Acclimatization)

When a normal subject is acutely exposed to low inspired oxygen tensions, there are stimulation of the peripheral chemoreceptors and an increase in ventilation. This causes a decrease in Pa_{CO_2}, an increase in plasma pH, and an increase in the pH of the CSF. After a few days, the increase in plasma pH is reversed by the excretion of an alkaline urine. The CSF pH is restored, somewhat more rapidly, with a decrease in bicarbonate concentration in the CSF. Ventilation gradually *increases* as the CSF pH is restored to normal. In this new state, with a normal CSF pH and a lowered CSF bicarbonate concentration, there is an increased sensitivity to changes in Pa_{CO_2}. If the hypoxia is removed by administration of oxygen or by descent, increased ventilation continues for several days. This is because as the hypoxic stimulus is removed and the ventilation begins to decrease, Pa_{CO_2} rises and maintains the ventilatory stimulus until the CSF pH and bicarbonate have returned to normal.

There is a gradual increase in red cell volume, leading to an increased hemoglobin concentration and an increased oxygen-carrying capacity of the blood. The increase occurs at a rate of about 1% per day so that in about 3 weeks there may be an increase in oxygen-carrying capacity of about 20%. Natives of high altitudes may have hemoglobin concentrations of 20 g/dL. There is also an increase in the concentration of 2,3-DPG in the red cells, which causes a decrease in oxygen affinity. The shift of the oxygen dissociation curve to the right favors the unloading of oxygen in the tissues. It may be noted (see later) that at very high altitude there may be a failure to correct the respiratory alkalosis, possibly because of reduced renal excretion, and the oxygen dissociation curve may then be shifted to the left. Under conditions of extreme hypoxia, this may be an appropriate response, because it aids oxygenation of the blood in the lungs in the presence of a very low alveolar P_{O_2}. In experimental animals an increased vascularity in muscle beds and an increased concentration of oxidative enzymes in muscle cells have been described. It is not certain that this occurs in humans.

The degree of acclimatization achieved by sea-level dwellers who go to high altitudes does not appear to be as complete as that found in individuals native to high altitudes.

The highest permanent human habitations are at approximately 5300 meters in the Andes of South America. But acute exposure to this altitude would require the inspired air to be enriched with oxygen. Above 12,000 meters, alveolar oxygen partial pressure is reduced, even when breathing 100% O_2. To maintain oxygenation above that altitude, pressurization is required.

Until recently, it was believed that it would be impossible to reach the summit of Mount Everest without supplemental oxygen.[5406] However, this feat was achieved in 1978 when two climbers did just that. The reasons for this success were examined during an expedition in 1981 and appeared to be related to three factors. The degree of hyperventilation was much greater than expected, with the Pa_{CO_2} decreasing to 7.5 mm Hg. The pH of the arterial blood was much higher than expected (between 7.7 and 7.8); the failure of the kidneys to excrete bicarbonate was thought to be due to reduced renal excretion, possibly secondary to dehydration. The high pH appears to be an advantage, because the left-shifted oxygen dissociation curve enhances loading of oxygen in the pulmonary capillaries under conditions of diffusion limitation more than it interferes with unloading in the tissue capillaries. Finally, the barometric pressure (253 mm Hg) was higher than expected at the summit. This is an important factor because it determines the inspired P_{O_2}. Measurements showed that on the summit of Mount Everest alveolar P_{O_2} was 35 mm Hg and the Pa_{O_2} was 28 mm Hg.

EXPOSURE TO HIGH BAROMETRIC PRESSURE

Individuals are exposed to higher than normal barometric pressure when under water or in the unusual circumstance of being in a hyperbaric chamber. The problems of functioning under water depend upon the fact that in air, at sea level, the atmospheric pressure is 1 atmosphere (At), and an additional similar pressure is generated by a depth of 10 meters of sea water. As a diver descends, the pressure exerted on the body therefore increases by 1 atmosphere for every 10 meters of descent. Thus, at 30 meters the total pressure is 4 At (3 At due to sea water plus 1 At surface pressure). The book by Bennett and Elliot[5407] provides a comprehensive review of the physiologic and medical aspects of diving.

Problems of Descent

Most of the tissues of the body are incompressible and are unaffected by the increasing pressure on decent. But the pressure is transmitted to any air-containing cavities and compresses them or, if they are not immediately compressible, establishes a marked pressure difference between the inside and the outside of the cavity. The lung is compressible up to a point. In free diving, if a maximum inspiration is taken before the dive, the chest wall is no longer compressible when the chest wall has decreased to about 25% of TLC (at 4 At). Further descent leads to damage to the pulmonary capillaries and alveolar tissue. To prevent this, air (or a gas mixture) has to be supplied at a pressure equal to that of the surrounding water. The nasal sinuses and the air spaces in the middle ear are incompressible, but so long as free communication is maintained between these spaces and the main airways, a pressure difference does not develop. If the eustachian tubes or ostia of the sinuses are blocked, a pressure difference develops, leading to pain and possible rupture of the tympanic membrane. Diving should not be undertaken when an upper respiratory tract infection is present.

Problems Encountered at Depth

The amount of a gas dissolved in a liquid is almost directly proportional to the partial pressure. Thus, as the diver descends, breathing air, there is an increase in the amounts of oxygen and nitrogen dissolved in the body fluids. Both gases have toxic effects as the partial pressure rises.

Nitrogen Narcosis

Breathing air, the diver may experience the symptoms of nitrogen narcosis when the total pressure reaches about 5 At (4 At N_2 pressure). Nitrogen at this pressure produces a true narcosis with euphoria, lack of concentration, and impairment of judgment (sometimes called "raptures of the deep"). Particularly striking is the lack of appreciation of the passage of time. The mechanisms by which nitrogen produces narcosis are not entirely clear but appear to be analogous to the action of some anesthetic agents.

Oxygen Toxicity

Perhaps surprisingly, oxygen becomes toxic when the partial pressure of oxygen in the tissues is increased. There are three major forms of oxygen toxicity.

When oxygen is breathed at partial pressures greater than 2 At, it is toxic to the central nervous system. There may be visual and auditory hallucinations, sensory disturbances, and convulsions. Thus, this can occur breathing air at 10 At (90 meters) or breathing 100% O_2 at 2 At (10 meters). The individual response to oxygen toxicity is very variable, but the average individual may develop convulsions after breathing O_2 at 2 At for 20 minutes.

If O_2 is breathed at 1 At (100% O_2 at sea level) for a longer period (24 to 48 hours), lung O_2 toxicity may occur. Oxygen acts as an irritant to the mucous membranes of the lung; causes a sterile inflammation, with increased production of mucus, leakage of fluid, and entry of cells into the alveoli; and produces a sterile pneumonia-like state. This effect is likely to be due to the presence of oxygen free radicals that cause tissue damage.

Newborn infants are particularly sensitive to the toxic effects of oxygen. If O_2 is administered to newborn infants in concentrations greater than 40%, they develop retrolental fibroplasia, which leads to permanent blindness. The high O_2 concentration appears to stimulate the growth of blood vessels in the eye, which are later replaced by fibrous tissue.

Because of the narcotic effects of nitrogen and the toxic effects of oxygen, divers must breathe gas mixtures with concentrations of O_2 appropriate for the depth of the dive. Nitrogen is usually replaced in these gas mixtures by helium. Although breathing helium removes the problem of narcosis, it does add two problems of its own. Helium is less dense than nitrogen, which is an advantage because it reduces the increase in the work of breathing that occurs as the pressure increases. However, it leads to a higher than normal frequency of vibration of the vocal cords and a "Donald Duck" voice. This interferes with good vocal communication between the diver and the surface. Helium has a high thermal conductivity so that the diver surrounded by helium in his suit loses heat extremely rapidly.

Problems of Ascent

As the diver ascends, air in the body cavities, which is now exposed to a lower pressure, expands. Unless the air is allowed to escape from the lungs, the nasal sinuses, and the inner ear, the expanding air may rupture tissues. Divers must exhale continuously while ascending.

If the diver has been subjected to high pressure for more than a few minutes, nitrogen (or helium) will have dissolved in the body tissues. Because nitrogen is more soluble in fat than in aqueous solutions, larger amounts will be contained in tissues with a high fat content (especially the brain and the loose fatty tissue around the joints). As the pressure is reduced, the dissolved gas may come out of solution in the form of bubbles. These bubbles may directly rupture cells or may occlude small blood vessels; some may be carried by the blood to the lungs, where they may block pulmonary capillaries. A wide variety of symptoms may be produced, depending on the site of bubble formation, but these symptoms may be grouped into three types. Pains in the limbs (particularly around the joints) produce stiffness and muscle cramps, which are referred to as the "bends." Disturbances of CNS functions lead to giddiness, paralysis, deafness, or loss of sensation, and almost any CNS symptom can be produced. Blockage of the pulmonary capillaries or rupture of the alveoli leads to breathlessness and hypoxia. These symptoms of "decompression sickness" do not necessarily appear immediately at the time of the ascent and may be first noticed several hours later.

Decompression sickness can be minimized by ascending slowly, so that time is allowed for the gas to leave the tissues without bubbles forming. The principles of decompression were first put forward by Haldane, who showed that if the change in pressure was one-half or less, decompression sickness was unlikely to occur. Thus, decompression can occur in stages; after each decompression to one-half the pressure, time must be allowed for equilibration of pressure to occur before the next decompression step. Some modifications of this original concept have occurred, and tables are available that give recommended decompression steps and equilibration times in relation to the depth of the dive and the time spent at depth.[5407] It should be understood that the use of such tables does not guarantee a zero incidence of decompression sickness.

Therapeutic Use of Oxygen

When oxygenation of the blood in the lungs is inadequate, it may usually be improved (except in the case of shunts) by increasing the oxygen concentration in the inspired air. Oxygen is usually administered through a mask that delivers O_2 at a known concentration and flow rate. Whenever O_2 rich air is administered, the problems of oxygen toxicity must be kept in mind. Another factor that must be considered is in the patient with chronic respiratory disease and CO_2 retention. When Pa_{CO_2} has been elevated for some time, the pH of the blood and the CSF will have been restored close to normal. At this time, the patient will be relatively insensitive to further increases in Pa_{CO_2} as a stimulus to breathe and may be maintaining ventilation largely because of a hypoxic drive from the peripheral chemoreceptors. Administration of supplemental oxygen may remove the hypoxic drive, depress breathing, and lead to a further increase in Pa_{CO_2}, which may reach narcotic levels. Depression of breathing on administration of O_2 may not be noticed unless the patient is closely monitored. An additional cause of the rise in Pa_{CO_2} during oxygen breathing may be a worsening of the $\dot{V}_A/\dot{Q}$ distribution.

PARTICLE DEPOSITION: MUCOCILIARY CLEARANCE: PHYSICAL SIGNS

Although a detailed discussion of the physics and physiology of particle deposition and aerosol penetration is beyond the scope of this book, there are several reasons why the chest physician should have some basic knowledge of these aspects of the exposure of the lung to inhaled material. Not only are these considerations basic to understanding dust deposition and other environmental influences on the lung, but the increasing use of inhaled aerosols in treatment and of inhaled aerosol challenges to the lung require similar background knowledge. Brain and Valberg[23] contributed an excellent review of this field in 1979. Other monographs[24] deal with different aspects or with attempts to model the respiratory tract for study of dust deposition.[28, 40, 42, 2944] Anatomic factors related to particle deposition are discussed in Chapter 1.

DEPOSITION IN THE NORMAL LUNG

As noted in Chapter 1, the proportion of inhaled particles deposited in different parts of the respiratory tract is affected by the geometry of the airways; the other main determinants are particle size and the pattern of breathing.

Under average conditions, the deposition fraction between the upper respiratory tract, which includes the nose and nasopharynx, and the lower tract, including the alveoli, varies with particle size, as shown in Figure 3–1. Particle size is expressed as the aerodynamic median diameter, which equates particles of non-spherical shape in terms of a similar settling rate for spherical particles.

Large smoke particles, such as those generated by open coal burning and those present in the air pollution to which this leads, have diameters between 10 and 100 microns. Such particles mostly impact the upper airway. About 40% of particles from automobile exhaust, which measure up to 5 microns, or from tobacco smoke, which are usually less than 2 microns, are deposited in the periphery of the lung. In studies of normal subjects, there is a fair concordance between deposition fractions predicted from physical theory and airway geometry and actual measurements. From cigarette smoke with particles between 0.2 and 0.5 microns, for example, between 70% and 90% of inhaled particles are deposited.[2940] The theoretical data are also consistent with clinical observations; as an example, bronchial cancer attributable to nickel sintering, which produces relatively large metallic particles, occurs in major bronchi, especially at bifurcations at which the particles impact.

In experiments on rats, 95% of chrysotile asbestos fibers less than 6 microns long and all less than 0.5 microns wide were found to impact at the bifurcation of alveolar ducts.[55] In other experiments, 17% of inhaled fibers 1 to 3 microns in size were found to be deposited in respiratory bronchioles.[30] Remarkable photographs of asbestos fibers deposited at bronchiolar bifurcations have been published by Brody and Roe.[2941]

Deposition is also influenced by breathing pattern, both by tidal volume and by breath holding between inspiration and expiration.[29, 49] With particles of aerodynamic diameter (MMAD) of 0.28 microns, deposition was greater at higher flow rates and was also influenced by the larynx.[28] It has been shown that pollen particles can penetrate to the alveoli.[37]

The persistence of aerosol with breath holding in normal subjects can be used to calculate the mean effective air space diameter in which the aerosol is resident during the period of the held breath. In such experiments, using an aerosol 0.55 micron in diameter, Lapp and his colleagues[29] concluded that in men, the diameters were between 0.3 and 0.79 millimeter, and in women, between 0.4 and 0.62 millimeter. The correlation with age of the subject or with lung volume was poor.

AEROSOL DEPOSITION IN DISEASE

Nebulizers used in therapy do not differ greatly in the size of particles they deliver[34]; these varied from 2.8 to 4.3 microns in comparisons of nine dispensers.[43] Some investigators have found that more deposition occurs if intermittent positive-pressure breathing (IPPB) rather than an ultrasonic nebulizer is used.[34] It has been suggested that interposition of a tube or cone between the nebulizer and the subject enhances deposition,[45] but the effect is not very great.[53, 58] Gayrard and Orehek[57] reported that only 25% of 69 untrained asthmatics were using a nebulizer correctly, and it is essential that proper instruction be given. Using response to judge the effectiveness of delivery, it appears that a given dose is best given in divided dosages 20 minutes apart, with the aerosol delivered when the lung volume is about 75% of total lung capacity (TLC).[32]

Studies of deposition fractions of pressurized aerosols using 2 micron diameter Teflon particles showed that eight cases of chronic airflow obstruction, 80% of the particles were in the mouth; only 8.8% were in the lungs; 5.8% were in the airways; and about 3% were in the alveoli.[45] Other data indicate that between 70% and 90% of the inhaled dose is deposited in the nasopharynx.[25] Some experimental data indicate that in severe chronic airflow limitation with a very low FEV_1, aerosol delivery is improved if a reservoir of aerosol is used, rather than direct inhalation from a metered inhaler.[2943]

Ruffin and his colleagues[44] reported that a given dose of histamine had a greater effect if delivered into central airways than more peripherally. A comparison of different techniques

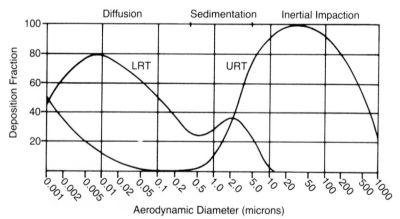

Figure 3–1. *Deposition Rate of Particles in the Human Lung*

This figure shows the fraction of inhaled particles, which will be deposited in either the upper respiratory tract (URT) or the lower respiratory tract (LRT) in human subjects. Notice that almost all particles between 10 and 100 microns in size will settle in the upper respiratory tract; many of these will be retained in the nose. It is also apparent that an increasing fraction of particles between 0.5 and 0.01 microns will be laid down deep in the lung in the lower respiratory tract. Particles smaller than 0.01 of a micron have a lower deposition rate in the lung. The aerodynamic diameter of the particle refers to its actual diameter which, in the presence of water vapor, may be rather larger than the physical size of the particle in dry air. (Figure courtesy of Prof. Paul Morrow, University of Rochester, N.Y.)

of aerosol generation and inhalation patterns conducted by the same laboratory showed that in 10 asthmatics the histamine response could be as reliably measured with a nebulizer and tidal breathing as with more complex dose-metering devices.[54]

There are important differences in aerosol deposition in the presence of lung disease. All those who have studied deposition in patients with chronic airflow obstruction have found it to occur more often in the central airways than in normal subjects. In a study of 50 patients with an FEV_1 averaging 38% of predicted, Pavia and associates[27] found that penetration was related to tidal volume and the FEV_1 and varied inversely with flow during inhalation. The relationship could be expressed by the following formula:

$$\text{Alveolar deposition}(\%) = 40.3(V_T) + 10.98(FEV_1) - [0.75(V_{flow}) + 40.4]$$

This relationship was simplified into a nomogram. Newhouse and Ruffin[33] compared distribution of ^{133}Xe gas and aerosols. In normal subjects, these were not discrepant, but major differences were found in patients with established chronic airflow obstruction in whom deposition of the aerosol was much more central. They concluded also that in symptomatic smokers with a normal FEV_1, aerosol deposition was reduced in small airways. Agnew, Pavia, and Clarke[50] concluded that aerosol deposition studies were not superior to other tests of small airway function. Bronchodilators have been shown to enhance the peripheral deposition of aerosols.[26]

In a small number of asthmatic subjects, aerosol penetration was shown to be very dependent on the speed with which a vital capacity was taken during inhalation.[33] Greening, Miniati, and Fazio[48] compared deposition of 1.2 micron diameter microspheres with ^{81m}Kr ventilation scanning, and in 20 cases of chronic airflow obstruction they found a strong correlation between FEV_1 and depth of aerosol penetration ($r = 0.91$). When the FEV_1 was less than 40% of predicted, the index of aerosol penetration was reduced by half. Zones of "hyperdeposition" were noted, some of which were central in location, but some of which were peripheral. Less penetration also occurred in those with a raised residual volume. More recently, the difference between regional ventilation measured with ^{81m}Kr and aerosol deposition measured with 5 micron polystyrene

particles tagged with ^{99m}Tc has been shown to widen in asthmatics as the maximal midexpiratory flow rate (FEF_{25-75}) falls.[2942] In these studies, aerosol penetration was generally reduced in non-smoking asthmatic patients but was normal in non-asthmatic smokers of the same age.[2942]

An increase in central deposition has also been noted in some cases of diffuse interstitial fibrosis.[56] Aerosol deposition was reduced in areas of bronchiectasis,[36] and deposition into consolidated pneumonic areas was only 10% of normal.[35] Experimental studies in Syrian hamsters have shown that aerosol deposition of 1.4- to 1.6-micron particles was reduced in the presence of papain-induced emphysema.[52] Aerosol deposition studies in 58 coal miners showed that deposition was significantly related to the $MEF_{50-75\%}VC$ ($r = 0.60$). However, it was not affected by the presence of simple coal workers' pneumoconiosis.[39] The data indicated that distortion or narrowing of peripheral airways in smokers might increase deposition.

Factors affecting the clearance of inhaled material are discussed later. Complex models have been studied to determine the balance between deposition and clearance. In one of these,[2944] it was calculated that in a continuous exposure to 4-micron particles, the equilibrium between retention and clearance would reach 95% of its final value after exposure for 293 days and that the whole lung burden after a year of exposure would amount to 9% of the total inspired mass.

MUCUS, MUCOCILIARY CLEARANCE, AND COUGHING

The mucociliary system is one of the lung's primary defense mechanisms. It protects the conducting airways by trapping and sweeping away bacteria, inhaled particles, and cellular debris. The system probably also serves as a reservoir of humidity for incoming air, and it may help to modify the airway response to inhaled agents. Useful reviews of pulmonary defense systems have been contributed[928-931] that deal with general clearance mechanisms.

The Mucociliary System

The airway epithelium consists of three strata. The surface stratum is composed largely of ciliated columnar cells, which are interspersed with non-ciliated, microvillus cells and goblet cells. The lower strata consist of intermediate and basal cells, from which the surface cells develop. As noted in Chapter 1, the cilia, whose structure is remarkably constant throughout the animal kingdom, beat in an asymmetric pattern, with a fast, forward stroke, during which the cilia are stiff and outstretched, and a slower return stroke, during which the cilia are flexed. The beating is coordinated in a metachronal pattern so that each cilium is slightly out of phase with its neighbor along the plane of motion. The direction of the forward stroke, and thus of fluid movement, is predominantly cephalad. Sanderson and Sleigh[890] have described in considerable detail the ciliary beat pattern and metachrony in rabbit tracheal epithelium.

In the human lung, the cilia are about 6 microns in length in the trachea, 4.7 microns in lobar bronchi, and 3.6 microns in segmental bronchi.[906] They comprise 53% of lining cells in the trachea, and this fraction diminishes to about 15% in fifth generation airways.[906] The beat frequency, 11 to 15 beats/sec, is essentially invariant between airway sites[369, 379] and varies little between individuals,[369, 379, 451, 905] except those with structurally abnormal cilia.[451]

As illustrated in Figure 3–2, the fluid lining the epithelium consists of two layers—the lower, a non-viscid serous fluid in which the cilia beat, and the upper, a visco-elastic material (the mucus), which lies on top of and is propelled by the cilia. This concept was first elaborated by Lucas and Douglas in 1934.[887] Mucus is secreted by both goblet cells and subepithelial glands. The source of serous fluid may also be in the glands, but this is not certain. Considerable evidence has been adduced to substantiate the essential validity of the two-layer model, although some of the fine details remain controversial. In morphologic studies in which care has been taken to preserve the epithelial lining, the existence of two distinct fluid layers has been seen—an electron-lucent material surrounding the cilia and an electron-dense material above it.[888, 889] The height of the serous layer is approximately that of the outstretched cilia, i.e., about 6 microns. Whether the tips of the cilia actually contact the mucus on their forward stroke is not absolutely certain, although evidence has been presented to support this view.[889, 890]

Mucus transport is theoretically possible whether the cilia contact the mucus or not; however, the exact nature of the relationship between the properties of mucus and mucociliary clearance would likely depend on the specific interactions that occur between the cilia and the mucus layer. Also, whether the mucus layer forms a more or less continuous blanket is open to question.[891] Evidence supporting a continuous mucus coating comes mainly from studies of trachea or large bronchi[2872]; other evidence supporting the notion that mucus moves in discontinuous islets and plaques comes from more distal bronchi.[933] It is possible that both views are correct and that the islands of mucus coalesce as they move in a cephalad direction.

Theoretical Model Studies

Two model studies, by Ross and Corrsin[892] and by Blake,[893] have identified several factors that control the rate of clearance (the mean linear velocity of the mucus layer). These may be grouped into ciliary, serous fluid, and mucus factors. The ciliary factors—beat frequency and amplitude—should both correlate positively with clearance rates. In fact, when the cilia are in firm contact with mucus during their forward stroke, mucus velocity should be directly proportional to the product of beat frequency and amplitude. The viscosity and depth of serous fluid should also be important to clearance. The mucus velocity should decrease with increasing serous fluid viscosity because of the negative influence of the latter on ciliary beat frequency (see later), and the velocity reaches an optimum when the serous fluid depth is approximately that of an outstretched cilium.[890, 893]

A mathematical analysis by Blake and Winet[529] further suggests that penetration of the cilia into the mucus layer during the forward stroke greatly enhances the net propulsion of the mucus. For a zone of penetration of 10% of the ciliary length (0.6 micron for human tracheal cilia), the mucus velocity would be a factor of two to 10 greater than when the mucus simply rides on top of the periciliary layer. Furthermore, this analysis predicted that there is little net flow in the serous sublayer; in other words, periciliary fluid is largely preserved.

The importance of the depth and physical properties of the mucus layer is less clear. The Ross and Corrsin study[892] predicts that the transport rate should decrease with increasing mucus depth, if constant serous fluid depth is assumed. Blake's model[893] suggests that mucus depth is unimportant to clearance by mucociliary transport but that movement by airflow and

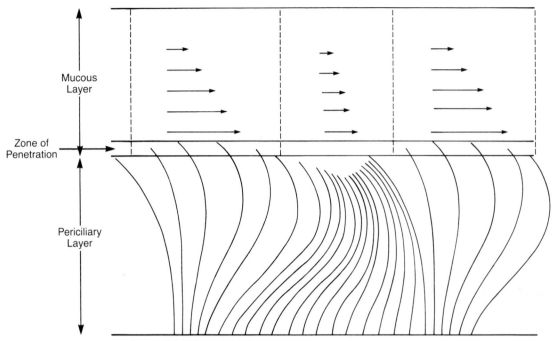

Figure 3–2. *Physical Model for Mucociliary Clearance*

The cilia beat in a non-viscid layer of serous fluid. The mucus lies on top of and is transported by the cilia, whose tips contact the mucus on their forward stroke. The arrows in the mucus layer represent potential flow profiles (exaggerated), which are due to mechanical energy dissipation between zones of ciliary contact.

gravity assumes increasing importance as mucus depth increases. Ross and Corrsin find that the visco-elastic properties of the mucus are unimportant *per se*, but predict that transport will decrease with an increasing viscosity/elasticity ratio (relaxation time). Blake concurs but suggests that even mucus relaxation times are not likely to be important at the usual ciliary beat frequency, mucus behaving essentially as an elastic solid. These factors are summarized in Table 3–1.

Table 3–1. EFFECT OF VARIOUS FACTORS ON MUCOCILIARY CLEARANCE IN TWO MODEL STUDIES

Factor	Effect on Clearance	
	Ross and Corrsin[592]	Blake[593]
Ciliary beat frequency and amplitude ↑	↑	↑
Serous fluid viscosity ↑	↓	↓
Serous fluid depth > or < ciliary length	—	↓
Mucus depth ↑	↓	→
Mucus visco-elasticity ↑ (rigidity)	→	→
Mucus relaxation time ↑ (viscosity/elasticity)	↓	→

Another experimental model has recently been described; it indicates that compression and expansion of a monomolecular film "permits a unidirectional transport of particles which are present on this film."[2953] This model is most appropriate for transport of alveolar surfactant but may have applicability to particle clearance, particularly in small airways in which mucus is absent or minimal.

Experimental Model Studies: Ciliary and Serous Fluid Factors

A large number of studies have examined factors that influence ciliary beat frequency (CBF). Isolated cilia preparations have been shown to respond to both cholinergic and adrenergic agents,[622, 894] with beta-adrenergic stimulation apparently exerting the strongest influence among the autonomic factors.[894, 895] A host of other factors have been shown to alter CBF, including chemical mediators of anaphylaxis,[896] temperature,[934] anesthetic agents,[894, 897] cigarette smoke,[898] and soluble components in sputum.[2951] If other parameters are unchanged, alterations in CBF should lead directly to alterations in mucociliary clearance rates (MCR). A few studies using intact preparations, with mucus present, have shown that changes in MCR correlated directly with changes in CBF.[898, 900] Whether a one to one correspondence between MCR and CBF occurs, as theory would predict,[892, 893] is not clear; in fact, this would be difficult to establish because most interventions that alter CBF in isolation also have the potential to alter the periciliary fluid and/or the mucous lining layer and, hence, to affect the MCR. Recent experiments indicate that sputum from asthma patients inhibits ciliary beating, the effect being greatest when the subject providing the sputum has more severe airflow limitation.[2951, 2956]

Alterations in depth and viscosity of periciliary fluid have not been examined directly. In isolation, increasing the viscosity of the medium bathing the cilia leads to a decrease in CBF.[901] Alterations in periciliary fluid depth would presumably alter the efficiency of mucus-cilia interaction, which appears to depend on actual contact between the mucus and the tips of the cilia.[890] The mechanism regulating periciliary fluid depth is unknown, but active ion transport across the epithelium[902] appears to be the most likely.

The interactive influence of mucus on cilia beating *in vivo* remains largely unexplored. Evidence from studies on excised frog palates suggests that CBF is not (very) dependent on the physical nature of the mucus overlying the cilia in that CBF, except for an initial effect, is the same whether mucus is present or not.[832, 903] If CBF were indeed independent of mucus rheology, the large variations in MCR with mucus rheology would be better explained by assuming that the amplitude of ciliary beating is dependent on other physical properties of the mucus. The amplitude in this case would be an effective amplitude, i.e., the arc length of the forward stroke during which cilia are in effective contact with the mucus. This factor is amenable to experimental analysis. Since both the linear velocity and frequency are measurable quantities, the effective amplitude can be computed from their ratio, assuming that the cilia actually penetrate the mucus during their forward stroke. In view of the large variability found in MCR, one should expect to find a wide variation in ciliary beat amplitudes.

Alterations in Ciliary Activity Induced by Disease

In isolation, the ciliary beat frequency, except in patients with ciliary dyskinesia, does not

seem to be altered in disease.[379, 451, 904, 905] However, the numbers of cilia and their distribution, as well as their length,[906] are altered, which also affects amplitude. In addition, there may be significant alterations in mucus-cilia interaction in disease, with increased loading and altered visco-elasticity adversely affecting ciliary function.

Experimental Model Studies: Mucus Factors

Both the depth of mucus and its physical properties could, in theory, affect clearance rate. There is little experimental evidence available on the influence of mucus depth on clearance, and theoretical model studies do not agree on its importance (Table 3–1). In frog palate epithelium, the depth of mucus or the particulate load has very little influence on transport, a phenomenon first demonstrated by Stewart in 1948[907] and confirmed by later studies.[908] It is not clear whether the respiratory tract epithelium has the same insensitivity to mucus depth, although in healthy dogs, mucus linear velocity and depth seem to be independent of each other.[909] The insensitivity to depth and load suggest the cilia have considerable reserve capacity for maintaining their frequency and amplitude.

Most of the information on the relationship between mucus rheology and clearance by cilia comes from studies using the frog palate model, principally because of its convenience. The frog palate epithelium is morphologically and functionally similar to that of mammalian respiratory mucosa. If solid particles (steel balls, carbon particles, etc.) are placed on a freshly excised palate, they are transported at rates similar to those observed in mammalian tracheas (about 20 mm/min at 30° C). Solid particle transport gradually decreases and then stops altogether as the epithelium becomes depleted of mucus, which occurs within a few hours of excision. That this is due to the lack of mucus and not to ciliary inactivity is evidenced by the fact that a drop of mucus taken from the cut edge of the palate and placed back on the surface will be transported and will clear particles at a velocity comparable to that initially observed.[908]

The mucus-depleted palate can be employed in two ways: (1) cilio-active agents can be added to the palate and their effect on clearance monitored by observing the change in the transport rate of control mucus,[834] or (2) variations in the rate at which samples of mucus from different sources are transported can be observed, assuming a constant beat frequency. The latter experiment is generally termed the "frog palate assay of mucociliary transportability."[910] The transport rate of exogenous mucus, expressed as a percentage of the frog palatal control rate, depends on differences in mucus rheology, provided that the passage of the test sample does not alter frog CBF. When dealing with sputum, or with mucus that may contain significant concentrations of cilio-active agents, this proviso may be important and may affect the interpretation of results.[911]

Optimal Rheologic Properties for Clearance

The optimal rheologic properties of mucus that lead to maximal clearance have been studied by a number of investigators. Figure 3–2 shows this relationship for gels prepared from guaran, a gel-forming polysaccharide. The optimum has been shown in terms of elasticity[912, 913] and elasticity and viscosity together,[914, 915] as well as solely in terms of gel concentration.[910] In the simplest terms, failure to attain the optimal rate may be due to mucus being either too watery or too rigid to be transported at the fastest rate on the frog palate. The optimum is located at the low end of the range of viscosity and elasticity values observed in whole mucus samples. With one important exception[914] (see later), the rheologic optimum has only been demonstrated in reconstituted gel systems, where gels of sufficient dilution can be prepared. Studies that have correlated the mucociliary clearance rate with mucus rheology in non-pathologic conditions[916, 917] have shown only a continuous decrease in clearance rate with increasing mucus elasticity; in other words, it appears that whole, non-infected mucus is well above the optimum in rheologic terms. Fortunately perhaps, the sensitivity of mucociliary transport to mucus rheology in the normal range is very low—a tenfold increase in mucus elasticity producing no more than a twofold decrease in clearance rate.[917]

With pathologic mucus (sputum), the optimal characteristics for transport are likely to be much more relevant than they are in the normal state. Figure 3–3 from the work of Puchelle and her colleagues[914] is a three-dimensional plot relating frog palate transport to viscosity and recoverable strain ([S_R], a measure of elasticity) for sputum samples from patients with chronic bronchitis. It shows that optimal transport oc-

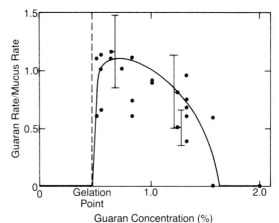

Figure 3–3. Ratio of ciliary transport rates of guaran gel and frog palate mucus versus guaran concentration in gel. Each point is derived from 5 to 10 readings each of guaran and mucus velocities on a single mucus-depleted palate. Representative standard deviations for 3 points shown. (Reprinted with permission from King, M., Gilboa, A., Meyer, F. A., and Silberberg, A. On the transport of mucus and its rheologic simulants in ciliated systems. Am. Rev. Respir. Dis. 110: 740–745, 1974.)

curs with samples with intermediate viscosity and S_R; sputum samples that lie outside the optimal range of visco-elastic properties are transported at slower rates. Although the majority of sputum samples exhibiting suboptimal frog palate transport rates do so because of their elevated viscosity or elasticity or both, it is clear that sputa can be found that are too low in viscosity and/or elasticity to be transported with maximal efficiency by ciliary action. The implication in these instances is that mucociliary clearance would be improved by an increase in viscosity, elasticity, or both. This aspect is discussed in more detail later.

Visco-elastic Properties and Clearance

As noted earlier, Ross and Corrsin[892] included mucus visco-elasticity in their model analysis of mucociliary clearance. They predicted that moderate changes in mucus viscosity would not affect the transport rate but that alterations in mucus relaxation time (the ratio of viscosity to elasticity in their simple visco-elastic model) were important in determining the clearance rate. The effect is such that an increase in viscosity at constant elasticity should result in a decrease in transport rate; a proportional increase in viscosity and elasticity should not result in any change in transport. This prediction is not readily tested because of the difficulty in inducing independent changes in viscosity and elasticity in whole mucus. A model study employing polysaccharide gels as mucus stimulants has shown the essential validity of the approach.[918] As illustrated in Figure 3–2, when elasticity and viscosity increase proportionately, the decrease in transport rate, although significant, is relatively minor. By contrast, when the ratio of viscosity to elasticity increases, the consequence is a much more rapid decrease in clearance rate.

The work with polysaccharide gels confirms similar conclusions based on the analysis of the frog palate transportability of whole canine tracheal mucus,[917] although in whole canine tracheal mucus the natural variations in the viscosity/elasticity ratio are greatly outweighed by the overall variations in viscosity or elasticity. Nevertheless, the two variables (viscosity/elasticity and elasticity alone) are of nearly equal importance over their naturally occurring ranges. Other studies of rheology and transport rate have not specifically examined this viscoelasticity factor, although in the studies by Puchelle and associates,[914, 924] for sputum samples in which the elastic properties were within the optimal range, submaximal transport was seen only for those samples in which the viscosity was elevated. Furthermore, as described later, reducing the viscosity of such material while maintaining constant elasticity results in an improvement in clearance rate.

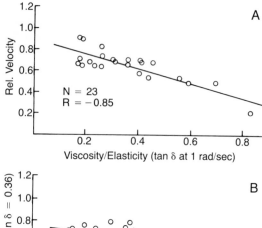

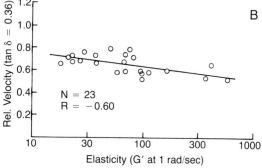

Figure 3–4. A, Ciliary transport rate of guaran gel (relative to frog palate mucus) versus viscosity/elasticity ratio of gel, expressed as tan δ and determined at 1 rad/sec. B, Relative ciliary transport rate of guaran gel, corrected for viscosity/elasticity correlation, versus logarithm of gel elasticity. (Reprinted with permission from Biorheology, vol. 17, King, M. Relationship between mucus viscoelasticity and ciliary transport in guaran gel/frog palate model system, Copyright 1980, Pergamon Journals, Ltd.)

A Physical Model for Mucociliary Clearance

The importance of both viscosity and elasticity to ciliary mucus clearance can be appreciated if one considers the energetics of mucociliary clearance. As they beat, the cilia contact the mucus layer during their rapid forward stroke, but not during the slower return stroke (Fig. 3–4). On the forward stroke, the mucus in immediate contact with the cilia moves at the rate of forward motion of the outstretched cilium. This linear motion is transmitted to other parts of the mucous gel (both vertically and horizontally). If the gel were perfectly elastic, the transmission would be instantaneous and without energy loss. Because mucus is viscoelastic, however, the transfer of momentum is retarded, and some of the ciliary energy is dissipated as heat. The visco-elastic parameter that governs this process is the mechanical loss factor, tan δ, the ratio of energy dissipated to energy stored per cycle (tan δ/frequency =

viscosity/elasticity). The higher the value of tan δ, the more energy dissipated and the less energy transformed into forward motion. Although energy dissipation might seem wasteful from a mechanical point of view, it is clearly necessary to some extent since a perfectly elastic mucus could not be permanently deformed and could never be expectorated or swallowed.

Although the nature of mucociliary clearance over the normal physiologic range is explained by the Ross and Corrsin model, the behavior at the extremes of gel concentration is not as readily explainable. The model study illustrated in Figure 3–5 suggests that the transportability optimum occurs very near the threshold for gelation. Although it has not been demonstrated, the most likely explanation for the failure of transport at low gel density is that interpenetration of macromolecular material between the cilia occurs, inhibiting their beating. At the other extreme, the gradual decrease in transport rate and its ultimate failure at high cross-link density, also unaccounted for by the simple model, could be due to the failure of

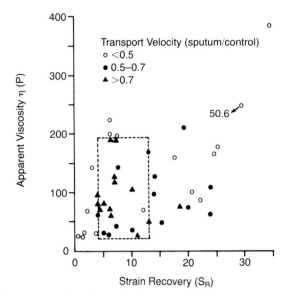

Figure 3–5. Relationships between mucociliary transport velocity and rheologic properties of sputum. The range of optimal viscosity and strain recovery (elasticity) is indicated (*dotted lines*). (Reprinted with permission from Bull. Eur. Physiopathol. Respir., vol. 12, Puchelle, E., et al., Rheologie des secretions bronchignes et transport muco-ciliaire, Copyright 1976, Pergamon Press plc.)

the tips of the cilia to penetrate the gel during the forward stroke.

Pharmacologic Alterations of Mucus Visco-elasticity

Although drugs are commonly given to patients with the aim of altering respiratory tract secretions, evidence on the *in vivo* pharmacologic control of mucus visco-elasticity has often been unconvincing or contradictory.[919] There are probably two reasons for this; the high variability in sputum visco-elasticity makes it difficult to draw conclusions from clinical trials, and the study of mucus rheology in animals requires the use of micro-methods, which have not been widely applied.

Mucus secretion in the lung is clearly under cholinergic control,[920] and cholinergic stimulation alters mucus visco-elasticity acutely. In dogs, the response to methacholine administration is biphasic.[921] With low doses, there is a fall in tracheal mucus viscosity and elasticity persisting for up to half an hour; with high doses, the viscosity and elasticity first increase, and then decrease before returning to control values. With both high and low doses of methacholine, tan δ increases. This accounts for the significant fall in ciliary transportability of the

mucus that is collected. Elevated levels of mucus flux are seen with all doses of methacholine. Furthermore, in awake dogs, resting vagal tone is likely to be responsible for some of the variability in baseline visco-elasticity. The conclusion is based on the observation that atropine increases mucus viscosity and elasticity when the control levels are low (consistent with moderate basal vagal tone) but does not alter visco-elasticity when the control levels are high.[922]

Tracheobronchial mucus secretion is also likely to be under adrenergic control. Studies in the ferret have shown that beta-adrenergic agents selectively stimulate secretion from mucous cells in the submucosal glands, whereas alpha-adrenergic agents stimulate secretion from serous cells.[923] Administration of methacholine stimulates both types of submucosal gland secretion. This suggests that beta-adrenergic stimulation leads to a thicker mucus secretion than that produced by cholinergic stimulation and alpha-adrenergic stimulation produces a more watery mucus. This has, in fact, been recently demonstrated by Leikauf, Ueki, and Nadel[932] using a cat tracheal gland preparation. Steroids may affect mucus by reducing protein transudation.[2957] Many studies have shown that proteins contained within the mucus, whether of local origin or due to transudation, contribute to the visco-elastic properties.[2499, 4973]

By comparison with *in vivo* effects on mucus visco-elasticity, the *in vitro* alteration of mucus is less problematic. Many studies have examined the efficacy of mucolytic agents in reducing the viscosity of sputum. Puchelle and her colleagues[924] have demonstrated the potential use of three types of mucolytic agent in their *in vivo* studies: (1) a mucolytic agent that reduces both viscosity and elasticity; (2) a mucospissic agent that increases both, which would be of value if sputum were too thin; and (3) a novel mucotropic agent, letosteine, which reduces viscosity but leaves elasticity essentially unaltered. This last agent would be of value for sputum with elevated viscosity but normal elasticity. It is clear that selective alteration of mucus visco-elasticity is possible, but in terms of effective therapy, the difficult problems of toxicity and delivery of the agent remain to be solved.

Alterations in Mucus Visco-elasticity Induced by Disease

The visco-elastic properties of mucus may be altered in disease, but this is much less certain than is the case with other factors that contribute to clearance, such as ciliary activity and the quantity of mucus. The main reason for this uncertainty is the lack of information on the normal state. Reid and her colleagues[925, 926] have surveyed many samples of sputum from patients with different hypersecretory diseases. They observed, as have others,[935, 2960] a great variability in the non-Newtonian viscosity of sputum samples, and their work shows that the most important parameter is the degree of purulence of the sample. Purulent samples in general tend to have a higher viscosity than non-purulent samples. Using chronic bronchitis cases as a quasi-control, Charman and Reid[925] suggest that only in asthma, and not in cystic fibrosis or bronchiectasis, does the viscosity of sputum appear to be consistently elevated. Dulfano and Adler[927] examined visco-elasticity and frog palate clearance rates in sputum from patients with chronic bronchitis. They reported that purulent sputum was generally of higher viscosity and elasticity than non-purulent sputum and that, consistent with this, the mucociliary transport rate of purulent sputum was slower.

In cystic fibrosis, we have found a minimal difference between sputum from clinically stable patients and tracheal mucus from healthy dogs, at least on average.[911] The range of visco-elastic properties was greater than that seen in dogs, however, and purulent samples tended to be of higher viscosity and elasticity than non-purulent samples. It was also found that ciliary transportability of cystic fibrosis sputum was slower than that of canine tracheal mucus for samples of equivalent visco-elasticity; this could indicate the presence of diffusible inhibitory factors, but this has not been confirmed.

The work of Puchelle and colleagues[914, 924] on sputum from chronic bronchitis patients makes it clear that the range of visco-elastic properties is so great that the sputum state of the individual patient must be considered. While most patients have "normal" or thickened mucus in terms of mucociliary transportability, there are individuals in whom the mucus is abnormally thin. Puchelle's experiments, which are illustrated in Figure 3–5, suggest that at least three different types of therapeutic approach would be necessary to improve mucociliary transportability, depending on the initial state. Unfortunately, neither the drugs nor the delivery system to effect these kinds of visco-elastic modification has yet been developed. There is no close association between pulmonary function status and measured sputum viscosity.[937–939]

Studies of Mucociliary Clearance Rate

Wanner[5250] and Pavia and associates[5251] have contributed useful reviews of this topic. Studies of radio-aerosol clearance show that in normal subjects 90% of radiolabeled particles are cleared from ciliated airways in the 6 hours following deposition and the remaining 10% are cleared between 6 and 24 hours.[952]

Mucociliary clearance rates decrease with increasing airway generation. In excised dog lungs, the rates for mucociliary clearance were 12.6 mm/min in the trachea, 8.3 mm/min in lobar bronchi, 4.0 mm/min in segmental bronchi, and 1.6 mm/min in more distal bronchi.[942] *In vivo* studies in dogs[943] and in humans[944] have noted similar regional differences.

Comparisons between nasal and tracheobronchial MCRs have yielded conflicting results. In one study there was a positive association between nasal and tracheobronchial particle clearance.[5252] Another study reported an inverse relationship,[940] and a third showed no correlation.[941] The reasons for these discrepancies are not apparent. The ciliary beat frequency appears to be comparable between nasal and pulmonary airways.[945]

The MCR decreases with age in normal adults.[645, 5253] Vastag and co-workers[5254] described an age prediction of MCR based on data from 80 normal subjects; whole lung MCR at age 60 was two-thirds of its value at age 20. In beagle dogs, it was found that tracheal clearance first increased with maturation, and then decreased thereafter.[5255] The MCR is reduced in normal subjects during sleep.[958]

Anesthesia generally decreases MCR,[5256, 5257] as does endotracheal intubation and oxygen.[950] Beta-adrenergic agonists are recognized to be potent stimulants of mucociliary clearance,[944, 947, 956, 5259] whereas the effects of cholinergic drugs are variable.[5259, 5260] There is some evidence that theophylline administration may enhance MCR,[943, 2947] although probably only in large airways. Drinking hot fluids caused a transient increase in tracheal mucus velocity, which was probably due to nasal inhalation of water vapor.[951] Hot chicken soup was slightly superior to hot water—a scientific validation of generations of maternal intuition.

A variety of airborne pollutants have deleterious effects on mucociliary clearance. These include sulfur dioxide, sulfuric acid mist, ozone, and nitrogen dioxide. Wolff[5261] has recently reviewed the literature in this field and has compiled 149 references up to 1986.

Effects of Smoking on Mucociliary Clearance

There is general agreement that tracheal or large airway clearance is impaired in smokers. In one study, the tracheal mucus velocity of non-smokers averaged 10.1 mm/min, while in age-matched smokers the rate was 3.4 mm/min.[645] Others have also found slower rates in smokers,[697] which is consistent with animal studies of slower mucociliary clearance after exposure to cigarette smoke.[946, 1109] In some smokers with chronic bronchitis, movement was noted to be almost absent in some zones of the trachea, presumably due to loss of organized ciliary function.[947]

Studies involving whole lung clearance, and particularly clearance from the lung periphery, have yielded conflicting results regarding the effect of smoking. Foster and co-workers[5262] found peripheral lung clearance to be impaired in young smokers (<5 pack-years of smoking) when compared with age-matched non-smoking controls. Central clearance rates in the two groups were similar. These findings fit with the conventional concept that small airway dysfunction preceded central airway involvement. Another recent study of 30 asymptomatic smokers, all with normal values of VC, RV, and FEV_1, found significant peripheral mucociliary clearance delay in those with abnormal closing measurements.[2952]

Vastag and his colleagues[5254] studied three groups of smokers with increasing degrees of clinical dysfunction. Group 1 consisted of smokers with no signs of large airway obstruction or chronic bronchitis; group 2 was made up of smokers with simple bronchitis but no central obstruction; and members of group 3 had both bronchitis and central airway obstruction.

Group 1 was similar in smoking history and age to the subjects in the study of Foster and co-workers.[5262] All three groups showed both central and peripheral clearance rates significantly lower than the predicted values established in normal non-smoking subjects. The functional impairment of clearance correlated positively with smoking history.

In contrast, Isawa and co-workers[1281] found that both whole lung and regional lung clearance was faster in smoking than in non-smoking subjects. For whole lung clearance, their finding was explicable by the fact that the non-smokers had deposited significantly more of their whole lung burden in the alveoli, based on a 24-hour count. Slower whole lung clearance in non-smokers is expected if slower moving particles from the periphery contribute proportionately more to the clearance curve. However, the faster clearance rates in the periphery of the lung are more difficult to understand when one considers that even young smokers show signs of small airway disease. Agnew and colleagues[5263] reported something similar in symptomless smokers—specifically an enhancement of peripheral mucus flux with no change in linear velocity—leading one to conclude that smokers may have a reserve potential that protects them from the effects of their smoking.

Other reports include a comparison of smoking and non-smoking twins, which showed no differences in mucociliary clearance rates[948] and one case of a normal rate of mucociliary clearance in a 100-year-old smoker.[949] Camner and his colleagues[641] reported that cessation of smoking resulted in improvement of mucociliary clearance after 3 months.

Mucociliary Clearance in Disease

The MCR is reduced following viral infections[953] and remains depressed for a week or so, returning to normal after 3 months. This depression may be due to acquired ciliary defects.[1341]

Cases of chronic bronchitis and emphysema generally have a reduced rate of clearance.[947, 954, 961, 5254] In one study of patients with chronic bronchitis, the rate was faster in those who produced more sputum and was unrelated to the FEV_1.[2954] Matthys and his colleagues[1417] have found a relationship between slowed mucociliary clearance and bronchial carcinoma.

Thirteen children with cystic fibrosis were found to have a normal clearance rate,[955] but it was significantly slowed in 14 adults with the same disease.[956] Tracheal MCRs in cases of cystic fibrosis have been found to range all the way from no detectable abnormality to a complete absence of transport.[5258] There was no good correlation with a clinical "score" of the severity of the disease.

Mucociliary clearance is impaired in asthma.[959, 5264] A particularly interesting finding by Mezey and co-workers[959] was that mucocili ary clearance was reduced to 72% of its baseline value in asthmatics after challenge testing, a finding consistent with the evidence noted earlier that various inflammatory mediators may adversely influence mucociliary clearance. The effect in asthma is apparently not related to either histamine release or cholinergic stimulation, since each of these enhance MCR.[5265] In allergic sheep, clearance rates were depressed from baseline values for more than a week following a single antigen challenge.[1462]

Effects of Coughing and Physiotherapy

Richardson and Peatfield[931] have contributed a useful review of coughing as part of lung defense mechanisms and have compiled 199 references up to 1981. Sutton and associates[2874] have recently reviewed the literature on chest physiotherapy.

As we have noted,[960] there is an important relationship between the characteristics of sputum and its behavior during coughing. During a cough, the mucus is exposed to higher shear stress because of interaction with airflow; the effective velocity (flow resistance) is low, and it flows easily forward. In quiet breathing after coughing, the shear stress is much lower, and the mucus viscosity is high again; therefore, it will not easily flow back into the lung. There may be a divergence between the rheologic properties of mucus that favor clearance by cough and those that favor mucociliary clearance. In our own in vitro studies, we have found that for transport by frog palate cilia, an elastic mucus is favored[918]; however, for transport by airflow interaction, a viscous rather than an elastic mucus led to more efficient clearance.[1280] A number of studies have shown the importance of coughing to clearance in chronic bronchitis.[961–963, 965]

A study of clearance by external counting of Teflon discs before and after 2 minutes of voluntary coughing showed that in six normal subjects the discs were not eliminated, but in six of eight patients with chronic bronchitis, they were all eliminated.[965] The authors noted that increased tracheobronchial secretions might be necessary to make the act of coughing effective. This observation has been made by others.[954, 963, 964] In vitro evidence[1280] suggests the same phenomenon.

The cough threshold is reduced in sleep and in older subjects, as noted in Chapter 4. It is

also reduced by ethanol blood levels between 80 and 100 mg/100 mL in normal subjects.[966] After a thoracotomy, the cough pressure was found to be reduced to 50% of its preoperative value for a week postoperatively, with a slow return to normal over the next 3 weeks. Pain was considered to be an important inhibitor.[967] It has been shown that a cough is followed by an effort-dependent forward flow phase in the arterial (systemic) circulation.[2958]

Various physiotherapeutic maneuvers have been shown to be of value in accelerating sputum removal. The forced expiration technique was valuable in cases of cystic fibrosis[968] and shown to be better than standard physiotherapy in a carefully controlled study.[5266] Others have reported that in cystic fibrosis, vigorous self-directed coughing is as effective as assisted methods in enhancing mucus clearance.[2955, 5267] An automatic vibration percussor has been designed,[969] and this and other methods have been shown to be effective in a variety of lung conditions.[970]

It has been shown that high-frequency chest wall compression (HFCWC) in dogs may lead to a threefold increase in clearance of mucus from the trachea.[2959] HFCWC was also shown to enhance clearance of mucus from the lung periphery,[2004] a region particularly difficult to deal with in patients with mucus hypersecretion. The role of the respiratory muscles in relation to coughing is discussed in Chapter 22.

PHYSICAL SIGNS AND FUNCTION

The remarkable story of Laennec's life[2, 2939] is generally well appreciated by chest physicians, but perhaps fewer realize that the stethoscope was the first introduction of any form of technology into the technique of medical diagnosis. Bishop[3] has pointed out that its introduction was generally received with enthusiasm by physicians, apart from a few traditionalists who derided its use. In a review of the history of progress of our understanding of breath sounds and added sounds and the origin, Murphy[4] notes that progress in theoretical knowledge has been slow; however, progress has undoubtedly been made in the last 20 years. Forgacs[12] has summarized his own interesting work and the literature on sound analysis in a recent editorial.

Normal Respiration

There is some doubt as to the origin of normal breath sounds. They do not appear to originate in the larynx or upper airway,[6] and some experiments indicate that the origin of inspiratory sounds may be located between airways about 3 millimeters in diameter and alveoli. There may be an expiratory component from larger airways.[7] Careful amplification and recording from normal subjects reveal that there is wide intra- and intersubject variation in breath sound intensity and little bilateral symmetry.[2938] White sound transmitted from the mouth to a recorder on the chest wall also shows wide variations in transmitted intensity in normal subjects, for reasons that are not clear.[2930] There is also commonly a significant difference in sound intensity, as that between the two bases of the lungs, and differences on either side of the sternum suggest that normal breath sounds do not originate in the trachea.[2936] Recent observations suggest that at frequencies below 200 hertz, musculoskeletal noise "seriously contaminates what is usually considered to be lung sound."[2931] The loudness of breath sounds correlates well with ventilation distribution in different body positions measured by ^{133}Xe.[8,9]

Auscultation in Lung Disease

An analysis of 663 cases reports in 1979 revealed the diversity of terminology still in common use to describe breath sound intensity and added sounds in disease.[10] The recent use of the term "Velcro" rales to describe the coarse rales usually heard at the end of inspiration in patients with alveolitis indicates that the terminology will continue to evolve. Because these rales occur at the same intrapleural pressure in consecutive inspirations, they are attributed to airway opening.[11]

In established chronic bronchitis and emphysema, 10 to 12% of patients are found to have crackles over the lungs[13]; these crackles usually occur early in inspiration and are usually also attributed to airway opening. Peaks of high frequency sound are especially found in chronic bronchitis.[14] No studies appear to have been conducted to establish whether smokers with a normal FEV_1 but with an elevated closing volume, presumably with respiratory bronchiolitis (see Chapter 6), have any audible abnormalities as compared with smokers with a normal closing volume.

Moran Campbell and colleagues[2932-2934] analyzed physical signs in cases of chronic bronchitis and emphysema 15 years ago; with Stubbing and others, Campbell has updated these observations in 48 cases of chronic obstructive lung disease examined by two observers.[2935] The physical signs evaluated were tracheal descent, sternomastoid contraction, scalene contraction, supraclavicular fossa excavation, supraclavicular fossa recession, intercostal recession, costal margin movement, upper rib cage movement, cardiac position, and tracheal length. Spirometry and lung volumes were measured in all cases. There was good agreement between the two observers. All the signs were related to the severity of airflow obstruction, but some were "due to large variations in intrathoracic pressure, some to hyperinflation, and some, possibly, to changes in the shape of the chest and the action of the respiratory muscles."

A number of studies have involved analyses of breath sound intensity in cases of chronic bronchitis and emphysema. The intensity of breath sounds heard over the lungs diminishes as airflow obstruction increases.[17] In one study using four examiners, there was a significant correlation between noted breath sound intensity and the FEV_1.[18] Using four signs—intensity of breath sounds in brisk inspiration, expiratory wheeze, moist crackling sounds in expiratory coughing, and palpable tensing of the scalene muscles during tidal ventilation—Pardee and his colleagues[20] found a close relationship to the FEV_1 if a weighting system of the signs was used.

Forgacs, Nathoo, and Richardson[19] reported a significant correlation between the FEV_1 and the intensity of breath sounds heard at the mouth in cases of chronic bronchitis; the louder the sound, the lower the FEV_1. The same relationship held in asthma but was not present in patients believed to have significant emphysema. In severely obstructed patients, breath sound intensity varies markedly over different regions of the lung. In general, conformity with results from radioactive gas studies[21] and from regional ventilation distribution seems to vary widely from breath to breath, perhaps being critically dependent on tidal volume. In recent studies of eight cases of emphysema,[2926] the recorded breath sound intensity was found to be closely related to ventilation distribution measured with ^{133}Xe. The low sound intensity in emphysema distinguishes it from asthma,[22] but in severe asthma the intensity of breath sounds may fall with the onset of respiratory failure and fatigue. Musical sounds are believed to be produced by bronchiolar wall oscillation.[16]

In 52 non-smoking normal subjects, 26 were found to have crackles when inspiration began from residual volume but not when it was started from functional residual capacity (FRC).[2937] However, if oxygen is breathed, they may be recorded when an inspiration begins from FRC.[2928] In cases of diffuse interstitial lung disease, there is often a musical sound in inspiration, and it is reported that in cases of extrinsic allergic alveolitis, this noise occurs later in inspiration, is of shorter duration, and is of higher frequency.[2929]

Ploysongsang[2980] has recently found evidence of differences in lung sounds between smokers and non-smokers. He studied 19 non-smokers and 15 normal smokers aged between 21 and 55 years. FEV/FVC, dynamic compliance (C_{dyn}), and FEF_{25-75} were significantly lower in the smokers but single-breath nitrogen (SBN_2/L) and CV/VC% were not different. The breath sounds were recorded during tidal breathing, and the phase angle (theta), compared between the same horizontal levels of the right lung at the start of the breath sounds, was no greater than 5 degrees in the normal subjects but was greater than 5 degrees in 11 of the 15 smokers. The phase angle correlated significantly with C_{dyn}. This is the first evidence that the respiratory bronchiolitis of smokers has an associated physical sign, but sound recording is required to elicit it.

Phonocardiographic added sound recording has been used in an epidemiologic study. 270 workers exposed to asbestos were compared with 222 controls. Thirty-two per cent of the asbestos-exposed group had fine crackles at the bases, compared with 4.5% in the control group.[15] Accurate recording of respiratory rate is important but is often not easy at the bedside. One study suggested that in patients over the age of 67, a respiratory rate of more than 26/min usually indicated the presence of a pulmonary infection,[5] but many other conditions may cause an elevated rate.

A recent advance of some importance in the physical examination of the patient with lung disease is the recognition that there are specific signs of respiratory and diaphragmatic muscle fatigue. These are discussed in detail in Chapter 22.

It is fair to conclude that there is still merit in teaching the careful inspection of the chest and the discriminating use of the stethoscope. The interpretation of abnormal findings has been sharpened by comparisons between studies of regional ventilation and recorded sound intensity and by sound recordings of added sounds. Indeed, Laennec might conclude that at last something is being added to his initial, but remarkably precise and comprehensive, observations.

ALTERED PHYSIOLOGIC STATES AND ASSOCIATED SYNDROMES

Another image of science, widely held within as well as outside the scientific community, but which I regard as an illusion, is the common taxonomy which differentiates the hard from the soft sciences, and the sciences from the humanities in a descending order of truth or validity. A far more important distinction is between the "more secure" and the "less secure" sections of the whole sphere of human knowledge.

K. E. BOULDING[4875]

AGING AND PULMONARY FUNCTION

In reviewing the data related to aging, the reader should be aware of the inherent difficulty in distinguishing between long-term environmental effects on the lung—such as those leading to slight degrees of emphysema—and effects directly attributable to aging. In spite of this difficulty, the topic is without doubt of major importance, since problems in managing elderly patients cannot be understood without background appreciation of the difference between the lung of a 20-year-old and that of an 80-year-old patient.

Changes in Chemistry and Morphology

If the collagen content of human lung is expressed as micrograms per milliliter of in-flated lung tissue, it is found to fall with increasing age,[95] in accordance with earlier observations.[1] More recent work has also confirmed previous data indicating that the elastin content—expressed as milligrams per gram of dry tissue—increases with age,[95] with a correlation coefficient of $+0.59$. However, this may indicate an increase in the elastic tissue of bronchi, blood vessels, and septae, and the elastin content of the parenchyma may be unchanged with age.[77] The lung content of mucopolysaccharides decreases with age,[2967] but the significance of this finding is unclear.

The morphologic changes in the human lung attributable to age are reasonably well defined:

1. The central core of the alveolar duct increases in size.[77] This change has also been noted to occur in dogs kept in environmentally clean surroundings.[104]

2. This leads to an increase in the average interalveolar wall distance (expressed as the mean chord, L_m) with increasing age.[77] The relationship is not a very tight one, but L_m appears to increase from a mean value of about 0.25 millimeter at age 20 to 0.30 at age 80. Expressed in a different way, the loss of alveolar surface represents about 2.7 square meters per decade of life.[1] Thurlbeck[77] has observed that the volume proportion of alveolar parenchyma falls with increasing age, with a correlation coefficient of 0.58.

3. In an autopsy study of 18 normal lungs from subjects aged 17 to 86, Pump[72] found that the area of the fenestrae of the lungs increased with increasing age and postulated that the pores of Kohn enlarged to become the expanding fenestrae. Recent studies have confirmed this finding.[2961]

4. Studies of isolated alveolar wall tissue have shown that the extension ratio of the tissue, which is the maximum length of the strip under stress divided by the resting length, falls with age ($r = -0.74$) from a value of 2.04 at age 20 to 1.74 at age 70. This occurs because the resting value increases, with a possible fall in extensibility.[78] Other workers have confirmed such a fall in distensibility in human lungs with age[71] but did not find any comparable changes in horses, rabbits, or rats.

5. At an inflation pressure of 25 cm H_2O, the volume of air contained in lungs studied at autopsy does not seem to be correlated with the age of the specimen, if a correction is applied for body length.[60]

6. Recent radiologic studies have documented the changes in the shape of the thorax and lungs that occur with age[2963]; these appear to be caused by an increase in the volume of the upper zones, with concomitant reduction in lower zone volume. These data were obtained from lifelong non-smokers.

Changes in Pulmonary Function

Resting Ventilation

The resting tidal volume is maximal at the age of 22 and is related linearly to body height. With aging, it slowly declines, and respiratory frequency increases.[5] The ratio of V_T to T_I (inspiratory time) remains constant with increasing age.[88]

Pulmonary Mechanics

As shown in Figure 4–1, aging is accompanied by a progressive reduction in maximal elastic recoil pressure, with displacement of the curve upward and to the left. Residual volume increases, as noted later.

In a study of 124 healthy lifetime non-smokers, aged from 17 to 82 years, 83 of whom were male, Colebatch, Greaves, and Ng[59] expressed the changes with age as a single exponential function:

$$V = (A - B) \exp(-kP)$$

where V is lung volume; P is recoil pressure; and A, B, and k are constants. k, called the index of compliance, is an index of curvature and was found to be independent of sex but to increase with age. The ratio B/A and recoil pressures at various lung volumes were higher in males than females, and in both sexes decreases with age were similar. Colebatch and his colleagues concluded that the loss of elasticity with age was consistent with an increase in the unstressed dimensions of alveoli and might be explained by loss of elastic fibers. All workers have not found these changes to be of the same order of magnitude,[80] but the differences may be accounted for by different selection criteria for the populations studied.

Knudson and Kaltenborn[2987] studied 110 normal non-smokers between the ages of 25 and 75. They concluded that the log of the k value was the best index of lung distensibility, being independent of sex and lung size and having a normal distribution. They calculated the following relationship:

$$\log k = (0.00406 \times \text{age}) - 2.19812$$

Some investigators have found that above the age of 40, women have lower recoil pressures than men at comparable lung volumes.[87] There are conflicting data in the literature, however, indicating that both total compliance and thoracic compliance are independent of age.[101]

Expiratory Flow Rates

The reduction in flow rates with age in lifetime non-smokers is represented by the age regressions of these measurements,[69] as derived from cross-sectional studies. There is evidence, however, that these may not be linear even in lifetime non-smokers.[62] The longitudinal study

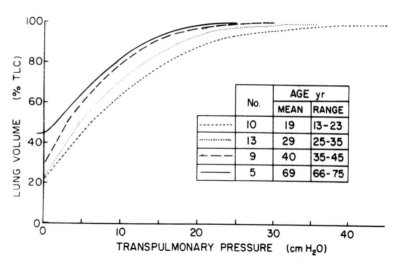

Figure 4–1. Changes in pulmonary pressure curves with age. Data for subjects of mean ages 19, 29, and 40 replotted from Turner, J. M., Mead, J., and Wohl, M. E. Elastic behaviour of lungs in patients with airway obstruction. J. Appl. Physiol. 26, 330–338, 1969. Data for subjects of mean age 69 replotted from Holland, J., Milic-Emili, J., Macklem, T. T., and Bates, D. V. Regional distribution of pulmonary ventilation and perfusion in elderly patients. J. Clin. Invest. 47: 81–92, 1968. Static deflection curves are shown. The subjects were predominately male.

| No. | AGE yr | |
	MEAN	RANGE
10	19	13-23
13	29	25-35
9	40	35-45
5	69	66-75

of 916 non-smokers published by Burrows and his colleagues from Tucson[2890] shows that the progressive decline in FVC and FEV_1 in that environment does not start until the mid-30's in either men or women. They found that after the age of 33, the FEV_1/FVC ratio declines with age, independent of the FVC value. A more recent summary of this study[5098] showed that delta FEV_1/year is a linear function in both men and women, and the authors noted: "Longitudinally determined delta FEV_1 showed much less decline in function and a later age of apparent onset of decline than suggested by cross-sectional analyses." Thus, prediction equations derived from cross-sectional studies may progressively underestimate FEV_1 as time elapses.

Other studies have shown that the rate of decline of expiratory flow rates in non-smokers is initially slow.[2968, 2969, 2971] Some studies have indicated that the rate of fall of FEV_1 may accelerate in older people. Studying men and women between the ages of 60 and 90, Milne[63] found that the 5-year fall in FEV_1 in men below the age of 70 was 11.5%, and in men over the age of 70 was 15.7%. However, Schmidt and his colleagues[67] studied 532 healthy subjects aged 55 to 94 (15% of the men were smokers) and noted no increase in rate of annual decline of FEV_1 with age.

Gelb and Zamel[65] found a reduction in flow (V_{max}) but little change in elastic pressure with age, and they concluded that there was probably increased airway collapsibility during maximal flow as age increased. Rea and his colleagues[2905] found that $\dot{V}max_{25\%}VC$ fell consistently with age in both black and white women and concluded that this measurement might

reflect tissue aging directly, as it could not be explained by any other factor. Airway resistance (R_L) does not change with age.[1] Miller, Grove, and Pincock[3832] studied 83 male and 143 female non-smokers and derived prediction equations for changes in time domain indices of the spirogram in relation to age.

Lung Volumes and Closing Volume

The reduction in vital capacity and the increases in residual volume and closing volume with age are documented by the age regressions for these values (see later discussion). Using the single-breath method of estimating the residual volume, increases in this value with age occur in non-smoking men and women.[2964] It is of interest that increases in residual volume were found to occur in beagle dogs kept in an environmentally clean atmosphere.[104] This is an important observation, since an increase in residual volume is an early change in function as a result of environmental influences (see Chapter 6). The increased closing volume with age has been confirmed by a variety of methods[105] and by a number of investigators.[85, 86] Holtz, Bake, and Winstedt[91] studied 64 subjects, aged 18 to 76 years, in the supine position and found that the closing volume measured with a maximal inspiration increased more with age than the value found if a submaximal inspiration was taken.[91] Other data[103] have confirmed earlier observations, indicating that the limitation of lung emptying with age is due to airway closure.[1]

Uniformity of Ventilation Distribution

The presence of increased airway closure with age in dependent regions means that measurements of uniformity of ventilation distribution will be greatly influenced by the depth of tidal volume during the measurements.[1] With nitrogen washout methods, 21% of normal subjects below the age of 30 are found to have two components to the washout curve, and this percentage increases with increasing age.[70] The single-breath nitrogen test shows that the slope of Phase III, expressed as the percentage change in nitrogen per liter expired, increases with age, but probably in a non-linear fashion.[1] This point is discussed in Chapter 5.

Studies of regional lung function using radioactive xenon[81] showed that the residual volume, expressed as a percentage of TLC, rose with age and that when the subject was seated upright, airway closure occurred in lower lung regions at a higher lung volume than in young subjects. It has been suggested that regional lung volume rises with age in all lung regions in women, but only in the upper lung zones in men.[90] Possibly, aging is accompanied by a loss of recoil in the upper zones and premature airway closure in the lower.[93] This would be compatible with the changes in thoracic volume measured by radiologic studies noted earlier.[963] The impact of this on indices of ventilation distribution will depend on tidal volume[1]; the overall effect may be minimal, however, as shown by Kronenberg and Drage[74] in comparisons of 21-year-old normal subjects and 26 non-smoking men aged between 63 and 77; the older subjects did not show significant non-uniformity of ventilation distribution in studies using radioactive xenon.

These somewhat conflicting conclusions are probably to be explained by the dependence of lung ventilation on the nature of the respiratory maneuver as the pressure volume characteristics change; by variable development of upper lobe emphysema in non-smokers over the age of 70; and by the general difficulty of defining the "normal" population over the age of 70—a group may be selected who have aged at a slower rate than the population as a whole (one investigator was heard to describe the population studied by another group as "geriatric athletes").

The Pulmonary Circulation

The resistance in the pulmonary circulation under resting conditions does not change much with increasing age. At a flow of 10 L/min in each group, the mean pulmonary artery pressure was 60 dynes cm^{-5}/sec in 20-year-olds and 70 dynes cm^{-5}/sec in normal subjects aged 70. The same equation relating pressure to age applied both at rest and on exercise.[83] Emirgil and his colleagues[2972] compared eight men of an average age of 66 with men of mean age 39; there were no differences at rest in cardiac index, arteriovenous oxygen difference, pulmonary arterial pressure, or resistance, but the resistance rose somewhat more on exercise with occlusion of one pulmonary artery in the older group. The distribution of pulmonary perfusion studied by the injection of radioactive microspheres was no different in 30 men of mean age 69 years than it was in young subjects.[76]

Blood Gas Tensions and $\dot{V}/\dot{Q}$ Distribution

It has been known for some years that arterial Pa_{CO_2} does not change with age (as noted in Chapter 5) but that arterial Pa_{O_2} falls (see Table 5–3). These data have been confirmed.[86] The explanation is probably that with aging, airway closure occurs in dependent units during tidal breathing, leading to development of low $\dot{V}/\dot{Q}$ zones.[81] Using the six inert gas method, Derks[92] found that at rest four normal subjects aged between 50 and 62 years had a wider $\dot{V}/\dot{Q}$ distribution than did younger subjects, but the distribution narrowed when the subjects exercised. Earlier results with this method[2973] showed a wider $\dot{V}/\dot{Q}$ distribution with age, apparently due to a wider standard deviation of blood flow distribution; ventilation distribution did not show much difference between young and older subjects. As the Pa_{O_2} falls with increasing age, the alveolar-arterial oxygen difference $[(A - a) D_{O_2}]$ widens,[125, 2975] and these changes are related to the closing volume (CV) in relation to the expired reserve volume (ERV).[2974]

The Diffusing Capacity

Although previous studies that showed a decline in diffusing capacity with increasing age did not take into account the smoking history of the subjects studied,[1] recent studies have shown beyond doubt that this function does decline with age in non-smokers. The regression equations are discussed in Chapter 5.

Georges, Saumon, and Loiseau[73] studied 70 adult non-smokers between the ages of 18 and 78 and measured the components of diffusing capacity, DM and V_c, using the single-breath method.[73] They found that DM began to decline after the age of 40, whereas the pulmonary capillary blood volume, V_c, was normally maintained up to the age of 60; thereafter, it fell off sharply. They concluded that their data were consistent with the anatomic changes described with aging. Similar results have been obtained using other techniques.[84] Both k_{CO} and the ratio of D_L to functional residual capacity decrease with age. The fractional uptake of CO also falls with age.[102] The change with age is probably attributable to the loss of alveolar surface area; a probable diminution in the capillary bed additional to this loss; and possibly a non-uniformity of the ratios between diffusing capacity and volume, ventilation, and flow parameters. It has recently been suggested that the decline of $D_{L_{CO}}SB$ with age might be partly accounted for by the greater weight of older subjects and the influence of this on lung emptying[2905]; however, this would not account for the same phenomenon observed under steady-state conditions.

Maximal Oxygen Uptake

Several interesting observations have been made on the phenomenon of decreasing maximal exercise performance with age. The maximal $\dot{V}O_2$ declines between 5% and 10% for every decade of life after the optimal age for performance is passed.[75] Reliable prediction formulae have been published, and the observed levels of maximal $\dot{V}O_2$ have been shown to be highly reproducible on different occasions.[97] Using treadmill exercise, Adams, McHenry, and Bernauer[97] found that the following formula applied:

$$\dot{V}max_{O_2} \text{ (mL/min/kg)} = 48.57 - 0.3225 \times \text{Age (years)} \pm 3.71$$

Patrick and his colleagues[2970] studied nine healthy men aged 64 to 70 over a 6-year interval and compared the results with those from 10 men aged 33. It was found that the ventilatory cost of submaximal work at a $\dot{V}O_2$ of one L/min rose from 24.3 L/min at age 64 to 31.8 L/min at age 70. The value at age 64 was no different from that found in the younger men. The rate of change in ventilation per unit of oxygen uptake appeared to be between 3% and 5%, greater than that deduced from cross-sectional data. Heart rate also increased, and the authors suggested that progressive anaerobiosis might account for part of the increased ventilation. The fact that different people age at different rates was vividly illustrated by observations on a man of 70 who took no systematic exercise until he was 60 and whose $\dot{V}max_{O_2}$ was as predicted for a 20-year-old.[66]

Control of Ventilation and Sleep

The unequivocal demonstration that the ventilation response to isocapnic hypoxia and to normoxic hypercapnia are both diminished with increasing age,[74, 100] falling by as much as 50%, is an important observation. It is probably explained by a reduction in central drive in response to these stimuli. It has been shown that threshold load detection declines with increasing age.[2966] Studies of monozygotic twins[4749] have indicated that variations in chemosensitivity to hypoxia and in P_{CO_2} response increase as age advances, the latter response becoming much more variable than the hypoxic response in the third and fourth decades of life.

Tracheobronchial Clearance and Coughing

The rate of tracheobronchial clearance has been shown to be diminished with increasing age, especially during sleep.[94] The rate of ciliary beating is slightly reduced in older subjects,[64] but probably not to a degree sufficient to explain the slower mucus transport. However, the cough response of older subjects to an irritant stimulus is reduced[82]; the mechanism for this is unclear.

Oxygen Combination in Blood

The P_{50} (Pa_{O_2} at 50% saturation) rises from 3.59 kPa or 26.56 mm Hg at age 20 to 3.96 kPa or 29.3 mm Hg at age 90.[99] The reason for this change is not clear, but the magnitude is small and unlikely to have a significant effect on function.

Summary

It is important to stress that age-related declines do not start at the same age for all functions.[61] The interrelationship between inherited factors controlling aging and long-term effects of the environment is clearly very complex, and more observations of different populations are required before precision can be given to general statements of these factors' comparative importance. A number of studies of older people include examples of individuals whose rate of aging is markedly slower than average.[66, 81]

Yet the data on lung aging are generally consistent. The 80-year-old who has aged normally but who has not been exposed to unusual environments and who has not smoked cigarettes, by comparison with a 20-year-old

- has reduced expiratory flow rates
- has a loss of lung recoil, with reduced VC and increased RV due to airway closure
- has an increase of poorly ventilated or low $\dot{V}/\dot{Q}$ units of the lung during tidal volume breathing as a result of mechanical changes in parenchyma or small airways
- has a lowered diffusing capacity
- has a lowered arterial oxygen tension and raised alveolar-arterial oxygen difference at rest
- has a diminished response to hypoxia and hypercapnia
- has a reduced rate of mucociliary clearance, especially during sleep
- has a diminished cough response

These factors go a long way to explain the differences in problems of managing the consequences of anesthesia combined with surgery or the effects of chest infection or trauma on the lung in older patients in comparison with younger individuals.

EFFECTS OF CHANGES IN BODY POSITION

The effects of body position on the distribution of pulmonary perfusion and ventilation in normal subjects have been described in Chapter 2. There are a number of additional observations that have been made in normal subjects under different circumstances, and these, together with observations of the effect of body position in a variety of clinical conditions, are conveniently considered together. The effects of position change in the presence of neurologic and neuromuscular disease are noted in Chapter 22.

Normal Subjects

Performance of ventilatory tests is very little affected in normal subjects by whether they are performed sitting or standing.[121] However, the mean FVC was about 70 milliliters greater in 90 middle-aged men when standing as compared with seated values.[4738]

The changes in the subdivisions of lung volume that occur with change from the upright to the supine position have been measured with the subject in a body plethysmograph when tilted from upright to supine[129] and also by the closed-circuit helium method.[112] Using the latter technique, Burki[112] studied six healthy subjects and recorded a mean reduction in FRC of 799 milliliters on going from the seated to the supine positions. The value of $P_{0.1}$, reflecting the neuromuscular drive to breathing, was unaffected by this change in FRC, but interpretation of this observation is complex. There are data suggesting that the fall in vital capacity when reclining occurs only in subjects younger than 60 years; it is not found in older normal individuals.[146] Changes in gastric, pleural, and transdiaphragmatic pressure (P_{di}) have been recorded in normal subjects when changing from a sitting to a supine position.[4760] Using CO_2 rebreathing to stimulate ventilation, the authors concluded that the seated position assisted diaphragmatic function "by placing the diaphragm in an advantageous pressure-generating configuration."[4760]

Forty-eight hours in the supine position did not change the $(A - a) D_{O_2}$ or the Pa_{O_2} in seven non-smoking men aged between 19 and 24 years.[126] Experiments we reported in 1969,[152] which indicated the possibility of a progressive diminution in ventilation of dependent lung zones after recumbency in older people, do not appear to have been repeated.

Recent radiographic studies of 15 young non-smoking normal individuals in different body positions[439] showed that in the left lateral decubitus position the apicothoracic dimension of the right (upper) lung increased and that of the left lung decreased. These findings confirmed the data on regional lung volumes obtained with ^{133}Xe, which showed that the two lungs were at different volumes and were on different parts of their pressure-volume curves in this position.[1] The increased perfusion and ventilation of the dependent lung has been confirmed[141] in recent experiments.

Hedenstierna and colleagues,[150] studying anesthetized normal subjects, found that in the left lateral position the FRC increased in the upper lung and decreased in the dependent lung, with no alteration in closing capacity (CC). Airway closure therefore became asynchronous between the upper and lower lungs, and pendelluft was possible between the two lungs. Their analysis of the effect of different vertical linear pleural pressure gradients on lung ventilation in the lateral decubitus position is of considerable interest.

Comparisons between natural breathing and IPPB breathing in normal individuals have shown that the magnitude of diaphragmatic tension is the main determinant of topographical ventilation distribution in the lateral position.[109] Radioactive xenon studies of normal paralyzed volunteers artificially ventilated and in the left lateral position showed that in comparison with natural breathing there was a more uniform distribution of inhaled gas between the two lungs.[139] In three awake and spontaneously breathing subjects, Froese and Bryan[2986] showed that in the lateral decubitus position the dependent part of the diaphragm had the greatest excursion. When these subjects were paralyzed, the dependent diaphragm moved toward the head, and on artificial ventilation under these conditions, the upper part of the diaphragm moved more than the most dependent part. The perfusion of the lower lung in the lateral decubitus position is increased by 100% O_2 breathing.[132, 148] However, in studies of five healthy volunteers, Aborelius, Lilja, and Zauner,[149] using a Carlens' bronchospirometric catheter and intravenous injection of krypton-85, showed that if the lower lung was breathing 10% O_2, 100% O_2 to the upper lung caused a large increase in flow to the upper lung. They concluded that gravitational factors alone could not explain the changes in perfusion distribution caused by oxygen breathing in the superior lung.

Rea and his colleagues[114] studied $(A - a) D_{O_2}$ with changes in posture in 24 healthy subjects aged between 23 and 72 years, four of whom were smokers. They documented the influence of airway closure in dependent regions, finding that the changes in $(A - a) D_{O_2}$ and $\dot{Q}_{va}/\dot{Q}_t$ from sitting to lying were related to the change in closing volume minus the ERV during both air and oxygen breathing. Marcq and Minette[135] studied the effect of changing body position between inspiration and expiration on the alveolar slope of Phase III, and Phase IV using nitrogen. They concluded that Phase IV was gravity-related but the slope of Phase III was independent of gravity. The effect of gravity on airway closure has been ingeniously demonstrated by Cumming and his colleagues[130] in experiments using argon boluses and measuring the oxygen saturation.

The gravity dependence of perfusion has been confirmed in a number of studies.[120, 2989] Prefaut and Engel[2989] measured perfusion distribution in six normal supine subjects and documented the preferential perfusion of the non-dependent zones, which was reversed by oxygen breathing. In a remarkable series of experiments, Lilja[140] found that apical perfusion declined for the first hour after sitting in eight normal subjects and that the effect of 100% oxygen or perfusion occurred only during the second hour. His results can be summarized as follows:

	First Hour	Second Hour
Apical perfusion	Decreased	No further decrease
Breathhold (40–60 secs)	Slight increase in apical perfusion	More marked increase in apical perfusion
Breathe 100% O_2	No effect	Increased perfusion of lung bases
Breathhold during 100% O_2 breathing	Increased apical perfusion	No effect

He concluded that the perfusion of lung bases increased up to the point at which relative alveolar hypoxia caused vasoconstriction. In other experiments[141, 142] he found that the decrease in apical perfusion during the first 10 to 20 minutes of adopting the upright position was accompanied by a fall in mean pulmonary artery pressure and that the fall in apical perfusion correlated well with a fall in cardiac output.

These observations are consistent with observed changes in total pulmonary blood volume in normal subjects with body tilting. In 12 normal subjects and making use of a new radionuclide method of determination, Muir found a coefficient of variation of 2.6%.[1754] When supine, the mean value of total pulmonary blood volume measured by this method was 430 milliliters which fell to 350 milliliters with a 45-degree tilt.

Earlier reports of changes in DL_{CO} with posture[1] have been confirmed by Jebavy and his colleagues[147] in studies of 18 normal subjects. The $DL_{CO}SB$ was 26.6% lower when upright than when supine. In a group of 40 patients similarly studied, they showed that this change did not occur in cases of mitral stenosis or post-pneumonectomy; the change in DL_{CO} closely correlated with the mean pulmonary arterial pressure and was found to lessen with higher pulmonary arterial pressures.

Using boluses of neon, carbon monoxide, and

acetylene, it has been shown that $\dot{Q}_c/\dot{V}A$ increases from apex to base in the seated subject.[111] The change in $DL/\dot{V}A$ is not so steep but is in the same direction. Hence, there is a vertical unevenness of the ratio $DL/\dot{Q}_c$. In nonsmokers, there is an 18.5% fall in k_{CO} from supine to sitting, but in smokers this change is much smaller, averaging only 3.5%.[136] This difference has been attributed to possible thickening of the walls of pulmonary vessels in the upper lobes of smokers.[110] In normal subjects, squatting leads to a fall in TLC of about 500 milliliters, the same fall in VC, no change in residual volume, and a small fall of 200 milliliters in FEV_1. The diffusing capacity is increased by about 6 mL/min/mm Hg in the squatting position, which is due to an increase in V_c from a mean of about 70 to 97 mL.[116]

In very obese patients, the $(A - a) D_{O_2}$ rises when the subject lies flat as soon as the ERV falls below the closing volume[134]; in the lateral decubitus position the upper lung becomes preferentially ventilated and the ERV is midway between its upright and supine values.[4761] It has been suggested that in very obese subjects, the diaphragm might be overstretched when supine.[4764] The transdiaphragmatic pressure was reduced in this position, although the diaphragmatic electromyogram (EMG) increased. The Pa_{O_2} has been noted to fall in obese supine subjects, and in one study of 10 patients, the Pa_{O_2} fell from 79.4 mm Hg sitting to 74.8 mm Hg supine.[134] It has also been noted that in such subjects, the fractional CO uptake (Fco) does not increase when the subject is supine as it does in normal subjects.

These data on normal subjects in different body positions are not only interesting but important in that the results confirm ideas about lung behavior in the gravitational field.

Effect of Body Position on Pulmonary Function in Disease

Several reports have appeared on changes in arterial Po_2 when patients with lung disease change position. With chronic airflow limitation, studies have been designed to explain why dyspnea may be greater in one position than another. Dyspnea on lying down (orthopnea) is not only characteristic of pulmonary congestion due to left ventricular failure (see Chapter 12) but is also the characteristic symptom of bilateral diaphragmatic paralysis (see Chapter 22).

In many cases of chronic airflow limitation,

the arterial Pa_{O_2} is the same in the sitting and supine positions,[2982] but $\dot{V}D/\dot{V}T$ rises and $\dot{Q}_s/\dot{Q}_t$ falls in the sitting position.[133, 138] There is a fall of about 4 mm Hg in the mixed venous Po_2.[138] However, it has been shown that in some of these cases, the Pa_{O_2} falls when the subject is recumbent[4767]; but in other individuals with greater body weight, it rose.[4767]

It is a common observation that some patients with advanced obstructive lung disease breathe more comfortably when leaning forward. Sharp and his colleagues[144] studied this phenomenon in 17 patients whose mean FEV_1 was only 0.56 liter, and whose $DL_{CO}SB$ averaged 26% of predicted. In seven patients, dyspnea was relieved by leaning forward; this was due to correction of a paradoxical (inward) movement of the abdomen on inspiration that occurred while standing or seated upright. The investigators concluded that diaphragmatic function was improved.

More recently, Druz and Sharp[2976] have suggested that in normal individuals the diaphragmatic EMG increases when standing or sitting as compared with supine values and that the transdiaphragmatic pressure also increases. But they found these changes did not occur in two of six severely disabled patients with chronic airflow limitation. O'Neill and McCarthy[2977] have recently reported on 40 patients with severe chronic airflow limitation studied in six different positions. They have shown that the leaning forward position was optimal for these patients, as the highest maximal inspiratory pressure could be generated when in that position. In contrast, the maximal expiratory pressure was unaffected by postural changes. In a 26-year-old woman with 40-degree thoracic scoliosis,[4769] the FVC rose from 1.84 liters to 3.57 liters when she flexed forward on sitting; the FRC increased by 1.4 liters. In asthmatics, 24 hours of recumbency lowers the peak expiratory flow rate (PEFR).[4246] In patients with cystic fibrosis and moderately severe lung disease, the Pa_{O_2} falls on recumbency,[4272] an effect possibly related to the more severe disease commonly found in the upper lobes.

The change in FRC that occurs in the presence of unilateral disease when the subject moves from the supine to the left or right lateral position has been used as an indicator of probable postoperative pulmonary function. Results of the test correlate well with data from ^{133}Xe studies,[122] and it has been claimed that the test is clinically valuable.[119, 123] However, in normal subjects its repeatability is poor,[145] and it is unlikely that a single measurement could be used reliably for the purpose for which it has been advocated.

The arterial Pa_{O_2} after thoracotomy is often higher when the unoperated side is dependent,[107] although most of the 12 patients in whom these measurements were made were smokers, which may have influenced the results. A patent foramen ovale may cause considerable postural shifts in Pa_{O_2} and occasionally cause diagnostic difficulty.[137] After abdominal surgery in 19 patients—upper abdominal surgery in nine patients and lower abdominal surgery in 10 patients—studied in the early postoperative period, surprisingly, a lower Pa_{O_2} was observed with the patients sitting rather than supine[151]; the sitting position conferred no advantage in terms of gas exchange.

The marked fall in vital capacity that occurs when a patient with diaphragmatic paralysis moves from the sitting to the recumbent position has been known for some years.[1] Recent data have shown that the average fall in unilateral paralysis was 19% in left-sided paralysis and 10% in right-sided lesions. The difference between ERV and CV often becomes negative in such patients. In one 55-year-old man with bilateral diaphragmatic paralysis of traumatic origin, the Pa_{O_2} fell from 58 mm Hg sitting to 39 mm Hg supine, and the VC fell from 1.87 liters to 0.66 liter. The $(A - a) D_{O_2}$ rose from 20 mm Hg to 44 mm Hg. This lesion is considered in more detail in Chapter 22.

In the presence of unilateral lung disease, the Pa_{O_2} is lower, often markedly so, when the diseased lung is dependent and the patient is in the lateral decubitus position.[2985] However, it cannot be assumed that it is always desirable for the patient to be nursed with the diseased lung uppermost, although the Pa_{O_2} is higher in that position, since other factors, like the possible spread of infection from the upper to the dependent lung, have to be considered.

Partial occlusion of a major bronchus may cause changes in Pa_{O_2} due to changes in the degree of bronchial obstruction with body position changes.[2979] It is of interest that experimental data suggest that a leak in the pleura may be lessened if the affected side is dependent.[2981] In eight patients with unilateral pleural effusions, the Pa_{O_2} was about 5 mm Hg higher when the side of the effusion was uppermost[2978]; another report on 10 patients with bilateral pleural effusions[4759] noted that in normoxic individuals the oxygen saturation fell by only 1% when the side with the larger effusion was dependent.

There are a number of reports of marked postural changes in Pa_{O_2} in patients with complex clinical disorders. In a 68-year-old man with an alveolar cell carcinoma, the tumor contained a shunt, and the Pa_{O_2} changed 16 mm Hg between the right and left lateral positions.[124] Changes between sitting and the supine position may be noted in the rare condition of pulmonary telangiectasia.[127] In two patients with complex disorders, worsening of the Pa_{O_2} when upright (orthodeoxia) and worsening of dyspnea when sitting up (platypnea) have been recorded.[117, 118] Increased intracardiac shunting through a patent foramen ovale can lead to decreased saturation when upright.[4737]

SLEEP AND SLEEP APNEA

Physiology of Sleep

Sleep is a temporary state of unconsciousness that can be interrupted by external stimuli. It is not a uniform state but is organized into a cyclic pattern of sequential stages. The stage of sleep is defined by a combination of electroencephalographic (EEG), electromyographic (EMG), and electro-oculographic (EOG) criteria.[5269]

Two separate phases of sleep are generally recognized: "quiet" or non–rapid eye movement sleep (non-REM) and "active" or rapid eye movement sleep (REM). During non-REM sleep, the EEG waves slow down progressively and increase in amplitude. Non-REM sleep is divided into four stages, representing progressively deeper stages of sleep. In stages 1 and 2, the EEG voltage is low and the frequency mixed. In stages 3 and 4, the EEG voltage is high and the frequency slow. Consequently, these latter two stages are often referred to as slow-wave sleep (SWS). Stage 2 is the predominant sleep stage and usually accounts for about half of an adult's sleep.

During REM sleep, the EEG is synchronized with low voltage and high frequency. REM sleep is characterized by two different patterns, one associated with muscle tone depression and the other with rapid eye movement and twitching movements of the face and limbs.[5270] Most dreams occur during REM sleep, and there is also increased autonomic and metabolic activity, with marked fluctuations in blood pressure, heart rate, and respiratory rate. REM sleep normally accounts for 20 to 25% of the total sleep time and occurs four to six times a night.

Increasing age, alcohol, and other sedatives all tend to decrease REM sleep.

A variety of terms are now commonly used when describing respiratory sleep disorders. Apnea is defined as cessation of airflow at the nose or mouth for more than 10 seconds during sleep. It is classified into three major types:

1. Central apnea is the cessation of airflow and of ventilatory effort.
2. Obstructive apnea is cessation of airflow despite the presence of ventilatory effort.
3. A mixed apnea is a central apnea that progresses to an obstructive apnea.

Hypopnea is a poorly defined term that refers to distinct periods of reduced airflow and is usually associated with an arousal or with a reduced arterial oxygen saturation. An arousal is a brief neurologic awakening; it may occur spontaneously or in response to various stimuli. It has been suggested that impairment of arousal responses may be a major mechanism in a variety of respiratory sleep disorders.[5271]

Effect of Sleep on the Respiratory System

In normal healthy adults, minute ventilation may decrease by 1 to 2 liters per minute during sleep as a result of a reduction in both tidal volume and respiratory frequency.[5272] Gas exchange is consequently affected, the Pa_{CO_2} increasing by 4 to 8 mm Hg and the Pa_{O_2} falling by 3 to 10 mm Hg. The pH decreases by 0.03 to 0.05 units.[5273] This hypoventilation is associated with changes in breathing pattern and in the chemical drive to breathe. In stages 1 and 2 of non-REM sleep, breathing tends to be periodic; whereas in stages 3 and 4, breathing is typically regular. REM sleep is characterized by an irregular breathing pattern that may include brief (<15 seconds) periods of apnea in normal adults.[5273] Studies in both animals and humans have demonstrated that the ventilatory response to CO_2 is lower in non-REM sleep than when awake.[5274, 5275] Ventilatory response to hypoxia is reduced but present in non-REM sleep and is reduced but not always present in REM sleep.[5276, 5277]

During sleep, the ability to arouse may be the most important response to a respiratory stimulus. In animal studies, arousal responses by hypercapnia,[5278] hypoxia,[5279] respiratory loads,[5280] and laryngeal[5281] and bronchopulmonary irritation[5282] are decreased in REM sleep as compared with non-REM sleep. Hypoxia was thought to be a powerful arousal-promoting stimulus; however, recent studies in humans have shown that hypoxia is a poor arousal stimulus in both non-REM and REM sleep.[5283]

During sleep, there is a progressive loss of tone in the respiratory muscles and muscles of the upper airway. This hypotonicity is maximal during REM sleep and partially spares the diaphragm.[5284] This dissociation of diaphragmatic and intercostal activity leads to increasing ventilation/perfusion inequality and is believed to be a major cause of arterial desaturation during sleep in some patients (as for example, in persons with cystic fibrosis).[5285] The mechanism is probably of less importance in older patients with reduced chest wall compliance.

Loss of tone in the muscles of the upper airway can result in airflow obstruction during sleep.[5286] Sleep also influences intrapulmonary receptor activity and lung defense mechanisms, predisposing to nocturnal sputum retention and aspiration. The cough reflex is depressed,[5287] and the mucociliary clearance rate slows during sleep,[958] as noted in Chapter 3. Sensitive radioactive tracer techniques have demonstrated that almost half of normal subjects aspirate during sleep.[5288] Both airway and pulmonary vasculature smooth muscle tone fluctuate markedly during REM sleep as a result of alterations in autonomic nervous activity.[5289]

Differences in normal respiratory changes between non-REM and REM sleep are summarized in Table 4–1.

Techniques for Evaluating Respiratory Sleep Disorders

Sleep studies (polysomnography) are usually performed at specialized referral centers; guidelines for the indications for cardiopulmonary sleep studies and standards for their performance have been developed.[5290] The studies are used to document the frequency, type, and duration of apnea and to record changes in cardiac rhythm, arterial oxygenation, and sleep pattern. Short daytime studies can provide a useful screening test for patients with respiratory sleep disorders. However, a complete overnight sleep study is usually required for a definitive diagnosis and to assess the full clinical significance of the sleep disorder.

Much of the current interest in respiratory sleep disorders has been stimulated by the

Table 4–1. NORMAL RESPIRATORY CHANGES DURING SLEEP

	Non-REM	REM
Ventilation	Decreased compared to awake	Marked fluctuations
Breathing pattern	Regular	Irregular with occasional apnea
Chemical drives to breathe	Decreased compared to awake	Markedly decreased
Arousal responses	Present	Decreased
Chest wall movement	In phase	Rib-cage paradox
Cough reflex	Decreased compared to awake	Decreased compared to awake
Airway smooth muscle tone	Stable	Marked fluctuations

development of non-invasive respiratory monitoring equipment. It is standard practice to document sleep and its various stages with an electroencephalogram, an electro-oculogram, and a submental electromyogram recorded by surface electrodes. A single electrocardiogram is routinely monitored to detect cardiac arrhythmias. Because of the periodic nature of gas exchange disturbances during sleep, continuous monitoring of arterial oxygen saturation (O_2Hb) and transcutaneous CO_2 (T_cPCO_2) is preferable to periodic blood gas measurements. Ear oximetry offers a stable, sensitive, and non-invasive method of monitoring the arterial saturation. T_cPCO_2 can be continuously measured by an infrared transducer applied over the skin stripped of the stratum corneum. T_cPCO_2 accurately reflects Pa_{CO_2} except during periods of acute hypoventilation, when it may be underestimated. Either thermistor probes or a CO_2 analyzer recording from the nose and mouth may be used to document periods of apnea and hypopnea. Tracheal breath sounds recorded by a microphone on the upper sternum provide an additional assessment of airflow and record the occurrence of snoring.

A variety of methods have been used to quantitate respiratory effort. Strain gauges have been used to monitor chest wall and abdominal movement, but they do not provide quantitative estimates of respiratory effort. Respiratory inductive plethysmography measures the cross-sectional area of the rib cage and abdomen through changes in electrical inductance.[5291] This technique gives accurate estimations of tidal volume, regardless of body position, and, by assessing paradoxical motion of the rib cage and abdomen, provides a further monitor of apnea. Esophageal pressure measurements provide the most accurate index of respiratory effort and are usually necessary for a definitive diagnosis of central sleep apnea.[5292] An overnight sleep study generates a vast amount of data. The introduction of microcomputers has enabled the development of on-line data collection, reduction, and analysis; microcomputers

have significantly improved the precision of sleep studies and have reduced the time needed for data analysis.[5293] A typical report is shown in Table 4–2.

Sleep Apnea Syndrome

Sleep apnea syndrome is defined as the presence of more than 30 apneas in a 7-hour sleep. In severe cases, the apneas may last for 60 to 90 seconds and may recur up to 500 times in a night. Although certain manifestations of the syndrome have been described for many years, a wider recognition of the pathophysiology and clinical features has been possible only over the last decade.[5294–5297]

Patients with sleep apnea syndrome exhibit a characteristic sequence of events. The patient stops breathing while asleep and develops progressive asphyxia. In response to the blood gas changes or other stimuli, the patient awakes and resumes breathing. He or she then falls asleep again and may repeat the cycle many times throughout the night. These recurrent periods of asphyxia are responsible for many of the clinical manifestations of the disease. Pulmonary vasoconstriction develops, which may progress to pulmonary hypertension and right heart failure. Systemic vasoconstriction ultimately results in sustained systemic hypertension. Erythropoiesis is stimulated by the periods of hypoxemia and may lead to a secondary polycythemia. Cardiac arrhythmias are not infrequent in these patients and are due to the combined effects of cardiac ischemia, discharge of sympathetic mediators, and vagal bradycardia.

Obstructive sleep apnea (OSA) occurs because of recurrent occlusion of the upper airway. Three general factors determine upper airway patency during sleep: airway size, neuromuscular activity, and neuromuscular co-ordination.[5286] OSA has been reported in patients with upper airway tumors,[5299] adenotonsillar hypertrophy,[5300] macroglossia,[5301] which may oc-

Table 4–2. OVERNIGHT SLEEP STUDY REPORT

Date: January 7, 1987

Age: 46   Weight 98 kg   Sex: M   BP: 130/104 mm Hg

Clinical Features: Habitual snoring, reported nocturnal apnea, nocturnal choking, unrefreshing sleep, morning headache, excessive daytime hypersomnolence, recent personality change, obesity.

Medications: None.

SUMMARY

Sleep Quality

Time in bed	429	min
Sleep period time (SPT)	407	min
Total sleep time (TST)	348	min
Efficiency index	81.12	%

Sleep Stages

	%SPT
Awake	14
1	26
2	43
SWS	5
REM	11

REM Latency:	Observed	187 min
	Predicted	72 min
Arousals:	Total	26
	Index	4.48/hour TST

Apneas

	Number	Mean (sec)	Max (sec)
		Duration	
Obstructive	271	28	68
Central	—	—	—
Mixed	—	—	—
Total	271	28	68

Apnea index:	46.72/hour TST	Hypopnea index:	14.48/hour TST
Total apnea time:	35.82% TST	Apnea and hypopnea index:	61.20/hour TST

Physiology

	Max	Mean	Min	
Oxygen saturation	99	87	59	(Sa_{O_2} %)
Transcutaneous CO_2	59	53	47	($T_cP_{CO_2}$ mm Hg)
Respiratory rate	28	12	0	(breaths/min)
Cardiac rate	108	69	35	(beats/min)
Esophageal pH				

Cardiac Rhythm: Marked cyclic variation in R-R interval (heart rate less than 40 bpm). One episode of 3 second sinus arrest.

Special Comments: Intermittent moderate snoring (maximum 64 decibels) with associated obstructive hypopnea. Awoke to urinate once. Restless sleep. Several episodes of subjective nocturnal choking, awoke in morning unrefreshed and confused.

Report: Severe obstructive sleep apnea with associated arterial oxygen desaturation, sleep fragmentation, and cardiac dysrhythmias.

cur in association with acromegaly, and significant retrognathia.[5302] Although most patients with OSA do not have these abnormalities, recent reports indicate that the airway in such patients is narrower[5303, 5304] and more compliant than in normal controls.[5305]

The oropharynx is the only collapsible segment of the upper airway, since its walls are not rigid enough to offer sufficient protection against negative transmural pressure. The walls of the oropharynx are lined by the soft palate, tongue, and pharyngeal muscles and do not include any bony or cartilaginous structures. It is considered that enlargement of the soft palate plays a major role in causing the upper airway narrowing present in many patients with OSA.[5306] The soft palate is a movable fold suspended from the posterior border of the bony palate, extending downward and backward into the oropharynx. Rodenstein and Stanescu[5307] recently reviewed the respiratory function of this structure. Riley and his co-workers[5308] reported that the soft palate was significantly longer in 10 patients with OSA as compared with five control subjects with similar sized posterior airway spaces. Shelton and Bosma[5309] noted over 20 years ago that apposition of the soft palate, tongue, and posterior pharyngeal wall results in upper airway obstruction. More recently, Suratt and his colleagues[5310] performed lateral fluoroscopy on six patients with obstructive sleep apnea and reported that upper airway obstruction first occurred when the soft palate touched the posterior pharyngeal wall and tongue.

Anch and his co-workers[5311] demonstrated, in a patient with OSA, that the onset of apneas coincided with cessation of tensor palatini EMG activity, despite continued genioglossus activity. They proposed that inhibition of tensor palatini activity results in posterior movement of the soft palate, increased oropharyngeal resistance, and ultimately upper airway obstruction. However, an enlarged and hypotonic soft palate is not the only determinant of the nocturnal upper airway obstruction seen in patients with OSA. Weitzman and his colleagues[5312] concluded from both endoscopic and fluoroscopic studies that upper airway closure was due to recurrent apposition of the superior lateral pharyngeal walls and posterior movement of the base of the tongue.

Patency of the upper airway depends on a balance of forces. The negative pressure produced when the thoracic inspiratory muscles contract tends to obstruct the upper airway unless adequately opposed by muscle activity in the upper airway dilating muscles, particularly the tongue.[5313] While awake, these muscles display a phasic inspiratory activity, which is reduced during non-REM sleep and virtually absent in REM sleep.[5314] By contrast, the muscle activity in the diaphragm changes little during sleep, shifting the balance toward upper airway closure. Remmers and his colleagues[5286] proposed that, for any upper airway configuration, the activity of the upper airway muscles relative to the thoracic inspiratory muscles determines upper airway patency. If the upper airway dilating muscle activity is selectively decreased, as occurs during sleep, after alcohol ingestion,[5316] and after hypnotic drugs,[5317] upper airway occlusion ensues. Similarly, any increase in inspiratory load due to a narrow airway requires increased upper airway activity relative to thoracic inspiratory muscle activity for the airway to remain patent.

Many of the same factors that stimulate thoracic inspiratory muscles also stimulate activity of the upper airway dilating muscles. In awake normal humans, genioglossus muscle activity progressively increases in response to hypoxia and hypercapnia and in a direct linear manner with the diaphragm.[5318] However, the two sets of muscles may differ in their sensitivity to these stimuli; in animal studies, the respiratory drive to the upper airway muscles has been shown to increase disproportionately to the thoracic inspiratory muscles.[5319] Thus, the upper airway is normally stabilized during increased ventilation. Recent studies in patients with OSA have suggested that the upper airways fail to stabilize in these persons during progressive asphyxia.[5320]

Clinical Presentation

Patients with obstructive sleep apnea may present with a wide variety of symptoms.[5321, 5322] Not infrequently, the patient is unaware of any problem, and the patient's bed partner draws attention to the nocturnal symptoms. Excessive daytime hypersomnolence is the commonest daytime symptom. The patient has an inappropriate urge to sleep during the day, which may be severe enough to result in motor vehicle accidents, disruption of family life, or termination of employment. Patients often complain that sleep is not a refreshing experience. They may awake with a morning headache (possibly induced by hypercapnia) and a sense of disorientation that gradually remits during the day. Although most patients are unaware of the recurrent apnea, some complain of insomnia or waking with a sense of choking. Other symptoms include intellectual deterioration and impotence.

In any patient suspected of having the sleep apnea syndrome, it is essential to obtain a history from his or her bed partner. A patient with obstructive apnea typically has a long history of snoring. The bed partner often reports that the patient stops breathing during sleep and that the resumption of breathing is signaled by sudden loud snoring. During the periods of upper airway obstruction, the patient is often very restless. Sleepwalking and assuming peculiar postures during sleep are other features of the syndrome. Family members often complain about a change in the patient's personality; he or she becomes aggressive, irritable, and even paranoid.

Obstructive sleep apnea may occur in children, especially in association with adenotonsillar hypertrophy.[5323] Daytime sleepiness, declining school performance, and nocturnal enuresis are the common symptoms of sleep apnea in children. Patients with a predominantly central apnea more often tend to present with a history of insomnia and daytime hypersomnolence.

Patients with obstructive apnea are often obese. However, at least 40% of them are not obese, and only a small proportion of overweight people develop sleep apnea. The majority of persons with sleep apnea have no associated disease, although as noted earlier, it is associated with some syndromes. Central apnea may occur in association with any infective, inflammatory, or neoplastic process involving the brain stem or cervical spinal cord.

Some patients with sleep apnea may have physical signs associated with the complications of the syndrome. In severe cases, clinical evidence of pulmonary hypertension may be present with right heart failure and peripheral edema. Systemic hypertension is reported to be present in 60% of patients. Secondary polycythemia is not uncommon, and the diagnosis of sleep apnea should be considered in any patient with an unexplained polycythemia.

Many conditions are associated with symptoms suggestive of sleep apnea. The majority can be distinguished on clinical grounds, but the definitive diagnosis of sleep apnea requires polysomnography. Narcolepsy, drug-related sleepiness, insufficient sleep, and neurologic and psychiatric disorders may all present with daytime hypersomnolence. Narcolepsy is most commonly misdiagnosed as sleep apnea. It is commonly associated with cataplexy (muscle weakness associated with intense emotion), sleep paralysis, and hypnagogic hallucinations.[5324] Narcolepsy is diagnosed by an EEG with a characteristic pattern of immediate onset of REM sleep. Nocturnal asthma (see Chapter 9), paroxysmal nocturnal dyspnea due to cardiac disease, bilateral diaphragmatic paralysis (see Chapter 22), and gastroesophageal reflux may all present with episodic nocturnal dyspnea and may be confused with sleep apnea.

Therapy of Sleep Apnea

The therapy of sleep apnea depends on the severity of symptoms and complications and the predominant type of the apnea. At present, it is not known whether asymptomatic patients with sleep apnea should be treated. It is important for patients to avoid sleep deprivation or any form of sedation, including alcohol, which may further depress breathing and predispose to upper airway occlusion. Similarly, patients should be advised to avoid sleeping in circumstances associated with reduced barometric pressure, such as long plane trips or sojourns at high altitudes, as these will further exacerbate hypoxemia during apneic periods. Treatment of chronic nasal obstruction secondary to allergic rhinitis with inhaled corticosteroid sprays may help to alleviate symptoms.[5325] In obese subjects, small reductions in weight may dramatically reduce the number and severity of apneic periods.[5326] This effect is inconsistent and unpredictable, however, but should be advised for every obese patient with sleep apnea. Respiratory stimulants, such as medroxyprogesterone, theophylline, and almitrine, have been tried with limited success.[5327] Protriptyline, a non-sedative tricyclic antidepressant, may benefit selected patients, but its use is often associated with significant anticholinergic side effects, such as urinary hesitancy and a dry mouth.[5328]

Nasal continuous positive airway pressure (nasal CPAP) is uniformly effective in the long-term treatment of OSA[5329] and in the prevention of snoring.[5330] Its efficacy is dependent on the degree of positive pressure applied to the upper airway, as this reduces the negative oropharyngeal pressure applied to the upper airway and, hence, reduces the negative oropharyngeal pressure generated during inspiration. It was originally proposed that CPAP acts as a "pneumatic splint," preventing upper airway collapse by pushing the soft palate and tongue forward and away from the posterior oropharyngeal wall.[5331] Although nasal CPAP might reflexly activate upper airway muscles, their activity seems to be reduced during nasal CPAP treatment.[5332]

The pressure applied during nasal CPAP must be determined for each patient during an overnight sleep study. After receiving short-term nasal CPAP therapy, patients often do not need treatment every night. Symptoms always reappear if nasal CPAP is completely withdrawn, but this occurs gradually over several days, so that short interruptions in therapy are usually well tolerated. This phenomenon may be due to the improvement in sleep pattern and gas exchange with relief of the recurrent upper airway occlusion. Sleep fragmentation has been demonstrated to reduce respiratory responses to chemical stimuli,[5333] and long-term nasal CPAP therapy improves hypercapnic ventilatory responses in patients with OSA.[5334]

Upon initiation of nasal CPAP, hypoventilation may occur during periods of REM sleep, requiring supplemental oxygen therapy. These periods of prolonged REM sleep with associated hypoxemia are not usually seen with continued use of nasal CPAP. Patients may require inhaled nasal corticosteroids or decongestants to dilate nasal passages for CPAP to be effective. There are no known contraindications to nasal CPAP therapy. In our experience, it is well accepted by many patients but is limited by the inherent cumbersomeness and restriction of movement during sleep. Five to 30% of patients are unable to tolerate nasal CPAP treatment on a long-term basis because of a feeling of suffocation, nasal drying or rhinitis, ear pain, or conjunctivitis. There are no reports of a pneumothorax, and pulmonary function does not deteriorate during nasal CPAP treatment.[5335] Nasal CPAP systems are now commercially available and may be rented from respiratory equipment suppliers. Nasal CPAP is now covered by some American medical insurance plans and some Canadian provincial medicare plans.

A surgical approach to the treatment of obstructive sleep apnea should always be preceded by a detailed evaluation of the patient's upper airway to locate the primary site of the nocturnal upper airway obstruction.[5336] In addition to clinical examination, this evaluation can be performed using such techniques as computerized tomography,[5337] cephalometry,[5338] nasopharyngoscopy, somnofluoroscopy, and acoustic reflection studies.[5339] Nasal surgery, such as removal of nasal polyps or septoplasty, may be indicated in patients with a predominantly nasal obstruction.

Uvulopalatopharyngoplasty (UPP) is a new surgical procedure[5340] that in terms of operative morbidity can be considered analogous to an extensive tonsillectomy and adenoidectomy. The operation enlarges the upper airway by removal of redundant oropharyngeal tissue from the lateral aspect of the posterior pharyngeal wall and pharyngopalatal arch while preserving the local musculature. The success of this operation is approximately 60% but varies considerably from center to center. Some of this variability may be accounted for by differences in the effect of the surgery performed or by differences in the period of follow-up or in the

actual site of occlusion during sleep. Maximal success is reported within 6 months of the procedure. Simmons and his associates[5341] have reported on presurgical and postsurgical polysomnographic evaluations of 20 patients' sleep apnea treated by UPP. Forty-five per cent had a successful result, but they were unable to predict, either prospectively or retrospectively, which patients would benefit. However, it should be noted that detailed anatomic studies were not performed on this group of patients, and no rejection criteria were established. The same authors have also presented results in another group of 35 patients[5342]; in 20 of these, retrognathia, excessive obesity, and absence of any clear anatomic abnormality in the oropharynx were taken as rejection criteria. The results from this study indicated that patients with mild to moderate sleep apnea and less than 30% excess weight were most likely to improve after UPP. The limited experience so far indicates that UPP is useful only in certain patients.

One approach proposed is to perform UPP only in those patients in whom the soft palate is the most likely cause of the oropharyngeal closure, i.e., in those persons with an abnormally thick (and perhaps long) soft palate that occupies an excessive space in the oropharynx. Older patients and those with macroglossia or retrognathia appear to respond less well. A low hyoid usually accompanies a small posterior airway space, and in such patients the results are also poor. Improvement following UPP continues during long-term follow-up, except in those patients who subsequently gain weight.[5343] UPP carries a less than 0.5% operative mortality; nasal regurgitation and a change in character of the voice are potential, but uncommon, side effects. A maxillofacial surgical approach has also been shown to be helpful in selecting patients with hypopharyngeal narrowing, emphasizing the need for a multidisciplinary approach in the optimal management of this condition.

In patients with central apnea, respiratory stimulants, such as medroxyprogesterone or theophylline, often result in a significant amelioration of symptoms. In more severe cases, some form of mechanical ventilation may be necessary during sleep. This can be provided by a rocking bed, a negative pressure ventilator, or a positive pressure ventilator in conjunction with a tracheostomy. Diaphragmatic pacing by electrical stimulation of the phrenic nerve is also an effective treatment for these patients and has the important social and psychologic advantage of obviating dependence on a mechanical ventilator.[5344]

Snoring

Snoring is caused by high-frequency oscillation of the soft palate,[5345] resulting in a partial upper airway obstruction. It is an important feature of the sleep apnea syndrome and is typically present for many years prior to the clinical manifestations of the disease. This has led some investigators to question whether snoring is more than a trivial complaint and whether it represents a risk factor of some significance.[5346, 5347] Approximately 45% of normal subjects occasionally snore, and 25% are considered habitual snorers. Predisposing factors include male sex, older age, menopause, obesity, and excessive alcohol ingestion. Heavy snorers tend to hypoventilate during sleep, with associated increases in pulmonary and systemic blood pressures.[5348] Patients who snore should be considered as part of the spectrum of respiratory sleep disorders, with those with severe sleep apnea representing one extreme of this spectrum.

Sleep Patterns in Association with Other Conditions

Obesity-Hypoventilation Syndrome

Primary hypoventilation syndromes and the effects of obesity on pulmonary function are noted later in this chapter. The syndrome of severe obesity associated with hypoventilation (originally dubbed the Pickwickian syndrome after the obese somnolent boy named Fat Joe in the *Pickwick Papers* of Charles Dickens) consists of obesity, hypersomnolence, hypoventilation, and eventually secondary polycythemia and right heart failure. Only a minority of obese subjects develop sleep apnea, and an even smaller number fulfill the complete description of the obesity-hypoventilation syndrome.

Why certain obese individuals develop the syndrome, whereas others of similar weight do not, has been the subject of considerable inquiry. Such patients have reduced ventilatory responses to hypoxia and to CO_2.[154] Consequently, it has been suggested that an interaction between the mass loading effect of the obesity and abnormal chemical drives to breathe (or being in the lowest 5% of the distribution of chemical responsiveness) may be responsible for the syndrome. However, it is possible that the reduced drive to breathe is acquired secondarily to the hypoventilation rather than antedating the onset of obesity.

The obesity-hypoventilation syndrome represents an uncommon special case of sleep apnea. The current hypothesis for the combined syndrome is that obesity produces fatty infiltration of the soft tissues of the oropharynx; this results in obstructive sleep apnea when it occurs in conjunction with decreased upper airway patency and perhaps reduced ventilatory drive. The nocturnal hypoventilation occurring during episodes of sleep apnea blunts the chemical drive further, in a manner analogous to the hypoventilation syndrome that may develop in dwellers at high altitudes. The depressed ventilatory drive in turn leads to more profound hypoventilation, initially during sleep, but later also during the day. Pulmonary and systemic hypertension develop concurrently, culminating in right heart failure and occasionally in biventricular failure.

Sudden Infant Death Syndrome

There is increasing evidence that the sudden infant death syndrome (SIDS) should also be considered as part of the spectrum of respiratory sleep disorders. Many of the infants have autopsy findings consistent with preceding hypoventilation.[5349] Babies often develop periodic breathing during viral infections of the upper airways, and many SIDS victims have historical and pathologic evidence of such infections.[5350] Some infants resuscitated from prolonged apnea (which has been termed "near miss" sudden infant death syndrome) have abnormal breathing patterns during sleep and decreased CO_2 ventilatory responses.[5351] These findings suggest that prolonged apnea is the final event in at least some sudden infant deaths.

"Near miss" SIDS and SIDS cases are often found in familial clusters, and there is one report in which a sudden infant death occurred in a family in whom four other members also had significant respiratory sleep disorders.[5352] Schiffman and co-workers[5353] showed that parents of victims of the syndrome had reduced ventilatory responsiveness to hypercapnia and reduced compensatory response to added resistive respiratory loads when compared with parents of normal infants. However, Zwillich and his colleagues[5354] conducted a similar study but could find no evidence of reduced chemical drives in the parents of SIDS victims. Polysomnography has also been performed on a group of parents of SIDS victims, but no significant difference in breathing patterns as compared with normal parents was demonstrable.[5355] Thus, although there is evidence that SIDS is partly due to an abnormality in ventilatory control during sleep, there is no consistent test available to identify families at risk; the exact nature of the abnormality remains to be identified.

Chronic Obstructive Pulmonary Disease

Some data on sleep studies in patients with chronic airflow limitation are noted in Chapter 8; in this section, these are placed in the context of other data on sleep.

Sleep is the period of greatest physiologic disturbance in patients with chronic airflow limitation and as such is the time of greatest danger in these patients. In these persons, sleep aggravates gas exchange abnormalities, resulting in secondary pulmonary hypertension, cardiac arrhythmias, and abnormal sleep patterns. It has recently become apparent that these patients may demonstrate striking gas exchange abnormalities while asleep.[5357-5359] Sleep desaturation occurs in all sleep stages, with maximal desaturation occurring during REM sleep.[1139]

The reduced alveolar ventilation (which occurs in normal subjects), when superimposed on the other defects present in cases of severe airflow limitation, is found to be the major mechanism causing desaturation. The magnitude of the sleep desaturation is related to the chemical drive to breathe when awake,[1139] and desaturation may be reduced by chronic ventilatory stimulation by medroxyprogesterone therapy.[5360] Because many of these patients are hypoxemic when awake and at rest, their arterial oxygen tension is near the steep portion of the oxyhemoglobin dissociation curve; hence, a given decrease in alveolar ventilation results in a greater decrease in saturation than it would in normal subjects. The sleep desaturation may also be due to a worsening of ventilation/perfusion matching.[5361, 5362] This may come about as a result of sudden changes in cardiac output or as a result of the dissociation of diaphragmatic and intercostal activity that occurs during REM sleep,[5284] or the $\dot{V}/\dot{Q}$ distribution may be worsened by small decreases in minute volume.

The episodes of sleep desaturation in patients with chronic airflow limitation are associated with increases in pulmonary arterial pressure.[1244, 5358] The magnitude of this pulmonary hypertension depends on the duration and severity of the desaturation and on the responsiveness of the pulmonary vessels; it may be prevented by nocturnal low flow oxygen.[5364, 5365] Sleep desaturation is more marked in the chronic bronchitic (or Type B) category of patient.[5359] It has been postulated that these transient episodes of hypoxemia and pulmonary hypertension cause the sustained pulmonary hypertension characteristic of this group of patients.[3233] Ventricular arrhythmias are twice as common in these persons during the night than during the daytime.[5366] The available data suggest that sleep desaturation is responsible for some of the arrhythmias and that nocturnal oxygen reduces their frequency.[5367] It is customary to prescribe nocturnal oxygen therapy for patients whose arterial oxygen saturation falls below 75% during sleep. Patients should be suspected of having significant sleep hypoxemia if (1) their Pa_{O_2} when awake is less than 55 mm Hg, (2) their Pa_{O_2} is higher than this but they are obese, (3) their Pa_{CO_2} is higher than 45 mm Hg, or (4) they have evidence of polycythemia or right ventricular failure.

Patients with chronic airflow limitation tend to have "poor quality" sleep, with decreased sleep duration, less REM sleep, and frequent awakenings.[3269] The reasons for the sleep disturbance are not yet clearly defined, but it may be that the periods of nocturnal desaturation cause their sleep to become fragmented, with multiple arousals analogous to what occurs in the sleep apnea syndrome. Theophylline and its salts have been widely used in the treatment of chronic airflow obstruction. Although usually administered for their bronchodilator effect, their other pharmacologic properties might influence sleep disorders. Recent studies have shown that theophylline improves gas exchange during sleep, although total sleep time and sleep quality are reduced.[5368]

Asthma

As noted in Chapter 9, some patients with asthma experience nocturnal symptoms, particularly in the early hours of the morning. Monitoring the peak expiratory flow rates demonstrates a diurnal pattern in over 30% of asthmatics, with the lowest values at night.[5369] Nocturnal cough and wheezing may be the first signs of an exacerbation of asthma and by fragmenting sleep may result in significant daytime intellectual impairment. Moreover, deaths from asthma usually occur during the night, and patients with excessive diurnal variation are thought to be at increased risk of sudden death.[1367]

The etiology of the diurnal rhythm of asthma appears to be clearly linked to sleep, although it is probably multifactorial in origin. In a study of asthmatic shift workers, reduction of expiratory flow rates was found to be closely related to their time of sleep and not to solar time.[5370] Depriving asthmatics of sleep late into the night does not prevent nocturnal wheezing.[1528] It has been shown in animal studies that airway smooth muscle tone varies considerably during REM sleep,[5289] and patients wakened during this stage of sleep have been found to have a greater degree of airflow obstruction than when they are wakened during non-REM sleep.[5372] Asthmatic patients with nocturnal symptoms sleep badly, with less REM sleep and episodes of arterial oxygen desaturation.[5373] The severity of sleep desaturation is related to their awake arterial oxygen saturation and, consequently, is not usually as marked as that seen in patients with chronic bronchitis and emphysema. The degree of sleep desaturation has been shown to be unrelated to the changes in expiratory flow rates that occur during the night.[3412]

A circadian variation in the endogenous production of both corticosteroids[1546] and catecholamines[5374] coincides with the changes in airflow limitation. But administration of both beta-agonists and systemic corticosteroids, which are sufficient to abolish these natural diurnal fluctuations, fail to prevent nocturnal wheezing. It has been suggested that gastroesophageal reflux, which occurs more frequently at night, might be the mechanism of early morning bronchospasm,[1356] but changing nighttime posture does not affect the cyclic nature of asthma.[5375] At the present time, there is no convincing explanation for the phenomenon; it may result from the interaction of a number of factors, including reduced mucociliary transport, which, as noted in Chapter 3, falls during sleep in normal subjects.

Summary

When sleep studies were first reported, it was unclear whether they would prove important in more than a small fraction of cases and whether a routine facility, which is not a simple matter to establish, was required in major cen-

ters. It has been shown beyond doubt that abnormalities occurring during sleep constitute an important segment of thoracic medicine and that events important to the clinical condition of many patients occur during the night, when their physicians are usually asleep.

PRIMARY ALVEOLAR HYPOVENTILATION SYNDROMES AND CHRONIC HYPERVENTILATION

Primary Alveolar Hypoventilation Syndromes

These syndromes consist essentially of respiratory failure in patients with normal lungs and normal chest walls. In most individuals, there is normal conscious control of ventilation but failure of automatic control, particularly during sleep. Syndromes of alveolar hypoventilation throw light on the complexity of the factors that may underlie the development of respiratory failure in a wide variety of circumstances. Hypoventilation may occur in association with obesity (see later section) and as a consequence of obstructive sleep apnea (see earlier section). Cases of primary hypoventilation have now been carefully studied and well described.

In a review written in 1974, Solliday and his colleagues[215] analyzed 39 cases of primary alveolar hypoventilation in the literature up to that date. The criteria for this diagnosis are

- abnormal arterial blood gases
- normal ventilatory and gas exchange function
- reduced ventilatory response to CO_2
- absence of neuromuscular disease of the chest wall

A reduced ventilatory response to normocapnic hypoxia is commonly but not invariably present.

The cases described can be conveniently divided into two categories:

1. Patients with cerebral disorders or significant history of neurologic disease

Solliday noted that in the 39 patients he analyzed, nine had a history of encephalitis, five had mental retardation, two had a history of head injury, two had parkinsonism, and one each had had meningitis, poliomyelitis, syringomyelia, and a vascular aneurysm, leaving 17 without any such history. Cases similar to these in the literature include: a 32-year-old farmer with a history of severe illness at the age of 9 characterized by headache and somnolence[200] but with a normal EEG and neurologic examination; two cases of narcolepsy[207] with normal pulmonary function and exercise Pa_{O_2} but in whom the Pa_{O_2} fell as low as 44 mm Hg during apneic periods that lasted from 20 to 90 seconds; a 39-year-old man with encephalopathy and parkinsonism with a greatly reduced CO_2 response[214]; a 14-year-old boy with a hypothalamic disorder, obesity, retarded sexual development, a normal ventilatory response to CO_2 but an abnormal exercise response (since the Pa_{CO_2} rose significantly on exercise[202]); and a 15-year-old boy, not obese, with normal resting pulmonary function but an abnormal EEG over the frontal lobes whose oxygen saturation fell on exercise due to an abnormal ventilatory response, whose Pa_{CO_2} was recorded as high as 87 mm Hg,[199] and whose hematocrit was 67%.

Carroll[168] collected nine cases of hypoventilation due to brain disease. In a number of these cases, although the neurologic deficits were recognized, the respiratory component of the illness was missed and the secondary polycythemia was thought to be a primary condition. In many of these cases, sleep apnea may well have been present, but their description antedated recognition of the importance of that syndrome.

2. Patients without a history of cerebral disorder

These cases, though rare, form a very interesting group. Several children, as well as two infants,[206] have been described with primary alveolar hypoventilation. One 10-year-old boy, slightly obese but normally athletic, had no chemical drive to ventilation, as measured with CO_2, or hypoxia.[195] Both his parents had reduced responses to CO_2 and hypoxia. Another 10-year-old boy had hypoventilation during sleep, when his Pa_{O_2} fell to 44 mm Hg. A 14-year-old girl had a complete absence of chemical drive with severe sleep apnea, necessitating respirator support at night.[187] Her parents and a sister all had normal responses. A 15-year-old boy had episodes of respiratory failure and had no chemical drive, but his ventilatory response to exercise was normal.[192] Although he had normal resting pulmonary function tests, he went into respiratory failure when an acute respiratory infection developed. A patient with this syndrome, fully studied at the age of 12,

died at the age of 20 after an anesthetic in the hospital. At autopsy, there was right ventricular hypertrophy and intimal thickening of the small pulmonary arteries, but no structural abnormality could be found in the brain. In contrast, a 5-month-old child with sleep apnea and no CO_2 response, whose ventilation fell on 100% O_2 (and who was, therefore, thought to have strong peripheral chemoreceptor input but weak central drive), was found at autopsy not to have an external arcuate nucleus; this may be involved in central chemoreceptor activity.[211]

Deficient central chemoreceptor response possibly due to previous poliomyelitis, with an absent CO_2 response but a normal hypoxic response, was found in a 41-year-old non-obese man.[215] His pulmonary function was normal, and his resting Pa_{O_2} was about 65 mm Hg, rising at once to 91 mm Hg on voluntary hyperventilation. During sleep it fell to 52 mm Hg. Few measurements of $P_{0.1}$ have been recorded, but in a 65-year-old Greek farmer, whose Pa_{O_2} was 34 mm Hg and whose FEV_1 and DL_{CO} were slightly reduced, the ventilatory response to CO_2 was about 25% of normal. The ratio of change in $P_{0.1}$ to change of Pa_{CO_2} was only 10% of normal.[217]

Patients in whom central primary alveolar hypoventilation is present with some degree of chronic airflow obstruction pose difficult diagnostic problems, requiring careful and critical evaluation.[194, 200, 212] Farmer, Glenn, and Gee[186] reported on the use of a diaphragm pacemaker in a case of alveolar hypoventilation and noted that obstructive defects and abnormalities of chemical control of ventilation can either occur independently or coexist. Although this method of treatment may well be indicated in some cases, there is some risk that it may induce obstructive sleep apnea. Equally difficult cases are the rare instances of a neurologic disorder, such as acid maltase deficiency (noted in Chapter 22), leading to muscle weakness and complicated by a central hypoventilation syndrome,[198] and instances of unexplained central hypoventilation, sleep apnea, and muscle wasting.[213] In another complex case, not wholly explained, a 56-year-old diabetic man with cor pulmonale showed an initial Pa_{O_2} of 37 mm Hg.[2983] No diaphragmatic paralysis was present, but severe muscular weakness was combined with a lack of response to both hypercapnia and hypoxemia.

Many of the reported cases presented difficult diagnostic challenges to the physician. The possibility of making measurements of the ventilatory response to normocapnic hypoxia and normoxic hypercapnia has greatly enhanced understanding of complex variants of this syndrome. Such cases raise very interesting and relevant questions concerning the normal control of ventilation, questions that cannot at this time be completely resolved within the context of existing physiologic knowledge.

It seems likely, however, that neurologic abnormalities, whether developmental or acquired, will be found to occupy a prominent place in the etiology of most of these cases. It is to be expected that studies of respiratory pattern during sleep will throw new light on their classification and etiology. There is a genetic basis for individual ventilatory response to blood gas changes; if normocapnic hypoxic and normoxic hypercapnic ventilatory responses are measured in twins, it is found that there is a significant correlation between identical twin pairs for the hypoxic response but not for the hypercapnic response.[191] Non-identical twins do not show this correlation.

Chronic Hyperventilation

Chronic hyperventilation has been recognized as a distinct syndrome for many years. In a remarkable review with 117 references, Brashear[2984] alleged that it occurred in between 6 to 11% of the general patient population; this does not accord with our experience that such patients in whom chronic hyperventilation causes significant symptoms are rarely encountered. Cluff[4732] has discussed its treatment by physiotherapy. In the last edition of this book,[1] we pointed out that a chronic lowering of arterial HCO_3, rather than a single determination of Pa_{CO_2}, may be useful in diagnosis if symptoms suggest that chronic hyperventilation may be occurring. It seems possible that the prevalence of this condition may vary widely in different populations, but no systematic comparison seems to have been reported.

EFFECTS OF OBESITY

The literature on the effects of obesity was reviewed in 1980 by Luce.[160] Several authors have suggested categorization of the stages of obesity and associated hypoventilation syndromes[163, 165] and have described as many as 10 variants.[168] Possibly the picturesque description of the syndrome of the fat boy in the *Pickwick Papers*[1] has outlived its usefulness, although it undoubtedly did much to direct the attention of physicians to this entity. Comroe[163] wrote an entertaining review of the classification of obesity and hypoventilation syndromes. Obesity may be associated with alveolar hypoventilation or with sleep apnea or may occur without either of these complications; in individual cases, careful blood gas studies and sleep studies are required, as well as an assessment of the ventilatory response to CO_2 or hypoxia before the clinical situation can be precisely defined. The obesity-hypoventilation syndrome was discussed earlier.

Although the complete pathophysiology of obesity may not yet be completely known, the following components in the syndrome are important:

- increased mass of chest wall, leading to a reduction in its outward recoil
- increased mass of abdominal wall and contents
- reduced FRC and particularly ERV, especially when recumbent
- basal airway closure, with resultant fall in Pa_{O_2}
- aggravation of all the adverse factors during sleep or recumbency
- reduced ventilatory response to CO_2
- ? reduced ventilatory response to hypoxemia and hypercapnia
- ? fatty infiltration of respiratory muscles

Engel and Prefaut[2990] studied ventilation and perfusion distribution in eight supine normal subjects (who would no doubt have indignantly denied they were obese) and were able to show that the ratio of abdominal girth to height (which varied from 0.48 to 0.56) was related to ventilation distribution. The higher the ratio (and particularly if it exceeded 0.5), the more the closing capacity supine increased from its value when the subject was upright and the more airway closure occurred in dependent regions. Ventilation was particularly reduced in paradiaphragmatic regions, which, since regional blood flow was not affected, became regions of lowered $\dot{V}/\dot{Q}$ distribution. The more obese the subject, the greater the volume of lung involved in this process.

For descriptive purposes, it is helpful to categorize the changes found in obesity into three stages, as follows:

Stage 1. Patients are moderately obese, with a ratio of weight to height (kg/cm) of less than 1.0. In these subjects, lung mechanics are usually normal,[180] airway resistance is normal, and the subdivisions of lung volume show only a small reduction in ERV.[180] Arterial blood gases at this stage are usually normal at rest. DL_{CO} is normal or only slightly increased.

Stage 2. Patients are more severely obese, with a ratio of weight to height of more than 1.0. The lung and chest wall compliance fall as the weight progressively increases.[166] The arterial Pa_{O_2} falls several millimeters when the subject goes from a sitting to a supine position,[179] and the increase in $(A - a) D_{O_2}$ when recumbent can be shown to correlate with the difference between ERV and closing volume.[134, 173] The arterial Pa_{O_2} may increase as much as 18 mm Hg if a few deep breaths are taken.[172] The ratio of FRC to TLC falls from a normal value of about 54 to 40%.[172] These patients have airway closure in dependent lung zones,[181] which is enhanced when supine,[2990] and a steady decline of $\dot{V}/\dot{Q}$ ratio from apex to base; this distribution may return to normal if deep breaths are taken.[93, 175] The low $\dot{V}/\dot{Q}$ regions account for the hypoxemia.[161] In this group, polycythemia may be present, and more severe blood gas changes may be demonstrated during sleep.

In some patients in this group, the dynamic compliance may be found to be frequency-dependent, even in lifelong non-smokers.[180] Both chest wall and static lung compliance may fall, the latter particularly if the hematocrit is increased.[156] A reduction in total thoracic compliance has generally been found but is not invariable.[4763] Respiratory frequency may be increased at rest, with a decrease in expiratory time; hence, T_i/T_e may be increased.[4736] $P_{0.1}$ has also been found to be increased, with an increased response to hypoxia but a decreased response to hypercapnia.[4736] However, it is unclear from the literature whether or not the ventilatory responses to hypoxia and hypercapnia are normal. In studies in Denver,[154] a group of 10 obese subjects with a mean weight of 122 kilograms and an arterial Pa_{O_2} of 48 mm Hg were found to have a hypoxic drive of only one-sixth normal and a CO_2 response about one-third normal. Other investigators have reported a normal hypoxic response both before and after weight loss[155, 171] or a reduced hypoxic response with a normal CO_2 response in individual patients.[153] It has also been noted that the ventilatory response to exercise may be normal in obese subjects whose hypercapnic response is depressed.[4762]

Stage 3. This stage is characterized by the changes noted in stage 2, plus hypersomnia and periods of severe arterial desaturation during sleep. Chronic hypercapnia is usually present. Both hematocrit and diffusing capacity may be increased in this stage; the increase in diffusing capacity is probably related to the increased blood volume and increased resting cardiac output.

The common association of sleep disorders with the hypoventilation of obesity was first noted by Gastaut, Tassinari, and Duron in 1966[182] and has been confirmed by other workers.[157, 178, 4758] Total sleep periods may be longer than normal.[169] These changes are discussed in more detail in an earlier section in this chapter. In one obese subject,[174] radiographic studies showed that the obstruction was due to the pharyngeal wall being sucked against the tongue root during inspiratory efforts, with resulting complete obstruction.[174] In another obese patient with enlarged tonsils, the Pa_{CO_2} rose to 71 mm Hg during sleep.[159] The mortality among severely obese patients with sleep disorders may be considerable, even during hospitalization.[158] As noted previously, it is possible that in recumbent, severely obese persons the diaphragm may be overstretched, leading to hypoventilation.[4764] The relationship among obesity, sleep apnea, and alveolar hypoventilation is complex. The syndrome of sleep apnea and primary alveolar hypoventilation are discussed in earlier sections of this chapter. The syndrome of obesity, hypersomnia, and sleep disorders may occur in severe hypothyroidism.[170]

In a comparison between hypercapnic and normocapnic obese subjects, Rochester and Enson[156] found that in both groups lung and chest wall compliance was reduced, airway resistance was normal, and the ratio between closing volume and FRC was increased. The hypercapnic group had higher pulmonary artery pressures and a decrease in inspiratory muscle strength to between 60% and 70% of normal. Hurewitz, Susskind, and Harold[4761] studied five obese patients with a mean weight of 154 kilograms and assessed ventilation distribution by the use of ^{81m}Kr when the patients were in supine and lateral positions. All the subjects preferentially ventilated non-dependent lung in both right and left lateral positions. The authors suggested that mechanical factors affected regional ventilation distribution in these patients, and they noted that the relative contributions of airway closure and changes in chest wall configuration were complex. The ERV in the lateral position was midway between its highest value when sitting upright and its lowest when supine. Ray and his colleagues[2991] recently studied 43 very obese subjects, all of whom were non-smokers. They found that VC, TLC, and maximal voluntary ventilation (MVV) changed only with extreme obesity and ERV and DL_{CO} changed in proportion to it. In all patients in whom the weight/height ratio (kg/cm) exceeded 1.0, weight reduction was followed by increases in lung volumes and falls in DL_{CO}. In the heaviest group, the value of DL_{CO}/VA was 140% of its predicted value, and ERV was only 32% of its normal value. They concluded that the presence of obesity did not preclude the use of the usual predicted values. Arterial blood gases were not recorded in this series.

Freyschuss and Melcher[176] studied 30 obese subjects, among whom the men were 94% overweight and the women 111% overweight, performing sitting and supine bicycle exercise and treadmill walking. It was found that the line relating $\dot{V}O_2$ to work output was displaced upward, but its slope was normal. Weight loss was followed by a return of the line to normal. Whipp and Davis[4735] considered that exercise limitation in obesity was due to a combination of three factors:

1. Increased metabolic rate and $\dot{V}E$ for a given work level.
2. Increased metabolic cost of breathing because of chest wall effects and increased breathing frequency.
3. Increased work of breathing and possibly pulmonary atelectasis.

$\dot{V}E$ is usually increased in relation to $\dot{V}O_2$. French investigators studied 63 obese subjects both at rest and at exercise[164] and noted that the arterial Pa_{O_2} generally rose on exercise, with little change in the Pa_{CO_2}. In several subjects, pulmonary hypertension was found on exercise.

Several authors have documented the changes toward normal that occur if weight is lost. The most remarkable instance of this would appear to be a 19-year-old man whose weight dropped by 160 kilograms after ileal bypass surgery.[177] Values before and after weight loss were as follows:

	Before	After
f (respirations/min)	20	13
V_T (mL)	360	946
VC (liters)	2.4	4.9
ERV (liters)	0.14	1.5
RV (liters)	1.2	1.6
TLC (liters)	3.6	6.5
FEV_1 (liters)	1.9	3.4
Pa_{O_2}	48.5	85.0
Pa_{CO_2}	55.5	42.0
$DL_{CO}SB$	24.4	23.9

Although the ERV nearly always increases with loss of weight in the obese, the closing volume appears not to change.[173, 179]

EFFECTS OF PREGNANCY ON PULMONARY FUNCTION

In pregnancy, the FRC falls by about 18%, the vital capacity is unchanged, and there is a slight reduction in TLC.[219] In studies on 10 healthy non-smoking women during the course of pregnancy, Garrard, Littler, and Redman[185] found rather inconstant changes in lung volumes; however, they found a progressive rise in closing volume as a percentage of vital capacity as pregnancy advanced. Airway closure occurs closer to the FRC.[219] In another report of 20 pregnant women studied sitting and supine at the thirty-sixth week, airway closure occurred within the tidal volume range in 10 women when upright and in six when supine.[201] One might have expected more airway closure when supine, but the reasons for the finding were not evident. The close relationship between closing volume and FRC may explain the variability in arterial Pa_{O_2} noted in pregnancy. An increase in $(A - a) D_{O_2}$ has been reported.[4765] In contrast, the Pa_{CO_2} almost always falls a few millimeters as pregnancy progresses.[219] In studies of 38 pregnant women in the first and third trimesters, Italian investigators[4739] reported that the $\dot{V}E$ response to Pa_{CO_2} was increased and delivery was followed by an abrupt decrease in this parameter.

The single-breath diffusing capacity ($DL_{CO}SB$) rises during the first trimester and then slowly declines until about 26 weeks, with no change thereafter.[218] These changes do not appear to be explained by changes in hemoglobin or in alveolar volume. The dyspnea commonly noted during the first trimester is unexplained but possibly relates to the increase in cardiac output or to the respiratory muscles.

In one group of 20 healthy women studied when 38 weeks pregnant and again when 3 months postpartum,[2992] an acceleration of $\dot{V}O_2$, $\dot{V}CO_2$, and $\dot{V}E$ was observed in the first 90 seconds of exercise. Six minutes of 50 watts of exercise were performed on each occasion. The authors concluded that the lower extremity muscles contracted on more distended veins in pregnancy and this led to an increased volume of venous blood through the lungs, with a consequent rise in $\dot{V}O_2$, $\dot{V}CO_2$, and $\dot{V}E$. $\dot{V}E$ followed $\dot{V}CO_2$ very precisely. Sleep studies have shown that the frequency of apnea and hypopnea are reduced during pregnancy, possibly due to increased progesterone levels.[4765]

There are several reports of pregnancies in patients with lung diseases. Patients with chronic airflow obstruction show slight evidence of worsening,[183] whereas those with sarcoidosis show little change or some improvement. One hundred ninety-six deliveries in 80 women after pneumonectomy were uneventful.[220] One patient who was recovering from severe adult respiratory distress syndrome with a predicted FEV_1 of 33%, a predicted VC of 35%, and a predicted diffusing capacity of 50% had a normal pregnancy and delivery.[203] Patients with alveolar proteinosis[4742] and diffuse interstitial lung disease[4733] have also had successful deliveries.

EFFECT OF INVESTIGATIVE PROCEDURES ON LUNG FUNCTION

Anesthesia

Gelb, Southorn, and Rehder[225] in 1981 reviewed the literature on the effects of anesthesia on lung function. There is usually a reduction in FRC and a fall in static lung compliance. Lung recoil pressure may be increased. The mechanism of these changes is unclear, but they are probably not attributable to alveolar collapse. Changes in surfactant, alterations in chest wall shape and motion, and impairment of the phasic activity of the respiratory muscles have all been suggested. There is a decrease in the efficiency of gas exchange, shown by an increased $\dot{V}D_{physiol}/\dot{V}T$ ratio and an increased venous admixture component. The increased $\dot{V}/\dot{Q}$ inequality is due to a decreased uniformity of ventilation distribution. Positional studies during anesthesia in normal subjects were described in an earlier section.

Experiments on dogs have shown that anesthesia and controlled ventilation delay mucus clearance from the lung,[204] particularly from more peripheral zones. The effect was independent of the tidal volume used.

Pulmonary Function Tests

The effect of breathing through a mouthpiece in 18 asthmatics was to cause an increase in minute volume of 2.7 L/min.[2994] Also in asthmatics, performance of an FEV_1 may induce airflow limitation. Gimeno and associates[193] found a fall of FEV_1 from a mean of 2.53 liters to a mean of 2.09 liters in 14 asthma patients of mean age 21 years.[193] Subsequent studies indicated that the inspiratory part of the FEV maneuver was responsible for the increased airway obstruction.

Rodenstein, Mercenier, and Stanescu[4746] recently studied 14 untrained subjects during unrestrained breathing; they were connected to a spirometer with and without a noseclip during unrestrained mouth and nose breathing. They concluded that changes in breathing pattern, previously attributed to the measuring device used, were in fact due to shifts in breathing route from nasal to oral breathing. Routine pulmonary function testing has been reported to cause an increase in atrial premature beats without clinical consequence.[189] Unanesthetized arterial puncture does not, of itself, affect the level of arterial Pa_{CO_2}.[205]

Fiberoptic Bronchoscopy and Lavage

A recent report gave the results of a questionnaire of 40,000 bronchoscopies, 87% of which were by fiberoptic bronchoscope.[4768] Major complications (pneumothorax, hemorrhage, respiratory depression, vasovagal episodes, and pulmonary edema in order of frequency) occurred in 0.12%; the mortality rate was 0.04%. Transbronchial biopsy was associated with a major complication rate of 2.7% and a mortality rate of 0.12%. (The authors noted that major resuscitation equipment was often inadequate.) Adverse reactions to lidocaine were very rare; the mean dose used was 342 milligrams.

If no oxygen is used, bronchoscopy leads to a significant fall in Pa_{O_2}[4745]; oxygen should be started before the procedure and continued for 30 minutes after withdrawal of the bronchoscope. During bronchoscopy, the FEV_1 has been noted to fall to 50% of its initial value in a group of patients whose average initial value was only 1.8 liters.[4741]

Another review of 4595 bronchoscopies, of which 1146 were performed with a fiberoptic bronchoscope,[2992] reported complications in

0.3% of those done with a fiberoptic instrument. None of the complications was fatal, and most were related to the anesthesia.

Studies of blood gases during transnasal fiberoptic bronchoscopy in 11 patients, all of whom had an arterial Pa_{O_2} above 75 mm Hg, showed that some hypoxemia occurred as soon as the bronchoscope entered the respiratory tract. A mean fall of 16 mm Hg in Pa_{O_2} was observed after the procedure; the largest observed fall was of 40 mm Hg at 15 minutes, the actual Pa_{O_2} being 48 mm Hg. In all cases the Pa_{CO_2} fell slightly.[228]

Bronchoalveolar lavage has been reviewed by a committee that concluded it was an acceptably safe research procedure.[4196] It has been conducted on 21 patients with chronic obstructive lung disease, in whom the FEV_1 was 43% of predicted, without major adverse effect.[4751] In asthmatics, no lowering of FEV_1 occurred after the procedure,[4740] although in instances of diffuse interstitial lung disease, a fall of PEFR of 24% was noted.[4492]

Studies of lavage in 10 non-smoking normal persons showed that hypoxemia was induced by the procedure if air was breathed, with the Pa_{O_2} returning to normal an hour later.[2993] Regional ventilation measurements using ^{133}Xe showed that all of the subjects developed abnormalities in the lavaged lung that persisted for 6 to 8 hours; all of these disappeared within 24 hours. Lavage with saline at body temperature caused no change in TLC, whereas lavage with saline at room temperature caused a 20% reduction.[2993]

Bronchography

In patients with chronic airflow obstruction, bronchography may cause a mild and reversible worsening of airway obstruction.[184] In 14 patients studied before and after unilateral bronchography, the maximal fall of Pa_{O_2} was 13 mm Hg immediately after the procedure[222]; the $(A - a) D_{O_2}$ increased. Normal values were regained 4 hours after the procedure. Five of the patients studied were normal; seven had restrictive impairment; and two had chronic airflow obstruction. Bronchography can lead to severe airflow obstruction and bronchospasm, and the procedure is contraindicated in cases of severe asthma or advanced chronic airflow limitation.

Thoracoscopy

In eight cases of pleural effusion, 15 minutes of thoracoscopy used to establish the diagnosis led to a fall in Pa_{O_2} of 8 mm Hg; the procedure was well tolerated.[2995]

Open-Lung Biopsy

A recent report on 101 patients who had a open-lung biopsy[4428] noted that in 92 a definitive diagnosis was made. Four patients died, all with very severe disease. All of these four were hypoxemic, with very poor pulmonary function before the operation (in one fatal case, the preoperative DL_{CO} was 8% of predicted).

Thoracentesis

In nine patients, removal of 600 to 1800 milliliters of fluid from the pleural cavity was followed by an increase in FRC from 2.63 to 2.95 and a 400 milliliter increase in TLC. RV and VC were not affected,[188] but the Pa_{O_2} rose by an average of 6 mm Hg after the procedure. In 11 patients with effusions due to cardiac failure, Karotsky and his colleagues[229] found that in some the Pa_{O_2} rose; in others the Pa_{O_2} fell after the procedure—in one patient by as much as 22 mm Hg, decreasing from 85 mm Hg to 63 mm Hg. They recommended that oxygen should be administered during and after the procedure as a precautionary measure.

Light, Stansbury, and Brown[4766] studied the effects of therapeutic thoracentesis in 26 cases. Changes in FVC averaged 410 milliliters, with a mean fluid removal of 1.744 liters (range 800–4400 mL). In nine cases the DL_{CO} rose from 13.4 mL/min/mm Hg before thoracentesis to 14.1 mL/min/mm Hg after the procedure.

Others have noted the improved $\dot{V}/\dot{Q}$ distribution and reduction in $(A - a) D_{O_2}$ that may follow immediately after thoracentesis and may last for 24 hours.[2996] In occasional cases of chronic airflow limitation with pleural effusion, a type of "tamponade" of the lung may occur, which is dramatically relieved after thoracentesis.

Injection of MIAA (Labeled albumin)

Studies on one series of 13 patients at rest and on exercise before and 2 hours after this procedure showed no changes in $\dot{V}D_{physiol}/V_T$ or $(A - a) D_{O_2}$.[223] Another study of nine cases using the same protocol showed an increase of $(A - a) D_{O_2}$ on moderate exercise, with a fall in Pa_{CO_2}. The changes were small, however, the exercise arterial Pa_{O_2} falling from 84.4 mm Hg to 81.3 mm Hg and the $(A - a) D_{O_2}$ increasing from 21.6 mm Hg to 27.5 mm Hg.[221]

The hazard of the procedure in severe cases of pulmonary thromboembolic disease is well recognized,[190] and occasional fatal outcomes have been reported.

Lymphangiography

The procedure has, on occasion, been reported as causing acute adult respiratory distress syndrome.[226] In one patient, the arterial Pa_{O_2} was 38 mm Hg, rising to a normal value of 78 mm Hg 3 weeks later. In a case described by other authors,[224] the $(A - a) D_{O_2}$ rose from 17 mm Hg to 40 mm Hg 3 days after the procedure, returning to normal 10 days later. A fall in the DL_{CO} has been noted to occur. This procedure is clearly attended by increased risk in patients whose function is already compromised.

Laparoscopy

In 32 patients undergoing this procedure, the arterial Pa_{O_2} fell 5 mm Hg, but there was no change in spirometric values.[227] The effects were ascribed to possible microatelectases of basal areas of the lung adjacent to the diaphragm.

5

NORMAL PULMONARY FUNCTION

The real purpose of scientific method is to make sure Nature hasn't misled you into thinking you know something you don't actually know. There's not a mechanic or scientist or technician alive who hasn't suffered from that one so much that he's not instinctively on guard. That's the main reason why so much scientific and mechanical information sounds so dull and cautious. If you get careless or go romanticizing scientific information, giving it a flourish here and there, Nature will soon make a complete fool out of you. It does it often enough anyway even when you don't give it opportunities.[5268]

R. M. PIRSIG

INTRODUCTION

The physiologic basis of pulmonary function tests was described in Chapter 2. This chapter deals with normal results in healthy people.

During the past 15 years, there has been an enormous expansion of the data base on normal pulmonary function; more than 700 papers were found that dealt with some aspect of normal function. This volume of work has clarified differences between people of different ethnic origin and between smokers and non-smokers. A sufficient body of data has now been accumulated that predicted normal data can be expressed for non-smokers—which was not previously the case. Differences in results between smokers and non-smokers are discussed in the next chapter.

Definitions of normality and the appropriateness of different criteria have also been commented upon in the literature. When the question is a matter of interpretation in an individual case, it is discussed in the section "Pulmonary Function Tests in the Hospital"; the interpretation of data from population surveys is dis-

cussed in detail in the section on the uses of pulmonary function tests in epidemiology. The recent publication by a working group of the European Community for Coal and Steel[2884] brings together all published regression equations on normal subjects; it should be consulted by all those interested in normal values. Factors that influence the choice of routine methods of testing pulmonary function are discussed in the last section of this chapter.

VENTILATORY FUNCTION: LUNG VOLUMES: INDICES OF GAS DISTRIBUTION

The Forced Expired Volume in One Second (FEV$_1$) and Forced Vital Capacity (FVC)

Methodology

Early work on the development of this test was summarized in the second edition[1] and need not be repeated. Recent studies have included evaluations of the performance of different spirometers* and the development of ingenious calibration devices† and testing procedures.[1157, 2881, 2921] Correction of the record to BTPS has been shown to increase the error of the measurement.[3022] Several reports have commented on the standardization of spirometry.[2923, 2998, 3817, 3818] It is recognized that the commonest source of error is failure to record a complete FVC.[3819] Townsend has studied the effect of a spirometer leak on the measurements of FEV_1 and FVC and has shown that a leak of between 34 to 46 mL/sec causes a decrement of about 350 milliliters in FVC in normal individuals and a fall of 790 milliliters in those with chronic airflow limitation.[3814] There was no decrement in FEV_1, however. This source of error has a considerable effect on the FEV_1/FVC ratio.

The usefulness of having a printed record of the expiration is generally recognized,[241] and it is agreed that the judgment of a trained technician as to the suitability of an individual record is satisfactory.[483] The FVC is not different from the vital capacity measured slowly in normal subjects, but considerable differences between the two values may be found in some patients with chronic airflow obstruction. A significant correlation has been shown to exist between the difference between the slow vital capacity and the fast FVC in cases of lung disease and the FEV_1/FVC ratio.[430]

Because the FEV_1 is related to height and age and is slightly different between men and women of the same age and height, separate regresssion formulae are used for men and women. It does not appear that much is gained by using the cube of height rather than actual height in the prediction formula.[3192] In a recent study of 2454 white adults aged between 25 and 74 years, Dockery and his colleagues[3821] have suggested that standardizing the FEV_1 and FVC by dividing by the square of standing height may be preferable. It appears that prediction formulae using height may be extrapolated for use for individuals at the extremes of height without significant error.[3824]

Reproducibility

Nathan, Lebowitz, and Knudson[278] found that there were no significant differences between (1) the average of the best two of five measurements, (2) the average of the best two of the first three tests, (3) the best of five tests, and (4) the best of the first three tests in the measurements of the FVC and FEV_1. Tager and associates[316] suggested that the largest three of five acceptable tracings should be preferred to the last three of five tests, since in 83% of comparisons the variance of the last three was greater than the variance of the best three. Sorenson and his colleagues[432] have recently suggested that the "best test" is the simplest and most practical result to record, and others have preferred maxima to means.[327, 3815]

Most investigators find the FEV_1 to be very reproducible in normal subjects,[235, 351] the coefficient of variation for the FVC and FEV_1 being less than 5%[388, 578, 3052, 3816] and in some studies less than 3%.[246, 386, 3051] In one study of adolescents, the coefficient of variation of the FVC was 3.1% if three curves were recorded and 2.6% if five curves were used.[3068] Whitaker, Chinn, and Lee,[388] after a detailed analysis of repeated flow curves, concluded that three test measurements were usually adequate. They also provided a formula for the calculation of the percentage change between test sessions based on the "within-subject" coefficient of variation, the standard deviation of the test, and the number of blows at each test session. The effect of the diurnal rhythm on pulmonary function is detectable, but small, in normal subjects.[340] Standardization of the time of day the test was performed might be important, however, in therapeutic trials or in abnormal subjects.

Altitude affects the results of FEV_1 tests; normal prediction data for Salt Lake City at 1400 meters' altitude have been published.[429] A study of white males living at 3100 meters found no differences in FVC but indicated higher values for FEV_1 and MMFR than in people at sea level,[326] although the differences were not great.

Normal Data

The predicted values given in Tables 5–1 and 5–2 are derived from studies of Caucasians. The FVC and FEV_1 have been noted to be lower in Malaysian aboriginal people[258]; in West Pakistani workers in the United Kingdom[255] (whose values were similar to black people in the United States, being about 12% below that of Caucasians[254]); in healthy adults in Pakistan[244]; in a group of normal persons in Canton[238]; in Maori soldiers (compared with Caucasians,[323]

---

*See references 342, 434, 1157, 2876, 3030.
†See references 435, 438, 3049, 3062, 3075.

Table 5–1. AGE- AND HEIGHT-DEPENDENT NORMAL VALUES FOR PULMONARY FUNCTION TESTS: NON-SMOKING MEN

1	2	3	4	5	6	7	8	9	10	11	12	13	14	15	16	17
									$FEF_{25-75\%}$				$DL_{CO}SB$	$DL_{CO}SS$	F_{CO}	
											$\dot{V}max_{50\%}$				(resp/min)	
HT (cm)	Age (yr)	VC (L)	FRC (L)	RV (L)	TLC (L)	FVC (L)	FEV_1 (L)	FEV/FVC%	VC (L/sec) A	B	(L/sec)	PEFR (L/sec)	(mL/min/mm Hg)	(mL/min/mm Hg)	10	30
155	20	4.07	2.73	1.04	5.11	4.22	3.74	87.4	4.35	4.85	4.90	8.82	28.90	23.8	0.52	0.29
	30	3.81	2.82	1.24	5.03	4.01	3.49	85.8	4.16	4.42	4.59	8.39	26.28	21.0	0.51	0.29
	40	3.55	2.91	1.44	4.99	3.79	3.25	84.3	3.78	3.99	4.28	7.96	23.66	18.2	0.50	0.28
	50	3.29	3.00	1.64	4.93	3.58	3.01	82.8	3.40	3.56	3.97	7.53	21.04	15.4	0.49	0.27
	60	3.03	3.09	1.84	4.87	3.37	2.76	81.3	3.02	3.13	3.66	7.10	18.42	12.6	0.49	0.26
	70	2.77	3.18	2.04	4.81	3.15	2.52	79.7	2.64	2.70	3.35	6.67	15.80	9.8	0.48	0.25
160	20	4.36	2.85	1.15	5.51	4.52	3.95	86.7	4.64	4.94	5.09	9.13	30.83	24.1	0.54	0.31
	30	4.10	2.94	1.35	5.45	4.31	3.70	85.2	4.26	4.51	4.78	8.70	28.21	21.3	0.53	0.30
	40	3.84	3.03	1.55	5.39	4.09	3.46	83.7	3.88	4.08	4.47	8.27	25.59	18.6	0.52	0.29
	50	3.58	3.12	1.75	5.33	3.88	3.21	82.1	3.50	3.65	4.16	7.84	22.97	15.8	0.51	0.28
	60	3.32	3.21	1.95	5.27	3.67	2.97	80.6	3.12	3.22	3.85	7.41	20.35	13.0	0.50	0.28
	70	3.06	3.30	2.15	5.21	3.45	2.73	79.1	2.74	2.79	3.54	6.98	17.73	10.1	0.49	0.27
165	20	4.64	2.97	1.25	5.89	4.82	4.15	86.1	4.74	5.04	5.28	9.44	32.76	24.5	0.55	0.33
	30	4.38	3.06	1.45	5.83	4.61	3.91	84.5	4.36	4.61	4.97	9.01	30.14	21.7	0.54	0.32
	40	4.12	3.15	1.65	5.77	4.39	3.66	83.0	3.98	4.18	4.66	8.58	27.52	18.9	0.53	0.31
	50	3.86	3.24	1.85	5.71	4.18	3.42	81.5	3.60	3.75	4.35	8.15	24.90	16.1	0.53	0.30
	60	3.60	3.33	2.05	5.65	3.97	3.18	80.0	3.22	3.32	4.04	7.72	22.28	13.3	0.52	0.29
	70	3.34	3.42	2.25	5.59	3.75	2.93	78.4	2.84	2.89	3.73	7.29	19.66	10.6	0.51	0.28
170	20	4.93	3.08	1.36	6.29	5.12	4.36	85.4	4.84	5.14	5.47	9.74	34.69	24.9	0.57	0.34
	30	4.67	3.17	1.56	6.23	4.91	4.12	83.9	4.46	4.71	5.16	9.31	32.07	22.1	0.56	0.33
	40	4.41	3.26	1.76	6.17	4.69	3.87	82.4	4.08	4.28	4.85	8.88	29.45	19.3	0.55	0.32
	50	4.15	3.35	1.96	6.11	4.48	3.63	80.8	3.70	3.85	4.54	8.45	26.83	16.5	0.54	0.31
	60	3.89	3.44	2.16	6.05	4.27	3.38	79.3	3.32	3.42	4.23	8.02	24.21	13.7	0.53	0.31
	70	3.63	3.53	2.36	5.99	4.05	3.14	77.8	2.94	2.99	3.92	7.59	21.59	10.9	0.52	0.30
175	20	5.22	3.20	1.46	6.68	5.42	4.57	84.8	4.94	5.23	5.66	10.05	36.62	25.2	0.58	0.36
	30	4.96	3.29	1.66	6.62	5.21	4.32	83.2	4.56	4.80	5.35	9.62	34.00	22.4	0.57	0.35
	40	4.70	3.38	1.86	6.56	4.99	4.08	81.7	4.18	4.37	5.04	9.19	31.38	19.6	0.56	0.34
	50	4.44	3.47	2.06	6.50	4.78	3.84	80.2	3.80	3.94	4.73	8.76	28.76	16.9	0.56	0.33
	60	4.18	3.56	2.26	6.44	4.57	3.59	78.7	3.42	3.51	4.42	8.33	26.14	14.1	0.55	0.32
	70	3.92	3.65	2.46	6.38	4.05	3.35	77.2	3.04	3.08	4.11	7.90	23.52	11.3	0.54	0.31
180	20	5.51	3.32	1.57	7.08	5.72	4.77	84.1	5.04	5.33	5.85	10.36	38.55	25.6	0.60	0.37
	30	5.25	3.41	1.77	7.02	5.51	4.53	82.6	4.66	4.90	5.54	9.93	35.93	22.8	0.59	0.36
	40	4.99	3.50	1.97	6.96	5.29	4.29	81.1	4.28	4.47	5.23	9.50	33.31	20.0	0.58	0.35
	50	4.73	3.59	2.17	6.90	5.08	4.04	79.5	3.90	4.04	4.92	9.07	30.69	17.2	0.57	0.35
	60	4.47	3.68	2.37	6.84	4.87	3.80	78.0	3.52	3.61	4.61	8.64	28.07	14.2	0.56	0.34
	70	4.21	3.77	2.57	6.78	4.65	3.55	76.5	3.14	3.18	4.30	8.21	25.45	11.6	0.55	0.33
185	20	5.80	3.44	1.67	7.47	6.02	4.98	83.5	5.15	5.43	6.04	10.67	40.48	25.9	0.61	0.39
	30	5.54	3.53	1.87	7.41	5.81	4.74	81.9	4.77	5.00	5.73	10.24	37.86	23.2	0.60	0.38
	40	5.28	3.62	2.07	7.35	5.59	4.49	80.4	4.39	4.57	5.42	9.81	35.24	20.4	0.59	0.37
	50	5.02	3.71	2.27	7.29	5.38	4.25	78.9	4.01	4.14	5.11	9.38	32.62	17.6	0.59	0.36
	60	4.76	3.80	2.47	7.23	5.17	4.01	77.4	3.63	3.71	4.80	8.85	30.00	14.8	0.58	0.35
	70	4.50	3.89	2.67	7.17	4.95	3.76	75.9	3.25	3.28	4.49	8.52	27.38	12.0	0.57	0.34

Table 5–2. AGE- AND HEIGHT-DEPENDENT NORMAL VALUES FOR PULMONARY FUNCTION TESTS: NON-SMOKING WOMEN

1	2	3	4	5	6	7	8	9	10	11	12	13	14	15	16	17
									FEF 25-75%						F_{CO}	
HT (cm)	Age (yr)	VC (L)	FRC (L)	RV (L)	TLC (L)	FVC (L)	FEV_1 (L)	FEV/FVC%	VC (L/sec) A	B	$\dot{V}max_{50\%}$ (L/sec)	PEFR (L/sec)	$DL_{CO}SB$ (mL/min/mm Hg)	$DL_{CO}SS$ (mL/min/mm Hg)	(resp/min) 10	30
145	20	3.01	2.28	0.95	3.96	3.09	2.87	92.9	3.99	4.08	4.21	6.26	24.25	20.7	0.59	0.40
	30	2.75	2.29	1.08	3.83	2.88	2.62	90.9	3.53	3.74	3.96	5.96	22.75	18.2	0.58	0.39
	40	2.49	2.30	1.21	3.70	2.67	2.37	88.8	3.07	3.40	3.71	5.66	21.25	15.7	0.57	0.37
	50	2.23	2.31	1.34	3.57	2.46	2.12	86.2	2.61	3.06	3.46	5.36	19.75	13.2	0.56	0.36
	60	1.97	2.32	1.47	3.44	2.25	1.87	83.1	2.15	2.72	3.21	5.06	18.25	10.7	0.55	0.34
	70	1.71	2.33	1.60	3.31	2.04	1.62	79.4	1.69	2.38	2.96	4.76	16.75	8.2	0.54	0.32
150	20	3.23	2.39	1.04	4.27	3.34	3.04	91.3	4.07	4.14	4.33	6.54	24.80	21.1	0.58	0.39
	30	2.97	2.40	1.17	4.14	3.13	2.79	88.8	3.61	3.80	4.08	6.24	23.30	18.6	0.57	0.38
	40	2.72	2.41	1.30	4.02	2.91	2.53	86.2	3.15	3.46	3.83	5.94	21.80	16.0	0.56	0.36
	50	2.45	2.42	1.43	3.88	2.69	2.28	83.7	2.69	3.12	3.59	5.64	19.75	13.5	0.55	0.35
	60	2.19	2.43	1.56	3.75	2.48	2.02	81.2	2.23	2.78	3.34	5.34	18.25	11.0	0.54	0.34
	70	1.93	2.44	1.69	3.62	2.26	1.77	78.7	1.77	2.44	3.09	5.04	17.30	8.5	0.53	0.32
155	20	3.46	2.51	1.13	4.59	3.59	3.21	90.3	4.15	4.20	4.46	6.81	25.35	21.5	0.58	0.38
	30	3.20	2.52	1.26	4.46	3.37	2.96	87.8	3.69	3.86	4.21	6.51	23.85	18.9	0.57	0.36
	40	2.94	2.53	1.39	4.33	3.16	2.70	85.2	3.23	3.52	3.96	6.21	22.35	16.4	0.55	0.35
	50	2.68	2.54	1.52	4.20	2.94	2.45	82.7	2.77	3.18	3.71	5.91	20.85	13.9	0.54	0.34
	60	2.42	2.55	1.65	4.07	2.72	2.19	80.2	2.31	2.84	3.46	5.61	19.35	11.4	0.53	0.33
	70	2.16	2.56	1.78	3.94	2.51	1.94	77.7	1.85	2.50	3.21	5.31	17.85	8.9	0.52	0.31
160	20	3.68	2.62	1.22	4.90	3.83	3.38	89.3	4.23	4.26	4.58	7.09	25.90	21.9	0.57	0.37
	30	3.42	2.63	1.35	4.77	3.62	3.13	86.7	3.77	3.92	4.33	6.79	24.40	19.4	0.56	0.36
	40	3.16	2.64	1.48	4.64	3.40	2.87	84.2	3.31	3.58	4.08	6.49	22.90	16.8	0.55	0.34
	50	2.90	2.65	1.61	4.51	3.19	2.62	81.7	2.85	3.24	3.83	6.19	21.40	14.3	0.53	0.33
	60	2.64	2.66	1.74	4.38	2.97	2.36	79.2	2.39	2.90	3.58	5.89	19.90	11.8	0.52	0.32
	70	2.38	2.67	1.87	4.25	2.75	2.11	76.7	1.93	2.56	3.33	5.59	18.40	9.2	0.51	0.31
165	20	3.90	2.73	1.31	5.21	4.08	3.55	88.3	4.30	4.33	4.70	7.36	26.45	22.2	0.56	0.36
	30	3.64	2.74	1.44	5.08	3.86	3.30	85.7	3.84	3.99	4.45	7.06	24.95	19.7	0.55	0.35
	40	3.38	2.75	1.57	4.95	3.65	3.05	83.2	3.38	3.65	4.20	6.76	23.45	17.2	0.54	0.34
	50	3.12	2.76	1.70	4.82	3.43	2.79	80.7	2.92	3.31	3.95	6.46	21.95	14.6	0.53	0.32
	60	2.86	2.77	1.83	4.69	3.22	2.53	78.2	2.46	2.97	3.70	6.16	20.45	12.1	0.51	0.31
	70	2.60	2.78	1.96	4.56	3.00	2.28	75.7	2.00	2.63	3.45	5.86	18.95	9.6	0.50	0.30
170	20	4.12	2.84	1.40	5.52	4.32	3.73	87.2	4.38	4.39	4.82	7.64	27.00	22.6	0.56	0.35
	30	3.86	2.85	1.53	5.39	4.11	3.47	84.7	3.92	4.05	4.57	7.34	25.50	20.1	0.54	0.34
	40	3.60	2.86	1.66	5.26	3.89	3.22	82.2	3.46	3.71	4.32	7.04	24.00	17.5	0.53	0.33
	50	3.34	2.87	1.79	5.13	3.68	2.96	79.7	3.00	3.37	4.07	6.74	22.50	15.0	0.52	0.32
	60	3.08	2.88	1.92	5.00	3.46	2.71	77.2	2.54	3.03	3.82	6.44	21.00	12.5	0.51	0.30
	70	2.82	2.89	2.05	4.87	3.24	2.45	74.7	2.08	2.69	3.57	6.14	19.50	9.9	0.49	0.29
175	20	4.34	2.96	1.49	5.83	4.57	3.90	86.2	4.46	4.45	4.95	7.91	27.55	23.0	0.55	0.35
	30	4.08	2.97	1.62	5.70	4.35	3.64	83.7	4.00	4.11	4.70	7.61	26.05	20.5	0.54	0.33
	40	3.82	2.98	1.75	5.57	4.14	3.39	81.2	3.54	3.77	4.45	7.32	24.55	17.9	0.52	0.32
	50	3.56	2.99	1.88	5.44	3.92	3.13	78.7	3.08	3.43	4.20	7.02	23.05	15.4	0.51	0.31
	60	3.30	3.00	2.01	5.31	3.71	2.88	76.2	2.62	3.09	3.95	6.72	21.55	12.9	0.50	0.30
	70	3.04	3.01	2.14	5.18	3.49	2.62	73.6	2.16	2.75	3.70	6.42	20.05	10.2	0.49	0.28

between whom the FEV_1 difference was 8%); and in Sudanese and Tanzanian people.[336] Men in North India had slightly lower values than Caucasian men but higher than these from South India.[447] Ethiopian women have lower values than Caucasian women but higher than those in Africans, Chinese, and Indians.[3820]

Prediction formulae have been derived for African and Indian adults in Guyana[307] and for Israelis.[262, 5044] The prediction formulae for Japanese adults are not different from those for Caucasians when the difference in height is allowed for.[287] In New Guinea, the highlanders have values that approximate European data, but lower values are found in coastal dwellers.[302] West African women have lower values for FEV_1 and FVC than Caucasian women.[3072] Studies on blacks in the United States have shown that the FEV_1 as a function of total lung capacity (TLC) is the same as in whites, although TLC, residual volume (RV), VC, and FEV_1 are all lower by about 12%.[2541] In one study it was found that the differences were greatest at the age of 25 and considerably less if 55-year-old age groups were compared.[273] By comparison with all these findings, a group of 139 adult Eskimos and 57 children living at Igloolik (latitude 60°20′ North) had values for FVC and FEV_1 that were higher than predicted values for Caucasians.[376] Most ethnic differences may depend on a different trunk length to body height ratio.

A study of 127 monozygotic and 141 dizygotic sets of twins aged 42 to 56 years showed significantly similar values for FEV_1 and FVC when smoking had been taken into account.[3010] Of interest is a recent study of twins from Japan,[3885] which found more similar flow curves and single-breath nitrogen (SBN_2/L) data between monozygotic than dizygotic twins; this demonstrates the influence of genetic factors on these function test parameters. There is also evidence that individual differences in FEV_1 may be explicable by different lung and airway geometry (dysynapsis)[3059, 3850] and by differences in tracheal diameter.[3849] In studies of normal persons, evidence has been found that another factor might be the relative predominance of fast-twitch muscle fibers.[3057, 3822] There has recently been convincing evidence that the expiratory flow curves are significantly different between boys and girls, probably reflecting different patterns of lung growth.[3823]

It is the very low coefficient of variation of the FEV_1 (3%), together with its ease of measurement, that accounts for its dominant place in pulmonary function testing.

Measurements of Expiratory Flow Rate and Flow-Volume Curves

In one study using computer-analyzed data, as many as 31 variables were measured from each recorded curve.[348] There are many studies that have attempted to assess the relative usefulness of measurements of flow over segments of the curve, measurements of flow at specific percentages of the vital capacity, and measurements of the time over which specific volume changes occur. The following sections provide no more than an introduction to a very extensive bibliography on this topic. It is useful to recognize that these data lead to two general conclusions: first, measurements of flow or time of the middle or terminal part of the flow-volume curve are generally more sensitive in detecting slight airflow differences between smokers and non-smokers than the overall FEV_1[305] (at least in restricted populations and under ideal testing circumstances); and second, the farther down the expiratory curve that measurements are made, the greater is the coefficient of variation[351] by comparison with that for the FEV_1.[386, 388] Measurements of flow at specific volumes include FEF_{25-75}, FEF_{75-85}, $\dot{V}max_{50\%}VC$, $\dot{V}max_{75\%}VC$, and so forth.

The first such measurement to be widely studied was the FEF_{25-75}, originally termed the maximal midexpiratory flow rate (MMFR).[1] This measurement is closely related to the $\dot{V}max_{50\%}VC$ by the following formula[399]:

$$FEF_{25-75} = 0.91 \times \dot{V}max_{50\%}VC$$

The reproducibility of the two tests is similar,[351] the coefficient of variation within individuals being at least 6% or nearly twice that of the FEV_1.[386, 578] Coefficients of variation for the $\dot{V}max_{50\%}VC$ vary between 6% and 8.7%.[3051, 3063]

The FEF_{25-75} is highly predictable from the VC and FEV_1, and the authors of one study of 2728 subjects[300] concluded that the FEF_{25-75} was redundant as a parameter for screening procedures but noted that their finding "does not necessarily detract from its usefulness as a relatively independent measurement in quantitating established airway obstruction." The FEF_{25-75} is also highly predictable from the FEV/FVC ratio.[300] It is noted later that there is considerable individual variation in the FEF_{25-75}, the lower limit of normal (2 SD) being almost 50% of the mean normal value.

In the previous edition of this book,[1] we recommended that the FEF_{25-75} be computed in addition to the FEV_1 because in the days of calculating each individual record by hand, it represented a useful check on the FEV_1, and also because in certain populations the FEF_{25-75} as a mean value was lower in respect to predicted values than the FEV_1. With automated calculation, the first requirement is not needed and the greater variability of the FEF_{25-75} as compared with the FEV_1 offsets the advantage in sensitivity. This question cannot be considered to be completely resolved, however, because there is recent evidence that the FEF_{25-75} may be a more sensitive indicator of the presence of morphologic change in the lung than the FEV_1.[353] The FEF_{25-75} is as sensitive as the FEV/FVC ratio in detecting abnormality (or is possibly slightly more sensitive) but is unsatisfactory in quantifying change in it. Thus, after bronchodilator administration, the FVC and FEV_1 may increase, but the FEF_{25-75} may be unchanged because the measurement being compared is made on the two very different flow volume curves. No test depending on the FVC is entirely satisfactory for quantifying the degree of abnormality; the measurements of terminal flow curve velocity are all influenced by the completion of the FVC.

The interpretation of data from survey studies is discussed below; data on individuals can be interpreted only in terms of probability of abnormality. In connection with the predicted normal FEF_{25-75} values given in column 10 of Table 5–1, the following data from Miller and associates[341] are of interest (see table at the bottom of this page).

In analyses of the same data, the authors concluded that the 75% prediction level was more useful than using the 95% confidence limit (calculated by multiplying the standard error of the estimate by 1.65) as an indicator of abnormality.[325] Knudson and Lebowitz[573] gave values for the predicted per cent value of FEF_{25-75} above which 95% of asymptomatic non-smokers

fall, as follows:

	Age: 16–35	Age: >36
Men	66.6% predicted	56.2% predicted
Women	63.6% predicted	57.2% predicted

The general problem of interpreting tests of different aspects of function in individual cases is discussed in a later section.

Some authors have stressed that the FEF_{75-85}, the more terminal part of the curve, might be useful for screening studies,[325] although the coefficient of variation of the $\dot{V}max_{75\%}VC$ was noted to be 16% by others.[388] In another population survey, the $\dot{V}max_{75\%}VC$ appeared to be more sensitive than the FEV_1 in older age groups, but not in younger, as an indicator of abnormality.[317]

Normal findings in different populations have been published.* Results of measurement of the $\dot{V}max_{50\%}VC$ in a population sample of 3115 people in Tucson, Arizona,[320] which were somewhat higher than previous data, have been the subject of subsequent discussion in the literature.[433] Table 5–1 shows two sets of data for the predicted values of FEF_{25-75}. Some authors stress the fact that the maximal expiratory flow volume (MEFV) curve is best expressed in terms of absolute lung volume.[301] Others have suggested that the area under the MEFV curve should be calculated.[472]

Analyses of Time Components

The simplest measurement of forced expiratory time (FET) is made with a stethoscope and stopwatch. Unfortunately, this has a coefficient of variation of 25% within subjects and is therefore unsuitable for use.[249] Measurements using more sophisticated instrumentation are not much better,[409] but it has been suggested that the ratio of FVC to FET may be useful.[409] The time for forced expiration of the volume FEF_{25-75} has been studied in a small group of

*See references 296, 325, 341, 351, 392, 425, 476, 483.

Age (yr)		Height (inches)					
		63	67	69	71	73	78
20	Predicted	4.65	4.82	4.91	5.00	5.09	5.30
	75% of predicted	3.49	3.62	3.68	3.75	3.82	3.98
	95% confidence limit	2.82	3.01	3.10	3.19	3.27	3.48
40	Predicted	3.73	3.91	4.00	4.08	4.17	4.30
	75% of predicted	2.80	2.93	3.00	3.06	3.13	3.29
	95% confidence limit	1.91	2.10	2.19	2.27	2.36	2.57

FEF_{25-75} (L/sec): Non-smoking Men

normal subjects[305]; comparison with 14 patients with chronic airflow obstruction suggested that this measurement was more highly correlated with specific conductance than was the FEV_1, FEV/FVC%, or FEF_{25-75}.[305]

The "effective time" (t_{eff}) has been calculated by dividing the area under the forced expiratory spirogram by the forced VC; this index has been claimed to be more sensitive than the FEV/FVC ratio in detecting abnormality.[239] A "partial effective time" has been computed by calculating the time for each 10% decrement of volume from TLC to RV.[234] In a study of 51 asthmatic children,[240] the mean transit time was significantly more sensitive in detecting abnormality than conventional indices but was no more sensitive in detecting change in airflow obstruction after salbutamol was given.

Permutt and Menkes[3070] have contributed a useful discussion of the technique of moment analysis of the spirogram. Miller and Pincock[348] have noted that if the spirogram is to be truncated for moment analysis, this should be done with respect to volume and not time. They suggest that the power of the moment ratio is maximal with truncation at 85% of the FVC and that either this or the ratio at 90% FVC might be the best measurement. Pride, Osmanliev, and Davies[398] discussed the topic of moment analysis and suggested that the square root of the second moment might be more sensitive than the FEV_1/FVC%. The first of these authors contributed a useful editorial in 1979 entitled "Analysis of forced expiration—a return to the recording spirometer?"[241] Jansen and his colleagues[583] concluded that analysis of the slope ratios of the forced expirogram was less useful than moment analysis in the detection of slight abnormalities in cigarette smokers.

It seems clear that time domain analyses[3832] of the spirogram involve the same problem as the measurements of flows at low lung volumes—the greater the influence of data collected at low lung volumes on the result, the more "sensitive" and the less reproducible are the indices. There may also be a major artifact in moment analysis due to gas compression, which the spirometer does not measure. The distortion of shape of the MEFV curve due to gas compression is greatest at low lung volumes, thereby enhancing its effect on moment analysis.

Osmanliev, Davies, and Pride have recently reviewed this method and the results obtained by studying 53 non-smoking men and 149 smokers.[3825] They showed that the square root of the second moment was slightly increased in smokers, without any abnormality in FEV_1/FVC ratio. They concluded by noting that "its usefulness in comparison with other available tests remains to be established." This paper was discussed in subsequent correspondence in the journal[3884] in which it was emphasized that errors in technique invalidated many of the findings; these errors included those due to comparing "time truncated" moments from different spirograms as well as errors due to cooling. However, the correspondence did not entirely resolve these issues. Using these methods, others[3832] have found evidence of abnormalities in smokers before the FEV_1 is abnormal. These findings are discussed in Chapter 6.

Peak Expiratory Flow Measurements

The peak expiratory flow rate (PEFR) can be measured by handy portable instruments that can be lent to patients and used by them in their homes. For survey purposes, the Peak Flow Gauge is as good as the less robust Peak Flow Meter,[251, 345] and the difference between the two instruments is less than 10%.[345] Application of a device to calibrate peak flow meters achieved a coefficient of variation of 2% in simulated PEFR trials.[3075]

In normal subjects, the coefficient of variation of the PEFR in different individuals has been found to vary between 2% and 14%.[3052] However, it has recently been noted that it is possible to produce deliberate errors using the miniature Wright Peak Flow Meter.[3826] Nigerians[259] and aboriginal people[258] have lower values for PEFR than do Caucasians. In studies of 37 asthmatic and 11 normal children using the Wright Peak Flow Meter, the average of the best three of 10 expirations was found to be the best index.[422] For adults, the regression of peak flow values with respect to age and height has been published,[338] and the resulting predicted data are given in Tables 5–1 and 5–2.

In studies of asthmatics, it has been shown that there is a significant correlation between PEFR and Pa_{O_2}, and it was concluded that the Pa_{O_2} was normal if the PEFR was 40% of the predicted value or greater.[346] As noted in Chapter 19, the ratio of FEV_1 to PEFR has been used to detect upper airway obstruction.[337]

Respiratory Muscle Force

Tests of respiratory muscle force and fatigue are described in detail in Chapter 22. Measurements of respiratory pressures in 924 healthy Caucasians between 13 and 35 years of age by Leech and colleagues[2864] gave the following mean data:

	Males			
Age (yr)	17–20	21–25	26–30	31–35
Number of subjects	77	54	90	108
PE_{max} (cm H_2O)	133	163	157	161
SD	41	37	41	32
PI_{max} (cm H_2O)	115	121	112	111
SD	38	32	42	34

	Females			
Age (yr)	15–20	21–25	26–30	31–35
Number of subjects	145	138	130	75
PE_{max} (cm H_2O)	95	95	93	92
SD	33	32	35	31
PI_{max} (cm H_2O)	80	70	65	66
SD	27	27	25	29

These authors noted that after taking height into consideration, respiratory pressures were the main determinants of FVC, FEV_1, and PEFR in both men and women, with age having no consistent effect within the span of age groups studied. Braun, Arora, and Rochester,[3023] in a comparison of maximal respiratory pressures in normal persons and patients with muscle weakness, reported similar values. Data and regression equations on 370 Caucasian children and adults have been published[3827]; another study of boys and girls found a coefficient of variation of about 10% in this measurement.[3828] Other data on normal values have been reported recently.[3829]

The maximal inspiratory and expiratory pressures recorded at the mouth are not correlated with static lung volumes.[426] The maximal inspiratory pressure is best correlated with the forced inspiratory volume in one second (FIV_1) (r value of 0.737 in 236 subjects[431]). It has also been shown that the use of the maximal inspiratory pressure improves the prediction of the relationship between the maximal voluntary ventilation and the FEV_1.[474]

Flow Curves on Helium/O_2 Mixtures and Air

Bonsignore and his colleagues[5412] found coefficients of variation of 5.3% for $\dot{V}max_{50\%}$ in air, 7.0% for $\dot{V}max_{50\%}$ of helium/oxygen, and 25% for the difference between the two flow measurements. While other authors have reported similarly high coefficients of variation for this measurement[576] (as high as 31%[3063]), it has been used to measure changes in small airway function after influenza infection[574] and to detect differences between smokers and non-smokers.[581] Standardization to TLC should be used as a reference point,[486] and each laboratory has to establish its own criteria of normality.[473] Even when observing all precautions, their variability makes the use of these tests in longitudinal studies difficult to evaluate.[414] Comparative studies of expiratory flow curves using helium/oxygen mixtures or SF_6/oxygen mixtures in patients with lung disease did not demonstrate any improvement in discrimination.[235]

The isoflow point between helium/O_2 and air has been used as an indication of small airway abnormality (V_{isoV}). Although this test does reflect changes in small airways,[638] its usefulness is also severely limited by a coefficient of variation found to be as high as 65.2% by one group of authors[3063] and above 100% by another.[3051]

Knudson and Schroter[3060] re-examined the basis of expiratory flow curves using helium or air and concluded that they were of little value as tests of peripheral airway function. MacNee and his colleagues,[3024] in studies of normal subjects and patients with chronic airflow limitation, concluded that tests using helium/oxygen mixtures were not useful in determining the site of airflow obstruction. Teculescu[3830] has reviewed the use of air/helium flow curves (with 84 references) and documented the high intersubject variability and coefficient of variation. Others have concluded that the variability is too great for these tests to be useful in survey studies.[3844] It seems clear that these tests have little usefulness when used on a routine basis.

Subdivisions of Lung Volume

Four principal methods have been used to measure the total lung capacity:

- open-circuit nitrogen washout
- closed-circuit helium equilibration
- body plethysmography
- planimetry of chest x-rays

A fifth method, helium dilution after a single inspiration and a period of breath holding, has also been studied. In normal subjects, all of these methods correlate closely.[3025] Reviews of all these methods have appeared.[397]

Comroe[331, 333] has written an entertaining account of the introduction of the body plethysmograph into respiratory research. Recent modifications of the older methods have included the development of a non-recirculating helium dilution method[279] and a closed-circuit nitrogen method.[291] The data from the body plethysmograph can be fully computerized,[349] and the mass spectrometer can be used for these estimates.[319, 321]

In normal subjects, all of these methods give results that are closely correlated, as indicated below:

1. Between planimetry and body plethysmography: r values of 0.955[257]; 0.96[236]; 0.87[322]; 0.89.[284]

2. Between planimetry and helium dilution: r value of 0.94[415] when a nasal thermistor signal was used to increase the accuracy of timing the respiratory phase during which the x-ray was exposed; another study found an r value of 0.93.[284]

3. Between body plethysmography and helium dilution: r value of 0.929.[359]

4. Between helium equilibration and single-breath estimate: r value of 0.99,[361] with no significant difference between estimates if the breath was held for 10 seconds or more[364]; in this study, estimates of RV were 120 milliliters higher by the single-breath method, and the difference between the two methods was greater in smokers over the age of 40 than in young non-smoking subjects.

McCarthy, Craig, and Cherniack[578] noted that the measurement of RV by the single-breath technique had a coefficient of variation of 12%. Crapo and his colleagues[2964] recently re-studied the single-breath method in 122 women and 123 men, all non-smokers, and published prediction formulae and 95% confidence limits. The results were very similar to those obtained by equilibration methods, as others have found in normal subjects.[3039] However, the single-breath method underestimates the TLC in subjects with airflow obstruction. Burns and Scheinhorn[3831] found that compared with the TLC measured by chest x-ray planimetry, the single-breath method underestimated TLC by 2.3% in normal persons and by 10.4%, 21.8%, and 38% in patients with mild, moderate, and severe airflow obstruction. They proposed a correction factor in such cases, based on the

FEV_1/FVC ratio, but the 95% confidence limit of such an estimate was 90 milliliters. The difference between the RV measured by helium equilibration and that measured by a single-breath determination in cases of lung disease is correlated with the FEV_1 as a percentage of the predicted value.[364] In children with severe asthma or cystic fibrosis, Motoyama and associates[3012] reported that lung volumes could be reliably measured with helium equilibration only if a positive pressure of 2.5 cm H_2O were applied at the mouth while the estimate was made.

The planimetric method has been applied to major radiologic surveys[3008] and has also been validated in children.[3002] Using both posteroanterior and lateral films, it was found to have a correlation coefficient of 0.93, as compared with the plethysmographic method, in a group of 52 cases of pulmonary disease of varying etiology,[267] but probably not including any subjects with severe airflow obstruction. Rodenstein and his colleagues[3834] have re-evaluated the planimetric method as described by Barnhard in 1960 and modified by Pierce[236]; 20 young adults were studied. Although an r value of 0.85 was found, there were individual divergences of as much as 800 milliliters. This method might be further improved by further standardization of the radiologic technique used.[3835]

The standard deviation for determinations of the functional residual capacity (FRC) in normal persons by the helium dilution or body plethysmographic method is about ±150 milliliters.[421] Different observers may have a variation of as much as 12%, however, in measurements of thoracic gas volume from the body plethysmograph,[248] but there is no systematic difference between manually computed values and those computed automatically.[247] The calculated thoracic gas volumes are larger when panting efforts are made with the intercostal and accessory muscles of respiration than when the diaphragm is used—an effect attributed to abdominal gas compression.[328] The magnitude of the error might be as great as 900 milliliters. Bohadana and his colleagues[354] recently described differences in the measurement related to panting frequency. Others have noted a difference of as much as 4.7% between the VC recorded spirometrically at the mouth and that measured in the body plethysmograph in smokers, as compared with a difference of 1.9% in non-smokers.[277] In 1973, Teculescu[295] pointed out that in some patients with severe airflow obstruction, the body plethysmograph gave erroneously high readings for TLC. Some of these values were far higher than could be explained by gas compression. Others have noted the same phenomenon.[3833]

In a remarkable series of experiments involving use of an endotracheal tube and induced bronchoconstriction in normal subjects, Stanescu and his colleagues[352] have demonstrated that considerable errors may result in these circumstances; these are partly due to compression of extrathoracic airways. Rodenstein and his colleagues,[3061, 3851] using a cineradiographic technique, demonstrated that marked changes in airway diameter occurred in normal individuals when panting against a closed shutter; the volume changes were closely related to the swings in mouth pressure. Knudson and Knudson[3843] conducted a series of model experiments and concluded from these that in the presence of lower airway obstruction, compliant extrathoracic airways act as a shunt impedance, mouth pressures being out of phase with (and underestimating) changes in pleural pressure. This produces overestimates of thoracic gas volume, particularly if rapid panting is used.

In some cases of chronic airflow obstruction, differences of as much as 2 liters have been reported between helium dilution and body plethysmographic values for RV,[359, 436] but in most cases the differences are smaller than this. Paré and his colleagues[3025] have reported mean differences of about 300 milliliters between helium and body plethysmographic volumes using esophageal pressure in 20 cases of chronic airflow limitation and of about 600 milliliters if mouth pressures were used. There is clearly a systematic difference between the two methods in cases with chronic airflow obstruction.[436] Brown and Slutsky[3836] found differences of about a liter between plethysmographic and helium dilution volumes in 10 cases of chronic airflow obstruction and suggested that interregional inhomogeneities during fast panting might contribute to the difference observed. Seven of their patients had FEV values of less than 56% of predicted normal.

In a review of the body plethysmographic method of measuring lung volumes, Begin and Peslin[3069] state that in normal subjects errors amount to only a few per cent but may be greater in non-uniform lungs. They conclude, "Solide il y a quelques années la position de la méthode plethysmographique s'est sensiblement dégradée."

When the plethysmographic method was found to give consistently higher readings in cases of chronic airflow obstruction than were found by the helium method, it was generally assumed that full gas equilibration in the helium dilution method was not occurring in such cases, although Teculescu had noted that some of the plethysmographic volumes were impossibly high.[295] It now appears that the values from the body plethysmograph can no longer be used as an absolute reference method under all circumstances; provided that the stability of the equilibrated helium concentration is carefully measured, it seems probable that this technique, or possibly x-ray planimetry, might provide the best estimate.

As noted in the second edition of this book,[1] the time for helium equilibration may have to be prolonged to 20 minutes in some cases of chronic airflow obstruction if the correct lung volume is to be measured on a helium circuit. Rodenstein and Stanescu,[356] using esophageal pressure instead of mouth pressure (which is believed to circumvent the major source of error in plethysmographic methods), have found that this lung volume in chronic airflow obstruction is underestimated by the 7-minute equilibration helium dilution method if the modified plethysmographic value is taken as correct; hence, a longer equilibration time may well be needed in some of these cases. Higenbottam and Payne[3029] studied the vocal folds via a fiberoptic bronchoscope in 34 patients with varying degrees of airflow limitation. Narrowing of the glottis during panting was observed to occur in 18 of the patients, and this might contribute to the overestimate in the plethysmographic method.

Closing Volume and Closing Capacity

The physiologic basis of these tests was described in Chapter 2. The conclusive demonstration by Engel and his colleagues[591] in 1975 that airway closure was actually occurring at the inflexion point between Phase III and Phase IV of the expiratory gas concentration curve ended a period during which closing volume was a more suitable designation than closing capacity. Methodology of the measurement has been discussed at a symposium[671] by Martin and his colleagues,[575] and by Buist and Ross.[570] Green and Travis[580] described a simplified method suitable for field use.[580] Becklake and her colleagues[2880] discussed methodology and precautions for using the test in the field.

Marcq and Minette[577] found a coefficient of 14% for CV/VC%, with evidence of slight diurnal variation. The measurements become abnormal in smokers,[265, 290, 312] as noted in Chapter 6, but some studies have shown that the slope of Phase III, the expired nitrogen plateau after inspiration of oxygen (SBN_2/L), is more often abnormal than the CV/VC% in population surveys.[276] The closing volume can be computer-calculated,[321] although some curves give rise to difficulty; the delivery of a bolus of helium can be made automatic.[283] Chinn and Lee[386] found that the "within-subject" coefficient of variation for closing volume was 13.99% ± 5.26% in replication studies and that for the CV/VC% was 14.27% ± 5.25%. Other data from the literature give ranges from about 9% to 36%.[386, 571, 575–579] These values have to be compared with values of about 3% for FEV_1 and 5.2% for the $\dot{V}max_{50\%}$, as noted previously.

If TLC is calculated from the single-breath dilution, any underestimate of RV by this method will result in an underestimate of the CC/TLC ratio.[487] The closing volume is not affected by holding the breath after the inspiration is taken, although the slope of Phase IV is changed.[488] Buist and Ross[570] measured the CV/VC% in 284 asymptomatic non-smokers and calculated the following regression equations (see also Chapter 4):

Men: CV/VC% = 0.375 × Age + 0.562

Women: CV/VC% = 0.293 × Age + 2.812

In routine applications, the usefulness of this test is limited by its high coefficient of variation. It is not of value in many patients with lung disease, because no definite transition between the alveolar slope (Phase III) and the change in concentration (Phase IV) can be detected in them. Until the significance of early change in this measurement in smokers is known, its routine use seems not to be of much value.

Single-Breath Nitrogen Test (Fowler) or Slope of Phase III (SBN_2/L)

The analysis of the slope of the expired alveolar plateau after a full inspiration of 100% oxygen* has been used as a test of uniformity of ventilation for many years.[1]

---

*See Table 5–3 for normal values.

A detailed model analysis by Engel and Paiva[3076, 3077, 3888] indicates that the geometry of the human lobule of itself, without the influence of any other factors, leads to non-uniformity of the slope of Phase III. Zwart, Jansen, and Luijendijk[3037] have recently analyzed factors affecting this slope in normal subjects. The test is affected by an increase in RV, and experiments using methacholine challenge testing in 10 normal persons, in which RV increased from a mean of 1.54 liters to a mean of 2.37 liters, found a concomitant increase in SBN_2/L from 0.88% to 2.84% after the challenge was administered.[3840]

The analysis of the test has been facilitated by use of the computer,[319, 321] and several studies have analyzed the factors affecting the slope of the plateau of alveolar concentration. It is not believed that stratification contributes significantly to the slope in normal individuals,[400] but it is affected by gas exchange as the expiration occurs—a conclusion drawn from the observation that the slope is steeper if expiration time is prolonged[488] and is also increased if it is recorded during exercise.[423, 3009] Cormier and Belanger[3066] have calculated that gas exchange at rest may contribute about 10% of the slope.

The use of an external resistance has been recommended to standardize measurements of the alveolar slope in patients[3071]; Hurst, Graham, and Cotton[3839] found that a fast exhalation decreased the value in normal subjects, but in 17 smokers with normal pulmonary function, the slope was increased by a fast expiration. They attributed this to increases in regional RV/TLC ratios distal to sites of small airway obstruction when expiratory flow was increased.

The test is affected by any factor that leads to non-uniformity of time constants in the lung or by alterations in ratios of ventilation to pre-existing volume. Horsfield, Barer, and Cumming[490] have published an interesting model analysis of centrilobular emphysema and its effect on the expired alveolar plateau. The analysis permits computation of the effects of varying compliance values for the centrilobular space and of varying tidal volumes on the measured slope of Phase III.

Experiments on nine normal non-smoking subjects comparing the results with the standard test and with a "reversed" technique[350] led to the conclusion that the nitrogen gradient within the lungs was responsible for the slope of Phase III and for the cardiogenic oscillations on the tracing. These were considered to be largely independent of the gradients that give rise to Phase IV and the slope of Phase IV.[350]

As noted in Chapter 6, this test has been used to compare smokers and non-smokers in population surveys. In one such study of the population of Humboldt in Saskatchewan, for example, the SBN_2/L test was abnormal in 24% of men and 28% of women and was more sensitive to abnormality than the closing volume.[276] A similar conclusion was reached in a study comparing 337 non-smoking men and women with 530 smokers.[294]

Measurements of SBN_2/L every day for 10 days in 20 subjects analyzed by two observers showed a correlation coefficient of 0.971 between them.[381] A line drawn through the largest possible part of the alveolar plateau provided the best measurement. Other authors have also reported correlation coefficients of 0.96 between duplicate measurements,[578] the 95% confidence limit being about 0.4% nitrogen/L.[578] McCarthy, Craig, and Cherniack[578] reported a coefficient of variation of 22% of the SBN_2/L.

Comparisons between the SBN_2/L, a forced expiration equilibration test, and the time to reach equilibration between inspired and expired nitrogen (to within 2%) indicated that the SBN_2/L was more sensitive to early changes but the other two parameters were more useful in established disease, as they deteriorated progressively, whereas the nitrogen slope did not.[310] Regression equations for the SBN_2/L based on age[268] and on age plus duration of smoking and smoking intensity[489] have been published. The prediction data in Table 5–3 were based on measurements made on 134 non-smoking men and 203 non-smoking women.[294] Sixt, Bake, and Oxhoj[3837] have recently published data on SBN_2/L on 178 lifetime non-smoking men aged between 30 and 70. They found that the slope increased with age over the age of 50 and published a curvilinear prediction equation. Data on adolescents have also been published.[3838]

As noted in Chapter 12, infusion of saline into normal subjects leads to changes in SBN_2/L as pulmonary extravascular lung water increases.[3486] Complex tests of gas distribution in cases of emphysema and involving gases of different densities[3036] are noted in Chapter 8.

In practical terms, this test may have some usefulness in providing objective (non-effort–dependent) evidence of abnormality in some patients or in providing evidence of abnormality before there has been a major change in expiratory flow data. Its value in the routine laboratory is limited by the fact that it is almost always abnormal in any case of established lung disease. However, it has recently been suggested that the SBN_2/L slope may predict a faster rate of longitudinal decline of FEV_1[3841] and may be related to the fall in FEV_1 in early cases of chronic obstructive lung disease.[3842]

Measurement of the Anatomic Dead Space (Fowler)

A computer program has been described for this measurement.[479] It has been found that the value of VD_{anat} increases by about 4 milliliters for every 100-milliliter increase in tidal volume.[477] The measurement has no value as an index of clinical function.

Inert Gas Measurements of Distribution

In 1974, Hatzfeld and Nury[372] summarized the literature on open-circuit clearance measurements in a review with 60 references. Analyses of the effect of tissue clearance of nitrogen or nitrogen washout curves have been published.[3040] Carefully controlled nitrogen clearance curves have been used to assess the effects of chest wall oscillation.[3845]

In an important contribution to the literature on nitrogen washin and washout methods, Mertens and colleagues[3041] showed that calculation of the moment ratio was the best method of analyzing the curves and that in normal persons there was no difference between washin and washout data. Fleming and his colleagues[445] applied digital computation to this method and calculated the moment ratio based on the number of volume turnovers. They agreed with Mertens and associates that this was superior to other indices, as the intrasubject variation was less than that for seven other indices derivable from the washout curve. Values were computed for normal individuals and persons with chronic airflow obstruction. Others have supported the use of moment analysis.[3027]

Cutillo and his colleagues[416] studied the reproducibility of the lung clearance index, the pulmonary clearance delay, and the mixing ratio—three different methods of quantitating gas distribution. The latter measurement, the mixing ratio, was found to be much better than the analysis of the ratio of slow space to fast space ventilation.

Chiang and colleagues[70] studied nitrogen washout curves from 225 normal subjects aged between 7 and 30 years and found that 21.3% of them had two exponential components to the curve; these were also found in half of the men in the sample between the ages of 25 and 30.

Cumming and Guyatt[339] analyzed the nitrogen recovered from the first expirations after switching to a 21% oxygen, 79% argon mixture. Four different methods of analysis were applied to 10 patients, in all of whom the FEV_1 was less than 1.18 liters. These did not yield significantly different results, and it was not clear whether the more rigorous methods of analysis yielded any additional information to that obtained from simpler test procedures.

The helium washin curve is only analyzable in terms of a two-component lung, and no more detailed analysis of it is possible in normal subjects.[450] Mathematical handling of the end-tidal nitrogen concentration during washout has been described.[480] This yielded a parameter significantly different between normal individuals and those with airflow obstruction, but it was not compared with simpler indices in the same patients. Thus, its advantages cannot be assessed. Nitrogen washout data in six normal subjects with controlled ventilation, using helium or SF_6 as the washout gas, have recently been reported.[3846] The data suggested that after the fifth breath, the increase in mean expired nitrogen plateau is due not to diffusion mixing but to convection-dependent inhomogeneity.

Paiva[455] in 1975 suggested on theoretical grounds that a more sensitive indicator of gas distribution inequality might be derived from a combination of nitrogen washout, during the course of which a single-breath alveolar plateau would be recorded. The slope of the alveolar plateau divided by the mean expired nitrogen concentration would provide a "normalized" slope; this would rise as a function of breath number, reach an asymptotic value, and provide an index of asynchronism. The best index of distribution would be not the slope of Phase III but the normalized slope of the alveolar plateau. It would be plotted as a function of the number of breaths and divided by the index of asynchronism. This interesting derivation does not appear to have been tested; modern computer technology would greatly simplify the calculations involved.

Smidt and Worth[491] have developed an analysis of gas distribution based on the differential rates of clearance of helium (fastest), argon (intermediate), and SF_6 (slowest). In normal subjects, the curves for helium and SF_6 cross after about five normal breaths. This crossover point is delayed in patients with chronic airflow obstruction.[491]

The helium closed-circuit mixing time, the SBN_2/L, and the RV/TLC% are highly correlated.[308] On grounds of simplicity, Hathirat, Renzetti, and Mitchell[308, 309] recommend the use of the helium mixing time as an index. Such an index does not compensate for differences in functional residual capacity and minute ventilation and is therefore bound to be less sensitive than an index that takes account of these factors.[1]

Recent studies of breath-by-breath analysis of seven gases (N_2, Ar, O_2, CO_2, He, SF_6, and N_2O) during closed-circuit breathing[3042] and at a fixed tidal volume showed that SF_6 reached equilibrium in normal persons 30% more slowly than helium when the subject was seated upright. Jones, Davies, and Hughes[3043] analyzed helium and SF_6 in a closed circuit, recording the number of breaths required to reach 99% equilibrium (a modification of the helium closed-circuit mixing index based on 90% equilibrium[1]). They demonstrated differences in equilibrium time for the two gases that were dependent on respiratory frequency. It is not known whether complex tests such as this might have any use in clinical investigation; it seems unlikely that they would be of much routine value.

All tests of inert gas distribution have only a very limited value in routine clinical application. It seems that, to this point, their usefulness is not enhanced by increasing the complexity of analysis. They do have some value in research methodology. Recent efforts to align quantitative descriptive morphometry of the human lung with observations of gas distribution have thrown new light on structure/function correlations.

MEASUREMENTS OF VENTILATORY RESPONSE TO HYPOXIA AND HYPERCAPNIA AND MEASUREMENTS OF RESPIRATORY CENTER DRIVE

As noted in Chapter 4, in some clinical cases it is very important to measure the ventilatory response to hypoxia (isocapnic) and hypercapnia (hyperoxic). Several papers have dealt with the methodology of such tests,[280–282, 293, 311] and in 1977 a report of a conference summarized advice on methodology.[314, 315] In Chapter 2, results of these tests were described.

There is still controversy as to whether sufficient time elapses in the rebreathing method for the increase in ventilation to be properly recorded after the change in inspired CO_2 has occurred.[335] Data on ventilatory responses were summarized up to 1973 by Strachova and Plum.[299] Repeat tests at intervals of 10, 20, and 30 minutes have shown satisfactory repeatability.[3848] The data for normal CO_2 response do not show a bimodal distribution, but the range of response is considerable, as indicated by the data of Irsigler[318]:

$\dot{V}E/Pa_{CO_2}$ (L/min/mm Hg)

105 Normal young men:	Mean: 2.73
	Range: 0.469–6.225
	SD: ±1.117
21 Normal young women:	Mean: 1.980
	Range: 0.85–4.926
	SD: ± 1.129

A repeat of the test several months after the initial results showed satisfactory repeatability. The CO_2 response had been noted to be greater in Europeans than in New Guinea natives[371]; recent data suggest that it may be lower in Chinese than in Caucasian persons.[3847]

In a mixed group of 16 normal individuals and 22 patients, the slope of the log of the breath-holding time correlated closely with the measured CO_2 response.[250] Hensley and Read[324] have measured the hypoxic response through the use of an ear oximeter and by giving five breaths of nitrogen while CO_2 is being rebreathed. This produces 15 to 20 seconds of hypoxia, and the recorded oxygen saturation is plotted against the ventilation.[324] It is claimed that this method possesses the advantage that the test is not affected by changes in the cerebral circulation. Shaw, Schonfield, and Whitcomb[3028] have described a progressive and transient hypoxic test that showed good reproducibility in 18 normal subjects.

The $P_{0.1}$ method of measuring respiratory center drive was introduced by Whitelaw, Derenne, and Milic-Emili in 1975.[355] This measurement of pressure during a tenth of a second interruption to airflow is believed to reflect the neurogenic drive to the respiratory muscles. It has been shown that the FRC does not change during measurement of the hypoxic and hypercapnic responses,[417] an important point since FRC change would affect the $P_{0.1}$ measurement.[314] The value of $P_{0.1}$ is doubled in hypoxia and increases several-fold during CO_2 breathing.[417] The normal value is about 1.5 cm H_2O; this can rise to 4.0 in cases of chronic airflow obstruction and may reach 8.0 in cases of respiratory failure.[484]

Measurements of Intrapleural Pressure, Compliance, and K Constant

In a study using the weighted spirometer method in 27 normal men aged 17 to 59 years,[101] mean respiratory compliance was 101 mL/cm H_2O, mean lung compliance was 360 mL/cm H_2O, and mean thoracic compliance was calculated to be 160 mL/cm H_2O. Total compliance is correlated with TLC (r = 0.808) and is related to body height by the formula[101]

$$C_{tot} = [6.24 \times Ht\ (cm)] - 997.07$$

It is independent of age, at least up to age 60. Other studies in normal subjects have given values for static lung compliance as follows[383]:

Men: C_{st} (mL/cm H_2O) = [36.6 × Ht (m^3)]
Women: C_{st} (mL/cm H_2O) = [33.3 × Ht (m^3)]

Several studies have been reported in which the compliance was indirectly computed from the MEFV curve and airway resistance was measured from the body plethysmograph.[405] These have shown that although in healthy subjects there is a fair correlation, this does not apply to patients with lung disease.[405, 458, 470]

Quasi-static measurements also indicated a significant correlation (r = 0.83) between static respiratory compliance and body height in 22 non-smoking normal subjects.[373] There was, however, considerable variation in P_{st} recorded at TLC; this varied from 23.8 cm H_2O to a single high value of 53.3 in one subject.

Yernault and his colleagues[3006] studied eight young normal persons on four occasions and reported coefficients of variation (within individuals) of 6.5% for pressure measured at 90% TLC, of 10.7% for static compliance, and of 10.2% for 1/EL indices. All these measurements were made from expiratory curves; slightly smaller values were recorded for pressure values from the inspiratory curve, but larger coefficients of variation were found for static compliance and 1/EL indices. Similar data on repeat studies were obtained from our laboratory. Ten healthy individuals—four static deflation curves per day measured on 5 separate days over a 2-month period were used—showed mean coefficients of variation of 11% for the K (shape) constant; 11% for PL_{max}; 13% for PL at 70% TLC; 15% for C_{st}; and 6% for TLC determinations.[3852]

As noted earlier, calculations of the K constant of the pressure-volume curve and its changes with age have been reported by a number of authors. Several studies have shown that careful balloon positioning is important if measurements are to be made in different body positions.[3013, 3017]

A number of studies have clarified the relationship between changes in lung recoil and ventilatory tests. An important finding has been that deviations in functional residual capacity and spirometric measurements are poorly predictive of loss of recoil.[492] It has also been shown that calculation of the compliance from the MEFV curve and measured airway resistance has a reasonable correlation with measured compliance in normal subjects but cannot be used in patients with lung disease.[405, 458, 470]

The physiologic basis of these measurements is described in Chapter 2.

Work of Breathing

The work of breathing was found to be independent of age or sex in studies of 93 healthy subjects.[457] It averaged 2.21 ± 0.92 g·cm/mL at a respiratory frequency of 15/minute. It was correlated with tidal volume. The highest single value observed was 5.38 g·cm/mL.[457] This is of physiologic interest, but such calculations have no routine clinical relevance.

Measurements of Specific Conductance (SGaw), Airway Resistance (RL), and Forced Oscillation Impedance

In studies of 29 men and 27 women, all non-smokers, using a very low resistance mouthpiece, a mean value of 0.407 was found for SGaw, somewhat higher than the previously recorded values of between 0.25 and 0.30 for this measurement.[420] Several techniques use computers on line to correct for thermal drift and to continuously adjust for changing lung volume.[412, 468] Graphical calculation of RL is recommended; average pressure points taken at 0.5 L/sec flow intervals are used.[468] Both manually calculated and automatically computed measurements of RL show considerable variability.[247] In one study with five observers working on pre-recorded signals, a variation of as much as 37% in calculated RL was noted.[248] The least variation of RL may occur when the slope is estimated over a wide interval of flow, such as 1 or 2 L/sec.[243] However, Allen[3078] studied four normal individuals on 4 consecutive days and noted a coefficient of variation in SGaw of between 7.5% and 13.8%. Estimates have ranged from values of about 5.5%[3853] to values of about 19.3%.[3858]

The oscillatory method of measurement of RL correlates well with the plethysmographic method at values of RL less than 9.0 cm H_2O/L/sec.[360, 482, 493] There is now extensive literature on the methodology and methods of analysis.* This method has the advantage that the subject breathes normally and quietly throughout. However, Landser and his colleagues,[3053] who have pioneered its development, have recently reported that in measurements on 407 healthy men, both smokers and non-smokers, no differences in values between the two groups could be demonstrated, although the mean FEV_1 was about 440 milliliters lower in the smokers. This suggests that the test is not as sensitive as flow rate or gas distribution indices. However, much may depend on technical details, since Peslin, Hannhart, and Pino,[582] using a slightly different oscillation method, did find differences between smokers and non-smokers. Pimmel and his colleagues[3079] studied 22 non-smokers before and after methacholine challenge and concluded that the forced oscillation method was detecting increases in peripheral rather than in central airway resistance.

Measurements of RL have been shown to be highest at about 7 A.M. in normal subjects[441] and to decline by 20% in the first hour; declines as high as 60% were noted in some patients with asthma and bronchitis.[441] In normal subjects studied with bronchoconstriction induced by histamine, a full inhalation reduced the value of RL significantly for 45 seconds.[413] Mathematical models dealing with calculated differences in mean airway resistance in inspiration and expiration have been described.[471] Predicted values for RL, taking length of smoking history and smoking intensity into account, have been published.[489]

MEASUREMENTS OF GAS EXCHANGE
Diffusing Capacity (Transfer Function)

No fewer than 11 different methods have been described for the measurement of the

---

*See references 582, 3053, 3078–3082, 3854–3857, 3881, 3882.

diffusing capacity and its components. The principal methods in use are the following:

1. Single-breath apnea method, which makes use of CO and helium ($DL_{CO}SB$). This may be corrected for Hb level ($DL_{CO}SB_{corr1}$) and/or for blood COHb level ($DL_{CO}SB_{corr2}$).

2. Steady-state CO uptake and computation of PA_{CO} from Pa_{CO_2} ($DL_{CO}SS_1$).

3. Steady-state CO uptake and measurement of end-tidal CO concentration ($DL_{CO}SS_2$).

4. Rebreathing CO methods ($DL_{CO}RB$).

5. Calculation of fractional uptake of CO (F_{CO}).

6. Methods using various isotopes of CO and oxygen.

During the past 10 years, much attention has been devoted to these methods in the European literature; by comparison, relatively little has appeared in North America. The single-breath method, available in North America with automated and computerized methodology, is, perhaps for that reason, most widely used in this region. Its development and use have recently been well reviewed by Forster and Ogilvie.[3026]

Calculation of $DL_{CO}SB$ has been facilitated by use of a nomogram,[256] and an automated apparatus has been described.[263] Computer handling of $DL_{CO}SB$ and $DL_{CO}SS_2$ methods[245] is now commercially available. Kindig and Hazlett[3873] have contributed a scholarly discussion of the differences between steady-state and single-breath methods of measurement.

Precise timing reduces the coefficient of variation with the single-breath technique.[263] The value for $DL_{CO}SB$ in normal persons is not much affected by using the helium equilibration measurement of RV instead of that computed from the single-breath dilution,[365] a conclusion in line with comparisons between the two methods in normal individuals noted earlier. It has been recommended that the apnea time should be reduced from 10 seconds to 4 seconds, as the $DL_{CO}SB$ calculated from this period of apnea corresponds closely to the $DL_{CO}SB$ measured on exercise[449]; this modification does not seem to have been widely adopted. Finley and his colleagues[494] suggested in 1974 that a "time constant" of CO disappearance should be calculated. In normal subjects, the time constant averaged 12 seconds and was more reproducible than the $DL_{CO}SB$. This modification, which would seem to have some advantages, does not appear to have been studied by other investigators.

A number of recent papers have analyzed reasons for differences in $DL_{CO}SB$ estimations, and a standardization conference has been held.[3859] It is clear that variations are introduced by differences in timing the held breath; differences in the alveolar sample taken or in correction for apparatus dead space[3864]; and possibly differences in expiratory velocity. To these variables must be added errors in helium estimation and, not least, errors in CO determination. Chinn, Naruse, and Cotes[3860] studied 50 pulmonary function laboratories in England and Wales and found that for CO analysis: "Percentage accuracy of the results was within 1% of the expected value in only 14% of determinations of CO concentration, 37% of helium determinations, and 48% of oxygen analyses." The coefficient of variation for the CO analyses was 9%. They concluded that analytic standards had declined over the past 20 years (the reasons for which were unclear).

A considerable number of papers have derived normal values for $DL_{CO}SB$,* and there has been an interesting correspondence on the reasons for differences between some of these regressions.[3861, 3862] Others have commented on the need for standardization.[3868] Graham, Mink, and Cotton[3869] have summarized their development of a refined method of calculation of $DL_{CO}SB$ based on fast CO analysis of expired gas. However, Rubin, Lewis, and Mittman,[3870] on the basis of model experiments, have suggested that CO waveform data require that a compartment of CO diffusion from part of the inert gas dead space is required to explain the data in normal and abnormal persons. Graham and his colleagues,[3883] by comparing their corrected method with others commonly used, showed that compared with their three-equation method, standard methods might be 30% higher or 10% lower in cases of emphysema. In normal individuals, differences were generally less than 10%.

The standard error of the estimate (SEE) of $D_{Lco}SB$ has varied from about 0.69 to 0.89.[231]

Miller and his colleagues[3000] recently measured the $D_{Lco}SB$ in 511 normal subjects and calculated the following regressions:

Non-smoking men:
$$DL_{CO}SB = [12.9113 - (0.2229 \times Age)] + [0.418 \times Ht \text{ (inches)}]$$

---

*See references 125, 231, 260, 303, 374, 384, 475, 3863.

Non-smoking women:
$$DL_{CO}SB = [2.2382 - (0.111 \times Age)] + [0.4068 \times Ht \text{ (inches)}]$$

There is a consensus that values of DL_{CO} measured by either single-breath or steady-state methods, when corrected for COHb and Hb, are about 10% lower in smokers than in non-smokers.[303, 374, 475] The significance of this finding is discussed in Chapter 6. In experiments in which the effect of increasing COHb on the measured $DL_{CO}SB$ were studied, it was found that there was about a 1% reduction in measured $DL_{CO}SB$ for each percentage increase in blood COHb.[495] If no correction is made in smokers, the $DL_{CO}SB$ is likely to be underestimated by about 5%.[3867] It has been suggested that DL_{CO} estimates should be corrected for variations in mean alveolar oxygen pressure,[3871] and standardization of measurements made during exercise has been proposed.[3872]

The coefficient of variation of $DL_{CO}SB$ is about 3.7%[384] and may be reduced if care is taken that timing is precise, as noted above, and that alveolar pressure is close to atmospheric during the period of apnea. This is particularly important if estimates of V_c and DM are being made, since attention to this point was found to reduce the coefficient of variability from 23% to 7% for V_c, and from 26% to 12% for DM.[384] Computation of these values has been facilitated by derivation of a formula[380]; correction for anemia is important.[3865]

The coefficient of variation of $DL_{CO}SS_2$ is about 6.9% in normal persons and 7.6% in patients with lung disease.[131, 427] The r value between double determinations was 0.951 in one large series.[440] Prediction formulae for $DL_{CO}SS_2$ per square meter of body surface area in relation to age have been published.[448] At rest, $DL_{CO}SS_2$ is correlated with tidal volume.[468]

It is important that in routine measurements of DL_{CO} a correction be applied for anemia. There is considerable literature on this effect,* and the DL_{CO} has been found to fall by between 6.0%[443] and 7%[306] for a change of hemoglobin of 1.0 g per 100 ml. $DL_{CO}SB$ and $DL_{CO}SS_2$ are both affected by body position.[147]

There is a good correlation between $DL_{CO}SB$ and $DL_{CO}SS_2$ in normal persons. In five normal individuals, five patients with chronic airflow obstruction, and five patients with diffuse interstitial fibrosis, the relationship between the

_____
*See references 230, 306, 406, 411, 443, 467, 3865.

results of the two methods was expressed by the formula[469]

$$DL_{CO}SB = 1.37 + (1.46\ DL_{CO}SS_2)$$

Although Stebbings[252] reported considerable variability in measurements of FCO others have found satisfactory repeatability.[375] It has long been known that this value is affected by respiratory rate and minute volume,[1] and recent data[375] confirm this. Harris and Whitlock[3073, 3074] have published a detailed analysis of actual and computer-calculated values for FCO consisting of different respiratory rates and tidal volumes—a very useful background to this measurement. Their data provide the normal predicted values shown in Tables 5–1 and 5–2.

Mastrangelo, Chau, and Pham,[102] in a study of 141 non-smokers, 60 ex-smokers, and 322 smokers, found that the variability of the FCO was less than that of $DL_{CO}SS_2$. It is not clear whether more complex refinements of FCO data provide much advantage.[462, 463] The calculated DL_{CO} has been corrected by a measured alveolar-arterial difference for CO_2,[461] but it has not been shown that this modification (or that using end-tidal CO_2 instead of CO) improves sensitivity or reduces variability.[84, 460]

A very detailed comparison between $DL_{CO}SS_1$, $DL_{CO}SS_2$, $DL_{CO}V_D$, and FCO in 28 normal persons and 91 patients with lung disease[131] found insignificant differences when the factor ($VD/VT + FCO$) was less than 0.7 but found considerable differences if this was 1.0 or greater.

Regression formulae for V_c and DM have been published from a study of 65 normal men, probably a mixed group of healthy smokers and non-smokers[374]:

$$V_c = [59.82 \times Ht \text{ (meters)}] - [(0.38 \times age) - 7.37]$$

$$DM = [55.8 \times Ht \text{ (meters)}] - [(0.33 \times age) - 33.19]$$

Normal values for these parameters according to smoking history were also derived from studies of the population in Berlin, New Hampshire.[303] Other studies contain useful notes on variability and normal values for these indices.[304, 378] Interestingly, a change of hemoglobin of 1 g/100 mL changes DM by 6.3% of the predicted value, but V_c and Hb are not correlated.[467] The value of V_c is very sensitive to the length of the held breath in the $DL_{CO}SB$

method, falling markedly if the apnea is prolonged.[467] It is clear that if these indices are to be used, very precise control of the conditions of measurement is required. There are several papers reporting the effect of differing carrier gases on CO uptake.*

Complex mixtures of isotopes have also been used to estimate both the CO and oxygen diffusing capacities. One of these studies, in which a mixture of 0.07% $^{18}O_2$, 0.07% $C^{18}O$, and 3% $^{16}O_2$ was used, found values of 42 mL/min/mm Hg for DL_{CO} and 48 for DL_{O_2}.[389] Slightly higher values of both indices, but with the same ratio between them (theoretically, 1.2), were found using $^{18}O_2$ and $C^{18}O$.[402] $C^{18}O$ has also been used for computation of DL_{CO} alone.[319, 385, 419] In one study using this method, DL_{CO} was found to be 28.8 when measured at FRC and 34.6 when measured at TLC; in both instances a rebreathing method was employed.[3866]

A useful simplification of the rebreathing technique in which the subject empties a bag containing 10% helium and 0.3% CO 10 times in 10 seconds has been described.[344, 3018] This method yielded a correlation coefficient with $DL_{CO}SB$ of 0.923 in 22 subjects.[344] It is particularly suitable for bedside use and might well be useful in detecting intrapulmonary hemorrhage.[313]

Predicted values have been described for the rebreathing method[363] used during bicycle exercise; these are based on the following relationship:

$$DL_{CO}RB = 0.5 \times [Ht\ (cm) - 120]$$

A rebreathing DL_{CO} method has also been adapted for use in patients on mechanical ventilation.[3874] Studies comparing results in different diseases using different methods of measurement of diffusing capacity† are discussed in later chapters in relation to the different diseases studied.

As noted in later chapters, it is important that the physician interpreting pulmonary function tests be fully aware of the factors that affect different methods of measuring the diffusing capacity (or "transfer coefficient" to use the term preferred by Europeans). The different methods correspond in normal persons, with the $DL_{CO}SB$ systematically giving higher values. No significant differences occur in cases of dif-

fuse interstitial fibrosis, but with asthma, the $DL_{CO}SB$ reads considerably higher than other methods (this is discussed in Chapter 6). No method is unaffected by variations in the distributions of ventilation, alveolar volume, and perfusion within the lung; what is important is that these useful tests be correctly interpreted in specific clinical situations. We are aware of difficulties in compensation or litigation cases arising because of different $DL_{CO}SB$ measurements from different laboratories.

The physiologic basis of this measurement is described in Chapter 2. Recent work on measuring the expired CO during different parts of the expiration and the effect of altering lung volume[358, 367, 3055] on the diffusing capacity in normal subjects are noted there.

Alveolar-Arterial Differences, End-Tidal–Arterial Differences, and V_D/V_T Ratios

West[332] reviewed the interrelationships between different components of the alveolar-arterial oxygen difference. Harris and his colleagues[114, 269-271] have measured these components in normal subjects of different ages, at rest and exercise, and breathing air and oxygen. The measured $(A - a)D_{O_2}$ at rest and breathing air in the sitting position rises from a value of about 4.3 mm Hg at age 25 to about 22.3 mm Hg at age 60. Values measured in the supine position are slightly lower. Values of the $(A - a)D_{O_2}$ are higher in smokers if measurements are made in hypoxic conditions[232]; this result is discussed in Chapter 6. The measured $(A - a)D_{O_2}$ decreases as the carrier gas density increases[424]; the mechanism of this effect is not yet well understood.

The V_D/V_T ratio is independent of age,[274] but in 240 duplicate measurements performed on 48 normal subjects aged 20 to 74, it was found to be poorly reproducible.[408] The actual value of $V_{D_{physiol}}$ in the same study had better reproducibility and could be calculated from the following equation:

$$V_{D_{physiol}} = (0.930 \times Age) + [1.725 \times Ht\ (cm)]$$

$$+ [(0.267 \times V_T\ (mL)) - (1291/f - 213)]$$

where f is the frequency of respiration. This equation applied to both men and women. Harris and his colleagues showed that precise

---

*See references 357, 368, 404, 437, 456.

†See references 235, 298, 367, 370, 387, 453, 469.

correction of the calculated pulmonary capillary mean CO_2 pressure for temperature is required if large errors in the measured $VD_{physiol}$ are to be avoided.[270] Vale[366] noted that the measured $VD_{physiol}$ fell on exercise in normal subjects.

The quick calculation of the $(A - a)D_{O_2}$ at the bedside has been facilitated by the development of nomograms.[288, 464] It has been suggested that if different inspired oxygen concentrations are being used, the ratio of arterial to calculated alveolar oxygen tensions may be useful in analyzing defects of gas exchange,[289] but detailed results of the application of this method to clinical problems have not been published. A recent comparison of gas tension measurements on the same sample at 11 different laboratories showed a coefficient of variation for Pa_{CO_2} of 4.5%.[3877]

In healthy subjects, the difference between arterial and end-tidal CO_2 averages 0.5 mm Hg,[261] but in disease may be much increased, reaching up to 17 mm Hg in some patients with chronic airflow obstruction.[261] This difference was originally proposed as useful in the diagnosis of pulmonary embolism[1]; other studies have confirmed that it is increased in that condition. By comparison, it was found not to exceed 3 mm Hg in a diverse group of persons with myocardial infarction, acute respiratory failure, and pneumonia.[285] In chronic airflow obstruction, the test could still be made useful if maximal expirations were taken and the CO_2 was measured at the end of the expiration.[285, 496] Thews and Schmidt[459] have shown that calculations of the components of the $(A - a)D_{O_2}$ can be made from studies of expiratory gas concentrations after hypoxic mixtures containing argon are inspired[442]—a method based on that of Vogel and Thews.[437] Calculations of $\dot{V}/\dot{Q}$ distributions by this method are noted later. A method of correction of the steady-state DL_{CO} by measurement of the $(A - a)D_{O_2}$ difference has been proposed by Pivoteau and Dechoux.[461]

Mixed Venous Oxygen Tension

Kelman[347] has recently published a useful theoretical analysis of the factors that affect the validity of an alveolar sample's being representative of mixed venous gas concentration. He shows that if the blood/gas partition coefficient exceeds 10.0, an alveolar sample with a prolonged expiration will be representative of mixed venous concentration and will be unaffected by $\dot{V}/\dot{Q}$ distribution abnormalities. If the coefficient is less than 3.0, it will be unreliable. The "plateau" method of equilibrating with different CO_2 mixtures so that there is no difference between inspired and expired CO_2 concentrations[410] allows the mixed venous CO_2 tension to be calculated to within ± 1.0 mm Hg in normal persons[407]; it is more accurate than calculation by extrapolation.[407] Expired gas can also be measured after 15 seconds of breath holding following inspiration of two gas mixtures.[329] The mixed venous tension can then be calculated from an exponential equation. This method has been successfully used in clinical cases and even in patients on respirators.[329] As noted later, relative hypoxemia of mixed venous blood is an important component of abnormality in some persons with chronic airflow obstruction and respiratory failure.[481] In spite of this fact, routine measurements probably would not greatly assist management.

Methods of Measuring $\dot{V}/\dot{Q}$ Distribution

The general (as opposed to regional) methods of measuring $\dot{V}/\dot{Q}$ distribution consist primarily of the six inert gas method and the indirect calculation technique of Thews. The methodology of the six inert gas method has been described,[330] although it has been modified by a different calculation method from that originally proposed.[396, 3046] This method has recently been excellently reviewed by Hlastala[3875]; Wagner and his colleagues[3876] have suggested that under certain circumstances, arterial sampling might not be necessary. Ratner and Wagner[3056] concluded that the method is subject to considerable variability if the spread of $\dot{V}/\dot{Q}$ distributions is very large. This technique cannot distinguish between parallel and series $\dot{V}/\dot{Q}$ inhomogeneity, but it has yielded interesting data on asthma and chronic airflow obstruction, which are discussed in the relevant chapters.

The method of Thews consists of complex analysis of expired gases after a few breaths of argon in low oxygen mixtures.[442, 459] The distribution of $\dot{V}/\dot{Q}$ ratios in normal individuals has been calculated by this method,[444] and abnormal spread of $\dot{V}/\dot{Q}$ distrbutions has been demonstrated in disease.

In our opinion, both of these methods are investigative tools of clinical research; it has not yet been shown that their routine availability would influence clinical management or decisions.

Measurement of Venous Admixture and Direct Shunt Fractions

Indirect calculation of the venous admixture component $(\dot{Q}_{va}/\dot{Q}_t)$ in normal subjects gives values of about 1.3% in subjects aged 20 to 30 years, rising to 4.98% in normal persons aged 60 to 74.[269] It is slightly lower when measured on oxygen. The shunt component is between 7% and 15% of $(A - a)DO_2$ by these indirect methods in normal individuals.[272] A different technique using dye dilution methods and ^{133}Xe in solution showed that the shunt component was about 8% of the $(A - a)DO_2$ in normal subjects.[266]

Normal Data on Regional Lung Function

Some additional data to that noted in Chapter 2 in normal subjects are pertinent to the interpretation of studies of regional lung function. The technique of ^{99}Tc-labeled MAA scans has been shown to yield normally distributed perfusion distribution data in normal subjects.[3005] The method is widely used for the diagnosis of pulmonary emboli. Comparisons of clearance measurements using ^{133}Xe from equilibration, perfusion delivery, or bolus inhalation have shown some evidence of delayed clearance from lower zones, which is possibly attributable to airway closure.[466] However, such experiments have to be interpreted with caution, as ^{133}Xe from the chest wall may interfere with the tail of such clearance curves[393] or with the calculation of FRC from ^{133}Xe data.[428] In general, such data in normal persons show very small differences.[264, 275] Using ^{133}Xe, Prefaut and Engel[3887] have refined earlier data on regional ventilation and perfusion distribution in recumbent subjects.

Differences in regional ventilation distribution in relation to different inspiratory flow rates[377] can be studied by a variety of methods. Using ^{133}Xe and a gamma camera, one group of investigators measured the "fractional exchange per second" as a percentage and noted values of 2.64% over the left upper lobe and 3.66% over the left lower lobe in normal persons during quiet breathing.[382] Studies in 57 nonsmoking subjects aged 20 to 82 years apparently showed an interesting difference between men and women with slow inspirations of [133]Xe. In women, the ratio of RV/TLC increased over all zones with increasing age, whereas in men this ratio only changed with age over the upper zones.[390] The reason for the difference was not clear. Xenon-133, [127]Xe, and ^{13}N have all been used for regional studies.[391, 394] Moving detectors have been used in supine subjects to quantitate regional differences.[418] Analyses have been simplified by on-line computer linkages.[452]

Drutel and his colleagues[362] studied normal elderly persons seated upright with the use of the Carlens bronchospirometric catheter; they found that the right lung accounted for 53% of $\dot{V}E$ and $\dot{V}O_2$ and the left lung accounted for 47%.[362] Measurements of lobar volumes have been reported using argon bolus dilution with bronchoscopic lobar sampling and radiographic estimation. The two methods gave closely comparable results.[233] By the argon method, the data were obtained in 10 normal subjects (see table at the bottom of this page).

Isotopes of CO—[11]CO or C[15]O—have been used to quantitate regional differences in CO uptake.[403] These experiments have shown that in normal seated subjects at rest, upper zone transit time averages 1.78 seconds and the lower zone averages 0.79 second. Calculations of regional differences in pulmonary capillary blood volume (V_c) showed that at rest the upper zone/lower zone ratio was 0.35 and on light exercise it was 0.56. Ratios of flow, upper/lower, were 0.17 at rest and 0.31 on exercise.[403] Comparisons between ventilation measured with ^{133}Xe and perfusion measured by ^{99}Tc-labeled MAA scans have been used to calculate "$\dot{V}/\dot{Q}$" regionally in normal subjects[454]; this method almost certainly diminishes significant differences. Denison and Waller[3045] have recently commented on the clinical usefulness of measurements of regional gas samples using fiberoptic bronchoscopy.

Apart from the importance of the physiologic studies that have depended on regional measurements, the clinical usefulness of these meth-

%TLC				
Right Upper	*Right Middle*	*Right Lower*	*Left Upper*	*Left Lower*
16.4%	9.6%	26.4%	27.1%	22.1%

ods has been confined to the study of regional function preoperatively in patients who might benefit from resection of lung bullae, or for whom thoracotomy represented a high risk, and in the diagnosis of pulmonary embolism.

Notes on Tables of Normal Data

As noted at the start of this chapter, the recent compilation of normal data published in Europe[2884] represents the most comprehensive attempt to date to derive standard normal values from the literature. In Tables 5–1 and 5–2 we give normal values for quick reference, all based on studies of non-smokers and all derived from recent surveys of normal subjects. Some comments on these data follow.

Tables 5–1 and 5–2: Columns 3, 4, 5, and 6

These columns give the subdivisions of lung volume. The data are from reference 425, which gives regression equations based on several series of measurements of normal subjects.

Tables 5–1 and 5–2: Columns 7, 8, and 9

These predictions for FVC, FEV_1, the ratio between them, and the $FEF_{25-75\%}VC$ are from data published by Crapo, Morris, and Gardner.[429] The FEV_1 data for men are somewhat higher than data published elsewhere, as the following comparison shows:

Subject Characteristics (Men)		FEV_1 Value	
Height	Age	Ref 429	Ref 320
160	20	3.74	3.32
175	20	4.57	4.36
175	70	3.35	3.01
185	20	4.98	4.88
185	70	3.76	3.53

It will be noted that the differences between the prediction data are greatest in short young men and diminish in older age groups and in taller men. Data collected by Milne and Williamson[98] are closer to those in reference 320 than to those in 429. There are smaller differences between predicted data for women between all three sets of data.

Data in column 7 for the FVC give values slightly higher than the slow VC values in column 1, although in normal subjects there is no discrepancy between fast and slow data. The FEV/FVC ratio given in column 9 shows good identity between all sets of data.

Tables 5–1 and 5–2: Columns 10 and 11

The $FEF_{25-75\%}VC$ data in column 10 are from reference 429 and were computed from the same curves as those used for the FEV_1. Column 11 is composite data from the regression equation given in reference 425. Although, as noted earlier, the FEV_1 values from reference 429 are in general somewhat higher than those in other references, the $FEF_{25-75\%}VC$ values in column 10 are lower than other data, particularly in relation to height in men. Thus, as can be seen from Table 5–1, there is a difference of 0.5 L/sec between the two sets of predicted data for a 20-year-old man 155 centimeters tall. For 70-year-old men of this height, the difference is only 0.06 L/sec. In women, however, the differences between the two sets of data are greatest between elderly women; for a 70-year-old woman 155 centimeters in height, this amounts to 0.65 L/sec.

Tables 5–1 and 5–2: Columns 12 and 13

These are both taken from reference 425.

Tables 5–1 and 5–2: Columns 14 and 15

Values for $DL_{CO}SB$ in column 14 in Table 5–1 are taken from Bradley and colleagues[475] and are slightly higher than those given in the second edition of this book. The data of Salorinne[387] for men are about 15% higher than these and those of Crapo and Morris[231] higher still. Teculescu and Stanescu's data[125] are intermediate between that in references 387 and 231, and their regression equation was expressed in relation to surface area.

In Table 5–2, the data for women are from Salorinne,[387] as these are similar to other sets of regressions for women. By contrast, the data of Bradley and associates[475] for women are for some reason lower than all other data. Thus, for a woman aged 70 and 145 centimeters in height, Salorinne's data, as shown in Table 5–2, predicts a $DL_{CO}SB$ of 16.75, whereas the regression equation in reference 475 predicts a value of only 7.63. Values for $DL_{CO}SS_2$ (end-tidal) in column 15 are from reference 1. They have been confirmed by the data of Mastrangelo and his colleagues[102] on 141 non-smokers and over 300 smokers and ex-smokers.

Tables 5–1 and 5–2: Columns 16 and 17

The predicted data of F_{CO} in these columns are from the regressions published by Harris and Whitlock[3073, 3074] for men or women seated upright. This varies with respiratory rate, but values can be interpolated between those shown for respiratory rates of 10 and 30 per minute. These data should improve the usefulness of this index. As noted later, the simple measurement of inspired and expired CO has only one of the sources of variation that contribute to differences in $DL_{CO}SB$ between laboratories.

Pulmonary Function Tests Independent of Height (Table 5–3)

The values for the slope of Phase III (single-breath nitrogen slope, SBN_2/L) are from Buist and Ross.[294] They noted that for normal women over the age of 60, a separate regression equation applied, and the values from this are shown in parentheses. The values of normal arterial oxygen tension are from the regression equation calculated by Hertle, Georg, and Lange[497] from measurements made in 323 supine subjects. They are very similar to earlier data from Sorbini quoted in reference 1.

Use of Normal Pulmonary Function Data

In the previous edition of this book,[1] we suggested as a rule of thumb that a value of less than 80% of predicted normal (or more than 120% if abnormality led to an increase, as in the RV) should be taken as an approximate indicator of abnormality. Such a criterion is open to several criticisms,[242] including the fact that it may over- or underestimate abnormality at different ends of the age range; it would accord different levels of significant abnormality to tests that have different standard errors and 95% confidence limits; and it may give a false sense of a definite cutoff between normality and abnormality.[3880] Any such criterion of "normality" has valid objections to it.[237] Some authors recommend the use of 75% of predicted for some function tests, preferring this to the 95% confidence limit or to 1.65 times the standard error of the estimate. Earlier, these two values were shown for the FEF_{25-75} to enable a comparison to be made between them. Several authors have discussed these and other problems of interpretation of normal values.[286, 388, 433] Pennock[3878] has suggested the use of deviation from the reference value (1.96 times the coefficient of variation) for the test.

In general these differences are small. As pointed out later, the physician interpreting function tests must always have in mind the coefficient of variation for the test when considering whether it indicates abnormality or not. This is why, in the previous sections, estimates of the coefficient of variation of each test have been given. In addition, it is important to recognize the following in relation to normal data:

1. Linear regressions are approximate only.[3879, 3886] Deviations are noted in the case of FVC[286] and FEV_1, but also apply to such measurements as the SBN_2/L in which, in women, one regression equation appears to fit up to the age of 60 and another equation seems to be applicable in women between 60 and 75 (as noted earlier). There are also some significant differences between normal regression equations. As noted in Chapter 4, there is longitudinal evidence that in non-smoking women the FEV_1 does not begin to decline before the age of 35.

2. There is, for most tests, a widening of confidence limits over the age of 60, partly because normal data for this age group may be deficient and partly because at extreme ages (such as 100 years old) survivors are unlikely to be representative of the populations tested at younger ages.

3. Interpretations are facilitated if several

Table 5–3. PULMONARY FUNCTION TESTS INDEPENDENT OF HEIGHT

Age (yr)	SBN₂/L (%/L) Non-Smokers		Arterial Oxygen Tension (Pa_O2 mm Hg)
	MEN	WOMEN	MEN AND WOMEN
20	0.91	1.22	88.20
30	1.01	1.31	84.20
40	1.11	1.40	80.20
50	1.21	1.49	76.20
60	1.31	1.58 (1.70)	72.20
70	1.41	(2.28)	68.20

different tests show consistency. Thus, an FEF_{25-75} in a 60-year-old patient of 65% of the predicted value might be taken as more likely to be significant if the SBN_2/L is elevated and the RV is increased.

4. As Vedal and Crapo[2922] have shown, false-positive rates may be found in healthy subjects if multiple tests of function are used. They tested 251 healthy non-smoking subjects. Each test used had an approximately 5% false-positive rate, defined as the percentage of normal subjects classified as abnormal by the test. With FVC, FEV_1, and FEV/FVC ratio, 10% had at least one abnormal test. This rose to 24% when a complete battery of 14 tests was performed. A normal test was defined as within the 95% confidence limits.

5. When automated equipment has a built-in range of predicted values, there is some hazard that the inexperienced physician will accord these numbers special (or even "absolute") significance. Differences in predicted normal values noted in the earlier section should correct the impression that there is only one set of definitive normal numbers. As Kauffman and Drovet[3016] have noted, the correct use of any reference set of values depends on the question being asked of the interpreter.

6. The interpretation of significant changes in tests in the same patient over time is simpler, because the error in interpretation introduced by not knowing the test value in the patient before some condition developed is diminished. This is why a simple test, such as VC, used serially to detect early adverse drug effect on the lung, is far more useful than an estimate of whether a single observation is significantly different from normal.

7. All single measurements should be interpreted in the light of the coefficient of variation that has been shown to apply to them. As noted above, these coefficients are much higher for measurements of the terminal part of the MEFV curve than for the FEV_1 by a factor of three or so. Some tests, such as the $\dot{V}_{iso}V$, have such a high coefficient that they are of little use in a routine setting.

8. Different technicians may interpret the same tracings differently,[414] which may be a source of difficulty in comparing earlier with later data on the same patient or the same population.

The interpretation of abnormality in popula-tion studies is a special problem and is discussed in the next section. General examples of the use and misuse of function tests are noted in the last section of this chapter, together with suggestions for a sequence of analysis applicable to individual patient data.

USES OF PULMONARY FUNCTION TESTS IN EPIDEMIOLOGY

Since the publication of the second edition of this book, there has been a spectacular increase in the use of pulmonary function tests as a measurement tool in epidemiologic studies of lung diseases and disorders.[723, 829, 2860-2864] Indeed, tests of lung function, perhaps more than all other clinical laboratory tests of organ function, have become a basic tool in epidemiologic studies of respiratory normality or abnormality. The reasons for this include the ease of their administration (compared, for instance, to tests of renal function); the increasing importance of chronic non-malignant disease associated with airflow limitation (which can best be measured by lung tests)[2865]; and the growing recognition of occupational exposures as potential and actual threats to respiratory health (as documented in Chapter 16). Statutory requirements for the use of pulmonary function tests in monitoring health status in those engaged in certain occupations have been introduced in some jurisdictions.[2866] This has also served to increase the use of lung function tests in population studies.

Epidemiology, defined as "the study of the distribution of health-related states and events in populations, and the application of this study to the control of health problems,"[2867] makes a contribution to our overall knowledge of respiratory disease at least equal to the contribution made by the study of disease mechanisms and diagnosis. The discussion that follows offers an introductory background to the methods and approaches of this discipline for the reader who is more familiar with the fields of chest medicine and/or respiratory physiology than with epidemiology. Examples are provided of the contribution that lung function tests have made as methods of measurement of response and outcome in such studies. No attempt will be made to provide a "recipe book" on how to develop and carry out epidemiologic studies; for this type of information the reader should consult one of the standard texts.[2868-2870] Nevertheless, it is important to emphasize that appropriate consultation, including statistical guidance, is best sought in the planning stage of an epidemiologic study, not when all the data have been gathered, and that the most successful studies are usually those in which the relevant expertise, epidemiologic, methodologic (in this instance, lung function), and statistical, is brought together at the outset to formulate the protocol.[2461, 2871, 2873]

Definitions used in this section are those provided by the Dictionary of Epidemiology recently updated.[2867] This extremely useful handbook, sponsored by the International Epidemiologic Association, is aimed at standardizing terminology in this discipline and is particularly valuable for those without formal or professional training in epidemiology. (Indeed, the varied terminology in different texts, even for basics such as study design, is reminiscent of the days before pulmonary function terminology was standardized.) In addition, the emphasis in this section is on methodology rather than on content; the latter, including information about the epidemiology of particular lung diseases, appears elsewhere in this volume. The references in this section are not exhaustive. They have been chosen to illustrate aspects of methodology, either in the design or execution of epidemiologic studies of respiratory disease in which lung function tests were used or to illustrate particular applications of lung function tests to address unusual or difficult epidemiologic issues. The emphasis is on chronic nonmalignant respiratory disease; in epidemiologic studies of malignant respiratory disease, lung function tests play little or no role.

Uses of Function Tests in Epidemiology

Epidemiologists, like clinicians, are concerned with describing health events or health status, explaining ill health, and assessing the usefulness of interventions such as treatment. The difference between the epidemiologist's and the clinician's approaches is that the epidemiologist regards the community or the population as the target for study, whereas the clinician is concerned with the individual patient.

Table 5–4, which gives parallel examples (clinical and epidemiologic) of each use, serves to illustrate the essential similarities between issues addressed by clinicians and epidemiologists. However, despite similarities in the issues addressed and in the methods of measurement used, there are important differences in approach and in the interpretation of the findings that need to be articulated; these form the substance of the rest of this section.

The Epidemiologic Approach

The procedure or protocol that a clinician follows in arriving at a diagnosis, planning management, and estimating the prognosis is individualized for each patient. As new information about the patient comes to light, the protocol may be changed, new tests may be performed, and treatment may be altered. The experienced clinician can usually be distinguished by the logic underlying each step taken in the gathering of data about the patient; each item of information gathered addresses a question (or hypothesis), the answer to which may determine the next step to be taken. By contrast, the procedure or protocol an epidemiologist follows in carrying out the study of a population, while infinitely fluid in the development stage, must be strictly adhered to in the executive or data-gathering phase. The protocol for such studies thus contains a clear statement of objectives (what is the hypothesis to be examined?); explicit definitions of the terms used (this is necessary because for most biologic events there are no universal definitions); and descriptions of the study design and target population, including whether the target population is to be studied *in toto* and, if not, the basis of sampling. In the light of this information, the methods of measurement to be used are also carefully detailed; because all measurements contain error, a good protocol usually includes plans to quantitate the error and/or minimize any bias it might exert on the study results (e.g., between observer error if there is more than one observer, between apparatus differences if more than one is used, etc.).

Thus, contrary to the belief sometimes expressed by some laboratory scientists, an epidemiologic study is not merely "a data-gathering exercise with at best a nebulously defined purpose and no hypothesis to test,"[2462] nor is it an exercise in which imprecise methodology is offset by large numbers of subjects. Protocol formulation and data-gathering must be carried out with as much precision as in studies exploring disease mechanisms. Indeed, imprecisions in methodology are more of a threat to the success of a population study than in the clinical context where other information is available,

Table 5–4. USES OF LUNG FUNCTION TESTS IN CLINICAL PRACTICE
AND IN EPIDEMIOLOGIC STUDIES

Uses (Issues)	Examples	
	Clinical Practice	*Epidemiologic Studies*
Description	To describe the functional status of a patient without known disease (e.g., preoperative), at risk for disease (e.g., smoker), or with lung disease	To describe the functional status in a population in relation to age, sex, race, etc. To record the evolution of disease To record the natural history of disease in a population
Explanation	To investigate the cause of dyspnea in a patient (e.g., respiratory versus cardiac origin) To characterize the pattern of lung function abnormality to suggest etiology	To investigate the cause of abnormality/dysfunction/ disease in a population in relation to suspected risk factors (e.g., smoking or occupational exposures)
Evaluation	To assess the effects of therapy, both intended (steroid effect) or toxic (e.g., the toxic effect of nitrofurantoin)	To assess the effects of therapy (randomized control trials) To assess the effects of other measures to protect health (e.g., dust control on silicosis rates)

enabling the experienced practitioner to ignore or appropriately weigh information that does not fit.

Design Options

The experimental design, illustrated in Figure 5–1, is the cornerstone of the scientific method. In its strict or complete sense, it requires that the researcher have complete control of all aspects of the study, including randomization of the population sample into study groups at the outset and no loss to follow-up. While feasible in animal studies, its main application in human populations has been in the form of randomized control trials (RCTs) of drugs, vaccines, and, more recently, health and social services.[2873] For example, in the field of lung disease, the usefulness of RCTs in evolving

and evaluating the drug regimes for the treatment of tuberculosis has been outstanding.

For the most part, however, non-experimental designs have to be used for studies in humans whether they are epidemiologic in nature or whether they are directed toward the study of disease mechanisms and make use of the methodology of the clinical laboratory sciences. The word "survey," recently defined as "an investigation in which the information is systematically collected but in which the experimental method is not used,"[2868] can thus be used to describe the bulk of published epidemiologic studies in humans in the last two decades. Such studies (or surveys) may have analysis or description as their objectives.

The analytic study, defined as "a hypothesis-testing method of investigating the association between a given disease and possible causative

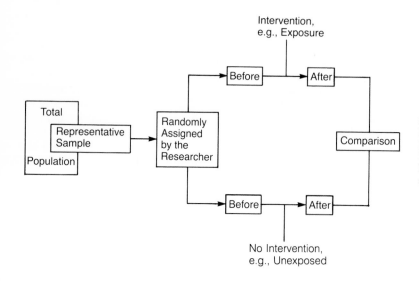

Figure 5–1. Basis of population studies. (After McDonald, J. C. Epidemiology. In: Occupational Lung Diseases. Eds: H. Weill and M. Turner-Warwick. Marcel Dekker, New York, 1981, with permission of the author and publisher.)

factors,"[2867] may be cross-sectional (prevalence), cohort (prospective), or case-control (retrospective). Cross-sectional studies, focusing as they do on a population or work force at a given point in time, have obvious shortcomings; as has been succinctly pointed out, at the time of study "the dead are buried and the sick are in hospital."[2461] Nevertheless, they are a valuable starting point, and, as in clinical medicine, a careful description of events at a given point in time is invariably a first step in understanding. Cohort or prospective studies[2867] are also called follow-up, longitudinal, or concurrent studies; these terms describe an essential factor in the study design, namely observation of the population for a sufficient period of time to generate reliable rates for the development of the health events studied, such as decline in lung function[1321, 2863] or the development of acute airway reactions to such substances as cotton dust.[2875] These studies usually involve large numbers of subjects, and the study period, which is usually measured in years or decades rather than in days or months, can start or end with the present.

Case-control studies,[2867] by contrast, start with identification of cases (persons who manifest the disease or other outcome variable of interest) and proceed to the selection of controls (persons who do not); the two groups are then compared for the exposures(s) or other attribute(s) thought to relate to the disease. The term "retrospective" has also been applied to this type of study because it starts "after the onset of illness and looks back to the postulated causal factors."[2867]

Descriptive studies may also be cross-sectional or prospective. However, in contrast to clinical studies (many of which are also descriptive in character), epidemiologic studies that fall into this category (i.e., in which there is no attempt to investigate an association between disease and a postulated causal factor) are infrequently reported; most at least record the influence of age and sex on disease rates, two usually important determinants of risk. Likewise, most studies of occupational disease consider the influence of some index of occupational exposure.[2873] This is presumably why the Dictionary of Epidemiology[2867] originally contained no entry under the title "descriptive studies"; most researchers would no doubt consider the returns on the time invested not sufficiently rewarding unless an etiologic hypothesis was investigated. An exception to this may be the description of changes in lung function with age.[2864, 2890]

Lung Function Tests as Measurement Tools in Epidemiologic Studies

In reply to the question what is the best test of lung function for use in epidemiologic studies, the answer is that there is no "best test"; a test is (or tests are) chosen for each study in the light of the defined objectives, as well as the nature of the expected abnormality, dysfunction, or disease in the study population. In addition, the choice should take into account study design, the population to be tested, resources available, numbers to be tested, duration of the study, and coefficients of variation of the different tests. However, although this point is incontestably correct at a conceptual level, it must be recognized that spirometric (i.e., volume/time) measurements have become so widely used in epidemiologic studies of chronic respiratory disease characterized by airflow limitation that in practice the questions to be asked at the beginning of a study are

1. Which of the following spirometric measurements should be selected for use in a given study—FEV, FEV_1, FEV_3, FEF_{25-75}, or others?

2. If the measurement apparatus also permits recording of flow rates, should any volume flow measurements ($\dot{V}max_{50\%}VC$, etc.) be included? Because they are readily available does not necessarily mean that additional measurements should be used in hypothesis testing even though they might provide useful descriptive information. It is important to note that the more tests that are used, the higher a percentage of "abnormal" results will be recorded.[2922, 5045]

3. Should any other function measurements besides spirometry be made? Here one may call upon the full range of available tests, most of which have been or could be adapted for epidemiologic use under field conditions. For instance, the single-breath diffusing capacity measurement is particularly useful for studies in which the outcome of interest is interstitial lung disease[2321, 2343, 4655]; tests of bronchial reactivity are important when the outcome of interest is asthma (see Chapter 5); exercise tests are useful for evaluating physical fitness[5052, 5054] or work capacity[2321, 2343]; and the single-breath nitrogen test is of benefit when small airway abnormality may be important.[3995] Detailed or complex tests may be particularly appropriate in carefully planned studies of selected subjects, for instance in case-control designs within a

cohort or prevalence study. They may also be appropriate to more precisely define the characteristics of the initial population to be followed in longitudinal studies.[1197, 2859]

Special mention must be made of studies in which the outcome of interest is asthma, whether induced by occupation or not. Because the essential feature of this condition is intermittent and variable airflow limitation, recording diurnal variation of airflow limitation (including, for instance, before, during, and after a workshift) is often called for, and measurement of peak flow carried out and recorded by the subject has proved a useful test.[511] Interpretation of the findings may not always be easy, however.[5056]

In adapting or selecting a lung function test (or tests) for use as a measurement tool in epidemiologic studies, a major challenge is to maximize and maintain precision (repeatability) of the measurement throughout a study, particularly if it is to last for weeks or months and is to take place under field conditions. Other requirements are acceptability and robustness. In addition, the standard rules for measurement in epidemiology should be observed.[2868] Thus, tests should, whenever possible, be administered and interpreted by technicians and readers unaware of the subject's status (diseased or not, exposed or not). Machine (computer) selection and reading of tests, nowadays the rule rather than the exception,[2876] obviates observer bias but is not without problems, particularly in curve selection. This is because of failure to recognize false starts or interrupted breaths—deficiencies in recordings that may be easily detected by a human observer. In addition, the number of trials to produce, for instance, an acceptable spirometric result (until recently regarded as a reflection of inadequate subject cooperation or comprehension) may of itself reflect impaired respiratory function[2877] and should be recorded.

Sources of Variation

An old proverb draws attention to the fact that variety is the spice of life; it is also the main subject for biologic study. Biologic variation is compounded by measurement error, and lung function tests are no exception.[2876, 2879] An essential preliminary to an epidemiologic study in which lung (or any other) function is to be measured is therefore to consider the sources

and magnitude of the variation in the biologic events under study; these include those that are the subject of study, the "signal," and those that are not, the "noise."[2873, 2879, 2880] In the present context, a convenient format for classifying sources of variation in lung function is illustrated in Table 5–5. Three broad categories are considered: within-individual, between-individual, and between-population.[2878, 2879] Since the essence of an epidemiologic study is the interpretation of between-population differences, this source of variation is almost always the "signal"; by the same token, within-individual variation is almost always "noise," and this

Table 5–5. SOURCES OF VARIATION IN MEASUREMENTS OF LUNG FUNCTION*

Variation		Source
Within-individual	Technical:	Within and between instruments
		Within and between observers in administration and reading of tests
		Curve selection
		Temperature†
	Biologic:	Comprehension and/or co-operation of the subject
		Circadian, weekly and seasonal effects
		Endocrine; other
Between-individual	All the above sources +	
	Subject:	Size, sex, age, respiratory muscularity
		Race and other genetic characteristics
		Past and present health
		Habits (e.g., smoking, physical activity)
	Environmental:	Residence (income, ambient pollution, etc.)
		Indoor pollution (smoking, gas stoves, etc.)
		Occupational exposures
Between-population	All the above sources +	
		Selection into or out of the target or study population

*Modified with permission from Becklake, M. R. Epidemiologic studies in human populations. In: Handbook of Experimental Pharmacology. Vol. 75. Toxicology of Inhaled Materials. Eds: H. P. Witschi and J. B. Brain. Springer-Verlag, Berlin, 1985, p 131. Reproduced with permission.

†Ambient temperature affects the accuracy of recording of certain spirometers.

must be held to the minimum possible for a successful study. Certain sources of between-individual variation, such as height, are usually "noise," and these must therefore be taken into account in some way before the size and significance of the "signal" can be evaluated. What is "noise" in one study may well be "signal" in another. For instance, the effects of smoking are frequently the objective of study, i.e., the "signal." However, in a study of the effects of an occupational exposure, smoking effects become "noise" to be taken into account before comparing exposed with non-exposed subjects—this comparison being the "signal." Sources of within-individual variation may be technical, related to variation within and between instruments, or it may result from variation within and between observers in the procedure for administering the tests or reading the results. They may also be biologic.

The publication of guidelines for instrument specification,[1157, 2876] testing procedure,[1157, 2881, 2923, 3817] technician training,[2882] and analysis of results[2459, 2878, 2883, 2884] has done much to minimize technical sources of variation; nevertheless, they remain a reality even in experienced hands.[2376, 8223] Townsend,[3814] for instance, has recently analyzed the effect of leaks in the spirometer on survey data.

Somewhat surprisingly, within-individual variation for spirometry (as measured by the coefficient of variation) is low,[2878] as noted in this chapter but does not appear to be further reduced by the use of computer-assisted methods for recording and analyzing tracings.[429, 2876] Another source of within-individual variation is less than optimal comprehension, cooperation, or muscular coordination[2864] on the part of the subject being tested. This can be diminished though not eliminated by coaching; indeed, the "learning effect" is thought to explain, at least in part, the not infrequent finding that on average, spirometric results in a second study in the same subjects are higher than they were in the first, even after a lapse of several months.[723, 2883, 2886] Likewise, physiologic (biologic) sources of variation must also be taken into account in planning an epidemiologic study. For example, failure to take into account circadian changes[1520] or weekly or seasonal effects[2886] would reduce the chances of detecting the effects of environmental exposure if all unexposed subjects were to be tested in the afternoon and all exposed subjects were tested in the morning. Testing schedules should therefore be planned so that all sources of within-

individual variation operate in such a way as not to bias the study results.

Attempts at standardizing procedures have also led to appreciation of the fact that the inability of a subject to achieve forced expiratory flow-volume curves that meet current reproducibility criteria may in itself be a measure of poor health.[2877] The explanation may be related to the fact that the maneuver of a forced expiratory flow-volume curve may, in a susceptible subject, induce a level of bronchoconstriction not relieved by a subsequent full inspiration (as noted in Chapter 9).

A useful preliminary to any field survey is an in-house exercise to quantitate measurement error.[2880] This should be partitioned into between-technician differences if more than one technician is to take part,[572] between-spirometer differences if more than one is to be used,[2887] and between-reader differences if there is more than one reader.[572] Such an exercise may reveal measurement differences that are correctable. Another check on quality control, particularly useful in a survey that lasts over several months, is to retest a small number of subjects during the course of the survey.[2885]

Sources of between-individual variation include, of course, all those accounting for within-individual variation just noted. For a test like the FEV_1, these probably account for between 3% and 5% of between-individual variation,[2879] as noted in the first section of this chapter. The major sources of between-individual variation are size, sex, and age, accounting for approximately 50%, 10%, and 5% (over the range from 20 to 70 years), respectively.[2878, 2879, 2904] Other sources of variation include ethnic differences,[2898] respiratory pressures,[2864] and a variety of environmental exposures, including active and passive smoking (Table 5–6).[2888] In all studies, a certain proportion of the between-individual variation, estimated as at least 20%, remains unexplained, inviting further study. Much of the research into the evolution of lung function with age has focused on the various recognized sources of between-individual variation as the signal. For example, Burrows and his colleagues[2890] in Tucson, Arizona trace the rise and fall of the FEV_1 with chronologic age through eight decades. On the other hand, in studies aimed at assessing the effects of environmental exposures, these sources of variation constitute "noise" and must be taken into account before the effects of environmental agents can be assessed.

A convenient method of taking into account

Table 5–6. ESTIMATES OF PROPORTION OF VARIATION IN FVC ATTRIBUTED TO IDENTIFIED FACTORS*

Factor	Attributable Variation (%)
Sex	up to 30
Age	8
Height	20
Weight	2
Race	10
Technical	3
Residual†	27
Total	100

*Modified from Becklake, M. R. Concepts of normality applied to the measurement of lung function. Am J Med 1986, 80:1158–1164. Reproduced with permission.

†Residual variation includes smoking (active and passive), childhood illnesses, and so forth, but a sizable proportion, perhaps about 20%, is unexplained.

the main determinants of between-individual variation in epidemiologic studies is to standardize the mean results of the different comparison groups to a common age, height, and (sometimes) weight for preference close to the mean values for the study.[2463]

There are choices to be made as to which method is to be used to compare values obtained in different study populations. Comparisons may be made in the following ways:

1. By using external reference standards.

2. By using recently reported reference standards developed for predictive purposes and tested in other sample populations.[2891]

3. By using height and age regressions derived from the study population itself,[2321, 2463] a method inappropriate in small studies (containing fewer than 100 subjects, for example).

4. By including age and height as a standardizing variable in a regression analysis.[2424, 2463]

5. By proportional standardization for height based on the demonstration that FEV_1 and FVC are proportional to the square of the height.[2893]

6. By dividing measured values by predicted values for the group as a whole based on their mean age and height furnished from some reference population.[2463, 2876]

Of these, the last is perhaps the least satisfactory method, given the wide range of reported predictions[2876, 2894] and the dilemma of selecting the most appropriate reference values.

Reference Values

In the first section of this chapter, we commented on the range of normal reference values in the literature. In epidemiologic studies, if reference values are to be used to take into account factors such as sex, age, and height, the choice of which values to use should be guided by methodologic considerations; thus, similar equipment and identical testing procedures and reading methods should have been used in the study which generated the reference values and in the epidemiologic study to which they are to be applied.[2876, 2879] A second requirement is that both study populations should be comparable in terms of age range and ethnic and social composition. The final criterion is conceptual[2879]: Is it more appropriate to compare a work force in Quebec with the male residents of Tucson, Arizona who do not smoke from choice[320, 2859] or with those from Portland, Oregon[2895] and Salt Lake City, Utah[429] who do not smoke from religious conviction? Alternatively, should data (of the type recently compiled in Europe[2884]) be used which is an aggregate from a large number of studies? It is for these reasons that the use of reference standards developed for the purposes of prediction rather than description[2890] may in the future become the accepted method for accounting for age and height differences. These criteria are also appropriate for the choice of reference values to be used in clinical laboratories, as indicated in the first section of this chapter.

In many epidemiologic studies, the design is such that the study objectives are met by comparing study groups, for example, exposed with non-exposed, smokers with non-smokers, and so forth. In these examples, the choice of reference values used to take into account age and height differences in the study groups is less critical than in the clinical context because both or all study groups are treated equally with respect to the adjustments for age and height (and any other confounding variables).

Under these circumstances, group differences are unlikely to be obscured or exaggerated by the choice of one set of reference values rather than another or one type of age/height adjustment rather than another. The same would probably be true if smoking and non-smoking reference values were used to take into account differences in smoking status between study groups.[629, 2892] An alternative approach is to analyze results from different smoking categories separately; the disadvantage of this is that numbers become small, particularly if there is a further subdivision into occupational exposure categories. It is more usual nowadays to use one of the forms of multivariate analysis that adjust for smoking internally, i.e., according to the smoking/lung function relationship shown in the data set under study. Thus, smoking may be considered as a continuous (pack/ year) or discrete (smoker/non-smoker) variable. However, it must be remembered that whatever adjustment is used, it is no better or worse than the quality of information upon which it is based, and it is wise to bear in mind that a subject's recall of his or her smoking may be neither accurate nor unbiased. How to adjust for smoking so that other environmental determinants of lung function status can be detected, remains a major challenge in all epidemiologic studies.

In certain instances, what is of interest is the prevalence rate of abnormality in a given population,[2896] an exercise similar to clinical case detection except that the clinician has other information by which to judge the significance of spirometric abnormality. Clearly, the prevalence of abnormality in a population depends on the criteria used to define it.[2896] It is also clear that not only is it unlikely that agreement could be reached on universal criteria or definitions of abnormality of lung function,* but it is probably also undesirable to promote the idea that a single set of criteria is appropriate for all circumstances or populations. On the other hand, specific definitions of normality or abnormality can be used to address specific issues.[2879] When comparisons are sought with other populations or studies, definitions used obviously must be identical or as close to identical as possible to those used in the populations with which comparisons are sought. For example, a recently published state-wide survey of Michigan[2896] reported on rates of spirometric abnormalities, defined as FVC or FEV_1 less than 80% predicted using Morris' prediction values.[2895] Others wishing to compare their data with data from Michigan should follow the same methodology for measurement and the same criteria for abnormality; for preference they should also compare rates at specific ages because abnormalities increased with age in the Michigan data,[2896] despite the fact that results were expressed as predicted percentage using the formulae of Morris and his colleagues,[2895] which took age into account.

In the field of chronic non-malignant disease, epidemiologic studies exploiting lung function tests as tools of measurement have contributed

to advances in knowledge in a number of different ways. In this section, several of these are described to illustrate the strength and versatility of epidemiologic approaches and methods.

Studies of Natural History of Chronic Airflow Limitation

These are described in a later section. The differentiation between the prognostic importance of the symptoms of chronic mucus hypersecretion on the one hand and a more rapid than predicted decline of FEV_1 on the other, summarized by Peto and his colleagues,[723, 1321, 2924] illustrates the kind of information that may be derived from longitudinal studies. Significant differences in survival between similar groups in different countries and the relative importance of different factors in relation to declining lung function, including the relevance of increased airway reactivity,[1235, 1276, 2863, 2891, 2897, 4063] may also be uncovered in such studies. Another way of approaching the same problem is to define risk factors for the development of severe chronic airflow limitation.

Higgins and her colleagues[2901] have used this approach to develop a risk index based on their own longitudinal data. The index was subsequently validated in several other populations.[4116] Large-scale prospective studies have also been carried out in Arizona,[2859] in Baltimore,[2902] and in Boston.[1394] The Tucson study was broadly based; covered all ages from childhood to adult life; usually carried out annual measurements; assessed smoking and occupational status by questionnaire; and collected information on hematologic and immunologic parameters for use as predictors of outcome.* The Baltimore study focused on familial and genetic determinants of natural history,[2902] and the Boston study concentrated on environmental factors, in particular active and passive smoking.[1394]

Identification of Long-Term Environmental Effects

Some of these studies are summarized in Chapter 6. Of particular interest is the Dutch study conducted by Van der Lende and his colleagues.[829, 2861, 2863, 2925] This began as an analytic cross-sectional population study of men and women aged 40 to 64 years living in three

---

*See references 1143, 2459, 2876, 2879, 2884, 2894, 2896, 5050.

*See references 320, 629, 1143, 2253, 2899.

communities with different pollution levels. The initial results showed higher symptom prevalences in the more polluted regions, but no differences in FVC or FEV_1. Longitudinal measurements were continued at 3-year intervals, and analysis after the fourth study cycle demonstrated the influence of both cigarette smoking and of residence in a more polluted area in the fall of FVC and FEV_1 with time. Increased airway reactivity also appeared to be a factor in increasing the rate of decline.[2863] This series of studies demonstrates the strength of the longitudinal study design in assessing the effect of environmental pollutants, using pulmonary function tests to measure the outcome. However, the most recent report of the results of follow-up[3990] indicate that with a longer period of observation, the difference first observed between the population in the clean region and that in the polluted area is less evident; the reason for this is obscure. Studies of this kind have the advantage that each subject is compared with his or her own initial data, so that between-individual variation due to size and age, which constitute much of the "noise" in the cross-sectional design, is replaced by within-individual variation, which is much smaller. But there are problems of instrument constancy over a long period and of the possibility that follow-up observations may be made at a time when function was, for some reason, fortuitously depressed or elevated.[2907]

Studies of the Effects of Occupational Exposures

Reference is made to a number of these studies, particularly in relation to coal miners, asbestos workers, and cotton textile workers, in Chapter 16. Extensive use has been made of epidemiologic methods in defining adverse health effects attributable to work exposures.[2461, 2873] The issues that can be addressed include:

1. The identification of poor health in the exposed; this may include long-term effects as in the decline of FEV_1 in coal miners or the acute effects of shift work on the FEV_1, for example, in firefighters or cotton textile workers.

2. The investigation of the relationship between poor health and the exposure in question; a key point here is to establish the nature of the exposure-response relationships, if any, since these form the scientific basis for the formulation of control strategies.

3. Once control strategies are in place, their effectiveness can be monitored by ongoing epidemiologic studies.

Most studies have addressed the first two issues; important as the third is, there have been few evaluation studies reported,[2873] perhaps because they are difficult to design and costly in terms of time and effort to carry out. McDonald[2461] has suggested that more serious consideration should be given to non-experimental designs, such as before-and-after studies and multiple time-series, giving appropriate attention to maximizing internal validity.

The precision with which the environmental or occupational exposure is measured is the main determinant of the quality of studies in this field. On the one hand, the tools for measuring poor health (in the present context, lung function tests) are relatively well understood and can be readily applied, and the measurement error involved either is known or can be quantitated. On the other hand, it is seldom possible to measure anything more than a subject's exposure to a given environment (often only very generally defined), and it is virtually never possible to quantitate the amount of the agent delivered to the lung (an exception to this may be the application of new techniques to measure lung dust burden in pathologic material, for example, in case-control studies of mesothelioma).[5049] Nor is it usually possible to identify, let alone quantitate, all other potentially noxious agents that may be present. Given these circumstances, it is surprising that the demonstration of exposure/response relationships is frequently achieved; indeed, it is far from being exceptional, provided that exposure assessment includes a measure of intensity as well as duration.[2889] As has been succinctly pointed out by McDonald,[2889] "failure to specify exposure, save in terms of duration, is the most common and serious weakness in occupational epidemiology," and he deplores the fact that investigators often show defeatism in this regard, allowing "the best to be the enemy of the better than nothing, always a mistake in epidemiology."

In the study of the ill-health effects of occupational exposures, the usual starting point is a prevalence or cross-sectional survey comparing exposed with non-exposed subjects (to address the question, "Is there an adverse health effect related to the exposure?"), or comparing more with the less exposed persons (to address the causal hypothesis that the occurrence of poor health is related to the duration or intensity of exposure.) Prevalence surveys are also the starting point for prospective studies, as well as providing a data base from which to select subpopulations with specific characteristics for further study (for instance, using a case-control design within a cohort[3603, 4633] to explore specific hypotheses). Prevalence studies are also often part of a broader research program into the health status of a given work force, which is likely to include mortality studies and industrial hygiene surveys of the workplace. The latter often permit the development of several indices of exposure, in keeping with the probability that different agents or different-sized particles in the working environment may be responsible for different adverse health effects.

In one such study of chrysotile asbestos workers in Quebec,[2321, 2911-2916] a cumulative exposure index was calculated for each subject based on his job history and measured or estimated dust levels at the time the job was held. Using this index, exposure/response relationships were demonstrable for most of the health outcomes studied; these included death from lung cancer and mesothelioma,[2912, 2913] as well as the prevalence of radiographic changes of pulmonary fibrosis and lung function abnormality, as recorded in cross-sectional studies.[2912, 2914] However, the development of new radiographic and function abnormality or the progression of these changes measured prospectively was not related to cumulative exposure;[2915] these effects related more closely to age and less strongly to smoking. This was thought to be due to the changing profile of exposure, which had fallen dramatically since the 1950's, with the result that age better reflected residence time of the dust in the lung (and presumably its pathogenic potential) than did the cumulative exposure index. Subsequent use of the components of the cumulative exposure index to develop mathematical models of the temporal profile of exposure of each subject has shown that whereas the cumulative index related best to radiologic evidence of interstitial disease, the duration of exposure was more important in the development of airflow limitation.[2916] Early exposures and heavy exposures were more closely related to wheezing syndromes.[2916] Finally, evidence that lung geometry was a risk factor in the development of asbestosis was obtained from a case-control study and was made possible because the data base of the prevalence study was sufficiently broad to permit matching for other potential risk factors such as age and dust exposure.[3603]

The study of workers in foundries in Finland[2917] provides an excellent model of an integrated, well-designed, and coherent multidisciplinary research program. This study had a broad base, with respiratory and cardiac effects being evaluated in relation to separate indices of dust, fume, and CO exposure; all indices were based on careful industrial hygiene surveys.

Questionnaires to ex-workers were used, an assessment of the turnover rates in the work force was made, and the disability status of ex-foundry workers was compared with that of the general population of Finland. Respiratory status, including lung function, was evaluated cross-sectionally[2918] and was supplemented by a systematic assessment of the "healthy worker effect" with potential underestimation of the effects of occupational exposure.[2919] The healthy worker effect derives from the fact that the health experience of working men and women is on average better than that of the general public, which includes the sick and the disabled. Originally described in relation to mortality experience,[2867] it is also evident in other health measurements reflecting organ function, including lung function.

The study of 556 Paris workers already referred to[2424] illustrated the insensitivity of cross-sectional as compared with longitudinal measurements of lung function in detecting the ill health effects of occupational exposures. When first studied in 1960 to 1961, there were no demonstrable differences between different exposure groups. But the decline in FEV_1 over the next 11 years (standardized for age, smoking, and function level) showed clear differences, with exposures to almost all the dusty atmospheres (silica, coal, iron, and grain) being associated with faster declines than those in less contaminated atmospheres. This study also gave evidence of health selection in the workplace, younger men with higher dust exposures having better initial function than those with little or no exposure. As Field[2462] has pointed out "a work force must always be treated as a biased sample of the general population and inhomogenous within itself." Indeed, it is increasingly coming to be recognized that an essential part of the study of the health of any work force must include some measure, direct or indirect, of the extent to which bias due to health selection may have led to an underestimate of any adverse health effects under study.

The evidence relating adverse health effects to ambient environmental pollutants discussed in Chapter 6 illustrates the difficulties of interpretation of data when large numbers must be studied and exposure data are imprecise.

The Use of Lung Function Tests in Screening Normal Populations

Screening programs that include lung function testing have usually one of two general objectives:

1. To detect disease or the precursors of disease as a guide to the medical care of the individuals.

2. To search for evidence of the impact of environmental factors on health in a defined population. Such evidence then becomes a guide for public health measures to reduce environmental exposures from whatever cause.

This section is concerned with the first of these objectives.

It must be emphasized at the outset that without adherence to sound principles such as those outlined by the World Health Organization,[3804] screening programs may well result in enhancing the perception of poor health, rather than improving the outlook for health and well-being.[3805] These principles include (1) scientific validity of the screening procedure used, and (2) evidence that early detection may result in a reduction in morbidity and mortality. In this context, a screening test or procedure refers to the means by which unselected populations can be classified into two groups: one with a high probability of morbidity or with a high risk of premature mortality, and the other with a low risk. (Note that a screening test is not meant to be a diagnostic test.) Early detection refers to the identification of a disorder before symptoms and signs become readily apparent to the individual or to his or her family. These definitions, formulated by the Canadian Task Force on the Periodic Health Examination,[3806] were used by the American Thoracic Society's statement on Screening for Adult Respiratory Disease.[2999]

Concern at their impotence in the face of the lack of effective treatment for severe chronic airflow limitation, together with the ease with which lung function tests can be performed and the availability of computerized equipment, led chest physicians in the late 1970's to use spirometry in what were described as screening programs for case-finding on a large scale. Implementation was often with less than careful consideration of the implications, ethical and otherwise.[2878]

These programs were based on current knowledge of the natural history of chronic airflow limitation, which held the disease to be primarily located in large airways, with smoking cessation as the only effective intervention. Interest in such screening procedures received a further boost with the accumulation of evidence that the small airways might be the location of early pathologic changes, which eventually led to chronic airflow limitation. Tests of small airway function were adapted and evaluated for field use.

In 1974, a workshop on early screening programs for the early diagnosis of airway obstruction was organized by the Division of Lung Diseases (NHLI) and the American Thoracic Society to evaluate potential screening tests.[3808] Although it was agreed that derivatives of the single-breath nitrogen test, in particular closing volume and closing capacity, were probably sensitive measures, it was felt that their validity in early diagnosis and their prognostic capacity had not been established. No doubt for these reasons, no recommendation in favor of large-scale screening was contained in the workshop report.

Subsequently, the use of spirometric screening as an aid to smoking cessation has been tested, with somewhat conflicting results.[2999] More recently, interest has been rekindled in the possibility of using tests of airway hyperreactivity as a screening test. After laying out the issues clearly, the American Thoracic Society statement on Screening for Adult Respiratory Disease issued in 1983 did not contain any recommendation for large-scale population screening for chronic airflow limitation on the basis of the current state of knowledge. However, the application of spirometric tests for clinical case-finding in apparently healthy subjects at high risk was recommended as part of the regular health examination (a policy we recommended in 1974[1263]). The high risk groups identified were heavy smokers; certain occupationally exposed groups (see later); and certain preoperative cases, such as those scheduled for thoracic or upper abdominal surgery, those with respiratory symptoms, and the elderly and the obese.[2999] These recommendations complement those of the Canadian Task Force on the Periodic Health Examination, which did not include respiratory function tests or lung disease in any of their 18 health protection packages for subjects 16 years and over.[3806]

Surveillance for respiratory hazards in the occupational setting was the subject of a separate American Thoracic Society statement[3595] that, in addition to outlining the general principles, draws attention to the particular requirements of screening programs to be applied in the workplace. These include employee education, industrial hygiene evaluation, assessment of respiratory protective devices, the maintenance of appropriate medical records, and plans for ongoing surveillance. Particular care should be given to the choice of respiratory function tests and their interpretation, with agreed-upon criteria for abnormality and handling abnormality so detected; these criteria included the availability of further diagnostic tests and/or treatment. This statement should be carefully studied by any physician about to embark on such a program. A recent detailed description of the respiratory surveillance program in place at the Aluminum Company of America[3809] serves as an excellent model for such programs.

Screening for asthma was dealt with separately in the American Thoracic Society statement on Screening for Adult Respiratory Diseases.[2999] It was felt that all subjects with cough, wheezing, or dyspnea should be tested with spirometry, and the same advice is obviously appropriate for those exposed persons at risk for occupational asthma.

From what has been said, it is evident that the background information underlying a sound screening program is essentially epidemiologic in nature and relates to knowledge of risk factors and the natural history of the disease in question, how it evolves, and what can diminish its progression. The principles outlined by the World Health Organization[3804] should be followed, and wherever possible, an evaluation of the program's effectiveness should be planned—another application of the epidemiologic method.[2873]

The role of lung function tests in screening is currently under study from many points of view. It is recognized that there is an important distinction between "the offering of a screening test to individuals whom the tester has solicited, versus offering to a patient who has presented for health care."[2999] Morris' lecture[3810] to the Royal Society of Medicine entitled "Four Cheers for Prevention" provides positive encouragement for more involvement in preventive strategies.

The screening of British civil servants for respiratory disease and diabetes, conducted by the late Donald Reid and his colleagues,[3811] represents an early initiative directed at a well-defined population group; there is some evidence that the demonstration of an abnormal FEV_1 in that study did lead to cessation of smoking in a significant percentage of those tested, but the follow-up data have not been published in detail.

No doubt the interesting argument will continue. One end of the spectrum of opinion is represented by Holland's cautious but largely negative conclusion[3813] and Colley's even more categorical statement that ". . . there is no clear evidence that intervention in chronic bronchitis confers any worthwhile benefit. For this reason alone, there can be no justification for introducing screening programmes aimed at detecting chronic bronchitis in the adult population."[3812] An alternative view is that the evidence to justify (or not) such a screening program can only be acquired by introducing it on a trial basis, with evaluation procedures built into the implementation plan. We feel that at the present time, screening tests as typified by the "spirometer in the supermarket" cannot be justified; indeed, they may properly be criticized as a thinly disguised attempt to "drum up business." But the use of spirometry in well-defined groups in whom effective counseling on the basis of test results (in the absence of symptoms severe enough to have led to previous medical consultation) may well be useful, as typified by Reid's survey of civil servants.[3811]

CHALLENGE TESTS TO THE LUNG

Since their development 15 years ago, and increasingly over the last 5 years, challenge tests of various kinds have been used in more laboratories and in a growing range of applications. The tests are designed to reproduce, in the laboratory, the clinical manifestations experienced by patients, and thereby to clarify the responsiveness of the subject's airway to specific or non-specific stimuli. The main purposes for which they are used are:

1. To establish an etiologic diagnosis in asthma and in extrinsic allergic alveolitis.
2. To investigate pathogenetic mechanisms in asthma, including evaluation of the role of immunologically or non-immunologically induced airway hyperreactivity.

3. To assess the effects of therapy on airway reactivity.

Basic aspects of airway reactivity were described in Chapter 1; here it may be noted that recent experimental work on sheep shows that there is a close relationship between the airway response when histamine is given by aerosol and when it is delivered by infusion.[3088] Data on asthmatic responses can be found in Chapter 9, and asthma of occupational origin is discussed in Chapter 16.

In this section, the methodology and results of challenge testing are described. Massey and his colleagues[3098] reported on the characteristics of different nebulizers,[3098] and several general reviews of airway challenge testing have appeared.[498, 514, 549, 561] An excellent symposium volume[535] deals with several important aspects of the subject.

A recent report from a European working group described standardization of bronchial challenge tests.[3107] A report in 1980 from the United States also dealt with technical standardization.[500] Techniques have been described in many papers[505, 506, 517, 523]; recently, attention has been paid to simplifying the method as much as possible for use in field surveys.[3091, 3102] Tattersfield[555] commented on uncertainties in testing bronchial reactivity. It should perhaps be pointed out that there are still many uncertainties in relation to airway response, and it has not been possible to show a significant relationship between *in vivo* response to histamine and the response of airway smooth muscle studied after surgical resection in the same subject.[3085]

Challenge tests can be carried out in several different ways:

1. Using non-antigenic pharmacologic agents, such as histamine and methacholine. These have been widely used to assess airway reactivity in normal subjects, among whom about 3% show hyperreactivity[535]; in population surveys[3106]; in suspected asthmatics (see Chapter 9); and in patients with occupational asthma.[518]

2. Using cold air, voluntary hyperventilation,[536] or exercise to induce bronchoconstriction. These are discussed in Chapter 9, but it may be noted here that comparative studies indicate that maximal exercise testing is not as good a screening test for detecting airway reactivity as are pharmacologic methods.[3095]

3. Using gases important in air pollution such as SO_2 and ozone.

4. Using challenge material encountered in a working environment. As noted in later sections, these include cotton dust, toluene diisocyanate, western red cedar dust, flour, spray paint, solder resin, formaldehyde, and so forth.

5. Using material to which the patient is believed to be exceptionally sensitive, such as aspirin.[546]

Types of Response to Challenge Tests

Three types of response may be noted following challenge tests:

1. Bronchial reactions; these are described in three forms—immediate, late, or combined immediate and late.

2. Alveolar response, as seen in hypersensitivity pneumonitis or extrinsic allergic alveolitis.

3. Systemic reactions, predominantly fever and leukocytosis.

Bronchial Reactions

Immediate bronchial reactions signaled by a decline in FEV_1 or in other tests of airflow can be induced by allergens[533, 537, 541] in sensitized subjects or by histamine or methacholine. When allergens are inhaled, the response is thought to be mediated by IgE antibodies, although short term sensitizing IgG antibodies have been implicated in some cases.[498] The response can be inhibited by pretreatment with beta-adrenergic stimulants and by cromolyn sodium but is unaffected by corticosteroids. Immediate responses are found to toluene diisocyanate in sensitized workers,[530] to cotton dust in subjects with byssinosis,[546] to formaldehyde,[515] and, in sensitized bakers, to flour.[550, 551] Falls in FEV_1 are induced within 2 hours of exposure to irritant gases such as SO_2[543, 557] and ozone[508] (see Chapter 6).

A late asthmatic reaction develops several hours after challenge; it is maximal at 5 to 8 hours and usually resolves within 24 hours, although it may persist for a few days. Such reactions are typically seen in patients with occupational asthma due to exposure to western red cedar dust when challenged with red cedar extract.[516, 519, 528, 566] Other patterns of late reaction have recently been described, and in one of these the response develops one hour after challenge and resolves in 4 hours. A second response develops much later, in the early hours of the morning, with a tendency to recur at approximately the same time on successive nights after a single exposure.[498] Late asthmatic reactions are commonly encountered after exposure to industrial materials and can be inhibited by prior administration of cromolyn sodium or corticosteroids (Figs. 5–2 and 5–3).

A dual response consists of an immediate component with spontaneous recovery, followed 4 to 6 hours later by the late component. Such a response to western red cedar extract is illustrated in Figure 5–4. It occurs commonly after antigen challenge and after challenge with industrial materials. The immunologic events underlying the late component of the dual reaction are not understood. It has been suggested that it is a Type III allergic reaction mediated by precipitating antibodies or that it may be part of an IgE-mediated response.[498]

In cases of extrinsic allergic alveolitis such as those due to farmer's lung or contact with birds, inhalation tests with the appropriate antigens reproduce the features of the disease. Hendrick and associates[510] reported on 144 challenge tests in 31 subjects with different types of extrinsic allergic alveolitis. In addition to declines in FEV_1, they noted significant increases in exercise ventilation and in respiratory frequency on exercise. FVC, body temperature, and circulating neutrophils and lymphocytes also changed. In 10 subjects, measurements of DL_{CO}, resting ventilation, and lung volumes were, by comparison, less affected. Lung auscultation and chest x-rays were not useful in assessing the

response. In a unique study, the same authors[559] tested the efficacy of a respirator in protecting against the antigen in patients with farmer's lung by assessing its ability to prevent these reactions when the subject was exposed.

Exposure to fungal antigens in a sawyer[521] led to a 50% decrease in FEV_1 and a fall in Pa_{O_2} from 85 mm Hg to 70 mm Hg on one occasion and to 55 mm Hg on another occasion. In a different study, 22 cases of farmer's lung showed an enhanced response to histamine during the acute phase of the disease, and in 16 of 20 subjects retested 2 months later, the challenge test with histamine had become negative.[552] There is controversy about the immunopathologic mechanisms in these diseases. The timing of onset and duration of the reaction, together with the ability of corticosteroids to block the reaction, are compatible with a Type III allergic reaction; but there is evidence that Type II, Type III, and Type IV immune reactions may play a part.

Factors Affecting Response to Inhalation Challenge

Drugs that affect the response to inhalation challenge include beta-adrenergic stimulants, cromolyn sodium, corticosteroids, antihistamines, atropine,[3096] and hydroxyzine.[500] Recent antigenic challenge, upper respiratory tract infections,[547] and influenza vaccination[500] may all increase bronchial responsiveness. In addition,

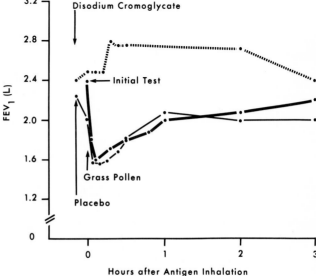

Figure 5–2. Immediate asthmatic reaction to grass pollen challenge. Administration of disodium cromoglycate before challenge inhibited the reaction.

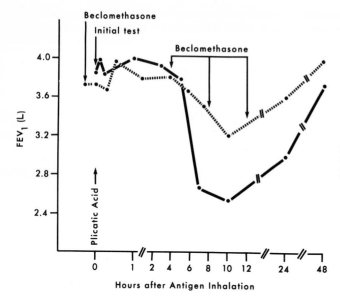

Figure 5–3. Late asthmatic reaction induced by plicatic acid challenge. Administration of beclomethasone before and at intervals after challenge partially inhibited the reaction.

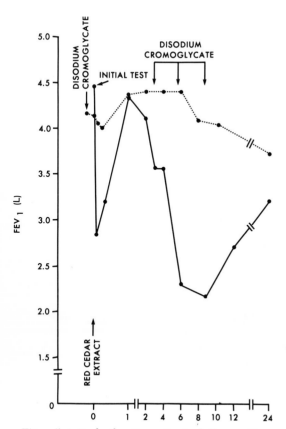

Figure 5–4. Dual asthmatic reaction to challenge with an extract of red cedar. Administration of disodium cromoglycate before and at intervals after challenge completely inhibited the immediate reaction and partially inhibited the late reaction.

both the rate of drug or antigen administration and breathing patterns are important factors. Tidal breathing favors deposition in smaller airways, whereas if fast vital capacity breaths are taken, more particles are deposited in larger airways.[502] For a given delivered dose of histamine, a greater fall in FEV_1 is observed if more of the drug is delivered centrally rather than peripherally.[44] The characteristics of the nebulizer and the delivery system determine the output and the particle size of the aerosol.[3098] Ryan and co-workers[501] noted that the output of the nebulizer, but not the particle size (if between 1.3 and 3.6 microns), altered the bronchial response. Consistent nebulizer output and breathing patterns are necessary for standardization of the test if consistent results are to be obtained.

Safety Procedures and Patient Preparation

Non-specific challenge tests may be safely carried out in the field (as noted later). Challenge tests using suspected allergens or materials encountered in the workplace should be carried out in a hospital setting where facilities for resuscitation or prolonged observation are available. Bronchial challenge tests should be performed by physicians with experience in these procedures and who are familiar with dealing with any complications. Inhaled and parenteral bronchodilators, corticosteroids, antihistamines, and oxygen should be available. It is important to ensure that adequate ventilation and exhaust fans are installed to protect laboratory staff. The staff administering the tests should have a normal bronchial reactivity. No inhalation challenge tests should be performed on subjects with an FEV_1 of less than 1.5 liters. Medications that might affect the response should be withheld for at least 4 hours before the procedure. Smoking and caffeine ingestions should be avoided for 6 hours before testing, and exercise and cold air exposure should be avoided for 2 hours before testing.[500]

Assessment of Response to Challenges

When challenge tests to dusts or chemicals are being performed, airflow measurements should be recorded before and immediately after the challenge; at 5, 10, 15, 30, and 60 minutes after the challenge; and then hourly for up to 8 or 10 hours. A further measurement at 24 hours is important, since this may reveal a late asthmatic reaction. The patient may be instructed to use a peak flow meter and record hourly measurements in the evening and during the night should he or she awake with dyspnea. In patients in whom alveolar or systemic reactions are anticipated, measurements of temperature, white cell count, lung volumes, and diffusing capacity should be included. The American Thoracic Society Subcommittee on Bronchial Inhalation Challenge[500] recommended that changes in lung function should exceed two standard deviations or be twice the coefficient of variation for repeated measurements in the same subject before a significant change can be said to have occurred. Minimal decreases were FEV_1—20%; VC—10%; PEFR—25%; FEF_{25-75}; VC—25%; and specific conductance—40%. However, when a late asthmatic reaction is observed, the results on the challenge day should be compared with those on the control test day, as noted later.

Control Tests

Control tests are important for three reasons: bronchial response may be affected by suggestion, very reactive patients may show a response to the diluent used for antigens or drugs, and the degree of diurnal variation in baseline function should be established. The diluent, usually phosphate-buffered saline, is used for the control test. The buffering is important, since it has been shown that if the pH is less than 5.0, the acidity alone may cause a response.[558] In testing exposure to occupational materials, the material selected for the control challenge depends on the nature of the material used for the challenge test. For example, challenge with an extract made from another species of wood serves as a good control test for a patient suspected of suffering from asthma due to western red cedar exposure (Fig. 5–5).

Methacholine and Histamine Challenge Tests

Bronchial hyperreactivity to these materials is the hallmark of bronchial asthma. Indeed, it may be stated that the diagnosis of asthma cannot be sustained if no hyperreactivity is present. The literature on this response is extensive.*

*See references 44, 500, 526, 531, 538–540, 553, 554, 556, 560, 562, 563, 3089, 3102, 3106, 3107.

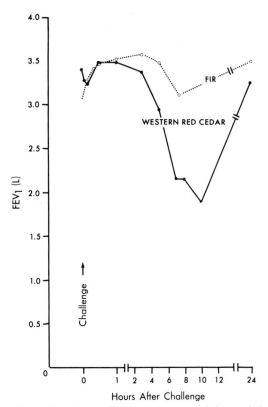

Figure 5–5. Late asthmatic reaction to inhalation challenge to western red cedar extract. No reaction to challenge with Douglas fir extract in a patient with red cedar asthma.

When a bronchial response alone is expected, measurements reflecting airflow obstruction, including spirometry, flow-volume curves, and body plethysmographic recordings of airflow reduction, are used. The peak expiratory flow rate (PEFR) has been successfully used in children,[3094] and 95% confidence limits for the dose needed to induce a 20% fall in PEFR have been published.

In adults, the FEV_1 is most commonly employed; but it has been suggested that the maximal flow at 40% of the vital capacity is a more sensitive indicator, and this has been used.[3101, 3103] It appears likely, however, that other flow tests, although more sensitive than the FEV_1, are less discriminatory.[3097]

The fall in SGaw has also been studied in relation to histamine challenges,[3090, 3099] and a new device has been described that permits a dose-response curve of R_L to be plotted during continuous methacholine inhalation.[3105] The slope of the response to histamine has been extensively studied,[3087] but Cockcroft and Berscheid[3093] showed that plotting a dose-response curve and calculating its slope was not superior to using the "PC20," or dose, to cause a 20% fall in FEV_1 and that this method is preferable in routine testing (Fig. 5–6). Increases in residual volume and SBN_2/L slope occur on challenge testing[527]; and in 10 normal subjects challenged with methacholine,[3108] a 20% fall in FEV_1 was accompanied by a mean increase in residual volume from 1.54 to 2.37 liters. The $SBN_2/L\%$ slope increased from 0.88% to 2.84%, and the authors concluded that the increase in residual volume accounted for 24% of the increased slope of Phase III.

It has been shown that sensitivity to an allergen is closely related to sensitivity to histamine[567]; if large numbers of patients are studied,[553] it is possible to show that there is a good correlation between the severity of asthma and the level of bronchial reactivity. However, this correspondence may not be demonstrable in smaller numbers of cases followed in detail.[525] There is a clear relationship between the mean wheal diameter on skin test to allergen and the dose of histamine required to lower the FEV_1 by 20%.[565] Bronchial reactivity is enhanced by exposure to ozone,[542] and asthmatics are more reactive than patients with chronic bronchitis[513] or cystic fibrosis.[568] Patients with bronchiectasis who are reactive to histamine do less well after surgery than those who are not.[532] Some patients with sarcoidosis are reactive to histamine,[544] as noted in Chapter 15.

Techniques used for histamine challenge are described by a number of authors.* The characteristics of the nebulizer used should be known and the output of it checked frequently. We have used a Bennett-Twin nebulizer with an output of about 0.25 mL/min at an airflow rate of 5 L/min. The mean particle size is 3.1 microns mass median diameter. As noted earlier, phosphate-buffered saline is used as the control solution. Methacholine (acetyl-beta-methylcholine chloride) and histamine acid phosphate are prepared at concentrations of 0.03, 0.06, 0.125, 0.25, 0.50, 1.0, 2.0, 4.0, 8.0, and 16.0 mg/mL. All solutions are stored at 4 degrees centigrade. Histamine solutions are renewed every 3 months and methacholine every 2 weeks (though data indicate that methacholine may remain stable for as long as 4 months[3086]). Aerosol of the control solution is delivered via a face mask loosely applied over the nose and mouth, and the subject is asked to breathe with a normal tidal volume for 2 minutes; then at 5-minute intervals the subject breathes histamine or methacholine in increasing concentrations

---

*See references 498, 500, 503, 505, 506, 517, 523.

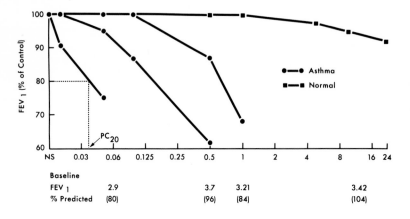

Figure 5–6. Dose-response curves of methacholine challenge tests on three patients with asthma and one normal subject. PC20 is the provocative concentration of methacholine that induced a 20% drop in FEV_1.

for 2 minutes at each level (in asthmatics the 2-minute inhalation time has been shown to give more reproducible results than a 30-second inhalation time[3104]). The FEV_1 is measured after each inhalation, at 30 seconds, and at 4 minutes. Inhalations are discontinued when the FEV_1 has fallen by 20% or more from the post-saline level. The response is expressed in terms of the provocative concentration of histamine or methacholine required to lower the FEV_1 by 20% and is known as the PC20. This method is based on that described by Cockcroft and his colleagues,[505] and like them, we have found it to be highly reproducible.[504] The r value in duplicate tests on the same individuals has been reported to be as high as 0.98.[3089]

The dose of histamine needed to induce a 20% fall in FEV_1 is usually found to be greater than 8.0 mg/mL in normal persons; in known asthmatics it varies from 0.06 mg/mL to 2.0 mg/mL—the two groups often being regarded as distinct.[3089] However, in an important paper, Cockcroft, Berscheid, and Murdock[3106] tested 300 randomly selected normal students and showed that the total distribution of response to histamine was unimodal—with those with a history of asthma being grouped at the higher sensitivity level but not distinct from normal subjects without any such history. Therefore, although the approximate differentiation of "normals" from "asthmatics" may be useful as a rule of thumb, the differentiation is not distinct as was formerly believed.

Using a simple screening procedure that took between 6 and 12 minutes per subject, a group of authors recently reported that the agreement between tests on two occasions showed an r value of 0.94.[3102] This simplified test will be useful in epidemiologic studies if it is standardized.

Antigen Challenge Testing

Sterile aqueous antigen extracts should be used. The diluent is usually phosphate-buffered saline with 0.4% phenol. Dilutions of antigen containing 10, 50, 100, 500, 1000 and 5000 protein nitrogen units/mL should be used. Skin tests by the prick method should be done using these dilutions. On the control day, the diluent is given by inhalation for 2 minutes. On the antigen challenge day, the starting dilution of antigen extract is that which on prior skin testing produced a wheal of less than 3 millimeters in diameter. Should the FEV_1 drop by less than 20% from the baseline value 20 minutes after the initial concentration has been given by 2-minute inhalation and if a late reaction is not expected, the next concentration may be given. If a new antigen is being investigated, or if a late reaction is expected, further inhalation is withheld until the following day. The FEV_1 should be monitored for 24 hours after both the control and antigen test days.

Exposure to a Simulated Working Environment

As noted in Chapter 16, measurements of decline of FEV_1 over a working shift constitute an important technique to establish the occurrence of airflow obstruction after exposure. Challenge tests refine this information and permit a more precise definition of the active substance, as exemplified by the demonstration that toluene di-isocyanate was the active material involved after exposure to a polyurethane varnish.[569]

Because these tests are becoming increasingly important, we feel that we should emphasize the fact that they are not easy to perform. Pepys and Hutchcroft[498] recommended that they should be conducted in a small cubicle or exposure chamber that can be well ventilated after the test. Chemical dusts, such as complex salts of platinum and piperazine hydrochloride, and antimicrobial drugs are highly allergenic. Well-dried lactose powder heated overnight to 105 degrees centigrade should be used as a vehicle for such dusts, and the concentration of dust in the lactose can be doubled on successive days. Exposure can be contrived by asking the patient to pour the dust from one container to another for a pre-set time. Wood dust, grain dust, and wheat flour can be used for such tests without dilution in lactose.

By such methods, sensitivity to the dust of western red cedar,[516, 519, 528, 566] baker's flour,[550, 551] toluene di-isocyanate (TDI) and diphenyl methane di-isocyanate (MDI),* solder used in electronics,[511] detergents,[522] spray starch,[520] spray paint,[524] ethylenediamine,[548] and cotton dust[509] has all been demonstrated.

It has been shown that sensitivity to TDI may not be accompanied by increased reactivity to methacholine[518] and that healthy subjects sensitive to cotton bract extract do not have an increased reactivity to histamine.[545] It is for

---

*See references 512, 518, 519, 530, 569.

these reasons that tests of actual response to material encountered in the working environment are important. The airway responses to voluntary hyperventilation and to exercise are discussed in Chapter 9.

Summary

Inhalation challenge tests have been shown to be important in the investigation of occupational lung diseases. The addition of histamine or methacholine tests to the work of a routine pulmonary function laboratory is too recent to permit a statistical evaluation of its usefulness. However, we have found this test to be of value in three clinical situations in addition to suspected occupational exposures:

1. When exercise bronchospasm is suspected in athletic young subjects.
2. When effort dyspnea and wheezing are noted by a non-atopic patient, either *de novo* or after a respiratory infection.
3. When response to therapy is evaluated.

The simplification of the test and its consequent use in field surveys is likely to provide an important insight into the meaning and definition of "asthma."

PULMONARY FUNCTION TESTING IN THE OFFICE

Although the use of the peak flow meter in following cases of asthma (when the instrument is used at home or in the office) has been documented, there have been few reports of spirometric tests being used in doctors' offices. We have argued that expiratory flow measurements should be part of the routine examination for life insurance purposes,[1263] since in this way the early effects of cigarette smoking might be detected and the individual warned of the hazard of continued smoking. However, we are not aware that this practice has become general. If a community physician is reasonably close to a hospital with a pulmonary function laboratory, there would be little reason for attempting any measurements in the office. On the other hand, if the practice has a large number of asthmatics or patients with occupational lung disease, it might well be convenient to be able to record a spirogram on follow-up visits. There are no publications as far as we are aware indicating the usefulness of making such measurements.

PULMONARY FUNCTION TESTS IN THE HOSPITAL

Choice of Equipment

Those setting up a new pulmonary function laboratory are offered a wide choice in automated and semi-automated equipment. It is advisable to consult with those who have had experience in operating whatever is to be selected before finally deciding what should be bought. The quality of maintenance service offered may affect the decision in different regions.

For measurement of the FEV_1, the equipment should meet the standards proposed by the American Thoracic Society. In our view it is always preferable for a written record to be obtained. We believe it is useful to record also the expiratory flow rates, such as FEF_{25-75} and the $\dot{V}max_{50\%}VC$.

In some laboratories, the body plethysmograph is used routinely to measure the FRC. More commonly, helium dilution is used; and if this is the method chosen, it is important that the circuit include a built-in method to ensure that some criterion of equilibration has been met.

In many laboratories, the same circuit will record the single-breath ($DL_{CO}SB$) and the end-tidal DL_{CO}, with collection of an alveolar gas sample during steady-state breathing. Such circuits can easily be used to measure the fractional CO uptake during steady-state conditions. A respiratory tracing should be obtained so that the respiratory rate can be recorded. As noted in an earlier section, the predicted value of F_{CO} can be calculated if the respiratory rate is known. The $DL_{CO}SB$ has the advantages of speed; of having been used in large series of normal subjects; and of being measurable with apparatus widely sold commercially and, hence, widely used. Among the factors that cause different readings in $DL_{CO}SB$ between different laboratories are:

- differences in timing of breath holding
- differences in the alveolar sample taken
- differences in apparatus dead space correction
- errors in helium analysis
- errors in CO analysis

By contrast, the F_{CO} involves no volume measurement and no sample timing, no dead space correction, and no helium analysis. In addition, it is a much easier method for those with a reduced vital capacity or difficulty in taking a deep breath and holding it. We would therefore recommend that both steady-state and single-breath methods should be available in most function laboratories. In many instances, the single-breath method is satisfactory, but on some occasions it is preferable to use a steady-state method.

Whatever methods are used, frequent routine calibration checks are essential. Quality control determinations on repeated occasions by laboratory staff are also helpful, and comparisons between neighboring laboratories are also useful in ensuring a high quality of measurement. Data on the accuracy of CO determinations, noted in an earlier section, suggest that inaccuracies are common in routine laboratory work.

Major Indications for Pulmonary Function Tests

If full advantage is to be taken of the results of pulmonary function tests, it is essential that some data be provided on the clinical problem, the smoking history, and the radiologic appearances. It is helpful if the point at issue is described, even if this is brief, as for example:

Old MI and some LV enlargement. Mod heavy smoker. Contribution of abnormal lung function to dyspnea?

Welder with multiple exposures. Linear streaking on chest x-ray. Occasional smoking only. Function?

Non-smoker; recently documented effort dyspnea after probable viral pneumonitis. Normal CXR. Cause?

COPD after 3 weeks of steroids. Improvement?

Obstructive sleep apnea with some bronchitis. No cigarettes for 15 years. Normal PF tests?

In our experience, the major indications for pulmonary function testing are the following:

1. To investigate the cause of dyspnea, particularly when the CXR is normal. Normal pulmonary function tests at rest may suggest the possibility of effort-induced airflow limitation or early pulmonary hypertension. Early pulmonary interstitial disease may be detected by an increased $(A - a)D_{O_2}$ on exercise or a lowered diffusing capacity.

2. To forewarn of early pulmonary toxicity of certain drugs, such as nitrofurantoin. A weekly VC reading gives earlier warning of serious pulmonary involvement than is given by a CXR. We note (in Chapter 14) that the importance of this use of simple pulmonary function tests is not yet generally appreciated.

3. To assess functional status, including airway reactivity, in cases of chronic airflow limitation.

4. To assess loss of function in cases of occupational lung disease.

5. To evaluate pulmonary function in smokers requiring upper abdominal, thoracic, or cardiac surgery.

6. To assess the indications for and effect of therapy in sarcoidosis, diffuse lupus erythematosus, and diffuse interstitial fibrosis syndromes.

7. To indicate a diagnosis, particularly in primary pulmonary hypertension, and in patients with both coronary arterial disease and chronic bronchitis (a common combination since both are found more commonly in cigarette smokers).

A Sequence for Examining Pulmonary Function Test Data

The following sequence may prove useful:

1. *Is ventilatory flow normal?*

   - Correction for a reduced FVC is important; the FEV/FVC ratio is of some value, but correction of FEF_{25-75} for volume changes is inexact.
   - If 80% of predicted is taken as the lower limit of normal for the FEV_1, 60% of predicted is the lower limit for the FEF_{25-75} and $\dot{V}max_{50\%}VC$ for equivalent deviation from normal (because of the higher coefficient of variation for the flow rate measurements).
   - The expiratory flow curve should be examined for flattening indicating possible airway obstruction.
   - A greater than 15% improvement in flow rates after a bronchodilator aerosol has been administered may indicate some reversibility, but note that the airflow limi-

tation may be reversible even if this criterion is not met.

2. *Are the lung volumes normal?*

- It is important to remember that a normal vital capacity can be found in severe emphysema.
- Also, early interstitial fibrosis may occur without any reduction in TLC (i.e., without "restriction").
- An increased residual volume with a normal FEV_1 may occur in asthma in remission or in chronic mucus hypersecretion.
- Obesity leads to a reduction in expiratory reserve volume.

3. *Is gas distribution normal?*

- The single-breath N_2 test may be useful as an indicator of abnormality that the patient cannot influence by expiratory effort.

4. *Is gas transfer normal?*

- The Pa_{O_2} and Pa_{CO_2} provide essential information in many cases. If discrepant with the FEV_1, alveolar hypoventilation as a result of a lowered minute volume (overall hypoventilation) may be suspected.
- A normal diffusing capacity excludes significant $\dot{V}/\dot{Q}$ abnormality or interstitial change.

5. *Are other tests indicated?*

- These may include exercise tests to clarify alleged dyspnea; studies of lung mechanics; measurement of the vital capacity sitting and lying if diaphragmatic paralysis is suspected; and measurements of nonspecific airway reactivity.

In an editorial entitled "The Pulmonary Function Test: Cautious Overinterpretation," Butler[5356] quoted K. P. Poirier who wrote in 1968: "The general tendency in pulmonary function testing at the clinical level is toward cautiously noncommittal overinterpretation expressed in language replete with modifiers." Caution is certainly called for in some situations—when the abnormality is marginal, for instance. On the other hand, confidence is engendered only by a detailed knowledge of the background literature and by comparison, over a long period of time, of function test results with lung biopsies or autopsy findings.

Pulmonary Function Test Reporting: Ten Examples

These cases are examples, either from the published literature or from our own laboratory. They illustrate "Level 2" pulmonary function test reporting (as noted in the Preface); a complete interpretation requires knowledge of background data in the literature.

Case 1

Sixty-six-year-old woman. "Asthma" since age of 45. Moderate smoker. Admitted through Emergency Room having flown back to Vancouver from Palm Springs, where she became acutely ill.

	Predicted	24 hours post admission	Post bronchodilator
FVC	2.81	2.08	2.63
FRC	2.65	3.09	—
VC (slow)	2.81	2.66	—
RV	1.80	2.18	—
TLC	4.61	4.84	—
FEV_1	2.03	1.20	1.55
FEV/FVC%	72%	58%	59%
FEF_{25-75} (L/sec)	2.35	0.53	0.72
$\dot{V}max_{50\%}VC$	3.70	0.64	0.90
PEFR (L/sec)	6.16	3.60	3.25
$DL_{CO}SS$	12.1	11.6	—
F_{CO} (f=20)	0.41	0.42	—

Comment?

Case 2

Forty-year-old woman. Smoked 5 cigarettes/day between ages of 18 and 25. Ht: 160 cm. Wt: 70 kg. Dyspnea with normal CXR.

	Predicted	Observed	% Predicted
VC	3.16	3.10	94.9
FRC	2.64	3.00	114
RV	1.48	1.90	128
TLC	4.64	5.00	108
FEV_1	2.87	2.50	87
FEV/FVC%	84.2	80.6	96
FEF_{25-75}	3.31	2.00	61
$\dot{V}max_{50\%}VC$	4.00	2.08	51
PEFR (L/sec)	6.49	1.80	27
SBN_2/L	1.40	1.40	100
$DL_{CO}SB$	22.9	21.8	95
Pa_{O_2}, at rest	80.2	83.0 mm Hg	
Pa_{O_2}, exercise	80.2	73.0 mm Hg	

Diagnosis? What additional test or examination recommended?

Case 3

Sixty-year-old man. Myocardial infarction (MI) 3 months ago, with normal recovery.

Smoked a pack a day for 30 years. Slightly obese with weight of 97 kg, c/o dyspnea. A few basal rales and occasional rhonchus. CXR LV 1+. Lung fields normal.

	Predicted	Observed	% Predicted
VC	3.89	1.80	43.3
FRC	3.44	4.25	123.5
RV	2.16	4.00	185
TLC	6.05	5.80	95.8
FEV_1	3.38	0.80	23.6
FEV/FVC%	79.3	44	55.4
FEF_{25-75}	3.32	0.90	27.1
$\dot{V}max_{50\%}VC$	4.23	1.10	26
PERF (L/sec)	8.02	4.00	50
SBN_2/L	1.31	3.90	×3
$DL_{CO}SB$	24.2	22.2	91.7

Are these findings compatible with
A. LV failure alone?
B. Chronic airway disease?
C. A + B?

Case 4

Forty-year-old man. Engineer. No specific dust exposure. Lifetime non-smoker. Normal CXR.

	Predicted	Observed	% Predicted
VC	5.6	4.4	78
RV	2.0	2.6	130
TLC	7.0	7.7	110
FEV_1	4.3	3.3	77
FEV_1/FVC%	77	75	97
FEF_{25-75}	4.39	3.10	71
$\dot{V}max_{50\%}VC$	5.5	4.3	78
$\dot{V}max_{25\%}VC$	2.0	0.8	40
SBN_2/L	1.1	4.0	×4
$DL_{CO}SB$	37.0	31.0	84
$DL_{CO}/\dot{V}_A$	3.4	3.5	103
Pa_{O_2}, at rest	80	72.2	
Pa_{O_2}, on 40 watts	80	66.9	
Pa_{O_2}, on 160 watts	80	60.9	

Can you suggest the diagnosis?

Case 5

Thirty-seven-year-old woman. Non-smoker. No sputum. C/o severe dyspnea. CXR overinflated.

	Predicted	Observed	% Predicted
VC	3.5	1.3	37
FRC*	2.9	2.9	100
RV	1.6	2.7	142
TLC	5.1	4.0	78
FEV_1	2.53	1.00	39.5
FEF_{25-75}	3.15	0.50	15.8

	Predicted	Observed	% Predicted
SBN_2/L	1.4	4.5	×3
$DL_{CO}SS$	17.2	3.5	20
F_{CO}	0.49	0.18	36
Pa_{O_2}	80.2	60.5	
Pa_{CO_2}	35	32	
HCO_3	24	24	

*Very slow equilibration with helium; probably incomplete.

Diagnosis?

Cases 6 and 7

Case 6. Thirty-two-year-old woman. "Flu" 2 months ago, and complaint of dyspnea since. No sputum. CXR normal. Non-smoker.
Case 7. Same sex, age, and history, except for slight sputum. Smokes 5 cigarettes/day.

		Observed	
	Predicted	Case 6	Case 7
VC	3.42	3.20	2.80
FRC	2.63	2.23	2.80
RV	1.35	1.50	2.35
TLC	4.77	4.50	5.15
FEV_1	3.13	3.10	2.70
FEV_1/FVC%	91.5	96.8	96.4
FEF_{25-75}	3.77	4.00	1.80
$\dot{V}max_{50\%}VC$	4.33	4.50	2.04
$DL_{CO}SB$	24.4	16.2	18.3
$DL_{CO}SS$	19.4	12.5	16.5
F_{CO}	0.52	0.36	0.48
Pa_{O_2}, at rest	80	80	80

What may be the diagnosis in each of these cases? What additional tests would you recommend and why?

Case 8

Thirty-year-old nurse with Stage II sarcoidosis. Non-smoker. Ht: 155 cm. Effort dyspnea noticed while jogging.

	Predicted	Observed	% Predicted
VC	3.2	2.7	84.3
FRC	2.52	2.00	79.3
RV	1.26	1.2	95
TLC	4.46	3.9	87.4
FEV_1	2.96	2.2	74.3
FEV_1/FVC%	92.5	81.5	88.1
FEF_{25-75}	3.69	1.92	52
$\dot{V}max_{50\%}VC$	4.21	2.50	59.3
SBN_2/L	1.4	3.0	214
$DL_{CO}SB$	23.8	18.7	78.6
$DL_{CO}/\dot{V}_A$	5.33	4.79	89.8

Why should bronchoscopy be performed on this patient? If this is negative, what is the likely distribution of the granulomata?

Case 9

Seventy-year-old woman. Ht: 145 cm. Mitral stenosis. Non-smoker.

	Predicted	Observed	% Predicted
VC	1.71	1.36	79.5
FRC	2.33	1.86	79.8
RV	1.60	1.60	100
TLC	3.31	2.96	89.4
FEV_1	1.62	1.29	79.6
FEV_1/FVC%	79.4	94.0	118
FEF_{25-75}	2.38	1.60	67
$\dot{V}max_{50\%}VC$	2.96	2.01	68
$DL_{CO}SB$	16.7	13.4	80

Are these findings compatible with mitral stenosis as the sole lesion?

Case 10

Fifty-seven-year-old maker of steel castings. Intermittent asbestos exposure. CXR shows evidence of pleural plaques. Recent chest discomfort and slight dyspnea. Lung fields clear. Light smoker.

	Predicted	April 1984	August 1986
VC	4.77	3.24	2.11
RV	2.38	2.91	3.21
FRC	4.02	3.97	3.91
TLC	7.23	6.34	6.00
FEV_1	3.40	2.32	1.77
FEV_1/FVC%	71.2	71.6	83.8
FEF_{25-75}	3.30	1.64	1.67
$\dot{V}max_{50\%}VC$	4.61	1.94	2.17
$DL_{CO}SB$	28.3	17.9	—
$DL_{CO}SS$	14.2	—	10.8
F_{CO}	0.40	—	0.34

Comment?

Answers and Commentary on Cases

Case 1

The normal CO exchange data when first seen exclude significant emphysema. Although the bronchodilator response was only moderate in the laboratory, after a week of steroids, her FEF_{25-75} had increased to 1.62 L/sec; her FVC was 2.83 liters; and the $\dot{V}max_{50\%}VC$ had doubled.

Case 2

The expiratory flow curve should be examined for evidence of upper airway obstruction.

Note that this diagnosis is suggested by airflow limitation, normal gas distribution, and normal gas transfer; it has been shown that in these cases, the arterial Pa_{O_2} commonly falls on exercise—one of the few examples in which this occurs in the presence of a normal DL_{CO}.

Case 3

The FEF_{25-75} falls to about 70% of its normal value after an uncomplicated myocardial infarction but has returned to normal after about 4 weeks. In this case, the depression is too great too long after the MI for the lowered FEF_{25-75} to be attributable to it. There must therefore be airway disease. Whether or not this is complicated by LV failure cannot be determined on a single set of tests. If it is, the FEF_{25-75} will improve after diuresis.

Case 4

Bronchoscopy was normal. Lung biopsy showed an obliterative bronchiolitis of unknown origin with normal alveoli. The pulmonary function test pattern suggests a predominant small airway lesion.

Case 5

Compare with Case 4. This is a case of severe obliterative bronchiolitis in association with rheumatoid arthritis. It was confirmed at autopsy after respiratory failure.

Cases 6 and 7

Two possible events after a "viral" infection are development of interstitial pneumonitis and the slow resolution of bronchiolitis. The findings in Case 6 would lead one to suspect early diffuse interstitial pneumonitis. An exercise $(A - a)$ D_{O_2} should be measured to show whether a gas transfer defect is present. In Case 7 the data suggest probable slowly resolving bronchiolitis. Expiratory flow tests should be repeated in 3 months.

Case 8

The impaired airflow is not uncommon in Stage II sarcoidosis. Bronchoscopy should be done to exclude intrabronchial sarcoidosis. The abnormal SBN_2/L indicates changes within the lung; hence, the reduced airflows are unlikely to be attributable to muscle weakness. There are probably granulomata in close association with small airways. A disproportionate fall in DL_{CO} in relation to the TLC should indicate the possibility of predominant small vessel involvement in this condition, which could lead to nonuniform perfusion distribution.

Case 9

A reduced FEF_{25-75} occurs in mitral stenosis, and the decrement is closely related to the increase in pulmonary artery pressure. No other lesion need be postulated.

Case 10

There has been a marked fall in VC between the two observations. A CT scan revealed a posterior lesion on the pleura the size of a golf ball, which was not visible on the posteroanterior film. At surgery, this was a rounded atelectasis with considerable infolding of lung tissue. The lung alveoli on the biopsy taken at the same time were normal.

6

EFFECTS OF SMOKING AND ENVIRONMENTAL POLLUTANTS

Effects of Cigarette Smoking

It is now recognized that cigarette smoking (1) causes changes in lung function that are potentially reversible, at least in part, within a few years in some individuals; (2) causes mucus hypersecretion (chronic bronchitis), after about 15 years in many individuals; (3) is almost certainly the chief cause of irreversible airway obstruction leading to chronic disability in the fifth and sixth decades of life; and (4) is responsible for most of the burden of lung cancer. This section deals with the acute effects of smoking and with the function changes found in asymptomatic smokers as compared with non-smokers when populations are surveyed. Comparisons between smokers and non-smokers that make use of more complex measurements than can be easily applied in field surveys are also discussed.

Discussion of the effects of cigarette smoke from a morphologic perspective can be found in Chapter 1. A synthesis of the known pathophysiology of chronic airflow limitation in smokers may be gained with data from that chapter, together with data from this chapter and Chapters 7 and 8 (which deal with chronic bronchitis and emphysema). This extensive coverage is needed of a topic that dominates so much clinical lung disease. A valuable discussion of many of the important issues raised with respect to cigarette smoking can be found in the recent volume entitled *The Lung in the Transition between Health and Disease*.[584] It has been claimed that cigarette smoking, before the development of significant bronchitis or emphysema, leads to identifiable changes in the chest x-ray,[3939] but this has been disputed.[3950]

Experimental Data

Recent advances in understanding the effects of cigarette smoke on alveolar macrophages form the basis of the proteolysis theory of emphysema. Bronchial lavage techniques have shown that smokers' lungs contain greater numbers of macrophages,[3117, 3977] which release more elastase,[3932] and neutrophils.[3951] Alpha-proteinase inhibitor levels are not affected,[3935] and alpha$_1$-antiprotease levels are not different in smokers.[3985] Immunologic elastase levels are increased in lavage fluid immediately after smoking.[3904] The macrophages release elastase and chemotactic factors,[3113, 3115] but it has not been possible to correlate their elastolytic activity with decrement in FEV$_1$.[3128] It has been shown that the total white count is elevated in smokers[3952, 3956, 3962] and that these individuals may have an increased release of toxic oxidant metabolites.[3123] The increased polymorphonuclear count appears to be related to plasma nicotine levels, rather than to increases in COHb.[3987]

Myeloperoxidase activity is increased in smokers,[3911] as are immunoreactive and functionally active alpha$_1$-proteinase inhibitor.[3944] Other data suggest that cigarette smoking causes "a partial inactivation of serum antioxidant activity accompanied by insufficient compensatory increase in ceruloplasmin concentration."[3981] Acute cigarette smoke inhalation in anesthetized dogs has been shown to lead to severe bronchoconstriction mediated mainly by extravagal mechanisms.[3986] In monkeys, exposure to cigarette smoke leads to a reduction in mast cells and an increase in degranulated cells in the lung,[3131] and elastase-induced emphysema in rats is enhanced by cigarette smoke exposure.[3946]

Of great interest have been the experiments indicating that cigarette smoke increases the penetration of horseradish peroxidase into the guinea pig lung.[3126] It also increases alveolar permeability.[3111] Increased airway permeability has also been demonstrated in human smokers,[3156] and it appears that the upper lobe may be more permeable than the lower lobe,[3154] for unexplained reasons. The increased airway permeability in smokers seems to be unrelated to increased airway reactivity as measured with histamine[3895, 3980] and is not directly related to airflow obstruction.[3966] Use of chewing gum containing nicotine did not affect permeability in five non-smokers who used it for 7 days,[3955] suggesting that the permeability changes are not attributable to nicotine. Cigarette smoking lowers the transbronchial cellular potential difference,[3138] which may relate to increased permeability. It has been suggested that there is a dose-response relationship between increased COHb and increased lung permeability in smokers.[3129]

Acute Effects of Cigarette Smoking in Humans

Cigarette smoking patterns vary among individuals, not only in frequency and depth of inhalations, but also in the time the breath is held after inhalation.[586, 3134] Smoke inhalation appears to be a learned act[3943] and is rare in pipe smokers. Smoking cigarettes with the burning end in the mouth—which seems to be fashionable in some societies—is not a good idea.[3961]

It is remarkable that smokers adjust the frequency of inhalations to the nicotine content of the cigarettes[648] and even adjust the depth of inhalation to the tar content.[3140] Substitution of lower tar cigarettes led to an increase in puffing in one study,[3973] but differences in nicotine content were not accompanied by observable changes in ventilation patterns in another study.[3968] Others have reported that switching to lower tar cigarettes produces less change in COHb than predicted,[3921] suggesting that the smokers are compensating for the lower tar and lower COHb inhalation by smoking more cigarettes.

What is not known is whether these different patterns of smoking are related to later effects, such as increases in closing volume (CV), changes in single-breath nitrogen $(SBN_2)/L$, or decreases in ventilatory function and development of mucus hypersecretion. Studies of time relationships during smoking have indicated differences in those with emphysema,[3933] but it is not clear whether this should be regarded as causal or an effect of the disease. It has been shown that smoking in normal subjects is followed by a reduction in the number of intact circulating basophils and an increase in degranulated cells, suggesting that histamine release has occurred.[3133]

The results of tests of function before and after smoking one or more cigarettes have been somewhat variable. Small changes in FEF_{25-75} of about 0.2 L/sec—with no changes in closing volume or SBN_2/L—have been reported,[596, 614, 615] changes in FEV_1 usually not reaching significance; small increases in airway resistance (R_L) have been observed[593] and increases in residual volume (RV) have been noted by some investigators.[606] Using air, helium/oxygen breathing, and maximal expiratory flow volume (MEFV) curves, Da Silva and Hamosh[3157] reported on studies of 12 normal subjects before and after smoking and found that flow became more dependent on gas density after smoking. The delta $\dot{V}max_{50\%}VC$ has also been noted to change after a cigarette is smoked.[3974]

Others have reported an increase in specific airway conductance (SGaw) and a fall in dynamic compliance in both smokers and non-smokers after smoking one cigarette.[3986] Significant prolongation of nitrogen washout times and indices of nitrogen clearance have also been reported.[606] In studies involving 82 smokers, McCarthy, Craig, and Cherniack[633] found a mean change in nitrogen slope (Phase III) of +11%, with no significant change in FEF_{25-75} but with a fall in effort-dependent tests such as the peak expiratory flow rate (PEFR) and FEV_1. In this study, however, cigarettes were inhaled deeply every 6 seconds until the subjects became nauseated, a procedure not followed in other experiments. Results in 508 men after smoking one cigarette showed a greater R_L change with deeper inhalation and in those who smoked more heavily.[607] Comparisons between the effects of cigarettes in asthmatic subjects and normal persons showed no differences if the asthmatic subjects were asymptomatic, but a greater increase in R_L in asthmatics with initial airway obstruction.[665] Anticholinergic drugs prevented the response in normal subjects and asthmatics, suggesting that a vagal reflex was responsible.

There is evidence that tidal volume increases after cigarette smoking, suggesting that irritant receptors are stimulated.[686] Comparisons were made between lit and unlit cigarettes. In seven smokers and 13 non-smokers, after 12 puffs of a cigarette reduced to a butt length of 30 millimeters, R_L increased after cigarettes with and without filters; $\dot{V}max_{50\%}VC$ fell only after non-filter cigarettes were smoked.[698] These experiments are difficult to standardize, since a deep inspiration before R_L is measured may reduce the bronchoconstrictor effect of cigarette smoke by as much as 30%.[705] If measurements are made frequently during cigarette smoking, the effect is found to occur after only one or two puffs and to be maximal after three.[705] In one study, decreases in specific conductance were found to be maximal 8 seconds after a single inhalation[651] and to be inhibited by salbutamol and ipratropium bromide; specific conductance was unaffected by sodium cromoglycate. Tests of non-tobacco smoking material have shown no effects from the new material, as compared with cigarettes.[650]

Although tracheal mucus velocity was slowed in dogs after exposure to cigarette smoke,[613] no change was produced in human subjects after smoking one cigarette.[645] There are some data to suggest that particle deposition may be greater in apical and central regions while smoking than it is with normal tidal breathing,[3982] a phenomenon that may be related to the common occurrence of upper lobar centrilobular emphysema in smokers.

The many papers on the effects of passive smoke inhalation have been summarized in two reports.[3988, 3989] There seems little doubt that maternal smoking causes more respiratory illness in children, has a small effect on lung function in later years,* and may even be related to an increased risk of lung cancer in later life.[3900] It is of interest to note that it has been shown that the particle deposition rate is lower (11%) from this smoke than from "mainstream" smoke (70%)[2940]; nicotine absorption from passive smoke is between a third and a tenth that of active smoking.[3135] Ten asthmatics and 10 controls inhaling cigarette smoke passively in a chamber[3153] were compared. In the asthmatics, after one hour, the FVC and FEV_1

*See references 2888, 3110, 3902, 3903, 3920, 3923, 3949, 3964, 3975, 3982, 3984.

had fallen 20% and the COHb had risen from 0.82% to 1.20%. No decrement in function occurred in the control subjects.

Pathologic Changes in the Lung in Asymptomatic Smokers

Although changes in small airways occurring as part of established chronic bronchitis had been recognized for many years as a result of the work of McLean and Reid,[585] strong evidence of pathologic changes in the small airways of young and probably asymptomatic smokers did not appear until 1974. In that year, Niewohner, Kleinerman, and Rice[599] published a study of the peripheral airways in 39 subjects—20 non-smokers and 19 smokers of average age 25 years—who had died from non-respiratory causes. The sections were interpreted without knowledge of the smoking history. All lungs with any significant emphysema were excluded. By comparison with non-smokers, they found that in smokers "the characteristic lesion observed was a respiratory bronchiolitis associated with clusters of pigmented alveolar macrophages . . . Lungs of smokers also showed small but significant increases in mural inflammatory cells and denuded epithelium in membranous bronchioles as compared with controls. We postulate that this respiratory bronchiolitis is a precursor of centriacinar emphysema and may be responsible for the subtle functional abnormalities observed in young smokers." In a later paper, they correlated these morphologic changes with observed function defects.[598] Confirmatory evidence of this association was published from McGill in 1978.[609, 625] As Thurlbeck noted,[626] a significant relationship between physiologic abnormality and morphologic change had been established.

This work was extended in 1980 when Cosio, Hale, and Niewohner[691] published morphologic studies on the lungs of 25 smokers and 14 lifetime non-smokers; all were over the age of 40 and had died from non-respiratory causes. The smokers' lungs had significantly higher scores for small airway disease, increased goblet cell metaplasia, and evidence of smooth muscle hypertrophy and inflammatory changes in the walls of respiratory bronchioles. However, the mean bronchiolar diameter was not different between the two groups, although the severity of the small airway disease correlated significantly with the percentage of airways less than 400 microns in diameter. The smokers' lungs had an increased proportion of bronchial gland mass, but this was not correlated with the severity of small airway changes nor with the extent of centrilobular emphysema (CLE). (Five of the smokers' lungs had >15 units of CLE.)

The same authors studied the small vessels of the same lungs.[692] In the lungs of smokers they noted an increased number of transected muscular arteries below 200 microns in diameter, an increase in medial smooth muscle, and an increased thickening of the intima of small vessels. These changes correlated significantly with the severity of the small airway disease and with the degree of CLE, but not with bronchial mucous gland enlargement.[692] They concluded that these arterial changes evolved in parallel with small airway changes and with the development of CLE but were independent of mucous gland enlargement. Auerbach and his colleagues[1624] have also reported on vascular changes in relation to smoking; they suggested that the severity of morphologic changes in relation to smoking history have diminished in lungs studied between 1970 and 1977, compared with lungs studied between 1955 and 1960.[3159] Increases in the number of goblet cells in the bronchioles of smokers, together with a reduction in Clara cells, have also been documented.[3976] It has also been suggested that the number of alveolar attachments to small airways may be reduced in smokers.[3947]

Wright and her colleagues[3118, 3160] have compared preoperative function tests with morphologic appearances in 96 patients undergoing lobectomy. In cases in whom the FEV_1 was greater than 80% of the predicted value, the severity of inflammatory changes in respiratory bronchioles was reflected in increasing numbers of abnormal small airway function test values. A more recent review of 150 cases similarly studied confirmed that cumulative abnormality in function test data correlated with a worsening airway score in respiratory bronchioles, and the SBN_2/L test was abnormal in some patients with respiratory bronchiolar pathology in whom the FEV_1 was still normal.[3893] These data are discussed in more detail in the next chapter.

Experimental data from the same laboratory on induced small airway lesions in dogs using HCl aerosol[3141] support the suggestion that inflammatory changes in small airways are closely related to abnormality of tests of small airway function. Berend and colleagues'[3146] data on 32 autopsy cases also support the conclusion that inflammatory airway changes are related to decrements in FEF_{25-75}.

These observations are related to function test changes below. The possible changes in the lungs of smokers that may have an impact on tests of lung function include:

- increased mucus in the small airways
- respiratory bronchiolitis
- reduction in lung recoil
- increased airway reactivity
- increased secretions in large airways
- vascular changes

In general, these changes might be expected to lead to non-uniformity of time constants in the lung, with consequent inhomogenous distribution of inspired gas and premature small airway closure, and to non-uniformity of ventilation, perfusion, and diffusion distributions. As noted in Chapter 1, the resistance normally contributed by small airways is a small fraction of the total, so that these constitute what has been described as the "quiet zone" of the lung.

The remarkable demonstration by Ploysongsang[2980] of differences in phase angle of recorded breath sounds measured in young non-smokers and young asymptomatic smokers was noted in Chapter 3. Although not detectable by stethoscope, these probably represent the only physical sign of respiratory bronchiolitis in this age group. It has been claimed that cigarette smoking alone leads to identifiable changes in the chest x-ray,[3939] but this has been disputed.[3950]

Differences in Lung Function Between Smokers and Non-smokers

There have been more than 70 survey studies of pulmonary function in very different populations over the past 10 years. The interpretation of these is made difficult by the fact that in some of them it is not clear whether normal subjects with symptoms of chronic bronchitis have been excluded, but some generalizations from the data are possible. Much of this literature has been concerned with the definition of the "most sensitive" test of function change in smokers. Of course, unless changes in such indices have some prognostic significance, there is little purpose in trying to devise tests that separate smokers from non-smokers, as this information can be directly obtained.

Differences in MEFV Curves

The MEFV curve has been found by some investigators to be the most sensitive indicator of difference between smokers and non-smokers. In 1971, Seely, Zuskin, and Bouhuys[659] found evidence of abnormalities of the flow-volume curve in smoking teenagers when they were compared with their non-smoking peers. In 50 smokers and 50 non-smoking high school students, Lim[618] found no differences in FEV_1, but 20% of the smokers had abnormalities of prolongation of the tail of the forced expiratory curve. It has been suggested that in asymptomatic smokers, convexity of the volume axis of MEFV curves is the most sensitive indicator of abnormality.[627] Some authors have reported that the $FEF_{25-75\%}VC$ shows a strong correlation with smoking history; but the RV shows the strongest correlation, with age and smoking considered as separate variables.[86] A follow-up survey of 10,989 school children in Sydney, Australia noted a slightly greater decline in $\dot{V}max_{50\%}VC$ in smokers as compared with non-smokers,[656] data that are consistent with the more detailed studies of teenage smokers noted earlier.

In one study of 725 subjects aged 25 to 54, the MEFV curves were as frequently abnormal as the closing volume (CV) tests or the SBN_2/L, and the authors concluded that there was little need to use the latter two indices.[647] Other authors have recommended the "$\dot{V}max_{25\%}VC$" (actually the $\dot{V}max_{75\%}VC$ as usually expressed) as the most useful test,[642] particularly in conjunction with the SBN_2/L value.[642] In a large random survey conducted by Knudson, Burrows, and Lebowitz[317] in Tucson, Arizona, the $\dot{V}max_{75\%}VC$ detected the greatest number of abnormalities. It was noted that although this index detected abnormalities more frequently in older people, the FEV_1 was more sensitive in younger age groups. In a rural population of 231 non-smokers and 95 smoking men and women aged between 17 and 82, more than half of the smokers had a value of $\dot{V}max_{50\%}VC$ within 1 SD of the non-smoking values,[483] but the rate of decline of $\dot{V}max_{50\%}$ was 0.055 L/sec/yr in nonsmokers and 0.062 L/sec/yr in smokers.

The $FEF_{25-75\%}VC$ is usually found to be significantly lowered in middle-aged smokers with between 20 and 40 pack-years of smoking,[605] when the mean value of the index may average about 72% of the value in non-smokers.[605] In measuring MEFV curves in survey work, the body plethysmograph appears to be inferior to the spirometer.[620] In the Tecumseh community survey of 6391 people, it was concluded that the $\dot{V}max_{50\%}VC$, the FEV_1, and the FEV_1/FVC ratio were the best spirometric indices to use and that there was little advantage in adding

other flow indices.[296] Among the 65,086 members of the Kaiser-Permanente medical scheme, the FEV_1 differences between smokers and non-smokers were greater in whites than in blacks or Asians[637]; it was not clear whether this was due to different smoking intensities or other factors. In one random sample of men over the age of 60, 1% of non-smokers and 44% of smokers had a $FEV_1/FVC\%$ less than 60%.[699]

In a recent comparison between non-smokers and 147 male and 212 female smokers, the flow indices (FEF_{25-75}, $\dot{V}max_{50\%}VC$, and $\dot{V}max_{75\%}VC$) were significantly different.[3949] This study also showed that this difference was not determined by large changes in a few smokers, but by a general difference in the majority of smokers. The FEV_1/FVC ratio and the moment analysis of the spirogram identified smokers with more marked changes. Another comparison between 86 women smokers and 100 female lifetime non-smokers showed differences in SRaw, CV, SBN_2/L, V_{isoV}, and mean transit times.[3914]

Knudson and his colleagues in Tucson, Arizona have recently compared 20 middle-aged smokers with 19 non-smokers of the same age (54 years).[3954] Subjects were excluded if they reported any heart trouble, physician-diagnosed asthma, chronic bronchitis, or emphysema or had a history of chest surgery. Significant differences in mean values were as follows:

	Smokers	Non-smokers
FEV_1 (% predicted)	94.4	105.9
RV (liters)	2.05	1.52
$DL_{CO}SB$	25.81	29.46
k (constant)	0.178	0.141
SBN_2/L	2.04	0.88

As a result of detailed regression analyses, the authors suggested that enlargement of terminal airspaces probably accounted for changes in DL, in k, and in their interrelationship. Moment analysis of the expiratory spirogram showed that in a comparison between 53 non-smokers and 149 regular smokers, the time for expiration of the FEF_{25-75} was significantly different between the two groups.[3825]

Spirometric changes in smokers are not closely related to indices of tar content of cigarettes and smoking history,[3114] indicating the importance of individual susceptibility and possibly differences in smoking patterns. One study of 5686 adult women suggested that cigarette tar content was related to cough and phlegm but that wheezing and dyspnea were more closely related to the vapor phase constituents of cigarette smoke.[3139]

A study of 45 pairs of identical twins, some of whom smoked and some of whom did not, found that $\dot{V}max_{60\%}VC$ was the best discriminator between smokers and non-smokers.[657] The variation between the twins was much less than in the population as a whole, a result that suggests the importance of host factors in the response to tobacco smoke.

Changes in Density-Dependent Flow Rates

While studying symptomatic smokers, Dosman and his colleagues[588] found clear evidence that the change in delta $\dot{V}max_{50\%}VC$ helium and air was related to tobacco consumption. Other authors have noted differences in $\dot{V}max_{75\%}VC$ on air and helium between smokers and non-smokers.[643] Teculescu[695] studied 26 asymptomatic smokers aged 35 to 55, all of whom had normal chest x-rays, FEV_1, and no physical signs. He noted that $\dot{V}max_{50\%}VC$ on air was related to tobacco history, as was the $\dot{V}max_{25\%}VC$ on helium, but he could not show a relationship between the delta $\dot{V}max_{50\%}VC$ helium and air and tobacco consumption. However, in more recent studies,[3142] he has reported on comparisons between 30 asymptomatic non-smokers, 22 asymptomatic smokers with a normal FEV_1, 17 smokers with chronic mucus hypersecretion but a normal FEV_1, and seven smokers with sputum and FEV/FVC% between 80% and 90% of predicted. All were men aged between 33 and 56 years. There was a poor correlation between helium/oxygen flow data and the FEV_1. He concluded that "it can be argued that density dependence and FEV_1 explore different aspects of respiratory function, and thus no correlation is to be expected." Other authors have noted the greater sensitivity of $\dot{V}_{iso}V$ and terminal flow measurements as compared with the FEV_1.[3148, 3149]

By the age of 30, the FEF_{25-75} in smokers is often significantly reduced, and differences are found in closing volume and in delta $\dot{V}max_{50\%}VC$ on helium and air.[636, 638] The $\dot{V}_{isoV}$ has also been observed to be a more sensitive discriminator than $\dot{V}max_{60\%}VC$ and CV/VC%,[635] but in a group of 22 asymptomatic healthy smokers of average age 32.5 years, it was noted to improve toward normal values after the administration of a bronchodilator in half of those in whom it was lowered. Fairshter and Wilson[702] studied 50 non-smokers and 30 comparable young smokers; they concluded that the $\dot{V}_{isoV}$ measurement was the best index for distinguishing the two

groups if the 95% confidence limit criterion was used. On this basis, they concluded that 40% of the young smokers were abnormal. The level of tobacco consumption was considerably lighter than in Dosman's group.[588] As noted in Chapter 5, all differential flow measurements with air and helium have a very high coefficient of variation, which limits their value in comparative studies. If the percentage decrease in time between 60% and 40% of the FVC is measured with air and with a helium/oxygen mixture, a significantly higher value may be found in non-smokers as compared with smokers.[581]

Differences in FEV_1

In asymptomatic smokers up to the age of 30 years, there is usually a significant difference in FEV_1,[636] and differences between smokers and non-smokers have been demonstrated in many studies.* It is invariably lower if symptoms are present.[317] By the fifth decade of life, the differences in FEV_1 between smokers and non-smokers are, as one would expect, greater.[623]

As noted later, other tests of function can demonstrate differences between smokers and non-smokers before the FEV_1 indicates differences between the two groups. The FEV/Ht^3 has been found to be a more sensitive discriminator between smokers and non-smokers than the FEV/FVC% index.[687] In 1056 20-year-old army recruits, the FEV_1 difference between smokers and non-smokers was only 0.1 liters, but significant differences were found in $FEF_{25-75\%}VC$ and $FEF_{75-85\%}VC$.[684] The investigators made the interesting observation that the differences between smokers and non-smokers were larger in taller men.

By the age of 50 years, differences in observed FEV_1 between smokers and non-smokers necessarily imply a faster rate of decline of FEV_1 in smokers; this has been a fairly consistent finding. Buist[3886] had contributed a useful review of longitudinal data in relation to smoking. Bande, Clement, and van de Woestijne[3998] have reported a follow-up study of 7123 men; they noted that the FEV_1 between smokers and non-smokers began to deviate at the age of 30, the difference becoming significant at the age of 40. The observed rates of FEV_1 decline were

	Annual Decline (mL/year)	
	Non-smokers	*Heavy Smokers*
Vital capacity	−32	−43
FEV_1	−27	−39

*See references 276, 296, 317, 595, 597, 605.

Values for moderate smokers were intermediate.

Woolf and Zamel[608] studied 302 women aged between 25 and 54 years after an interval of 5 years and noted the following declines expressed as a percentage of the initial value:

	FEV_1	$FEF_{25-75\%}$ VC
Non-smokers	−1.1%	−13.2%
Smokers with no symptoms	−1.7%	−17.3%
Smokers with symptoms	−5.0%	−23.9%

In another study of a group of 556 men, non-smokers had a decline of −38 mL/year in FEV_1, whereas these values in smokers were declining at a rate of −51 mL/year.[89] A rather larger difference was noted in a Polish study of 2572 people in an urban environment studied at an interval of 5 years. The FEV_1 of these smokers was declining at a rate of −70 mL/year and that of the non-smokers at −48 mL/year in groups of men aged between 31 and 50 years.[679] In another group studied in Finland at an interval of 10 years, the FEV_1 decline in male non-smokers was −33 mL/year and in smokers was −51 mL/year. A follow-up of a cohort in the Framingham study noted a lower rate of decline in FVC in non-smokers as compared with smokers.[649]

Data from Baltimore indicate an annual rate of decline of −41.7 mL/year in FEV_1 in smoking men below the age of 45.[3152] Other studies have documented the faster decline in FEV_1 in smokers.[3912] In 1912 adults tested twice at an interval of 4.7 years,[3842] the differences in rates of decline between smokers and non-smokers increased as age increased, so that in men aged over 60 the annual rate of decline was −30.5 mL/year in lifetime non-smokers but −79 mL/year in heavy smokers. In this study it was shown that an increased closing capacity (CC) at the initial visit was associated with a faster rate of FEV_1 decline.

In a significant study, Tager and his colleagues[3999] followed 669 children aged between 5 and 19. They concluded that children who started to smoke at the age of 15 and continued to smoke would achieve only 92% of their expected FEV_1 and 90% of their expected FEF_{25-75} at the age of 20. Five-year declines in FEV_1 in 1092 men and 1309 women in Los Angeles were increased above usual values in non-smokers but were even higher in smokers.[3967] Passive smoking was not related to faster FEV_1 decline in a study from Holland.[3963]

Differences in Lung Volumes

The residual volume has been less often measured but is increased as a percentage of total lung capacity (TLC) when older smokers and non-smokers are compared.[676, 3954] A study of 118 army recruits suggested that the RV/TLC (measured by the multiple-breath method) and the FEV_1 were the most useful indices and were better than the CV/VC%.[682, 683] These two indices were found to have a correlation coefficient (r) of 0.50 in those in whom either index was abnormal. Some authors have found the RV to be normal at the earliest stage of change in MEFV curves,[636, 638] but others have found an increase.[592] As noted earlier, Knudson and his colleagues[3954] found a significant elevation in RV in middle-aged smokers as compared with non-smokers. There is evidence from careful radiologic comparisons that the volume of the lower lobes is increased in smokers as compared with non-smokers.[2963]

Differences in Ventilation Distribution

The slope of the alveolar plateau (SBN_2/L) is influenced by an increase in RV. In a significant number of studies, the SBN_2/L is the test that best discriminated between smokers and non-smokers. With 134 non-smoking men and 203 non-smoking women as controls for 530 current smokers, the percentages of abnormal tests were as follows[294]:

SBN_2/L slope	47%
CC/TLC%	44%
FEV_1	11%

In this series, if the SBN_2/L slope and the CV and CC data were combined, 64% of the smokers had an abnormality as compared with the controls. In another group of 101 asymptomatic smokers between the ages of 18 and 39, the SBN_2/L was significantly reduced in 28% of light smokers and 56% of heavy smokers[634]; by contrast, only 4% of the smokers had an abnormal FEV_1 or $FEF_{25-75\%}$. However, other authors have noted that although the SBN_2/L identifies a larger group of smokers as abnormal than other indices, a normal value in this index may be found in some with evidence of ventilatory abnormality.[610]

In 1900 subjects selected randomly in Tucson, Arizona, the SBN_2/L test was the most sensitive discriminator between smokers and non-smokers.[628, 3954] Other data have shown the

	Number	Age	FEV_1	FEV_1 (% predicted)	FEV/FVC%	$\dot{V}max_{50\%}$	SBN_2/L	CV/VC%
Non-smokers	43	51.6	3.84	110.3	74.8	4.6	0.59	20.7
Smokers	46	51.7	3.10	91.9	65.6	4.1	1.52	27.3

same phenomenon.* There is some evidence that the SBN_2/L changes less with age in women smokers than in men.[674]

In an interesting longitudinal study of 405 school children in Britain given yearly pulmonary function tests between 1975 and 1979, it was shown that cigarette smoking led to differences in $\dot{V}max_{50\%}VC$ and SBN_2/L after 2 years of smoking. The FVC was larger in the smokers, and a small decrement of about 240 milliliters in mean FEV_1 was observed.[3972]

Differences in pulmonary function between smokers and lifetime non-smokers become wider as older age groups are studied, as one would expect. In one study,[672] the following data were obtained from 51 young smokers and 214 older smokers as compared with lifetime non-smokers:

	Percentage of Smokers with Abnormal Tests			
Age	FEV/Ht^3	CV/VC%	SBN_2/L	Pa_{O_2}
20–30	4%	12%	6%	26%
40–55	20%	34%	21%	36%

In a report on the same data (which was drawn from a survey of 500 working men), the authors further concluded that it was not possible to draw conclusions as to the prognostic value of the different measurements.[668] Other investigators in a 10-year follow-up of 120 subjects[669] concluded that the CV data did not add additional information to the SBN_2/L and FEV_1.

DIFFERENCES IN REGIONAL VENTILATION

Measurements of regional ventilation distribution have been used to illustrate the non-uniformity of time constants in smokers. Using radioactive ^{133}Xe in studies of regional function in a subgroup of smokers from an epidemiologic study, ventilation distribution was abnormal in all those with either an abnormal FEV_1 or with an elevated CV or RV. Five of 8 subjects in whom these tests were normal and who were asymptomatic[670] were found to have significant regional abnormalities. Regional differences in the ratio of RV to TLC have also been demonstrated in smokers through the use of ^{133}Xe.[644, 685]

*See references 276, 612, 628, 646, 655, 673, 674, 676, 682, 687, 694.

Martin and his colleagues[685] showed that regional ^{133}Xe distribution was more influenced by inspiratory flow rate in young smokers than in non-smokers. Marcq and Minette,[135] in ingenious experiments using helium boluses and the residual nitrogen method in different body positions in eight smokers whose SBN_2/L was at least 3.2%, found changes that were explicable on the basis of regional differences.

Recent ^{133}Xe data on 11 non-smokers and 20 smokers of average age 23.8 years showed that although overall tests of function were not different, there was an increased RV in the lower zones of the smokers.[3145] Anterior and posterior detectors, five in each lung, were used, and all experiments were performed with the subjects seated. Barter and his colleagues,[4000] using inhaled ^{81m}Kr, compared 46 current male smokers, aged 44 to 61, with mild or no respiratory symptoms with 43 male lifetime non-smokers. All chest x-rays were normal. Routine tests of lung function were as shown in the table at the top of this page.

The regional $\dot{V}$ distribution data showed that diffuse abnormalities were present in 46% of the smokers but in none of the non-smokers. In the smokers there was a weak relationship between the occurrence of $\dot{V}$ distribution defects and overall ventilation tests, so that abnormal scans were found with normal pulmonary function test data and normal scans found in some cases with abnormal resting tests. There was no correlation between abnormal scans and the presence of chronic expectoration. The authors noted that "the prognostic significance of an abnormal ventilation scan in such smokers remains to be established."

A comparison of radioactive aerosol deposition with ^{133}Xe showed more central deposition in smokers,[33] but this test is not a sensitive indicator of small airway abnormality.[50] However, a comparison between nine non-smokers and 11 smokers showed less distal aerosol penetration in the smokers; there was also a difference in $\dot{V}max_{50\%}VC$ between the two groups, and the mean FEV_1 was 106% predicted in the non-smokers and 92% predicted in the smokers.[3960]

Teculescu, Pham, and Hannhart[3996] compared three groups of men aged 35 to 55: healthy non-smokers, asymptomatic smokers with normal spirometry values, and smokers with mild bronchitis with or without airflow changes. They found that in non-smokers, there was no correlation between the FEV_1 and RV/TLC, SBN_2/L, or DL_{CO}. In asymptomatic smokers, there was a significant relationship between SBN_2/L and CV on the one hand, and the FEV_1, RV/TLC%, and DL_{CO} on the other. In symptomatic smokers, all the "sensitive" tests were related to the FEV_1. They suggested that their results probably indicated the development of early emphysema in some cases.

Changes in Closing Volume

Closing volume, like the SBN_2/L, is also affected by an increase in RV. Most studies have found evidence of an increased CV in young smokers before the FEV_1 has become abnormal.[578, 663, 666] In some studies, significant abnormalities in asymptomatic smokers in CV/VC%, CC/TLC and $\dot{V}_{isoV}$ have been found without abnormality of $FEF_{25-75\%}$VC, RV, or SBN_2/L.[696] In one study of 100 male smokers, only 13 had an abnormal FEV_1, but 56% had a CC/TLC% more than 2 SEE different from non-smokers of the same age.[617] Others have noted that although there is a relationship between CV/VC and FEV_1 among smokers, the predictive value of CV/VC is not great.[3969] A review of 1073 people who attended an emphysema screening center showed that in 524 cigarette smokers CC/TLC% was abnormal in 44%, $FEF_{25-75\%}$VC was abnormal in 21%, and the FEV_1 was abnormal in 11%. In smokers aged 50 to 60, many with symptoms, the FEV_1 was abnormal in 22%.[621]

In some series, the percentage of smokers with an abnormal CC/TLC% has been somewhat lower (20% in one survey of 336 urban and 287 rural inhabitants).[646] Others have not found the CV/VC ratio to be a sensitive discriminator when compared with the SBN_2/L or the RV.[3954] There are some longitudinal data indicating that CV/VC% does not change progressively in smokers,[611] but baseline differences may be found that relate to a faster rate of decline of FEV_1.[3842] Dosman and his colleagues[3144] have updated their review of the population in Humboldt, Saskatchewan.[3144] They reported the following percentage abnormalities in 241 male smokers (as defined by a more than 2 SD difference from non-smokers) (see the table at the bottom of this page).

One pack-year was defined as 20 cigarettes/day for one year. Data from 215 women were not much different. Values in non-smokers were similar to most other series.

Changes in C_{dyn}/f

Several authors have found that the change in dynamic compliance with frequency (C_{dyn}/f) is the most frequently abnormal test when smokers and non-smokers are compared.[660, 675] In one study of 52 smokers whose FEV_1 and FVC were greater than 70% of predicted, 29 had a reduced C_{dyn}/f. Of these, 23 had demonstrable regional abnormalities of gas distribution with the use of ^{133}Xe; 20 had an increased CV; 13 had a reduced $FEF_{25-75\%}$VC; and eight had an increased RV.[688] In another group of 10 smokers aged between 38 and 52 years, all had a decreased C_{dyn}/f. Of these, seven had an $FEF_{25-75\%}$VC less than 80% of predicted; six had a fall of $\dot{V}max$ as a function of recoil pressure; and four had an abnormal SBN_2/L.[701]

Changes in Lung Recoil

There is some conflict of evidence relating to lung recoil and the effect of smoking. Corbin and his colleagues[654] reported a major decline in Pst at 50% TLC over a 4-year period in 21 smokers of mean age 44.5 years. This value fell from 5.51 cm H_2O to 2.80 cm H_2O. Over the same period, the value fell from 7.28 cm H_2O to 5.52 cm H_2O in 12 non-smokers of similar age. The smokers had a significant fall in flow at low lung volumes, but the $\dot{V}max_{50\%}$VC and FEV_1 did not change between the two studies. Other authors have found evidence of a loss of

		Percentage Abnormalities in Male Smokers			
Age	Mean Pack-year	FEV/FVC(%)	SBN_2/L(%)	CV/VC(%)	SBN_2/L + CV/VC(%)
25–29	9.9	5.6	11.1	13.0	5.6
30–34	17.0	2.9	11.4	8.6	5.7
35–39	20.0	8.7	21.7	13.0	6.5
40–44	23.8	6.7	20.0	10.0	0
45–49	30.1	6.1	45.5	6.1	6.1
50–54	38.9	11.8	29.4	5.9	0
55–59	39.6	19.2	46.2	7.7	7.7

recoil associated either with an early increase in RV^{592} or with no change in R_L or RV.[707]

A normal C_{stat} in smokers has been reported[601, 635] with normal recoil pressures, although C_{dyn}/f was abnormal.[602] Other authors have concluded that the quasi-static pressure volume curves show no detectable effect of smoking on lung recoil in men.[87] It has been reported that the Pel_{max} was 10% greater in 86 smoking women as compared with 100 lifetime non-smoking women of the same age.[3914] This might be a reason for a larger FVC in smokers.

In a comparison between 46 smokers and 41 non-smokers ranging in age from 16 to 60, Hoeppner and his colleagues[290] concluded that the elevated CV in the smokers was due to loss of recoil. At 60% TLC the recoil pressure was 5.7 ± 1.7 cm H_2O in the smokers and 6.8 ± 2.1 cm H_2O in non-smokers. Other authors have reported an increase in C_{stat} in smokers, with no significant change in the coefficient of retraction.[661, 662] Colebatch and Greaves[3894] studied 73 male smokers, aged 18 to 60, whose mean FEV_1 was 97% predicted. They found that the k constant increased with age at a faster rate than in non-smokers and that in 18 of the smokers it was more than 2 SD above the normal range. They concluded that k increased long before significant airflow developed. The same authors in a more recent report[4754] noted that in smokers TLC increases as the k constant increases. They attribute the k constant increase to an increase in size of air spaces, without an effect on flow rates. The slope of the maximal negative intrapleural pressure with age was similar between smokers and non-smokers but consistently lower in the smokers.

Other Differences in Function Between Smokers and Non-smokers

The oscillatory airflow measurement of R_L has, in some studies, shown differences between non-smokers and asymptomatic smokers.[630] The ratio between low-frequency R_L and high-frequency R_L was different between smokers and non-smokers.[652] However, a more recent study could not find differences with this technique between smokers and non-smokers, although there was a different mean FEV_1 between the groups.[3147] Measurements of mechanical impedance of the respiratory system at different frequencies have been noted to show differences between smokers and non-smokers.[681]

AIRWAY REACTIVITY

In a comparison between 17 smokers and 17 lifetime non-smokers of average age 50, there was a highly significant difference in airway reactivity as shown by a histamine challenge test[693]; the $FEF_{25-75\%}VC$ was 0.6 L/sec lower in the smokers than in the non-smokers, but this difference did not attain significance. Data also show that smokers are more sensitive to methacholine.[3121] However, in another study of subjects aged 20 to 36, no difference was demonstrable in histamine reactivity between 17 smokers and 21 non-smokers; the response to histamine was shown to be related to baseline expiratory flow measurements.[3910] There were no differences in SBN_2/L data between the two groups. There seems little doubt that smoking is associated with a positive response to a eucapnic hyperventilation test with subfreezing air.[3957, 3965]

In a comparison between 18 non-allergic non-smokers and 18 non-allergic smokers matched for age, there was no difference in methacholine reactivity.[3978] The authors noted that if nine matched pairs were compared with the smokers having a greater than 10 pack-year consumption, the methacholine reactivity was significantly greater in the smokers as compared with the non-smokers. In this study, the FEV_1 was not different between the two groups, but the $\dot{V}max_{75\%}$ VC was lower in the smokers. However, if allergic rhinitis is present in smokers, the two factors seem to interact to lower the methacholine threshold.[3979] Other data suggest that methacholine reactivity is elevated in smokers only if the RV is elevated[3958]; in this study, the FEV_1 in the smokers was 107% predicted, and reactivity was unrelated to CV/VC%, SBN_2/L. The $DL_{CO}SB$ was lower in those smokers who were reactive.

In a recent follow-up of 117 smokers, Taylor and his colleagues[4001] found that the decline in FEV_1 was faster over a 7-year interval in those smokers whose PC20 to histamine was <16 mg/mL as compared with those in whom it was above this level initially. Thirty per cent of the smokers were in this category as compared with 5% of non-smokers.

TRACHEAL MUCUS VELOCITY AND CLEARANCE

Some investigators have found that the tracheal mucus velocity is reduced in smokers[641, 697] and ex-smokers.[645] As noted earlier, an acute reduction has been reported in dogs after cigarette smoke inhalation[613] and in cats[624]; in human subjects the mucus velocity was unaffected by one cigarette.[645] Other investigators found no differences between smokers and non-smokers.[640] Cohen, Aria, and Brain,[3158] using a new technique, have reported that clearance of iron oxide particles from the lung over a period of 11 months was one-fifth as rapid in three smokers as in nine non-smokers. These and other findings are discussed in Chapter 3.

DIFFERENCES IN CONTROL OF BREATHING

In a study of 23 pairs of monozygotic twins,[3124] a significant difference was shown between the ventilatory response to Pa_{O_2}, with the smokers having a greater ventilatory increase. No difference in response to Pa_{CO_2} was present. It has been suggested that nicotine-mediated endorphin release may have the effect of blunting the respiratory drive in some smokers,[3150, 3155] but these data are still preliminary. An increase of V_T/T_I has been noted to follow smoking a cigarette and has been attributed to nicotine stimulation.[3143] A study on the effect of changes in body position on ventilation pattern, interpreted as possibly indicating differences in respiratory control between smokers and non-smokers,[3925] was criticized in later correspondence.[3926]

DIFFERENCES IN GAS EXCHANGE

By contrast with the somewhat conflicting data on all these indices of mechanical, ventilatory, and distributional aspects of lung function, the gas exchange data between smokers and non-smokers show remarkable unanimity. As noted in the second edition of this book,[1] Strieder and Kazemi found an increased $(A - a) D_{O_2}$ in supine smokers. More recently, Frans and his colleagues[590, 667] demonstrated such differences in asymptomatic smokers on exercise (when it was 5.5 mm Hg in non-smokers and 11.9 mm Hg in smokers) and under hypoxic conditions. The exercise $(A - a) D_{O_2}$ correlated with the DL_{CO} (r = -0.63). Some authors have found no differences between the Pa_{O_2} in seated subjects between smokers and non-smokers[700] but noted that in smokers there was a bimodal distribution, suggesting significant impairment in small fractions. Another study apparently demonstrated a greater effect of nitroglycerine on arterial oxygen tension in smokers as compared with non-smokers.[604]

The early studies of diffusing capacity between smokers and non-smokers[1] showed some differences, but there was doubt concerning the reliability of these, as COHb blood levels might have influenced the results. During the last 10 years, however, a number of very carefully conducted studies have shown beyond doubt that whatever method of measurement is used, and independently of any COHb effect, values of DL_{CO} are between 6% and 20% lower in smokers than in age-matched non-smokers. Comparisons at rest by the $DL_{CO}SB$ method,* by calculation of k_{CO} or $DL_{CO}/\dot{V}_A$,† or by $DL_{CO}SS$ end-tidal methods or measurement of F_{CO},[102, 638, 643, 664] all show lower values in smokers as compared with non-smokers matched for age. In one study of subjects in their mid-40s, F_{CO} was 0.492 in non-smokers and 0.466 in smokers, a difference of 6%.[102] The diffusing capacity has also been noted to be lower in smokers when groups of smokers and non-smokers, between whom there was no significant difference in SBN_2/L or CV/VC%,[643] were studied. There is some indication that DL_{CO} differences are greater between non-smokers and smokers in women than in men.[643]

In one recent survey of 511 randomly selected subjects from a population in Michigan, Miller and his colleagues[3000] noted the effect of smoking on the $DL_{CO}SB$ in all groups studied. In men, the difference averaged 5 mL CO/min/mm Hg. Exercise diffusing capacity is also lower in smokers.[303, 378, 589] An interesting point has been made that changes in DL_{CO} with changes in posture are different between non-smokers and smokers. In one study, smokers were found to have only a 3.5% change in DL_{CO} and k_{co} between supine and sitting positions as compared with an 18.5% change in non-smokers of comparable age.[136]

Measurements of pulmonary capillary blood volume (V_c) and DM, through the use of different oxygen tensions in inspired gas, apparently show that V_c is generally the same as in non-smokers but DM is reduced, leading to the reduced DL.[303, 378, 589, 704] Differences in diffusing capacity have also been found by using a technique of calculating the DL_{O_2} using hypoxic and hyperoxic gas mixtures.[667] In studies of 40 smokers aged 18 to 29 using $^{99}TcMIAA$ scans, no abnormalities of perfusion distribution were demonstrated.[3120] On maximal exercise, the

---

*See references 110, 125, 303, 589, 623, 639, 643, 644, 704, 3954.

†See references 110, 125, 136, 704, 3954.

$\dot{V}O_2$max measured in 61 young men was about 300 milliliters higher in non-smokers than in smokers,[690] a difference of about 3.0 mL/min/kg body weight.

In a comparison between 114 non-smokers, 66 light smokers, and 50 heavy smokers,[3130] it was noted that the O_2Hb was lower in smokers and that the lowering of O_2Hb occurred before there were significant changes in Hb or packed cell volume; these were noted in older smokers.

Effects of Smoking Cessation

There have been several studies of changes in pulmonary function when subjects stop smoking; these are important because they may assist in distinguishing between reversible and irreversible differences in smokers and non-smokers. A week after smoking cessation there was no change in tracheal mucus velocity, but this had increased when the subjects were re-studied 3 months later after abstinence.[641] Seventeen smokers studied 5 months after quitting were found to have significant increases in VC and FEV_1 (by about 4.4% of the predicted value) but no significant improvement in CV, CC, or MEFV curves. The SBN_2/L did fall but did not reach significance.[677]

Ventilation distribution measured by open-circuit nitrogen clearance improved in 19 heavy smokers studied before and one week after smoking cessation.[3161] Detailed studies in five men and five women before and 60 days after stopping[3953] found no changes in $\dot{V}max_{60\%}$TLC on helium or air, no change in FEV_1 or FVC, and no change in the maximum flow-static recoil curve; there was a significant fall in Pst at 60% TLC from a mean of 6.1 cm H_2O to a mean of 4.9 cm H_2O. The authors concluded that there might have been a decrease in small airway muscle tone to account for these findings.

In another study of 26 healthy smokers who stopped smoking, VC, FEV_1, and C_{dyn}/f all improved, but changes in SBN_2/L and delta $\dot{V}max_{50\%}$VC on air and helium were borderline.[658] Lung recoil apparently declined significantly, leading the authors to suggest that decreases in lung recoil were "even more accentuated after cessation of smoking." In four subjects who stopped smoking, the $(A - a)\,D_{O_2}$ fell significantly.[601] Ten subjects studied before and 10 to 14 weeks after smoking cessation had improved flow rates at 50% and 25% VC on helium; the CV fell. FEV_1, $FEF_{25-75\%}$VC, and VC were unchanged.[603] Other investigators

have found no change in CV/VC% after smoking cessation.[611] Buist, Van Fleet, and Ross[621] noted small changes in CC/TLC% in ex-smokers after 6 months of abstinence and a larger and more significant fall in those who had stopped smoking for between 6 and 14 years. Other data suggest that improvement occurs in FVC, FEV_1, CV/VC%, CC/TLC%, and SBN_2/L for up to 8 months after smoking and function is thereafter relatively stable.[653]

McCarthy, Craig, and Cherniack[631] studied 131 smokers aged between 17 and 66 years and noted improvement in SBN_2/L, CV, CC/TLC, FVC, FEV_1, and PEFR, together with a reduction in RV in those who stopped smoking or reduced their cigarette consumption significantly. Resumption of smoking led to a significant (22%) increase in SBN_2/L. Others have also documented improvement in CV/VC%, CC/TLC%, and SBN_2/L some months after smoking cessation.[632] In 12 subjects studied 2 months after smoking cessation, regional lung function data studied with ^{133}Xe showed improvement, and the fall of C_{dyn} with frequency was significantly reduced.[688]

It may be noted that most studies find significant differences in most of these tests of function between smokers and ex-smokers,[676] probably indicating an improvement in function or at least a modification in the rate of decline of function. The latter phenomenon was shown to occur in one longitudinal study over a 10-year interval in which the rate of FEV decline in those who had stopped smoking was lower than in those who continued smoking, but interestingly the rate had not declined to the values found in non-smokers.[680]

Nemery and colleagues[3137] reported data on 51 ex-smokers who had stopped for a mean of 8 years and compared them with 54 non-smokers and 105 current smokers; all the men were steelworkers aged 45 to 55 years. The data suggested that stopping smoking led to slower rates of decline of FEV_1, VC, and PEFR; values of RV, SBN_2/L, and CV/VC% were all more favorable in the ex-smokers than would have been predicted to have occurred if they had continued smoking. Similar data have been reported from a Los Angeles study; smoking cessation led to a slower rate of decline in small airway tests.[3967]

Summary of Effects of Cigarette Smoking

With so much information now at our disposal concerning differences between smokers and non-smokers, it might be thought that it would be simple to write a definitive description of the early effects of cigarette smoking on the lung and closely linking pathology and function. Yet it has to be admitted that although our understanding of this question has advanced substantially since 1970, many questions have only tentative answers. In the following paragraphs, an attempt is made to identify the solid ground in the morass of data.

1. The acute effects of cigarette smoking are to cause changes in airflow resistance, probably as a consequence of stimulation of irritant receptors. Although there are considerable individual differences in the pattern of cigarette smoking, it is unclear whether these determine later effects.

2. Early changes in CV/VC%, CC/TLC%, SBN_2/L, and the flow measurements of the later part of the flow volume curve could all be caused by the respiratory bronchiolitis of non-bronchitic (no sputum) cigarette smokers. Presumably, the inflammatory component of this bronchiolitis may slowly resolve and lead to improvement in these aspects of function. These tests are a great deal more sensitive than the FEV_1 in distinguishing smokers from non-smokers. Changes in regional function are early, suggesting that the impact of cigarette smoke is not uniform throughout the lung.

3. Although loss of lung recoil may lead to an increase in CV/VC% and in RV (as it does in normal aging), it is not clear whether an early loss of recoil in smokers is responsible for changes in these indices. Possibly, it first occurs regionally, but whether in upper or lower lobes is unknown. We do not know whether a change of lung recoil without the destructive lesions of emphysema may be capable of reversal over time.

4. Excess mucus production in small airways at a stage before hypertrophy of bronchial mucous glands has led to overt chronic bronchitis; may lead to non-uniform gas distribution and to increases in CV/VC%, CC/TLC%, RV, and SBN_2/L slope; and presumably may reverse with time. It is not clear to what extent this factor, which would presumably be closely associated with the inflammatory bronchiolar wall changes of respiratory bronchiolitis, may influence function.

5. The FEV_1 is a relatively late indicator of changes due to smoking. The timing of its decline in continuing smokers relative to non-smokers suggests the possibility that it only becomes significantly lower in smokers after the development of upper lobe emphysema.

6. It is not easy to suggest the most likely explanation for the consistently demonstrated reduction in diffusing capacity in smokers. It is tempting to relate the lowered DL to the vascular changes that accompany respiratory bronchiolitis. Possibly, non-uniform vascular changes in the lungs may lead to changes in the relationship between DL and flow. It seems unlikely that $\dot{V}/\dot{Q}$ disturbances, which do occur in chronic bronchitis before the FEV_1 is very abnormal, could explain the differences, since all methods of measurement of diffusing capacity show about the same differences. There is no evidence of thickening of the capillary membrane in smokers, but it is marginally possible that some decrease in DL may be caused by the increased numbers of cells between alveolar gas and capillaries. Alternatively, the respiratory bronchiolitis may diminish the gas exchange that normally occurs in alveoli adjacent to small airways. It would be very interesting to know whether DL improves if smoking ceases, and if so, after what time interval.

7. As will be noted later, since the effects of cigarettes in causing early respiratory bronchiolitis, later mucus hypersecretion, and eventual emphysema may well be due to different host responses and/or different constituents of cigarette smoke, there is no reason to assume that these effects are necessarily sequential. Presumably, each could occur independently of the others. Therefore, one must be very cautious in assuming that demonstrable early function test changes related to respiratory bronchiolitis can be assumed to mean that earlier mucus hypersecretion or emphysema will occur (though prudence would suggest that a demonstrated early respiratory bronchiolitis would be a good reason to stop smoking). There is preliminary evidence suggesting that those with early small airway changes may have larger falls in FEV_1 when studied longitudinally.[687, 706, 3983] However, the early detection of the "sensitive" smoker is still poorly understood.

EFFECTS OF OPIUM

Da Costa, Tock, and Boey[708] described 54 opium smokers in Singapore, with nine autopsies. There was radiologic evidence of bronchiolitis in 45 of them, and 25 were thought to have radiologic evidence of generalized emphysema. The lungs were heavily pigmented, with bronchiolitis, bronchiolectasia, and centrilobular emphysema. The FEV_1 ranged between 11% and 77% of predicted, the vital capacity was reduced, and residual volumes were elevated. The arterial saturation averaged 89%. Cor pulmonale and right ventricular hypertrophy were said to be common. Poh[390] described earlier cases, still asymptomatic. Those with a normal FEV_1 had a mean DL_{CO} of 83.6% of predicted and were considered to have peripheral disease. Eleven persons with a mean FEV_1 of 54% predicted had an elevated residual volume and a DL_{CO} of only 54% predicted.

This condition therefore seems to be characterized by a severe bronchiolitis leading to centrilobular emphysema and provides an interesting parallel case to that of tobacco smoking. From the descriptions it would appear that chronic sputum production (and presumably chronic mucus hypersecretion) is a less characteristic part of the syndrome following opium smoking than following tobacco smoking.

EFFECTS OF MARIJUANA

Studies on 74 regular marijuana smokers showed a slight increase in RL, but no effect on closing volume, SBN_2/L, or FEV_1.[884] It has a slight bronchodilator effect that lasts for about an hour[478, 3182] and does not depress the respiratory center.[3182] In one study, it increased the $\dot{V}E/Pco_2$ response.[709] The bronchodilator effect has been demonstrated in asthmatics.[710]

Effects of Air Pollutants on the Lung

We were perhaps misled by the example of smoking and lung cancer, which has been taken as a general model for the epidemiological study of causes. It was in fact an exceptional situation, in which there was large heterogeneity of exposure both within and between populations. If everyone in the country had smoked 20 cigarettes a day then clinical, case-control, and cohort studies alike would have led us to conclude that lung cancer was a genetic disease; and in one sense that would have been true, since if everyone is exposed to the necessary external agent then the distribution of cases becomes wholly determined by individual susceptibility.

We reach then this paradox, that the more widespread is a particular environmental hazard, the less it explains the distribution of cases. The cause that is universally present has no influence at all on the distribution of disease, and it may be quite unfindable by the traditional methods of clinical impression and case-control and cohort studies; for all of these depend on heterogeneity of exposure.

The second problem is in the interpretation of low order risks, owing to the complexity of study situations. In examining the relation of cigarettes to lung cancer we were dealing with an almost unifactorial aetiology and the answer came out clearly. In a multifactorial disease a factor which increases the risk by less than half will almost certainly be undetectable. We must learn to live with uncertainty and to make room for it in policy judgements. This will not be popular.

In summary, to seek to limit the hazards for high risk workers and critical population groups is admirable; but for the population as a whole it may have little relevance in circumstances where the dose response curve has no threshold and low level exposure is widespread. In that case the only effective control is mass control. The problem then arises that an order of risk which might be important for the population is likely to be undetectable. In that state of uncertainty we have to avoid both the panic of the professional protesters and the unfounded but seemingly unshakeable confidence of the professional experts.

GEOFFREY ROSE[196]

The literature on air pollution is now so extensive that in this section it is not possible to attempt more than a review of main issues and references. The search for proof of adverse health effects has been difficult, largely because of the preponderant effect of cigarette smoking in the genesis of lung disease and the presence of other confounding factors such as socioeconomic status and climate. General reviews of the health effects of air pollutants include some books,[711, 712] reviews by individual authors,[729] and a statement by the American Thoracic Society.[763] Guidelines as to what should be considered an "adverse health effect" have recently been published.[3200, 3936, 3938]

Sulfur Dioxide, Sulfates, and Particulate Pollution

This reducing and acidic type of air pollution, which in extreme form was responsible for the London episode of December 1952 that caused the death of 4000 people, is associated with the "pea-soup" fogs of the Industrial Revolution. The sulfur dioxide was produced from the uncontrolled combustion of high sulfur coal with no smoke control, and the particles included a considerable proportion of relatively large size (20 to 50 microns). Such episodes produced excess mortality, largely among those with compromised pulmonary or cardiac function, but also among infants and children. A great deal of research over the last 20 years has established that a combination of high SO_2 and particulate pollution has the following effects[3221]

1. When increased episodes of both pollutants occur, hospital emergency visits for respiratory illness are increased,[814, 3899] FEV_1 levels decline,[819] and patients with chronic lung disease note a worsening of symptoms.[3213, 3223]

2. Higher levels of both pollutants are associated with increased lower respiratory tract illness in children.[711, 794, 3218–3220] Barker and Osmond[4867] have reported from the United Kingdom that there was a strong geographical relationship between death rates from chronic bronchitis and emphysema in the period 1959 to 1978 and between the infant mortality from bronchitis and pneumonia in the period 1921 to 1925. From the United States, the six-city study of 10,106 white pre-adolescent children found that average particulate concentrations were related to bronchitis and a composite measure of lower respiratory tract illness.[4860]

3. When smoking and socioeconomic factors are taken into account, areas of higher SO_2 and particulate pollution are associated with more respiratory symptoms, an increase of bronchitis, and a lowered level of FEV_1.* These effects are seen in non-smokers but are more prominent in smokers. They have also been documented in children[3924, 3931] and adolescents.[3942] However, one study of the population living near a coal-fired power plant found no relationship between pollutant levels and symptoms.[5093]

4. There is some evidence that reduction in levels of these pollutants may be followed by some improvement in function and a lessening of symptoms of chronic bronchitis.[723, 728, 745, 3186]

5. Necropsy studies have provided some indication of a greater degree of mucous gland hypertrophy in areas of higher pollution[767] and some indication of a possible relationship between the degree of emphysema and ambient pollutant levels,[711, 764, 815, 1754] but only in a comparison between autopsy data from St. Louis and Winnipeg was the effect considerable.[815] Mostly, it has been of a low order of significance.[3222, 3229]

6. There is evidence of a slight general effect of these pollutants on pulmonary function, especially in children.[766, 3191, 3224] In some of these studies, the influence of socioeconomic effects or parental smoking were not taken into account, and it is not easy to be confident that the data are to be explained by the air pollution.† In other studies, a differential effect is present.[3191] In a study of three communities near Montreal in Quebec, there was some evidence of a relationship in children between the closing volume and higher levels of particulate pollution.[739, 824, 831] It is worth noting that although no significant difference in closing volume, RV, and SBN_2/L were found between inhabitants of three cities with different levels of air pollution participating in a collaborative study,[655] McCarthy and Craig[853] observed that closing volumes were higher in women living in London than they were in women in Winnipeg with comparable smoking histories; this raised the possibility that the difference might be due to air pollution. This suggestion would be supported by the observation that the closing volumes in an unpolluted town in Western Australia were lower than those in Sydney as measured by the same research group.[823]

---

*See references 742, 854, 3190, 3191, 3209, 3225.
†See references 811, 820, 821, 826, 827.

7. It may be that longitudinal—rather than cross-sectional—studies are required to demonstrate small effects at low concentrations.[821, 829] Van der Lende and his colleagues[3193] reported that FEV_1 declines in a population in rural Holland were 9.2 mL/year, whereas in a population in a suburb of Rotterdam they averaged 22.9 mL/year. Cross-sectional studies of the same populations by the same laboratory showed no significant differences. However, an update of these data in a recent symposium volume indicated that with a longer review the differences were less marked.[3990]

Controlled exposures in asthmatics have shown that they may react with bronchoconstriction to less than 0.5 parts per million (ppm) of SO_2* and that they are more sensitive to sulfate aerosols than other normal subjects.[855, 3177, 3216] The SO_2-induced airflow reduction in asthmatics is inhibited by the prior administration of disodium cromoglycate.[543]

The effect of SO_2 is potentiated if a saline aerosol is breathed at the same time as the gas[816]; nasal breathing reduces the effect.[3187] Non-asthmatic subjects also respond, but to higher concentrations.[788, 833, 845, 852] However, patients with chronic obstructive lung disease do not seem especially sensitive.[3922]

In humans, tracheal mucus velocity was unaffected by breathing 5 ppm of SO_2,[779] but it was slower in dogs at higher concentrations.[782] SO_2 may produce changes through a vagal reflex but may also involve mediator release.[852] It is not known whether glottal narrowing plays any part in the effect.[3029]

Experimental animal exposures have been of limited use in clarifying long-term effects. Sulfate aerosols increase mortality from subsequent bacterial aerosols, however,[732] and morphologic changes have been observed with repetitive exposures.[730] Humidity has been shown to increase the effect of sulfate aerosols in guinea pigs.[773] Concentrations of 500 ppm of SO_2 for 2 hours twice a week for 5 months in dogs[778] produced squamous metaplasia, goblet cell hyperplasia, and areas of alveolar dilatation. Lower concentrations have affected pulmonary function in dogs.[800] Concentrations of 200 ppm produce chronic changes in the mucous glands of dogs,[3185] but these are more than 400 times greater than ambient levels encountered. Even with exposure to sulfuric acid mist rather than

SO_2, high concentration exposures in monkeys led to relatively minor effects.[799]

An intriguing but unexplained observation by Davies and his colleagues[885] was that rabbits exposed to 150 ppm of SO_2 for 12 3-hour periods showed evidence of altered reflex activity. They noted that "the results indicate that chronic exposure to SO_2 inhibits pulmonary stretch receptor activity and its reflex effects and raises the question whether this mechanism may play a part in the control of breathing in human patients with chronic bronchitis."

It is perhaps surprising that 32 years after the London smog episode, there should still be lively controversy over the levels of particulates and SO_2 that may be responsible for short-term and long-term effects. Whittemore[3199] has pointed out that earlier epidemiologic studies did not permit any kind of precise "dose-response" conclusions to be drawn. Some investigators believe that effects at present levels are probably very minor[3203]; an extension of our studies of southern Ontario[713] has shown that sulfates account for the largest part of the variance in respiratory admissions in the summer in that region, indicating the possible importance of acid rain in that context.[3198] Portnoy and Mullahy[3908] have shown some relationship between the recording of "reduced activity days" in large scale surveys and air pollution levels in the United States. Chappie and Lave[3230] have shown that the significant relationship between average sulfate levels and mortality across the United States still exists, even when all confounding factors have been eliminated. No doubt the controversy will continue.* It has recently been found that there is a significant relationship between mortality from short-term exposure and the level of air pollutants in Athens,[3928] where general climatic conditions are very different from London.

Photochemical Oxidant Pollution (Ozone)

The chemical reactions that occur in the presence of sunlight and hydrocarbons to form oxidants from nitrogen dioxide were first described by Haagen-Smit in 1952.[720] These reactions are now known to be very complex, and many different compounds appear, some of them very transiently. The eye irritation of

---

*See references 3163, 3173, 3175, 3177, 3183, 3184, 3216, 3890, 3929, 3930, 3937.

*See references 715, 717, 721, 729, 734, 737, 742, 763, 795, 846, 847, 872, 3203.

photochemical smog is attributable to peroxyacetyl nitrite (PAN) compounds, and the principal oxidant is ozone. This smog reaches a peak some hours after the maximal emissions of nitrogen dioxide and then may drift hundreds of miles before being reduced to oxygen. The meteorologic and chemical factors that cause increased levels of ozone are complex.* It was once thought that this type of pollution was only important in Los Angeles, but it is now realized that large areas of North America are affected by it, including southern Ontario[3897] and New England. Episodes of ozone formation and drift have also been recorded in Europe.[741] Levels of 120 parts per billion (ppb) occur over widespread regions during the summer months,[856] but the levels are still highest downwind from Los Angeles, where peak values of over 700 parts per billion have been recorded.[740]

Ozone is the most irritant gas to which we may be exposed. Normal subjects have severe irritant symptoms and major declines in ventilatory function when exercising intermittently in 750 ppb; ventilatory function is adversely affected by exercising in 500 ppb[774] and is significantly reduced after 2 hours of intermittent exercise in 350 ppb.[859, 3913, 3941, 3992]

If very heavy exercise is performed with ventilation rates of 55 L/min, significant declines in FVC and FEV_1 are noted in concentrations as low as 120 ppb.† Under these conditions, women may be more sensitive than men.[3891] The fall in FVC is highly reproducible in normal subjects, but all investigators have noticed that there is wide individual variation.[3934]

The decline in FEV_1 is proportional to the delivered amount of ozone, calculated from minute volume and concentration.[751] Ozone also lowers the maximal $\dot{V}O_2$ attainable in normal subjects; the mechanism of this effect is probably complex.[873]

A careful comparison between chamber studies and observations in ambient pollution in Los Angeles indicated that when the ozone levels were similar in the two locations the effects were the same.[3202] Adaptation to ozone occurs, so that if breathed for 2 hours or 5 consecutive days, by the fourth day the ventilatory response is much reduced; this effect lasts for a week or so.‡ Whether this adaptation is "protective" is

unclear,[863, 871] but Linn and his colleagues[863] have recently concluded that it would not confer much protection.[863] Animal studies[886] have indicated that ozone-induced particle clearance delay in rats may be modified by pre-exposure to ozone 3 days before, but the cellular basis of ozone tolerance is not yet understood.[3180] There is some evidence that those living in Los Angeles may be less reactive to ozone than those not habitually exposed.[835]

An important effect of ozone is to cause increased bronchial reactivity,[716, 738, 3171] a laboratory observation that may explain the relationship between attacks of asthma and ozone concentration noted later. It must be noted, however, that neither asthmatics[3993] nor patients with chronic obstructive lung disease[867, 3940] are more sensitive to ozone than normal subjects. Experimental studies have indicated the possibility that increased reactivity may be related to inflammation,[3167] and this may indicate that ozone invariably causes an inflammatory response.

These laboratory observations have been confirmed by field studies. Children exercising in Arizona had a decrement of FEV_1 on high oxidant days.[762] Lippmann and his colleagues[856] have recently documented an average fall of FEV_1 of 150 milliliters in 83 school children at a summer camp in Pennsylvania when ozone levels reached a maximum of 110 ppb. This observation confirms data from Japan indicating an effect of ozone at low concentrations on school children there.[784]

Acute symptoms of ozone toxicity have occurred in flight attendants,[850] and concentrations of ozone of one ppm have been recorded in aircraft in flight on some occasions.[3227] The symptoms noted exactly mimicked those observed in controlled exposures.[858] Respiratory symptoms in Los Angeles also parallel the ozone concentrations.[790, 791, 876] Early data showing a relationship between acute respiratory admissions and oxidant concentrations[746, 747] have been superceded by the careful analyses of Whittemore and Korn,[743, 3898] who concluded that a level of ozone as low as 120 ppb resulted in a 20% increase in risk of an asthmatic attack. These data have recently been confirmed by similar studies in Houston, Texas.[3994]

We have published evidence that hospital admissions for respiratory disorders in southern Ontario are associated with increased levels of ozone during the summer months.[713] In a more recent analysis,[3991] we have been able to add aerosol sulfate levels over the region into the

---

*See references 718, 740, 741, 748, 857.

†See references 3169, 3202, 3228, 3901, 3915, 3945.

‡See references 542, 725, 863, 874, 875, 3166, 3180, 3916.

analysis; we found that in terms of asthma, both ozone and aerosol sulfates are important causes of variance. In hospital respiratory admissions, aerosol sulfate levels appear to be the most important single factor. A large population is required to demonstrate consistent relationships of this kind, and some studies have not found similar evidence.[721, 877, 878, 3889]

Although there is some evidence of chronic effects, as indicated by lowered ventilatory function in cross-sectional studies, their magnitude is very small,[841, 879] and symptom prevalence does not seem much different between populations in the same region with somewhat different concentrations of oxidants.[770, 880] However, Hodgkin and his colleagues[5094] recently found a higher prevalence of symptoms in more polluted regions, but the pollutants were not only oxidant.

Data have indicated that there may be a faster rate of decline of FEV_1 and of SBN_2/L in more polluted regions of Los Angeles.[3195, 3197] These data have not yet been published in full, and the period of follow-up is probably too short for a definitive answer to this very important question. There are data suggesting that respiratory mortality for the Los Angeles basin follows windflow direction,[881] but it is difficult to exclude other variables from influencing such studies.

There is a great deal of animal data on the effects of ozone exposure. These data show that the earliest effect occurs at the region of the terminal bronchiole,[882] where theoretical calculations indicate that the dose may be highest.[802] Pre-exposure to ozone at concentrations as low as 200 ppb increases the mortality of mice from subsequent bacterial aerosol challenge,[722, 731] possibly as a result of interference with macrophage function. Particle clearance is also adversely affected.[844] Inflammatory changes[3167] and interference with collagen synthesis[3196] also occur. In dogs, there are unexplained effects on cardiac output.[3170] Morphologic changes in the airways are well documented in a variety of species and by many different investigators*; summaries of these extensive data can be found in the EPA criteria document for oxidants.[740]

Ozone and oxygen radicals have profound tissue effects,[755, 837, 849, 3196] but their long-term significance is not known. It has been sug-

gested, however, that ozone may interfere with human alpha$_1$-proteinase inhibitor[848]; whether this is significant in terms of human disease is also unknown. Data on whether ozone and SO_2 or sulfates together have a greater effect than either singly are conflicting. In animal studies, there is evidence of enhancement when both are present.[3179] In human studies, our original data indicating such an effect[860] have not been confirmed[714, 833, 868, 3917]; sulfate formation in the chamber may possibly explain the discrepant results.[862] Stacy and his colleagues[3204] noted a considerably greater decline in FVC and FEV_1 when both O_3 and acid sulfates were present,[3204] but the differences did not reach significance. However, ozone and SO_2 have been found to have greater effects on mucociliary clearance together than either pollutant at the same concentration alone.[3907]

To a much greater extent than with SO_2 and particulates, the oxidant data show good internal consistency. Field observations have confirmed controlled laboratory exposures, and effects in animals are caused by similar concentrations to those producing acute effects in humans. However, we still lack detailed understanding of the effects at the cellular level, and there are insufficient epidemiologic data to confirm or exclude long-term effects in exposed populations.

Oxides of Nitrogen

A recent symposium volume has summarized data on nitrogen oxides.[3919] They are the precursors of oxidant air pollution. Adverse effects occur at about 10 times the concentrations of ozone needed to produce them; the effects of nitrogen oxides and ozone are in general similar.[719, 3927]

Acute poisoning has been known for many years (see Chapter 16), but only recently has it been suspected that low levels might cause adverse effects. Supporting data have come from the finding that more respiratory infections may occur in young children in homes with gas cooking as compared with electric cooking when all other factors, such as socioeconomic, regional pollution, and parental smoking, have been taken into account.[745, 828, 869] This phenomenon is not yet definitively established, however,[883, 3201] and Melia and his colleagues[5095, 5096] could find no clear relationship between respiratory conditions in children and NO_2 levels measured in the home. There is no doubt that

---

*See references 731, 735, 736, 744, 755, 758, 760, 761, 769, 772, 777, 786, 787, 789, 798, 805, 806, 808, 811, 813, 818, 836, 837.

significantly higher levels of NO_2 often occur in homes with gas cooking, particularly in winter.* Whether urban levels of NO_2 account for the increased incidence of respiratory syncytial virus infections in city children as compared with rural children is not clear,[752] since other factors make comparisons difficult. A report that NO_2 at low levels increased the airway reactivity in asthmatics[776] has not been confirmed in replicate studies.[3207]

The effects of nitrogen oxides on animals are similar to those of ozone, except that higher concentrations are required† and bronchiolar lesions may be commoner.[3174, 3178] Guidotti[719] has summarized much of these data. Nitrogen oxides may interfere with immunologic processes in the lung[756] and have been reported to increase the spread of cancer to the lung in experimental animals.[753] Bronchial permeability is increased[830, 843] and a few reports have indicated that emphysema may follow long-term exposure.[768]

Carbon Monoxide

The main effects of carbon monoxide at the low levels generally encountered in ambient air are on the cardiovascular system. It has been reported that small increases in COHb shorten the distance walked before the onset of pain in patients with coronary artery disease.[757] Such a result might be expected, since the oxygen tension of working muscle would be lowered if COHb was present. However, the exact level at which this effect becomes important in patients with coronary artery disease has not yet been identified.

Volcanic Ash

The eruption of Mount St. Helens led to studies of the effects of volcanic ash on experimental animals and on children who had been tested before and immediately after the eruption.[3168, 3172] No adverse effects were recorded in these studies. In one of them,[3172] a decline of FEV_1 was noted after 3 days of high ambient air pollution (440 μ/m^3) not attributable to the eruption. A longitudinal follow-up of forestry workers exposed to the ash[4696] indicated that transient declines in FEV_1 had occurred.

---

*See references 828, 840, 842, 883, 3181, 3214.
†See references 731, 759, 768, 771, 792, 793, 803, 804, 807, 809, 817, 822, 825, 838.

Fluoride Pollution

Ernst and his colleagues[3995] have documented differences between the CV/VC% in boys living close to an aluminum smelter and that of others of the same ethnic origin and socioeconomic status living farther away. This study indicates the importance of considering effects other than those on the FEV_1, although there is as yet no definitive answer to the question of long-term significance.

Indoor Air Pollution

As noted previously, it is now known that gas cooking results in raised NO_2 levels indoors. As also noted earlier in this chapter, respiratory infections have been shown to be commoner in households in which the mother, but not the father, smokes, and there is evidence of lower FVC values in children in those households.[3231] Other important indoor problems are radon, which may influence lung cancer rates, organic chemicals, such as formaldehyde and resins used in insulation, and other materials. A recent volume on indoor air pollution summarizes what is known of these hazards.[3909]

Summary of General Issues

The main unresolved issues concerning contemporary levels of air pollution are

- the relationship of air pollution to long-term adverse changes in populations
- the influence of air pollution on morbidity
- the significance of short-term effects, such as FEV_1 decline in exercising children, on long-term function

Acute episodes of high SO_2 and particulate pollution are unlikely to recur, but occasional high levels of oxidant pollution may be expected in certain regions when meteorologic conditions are favorable to smog formation. Further epidemiologic work is required to decide whether or not transient phenomena can be dismissed or whether costly control strategies should be implemented. With ozone, there appears to be very little, if any, margin of safety between current ambient levels and acute adverse effects on adults and children. It is not known whether we should be concerned about long-term exposure to sulfates, which occurs over large areas of North America and Europe in the summer.

It is important that chest physicians should be well informed on the state of evidence on these problems if they are to give intelligent answers to questions from patients with increased airway reactivity and if they are to provide informed leadership on matters of community health related to environmental problems. Should they occasionally be surprised at the complexity of political decision-making in this field, they would do well to read Lord Ashby's remarkable account of the series of events that led up to the adoption of legislation against open coal burning in Britain, *The Politics of Clean Air*.[3212]

7

SYNDROMES OF CHRONIC AIRFLOW LIMITATION

> One might expect, accordingly, that parenchymal function tests should be specifically sensitive to intrinsic diseases of the parenchyma, and airway function tests to intrinsic disease of airways. But this leaves out of consideration the fact that the parenchyma depends entirely on the airways for the gas that expands it, while the airways depend on the parenchyma to supply the retractive forces which help maintain their patency. These important interdependencies of supply and support mean that primary changes in one part can have secondary influences on the function of the other...
>
> JERE MEAD[989]

> There will be no simple solution to the puzzle of COPD.
>
> G.L. SNIDER[4018]

INTRODUCTION

The problem of classification and definition of the syndromes that lead to chronic airflow limitation is made complex by many factors:

1. Chronic airflow limitation is a physiologic term and requires a measurement of function for diagnosis ("chronic" is a word requiring some definition).

2. Chronic mucus hypersecretion is diagnosed by a history of persistent cough and sputum that is sometimes defined by responses to a standard questionnaire. Although such a definition leads to a division between "positive" and "negative," the distribution of morphologic bronchial mucous gland size in the population is unimodal[988]; thus, differentiation rests on an insecure morphologic foundation.

3. Emphysema is a morphologically defined entity and, strictly speaking, can only be diagnosed post mortem or after surgical intervention.

4. Accurate diagnosis during life is therefore problematical.

5. The fact that methods (or fashions) of classification predetermine conclusions has, in the past, hampered understanding. Thus, if radiologic criteria are taken to be the sole determinants of the presence of morphologic emphysema, it is easy to conclude that chronic bronchitis causes most of the disability. As Thurlbeck has pointed out,[1250] if chronic bron-

172

chitis is defined as chronic mucus hypersecretion, "more severe" chronic bronchitis would logically imply more severe mucus hypersecretion, whereas what is often meant is worsening airflow limitation or the development of gas exchange abnormalities.

6. The effects of inhalation of cigarette smoke over a lifetime are very complex. The same components of the smoke may cause different effects at all levels of the airway, sometimes in varied sequences among individuals. In some individuals, these components may have no effect at all.

7. The lure of convenient short-hand phrases such as COPD, chronic lunger, and so on is to be avoided. These phrases may serve an immediate purpose but militate against a critical approach to this group of syndromes. This in turn leads to poor management.

All of this may lead to descriptions of this group of diseases, if properly qualified and accurately delineated, that read more like legal contracts between hostile parties than broad descriptions of disease. The logistic problems of arranging the different aspects of information about these disease are formidable. However, these difficulties should not obscure the fact that we have made major advances in understanding the components of the syndrome, and in many ways the description of the function defects associated with it is simpler than it was in 1970[1] and certainly is much more informative. The literature on the syndrome continues to expand at the rate of about a hundred papers a year.

In the previous edition of this book,[1] we noted the attempt to classify these syndromes into a Type A (predominantly emphysema), Type B (predominantly chronic bronchitis) and mixed types; or more picturesquely into "pink puffers and blue bloaters" and others. Although embodying some elements of reality, these simplistic categories do not, in our opinion, any longer serve a useful purpose. However, since a considerable body of literature uses these categories for classification, the differentiation cannot be ignored.

This chapter and the next are based on an alternative approach. Those readers interested in following the history of the classification of chronic airflow limitation diseases will find useful starting points in Thurlbeck's book on these syndromes,[585] in his discussion in more recent volumes,[584, 3229] and in Burrows' overview,[1143] as

well as letters and editorials in respiratory journals.* Fletcher and Pride[4120] have recently reviewed problems of definition. In Chapter 8, the very extensive literature on changes in severe cases of chronic airflow limitation is summarized, without attempting any differentiation between different categories of disease. The problem of describing reported pulmonary function changes in this syndrome may be illustrated by reference to one paper[1084] reporting on 24 cases of "chronic obstructive pulmonary disease" comprised of 10 persons with asthma; three with bronchitis; two with bronchitis with cor pulmonale; two with asthmatic bronchitis; two with asthmatic emphysema; four with emphysema; and one with emphysema with cor pulmonale. Other authors have suggested classification based on severity as judged by pulmonary function tests.[4112] The difficulty with this approach is the reversibility of apparently "irreversible" air flow obstruction in some patients.[3997]

COMPONENTS OF THE SYNDROME

The syndrome of chronic airflow limitation consists of four potential major components (Table 7–1):

1. Chronic mucus hypersecretion (a clinical diagnosis based on history).
2. Pulmonary emphysema (destruction of parenchyma).
3. Airway hyperreactivity ("asthma," "reversible airflow limitation").
4. Changes in small airways (including respiratory bronchiolitis).

It may also result from five less common clinical entities:

1. Bronchiectasis and cystic fibrosis (see Chapter 10).
2. Airflow limitation in association with parenchymal fibrosis or granulomatosis (see Chapters 13, 14, 15, and 16).
3. Pulmonary lymphangiomyomatosis (see Chapter 17).
4. Tracheal stenosis (see Chapter 19) and other large airway obstructive lesions.
5. Syndrome of chronic bronchiolitis, either

*See references 1001, 1006, 1140, 1200, 1206, 1257, 4095.

Table 7–1. DIFFERENTIATION OF CHRONIC AIRFLOW LIMITATION SYNDROMES*

Syndrome	Sputum	Chest X-Ray Over-inflated	Vascular	SBN$_2$L	He Mixing Delay	RV Incr	FEV$_1$ Decr	DL$_{CO}$ Decr	K	Pa$_{O_2}$ Decr
Single (pure) forms:										
A Generalized emphysema	0	+ +	Def	Incr	+ + +	+ +	+ + +	+ + +	+ +	+/−
B Mucus hypersecretion	+ +	+	N	Incr	+	+	+ +	+/−	N	+/−
C Increased airway reactivity	0	+ + +	N	Incr	+ +	+ +	+ +	−	N	−†
D Small airway disease	0	+ +	N	Incr	+ + +	+	+ + +	+	N	+/−
Mixed forms:										
B + A	+ +	+ +	Def	Incr	+ +	+	+ +	+ +	+ +	+
B + D	+ +	+ +	N	Incr	+ +	+	+ +	+/−	N	+
C + B	+ +	+ +	N	Incr	+ +	+	+ +	−	N	+/−
A + D	0	+ +	Def	Incr	+ + +	+ +	+ + +	+ + +	+ +	+/−
A + B + D (+ C)	+ +	+	Def	Incr	+ + +	+ +	+ + +	+ + +	+ +	+

*Def, deficiency; N, normal; Incr, increase; Decr, decrease.
†Only in severe asthma.

in association with rheumatoid disease (see Chapter 13) or as a primary condition (see Chapter 19).

In the following sections, each of the four major components of "chronic obstructive lung disease" is discussed in terms of a complete dissociation between them—that is, the information that exists on pulmonary function in "pure" forms is discussed, the factors and responses that influence outcome are analyzed, and the role of pulmonary function tests in management is summarized. Such an approach is now possible because we have detailed studies of function in cases of alpha$_1$-antitrypsin (AT) deficiency emphysema without mucus hypersecretion, and of disease of small airways occurring as the only lesion.

Each major component may exist alone, but usually they exist concomitantly. It is for this reason that some physicians use the term COPD for any combination of them. In our view, discussion of these entities should not be confined to discussing a lowered FEV$_1$ as if this was, in itself, a disease entity. (This is a temptation, and one deservedly well-known text entitled *The Natural History of Chronic Bronchitis and Emphysema*[723] is primarily an account of longitudinal FEV$_1$ decline.)

In Chapter 8, the extensive literature on functional components of the developed syndrome of severe chronic airflow limitation is analyzed. In most of the work reviewed in that chapter, no attempt was made by the authors to assign the patients studied to any category other than chronic airflow limitation; the resulting data can therefore be discussed only in those terms. Useful reviews of the total syndrome have appeared recently.[4106, 4109]

Chronic Mucus Hypersecretion

This diagnosis is made clinically or from questionnaire data. It is commonly made when a cough with sputum is present for more than 3 months a year and when other causes can be excluded.

As noted in Chapter 6, there are morphologic changes in the small airways of smokers and concomitant changes in pulmonary function before chronic mucus hypersecretion and, presumably, before mucus gland hyperplasia, as indicated by the presence of a productive cough, have occurred. A chronic productive cough probably begins about 15 years after starting regular smoking.[972, 973] Although it cannot be assumed that at this stage there is no morphologic emphysema, the changes in pulmonary function commonly found in patients between the ages of 30 and about 45 with chronic mucous hypersecretion can be described.

Incidence

The introduction of the tested questionnaire has greatly expanded our knowledge of the incidence of respiratory symptoms. Several comparative tests have been conducted of four slightly different questionnaires[1157, 1177]; the differences between them are small. However, there is some question as to how constant the findings are over time. In 1973, Sharp and his colleagues[1312] noted that individuals diagnosed as having chronic bronchitis on one occasion would not have fitted the criteria when questionnaires were re-administered a few years later. More recently, Pham and his colleagues[2355, 2378] recorded "switches" in diagnosis in as many as 25% of men originally surveyed. Recent studies show the importance of using different inputs in relation to symptomatic enquiries,[4122] that is, it is necessary to check the information by different methods.

There are considerable differences in the apparent occurrence of respiratory symptoms in different countries. A complete analysis of this literature is beyond the scope of this volume, but an idea of the prevalence of these symptoms is given by noting the countries from which such data have been reported over the past 10 years: Rhodesia,[1295] India,[1247, 1302] New Guinea,[1172] Norway,[1101, 1102, 1181] Sweden,[1021] Switzerland,[1119] Great Britain,[1131, 1180, 1307] Denmark,[319] Rumania,[1111] and different regions of the United States—Arizona,[1184] Colorado,[1324] Boston,[2187] Michigan,[1169, 1183, 1224] and the Hispanic population in New Mexico.[3295] A careful comparison between data from the United States and the United Kingdom suggests that the syndrome of chronic airflow limitation is about four times more common in the United Kingdom than in the United States.[3186]

The incidence of chronic respiratory symptoms is very closely related to environmental factors, of which cigarette smoking is dominant. However, it seems probable that other factors play a part, particularly climate, presence or absence of air pollution, special local environmental factors (as in New Guinea), and socioeconomic status. In one study conducted in Copenhagen, respiratory symptoms were more closely correlated with the quality of housing than with smoking or alcohol consumption.[1319] Respiratory symptoms and lowered pulmonary function have also been noted to be associated with the number of years spent in dwellings without central heating in cool damp climates.[1063]

In Glasgow, a survey of 83 men and 217 women over the age of 65[1307] found that 26% of the men and 13% of the women had symptoms of chronic bronchitis. The mean FEV_1 in the men with symptoms was 1.35 liters and 2.04 liters in those without symptoms. The warm dry climate of Arizona apparently causes less sputum production with a chronic cough, but wheezing is commoner.[1184] In that climate, 29% of persons with chronic bronchitis had never smoked cigarettes. Chronic mucus hypersecretion and airflow obstruction are not uncommon in warmer climates,[1035] but in some native people the disease may be related to special local factors (of which indoor air pollution may well

be important[4122, 4123]). In others, such as the aboriginal people of Australia, different factors must be relevant; a survey of 1287 aborigines showed that 29% had lower respiratory illness.[4092] The role of dusty occupations in causing bronchitis is discussed in Chapter 16.

In Rhodesia, the prevalence of chronic bronchitis in white men over the age of 20 was only 1.2%. There was no evidence that it increased with age, a finding the authors attributed to lack of air pollution.[1295] There is clear evidence that respiratory symptoms and the occurrence of respiratory infections in children are related to parental smoking (particularly whether the mother smokes), as well as to other environmental factors, such as mode of cooking (see Chapter 6) and air pollution. A review by Kauffmann[4080] concluded that there was "strong evidence in favor of genetic factors explaining the association of COPD in relatives." Although the dominance of cigarette smoking in the genesis of mucus hypersecretion is evident in many studies and therefore dominates risk factor analysis,[4116] it does occur in non-smokers (a topic that was the subject of a recent symposium.[3312]

Pathology

The complete reviews by Thurlbeck[585, 988] of the morphologic changes that occur with chronic mucus hypersecretion indicate the complexity of these events in both large and small airways. Bignon[1152] has reviewed the relationship between changes in large and small airways and has provided striking illustrations of these.[1130] Mucous gland hypertrophy may be more prominent in segmental than in major bronchi[1214]; this is due to an increase in the number of cells.[1287] There is narrowing of small airways and mucus plugging,[1202] and the number of Clara cells is reduced.[1189] The cilia in patients with chronic bronchitis are commonly atypical[3358, 4117]; this may be linked to delayed mucociliary clearance. It has been reported that goblet cell metaplasia is found only when airflow limitation has been present[1185], but in a recent study the goblet cell "score" was higher in the lungs of 25 regular smokers without severe disease than it was in non-smokers or in persons with chronic airflow limitation.[4103] Distortion and actual stenoses of bronchioles become features of more chronic stages of the disease, and these are reminiscent of the changes in experimental animals after long-term exposure to oxides of nitrogen (see Chapter 6).

Berend[1149] found that inflammatory changes

in respiratory bronchioles were more common in the lower lobes than in the upper, but there is no close correspondence between the regional distribution of the airway changes and the extent of emphysema peripherally. Although cases of morphologic emphysema have a greater than normal degree of mucous gland hypertrophy, extensive emphysema may be found at autopsy with no mucous gland hyperplasia.[1273] Taking the data as a whole, it is important to stress that chronic mucus hypersecretion is often, but probably not invariably, accompanied by widespread airway changes. It is likely, but cannot be taken as strictly proved, that when chronic productive cough is present with mucous gland enlargement, there are also changes in small airways. Correlative studies between function and morphologic changes are discussed later in this chapter.

Physical Signs and Radiology in Chronic Mucus Hypersecretion

Inspiratory crackles (rales) may be heard in patients with mucus hypersecretion, and these have been attributed to mucus in small airways.[16] In other patients, the inspiratory crackles may occur late in inspiration and are then attributed to explosive opening of airways. Rhonchi are thought to originate in larger airways, and their presence may indicate associated increased airway reactivity; they are not affected by breathing a helium/oxygen mixture.[16] Gross variations in regional ventilation, which occur in emphysema, should not be present. The principal finding on plain radiography is overinflation of the lungs[973], that is, in these patients overinflation is noted with mucus hypersecretion, only slight flow rate impairment, and normal diffusing capacity. It is not clear whether it is to be ascribed to airway changes or to concomitant (but essentially independent) loss of recoil. Bronchography may reveal loss of peripheral filling, probably due to mucus, causing small bronchioles to end abruptly like broken twigs. Filling of enlarged mucous glands is seen only in long-standing cases. The pulmonary vasculature should be normal. Individuals are described in whom the bronchitis is so severe that gross atrophy has occurred and bronchial collapse is present.[3340]

Pulmonary Function

Chronic mucus hypersecretion may be present with no alteration in any of the general tests of pulmonary function. In one survey of 374 men and 377 women aged between 60 and 85 years, 39% of the smokers with persistent coughs had normal spirometry values.[1111] Tests of small airways, such as the closing capacity, may also be normal. As noted in Chapter 6, cigarette smokers are commonly found to have an increased closing capacity and increases in SBN_2/L. These changes occur in smokers both with and without mucus hypersecretion.[265]

There is convincing evidence that tests of pulmonary function are more commonly abnormal in those with symptoms than in those without. Knudson, Burrows, and Lebowitz in Tucson, Arizona[317] in a random population sample noted that twice as many symptomatic smokers had an abnormal $\dot{V}max_{75\%}VC$ (23.9%) as did asymptomatic smokers of the same age (11.9%). This test was the most sensitive of those used. Specific airway conductance (SGaw) has also been noted to be more often abnormal than the FEV_1.[1066] Differences in helium and air $\dot{V}max_{50\%}VC$ appear to occur only in symptomatic smokers.[695] When a series of such cases are studied, it is common to find airflow changes, not usually very severe, and an increased residual volume (RV).

We studied 216 Canadian veterans in four different cities with chronic mucus hypersecretion (as defined by the United Kingdom MRC questionnaire). The participants were of average age 45, were fully employed, and were without evidence of cardiovascular disease. The FEV_1 level averaged between 70% and 80% of predicted, and the FEF_{25-75} was between 70% and 60% of predicted.[973] The residual volume was increased by between 600 and 1200 milliliters, and CO gas exchange values were normal.[972, 973] Other authors have noted the normality of F_{CO} in cases of chronic mucus hypersecretion and have suggested its use in screening patients.[1020] Both the residual volume and MMFR may be abnormal when the FEV_1 is still within normal limits,[601, 701] but some authors do not find evidence that the FEF_{25-75} is a more sensitive indicator than the $FEV_1/FVC\%$.[300] When the FEV_1/FVC ratio is still normal, the effective time (t_{eff}) of the expiratory spirogram is prolonged.[234, 239]

In one study, 19 men aged between 30 and 40 years with mucus hypersecretion had a mean FEV_1 of 74% of predicted and an increased RV/TLC ratio, with possibly a slight reduction in P_{stat} measured at TLC.[1219] In an interesting comparison between 17 asthmatics in remission and 21 subjects with mucus hypersecretion, all

38 subjects had a normal FEV_1. The study showed comparable reductions in FEF_{25-75} in both groups and abnormal SBN_2/L tests in four asthmatic and nine bronchitis individuals.[1188] C_{dyn}/f was reduced to below 80% of control values in all subjects of both groups. Penman, O'Neill, and Begley[1234] studied 200 patients and grouped them into four categories, depending on measured increased RL and normality or loss of lung recoil. Their data suggest that an increased RV is related predominantly to loss of recoil.

We[1175] addressed the question of whether symptoms can be relied on to indicate changes in cigarette smokers and concluded that function test derangements were more useful, confirming a similar conclusion we noted previously.[983] As noted in the previous chapter, Teculescu, Pham, and Hannhart[3996] have published a detailed comparison between asymptomatic smokers with normal spirometry and smokers with mild airflow limitation. In the first group, there was no relationship between the FEV_1 and tests such as SBN_2/L, RV/TLC%, and closing volume (CV). But in the second group, these were related and were also associated with changes in DL_{CO}, leading the authors to suggest that some instances of emphysema had developed in the second group.

Exercise-induced falls in FEV_1 are less common in persons with chronic bronchitis than in those of comparable age with asthma.[1028] The response to bronchodilators is greater in asthmatics than in patients with mucus hypersecretion.[1070] In general, bronchial reactivity as measured with histamine or mecholyl is not greatly increased[513] and is very much less than in persons of comparable age with asthma. Recent comparisons between individuals with asthma and chronic bronchitis have indicated that the mechanisms of the response are different in the two conditions.[4029, 4070] However, as noted later, there is an association between chronic mucus hypersecretion and greatly increased airway reactivity in some patients; these constitute the group designated as having "asthmatic bronchitis." In a recent study of 27 smokers, several instances of increased reactivity were found in those with normal FEV_1 data and mild symptoms,[4124] although increased reactivity is commoner in those with airflow limitation.[4143] Increased reactivity is demonstrable with histamine, or mecholyl, or cold air breathing.[3965]

Studies of regional ventilation using ^{133}Xe show abnormalities in most symptomatic smokers in whom CV or RV is increased.[670] We

found evidence that the lower zones of the lungs were more often abnormal than the upper zones,[984] a finding others have confirmed.[1019, 1082, 1129] It has been suggested that there may be a reduction of compliance in the lower zones.[1082] In studies of ventilation and perfusion using ^{133}Xe it is possible to demonstrate that low $\dot{V}/\dot{Q}$ regions exist even when the FEV_1 is still within normal limits.[984] The increase in measured $(A - a) D_{O_2}$ in these cases is consistent with this finding. A detailed study in which 43 non-smokers and 46 smokers of comparable age inhaled krypton-81m showed evidence of regional abnormalities in 46% of the smokers (whose mean FEV_1 was 92% of predicted).[4000]

It may of course be argued that all these changes indicate loss of recoil or beginning emphysema and that they cannot be ascribed to chronic mucus hypersecretion *per se*. This may well be the case (though very difficult to prove); the point being made here, however, is that these changes are described not infrequently in patients without chronic airflow limitation, but with chronic productive cough. In a study of 109 patients with normal or stable radiologic findings and referred for examination because of chronic cough, the value of bronchial challenge testing in establishing airway reactivity was noted.[3302] The authors stressed that pulmonary function testing was usually more useful than bronchoscopy in the investigation of such cases. Sweat tests have been shown to be negative in cases of chronic mucus hypersecretion without cystic fibrosis.[3234]

Other changes in patients at this stage in the evolution of their disease include a decrease of peripheral penetration of aerosol[33] when the FEV_1 is still normal. However, there is a relationship between the depth of penetration and the FEV_1.[48, 51] Clearance is delayed, often to a considerable degree[645] if there is no coughing.[961] This greatly accelerates clearance, as might be expected.[963, 2954]

Hemodynamic Data and Mild Airflow Obstruction

The cardiac output on exercise in persons with mucus hypersecretion but without emphysema is probably normal.[1283] The only clearly relevant hemodynamic data are these in the study by Ravez and his colleagues.[1091] They selected 77 persons of average age 52 in whom the mean VC was 101% of predicted, the RV/TLC was 29% of predicted, and the FEV/FVC ratio averaged 65% of predicted. In all of them the resting Pa_{O_2} was greater than 70 mm Hg, and the Pa_{CO_2} was less than 45 mm Hg. Forty-four of these subjects had a pulmonary artery pressure at rest less than 10 mm Hg, but in 33 it exceeded this. The group with the higher pulmonary artery pressure had lower VC (96.5%P vs 104%P), lower FEV_1 (81.9%P vs 97.4%P), higher RV/TLC (31.2% vs 27.1%), and a lower Pa_{O_2} at rest (66.9 mm Hg vs 72.7 mm Hg). Gas exchange data, including the fractional uptake of CO, was not different between the two groups. This study suggests that a slight rise of pulmonary artery pressure may accompany the early stages of the syndrome. This observation fits with the finding of early evidence of vascular change in the lungs of smokers, as noted in Chapter 6. Other authors have noted a slight reduction in ventilatory response to exercise at this stage.[1210]

Chronic Mucus Hypersecretion of Long Duration

It is clear that a chronic productive cough may be present for a lifetime without leading to significant airflow limitation. Although the annual decline in FEV_1 is greater than normal in most of these patients, in many it closely follows the expected age regression. In such subjects, there is no development of significant emphysema and, what is probably just as important, no continuing development of progressive small airway changes. Probably, there is also no development of significant airway hyperreactivity, although the point is not established.

Clement and Van de Woestijne[3305] have reported on a longitudinal study of 2406 members of the Belgian Air Force. Accelerated annual FEV_1 declines were noted in smokers, but these authors also document an annual loss of FEV_1 of -43 mL/year more than that occurring in 720 non-smokers in a man who was also a non-smoker but suffered from "wheezy bronchitis." This compared with an annual FEV_1 loss of -12.6 mL/year more in heavy smokers than in non-smokers in this population.

Severe cases of long-standing chronic mucus hypersecretion are occasionally encountered. These "advanced" cases of "chronic bronchitis" with gas exchange abnormalities and unrelievable severe airflow limitation have severe V/Q disturbances, probably with abnormalities of ventilatory control (see Case 61, pp 466–467, in the second edition of this book).

EMPHYSEMA WITHOUT CHRONIC MUCUS HYPERSECRETION

In the second edition of this book, we stressed the importance of the $alpha_1$-AT deficiency syndrome in relation to the genesis of emphysema,[1] but at that time relatively few cases had been identified and studied. In the past 12 years, many hundreds of cases have been reported, and the syndrome is well understood. Mittman[1298] has contributed a useful review of all aspects of it,[1298] and other reviews have also appeared.[1226]

In Laurell and Eriksson's original description of the syndrome, there were several cases with chronic mucus hypersecretion; however, some non-smokers and some smokers also had mucus hypersecretion.

This syndrome has led directly to the development of the "protease-antiprotease" theory of the development of emphysema—a major advance in understanding. Detailed discussion of this is beyond the scope of this volume. Janoff's[4069] excellent review and that of Hoidal and Niewohner[3350] provide excellent starting points, and there are other useful references.*

There are still areas of uncertainty. For example, careful histologic studies of seven cases of severe panlobular emphysema (PLE) matched by age and sex with seven cases of severe centrilobular emphysema (CLE) showed that generalized thickening of the wall of bronchioles was as common in the PLE group as in the CLE group[3246] and that these changes may be important in limiting airflow.

The evolution of changes in pulmonary function in persons with $alpha_1$-AT deficiency is reasonably well established. In children between the ages of 3 and 7 years with $alpha_1$-AT deficiency, defects in pulmonary function are usually absent,[1262] but one 13-year-old boy with the condition had reduced blood flow and ventilation to the left lower lobe as measured with ^{133}Xe.[1262] Impaired FEF_{25-75} has also been recorded in a 15-year-old; at autopsy there was some increase in mean alveolar diameter (L_m) but no overt emphysema. Cigarette smoking usually precedes the development of disease[1271] and is clearly a severe risk in these patients.[1095, 1114] Even with minimal smoking, defects in pulmonary function begin to appear when the subjects are in their twenties and may be ad-

---

*See references 3239, 3262, 3283, 3298, 3299, 3311, 3320, 3361, 4098, 4119.

vanced by the age of 40.[3364] Changes in pulmonary function occur in the following sequence:

1. Decreased clearance of perfused ^{133}Xe through the affected zone, usually the lower lobe. This is a more sensitive test than nitrogen clearance data.[1322] There is no mucus hypersecretion, and the patient may be asymptomatic.[600]

2. Loss of lung recoil,[994, 1207, 1208, 1243] with changes in the MEFV curve and a lowered diffusing capacity.*

3. A falling FEV_1 and FEF_{25-75}, and a slight reduction in Pa_{O_2}.[1193]

These changes progress at different rates in different subjects. All three of the changes may be present by the age of 40, and FEV_1 values of 0.4 liters have been recorded in smokers with severe alpha$_1$-AT deficiency by this age. We have recorded severe ventilatory defects in one such patient with a minimal smoking history and no sputum.[3364]

In some cases, progress of the condition is slower. One group of investigators reported that of 18 lifetime non-smokers of PiZ phenotype not exposed to dust or pollution, several lived into their sixth and seventh decade.[1324] Pulmonary function tests showed expected reductions in FEF_{25-75}, DL_{CO}, and PmaxTLC. It is interesting that half of these subjects developed chronic cough and sputum in later life.[1324] Galdston and his colleagues[1166] have derived a composite index based on trypsin inhibitory capacity (TIA), pack-years of smoking (PKY), and elastase-like esterolytic activity (E-LEA) as predictors of a pulmonary function (PF) score:

$$PF\ Score = 18.5 + 0.176(TIA) + 0.0031611\ (PKY \times E\text{-}LEA)$$

Studies of 78 members of a large family of phenotype PiZ with M-malton–deficient allele for alpha$_1$-AT showed that four of these members whose alpha$_1$-AT was only 16% of normal had severe emphysema. In this series, pulmonary function tests (including ^{133}Xe data) appeared to be normal when the serum alpha$_1$-AT was at least 63% of normal.[3275]

There is no doubt that severe deficiency combined with even minimal cigarette smoking can cause remarkable declines in FEV_1.

Mittman[1298] noted an average fall of -60 mL/yr in 163 MZ phenotypes followed for 6 years and noted larger falls in individuals.[971] It may be noted that if an FEV_1 is normal at age 20 and is reduced to 0.5 liters by age 40, an annual fall of -175 mL/year may have occurred.[3364] One study of non-smokers found no differences in lung volumes, FEV_1, or DL_{CO} but significantly lower flow rates in MZ phenotypes.[1192] The authors suggested that generalized changes in structure and function, rather than regional loss of recoil or basal emphysema, might be the earliest change in these subjects when other environmental factors are not present.

These observations lead to an important conclusion, namely, that panlobular emphysema without chronic mucus hypersecretion may cause severe declines in pulmonary function over a relatively short period of time. Presumably, this is predominantly due to loss of recoil, but as noted above, there may also be concomitant structural changes in small airways. In smokers, a respiratory bronchiolitis may well accelerate the airflow limitation if lung recoil is also much reduced.

In one subject followed by us over a 20-year period,[3364] it seemed probable that the FEV_1 must have fallen by over 200 mL/year from the age of 20 (when the patient was physically active) to the age of 40, when it was only 600 milliliters. No change occurred between the age of 40 and 60, when respiratory failure developed. Similar cases have been recorded by others.[1298]

The fact that much remains to be learned of the factors responsible for maintaining lung integrity is indicated by the three cases reported by Martelli, Goldman, and Roncoroni.[1304] The subjects were aged 22, 30, and 34, and one was a non-smoker. They had FEV_1 values of 1.07, 0.9, and 0.6 liters. Alpha$_1$-AT levels were normal, but severe lower lobe panlobular emphysema was present (proved at autopsy in one of the subjects).

SMALL AIRWAY CHANGES WITHOUT MUCUS HYPERSECRETION OR EMPHYSEMA

The respiratory bronchiolitis of smokers, described in Chapter 6, presumably exists in many persons with no associated emphysema; sputum is often not present, so that mucous gland

---

*See references 1007, 1018, 1064, 1107, 1171, 1208, 1228, 1229, 1242, 1311, 1316.

enlargement has presumably not yet occurred. The functional changes associated with this stage were fully described in Chapter 6.

A clearer idea of the functional consequences of severe and widespread bronchiolitis as an isolated lesion has become possible through the identification of severe small airway disease in association with rheumatoid arthritis, a syndrome first described by Geddes and his colleagues.[1320] An analysis of this syndrome will be found in Chapter 13. In 1971, Macklem and his colleagues described cases of small airway disease in adults as a recognizable clinical entity.[2855] Some cases were associated with bronchiectasis, but in others the disease was apparently a primary entity. This "non-occupational" bronchiolitis is discussed in Chapter 19.

As follows, these cases provide a basis for describing the functional consequences of disease limited to the small airways, without either emphysema or mucus hypersecretion[975, 976, 2855, 3367]:

1. There is usually overinflation of the lungs with an increased TLC and FRC. Lung recoil is normal. The vital capacity is reduced.

2. There is severe chronic (unrelievable) airflow limitation, with FEV_1 values of less than 25% of predicted and FEF_{25-75} values less than 20% of predicted.[975]

3. There is very delayed helium equilibration on closed-circuit measurement[1320] or very delayed nitrogen clearance.

4. The $DL_{CO}SB$ and $DL_{CO}SS$ values are reduced to between 40% and 60% of predicted values,[975] but DL_{CO}/VA may be relatively normal.[976]

5. Hypoxemia, with Pa_{O_2} values between 42 mm Hg and 62 mm Hg, and mild chronic hypercapnia occur during the later stages, and death is common in respiratory failure.

As noted in Chapter 1, because the cross-sectional area of the small airways is large, considerable generalized change must occur in them before the FEV_1 is reduced to low levels. This occurs in this syndrome, however, and presumably occurs in any case in which the lesions are widespread.

SEVERE AIRWAY HYPERREACTIVITY

As noted in Chapter 9, it is not possible to define "asthma" in terms of complete reversibility of airflow limitation—problems of definition would be simplified if this were not the case. The pathologic changes noted in patients dying in status asthmaticus after many years of severe episodes of asthma, particularly bronchial muscle hypertrophy, small areas of bronchiectasis, excessive mucus retained in small airways, and so forth might all contribute to chronic airflow limitation.

Patients with chronic mucus hypersecretion who are not atopic may acquire increased airway reactivity. Airway reactivity is not increased in association with alpha$_1$-AT–deficient emphysema[3122] as one would expect, but in cases of "chronic obstructive lung disease," it is increased. In one study of 26 cases in which the FEV_1 response to cold air was studied, the authors concluded that airway reactivity could not be described accurately as "non-specific" because it depended on the agent used.[3244]

In another study of 22 cases of "chronic obstructive bronchitis,"[3260] from which persons with asthma were excluded, airway reactivity to methacholine was shown to be increased. The authors concluded that "airway hyperreactivity may contribute to acute, transient exacerbations experienced by patients with chronic obstructive bronchitis even in the absence of acute improvement in pulmonary function after the administration of sympathomimetics, and may warrant chronic bronchodilator therapy." The initial FEV_1 in the cases studied was 0.96 liters ±0.44.

Persons with mucus hypersecretion and increased airway reactivity are often classified as having "asthmatic bronchitis" or "chronic infective asthma" (see Case 6, p 140, in the second edition of this book). There is very little detailed morphologic information on such cases, although it has been suggested that there is no hypertrophy of bronchial muscle in asthmatic bronchitis, in contrast to what is found in cases of asthma.[1213] It is possible that later hyperreactivity is commoner if multiple respiratory infections have occurred in childhood.[4049]

Yan, Salome, and Woolcock[4051] have reported their results of surveying the community of Busselton in Western Australia, an area where there are no occupational respiratory hazards and no air pollution in terms of airway reactivity. They found that although 27 out of 59 cases of chronic obstructive pulmonary disease had increased reactivity, this was less severe than that observed in asthmatics. The fall in FEV_1 on histamine had a general relationship to the initial FEV_1 as a percentage of predicted across all the groups tested.

The role of airway hyperreactivity in chronic mucus hypersecretion is complex, and the existing data do not permit quantitative estimates of its relative importance[1142]; its role in relation to the rapidity of decline of FEV$_1$ is discussed later. There is little doubt that increasing airway reactivity occurring in association with chronic mucus hypersecretion or as a new component in a patient with emphysema may be responsible for abrupt decreases in FEV$_1$ or for a faster than normal rate of decline in this measurement. This has important implications for management, as noted later.

FACTORS AND RESPONSES THAT INFLUENCE OUTCOME

The syndrome of chronic airflow limitation is caused by four principal external causative factors, is mediated by four principal tissue responses, and is modified by four principal "physiologic" responses.

Principal "External" Causative Factors
1. *Irritants:* Cigarette smoke; gases; dusts; cadmium; proteolytic enzymes
2. *Allergens:* Pollens; chemicals?
3. *Infections:* Viral (sequelae of episodes in childhood?)
4. *Climatic:* Effect on sputum?

Principal Tissue Sequelae
1. *Large Airway Changes:* Mucous gland hypertrophy; loss of cilia
2. *Small Airway Changes:* Goblet cell hyperplasia (loss of surfactant?); inflammatory changes; reduction in numbers of goblet cells
3. *Acquired Airway Hyperreactivity:* Morphologic counterpart?
4. *Alveolar Destruction:* Emphysema

Principal "Physiologic" Responses
1. *Airway Reactivity* (insofar as this is reversible)
2. *Pulmonary Vascular Response to Alveolar Hypoventilation* (relationship between Pa$_{O_2}$ and pulmonary arterial pressure)
3. *Control of Breathing Response to* $\dot{V}/\dot{Q}$ *Imbalance and Hypoxemia*
4. *Tissue Defenses Against Elastase*

The rate of decline of function in an individual patient and the slow or rapid evolution of the syndrome depend on the particular combination of causative factors and individual responses present in that particular patient.

Aspects of the Natural History

RESPIRATORY BRONCHIOLITIS IN SMOKERS

As noted in Chapter 6, changes in small airway function may be detected in a considerable fraction of symptomless (without chronic mucus hypersecretion) smokers. Whether these individuals are any more likely to develop emphysema or acquire airway hyperreactivity is not known. Pride and Connellan[3296] have noted that an increased closing capacity in a group of smokers was not associated with an accelerated FEV$_1$ decline in subsequent years, but this was based on observation of a small number of cases. As noted in Chapter 6, Olofsson and his colleagues[3841] have published more comprehensive data on 460 men followed for 7 years and showed that initial abnormality of SBN$_2$/L was associated with a subsequently faster decline in FEV$_1$.

CHRONIC MUCUS HYPERSECRETION

When symptoms of chronic cough and sputum production have developed—so that the patient is classifiable as having chronic bronchitis as defined by questionnaire responses—but no extensive morphologic emphysema is present (excluded either by radiologic criteria, which as Thurlbeck has noted[988] are unreliable, or by the presence of a normal DL$_{CO}$[1344]), there is no general rapid progression of the disease.[1197] When the FEV$_1$ is more than 70% of predicted in such cases, the rate of decline is not much different from that in the general population.[977] Rapid episodic declines in function, which later reverse, may well be due to airway hyperreactivity during periods of infection. It seems very likely that more severe airflow limitation in this syndrome without emphysema is to be attributed, as Thurlbeck suggests,[1250] to progressively more severe changes in small airways. Peto and his colleagues[2924] have brought together a great deal of data indicating that outcome is determined not by the presence of chronic mucus hypersecretion but by the rate of decline of the FEV$_1$.

The falling FEV$_1$ may well be accompanied by a worsening of the $\dot{V}/\dot{Q}$ distribution, leading to increasing hypoxemia and pulmonary hypertension,[1091] so that chronic cor pulmonale may occur without any emphysema. These cases are exceptional, however, and may occur only when ventilatory control is abnormal, that is, when developing hypoxemia and hypercapnia are not followed by increased ventilation or, possibly, when this phenomenon is aggravated during sleep or by obesity or by both.

AIRWAY HYPERREACTIVITY

As noted later, there is some, but not conclusive, evidence that increased airway reactivity may be followed by a faster rate of FEV_1 decline.

PULMONARY EMPHYSEMA

It is clear that if a person has alpha$_1$-AT deficiency and is exposed to cigarette smoke, severe chronic airflow limitation may develop. However, there are still many uncertainties in describing the role of emphysema in determining outcome in patients not deficient in alpha$_1$-AT.

Upper lobe CLE is characteristically found in smokers at autopsy.[585] Does this cause progressive FEV_1 decline and is it related to prognosis? Is the loss of recoil associated with the development of emphysema responsible for premature closure of small airways and airflow limitation? Is the principal effect of emphysema to cause $\dot{V}/\dot{Q}$ imbalance and hence affect gas exchange?

Perhaps the most important generalization that can be made is the variability of all these factors in different patients. It is for this reason that many physicians prefer to group these conditions together (as "COPD") and not attempt any further differentiation. It is clear that the components of this syndrome are loosely linked by being related to a common (but very complex) agent—cigarette smoke—but various patterns of effect and evolution occur in different patients. The point is made later that it is because of this variability that pulmonary function tests are important in the management of patients with this group of conditions.

STRUCTURE AND FUNCTION CORRELATIONS IN THE "COPD" SYNDROME

It might naturally be supposed that the resolution of the problem of relating function test changes to morphology would be to compare test results in life with morphology at autopsy or from surgically removed specimens. These studies have been excellently summarized by Thurlbeck[584, 585] and more recently by Berend.[3359]

Some of the more important conclusions that have been drawn from such studies are the following:

1. Nagai and his colleagues, including Thurlbeck, have reviewed the findings in 48 autopsies of cases of hypoxemic chronic obstructive lung disease from the NIH Intermittent Positive-Pressure Breathing Trial.[4059, 4060] They noted that (1) bronchial muscle was not related to either clinical features or airflow measurements; (2) the degree of emphysema was related to body weight and to right ventricular hypertrophy and was the major correlate of airflow abnormality and of increased RV and SBN_2L; (3) goblet cell metaplasia was related to airway resistance; and (4) surprisingly, increased muscle and fibrosis in the bronchioles was related to better Pa_{O_2}, lower Pa_{CO_2}, less edema, less right ventricular hypertrophy, and better airflow and lower residual volumes. They concluded that the results "substantiate the importance of emphysema as a cause of chronic air-flow obstruction."

2. Petty, Silvers and Stanford[4136] studied 54 excised lungs with varying degrees of emphysema and concluded that there was a relationship between elastic recoil at 70% of TLC and bronchiolar diameter; loss of recoil and fibrosis of small airways might be related by a common inflammatory process.

3. The extent of emphysema is best related to loss of recoil and to the diffusing capacity. In 1973, Teculescu and his colleagues noted that up to that date the literature contained data on 226 cases studied during life with autopsy assessment. The relationship between severity of emphysema and DL_{CO} had r values between 0.57 and 0.91.[1121] This confirmed our own conclusions.[1] Berend[3359] concluded that "the current evidence suggests that the best single test for diagnosis and assessment of emphysema is a test for the diffusion capacity of carbon monoxide." The relationship to F_{CO} might be even stronger if corrections were applied for the respiratory rate, as suggested in Chapter 5.

4. Loss of recoil is also closely related to extent of emphysema, with an r value of 0.71 reported in one series of 26 cases.[1222] In another series of 24 cases, the r value was 0.489.[1148] The computed k value from the pressure-volume curve is closely related to alveolar size.[1137] The elastic recoil at 90% TLC, expressed as a percentage of predicted, had an r value of -0.696 with extent of emphysema in 65 excised lungs.[1286] The value of k in the diagnosis of emphysema has been discussed by Colebatch

and Greaves[1124]; they have summarized and updated this information.[3894] They have also noted conflicting data on the importance of small airway disease.[4144]

5. The DL_{CO} and the elastic recoil have comparable predictive capability, and this is enhanced if both are used.[1326] Loss of vascularity on the chest x-ray is also useful. This was noted by Simon and his colleagues[1308] who compared the DL_{CO} with radiologic appearances and wrote that "the radiological diagnosis of widespread emphysema can be made with confidence only when there is evidence of alveolar destruction— as indicated by attenuation of medium-sized pulmonary arteries—as well as overinflation." In a recent paper from Japan,[4132] detailed studies of "ring shadows" on alveolobronchograms in cases of chronic airflow limitation were reported. The 64 subjects were divided into two groups: Group A, with a mean diameter of ring shadows greater than 90 microns, and Group B, with a mean diameter less than 90 microns. Group A subjects were 10 years older, had an FEV/FVC ratio of 40 (versus 54 in Group B), had a $DL_{CO}/\dot{V}A$ of 3.6 (versus 6.4 in Group B), and had a higher residual volume. There were no differences in vital capacity or in Pa_{O_2} between the two groups. The authors considered that the ring shadows reflected the presence of emphysema.

6. The SBN_2/L test and the MEFV curve are poorly related to extent of emphysema.

7. Deaths in acute respiratory failure are associated with a severe degree of goblet cell metaplasia.[1009] Studies of function of lungs removed at autopsy confirm the importance of peripheral airway disease in determining airflow.[1190, 3304]

8. Several studies have confirmed the observation that a normal DL_{CO} indicates a normal parenchyma when the MEFV curve is abnormal.[1203]

9. In 1981, from 22 surgical specimens and 32 autopsy specimens, Berend[3146] concluded that in such studies a "total pathologic score" of small airway changes was more useful than measured internal diameter and that such a score correlated with the FEF_{25-75} and $\dot{V}max_{50\%}VC$ with an r value of -0.46. The FEV_1 was more closely related to the Reid index of bronchial mucous gland enlargement. He has also pointed out that small airways are narrower in surgically removed specimens than in autopsy specimens, possibly because of persistence of muscle tone in the former.[3146]

10. Wright, Pare, Hogg, and their colleagues have been sequentially publishing a series of function and morphology correlations from resected lung specimens. Wright and colleagues[4017] have presented evidence that the extent of emphysema can be reliably deduced from lobar specimens—an important point in relation to the data.

They initially reported observations on 17 cases[3240]:

	Non-smokers	Smokers Minimal E	Smokers Moderate E
Sex: M/F	0/3	7/0	6/0
Age: Mean	60	59	62
Smoking (pack-years)	0	65	63
Pa_{O_2} (mm Hg)	—	71	79
TLC (%P)	97	119	113
VC (%P)	98	103	95
RV (%F)	95	146	134
$FEV_1/FVC\%$	88	63	68
FEF_{25-75} (%P)	119	43	48
DL_{CO} (%P)	115	87	58
k (%P)	—	112	154
Emphysema grade	0	7	28
Airway score	97	140	222
PaP (mm Hg):			
Rest		17	13
Exercise (n = 13)		27	34
Vessel morphology			
% Intima	14	18	21
% Media	17	18	19
% Adventitia	69	64	60
Area of wall mm	0.12	0.26	0.34

They later updated this to include 45 surgically removed lobes or lungs[3368]:

	Emphysema Score 0	Emphysema Score 3–15	Emphysema Score 20–80
Number	19	20	16
Age:			
Mean	56	66	64
Range	23–81	47–79	55–79
Pack-years:			
Mean	39	55	58
Range	0–108	0–133	16–91.5
$\dot{V}max_{50\%}$ (%P):			
Mean	82	56	47
Range	18–123	22–113	14–95
FEF_{25-75} (%P):			
Mean	72	38	39
Range	8–116	17–56	9–80
DL_{CO} (%P):			
Mean	87	91	63
Range	54–155	60–131	41–92
F_{CO} (%P):			
Mean	93	98	74
Range	65–108	70–144	45–100
P_Lmax (cm H_2O):			
Mean	26	23	19
Range	12.5–40	11–32	10–35
k (cm H_2O):			
Mean	0.179	0.181	0.245
Range	0.104–0.377	0.105–0.284	0.097–0.432

Wright and her colleagues concluded that "minimal emphysema may be detected by exponential analysis of the lung pressure volume curve." However, they also concluded that k "did not distinguish those with mild emphysema from those without." The data also indicate the probability that mild to moderate degrees of emphysema would be best detected by the consistency of change in several indices, rather than in one, since every test showed at least one individual at marked variance from the others. This is true for all indices noted. Reviewing their data when 96 cases had been collected,[4135] they stressed the importance of inflammatory changes in the bronchioles and the close correspondence among FEF_{25-75}, $\dot{V}_{isoV}$, and SBN_2/L with progressive small airway pathology. They concluded that when the FEV_1 was greater than 80% predicted, these tests accurately reflected small airway changes.

Reviewing 110 cases,[4048] they could find little relationship between the density-dependence of flow rates and the severity of peripheral airway abnormality or emphysema. The group with more than 15 units of emphysema, compared with groups with less than 10 units, were noted to have a lower $P_L$max, a higher k constant, a lower $DL_{CO}SS$ and F_{CO}, and a higher SBN_2/L slope.

More recently, Hogg and colleagues[3893] reviewed this series, now consisting of 150 cases, and concluded:

1. That the FEV_1 as a predicted percentage correlated with smoking history in cigarette-years but that this relationship was weak if non-smokers were excluded.
2. That the TLC and FRC were close to predicted values when the FEV_1 had fallen to less than 50% predicted.
3. That the RV increased when the FEV_1 fell below 60% of predicted and in some instances was increased when the FEV_1 was still 80% of predicted.
4. That the DL_{CO} fell as the FEV_1 dropped from 100% to 80% predicted and continued to decline as the FEV_1 fell.
5. That cumulative abnormality in test results correlated with worsening airway score in the respiratory bronchioles.
6. That the SBN_2/L was often abnormal in persons with respiratory bronchiolar pathology but with a normal FEV_1.
7. That significant emphysema could be present when the FEV_1 was 80% predicted and there was very considerable variation in emphysema score versus FEV_1.

In spite of these general relationships, there is considerable variation in all the data. Thurlbeck[3229] has pointed out that emphysema of moderate severity (a maximal score of 15 out of 30) occurs with DL_{CO} values and recoil pressure only marginally abnormal. However, it must be noted that although it is often stated that considerable degrees of emphysema are associated with "no disability," it is often not clear whether the actual physical limitation of the patients has been as carefully assessed during life as was the quantitative morphometry of the lung when it was available for examination. Some loss of recoil may be found without morphologic emphysema, leading Thurlbeck[584] to suggest that a qualitative loss of recoil may antedate morphologic changes.

RELATIONSHIPS BETWEEN CLINICAL AND FUNCTIONAL STATUS AND BETWEEN FUNCTION TESTS

Much of the pulmonary function literature has been concerned with the differentiation between Type A and Type B chronic airflow limitation. Although this differentiation is not, we believe, of much value (since it represents two ends of a continuous spectrum and most cases fall in the middle), some of these distinctions are summarized.

Type A cases (predominantly emphysema) are generally characterized by:

- a larger TLC than Type B cases,[1040, 1041, 1044] and a larger RV[1040, 1135] and FRC[1039]
- reduced lung recoil[1044, 1045, 1326] and an increased C_{stat}[1126]
- possibly slower nitrogen washout[310]
- lower DL_{CO} values* possibly due to a lower DM component[1037, 1209]
- regions of high $\dot{V}/\dot{Q}$, as determined by the six-inert gas technique,[1332] with a bimodal pattern of $\dot{V}$ distribution
- slowly ventilating spaces of large volume and poor ventilation, with a low diffusing capacity and a low $\dot{V}/\dot{Q}$ ratio[1039, 1279] as determined by Bohr isopleth analysis and nitrogen washout data

Type B cases are generally characterized by:

- large volumes of low $\dot{V}/\dot{Q}$ regions as noted by

---

*See references 992, 1041, 1097, 1153, 1303, 1326.

the six-gas method, with substantial perfusion to them[332]

- slowly ventilating spaces, which are smaller and have a relatively good DL but a very low $\dot{V}/\dot{Q}$ ratio as determined by nitrogen washout and Bohr isopleth analysis[1279]
- more severe hypercapnia and hypoxemia in some series[1040, 1126, 1135] (in other series,[1041, 1044] there is not much difference in this respect between the two types)

In any other studies, overlap of findings and contradictions have been noted.*

Exercise results are also discrepant, as noted later. Although Jones noted that a fall of Pa_{O_2} on exercise more often occurred in Type A than Type B cases (see 1984 Clinics in Chest Med), others have not found consistent differences in tidal volume or Pa_{O_2} on exercise.[1017, 1041] It has been noted, however, that if patients are divided into A and B categories on the basis of loss of recoil in A, and increased RL in B, there are differences in ventilatory response to exercise and CO_2, as discussed later.[1210] We originally suggested that emphysema was characterized by loss of recoil combined with a lowered $DL_{CO}SS$.[985] Duffell, Marcus, and Ingram[1010] confirmed this, finding a linear relationship between the $DL_{CO}SS$ measured on exercise and loss of lung recoil in a group of 25 patients.

It is important to note that changes in FRC and airflow measurements are very poorly predictive of measured loss of recoil.[1205] Colp, Park, and Williams[1232] have described persons with considerable emphysema ($DL_{CO}SB$ from 40% to 71% of predicted and lung recoil reduced to half normal) in whom the FEV_1 was remarkably preserved, varying between 60% to 120% of predicted. Of the six subjects described, all were male smokers, and the chest x-rays and tomograms were abnormal in five. There do not appear to be any obvious differences clinically between those in whom the slow VC is or is not more than 350 milliliters larger than the fast FVC.[1232] It has been suggested that comparisons of rate of washout of helium and sulfur hexafluoride may distinguish individuals with emphysema from those with airway disease but without emphysema,[334, 1094, 1106] but others have not found this test to be more useful than measurements of recoil and $DL_{CO}SB$.[1002]

Schrijen and Jezek[1069] classified 47 persons into two groups of comparable age, depending on whether less than or more than 50% of

wedge angiograms showed abnormalities.[1069] The group with more than 50% showing abnormalities had a slightly higher RV/TLC ratio and exercise pulmonary arterial pressure than the other group, but the cardiac outputs and FEV_1/FVC ratios were not different.

Measurements of recoil pressure and airflow in 62 cases of chronic airflow limitation led one group of authors to conclude that "airway disease limits expiratory forced flows in most patients with chronic obstructive pulmonary disease regardless of whether morphologic emphysema is present,"[1198] but others have concluded that loss of recoil is important in a considerable fraction of cases.[1165] However, there is an overlap of measurements of recoil between Type A and Type B cases when the FEV_1 levels are comparable.[356]

In an interesting recent study of 27 subjects with chronic airflow limitation, all with chronic bronchitis, Gelb and his colleagues[3325] divided them into two groups according to the $DL_{CO}SB$ data as follows:

	Number	Mean Age	$FEV_1/FVC\%$	$DL_{CO}SB$ (%P)
Group 1	14	63	43	125
Group 2	13	60	33	55

Elastic recoil was reduced only in those cases with a lowered DL_{CO}. Studies of MEFV curves indicated that in both groups "limitation of airflow occurs primarily in the small (<2 mm in internal diameter) and not in the large airways." This study confirms the original experimental evidence indicating the same phenomenon.[1] Some authors have found that groups categorized into Types A and B are not different in respect to pulmonary artery pressure levels,[1249] but others have noted higher levels in Type B cases.[1040, 1126, 1135]

The effects on function of emphysema involving different lobes are a matter of some interest. Martelli, Hutchison, and Barter[1327] studied 50 persons with emphysema, excluding anyone with alpha$_1$-AT deficiency. They divided the cases into predominantly upper lobe emphysema (n = 31) and predominantly lower lobe emphysema (n = 19) using radiologic criteria. They found that lower zone disease was associated with a lower FEV_1 (30%P vs 44%P), more severe hypoxemia (Pa_{O_2} of 69 mm Hg vs 77 mm Hg), and hypercapnia (Pa_{CO_2} of 46 mm Hg vs 39 mm Hg). The mean ages of the two groups were 52.4 years and 54.9 years.

The FEV_1 correlates poorly with the ability

---

*See references 310, 356, 1040, 1042, 1045, 1126, 1135, 1165, 1198, 1219, 1220, 1248, 1256.

to lower arterial Pa_{CO_2} by voluntary hyperventilation,[1016, 1267] but the worse the FEV_1, the greater is the discrepancy between end tidal CO_2 tension and arterial Pa_{CO_2}.[1221] However, this difference is much reduced if a maximal expiration is made.[1221] Correlations between FEV_1 and Pa_{CO_2} are weak, with r values varying from about -0.35 to -0.56.[1072, 1118, 1125] With Pa_{O_2}, the FEV_1 correlated with an r value in one series of 152 cases of $+0.52$.[1118] In a recent study of 651 ambulatory men with chronic airflow limitation,[3263] a loose correlation was noted between spirometry, studies of mechanics, and gas tensions. Isolated hypoxemia was accompanied by an increased respiratory rate, without differences in tidal volume, whereas isolated hypercapnia was accompanied by an increase in frequency, together with a decrease in tidal volume. This had the effect of increasing the $\dot{V}D/\dot{V}T$ ratio and causing a drop in alveolar ventilation. Other aspects of the control of breathing in this condition are discussed in the next chapter.

Several authors have noted a poor relationship between clinical and radiologic "scores" and function test results. This confusion was eloquently (but unintentionally) expressed by the translator of the English abstract of an article written in French: "The clinical score is not dominant for the clustering of the patients into the dynamic clouds."[1078] One knows exactly what he meant.

Role of Function Tests

The pulmonary function laboratory is valuable in the management of cases of chronic airflow limitation in five different ways:

1. Assessing status. When a new patient is seen for the first time, the probable extent of emphysema can be gauged by measurement of DL_{CO} and elastic recoil, together with assessment of vascular changes on the chest film or tomogram.

2. Monitoring the effect of treatment, particularly steroids. In general, a trial of steroids with assessment of change is often indicated, and always if there is severe airflow limitation but relative preservation of DL_{CO} and recoil pressure. Studies by Mendella and her colleagues[982] have shown that significant FEV_1 improvement may follow the use of steroids in cases in whom no improvement occurred after routine bronchodilators.

3. Determining discrepancies between arterial blood gas changes and the FEV_1. Such discrepancies should lead to a suspicion that control of breathing is disordered.

4. Verifying the actual cause of dyspnea. Since mucus hypersecretion and emphysema and coronary artery disease are all related to cigarette smoking, dyspnea may be attributed to left ventricular failure when it is in reality due to primary lung disease, or it may be attributed to chronic bronchitis when it is actually due to pulmonary congestion.

5. Assessing preoperative status (see Chapter 17).

6. Assessing functional status in alpha$_1$-AT–deficient patients and their relatives. This may be important in relation to advice on occupation or to reinforce advice on smoking cessation.

Of the four major components of the syndrome of chronic airflow limitation—mucus hypersecretion, small airway changes, emphysema, and airway hyperreactivity—the following generalizations may be made:

1. It is doubtful if mucous gland hyperplasia of itself can cause irreversible airflow limitation. (Indeed, one might take an extreme but unproven position that the effect, *per se*, on function is very slight.) It is probable that associated small airway changes are always present when severe chronic airflow limitation is present and morphologic emphysema is absent. Small airway changes, emphysema, and airway reactivity may all cause chronic airflow limitation when present as the sole lesion. All may cause an increased residual volume.

2. Severe $\dot{V}/\dot{Q}$ disturbance may lower CO transfer (however this is measured) and widen the $(A-a) D_{O_2}$.

3. Emphysema is particularly associated with loss of recoil and loss of DL_{CO}.

4. Severe airflow limitation with a normal DL_{CO} indicates airway changes that may be reversible.

5. When chronic hypercapnia is present, but ventilatory flow rates are not severely impaired and the $DL_{CO}SB$ is also not grossly reduced, the probability of an abnormality in ventilatory control increases.

TYPICAL LIFETIME HISTORY OF PATIENT WITH CHRONIC AIRFLOW LIMITATION

Our present understanding of the probable sequence of events in the common form of the developed syndrome of chronic airflow limitation in a cigarette smoker may be summarized as follows:

1. The earliest change, partially reversible, is respiratory bronchiolitis with changes in SBN_2/L and flow rates; possibly these changes begin in the lower lobes.

2. Mucus hypersecretion at a stage when DL_{CO} and recoil are still normal is associated with an increased residual volume; it is not clear if this is due to loss of recoil, the development of CLE, or mucus in small airways.

3. It is not known whether Stages 1 and 2 invariably antedate the development of emphysema, but if the FEV_1 or FEF_{25-75} is significantly lowered by the time a subject reaches the age of 40 years, the airways have become hyperreactive, considerable small airway disease has developed, or there is loss of recoil and beginning emphysema (probably upper lobe CLE at this stage).

4. Significant worsening of the $\dot{V}/\dot{Q}$ distribution, as shown by the arterial gas tensions, in association with a fast decline of FEV_1 and DL_{CO}, signal the imminent development of pulmonary hypertension. This stage is discussed in the next chapter.

8 SEVERE CHRONIC AIRFLOW LIMITATION

> When we remember that we have as yet no adequate study of prognosis in chronic bronchitis, no adequate data on the changes in respiratory function that occur day by day and week by week in this disease in relation to atmospheric conditions and respiratory infection, no detailed study of the effect of treatment on respiratory function, and very little information on the value of function tests in grading such patients, it must be evident that the major part of the work remains to be done.[5418]
>
> D. V. BATES (WRITTEN IN 1958)

INTRODUCTION

In many important contributions to the understanding of the syndrome of chronic airflow limitation, no attempt is made by the authors to separate the cases into any kind of subdivision; usually such cases are selected on the basis of an FEV_1 of less than 1.2 liters or so. This chapter summarizes these data, which are important for a full understanding of the condition.

Incidence

A recent publication on the Health Consequences of Smoking[3369] contains a useful summary of differences in mortality from chronic obstructive respiratory disease in the United States and other countries. In white males in the United States, the age-adjusted mortality rate rose from 10 per 100,000 in 1960, to 23 per 100,000 in 1970, and to 26 per 100,000 in 1980. The rate has also increased in women,

particularly since 1975, as shown by the following actual numbers of deaths:

	Men	Women	M/F Ratio
1970	26,784	6227	4.30
1975	31,520	9580	3.29
1980	37,333	15,826	2.36

Another review[1036] included the following table of reported death rates per 100,000 population for persons between the ages of 55 and 64:

Country	Male	Female	Ratio
Japan	16	8	2.0
Sweden	16	6	2.7
France	60	14	4.3
Canada	61	15	4.1
USA	77	15	5.1
Italy	108	24	4.5
England and Wales	202	37	5.5
Scotland	205	40	5.1
Northern Ireland	222	49	4.5

A table with slightly different data was recently published by Catford and Ford[4107] for

1980 for European countries (mortality per 100,000 aged 55 to 64 years):

Country	Circulatory		Respiratory		Neoplasms	
	M	F	M	F	M	F
England and Wales	946	359	147	72	562	417
Scotland	1152	515	176	84	633	451
Northern Ireland	1248	505	170	111	513	433
Belgium	663	236	136	27	597	312
Denmark	774	262	93	54	546	431
Netherlands	669	206	53	17	550	316
France	428	141	68	19	620	275
West Germany	728	246	78	26	505	348
Norway	773	201	58	26	392	304
Sweden	721	204	54	34	372	330
Finland	1133	291	113	30	506	281

It is not at all clear why such large differences should exist. As noted earlier, there is convincing evidence that the difference between the mortality in the United States and Canada and that in the British Isles from these diseases is real.[3186] Williams and Nicholl[4014] have recently surveyed the city of Sheffield in the United Kingdom (population 542,700). They drew one of 12 random samples obtained each month from family physicians and drew a 1 in 50 sample of their records. They then administered a questionnaire, recording the FEV_1 if this was positive. Finally, they referred all patients with an FEV_1 less than 70% of predicted to a pulmonary physician's clinic. The data show that 0.3% of the city population (confidence interval 0.06 to 0.5%) had a Pa_{O_2} less than 60 mm Hg and an FEV_1 less than 50% of predicted. They estimated that 603 cases would be eligible for domiciliary oxygen and that 60,000 such cases existed in England and Wales. The data also showed that family physicians were unlikely to be able to assess a patient's need for oxygen without specialized advice. There are no comparable studies published that one can use for comparisons. Risk factors for the development of chronic airflow limitation are discussed in a later section.

Pathology

Thurlbeck[585] has reviewed in detail the pathology of chronic mucus hyperplasia and emphysema. He documents the fact that detailed quantitative studies (1) do not support the differentiation of lungs into strict "bronchitis" and "no bronchitis," categories, and (2) do not support categorization into Type A and Type B, since most cases are mixed. These conclusions are supported by other studies.[1298] In this section, no attempt is made to duplicate that information, but observations relevant to the relationship between morphology and function status are noted.

The incidence of emphysema in non-smokers was studied by means of macrosections by Anderson and his colleagues.[1233] The study consisted of 68 women and 12 men.

Severity of Emphysema (0 to 6)	Age		Sex		Type	
	< 60	> 60	M	F	PLE	CLE
0	18	38	6	50	0	0
1	0	12	5	7	10	2
2	0	7	0	7	5	2
3	0	5	1	4	5	0

No cases of more severe grades of emphysema (4, 5, and 6) were encountered.

The impact of smoking on emphysema incidence is shown by data from Auerbach and his colleagues on a large sample of 1015 men[1231]:

		Percentages			
	Number	No E	Minimal E	Moderate E	Severe E
Non-smoking	176	90.0	3.8	2.9	0
1–19 cigs/day	181	13.1	16–34	25.1	11.7
20 + cigs/day	658	0.3	5–40	32.7	19.2

Data from studies of the lungs of 388 women were similar. These data complement a very similar series published by Dunnill.[1273] Correlative morphology/function data were reviewed in Chapter 7.

The loss of recoil is related to the degree of emphysema and measurements of internal surface area.[1174] Although elastic fibers appear to be of normal diameter in cases of emphysema,[1168] there is a loss of elastin in subjects with panlobular emphysema (PLE)[1329] Cosio and his colleagues[4019] have studied the lungs of 12 smokers with the use of scanning electron microscopy. They noted that alveolar fenestrae near terminal airways were consistently larger than those in the periphery and that the overall area of these fenestrae correlated with the FEV_1, FEF_{25-75}, and the PL at 90% TLC. They concluded that in smokers with mild to moderate emphysema "destruction affects preferentially the areas round the terminal airways, and these changes, although small, might play an important role in lung function." In eight of the cases, the FEV_1 was between 78% and 100% of the predicted value. Petty, Silvers, and Stanford,[4020] in studies of 47 excised human lungs in which the alveolar attachments to the outside of bronchioles were counted, concluded that "alveolar attachments and elastic recoil are related to the size and function of the small airways."

Other studies have confirmed that upper lobe centrilobular emphysema (CLE) is a characteristic finding in smokers.[1305] In lungs with emphysema, there is a reduction in the number of small airways, and they are reduced in diameter.[1202, 1212] Berend[1149] graded inflammation in bronchioles of 37 excised lungs and found that in 17 lungs without emphysema there was more inflammation in lower lobes than in upper. In 17 lungs with a greater degree of emphysema in the upper lobes than the lower, there was also greater inflammatory change in lower lobe bronchi. He concluded that inflammatory changes and emphysema were not regionally associated. There is also a dissociation between the severity of emphysema peripherally and the percentage mucous gland volume.[1328] Mullen and his colleagues[4050] recently reassessed the role of inflammation in airways in subjects with chronic bronchitis in 45 resected lungs. There were no differences in Reid index, in proportions of mucous glands, in pulmonary function tests, in the morphology of the small airways, or in the degree of emphysema between 20 of the patients who had clinical bronchitis and 25 who did not.

Butler and Kleinerman[1223] pointed out that capillary density in the lung increases from apex to base and that alveolar diameter decreases. The ratio of capillary density to alveolar diameter must increase from apex to base. They noted that this ratio was markedly reduced in areas of emphysema because of both air space enlargement and capillary loss. They computed that the ratio was only one-tenth of normal in many lung areas with emphysema. Vascular changes are present in lungs with mild degrees of CLE.[1085] Loss of bronchial cartilage in emphysema is related to the degree of emphysema and is usually most evident in the lower lobes and in segmental and first and second order subsegmental bronchi.[1195]

Horsfield, Barer, and Cumming[490] attempted to relate morphologic changes to functional consequences by modeling the lesions of CLE. It seems clear that these lesions may have distinctive effects on gas exchange (as we suggested in the first edition of this book). Other observations on cases of emphysema have included apparent hyperplasia of the carotid body[3282] and a reduction in the number of muscarinic cholinergic receptor binding sites.[3270]

There are discrepancies in observations made of the diaphragm in patients with emphysema.

It has been noted to be smaller in area, thickness, and volume in these subjects,[1330] but normal in asthmatics. Careful comparisons with body weight in 51 subjects without emphysema, 51 with mild, 19 with moderate, and nine with severe emphysema showed that the ratio of diaphragm weight to body weight decreased as the degree of emphysema became more severe.[1294] In another series of 95 cases, the area of the diaphragm significantly correlated inversely with the percentage of the lung occupied by emphysema.[1176] The authors concluded that the thickness was not much affected and the altered area was related to altered thoracic shape, which represented contracture rather than atrophy. One study reported an increased diaphragm weight in emphysema,[1199] but in this series the mean may have been influenced by one case with a recorded diaphragmatic weight of 855 grams.

Thurlbeck[85] has documented the differences between reported correlations between right ventricular weight and the degree of emphysema in different series of autopsy studies. Scott's[1313] studies on 50 cases support previous evidence relating extent of emphysema to right ventricular hypertrophy. As noted in the previous chapter, Nagai and his colleagues[4059, 4060] have recently reported the same relationship.

Others have found that this hypertrophy is more closely related to the presence of CLE and bronchiolar stenoses[1265, 1310] or to other bronchiolar abnormalities.[1331] Some authors find little relationship either to extent of emphysema or to bronchial changes.[1326] In one series of 52 patients, 86% had evidence of pulmonary thromboembolism, but this bore no relation to right ventricular hypertrophy.[1046] A comparison between x-ray evaluation of cardiac chamber size and autopsy measurement in 72 cases showed that "the inaccuracy and interobserver variability in the detection of enlargement of specific chambers make it evident that the criteria are not valid, and that roentgenographic appraisal of cardiac size in these patients is limited to findings of normality or cardiomegaly.[1251]

A recent pathologic study compared the kidneys in 16 patients dying in respiratory failure[3287] with seven similar cases without renal or lung disease. The patients with chronic obstructive pulmonary disease (COPD) showed a significant increase in glomerular tuft area, a finding unrelated to whether they had or had not received domiciliary oxygen. There appeared to be a relationship between arterial

Pa_{O_2} and glomerular size. The authors considered that these changes probably reflected changes in salt and water handling.

Symptoms

The cardinal symptom is dyspnea, which is of varying intensity in some patients whose airflow limitation varies, but which is progressive and unvarying in those with advanced emphysema. Only recently have systematic studies of these been reported. Kinsman and colleagues[3352] asked 146 patients with mixed chronic bronchitis and emphysema to rate the frequency of 89 symptoms and experiences. Following dyspnea, in decreasing order of frequency were fatigue, sleep disturbance, congestion, irritability, anxiety, decathexis (loss of interest in things and poor appetite), helplessness-hopelessness, poor memory, and alienation.

Although many of these symptoms are caused by hypoxemia, particularly loss of memory,[3277] sexual dysfunction,[3331] and loss of weight,[3337, 3342] in this large series no close association was found between the symptoms and the arterial Pa_{O_2}. However, differentiation of the cases by clinical criteria into those with more emphysema indicated that the greater the degree of emphysema, the more severe were the symptoms relating to loss of interest in life. A recent study[4047] defined the psychiatric characteristics in these patients, documenting significant depression (which was more closely related to the DL_{CO} than to effort tolerance).

Physical Examination and Radiology

Godfrey and his colleagues[979] studied observer variation with respect to six classic signs and seven unfamiliar signs (previously described by Campbell[4875]) in patients with chronic airflow limitation. They found that the repeatability of all the signs "fell about midway between that expected by chance and the maximum possible." There was no difference between the familiar and unfamiliar signs. In a second study,[980] Godfrey and colleagues found that only the forced expiratory time correlated with the degree of obstruction.

The physical signs associated with respiratory muscle and diaphragmatic fatigue are described in Chapter 22.

There is little to add to the interpretation of conventional radiographs since the last edition.[1] Thurlbeck and Simon[4089] reviewed 696 cases. Sixty-six percent of those with the most severe grade of emphysema were diagnosed radiologically. In those with moderate emphysema, only 41% were recognized. They confirmed the importance of noting the arterial pattern, a point to which we drew attention in earlier editions of this book.

Recent work from Japan that studied selective alveolobronchograms in relation to emphysema has been noted earlier.[4132] This has been taken a step further by Bergin and her colleagues.[4008] They have shown that a CAT scan of the lungs permits accurate identification of the bullae and avascular spaces characteristic of emphysema. This method should be used in the future in studies in which it is important to establish the presence or absence of emphysema.

CHANGES IN PULMONARY FUNCTION

Airflow Limitation, Mechanics, and Lung Volumes

The very severe airflow limitation that may be found has been well documented, as have the changes in lung volume.[1] Many published studies include cases in whom the FEV_1 is between 800 milliliters and 1 liter, and in whom the residual volume is more than twice the predicted value.

Preservation of the vital capacity is occasionally encountered in severe cases—an important observation since changes in this volume are unreliable indicators of severity. However, differences between FVC and VC may be important in routine function testing.[3048] Several studies of chest wall motion have been published; in one study of 40 cases (with a mean FEV_1 of 28% of predicted) that made use of chest wall magnetometers, abnormalities of motion were common, but the quantitative relationship between abnormal motion and disease severity was weak.[4121] In general, the greater the hyperinflation, the less was the degree of abdominal movement. Other data[4100] confirm the observation that indices of synchronous or paradoxic motion do not correlate with the severity of the airways obstruction.

Studies of chest strapping in severe cases (with a mean FEV_1 of 930 milliliters) indicated that the cause of dyspnea under these conditions was not respiratory muscle fatigue but possibly the configurational change of the chest wall.[4045] Data on nine cases with a mean FEV_1 of 1.4 liters indicated that if abdominal breathing was voluntarily adopted, the ventilatory drive as measured by the V_T/T_I ratio was reduced.[4145]

The problem of measurement of lung volumes in these patients is discussed in Chapter 5. Additional data will also be found in references 4013 and 4076. Respiratory impedance measurements by forced oscillations are unreliable in cases with severe airflow limitation.[4057] The finding that in some cases severe airway narrowing occurs during expiration[1] has been confirmed in more recent studies.[4075] It has been shown that measuring flow rates by means of helium/oxygen or neon/oxygen mixtures in these subjects is not a reliable way to differentiate the site of airflow obstruction.[3024] Rochester and Braun[4052] found abnormally low maximal expiratory mouth pressures in half of the 32 patients with chronic airflow limitation they studied. It did not bear a close relationship to other indices.

Kimball, Leith, and Robins[3266] have reported detailed studies on a 70-year-old man with advanced chronic obstructive lung disease. In 1964, his FEV_1 was 900 milliliters, and studies were done in 1979 when he was respirator-dependent. They showed that his relaxed expiration was flow-limited. Recoil pressures were 6.5 cm H_2O at end-inspiration and 1.5 cm H_2O at end-expiration. His chest wall recoiled inward at all times. Consequently, the pleural pressure was always substantially positive (11 to 33 cm H_2O). Resting expiratory flow was maximal, and the jugular veins were full. Inspiratory work was measured at 0.27 kg/meters per breath, about seven times the normal value. Most of this was elastic work done on the chest wall.

As noted earlier in Chapter 4, important observations have been made on the effect of body position on lung mechanics in these patients. The effect of glottal changes in determining airflow or influencing lung volume may be important but has yet to be precisely defined.[3188]

Comparisons between FEV_1 and changes in C_{dyn} in 14 cases showed that when its frequency was increased, C_{dyn} fell more significantly than the measured R_L rose.[3318] C_{dyn} correlated with FEV_1 (a greater change in C_{dyn}/f occurred the more impaired the FEV_1).

Ventilation/Perfusion Imbalance

The physiologic basis of the impact of the constancy of the ratio between ventilation and perfusion throughout the lung on gas exchange was described in Chapter 2. Since worsening $\dot{V}/\dot{Q}$ ratios have an adverse effect on arterial gas tensions (which in turn are related to prognosis), this aspect of pulmonary function in this disease assumes major importance.

In reversible airflow obstruction, as in airway hyperreactivity, an FEV_1 of less than 50% of predicted may commonly be found in the absence of evidence of significant $\dot{V}/\dot{Q}$ imbalance. In the syndrome of chronic airflow limitation, the widening of the distribution of $\dot{V}/\dot{Q}$ ratios is a very significant event, since the consequent disturbance of gas tensions is associated with increased mortality.

Simple tests of abnormal $\dot{V}/\dot{Q}$ distribution include:

- Detection of hypoxemia and hypercapnia in the presence of a normal minute volume
- Widening of calculated $(A-a) O_2$ difference
- Calculation of V_D/V_T ratio
- Comparisons between end tidal and arterial CO_2 tensions

In addition to these, more complex procedures have been used in the study of $\dot{V}/\dot{Q}$ imbalance in these syndromes. These methods include:

- Studies of nitrogen clearance and analyses of Bohr isopleths (dividing the lung into two "compartments," each with a certain volume, ventilation, blood flow, and diffusing capacity)
- Studies of $\dot{V}/\dot{Q}$ distribution using the six inert gas method
- Regional studies with radioactive gases
- Studies of the shunt component

The divergence between end-tidal and arterial Pa_{CO_2} is reduced to no more than 2 mm Hg if deep expirations are made.[1221]

As noted earlier, the six inert gas method shows that some cases of chronic airflow limitation have regions of high $\dot{V}/\dot{Q}$, others have large volumes of low $\dot{V}/\dot{Q}$ regions, and others have some mixture of these two patterns.[1332] These data should be interpreted in the light of the difficulty that the wider the distribution the less certain are the results from the method.[3056] A recent study[4033] using the six inert gas method in 51 cases of severe chronic airflow obstruction (mean FEV_1 of 840 milliliters, mean Pa_{O_2} of

58.5 mm Hg, mean pulmonary arterial pressure at rest of 22 mm Hg) found that 24 cases had a pattern of high ventilation in high $\dot{V}/\dot{Q}$ regions; nine had a pattern of high flow through low $\dot{V}/\dot{Q}$ units; and 16 had a pattern intermediate between these two. Two cases had a high shunt fraction. No relationships were detectable between the $\dot{V}/\dot{Q}$ pattern and the Type "A" or "B" clinical differentiation. Also, no relationship between $\dot{V}/\dot{Q}$ and Pa_{O_2}, FEV_1, or TLC were found. An r value of 0.895 existed between the calculated and observed Pa_{O_2}. No DL_{CO} data were reported.

By contrast, regional studies with ^{133}Xe do not reveal any regions of high $\dot{V}/\dot{Q}$.[1038] It can be concluded that there must be great variations in perfusion per unit volume within individual counter fields. Possibly, normal lung lobules are arranged in parallel with diseased units, or possibly proximal parts of diseased lung lobules constitute high $\dot{V}/\dot{Q}$ zones, with poorly ventilated low $\dot{V}/\dot{Q}$ zones distally. These differences within counter fields are also shown by differences between ^{133}Xe clearance, as between perfusion delivered and equilibrated gas.[981, 1116] Studies with [81]Kr do show high $\dot{V}/\dot{Q}$ zones in some cases.[1098, 1099] When the disease is localized (as it may be initially in cases with alpha$_1$-antitrypsin deficiency), both ventilation and perfusion are reduced to the region. As noted earlier, chronic mucus hypersecretion may be characterized by a reduction of both ventilation and perfusion to the lung bases,[1019] and some reduction of flow in lower zones as compared with the upper is commonly seen in general cases of airflow limitation.[1117] With the use of ^{133}Xe for ventilation measurement and ^{99}Tc-labeled scans for perfusion, patients with chronic airflow limitation show reductions in both measurements over affected zones.[454]

Staub and Conhaim[1093] have suggested that single preserved arterioles traversing an emphysema space (which is not uncommonly seen) might constitute a low $\dot{V}/\dot{Q}$ zone. They calculated that a 190-micron vessel with a transit time of 1 second would have an apparent $\dot{V}/\dot{Q}$ ratio of 0.01. In many cases, delay in gaseous equilibrium is indicated by comparative studies of helium and SF6.[401]

In 10 subjects breathing air or helium and studied by the six inert gas method,[3354] the only significant effect was to widen the $(A-a)D_{O_2}$ by a mean increase of 6.5 mm Hg. This was interpreted to indicate "an impairment of series heterogeneity and O_2 diffusion during helium breathing." These patients averaged 58 years of age, their Pa_{O_2} averaged 61.4 mm Hg, and their mean FEV_1 was 920 milliliters. As noted in Chapter 4, changes of body position in these patients may affect the $\dot{V}/\dot{Q}$ distribution.[4128]

Previous work showing no major shunt component in cases of chronic airflow limitation[1] has been confirmed.[266, 1245] However, 27 cases of chronic airflow limitation (mean age 63 years, with FEV_1 less than 50% of predicted) studied with macroaggregated albumin particles tagged with [99m]Tc[4087] and compared with 10 controls of mean age 58 years showed that shunt values were slightly higher as compared with the controls. In the COPD cases, the shunt was from 3% to a single high value of 27%, with most values between 6% and 19%. In the controls, values scattered between 2% and 11%, with most not more than 7%. The shunt was not related to the FEV_1 but was related to the $DL_{CO}SB$. The data raise the question of whether an actual shunt is being measured or whether the increased particle passage through the lungs is occurring through dilated capillaries and remaining arterioles (see Staub's suggestion noted earlier).

Injection scans in 100 subjects with chronic airflow limitation[1269] (with quantitative analysis of perfusion defects in four planes) showed that there were relationships among the extent of these defects, abnormality in FEV_1, elevation of RV/TLC%, and exercise capability. The DL_{CO} correlated poorly with the degree of perfusion abnormality. However, in another series of 72 cases, the ratio of DL_{CO} to TLC was correlated to perfusion defects, with an r value of -0.632.[1268] The reason for the discrepancy between these two studies is unclear.

The ability to lower the Pa_{CO_2} with voluntary hyperventilation correlated best with the VD/VT ratio[1267] but correlated poorly with the FEV_1. Education of nine subjects so that respiratory frequency was reduced from an average of 16.7/min to 8.3/min, led to an increase in arterial saturation from 82.2% to 89.7% and a lowering of Pa_{CO_2}.[1333] A detailed study of 14 cases of chronic airflow limitation[1100] showed that increasing the tidal volume and lowering the frequency could increase the Pa_{O_2} (as it does in elderly normal subjects) or that the Pa_{O_2} could remain unaffected. Increases of more than 4 mm Hg were noted in five patients, with one subject showing an 18 mm Hg increase. Recent studies reported that the capacity of six subjects with a mean age of 61.8 years and chronic hypercapnia to sustain ventilation to lower end-tidal PCO_2 was related to the lowest VD/VT

ratio. Electromyographic evidence of respiratory muscle fatigue developed in four of the six subjects. Their mean FEV_1 averaged only 690 milliliters (the range was 350 to 1100 milliliters).

Oxygen breathing in cases of chronic airflow limitation has been suspected of altering $\dot{V}/\dot{Q}$ distribution.[1334] In one study, the mean $(A-a)$ D_{O_2} increased from 30 mm Hg on air to 135 mm Hg on 10 minutes of 100% O_2 breathing,[4038] with the calculated shunt component increasing from 2.8% to 7.5%. The authors concluded that oxygen breathing in these cases could convert low $\dot{V}/\dot{Q}$ units to a shunt and could cause atelectasis of low $\dot{V}/\dot{Q}$ units. The authors also found that this atelectasis was not prevented by an increase in tidal volume.

Studies of 16 patients made use of injected ^{13}N and clearance measurements from four lung zones. The reports showed that 30% oxygen produced significant delay in clearance from 23 zones in 10 of the cases. No systematic change in clearance occurred in inhaled ^{13}N.[1335] The authors concluded that local hypoxic vasoconstriction was present in these cases and that the oxygen resulted in "a diversion of local blood flow from well-ventilated to more poorly ventilated areas." As noted previously, others have found that oxygen breathing in patients with chronic airflow limitation reduces the ventilation to already poorly ventilated regions. A more recent study that made use of ^{13}N[3293] for ventilation distribution measurement found that oxygen breathing in hypoxemic cases reduced still further the ventilation to poorly ventilated lung regions. In severe cases of airflow limitation, it may take as long as 20 minutes after the withdrawal of oxygen for the arterial Pa_{O_2} to return to a stable baseline level.[1259]

The six inert gas method has also been used to study the effect of oxygen breathing in these cases. A recent study[4027] of 14 patients with severe disease (mean age of 59 years; mean FEV/FVC% of 27%; mean Pa_{O_2} of 54.9 mm Hg)—in whom the Pa_{O_2} rose 20 mm Hg and the mixed venous P_{O_2} rose 4.2 mm Hg—found that oxygen increased the flow through low $\dot{V}/\dot{Q}$ regions. No change in Pa_{CO_2}, $\dot{V}E$, or respiratory frequency occurred during the oxygen breathing. In these patients, three had the pattern of high $\dot{V}$ to high $\dot{V}/\dot{Q}$ regions; three had high perfusion to low $\dot{V}/\dot{Q}$ regions; and six were intermediate. The effects of oxygen are also discussed in Chapter 23.

The evolution of changes in blood gases has been inferred, from cross-sectional studies, to follow worsening ventilatory function. However, in 151 ambulatory men with chronic airflow limitation studied at intervals of up to 36 months, variations in Pa_{CO_2} seemed to be independent of evolution of FEV_1, FVC, or RV/TLC.[3314] Increases in Pa_{CO_2} were associated with decreases in VT, however, with a consequent increase in VD/VT ratio. In this series from France, the Pa_{CO_2} in the severely hypercapnic group averaged 58.9 mm Hg, but the FEV_1 in the same group was reported to be 77.3% of predicted; this is a very high value and suggests that significant hypoventilation was present.

The influence of mixed venous gas tensions on the resulting arterial pressures may be considerable if very low $\dot{V}/\dot{Q}$ units are present. These interrelationships have been explored in 55 cases of chronic airflow limitation.[1163] In one series of 56 cases,[481] a mixed venous P_{O_2} of less than 34 mm Hg (the lower limit of normal) was found in about a third of the subjects. Breathing 40% O_2 raised the mixed venous P_{O_2} from 40 to 43 mm Hg in normal subjects and from 31 mm Hg to 37 mm Hg in those with chronic airflow limitation.[1261] Tenny and Mithoefer[3255] have compared the status of persons with respiratory failure with normal subjects at altitude; the importance of oxygen capacity and cardiac output to total oxygen delivery is evident in both circumstances. The mixed venous oxygen tension may be a better indicator of body oxygenation than the arterial P_{O_2}.

Changes in arterial blood gas tensions have been studied in chronic airflow limitation when the patient is switched to 80% helium and 20% oxygen.[1049] In 24 cases, the Pa_{CO_2} fell by about 1 mm Hg, but the Pa_{O_2} also fell (by 1.5 mm Hg). The authors concluded that the fall in Pa_{O_2} was greater in patients with more radiologic evidence of emphysema. The FEV_1 averaged 0.86 liters in the cases studied. The fall in arterial oxygen tension was attributed to interference with diffusion-mixing in the gas phase, a conclusion confirmed by studies on the $(A - a)$ D_{O_2} on helium breathing noted earlier.

Recent data indicate that almitrine is without effect on lung mechanics or ventilation distribution in normal subjects,[3363] but it does affect the hypoxic ventilatory response.[3322] In patients with chronic airflow limitation, it appears to improve the $\dot{V}/\dot{Q}$ distribution and to increase VA. Hence, the arterial Pa_{O_2} rises,[3243, 3349] T_i/T_{tot} falls, and VT/T_i rises.[3271] Almitrine is believed to act by chemoreceptor stimulation.

It is evident from all these observations that

1. Significant $\dot{V}/\dot{Q}$ differences exist within small regions of the lung in many cases.

2. Both ventilation and perfusion are reduced within the region where the disease process is localized, so that disturbance of $\dot{V}/\dot{Q}$ ratios is minimized.

3. Gas exchange is very dependent on tidal volume in some cases of chronic airflow limitation (those with CLE?), suggesting the importance of an increased tidal volume in improving gas exchange at the periphery of the lobule in some patients, but not in others.

4. No precise relationship can yet be adduced between morphologic change and the pattern of $\dot{V}/\dot{Q}$ abnormality.

Factors Lowering the $D_{L_{CO}}$ in Chronic Airflow Limitation

In an unusual study of the rate of uptake of CO, 20 normal subjects and 20 patients with chronic airflow limitation breathed 0.03% CO for 45 minutes. In the normal subjects, this led to an increase in COHb of 4.27% and an increase of 3.48% in the patients with disease.[1083] The rate of uptake is reduced in emphysema by some combination of the following factors:

1. Wider than normal distribution of $\dot{V}/\dot{Q}$ ratios.

2. Variation in the ratio between ventilation and diffusing capacity (in steady-state methods) or between ventilated volume and diffusing capacity (in the single-breath method).

3. Non-uniformity of the ratios between diffusing capacity and flow within the lung.

4. Decrease of capillary blood volume and reduced surface area.

5. Reduced rate of equilibration in the gas phase within the lung (slowed gas phase equilibrium due to disordered architecture).

In many patients with severe airflow limitation, no doubt all these factors exist to some degree. Attempts to assign a major component in individual cases are necessarily very approximate. However, patients are occasionally seen with a very low CO uptake (however measured), minimal hypoxemia, and a near normal $(A - a) D_{O_2}$. Such patients may be found to have evidence of considerable vascular abnormality on the chest x-ray and a markedly reduced lung recoil. It is fair to conclude that in those patients factors 4 and 5 are dominant. However, most cases do not present this picture.

Although a method of quantitating D_L from precise morphometric measurements of the lung has been described,[1202] it has not yet been applied to patients with emphysema studied during life. The increase of $D_{L_{CO}}$ with breath-holding time in emphysema but not in reversible airway obstruction[1113] presumably indicates the importance of mechanism 5 above, as does the widening of $(A - a) D_{O_2}$ on helium breathing. Knudson and his colleagues[3954] noted that in patients with emphysema, the distance for gas diffusion in the gas phase may increase from 2 millimeters to 10 millimeters. In smokers, they found that the $D_{L_{CO}}SB$ correlated with the SBN_2/L, which explained 17% of the variance in $D_{L_{CO}}SB$. They concluded that air space enlargement was an important determinant of both indices.

Recent data obtained through the use of fast response gas analysis methods have indicated the sources of variation between different measurements of the single-breath $D_{L_{CO}}$.[3883] These were noted in Chapter 5. Using this method, Graham, Mink, and Cotton[3869] developed a "three equation" method of calculating $D_{L_{CO}}SB$. They showed that in patients with emphysema this value increases with increasing breath-holding time but does not do so in normal subjects. They suggested that the $D_{L_{CO}}SB$ might be decreased in some patients if the breathing-holding time is short "because overall diffusion is limited by the reduced transport of CO from the inspired gas through the alveolar gas prior to alveolar-capillary gas exchange."

The ratio of $D_{L_{CO}}SB$ to $D_{L_{CO}}SS$ in emphysema is about 1.0,[1097] whereas in reversible airway disease it is nearer 2.0. This probably indicates that in emphysema the ratio of the distribution of ventilation to diffusing capacity is not much different from the ratio of volume distribution to diffusing capacity. Analysis of models indicates that $D_{L_{CO}}SB$ will overestimate the diffusing capacity if the fast ventilating compartment has a higher k_{CO} than the slowly ventilating regions.[469] It is to be noted that lung models can be devised in which both methods underestimate the true D_L of the system or in which the $D_{L_{CO}}SB$ is correct and the $D_{L_{CO}}SS$ is low.[469]

BREATHING PATTERN AND CONTROL OF BREATHING

In this volume, no comprehensive discussion of the control of breathing in chronic airflow limitation is possible. However, the past few years have seen substantial advances in this field, which at the time of the last edition[1] was limited to studies of response to CO_2 breathing. The introduction of the $P_{0.1}$ technique, briefly noted in Chapter 5, has stimulated a great deal of recent work. This measurement, reflecting the neural drive to ventilation, is increased in chronic airflow limitation,[4141] especially if the FEV_1 is less than 50% of predicted. With hypercapnia, T_I is shortened and the tidal volume is reduced.[4138] The $P_{0.1}$ and threshold perception in hypercapnia are similar in both patients with disease and normal subjects, but the responses differ under load conditions.[4040] These experiments indicated that the lower the threshold of perception, the higher was the respiratory drive during loaded ventilation. In general, the perception of added loads is not abnormal in these patients.[4055]

The resting breathing pattern of 12 patients with chronic airflow obstruction (mean FEV_1 of 31% of predicted; mean Pa_{O_2} of 70 mm Hg) was compared with eight age-matched controls.[4105] The V_T was shown to be similar between patients and controls, but both the frequency and the minute ventilation were greater in the patients. Also, in the patients the inspiratory and expiratory times were both shorter, and inspiratory flow rates were faster than in the controls. In this study, a mean of 702 breaths per subject were measured. The results of studies to elucidate the role of opioids have been conflicting. Results from a study that used naloxone, an opioid antagonist, indicate that this increases the $P_{0.1}$ response to hypoxia[4097] or hypercapnia. However, other experiments have shown negative results.[4142]

In studies of 15 subjects with chronic airflow limitation who had a mean FEV_1 of 1.46 liters and a k_{CO} of 67% of predicted[1089] an increase of V_T/T_I and f was noted, but V_T, T_I, and T_E were all smaller than in controls (a finding confirmed by others[1337]). The value of $P_{0.1}/\dot{V}_{CO_2}$ at maximal load correlated significantly with the FEV_1 and Pa_{O_2}, but not with the Pa_{CO_2}, and increased when arterial pH fell below 7.3.[1089] The authors concluded that chemoreceptors and increased chest wall and lung afferent signals were mainly responsible for the increased drive.

Studies of the consequences of increased airflow obstruction by methacholine in 12 subjects with moderately severe airflow obstruction[4047] showed that a progressive rise in Pa_{CO_2} occurred. Although $\dot{V}_E$ increased, the degree of CO_2 retention was inversely related to changes in V_T and inspiratory time. The authors concluded "that COPD cases retain CO_2 during acutely increased airway obstruction induced by bronchoconstriction partly because of a rapid shallow breathing pattern that reduces alveolar ventilation."

Studies of cerebral blood flow in 15 patients with chronic airflow obstruction (five of whom were hypercapnic) suggested that this was one of the determinants of the drive and timing of respiration.[4115]

As was noted in an earlier section, almitrine administration improves both alveolar ventilation and $\dot{V}/\dot{Q}$ balance, increasing the output of peripheral chemoreceptors[3997] to hypoxia. The Pa_{O_2} rises,[3243, 3349] and the T_I/T_{tot} ratio falls.[3271] It has been shown that none of these effects occurs when almitrine is administered to patients who have had a bilateral carotid body resection.[4030] Airway anesthesia has been shown to cause a fall in respiratory rate and an increased tidal volume.[4068] Particularly in acute respiratory failure, this has been interpreted to indicate that irritant receptor stimulation, in some cases at least, may be responsible for the increased respiratory rate and reduced tidal volume often observed.[4137] The action of histamine in shortening T_I and reducing the tidal volume in response to hypercapnia[4138] may be related to the same mechanism. In this connection, it may be noted that the early effect of ozone is to cause an increased respiratory rate and reduced FVC (see Chapter 6), presumably as a result of irritant receptor stimulation. Hydralazine has been shown to increase dyspnea and to accentuate the pulmonary hypertension in nine patients whose mean FEV_1 was 1.2 liters.[4131] A potent synthetic progesterone has been shown to augment the neuromuscular response to hypercapnia and hypoxia in 12 subjects with severe airflow limitation.[4009]

A recent finding of great interest has been the observation that there is a close correlation between the ventilatory response of persons with chronic airflow limitation to hypercapnia and hypoxia and the $P_{0.1}$ response of the offspring of these patients.[4126] As noted later, the individual ventilatory response to hypoxemia and hypercapnia due to increasing $\dot{V}/\dot{Q}$ abnormality in these patients plays an important role in determining survival. If the response is diminished, pulmonary arterial hypertension and cor pulmonale occurs earlier than in those with a normal or better than normal response.

EXERCISE LIMITATION

After noting the proven value of exercise tests in cardiac conditions, Denolin commented: "Beaucoup plus complexe est, malheureusement, la situation dans les pneumopathies chroniques."[1075] However, over the last 12 years, more than 150 papers have been published that contain data from exercise studies in patients with chronic airflow limitation. Although difficulties have arisen because of the non-standardization of exercise tests, in fact, three protocols were recently shown by the group at Nancy[3355] to give closely comparable results:

- Progressive incremental bicycle exercise (30 watts every 3 minutes)
- Constant exercise at near maximal work
- Trapezoidal (10 minutes or 40 watts + 30 watts every 3 minutes)

The $\dot{V}O_2$ maxima attained were shown to be similar with all three methods in 26 patients with chronic airflow limitation, in whom the maximal $\dot{V}O_2$ ranged from 14.7 to 46.2 mL/kg/min. Additional data[4113] on 21 cases showed similar findings from constant versus progressive exercise protocols. The authors noted that pain in the legs was a common reason for stopping the exercise but the actual $\dot{V}O_2$ max was believed to have been attained in 81% of the cases.

The time course of ventilatory adaptation at the start of bicycle ergometer exercise in 20 subjects with a mean FEV_1 of 1.45 liters and in 20 subjects with a mean FEV_1 of 0.62 liters was not related to the FEV_1.[1081] The Pa_{O_2} falls less rapidly in these subjects than in normal persons at the start of exercise; this is probably due to a slower increase in tissue consumption of oxygen.[990] In two groups—one of 20 subjects with a mean FEV_1 of 1.45 liters and another of 20 subjects with a mean FEV_1 of 0.62 —that were compared with normal subjects, the $\dot{V}E$ at a $\dot{V}O_2$ of 0.75 and 1.0 L/min was significantly raised in both patient groups, with no mean difference between them. All the cases had tachycardia on exercise. The lactate level was not important in limiting the exercise,[120] but

others have noted a relationship between hydrogen ion concentration in arterial blood and pulmonary artery pressure on exercise.[1034] Arterial blood samples must be withdrawn during exercise for reliable data to be obtained.[3346] It has been shown that the Pa_{O_2} may rise in some subjects within 20 seconds after stopping exercise. In general, exercise capability is related to the FEV_1, but different levels of oxygen uptake are noted in patients with similar degrees of FEV_1 impairment.

In exercise studies of 152 subjects, studied during 5 minutes of 40-watt exercise on a bicycle ergometer, the following relationship was adduced[1120]

$$\text{Exercise } Pa_{O_2} = [0.06(VC) + 0.276(FEV_1)] - [0.185(Age) + 68.5]$$

Sergysels and his colleagues[1133] reported the following relationships between maximal work and respiratory variables (see table at the bottom of this page).

For the same FEV_1, the maximal $\dot{V}O_2$ varied by at least a factor of two. Other studies have confirmed this variability in severely disabled persons.[4071]

A recent study of exercise in 92 patients with chronic airflow limitation showed that the r value between maximal power output and FEV_1 was 0.79,[4130] but the spread was considerable at any given FEV_1 level. Other studies have confirmed the general relationship between airflow indices and exercise capability.[4086] A complex nomogram involving DL_{CO} at rest, FEV_1, and VD/VT ratio predicted the measured maximal $\dot{V}O_2$ in a group of subjects, including six with chronic airflow limitation.[1191]

When 20 patients (seven had emphysema, six had chronic bronchitis, and seven had mixed forms[4064]) were tested with incremental cycle exercise, a regression formula was adduced:

$$\dot{V}E_{max} = 21.34 \times FEV_1 \text{ (liters)} + 6.28 \times PIFR \text{ (L/sec)}$$

This equation embodies a test related to muscle

Maximum Effort (Watts)	Number	Pa_{O_2}	Pa_{CO_2}	FEV_1	$\dot{V}O_2$ max	$\dot{V}E_{max}$
40	6	57.4	50.0	0.94	0.73	23.5
60	4	55.0	53.4	0.82	1.16	33.4
80	6	61.5	47.7	0.97	1.28	34.4
100	3	66.3	46.7	1.13	1.62	51.3
120	1	65.8	45.8	1.40	1.83	67.2

strength, the peak inspiratory flow rate (PIFR). This factor improves the relationship.

Performance of the 12-minute walking test correlated better with FVC, with maximal $\dot{V}_{O_2}$, and with maximal $\dot{V}_E$ than with FEV_1 in studies of 35 subjects aged 40 to 70 years with a mean FEV_1 of 1.05 and an FVC of 2.84.[1015] The average power output in stair climbing was 66 watts in 10 men similarly disabled, which compared with 154 watts in normal men of similar age. The power output was related to the FEV_1.[1290]

The aerobic capacity correlates well with DL_{CO}, and the $\dot{V}_{O_2}$ max is related to the vital capacity.[1054] Resting variables related to maximal $\dot{V}_{O_2}$ in one study[1023] were (1) non-invasive tests (RV/TLC, Pa_{CO_2}, $(A - a) D_{O_2}$, FRC, and arterial pH), and (2) invasive tests (diastolic pulmonary artery pressure). Twenty-four subjects were studied, with supine bicycle exercise increasing in increments of 25 watts.[1023]

There is evidence that the Pa_{O_2} falls more in patients with chronic airflow limitation during walking than during bicycle exercise, at comparable levels of $\dot{V}_{O_2}$.[4031] The data from this study of nine subjects with severe disease indicated that possibly there was greater anaerobiosis on bicycle exercise and the resulting acidosis led to increased ventilation and to a reduced fall in Pa_{O_2}. The largest observed difference in Pa_{O_2} between bicycle and treadmill exercise was 12 mm Hg.[4031] In 50 men with chronic airflow limitation studied at 60% of maximal work capacity,[1215] work capacity correlated significantly with the grade of dyspnea, the observer's assessment of a step test, the FEV_1, and the DL_{CO}, but the prediction value of all these indices was imprecise.

Studies on Type A, Type B, and mixed (Type C) patients of comparable ages and FEV_1 showed that Type C individuals had most impaired performance; Type A patients had an increased ventilation for a given $\dot{V}_{O_2}$; and DL_{CO} increased less on exercise in Types A and C than in Type B individuals. The cardiac output was not different between the two groups and was essentially normal.[1283] The maximal $\dot{V}_{O_2}$ was predictable from the FEV_1 and FVC, or from the Pa_{CO_2} and $DL_{CO}SB$, but was not closely related to the degree of emphysema in one series of 14 cases.[1217] In the group of patients studied, the DL_{CO} values at rest varied from 34% of predicted to 139% of predicted.

In a study of maximal exercise in 14 Type A and 20 Type B subjects, $\dot{V}_{O_2}$ max correlated well with VC, $\dot{V}_E$ and V_T, but poorly with FEV_1.[1017] In most cases, V_T was 50% of VC at maximal effort. In both groups, the Pa_{O_2} rose on exercise. The Type A subjects averaged 61 years of age, with a mean FEV_1 of 45% predicted, and managed 88 watts of exercise. The Type B cases were 48 years of age, with a mean FEV_1 of 68% of predicted, and managed 112 watts output. Neither group was hypoxemic at rest or on exercise.[1017] Another group, also divided into Type A and Type B subjects, when compared with normal individuals of the same age at comparable work loads, had a higher $\dot{V}_E$ and a shorter T_{tot}. T_i/T_{tot} was the same in patients and normal subjects, with T_i and T_e shortened to a similar extent. There were no differences between the Type A and Type B groups,[1062] a finding supported by other data.[1090] However, there are data suggesting that swings in Pa_{CO_2} during exercise may be lower in Type B individuals than those of Type A studied during exercise.[4003] It has recently been reported that exercise falls in Pa_{O_2} are commoner in Type A cases than in Type B.[4130]

In 12 men with severe chronic airflow limitation and in whom the FEF_{25-75} was below 0.8 L/sec, maximal expiratory flow predicted from the flow volume curve was reached in 10 subjects when their heart rate was not maximal.[3232] In another group of 11 severely impaired patients[3308] (whose mean FEV_1 was 570 milliliters, mean DL_{CO} was 6.0 mL/min/mm Hg, and Pa_{O_2} was 58 mm Hg), asymmetric movement of the chest wall and abdomen was observed; the subjects could walk further when exercising partially flexed at the waist.

Studies of the effect of adding an external resistance in normal individuals, in 19 men with mild airflow resistance, and in 10 men with more severe impairment ($FEV_1/FVC\% = 53.7\%$) showed that the cardiopulmonary and subjective responses to the added resistances were not different in these groups.[3248] The effect of adding a dead space of 250 milliters if the FEV_1 was less than 800 milliliters and of adding 500 milliliters if it were greater than this was recently studied in 22 subjects with severe chronic airflow limitation whose mean FEV_1 was 960 milliliters.[4012] Their mean RV was three times the predicted level. On exercise, the added V_D caused $\dot{V}_E$ to rise 12.2%, with the increase being in tidal volume and not in respiratory rate. The added dead space caused a further fall of 6 mm Hg in exercise Pa_{O_2}. From these studies, the authors concluded that exercise performance in these subjects was limited "primarily by impaired ventilatory mechanics."

Recently, it has become clear that respiratory muscle fatigue may be a major component in exercise limitation, and the impact of increased RV on the mechanical efficiency may be a very important component of the early development of diaphragm or respiratory muscle fatigue.[1047, 1050] Macklem[4125] has commented on the adverse effects of an increase in residual volume during exercise (hyperinflation) on respiratory muscle function. Increases of 630 milliliters commonly occur in these patients,[4127] particularly in those whose FEV_1 is less than 1 liter. Macklem[4125] notes that the increasing ventilation on exercise is associated with an increase in the passive outward displacement of the abdomen relative to the total volume change. On exercise, the expiratory intercostal and abdominal muscles contract forcefully during expiration, resulting in a marked increase in pleural pressure and a change in the thoracoabdominal configuration. The diaphragm is of major importance in generating the greater inspiratory pleural pressure on exercise.

It is clear that the end-expiratory level may increase significantly in patients with chronic airflow limitation on exercise.[1060, 1061] In one series,[1150] the increase of end-expiratory volume on exercise was between 10% and 20% of VC (300 to 800 milliliters) in seven cases. The end-expiratory level was unchanged in one subject, and it decreased slightly in four. The shortening of V_T and tachypnea has been attributed to a pulmonary reflex.[1061] The $V_T/FEV\%$ for a given $\dot{V}O_2$ is much higher in these cases, and the $P_{0.1}$ versus $\dot{V}O_2$ is increased.[1061] It has recently been shown that fatigue in the sternomastoid muscle can be detected in patients with severe airflow limitation when stressed by exercise.[4133] General concepts of muscle fatigue are discussed in Chapter 22.

In light of this thinking, the effect of respiratory muscle training becomes of great interest. Flenley[4022] has recently written a useful summary of the reported effects of respiratory muscle training, noting the many unanswered questions that exist. He concluded that a large multicenter trial might be needed to establish benefit. Although not a controlled experiment, inspiratory muscle training improved tolerance of an added inspiratory resistance in 10 subjects with severe airflow limitation.[1104] Inspiratory muscle training also improved the endurance time at two-thirds of maximal exercise in nine subjects with a mean FEV_1 of 25% of normal as compared with eight subjects who received physiotherapy only. The FEV_1 of both groups

were comparable.[1145] This effect occurred only in those persons in whom the EMG changes heralding fatigue occurred during exercise.[1144]

Respiratory muscle training has been found to increase exercise endurance, increasing the 12-minute walking distance from 1058 to 1188 meters in 10 severe patients.[1136] However, a recent study of 16 subjects given a month of training by means of resistive breathing[4114] found no improvement in pulmonary function tests or in 12-minute walking performance. Negative results[4007, 4023, 4088] or only slight improvements in exercise performance have been reported.[4024] There is a relationship between the point of onset of fatigue and the maximal ventilation recorded on bicycle ergometry.[1096] Added airway resistance in six patients with severe chronic airflow limitation produced earlier respiratory muscle fatigue.[1104]

In 50 patients with chronic respiratory disorders, including some with pneumoconiosis and some with chronic airflow limitation, there was a significant relationship ($r = 0.744$) between the onset of respiratory muscle fatigue and the maximal breathing capacity (MBC) in liters.[1058] This group of patients had a mean FEV_1 of 68% of predicted, a DL_{CO} of 61% of predicted, and a Pa_{O_2} of 91% of predicted normal values. Comparisons of the effect of maximal voluntary ventilation (MVV) and the 12-minute walking test in five men whose FEV_1 ranged from 0.72 to 1.34 liters[3272] showed that although the voluntary hyperventilation produced evidence of fatigue in the sternomastoid muscle, blood lactate did not increase. On walking, however, three had significant lactate increases.

In 10 severely hypoxic patients with a mean FEV_1 of 0.76 liters, breathing 30% oxygen on exercise decreased the arterial lactate and consistently lowered both $\dot{V}E$ and $\dot{V}CO_2$, the latter effect being unexplained.[1336] Fifty per cent oxygen breathing lowers the PAP on exercise.[1122] Most studies have found that oxygen improves exercise performance, possibly by postponing the onset of respiratory muscle fatigue.[4065]

If subjects with chronic airflow limitation are divided into a group who develop hypoxemia on exercise and a group who do not, both groups being of comparable age, there are no differences in cardiac output or in mixed venous oxygen tension, and there is overlap between the FEV_1 values.[993] The hypoxemic group have a higher RV and a significantly lower FEF_{25-75}. In some cases of chronic airflow limitation, the Pa_{O_2} rises on exercise, and in others it falls. In both cases the differences from resting values may exceed 20 mm Hg.[3346] The transcutaneous Po_2 in 23 subjects with emphysema was measured on exercise, and the fall in this value was correlated with the FEV_1, the TL_{CO}, and the resting Pa_{O_2}.[4146] One of the patients showed a continuous increase in the value during exercise. It has also been shown that the ear oximeter can be used in studying the changes in oxygen saturation on exercise.[4056] In reading a change in saturation, a variation of between 2.5 and 3.5% represented twice the standard error of the estimate as compared with simultaneous arterial blood determinations.

A recent, unexplained finding has been the demonstration, in a carefully controlled blind study, that oxygen relieves the dyspnea of some patients with chronic airflow limitation who are not hypoxemic.[1004, 3360] Oxygen breathing probably acts by reducing the ventilatory requirements for the same work load, and the relief of anaerobiosis is less important.[4839] It may also delay the onset of respiratory muscle fatigue. The beneficial effect of oxygen was clearly demonstrated in a study of 20 subjects with severe chronic airflow limitation (mean age of 61 years, mean FEV_1 of 920 milliliters, and Pa_{O_2} of 66.7 mm Hg) breathing air or oxygen at different flow rates through nasal catheters. A placebo effect was shown to account for a fraction of the improvement observed.

In another study that used either compressed air or oxygen in a tank, 26 patients with an FEV_1 <35% of predicted improved their endurance on oxygen, but not their maximal work rate.[1161] Surprisingly, there was no relationship between increased endurance and the degree of hypoxemia, hypercapnia, or acidosis during exercise. In a recent study of exercise in 12 patients with severe disease and a mean FEV_1 of only 730 milliliters,[4118] the breathlessness level was scored. It was found that dihydrocodeine reduced breathlessness by 18%; 100% oxygen reduced it by 22%; and if both were administered together, there was a 32% reduction in dyspnea. Caffeine had no effect, but alcohol increased the FVC by 9% and exercise tolerance by 7%. The onset of anaerobic metabolism is associated with a sharp rise in the pulse deficit (total heart beats in last 4 minutes of exercise minus total heart beats in first 4 minutes).[1211]

There have been a number of studies of the effect of exercise training, and it has been shown that the maximal sustained speed on a treadmill can be reliably calculated from the results of a rapid incremental test on a bicycle ergometer.[3265] This information is useful in planning a training program. Hughes and Davison[3345] have written a useful review of exercise training programs in patients with chronic airflow limitation.

In a well controlled trial of exercise training, the following two groups were selected[3326]:

	Group 1	Group 2
Number	12	10
Age	58.6	59.7
FEV_1	0.66	0.68
Raw (cm/L/sec)	6.0	6.1
VC	2.6	2.4
$DL_{CO}SB$	11.1	10.9
SBN_2/L	11.2	11.3
Pa_{O_2} (mm Hg)	69.3	65.3

The first group had intensive exercise retraining on a treadmill, together with breathing retraining, and the second group did not. There were no differences after 5 weeks of the training period when only exercise retraining was done, but when breathing retraining was then added to the protocol, the maximal $\dot{V}O_2$ of Group 1 steadily improved, being about 500 milliliters greater than that of Group 2 at the end of retraining. The Pa_{O_2} on exercise in Group 1 after 9 weeks was 77.5 mm Hg and in Group 2 was 60.0 mm Hg.

Arm and leg exercise training is of little use,[3333] and theophylline administration does not improve performance.[3336] In a small group of patients[4037] steroid therapy did not improve performance. Exercise training does not change muscle enzymes on muscle biopsy studies, probably because the level of exercise achieved is insufficient.[1147]

The effects of unsupervised training at home on 24 patients with a mean FEV_1 of 0.97 liters were to improve well-being and to reduce the level of dyspnea; FEV_1 and tachycardia were unaffected.[1297] Some slight fall in $\dot{V}E$ and $\dot{V}O_2$ for comparable exercise has been noted by some observers,[1090, 1248] as well as an increase in $\dot{V}O_2$max of about 10%.[1112, 1194, 1217] In a randomized controlled study of 39 subjects, the 12-minute walking distance was significantly increased by training.[1003]

In another study, 12-minute walking distance increased after training from 960 to 1028 meters. In this study, TL_{CO} increased, but no change was noted in other parameters.[1284] A controlled study of 33 patients followed for 10 months showed that stair climbing training improved the 12-minute exercise test by 203 meters; the control group showed no differences.[1014]

Patients with and without a history of respiratory failure, but with evidence of coronary insufficiency, responded similarly to one exercise training program. This was followed by modest improvements in exercise capacity and sense of well-being.[1024] In three cases, the exercise Pa_{O_2} improved, but in three it fell after training.[1023] DL_{CO} was not changed.[1023] Most studies report an improvement in well-being and an increase of daily activity as a result of training,[1065, 1073, 1090] and some have noted a decrease in metabolic acidosis.[1056] Breathing helium/oxygen mixtures during training has not been found to be useful.[1108]

After training, the mean maximal work increased by 60 kilopond-meters in 12 men with a mean FEV_1 of 096 liters, VC of 2.56, and a Pa_{O_2} of 66 mm Hg. FEV_1 and Pa_{O_2} were unaffected.[1293] Others have reported similar findings.[1056, 1065] The cardiac output is not changed by training.[1249] A lowering of breathing frequency during exercise is not beneficial and may reduce effort tolerance.[1288]

There is a vicious circle of loss of muscle tone, poor mechanical efficiency, and discouragement in many of the seriously disabled patients.[1071] The importance of graduated rehabilitation and careful follow-up of these patients, especially if elderly, has been shown by one report of 50 patients studied after discharge from the hospital.[1011] Ninety per cent of these were unable to do previously performed chores, and 30% could do less than before the acute episode that led to hospital admission. A "quality of well-being" index bore a general relationship to the FEV_1 in 28 men and 47 women with chronic airflow limitation. A mean FEV_1 of about 64% of predicted was obtained,[4090] but changes in the two indices over time correlated poorly. Gas distribution, as measured by the nitrogen lung clearance index, is not changed on exercise.[1086]

In a double-blind controlled trial of 24 men with a mean FEV_1 of 0.83 liters, salbutamol increased the 12-minute walking distance by an average of 62 meters from an initial mean value of 876 meters.[1292] In another study, carbimazole did not improve exercise performance.[1000] Promethazine has been reported to improve exercise performance and reduce dyspnea.[1013] Nifedipine[4062] reduces pulmonary vascular resistance on exercise.

When the ventilatory capacity improves with therapy, especially in relation to steroids, exercise tolerance improves. In 18 patients with a mean increase of FEV_1 from 1.07 liters to 1.54 liters, the walking tolerance increased from 593 feet to 1525 feet.[1272] However, as this group contained four non-smokers, it may have been influenced by cases of asthma.

Hemodynamic Data

In normal men at a $\dot{V}O_2$ of 1 L/min, the $\dot{Q}_c$ at sea level is about 11 L/min and at 3100 meters altitude is 9 L/min. The equivalently hypoxic patient with airflow limitation and hypercapnia has no reduction of $\dot{Q}_c$; there are thus differences between the normal subject at altitude and the hypoxemic patient at sea level in this respect.[1338] In a study of 92 patients with chronic airflow limitation without heart failure,[1043] 30 to 40 watts of supine bicycle exercise were used to show that there was a significant relationship between resting and exercise pulmonary artery pressure (PAP) (r = 0.719) and between Pa_{O_2} and PAP when both are measured on exercise (r = −0.46). The FEV_1 was weakly related to exercise PAP (r = −0.31). In 23 of the subjects with no rise in PAP on exercise, the Pa_{O_2} was a mean of 67 mm Hg at rest and rose to 81 mm Hg on exercise. In the group of 29 subjects with a resting PAP of more than 20 mm Hg, the arterial Pa_{O_2} was 57 mm Hg at rest and on exercise.[1043] The weak association of FEV_1 or MVV with exercise capability has been noted by others.[1074] It is interesting that in a second exercise period (after the first and after a rest period), PAP and wedge pressures have both been noted to be lower than on the first occasion.[1155]

Although there is some uncertainty about the accuracy of wedge pressures, in one exercise study of eight patients with FEV_1 lower than 60% of predicted,[4044] increases in left ventricular end-diastolic pressure were observed on exercise. In these patients, the Pa_{O_2} fell from 61 mm Hg at rest to 51.4 mm Hg on exercise. Other authors have concluded that although evidence of left ventricular malfunction is seen in some patients with severe disease,[1275] it is most commonly normal.[1237] The right ventricular ejection fraction is commonly reduced,[1275] but this reduction does not correlate either with FEV_1 or with Pa_{O_2}.[1237]

Studies of transient changes in $\dot{V}E$, $\dot{V}O_2$, and $\dot{V}CO_2$ at the start of exercise in nine patients whose mean FEV_1 was 1.1 liters[4171] showed that differences from normal subjects were probably to be ascribed to circulatory factors. However, it is not clear how far these data are generally applicable, since the mean $DL_{CO}SB$ of the cases studied was reported as 89% of predicted.

In studies on 14 men whose resting PAP was more than 33 mm Hg and whose mean FEV_1 was 33% of predicted, hydralazine was shown to improve oxygen transport by increasing alveolar ventilation and cardiac index[4101]; however, side effects were noted in three of the patients. As noted earlier, others have reported that this drug increases the level of dyspnea.

In 12 men with a mean FEV_1 of 33% of predicted and a mean resting Pa_{O_2} of 77 mm Hg,[4104] exercise produced a considerable increase in PAP, but the right ventricular ejection fraction failed to increase normally. The end-diastolic volume index increased significantly. The authors noted that right ventricular dysfunction was important in exercise limitation. The importance of the right ventricular ejection fraction in these patients has been noted by others.[4072] There is no evidence that cardiac performance in cases of chronic airflow limitation is improved by digoxin administration.[4096] Aminophylline appears to improve exercise performance by mechanisms other than bronchodilation,[4084] but it is unclear whether these are related to respiratory muscle fatigue or to circulatory factors.

Reduced exercise tolerance was found to be related to prevalence of perfusion defects in lung scans in 100 subjects[1269] who were divided by mean FEV_1 into four groups of 2.28, 1.39, 0.89, and 0.69 liters, with progressively more perfusion defects visualized as the FEV_1 fell. In 41 patients aged 56 with stable airflow limitation and a mean FEV_1 of 37% of predicted, the mean mixed venous Po_2 fell from 29.5 mm Hg standing at rest to 22.4 mm Hg on maximal upright exercise.[138] In this group, PaO_2 was found to be related to $\dot{Q}_{va}/\dot{Q}_t$.

Since the linear relationship between $\dot{Q}c$ and $\dot{V}o_2$ is the same in patients with chronic airflow limitation as in normal individuals, it has been inferred that exercise is not limited by circulatory factors.[1055] However, other studies have suggested that poor filling of the left ventricle and limitation of stroke volume (attributed to loss of capillary bed) are important in many cases of chronic airflow limitation.[1054] A lowered baroreceptor response on exercise that limits heart rate response has also been noted.[1339]

There was a close relationship between pulmonary vascular resistance (PVR) and DL_{CO} on exercise (r = −0.87) in 18 subjects.[1282] Between exercise PVR and resting DL_{CO}, r was −0.78. There are no differences in measured PVR on exercise between patients categorized as Type A, Type B, or mixed,[1040] but there appears to be a relationship between the logarithm of PVR and oxygen uptake at a maximal tolerated power output.[1033] Other authors have found no relationship between severity of emphysema, as judged by loss of recoil and lowered $DL_{CO}SB$, and the rise of PAP on exercise.[1249] It was also unrelated to swings in intrathoracic pressure.[1052] Propanolol intravenously was found not to impair exercise performance.[1216, 1258] An increase in COHb from 1.43% to 4.08% in a double-blind randomized crossover study of 10 patients[1278] lowered the mean exercise time from 218 seconds to 146 seconds. Heart rates were unaffected.

The important observations of Ravez and his colleagues[1091] on pulmonary hypertension in chronic mucus hypersecretion without severe airflow limitation are noted in Chapter 7.

Summary

From all this data, one can draw the following conclusions:

1. It seems very likely that respiratory muscle fatigue limits exercise in many of these patients. Its onset may be related to increased residual volume and hypoxemia; this factor may well account for the poor relationship between the achievable maximal $\dot{V}o_2$ and the resting FEV_1. General physical "de-conditioning" is also important.

2. Complex shifts in $\dot{V}/\dot{Q}$ distribution coupled with impacts of increasing respiratory frequency on gas exchange probably lie behind the variability observed on the effect of exercise on arterial blood gas tensions. Failure of gas equilibration due to increased cardiac output and shortened capillary transit time may be a factor in some cases.

3. The value of careful exercise rehabilitation programs has been clearly demonstrated; the favorable effects are not related to improvement in pulmonary function tests but to a general improvement in condition.

4. Pulmonary hypertension is related to arterial hypoxemia and is partially reversible in many cases. In patients with advanced severe chronic airflow limitation, right ventricular dysfunction may well be an important limiting factor. The roles of myocardial disease and of

some degree of left ventricular failure coexisting with chronic airflow limitation are difficult to assess, but pulmonary hypertension in some patients may be caused by this mechanism rather than by hypoxemia or loss of capillary bed.

In this section, no analysis of dyspnea has been attempted, but two remarkable observations have been noted. The first is that oxygen relieves the dyspnea in patients with chronic airflow limitation who are not hypoxemic.[1004] The second is that venesection relieves dyspnea without changing pulmonary function tests[1254]; this study is described later. These two observations not only indicate how much remains to be learned of the nature of dyspnea in these patients but also suggest that pulmonary hypertension may be an important component of the sensation of dyspnea, even if actual exercise performance is limited by muscle fatigue.

ADAPTATIONS AND SECONDARY EFFECTS OF CHRONIC AIRFLOW LIMITATION AND RESPIRATORY FAILURE

Secondary Polycythemia and Changes in the Blood

During the past 12 years, several important observations have been added to those previously made relating to the changes in the blood in patients with chronic airflow limitation. In chronic hypercapnia,[1110] the total body buffering capacity $(dH + a/dPa_{CO_2})$ is an inverse function of the chronic Pa_{CO_2} level:

$$H^+ a \text{ (nmol/L)} = 0.19 \times P_{CO_2} + 32.3$$

The close relationship between oxygen saturation and red cell volume has been confirmed.[1309] Venous hematocrit and red cell count may be normal even though red cell volume is increased. The polycythemic response to hypoxia is generally found to be "subnormal" (that is less than in normal subjects at altitude). This has been attributed to iron deficiency and chronic infection.[1309]

A comparison between 33 patients with chronic airflow limitation with RBC volumes <120% of predicted and 12 patients in whom RBC levels exceeded this showed no differences in age, FEV_1, or $DL_{CO}SB$. Pa_{O_2} at rest and on exercise was lower in the polycythemic group.[1342]

There is little doubt that in patients with chronic airflow limitation, the polycythemia is related to the level of carboxyhemoglobin in the blood (and hence to the intensity of current smoking).[1246] In one study[3303] of 47 chronically hypoxemic patients in whom the mean Pa_{O_2} was 52.5 mm Hg, red cell mass was found to correlate with COHb levels (r = 0.73) but not with the Pa_{O_2}. In 15 subjects given long-term oxygen, red cell mass decreased only in those who stopped smoking, as shown by a fall in COHb.[3303]

Wedzicha and colleagues[5097] compared 16 patients with chronic airflow limitation (aged 60 years and with a mean FEV_1 of 880 milliliters) with a control group of similarly hypoxemic, but not polycythemic, patients. The pulmonary capillary blood volume, V_c, was 65 milliliters in the controls, but only 32 milliliters in the subjects with polycythemia. After erythropheresis, which reduced the packed-cell volume from 58% to 47% and lowered the blood viscosity, the V_c rose to a mean of 49 milliliters.

In a remarkable study, Dayton and colleagues[1254] organized a protocol in which some polycythemic patients had blood removed and some did not. The protocol was such that all patients were unaware whether venesection had actually occurred. In 18 patients with chronic airflow limitation, all those who actually had blood removed said they were less dyspneic for 48 hours afterward. All those in whom blood was not removed said their dyspnea was unchanged. Phlebotomy did not change any of the pulmonary function parameters. There are also detectable abnormalities in blood platelets, as shown by studies of their metabolism, that are attributed to overstimulation.[3317]

In six patients in whom the blood volume was increased by more than a liter from normal, long-term diuretic therapy led to a fall in PAP, a rise in Pa_{O_2}, an 8% fall in hematocrit, and a reduction of total blood volume.[1238] These favorable results suggest that this form of therapy should be more widely used.

A recent finding may explain the increased frequency of pulmonary thromboses found at autopsy in patients with chronic airflow limitation. By means of autologous platelet labeling, deep venous thromboses were detected in 13 of 29 patients with exacerbations of severe chronic airflow limitation.[3285] In nine of these, the thromboses were proximal to the knee, a location known to be associated with increased risk of pulmonary embolism.

Patients with chronic airflow limitation and hypoxemia have been shown to have severe neuropsychiatric defects as a consequence of the hypoxemia.[1240] Mental tests have shown that memory is principally involved.[3277] In men, sexual dysfunction worsens as the disease becomes more severe.[3331]

Other Changes

Studies of mucociliary clearance in patients with chronic airflow limitation give variable results. In patients with mild to moderate disease, mucociliary clearance by coughing may be better than in controls. However, when blood gases are abnormal, delayed clearance even with coughing is often observed.[4079]

Semple and Macpherson[3278] have described changes in the pituitary fossa in patients with chronic airflow limitation and hypoxemia, which they have ascribed to increased cerebral blood flow rather than to increased intracerebral pressure. In other reports of seven subjects with severe airflow limitation studied during recovery from an exacerbation, Semple and his colleagues[3286] noted that serum testosterone, follicle-stimulating hormone, luteinizing hormone, dihydroepiandrosterone, and urinary 17-ketosteroids all rose significantly.

The loss of weight from which many suffer[3337, 3342] appears to be associated with an increased resting metabolism rather than with a reduced caloric intake. Wilson, Rogers, and Hoffmann[4066] have recently reviewed the problem of nutrition in patients with chronic airflow limitation. In one study,[4085] 27% of 60 outpatients with chronic airflow limitation reported weight loss. Five per cent had a body weight of less than 60% of the ideal. This correlated with the FEV and the $DL_{CO}SB$ as per cent of predicted but not with the resting Pa_{O_2}. Caloric intake appeared to be normal. The prognosis has been noted to be worse in those whose body weight is below the ideal, but survival is not improved by an increased caloric intake.[4073] It has been suggested that parenteral hyperalimentation may improve ventilatory function in some patients.[4074]

CHANGES DURING SLEEP

This section should be read in conjunction with the section on sleep disorders in Chapter 4.

Sleep disorders in patients with chronic airflow limitation have recently been reviewed by Fleetham and Kryger.[1141] These patients have a shorter total sleep time and increased shifts in sleep stage, and they get less REM sleep than normal subjects.[1141] The reasons for these changes are not known, but it is well established that falls in arterial oxygen tension during sleep are common and are accompanied by an increase in PAP. The relationship between saturation and PAP is linear and directly related in individual cases,[1105] however, some patients are encountered in whom the relationship is less direct,[1105] probably because the constrictive response to hypoxia varies. The greatest falls in saturation, which have been documented to be as large as 36%,[1277] occur in REM sleep. In four patients with very severe disease who had FEV_1 values of 0.54, 0.88, 0.97, and 0.98 liters and $DL_{CO}SS$ values of 3.9, 4.4, 8.2, and 3.6 mL/CO/mm Hg, documented episodes of a fall in $O_2Hb\%$ were invariably accompanied by a rise in PAP.[1244] In a recent study of 20 patients, falls of more than 10% in O_2Hb occurred in all patients who were hypoxemic while awake and at rest and in three of seven non-hypoxemic patients.[3233] Others have noted greater falls in hypoxemic subjects.[3328]

In another study,[3269] 24 patients spent 24% of the night with O_2Hb levels more than 5% lower than when awake. Relief of hypoxemia did not affect their arousal frequency.[3269] Others[1141] have noted that the abnormal sleep profile is unaffected. However, it has also been reported that nocturnal oxygen improves sleep duration,[3309] as well as arterial saturation.[1236] The maximal and mean nocturnal fall in saturation correlates negatively with the level of oxygen saturation when awake.[1139] The nocturnal saturation change also correlates negatively with the ΔP_{CO_2} response.[1139]

It seems likely that these changes should be regarded as a consequence of the physiologic changes occurring in REM sleep and that these changes are superimposed on the physiologic abnormalities—particularly the mechanical and $\dot{V}/\dot{Q}$ abnormalities—of those with chronic airflow limitation. Classic obstructive sleep apnea is believed to be rare in these cases,[1141] although some authors have suggested that sleep-related partial upper airway obstruction may occur.[1138] Short desaturation episodes associated with upper airway occlusion are sometimes documented.[3338] Because chronic airflow limitation and obstructive sleep apnea are not rare conditions, one can expect that they might by chance occur in combination fairly frequently.

An important recent observation was that alcohol (producing a blood level of 40 mg/dL) in 20 patients with chronic airflow limitation increased episodes of apnea, total apnea duration, and the number of episodes per hour of sleep time, although its effect on oxygen desaturation was not significant. However, it also produced a significant increase in premature ventricular contractions.[3348]

In an interesting comparison between six patients with chronic airflow limitation and six patients with right to left intracardiac shunts, both groups being equally hypoxemic, it was found that significant episodes of hypoxemia occurred in all those with airflow limitation but in none of those with shunts.[3279]

The long-term consequences of intermittent pulmonary hypertension occurring during sleep in these patients, are not known. Whether this represents a stage in the development of pulmonary hypertension when awake cannot be answered until more information is available. However, there is no doubt that nocturnal oxygen improves survival in these cases, postponing the onset of cor pulmonale.* Anthonisen's comprehensive review of hypoxemia and oxygen therapy in patients with chronic airflow limitation summarizes what has been learned from domiciliary oxygen therapy.[3257]

EFFECTS OF BRONCHODILATORS

There have been a number of studies of the effects of bronchodilator therapy.† Mendella and her colleagues[982] have contributed the important point that a number of patients with severe airflow limitation (perhaps as many as 10% of the total) may have significant improvement on steroids, even though conventional bronchodilators have been without effect. It follows from this that errors in management can occur both from continued use of steroids when no benefit results and from not using them on a trial basis.

FACTORS INFLUENCING PROGNOSIS IN CHRONIC AIRFLOW LIMITATION
Studies of FEV₁ Decline

Cross-sectional data summarized in Chapter 5 and in Tables 5–1 and 5–2 predict a fall of

FEV_1 with age of about 30 mL/year in normal non-smokers on the basis of linear regressions. During the past 15 years, a considerable volume of longitudinal data has been collected. Berry[1031] has contributed a valuable review of the statistics of cross-sectional and longitudinal studies of FEV_1. These statistical considerations have recently been reviewed by Cook and Ware[4094]; by Schulzer and his colleagues[4093]; by Ware[4043]; and by Woodbury, Manton, and Stallard.[4091]

Schlesselman has reviewed the design of longitudinal studies.[1182] Burrows[1143] has contributed very useful data from a retrospective review of longitudinal FEV_1 measurements in patients with chronic airflow limitation. These papers show that the SD of FEV_1 decline being observed longitudinally in a population decreases as the follow-up time lengthens and stabilizes after 5 years or so:

SEE Values of delta FEV₁ (mL/year)	Years of Follow-up
270	1
100	3
60	5
45	7
40	9
35	11

Burrows concluded from this data that the "longitudinally determined delta FEV_1 showed much less decline in function and a later age of apparent onset of decline than suggested by cross-sectional analysis."

One of the few studies to follow normal subjects was reported by Lawther, who measured the VC and FEV_1 in 47 medical students when they were 19 years of age and again 10 years later. They were light smokers, and the mean VC and FEV_1 both increased over this period.[1291] As noted in Chapter 5, there are reasons to doubt that linear regressions beginning at age 20 accurately represent the normal course of events up to the age of 35. A considerable body of information now indicates the importance of longitudinal data in patients with chronic airflow limitation. Evidence that the rate of decline may be accelerated in different industrial settings is noted in Chapter 16.

In a pioneer study in this field, Fletcher and his colleagues followed a stratified random sample of 1136 men selected in 1961, of whom 792 were seen regularly enough over the next 8 years to provide data for analysis. The results have been described in a book[723] and summarised in a journal article.[1321] At selection, the men were between 30 and 59 years of age and were skilled manual or clerical workers in Lon-

---

*See references 1005, 1008, 1169, 3249, 3257.
†See references 4016, 4026, 4058, 4134.

don. The mean FEV_1 decline in smokers was −54 ml/year. The authors concluded that sharp falls in FEV_1 were not present (though their complex method of statistical analysis might have obscured them) and noted that chronic mucus hypersecretion and the obstructive disorder whose progress they were following were separate conditions linked to common etiologic factors. As Fletcher noted,[1035] and as indicated by the wide range of DL_{CO} measurements obtained in a small subsample,[723] the patients had some combination of chronic mucus hypersecretion without airflow limitation, already-developed emphysema, and small airway involvement and $\dot{V}/\dot{Q}$ disturbance. The data showed that faster decline occurred in those with initially lower values (a phenomenon described as the "horse race" effect), but the scatter of individual data on which this conclusion is based is more impressive than the relationship (see data in the Appendix of reference 723). We have noted the same variability in the relationship between initial deviation from predicted FEF_{25-75} and subsequent change.[1197] Others have noted the large scatter in such data.[1092] However, the fact that faster decline occurs in those who in middle life already have a significantly lowered value is important in preventive strategy, as we have pointed out.[1263] It is also confirmed by the analysis of risk factors noted later.

A group of 54 men of average age 52 and with mean initial FEV_1 of 50% of predicted, normal blood pressures, and a productive cough were followed between 1963 and 1974 in Dundee.[1317] They were found to have a mean FEV_1 decline of −34 mL/year. The authors noted that "where the FEV_1 is 70% of predicted or more, the prognosis approaches that of the population at large, but where it falls to 50% or less, there is a higher risk of cardiorespiratory failure and a considerable mortality." They concluded that emphysema, defined radiologically, progresses slowly and that heavy smoking seemed more closely related to falls in $DL_{CO}SB$ than to changes in ventilatory tests.

Many studies are influenced by declines in cigarette smoking over the period. Of 1263 people surveyed in 1961 and again in 1968, 19% had improved FEV/FVC ratios over this interval,[1312] possibly due to changes in smoking. A study of 67 men over a 9-year interval by Ogilvie[1300] in Newcastle indicated a fall of FEV_1 of −51 mL/year in the least severe group, whose mean FEV_1 was 2.26 at the start, and a fall of −80 mL/year in a more severe group

over the same period. The smoking history was similar in the two groups.

Howard and Astin,[1318] who originally documented the occurrence of sharp falls in FEV_1 in one or two patients, confirmed this phenomenon in longitudinal studies of 159 men in an engineering works in Sheffield between 1956 and 1967.[1285] The mean FEV_1 decline was −34 mL/year, but the FVC decline observed was −64 mL/year. Men with sputum had higher rates of decline. Twenty-seven episodes of a fall in FEV_1 of more than four times 34 milliliters with no subsequent recovery were recorded in 25 of the men. This observation might have been influenced by occupational exposure or air pollution. However, Clement and van de Woestijne[3305] also observed very rapid rates of decline in FEV_1 in some cases. As noted earlier, this phenomenon was not observed in Fletcher's series, possibly because the statistical method used had the effect of eliminating such observations.

Kanner and his colleagues from Salt Lake City observed high rates of decline in a 6-year study. Overall, the FVC declined by −94.3 mL/year and the FEV_1 by −69 mL/year. Faster declines were associated with age, years of smoking, airway reactivity (assessed by response to bronchodilators), and frequency of lower tract illness. This last factor has not been found to be associated with worsening in other series.[977]

From Australia, Barter and Campbell[1235] reported a faster rate of decline in smokers than in non-smokers (−60 mL/year versus −30 mL/year) and suggested that increased bronchial reactivity might be related to a faster decline. The same group has recently[4067] reported on a follow-up of 66 men with chronic bronchitis from different parts of Australia:

	Number	Age	Height (cm)	FEV_1 (%P)	Mean Annual FEV_1 Decline (mL/year)
Queensland	20	51.2	171.7	84.2	−25.8
NSW	17	50.4	172.4	86.9	−65.8
Victoria	29	56.6	171.3	86.5	−77.1

They suggested that the warmer climate of Queensland was responsible for the slower rate of decline. Details of the smoking history over the period of the follow-up were not given, but the differential rates were not thought to be attributable to smoking differences.

Kanner[4083] studied a varied group of patients and assessed the airway responsiveness by the change in FEV_1 after a bronchodilator was administered. He concluded that airway re-

Diagnosis	Number	Age	FEV$_1$ (post/pre-Bronchodilator)	Annual Decline (mL/year)	
				FVC	FEV$_1$
Chronic bronchitis + emphysema	49	54.1	1.17	− 129.7	− 90.0
Emphysema	6	46.8	1.08	− 90.6	− 62.5
Chronic bronchitis	14	50.9	1.08	− 8.6	− 12.2
Asthma	10	51.4	1.17	− 86.0	− 70.8
Bronchiectasis	5	46.6	1.14	+ 15.8	− 30.5

sponsiveness is related to the rate of decline of FEV$_1$, although it is unlikely to be a causal relation (see table at the top of this page).

Weiss and Speizer[4081] commented on this study in an editorial.

A follow-up of 117 people in Colorado[1340] over a 6-year period originally classified as abnormal (by symptoms or an FEV$_1$/FVC ratio of <60%) and 111 subjects classified as normal gave the following data:

FEV/FVC (original)		Number	FEV$_1$ Decline (mL/year)	FVC Decline (mL/year)
MEN:	<60%	25	− 41	− 106
	60–74%	34	− 17	− 27
	>75%	34	− 4	+ 3
WOMEN:	<60%	2	—	—
	60–74%	44	− 16	− 32
	>75%	40	− 2	− 2

These data show a faster rate of decline in association with lower initial values.

A 1964 study by Mitchell, Webb, and Filley[4111] reported on a follow-up of 150 patients not seriously disabled initially (35% could still climb one flight of stairs without stopping). Ten years later, 30% had died, 30% were severely disabled, and "only 40% were still able to climb a flight of stairs without stopping." Their initial maximal breathing capacity was about 30% of predicted. Survival related better to the O$_2$Hb than to the DL$_{CO}$.

Vollmer, Johnson, and Buist[4063] have recently reported on 795 subjects drawn from two cohorts in Portland and followed over a 9 to 11 year interval. The mean age of the Portland cohort was 49 years on entry, and the mean age of the screening cohort was 59 years. They compared 44 bronchodilator responders with 132 non-responders and showed that the annual rate of decline in the responders was greater than in the non-responders, regardless of whether bronchitis was present (see table at the bottom of this page).

A 5-year follow-up of 2539 adults in Baltimore who initially had FEV$_1$, SBN$_2$/L, and DL$_{CO}$SB tests showed that 115 died, three from respiratory causes. When adjustments were made for age and smoking, the SBN$_2$/L was found to be most strongly associated with mortality.[4053] The authors suggested that either the lungs may serve to protect other systems (and, hence, poor function may contribute to other causes of death) or, alternatively, lung function tests may reflect existing disorders in other systems. Noting that saline infusion in normal subjects alters the SBN$_2$/L, they suggested that possibly an increased SBN$_2$/L reflected an increase in left atrial pressure.

The possibility that the close relationship of the FEV$_1$ to survival partly depends on its lowering in patients who will die later of cardiovascular disease is supported by data from the Cracow study in Poland.[4042] Presumably, this effect would be mediated by reductions in FVC that result from left ventricular failure or an increase in left atrial pressure. Bloom[4493] has also suggested that cardiovascular factors may be important in relation to FEV$_1$ decline. This question is discussed further in Chapter 12.

Postma and her colleagues in Sweden[4021] followed 65 patients with severe airflow obstruction. The mean age of the subjects was 54 years. Eighty-one per cent were men, and 64% were

	Number of Pairs	FEV$_1$ (mL/year)			FVC (mL/year)		
		R*	NR	p	R	NR	p
Portland Cohort							
Current smokers	4	− 67	− 45	0.46	− 34	− 32	0.28
Ex-smokers	7	− 89	− 43	0.01	− 84	− 27	0.005
Non-smokers	1	− 38	− 43		− 17	− 16	
Screening Cohort							
Current smokers	17	− 70	− 60	0.02	− 72	− 45	0.02
Ex-smokers	8	− 70	− 56	0.20	− 68	− 51	0.06
Non-smokers	7	− 49	− 37	0.03	− 43	− 33	0.09

*R = Responsive to bronchodilator; NR = non-responsive to bronchodilator.

current smokers. FEV_1 was 25% of predicted, and VC was 62.4% predicted. There were seven serial observations of each patient over a period of at least 10 years. Prednisone (10 to 15 mg/day) administration was started at the beginning of the study. Three distinct patterns of FEV_1 were noted—no change; no initial fall; and linear decline. All the patients who died and had autopsies were found to have emphysema.

Studies over a 4-year period of 366 men in Holland showed an FEV_1 decline of -47 mL/year and an FEF_{25-75} decline of -0.13 L/sec/year.[821] In this series, there was not a close relationship to smoking, an unusual finding.

In Sweden, a 10-year follow-up of 269 men who were 50 years of age at the start of the study showed that the percentage of non-smokers with symptoms increased from 9.5% to 23%. In smokers, the percentage rose from 40.1% to 55.2%.[1079] Rates of FEV_1 decline of -40 mL/year were seen in non-smokers and of -57 mL/year in smokers; FVC declines were similar. In the non-smoking group, the mean VC decline in those without symptoms was -35 mL/year, but in those with symptoms it was -95 mL/year.

In Paris, 556 men aged 30 to 54 were resurveyed after an interval of 12 years; the FEV_1 decline in heavy smokers was -51 mL/year and in non-smokers was -38 mL/year.[89] The FEV_1 decline decelerated in those who gave up smoking. Those who were ex-smokers at the start of the study and did not smoke over the 12-year period were found to have the same rate of decline as the non-smokers.

In a population of 2572 people studied in Cracow between 1968 and 1973, FEV_1 declines of -78 mL/year in smokers and -48 mL/year in non-smokers were noted.[679] The level of education as an index of socioeconomic conditions was as strongly related to FEV_1 decline, as was smoking.

Huhti and Ikkala[1092] observed 492 men and 671 women in Finland over a 10-year period. The FEV_1 decline in male non-smokers was -33 mL/year ($\pm$ 30), and in smokers it was -51 mL/year ($\pm$ 33). In women, the figures were -27 mL/year for non-smokers and -35 mL/year in smokers. In this series, stopping smoking did not lower the rate of decline to the non-smoker level. Larger FEV_1 declines were noted in those with initially lower values, but these authors stress the large scatter in the data.

A comparison of two communities in Holland, one with high air pollution and one rural, showed rates of decline of -24 mL/year in the polluted and -15 mL/year in the unpolluted regions.[829] Cross-sectional studies of the same communities had not shown a significant difference. As noted in Chapter 6, later reports have indicated that further follow-up may modify these results.

Madison and colleagues[1151] have published an interesting follow-up of 163 subjects with alpha$_1$-AT deficiency or relatives of those with this condition who were studied over a 6-year period. Their extensive data showed FEV_1 declines of -72 mL/year in MZ phenotype subjects—in both smokers and non-smokers—when a family history of respiratory disease existed. The FEV_1 decline was -30 mL/year in non-smokers and -43 mL/year in smokers without such a history. Rates of decline of M phenotypes were not much different from expected rates, but faster rates were found in those with a family history of respiratory disease and also in smokers. The authors concluded that phenotypes, family history, and smoking were all risk factors.

In a 20-year follow-up of men with chronic bronchitis, we have found a difference between the rate of FEV_1 decline in 15 men in Halifax (-56 mL/year) and 34 men in Winnipeg (-46 mL/year); a similar difference in rate of decline was observed in vital capacity, which was measured independently. The Winnipeg group had smoked more heavily over the period than the Halifax group. Although the numbers are small in each group, their initial FEV_1 and DL_{CO} data were no different from those of the larger groups from which they were drawn.[986] Environmental factors that may explain this difference include very different winter climates and high levels of aerosol sulfates in Halifax (about fourfold greater than in Winnipeg).

As noted in Chapter 4, Burrows and his colleagues have reported on an 11-year follow-up of 466 subjects in Tucson. All were non-smokers, randomly selected, and studied an average of seven times. They were between 30 and 70 years old. Rates of FEV_1 decline were only -8 mL/year up to the age of 50, increasing to about -20 mL/year at 70. The authors noted that the longitudinally determined FEV_1 declines were much less, and the decline started later in life than would be predicted from cross-sectional studies.[5098]

In a study from Holland of 129 subjects, all had an initial FEV_1 of less than 1 liter.[991] In those who survived less than 5 years, the rate of FEV_1 decline was -162 mL/year, and in those who survived more than 5 years, it was +25 mL/year. The changes in VC were −163 mL/year and −40 mL/year, respectively.

A 5-year follow-up of 27 patients with severe chronic airflow limitation showed that the mean FEV decline was from an initial value of 1.18 to a value of 0.935, a rate of change of about −30 mL/year. Over the same period, the VC declined at a rate of −76 mL/year. All subjects exhibited EKG changes,[1128] and 12 died during the period of observation.

A group of 65 subjects with severe airflow limitation and with initial FEV_1 between 0.625 and 1.98 liters was studied over 5 years. The rate of decline of VC was −103 mL/year and that of FEV_1 was −47 mL/year.[1115] All these subjects were hypoxemic. Thirty-eight had one or more episodes of right ventricular failure, and 25 died during the course of the follow-up. At this advanced stage of the disease, the rate of FEV_1 decline is probably a poor indicator of adverse change. However, it has recently been shown that in patients with established emphysema[996] the annual rates of decline in smokers (−53.5 mL/year) were greater than in those who had stopped smoking (−16.4 mL/year). In these subjects, the decline in VC was the same as the decline in FEV_1.

To what is a decline of FEV_1 attributable? From our knowledge of the separate components of the syndrome of chronic airflow limitation, we can draw the following conclusions:

1. There are five possible components associated with major progressive declines in FEV_1 in patients with chronic airflow limitation:

- A faster than normal loss of lung recoil
- Progressive changes in small airways and increase in peripheral airflow resistance
- Progression of emphysema
- Increase in airway hyperreactivity
- Reduction in FVC for cardiovascular reasons

2. The detailed analysis of several different data sets by Peto and colleagues[2924] indicates that chronic mucus hypersecretion probably plays a minor role in increasing FEV_1 decline.

3. Episodes of reversible bronchospasm are important. In some patients with apparently stable chronic airflow limitation, changes reversed by steroid therapy may be responsible for FEV_1 decline. Data from Mendella and colleagues[982] indicate that this factor played a major role in lowering the FEV_1 in six of 46 subjects studied, even when bronchodilators had been given.

4. The decline in FEV_1 may be "driven" by a decline in FVC in the later stages of the disease. When both of these have reached low levels, circulatory factors become closely related to prognosis, as noted later.

5. Longitudinal studies, and the continued observation of individual patients, are of the greatest value in understanding the natural history of these conditions.

Factors Related to Reduced Survival: Risk Factor Analysis

The relationship between FEV_1 and mortality has been shown in a variety of studies; in some data it is extremely close. It is a predictor of mortality in community studies, such as that in Tecumseh, Michigan.[1224, 2901] A summary of risk factors is provided in Table 8–1.

In several series, the FEV_1 has been shown to be significantly lower in groups with a lower 5-year survival.[1030] It is also a predictor within the spectrum of chronic airflow limitation. One such report from Sweden studied 339 patients 40 to 69 years of age, all with an FEV_1 of 1.5 liters or less. The following data were obtained for 5-year survival rates,[1315] as compared with a predicted mean survival of 90% for the population as a whole:

FEV_1	Number	5-Year Survival
1.25–1.50	47	82%
0.95–1.24	111	67%
0.65–0.94	123	52%
<0.65	58	40%

In another series of 1487 men 45 to 49 years old,[1025] the FEV_1 ranged between 3.2 liters and 2.9 liters and was significantly related to survival over a 10-year period. In this study, it was noted that the presence of cough and sputum were not related to survival.

Survival in Groningen, Holland is apparently better than in the United States, as the following comparison shows[1132] (see table at the bottom of the following page).

The data obtained in the United States were from the study by Diener and Burrows.[1323] The reasons for the difference are not known.

As was noted earlier, the recent comprehensive analysis of several data sets by Peto and his colleagues[2924] indicates that it is the FEV_1 that is related to survival and not the presence of chronic mucus hypersecretion. This finding supports the view that of the factors lowering the FEV_1 noted in the previous section it is not

Table 8–1. RISK FACTORS FOR CHRONIC AIRFLOW LIMITATION*

Factor	EMPH	CMH	RB	CAB
Host Factors				
Pi type Z	Proven	No	No	No
Immune	No	Proven	?	Proven
Br. reactivity	No	No	No	Probable†
Other	Probable	??	?	??
Exposures				
Cigarettes	Proven	Proven	Proven	Aggravator
SO$_2$ and TSP (particulates)	?	Proven	Probable	Aggravator
Oxidants (O$_3$)	?	?	?	Aggravator
Coal dust	Proven	Proven	Probable	Aggravator
Cadmium	Proven	?	?	?
Allergens	No	‡	HS‡	Proven
Climate and SES				
Climate	?	Probable	?	Aggravator
Socio-economic status (poor housing)	?	Proven	?	Aggravator

*EMPH, emphysema; CMH, chronic mucous hypersecretion; RB, respiratory bronchiolitis; CAB, chronic asthmatic bronchitis (? eosinophilic bronchitis); HS, hypersensitivity pneumonitis; ?, unknown; ??, unlikely.

†Proven feature but not proved to be a preceding risk factor.

‡In susceptible subjects only.

mucus hypersecretion that determines prognosis. However, it does leave the question open.

Higgins, using Tecumseh data, has developed a detailed risk factor analysis, which is based on initial ventilatory flow rates and age and assumes no change in smoking history.[2901, 4116] She concluded from this: "For example, the risk of developing obstructive airways disease in the next 15 years is about 1 in 200 for a 45 year old male nonsmoker whose $\dot{V}max_{50\%}$ is 100% of predicted, if he doesn't take up smoking. The risk for a man of the same age who smokes 40 cigs/day and whose $\dot{V}max_{50\%}$ is 80% of predicted, is 1 in 5 or 6 if he doesn't cut down on his smoking, and about 1 in 15 if he stops smoking. . ." This information was based on observations of 1358 men and 1596 women; social class did not affect the risk factors. Genetic markers were unimportant in men but were possibly related in women. The same risk factor analysis has been applied to other populations and has been shown to apply to them also.[3357] Others have not been able to identify significant genetic risk factors,[3268] apart from

alpha$_1$-AT deficiency. Alcohol does not appear to accelerate decline.[3247]

The level of Pa$_{O_2}$ is linked to survival. In one series of 93 subjects observed for 7 to 10 years, the mortality among those with normal blood gases at rest and exercise was 9.1%; in those with abnormal blood gases it was 34.6%.[1127] This fits in with the observation that living at high altitudes reduces survival.[3310]

Keller, Ragaz, and Borer[4041] reported on 87 patients on long-term domiciliary oxygen therapy who were observed for 3 years. Their mean age was 62.9 years. Initial Pa$_{O_2}$ was 46.4 mm Hg, VC was 57.6% of predicted, and FEV$_1$ was 32.6% of predicted. Fourteen hours of oxygen were administered each day. Of these patients, 23.7% died in the first year, 37.4% died after 2 years, and 45% after 3 years. In the early death group, the mean PAP had been 40 mm Hg; in the survivors it was 29.4 mm Hg. Severe airway obstruction and worse hypoxemia were not related to early death in these patients, but the response of the pulmonary vascular resistance to oxygen breathing was found to be related.

In a recent report on 985 subjects with

Initial FEV$_1$ (%P)	Cumulative Survival (%)			
	5-Year		10-Year	
	Holland	USA	Holland	USA
20	60	11	19	11
20–29	52	30	22	10
30–39	74	47	41	21
40–49	70	89	47	39
50–59	87	95	87	57
60+	88	89	74	89

chronic airflow limitation without hypoxemia who were observed for 3 years,[4015] Anthonisen, Wright, and Hodgkin noted that overall mortality was 23% over this period and the patient's age and FEV_1 were the most accurate predictors of death. The initial characteristics were mean age 60.9, 20.9% were females, 86.9% were white, 96.5% were smokers, and mean FEV_1 was 36.1% of predicted before any bronchodilator therapy and 41.0% of predicted after bronchodilators were administered. The $DL_{CO}SB$ averaged 49% of predicted, the Pa_{O_2} was 70 mm Hg, and the Pa_{CO_2} was 37 mm Hg. They noted that the level of mortality was lower than in other reports and about the same as in that of hypoxemic cases receiving domiciliary oxygen. The rate of decline of FEV_1 was -44 mL/year, but the SD was large. In those with a good initial FEV_1, the rate of decline correlated negatively with bronchodilator response, symptomatic wheezing, and psychologic disturbances. It was believed that cases of asthma had been excluded.

The presence of cor pulmonale significantly worsens the rate of survival when the FEV_1 levels are similar.[1022] In one series, 66% of patients were noted to die within 2 years of the first episode of respiratory failure.[1266] Electrocardiographic changes are also indicative of a poorer prognosis. In 228 patients with an FEV_1 of 1.5 liters or less, the 4-year survival rate was significantly lower in those with a QRS axis of $+90$ to $+180$ degrees or with a P_2 amplitude of 0.2 millivolts or more.[1314] Only about 40% of those with these changes were alive after 4 years. The same two signs were associated with a poorer prognosis in another series,[1026] and the authors pointed out that this was true even if the precordial leads were normal. Not only are these criteria important, but survival is also related to visual grading of enlargement of the pulmonary arteries.[1068] A relationship between EKG changes and FEV_1/FVC ratio[1264] has been found.

Although the measured rise in PAP over a 2-year period has been observed to be small (about 7%),[1249] the survival rate is significantly lowered in those with a PAP above 20 mm Hg.[998] In this series of 175 patients, 45.9% of those with an FEV_1 of less than 1.2 liters survived 4 years; 69.8% of those in whom it was above this level survived 4 years. The FEV_1 decline was -67 mL/year in those who died within 7 years and -47 mL/year in those who survived longer than this. The VC declines were -150 mL/year and -79 mL/year, respectively.

The annual rate of increase of PAP was 0.8 mm Hg/year over a 3-year period in those who did not survive 7 years and 0.5 mm Hg/year in those who did.[998] In another series of 65 subjects,[4163] the resting PAP rose by more than 5 mm Hg in 19 of those studied over a mean interval of 57 months, a rate of increase of about 1 mm Hg per year.

In 195 patients with chronic airflow limitation who were studied at rest and on exercise,[1051] the rate of survival was significantly lower in those with a resting PAP of more than 30 mm Hg and in those in whom the pressure rose more than 10 mm Hg on exercise. These subjects were observed for up to 12 years. In half the patients the FEV_1/FVC ratio was less than 65% and the RV/TLC ratio was more than 30%. The relationship between resting PAP and survival was as follows:

Resting PAP (mm Hg)		5-Year Survival
<20	(n = 88)	86%
20–30	(n = 103)	75%
>30	(n = 24)	35%

However, in a series of 27 patients with more severe disease who were followed for 5 years, survival did not appear to be related to the PAP.[1128]

Weitzenblum and Jizek[4077] have reviewed the evolution of patients with chronic airflow limitation in terms of hemodynamic data. On the basis of repeat catheterization studies after an interval of about 5 years, they conclude that PAP increases about 0.6 mm Hg per year. Other data[4110] on 50 randomly selected subjects observed for 4 years suggested the level of mixed venous oxygenation, rather than the initial PAP or vascular resistance, was related to survival. Twenty-seven of the initial group of 50 died over the interval.

In another series of 54 subjects in Japan who were randomly selected from 119 patients with chronic airflow limitation, 19 had died from respiratory failure after 4 years of follow-up.[3330] Indicators of poor prognosis were

• resting arterial hypoxemia
• a fall in Pa_{O_2} during exercise
• a lower Pa_{O_2} on oxygen breathing during exercise
• a higher Pa_{CO_2}

This group averaged 61.3 years of age; the mean FEV_1 was 1.02 liters; the RV was 134% of predicted; and the $DL_{CO}SB$ averaged 56% of predicted. The mean Pa_{O_2} was 71 mm Hg. The

$DL_{CO}SB$ was not related to survival, but the level of FEV_1 was found to be related.

The distribution of emphysema may be related to prognosis. Hughes and his colleagues[999] observed a group of patients between 3 and 13 years. The emphysema was classified radiologically as mainly upper zone (UZ), mainly lower zone (LZ), or generalized (G). All had normal alpha$_1$-antitrypsin levels (see table at the bottom of this page).

From these data, upper zone disease appears to be associated with a faster rate of decline in both smokers and ex-smokers.

Some studies have shown that combinations of abnormal tests can be used to predict survival. In one such study, those patients with an FEV_1 <0.75 and a $DL_{CO}SB$ <3.0 had a 5-year mortality rate of 90%.[1196] Radiologic evidence of emphysema also worsened the prognosis in this series of 663 subjects.

Acute exacerbations of chronic airflow limitation, usually attributed to infections, are a common cause of death in these patients. Thirty-six consecutive patients admitted to the hospital with acute exacerbations of their disease[3334] have been studied. Their mean age was 61 years, and the FEV_1 when stable was 990 milliliters. The mean Pa_{O_2} was 47 mm Hg, and the Pa_{CO_2} was 48 mm Hg. Their 2-year survival after the acute episode was 72%. The authors noted that this was somewhat better than in some other series, which have noted 1-year survival rates of between 30% and 60% for such patients. However, the findings were similar to four other studies showing 2-year survival rates of between 60% and 85%.

A recent study indicated (rather surprisingly) that the use of tetracycline in such exacerbations has little favorable effect on their course.[3290] However, a more recent detailed report compared a placebo and an antibiotic given to 173 subjects over a period of 3 and a half years, in which 362 exacerbations occurred.[4314] The study clearly indicated that the course was shorter, the outcome more favorable, and the PEFR returned more quickly to its previous value if antibiotics were used.

Summary

All these observations permit some general conclusions to be drawn:

1. The rate of decline of FEV_1, or its deviation from normal by middle life, is related to prognosis. However, this may become less reliable as very low levels are reached. When this has occurred, cardiovascular factors become more closely related to survival.

2. A worsening $\dot{V}/\dot{Q}$ distribution loosely accompanying the fall in FEV_1 leads to arterial hypoxemia and hypercapnia. The magnitude of the hypoxemia is probably related to the anatomic changes within the lung and to the ventilatory drive.

3. Hypoxemia is accompanied by elevation of PAP with some variation in degree; this often worsens episodically at night.

4. Elevation of PAP, which usually occurs only when the FEV_1 value approaches a liter, is associated with a reduced survival rate. Possibly, the mixed venous oxygen tension is an important prognostic factor once pulmonary hypertension has developed.

These generalizations should not obscure the fact that very considerable variation exists in the following relationships:

- between morphologic changes and function tests
- between loss of recoil and extent of emphysema
- between initial FEV_1 and later decline
- between FEV_1 and arterial blood gases
- between hypoxemia and pulmonary hypertension
- between maximal $\dot{V}O_2$ and FEV_1

FEV$_1$ DECLINE IN RELATION TO REGIONAL EMPHYSEMA DISTRIBUTION

	Smokers			Ex-smokers		
	UZ	LZ	G	UZ	LZ	G
Number	11	4	22	6	5	8
Age	48	62.5	55.2	54.4	59.2	56.6
FEV$_1$ (%P)	64	68	60	65	50	46
TL$_{CO}$ (%P)	61	66	56	78	53	63
PaO_2 (mm Hg)	74	77	69	73	66	69
VC decline	− 104	− 30	− 26	− 1	− 2	+ 5
FEV$_1$ decline	− 86	− 38	− 43	− 46	− 3	− 1

- between perceived level of dyspnea and function status
- between resting function tests and maximal $\dot{V}O_2$

The course of this syndrome in any one patient can thus be seen to depend on a very complex interrelationship between risk factors and responses.

CLINICAL ASPECTS OF PATIENTS WITH CHRONIC AIRFLOW LIMITATION

Important Questions

A complete approach to the patient with chronic airflow limitation, when seen for the first time, can be sketched by describing those questions that must be answered before a detailed management plan can be proposed.

History

- Duration of cough?
- Amount of sputum? Constancy? Characteristics?
- Attacks of wheezing?
- Family history? (alpha$_1$-AT or cystic fibrosis?)
- Smoking history? Other family members?
- Occupation? (present and previous)
- Time course of dyspnea? Episodic or constant?
- Severity of dyspnea?
- Evidence of right ventricular failure?
- Systemic symptoms—loss of weight, memory changes, etc.?

- Sleep pattern? Daytime somnolence?

Physical Examination

- Uniformity of air entry?
- Rhonchi or rales?
- Use of accessory muscles?
- Evidence of respiratory fatigue?
- JVP increase? Liver enlargement? Peripheral edema?

Radiologic Examination

- Hyperinflation?
- Evidence of loss of vascularity?
- Large or very large bullae?
- Is disease "localized"? (Possibility of resectional surgery?)
- Cardiac hypertrophy?

Pulmonary Function Test Report

- Hyperinflation?
- Severity of flow limitation?
- Abnormality of DL_{CO} measurement?
- Hypoxemia or hypercapnia?
- Is blood gas data "compatible" with flow limitation?
- Need for other tests (mechanics; regional function; ventilatory control)?
- Need for sleep studies?
- Previous FEV_1 data? Rate of decline?
- Response to bronchodilator?

Other Laboratory Data

- Is a sweat test indicated?
- Polycythemia?
- EKG evidence of RV hypertrophy?

CHAPTER

9

ASTHMA

"His asthma, I think, is not of the same kind as mine."

INTRODUCTION

At our present stage of knowledge, asthma is very difficult to define. A good case can be made for a definition based only on measured airway reactivity; if this is adopted, perhaps the syndrome should be called "non-specific airway reactivity," and the word "asthma" reserved for situations in which specific antigens or inducing agents have been identified. Reynolds[3437] has noted that "asthma represents at least five clinical entities that no longer can be lumped together for diagnostic purposes under a common syndrome, but must be differentiated." Atopic patients can be differentiated by family history, by evidence of skin sensitivity, and by an elevated IgE level. Clinical manifestations of asthma and airflow limitation vary considerably in patients with the same degree of airway reactivity.[525] A definition containing the word "reversible" is inappropriate, since the airflow limitation is not reversible in many patients; hence, reversibility, however defined, is an unsatisfactory criterion.[4156]

In one study in which the response to bron-

chodilators of 60 "asthmatics" and 28 normal subjects was compared, it was not possible to make an exclusive separation between the two groups.[1556] Another group of authors found a greater response to salbutamol in asthmatics than in chronic bronchitis patients, but they noted that the presence of "irreversible" airflow limitation did not disprove the diagnosis of asthma.[1070] Dodge, Cline, and Burrows[4158] surveyed 3504 subjects (of whom 628 were younger than 15) in Tucson, Arizona. Those subjects were studied again 8 years after the initial study. All were from households other than Mexican-American ones. The authors noted that physicians tended to label men as having emphysema and women as having asthma. The study concluded: "While the labels of asthma, emphysema, and chronic bronchitis do identify subjects with high rates of respiratory symptoms and laboratory abnormalities, these labels do not isolate specific syndromes in cross-sectional analyses of our population." These difficulties will only be resolved when our understanding of the cellular basis of airway reactivity has advanced beyond its present stage, and little is to be gained by semantic refinement in its absence. One editorial writer concluded that "a precise definition of asthma remains elusive, despite the labours of a distinguished international panel, but in functional terms the most

---

*Sakula's historical notes on Sir John Floyer's book *A Treatise of the Asthma*, which dates from 1698, should be consulted by anyone interested in the history of this condition.[4241]

generally accepted is that asthma is variable airways obstruction."[1354]

It is easy to take the basic concepts of the meaning of airway narrowing and its relationship to airflow limitation for granted. Moreno, Hogg, and Pare's detailed analysis of this interrelationship[4161] is a valuable corrective to simplistic ideas. The question of whether induced airflow limitation is bound to be higher in the presence of an initially lowered FEV_1 is an important one and in many of the reported studies has been insufficiently considered. In asthmatics, there is a linear relationship between response to methacholine and baseline FEV_1.[4070] Inhalational bronchial challenge testing is described in Chapter 5.

A recent volume on asthma edited by Clark and Godfrey[4247] contains particularly good reviews of the epidemiology of asthma and of exercise-induced airflow limitation.

Incidence

A random sample of the population of Oslo, Norway, aged between 16 and 69 years, was studied by questionnaires, physical examination, chest x-rays, and spirometry. Of the population, 1.4% were considered to be asthmatic.[1101] Of a random sample of 485 people in South Wales, 2.9% were considered to have current asthma[1366]; an additional 3.6% had mild asthma, as determined by history. These categories were noted to include both those with sputum eosinophilia without chronic bronchitis and those with chronic bronchitis and reversible airflow obstruction. Although these are distinct categories,[1545] they may be difficult to separate. A study of 2311 people in Tucson, Arizona showed that eosinophil percentage was related to decreased airflow in older subjects, and a group of elderly non-smokers with asthmatic bronchitis could be clearly identified.[1393] In a population of 134 adults and 213 children in East Boston,[4251] eucapnic hyperpnea with cold air indicated that children with a doctor's diagnosis of "asthma" were twice as likely to respond as others and that 92% of current asthmatics were responders. However, 18.9% of asymptomatic children also responded to the test. In a similar study by the same authors of 171 adults who were also tested with eucapnic hyperventilation with subfreezing air,[3965] a positive response was associated with a history of asthma. Data from this study suggested that

airway hyperresponsiveness and atopy were independent traits.

A survey of 1303 white residents of Lebanon, Connecticut[4210]—the participants were 7 years and older and were examined in 1972 and again 6 years later—showed that in the interval 50% of the asthmatics were in remission and 19 new asthmatics were identified. Seventy-seven per cent of those who complained of wheezing had improved and only 4.6% were worse. The mean FEV_1 declines in the non-asthmatics were -6.3 mL/year, but the declines were four times higher than this in the asthmatic individuals.

Cockcroft, Berscheid, and Murcock[3106] have recently conducted a survey of 300 randomly selected college students (131 men and 169 women) aged between 20 and 29. In this group, 2.7% had current asthma, 3.3% had asthma on occasion, and 3.3% had a history of past episodes, making a total incidence of 9.3%. The histamine threshold was measured and found to be unimodal, "the asthmatic patients representing a subgroup within the hyperresponsive distribution tail rather than a separate distribution peak." In a later report based on 400 randomly selected college students, the same authors[4216] noted a PC20 of less than 8 mg/mL of histamine in 10.3% of the population. In nonatopic subjects, the rate was 6.1%, but reached 33% in markedly atopic subjects.

In another series, 3% of "normal" people had an increased reactivity to histamine or methacholine.[535] Malo and his colleagues[3083] evaluated 100 non-smokers who were between 20 and 60 years old (50 men and 50 women). Using the PC20 (the dose of methacholine required to lower the FEV_1 by 20%), they found that 34 subjects had a PC20 <128 mg/mL. Four of the eight subjects in whom it was <16 mg/mL had lower initial values of FEF_{25-75}.

Asthma is particularly important in children. In Boston, a survey of 650 children revealed that 9.2% had a persistent wheeze.[1394] These children had more frequent coughing, more phlegm, more past hospital admissions for respiratory disorders, and a higher incidence of a history of asthma. There was also a higher level of maternal cigarette smoking in the households from which they came.

Another survey of 4000 elementary school children in western Pennsylvania[3964] found that the FEF_{25-75} averaged 92.1% of predicted in 107 children with doctor-diagnosed asthma and about the same in 225 children with a persistent wheeze. By comparison, it averaged 99.4% of predicted in children who had had a chest illness before the age of 2 years. A complete review of childhood illness associated with wheezing cannot be attempted here, but it may be noted that prospective studies of these children seem to indicate that about half of those whose wheezing started before the age of 7 and stopped before adolescence remain wheeze-free.[4227] However, it is commoner for children who wheezed before the age of 7 to continue doing so during adolescence. A recent survey of school children between the ages of 7 and 11 around Lewes in Britain found that 5% were using inhaled medication.[5298]

It has been established that growth delay occurs in asthmatic children[4228] but by age 21 their height and weight are not different from controls. The syndrome of asthma is an important cause of disability in children, as noted earlier, and in adults. In observations of 1849 men over an 8-year period, "asthma" was a high risk factor for days lost from work, this number being six times higher in those with an "asthma" designation.[1551] In another study of 277 subjects aged 21 and who all suffered from wheezing before the age of 7, it was found that those who had been free of symptoms for 3 years were not distinguishable from a control group.[1395] However, 60% of the subjects who had ceased wheezing had an increased reactivity to histamine.

There has been clear evidence that hospital admissions for asthma have increased considerably in the past few years. Halfon and Newacheck[4169] estimate that hospital admissions for childhood asthma increased by 45% from 1979 to 1984 in the United States. Similar increases have been documented in the United Kingdom,[4230–4232] in Auckland in New Zealand,[4220] and in Canada. At a recent workshop on this question, we noted the following data from Canada[4170]:

Hospital Discharges for Asthma According to Patient Age (per 100,000)

	0–14 Years		15–64 Years		>65 Years		Total	
	M	F	M	F	M	F	M	F
1974	286	183	77	112	307	225	152	142
1976	310	187	62	100	267	207	143	132
1978	369	237	70	119	256	212	159	152
1980	551	343	83	135	343	296	215	198
1982	542	326	82	134	314	284	208	192
1983	659	385	92	150	351	328	244	220

The change in classification categories between International Classification of Disease (ICD) 8 and ICD 9, which occurred in 1979, complicates the analysis, but there is little doubt that hospital admissions for asthma have generally been increasing, although admissions for all respiratory causes and total hospital admissions have fallen (in Canada by about 15%) over the same period. A more recent and comprehensive review of asthma mortality and hospital admission rates for asthma for the different provinces of Canada[5363] indicates that both of these have increased over the last 10 years.

In a prospective study of 261 consecutive episodes of severe acute asthma in 1 year in the United Kingdom, Arnold, Lane, and Zapata[4215] noted that 67 episodes were treated at home by 34 family physicians, 148 episodes were treated in the hospital after referral from family physicians, and 46 were treated in the hospital as a result of self-referral by the patient. Comparisons indicated that those cases treated in the hospital were more severe, as judged by PEFR data and tachycardia, than those treated at home. Children and those living near a hospital were more likely to be treated in the hospital. Self-referrals occurred in all age groups.

There have been a number of studies of seasonal variations in asthma morbidity. Goldstein and Currie[4239] concluded that in New York City, emergency visits for asthma increased in September, reached a peak in October and November, and declined in December. They contrasted this with data from New Orleans, where no regular autumnal increase occurred. In that city, higher levels were found in April, May, and June. On the basis of their studies,[2534, 3165] it seems possible that such diverse factors as seasonal allergens and exposure to indoor air pollutants play a part in determining the variability of asthma.

A detailed study conducted between 1976 and 1983 by the Royal College of Family Practice in Britain[4162, 4163] shows that the autumn peak coincided with a rise in the attack rate of acute bronchitis, "suggesting that autumnal asthma may be due to viral infections occurring against the background of bronchial hyperreactivity induced by summer pollen exposure." In a study of 10 pollen-sensitive asthmatics,[4253] it was shown that their mecholyl sensitivity increased in the pollen season of May and June. Packe and Ayers[5099] analyzed a remarkable increase in acute asthma episodes in a town in Britain that coincided with a thunderstorm. They concluded that this was possibly attributable to an increase in airborne fungal spores.

There is convincing clinical evidence that viral infections in children are associated with increased wheezing in asthmatics,[1552] and live attenuated influenza A virus has been shown to increase histamine reactivity in asthmatics 14 to 28 days after inoculation.[1418] However, in one study, only about 10% of exacerbations of asthma could be attributed to infection.[1553] In another study, viral but not bacterial infections were associated with increased wheezing.[1345] High humidity encourages the growth of house mites (Pyroglyphidae). One study showed these to be commoner in 23 homes of asthmatics as compared with 75 control homes.[3414] Among the many unexplained features of asthma is the recent observation that the PEFR is lower in children in Britain if they were born in July and August.[3430]

It is clear that a great deal more comparative study is required before this problem will be fully understood. As noted in Chapter 6, we have observed that hospital admissions due to acute respiratory episodes in the summer in southern Ontario are related to sulfate aerosol and ozone levels; ozone increases airway reactivity. Whether these environmental factors are generally important remains to be established.

Occupational asthma is discussed in Chapter 16. In one subject with increased airway reactivity, alcohol produced acute airflow limitation,[3441] and passive exposure to cigarette smoke also induced airflow limitation, which was reversed by metaproterenol.[3153] Asthma mortality is discussed later in this chapter.

Pathology

It is not surprising that there are no detailed pathologic studies of the lungs of mild asthmatics and that their relationship to the changes found in status asthmaticus is not clear. Thurlbeck[585] has summarized the morphologic changes found in patients dying in status asthmaticus. The increase in bronchial smooth muscle is well documented,[1213, 1474] amounting to a threefold increase in both area and volume and consisting of hyperplasia of muscle cells rather than hypertrophy.[1474] Severe small airway disease and mucus blockage have been noted in some fatal cases.[1507] The pathogenesis of these changes is discussed in Chapter 1.

Sobonya[4223] reported on pathologic findings in six elderly asthmatics (mean age of 64 years) with severe long-standing allergic asthma of mean duration of 45 years. They were compared with seven controls of similar age. The FEV_1 levels in the subjects with asthma had been usually between 17% and 58% of predicted and was never better than 83% of predicted. All were symptomatic, and all were on steroids. The area of bronchial muscle was increased, and the basement membrane was thicker in these subjects. In two of the asthmatics, the small airway diameter was decreased. In one, L_m was increased and very mild emphysema was present, but there was no emphysema in the other six.

A new dimension to the understanding of the pathology of asthma has been added by Laitinen and colleagues' studies of bronchial biopsies in eight non-smoking asthmatics.[4192] None had had a respiratory infection within 2 months of the study; two had mild disease, three moderately severe disease, and three severe disease. The light and electron microscopy studies showed epithelial destruction at all levels sampled, with involvement of ciliated cells and increase in intraepithelial cells and mast cells. The authors concluded that "Epithelial destruction in the respiratory tract of the asthma patients with mild to severe bronchial hyperresponsiveness was prominent enough to expose the epithelial nerves for specific or nonspecific stimuli." There was no close correlation between the degree of ciliary damage observed and the increase in bronchial hyperresponsiveness measured.

There have been many studies of bronchoalveolar lavage in human asthmatics and in animal models of asthma. A workshop concluded that the technique was safe as a research procedure in asthmatics.[4196] The data from humans show an increase in mast cells,[4181, 4252] changes in alveolar macrophage function,[4225] and evidence of inflammatory changes in animal models with increased airway reactivity,[4193, 4195] but the increased airway responsiveness seems to be more closely related to the edema produced by inflammation than to the infiltration of neutrophils. Bronchoalveolar lavage has also shown that eosinophilia is an important component of the late asthmatic reaction after allergen inhalation.[5100]

Physical Signs and Radiology

As noted in Chapter 3, Kraman[4237] has studied the wheeze that may be heard in normal subjects on forced expiration and concluded from the components of frequency within it that it originates from large airways and may be related to recoil pressure. Detailed study of the wheezes of asthma that make use of sophisticated sound recording equipment suggest that they originate either from vortex-induced wall resonance or dynamic fluid flutter.[4151] Continuous nocturnal recording showed that maximal wheezing occurred between 4 and 4:30 AM. The degree of wheezing correlated well with the simultaneously measured FEV_1.[4186] The degree of hyperinflation seen on the chest film is related to the decline in FEV_1.[1314] The pulmonary vasculature remains normal in asthma, an important feature that distinguishes it from pulmonary emphysema.

Pathophysiology

Although some experimental studies indicated that antigen challenge was followed by increased permeability in the lung,[2215] we found no relationship between permeability measured with ^{99m}Tc-DTPA and airway reactivity in 10 clinically stable asthmatics and nine non-asthmatic controls.[2201] As noted in Chapter 5, there is no correlation between *in vivo* reactivity and *in vitro* muscle response to histamine.[3085] Atropine has no antihistamine effect *in vitro*.[2346] We have recently summarized the evidence and have suggested that the primary defect in asthma may be an inability to control the osmolarity and ion concentration of the fluid lining the airway surface.[4248]

A recent and important area of study has been the changes in pulmonary mechanics and respiratory muscle function that follow induced airflow limitation. In seven asymptomatic asthmatics who were between 21 and 46 years old and had baseline flow values only slightly abnormal, it was found[2750] that a fall in FEV_1 with histamine to 49% of the control value led to a 10.7-fold increase in the inspiratory work rate of inspiratory muscles—from 6.7 to 71.4 joules/min. Elastic work accounted for 69% of total work during the control period and for 57% of work during bronchoconstriction. The authors of this study concluded that during induced asthma the increased work is largely the result of hyperinflation and that recruitment of intercostal muscles exceeded that of the diaphragm. In one subject, the relationship between FEV_1 change and esophageal pressure changes was as follows:

FEV_1	FRC	f*	P_{pl} (cm H_2O swings)
2.70	2.68	5	10
2.34	2.92	5	20
1.35	3.88	7	45

The doubling of the pressure swing for a reduction of FEV_1 of 360 milliliters should be noted. In further experiments on respiratory muscle activity in normal subjects during inspiratory resistive loading and elastic loading,[3417] the same group concluded that both influence respiratory muscle behavior during expiration by diminishing expiratory braking by inspiratory muscles, and also by recruiting expiratory muscles.

The increased RV after histamine administration has been attributed to a loss of recoil,[1437] but Martin and his colleagues have recently confirmed that persistent inspiratory muscle tone in intercostal muscles during expiration may account for the rise in FRC, which they noted was linearly related to an increase in RL in seven asymptomatic asthmatics challenged with histamine.[1388] In experiments on five normal subjects with hyperinflation to between 78% and 83% of VC by external resistance, they showed that persistent activity of intercostal inspiratory muscles, rather than the diaphragm, during expiration was responsible for the hyperinflation.[4238]

Another important area of research has been the analysis of upper airway changes. Collett, Brancatisano, and Engel[2637] have reported that airflow limitation induced in 12 asymptomatic asthmatics by histamine or water aerosol (in which expiratory flow rates fell to 36% of their control value) led to a fall of cross-sectional area of the glottis of as much as 45% in some subjects. Five also showed mild glottal constriction during inspiration. Ten centimeters of CPAP during the induced asthma temporarily abolished the glottal constriction. In a more recent series of similar experiments, the same authors[4159] studied eight seated asthmatics. They measured the diameter and vertical displacement of the laryngeal and oropharyngeal airways in two planes by an x-ray fluoroscope attached to a videotape recorder that also recorded flow and volume. After histamine-induced bronchoconstriction, which reduced the FEV_1 to 35% of its initial value, the lateral diameter of the larynx at mid-expiration narrowed over a distance of 10 centimeters above the glottis, and the glottal lateral diameter fell by 46%. They concluded that in asthma "upper airway muscles take part in the co-ordinated increase in respiratory muscle activity and act as accessory organs of ventilatory control." The implications of these results in challenge testing and in response to ozone or SO_2 have not yet been fully studied.

Others have noted changes in glottal area in asthma.[2651, 3029] In one set of experiments, it was concluded that laryngeal resistance increased less on provocation of bronchoconstriction than it did during a spontaneous attack.[4198] However, the role of this factor in airflow limitation has yet to be precisely determined. It may combine with increased inspiratory muscle recruitment to cause the increased FRC that follows histamine challenge.

Any review of the enormous literature on the comparative effects of different bronchodilators in asthma is beyond the scope of this volume. However, Paterson, Woolcock, and Shenfield[1347] have contributed an excellent review of bronchodilators with 292 references. Sourk and Nugent[3237] have restudied the response of normal subjects to bronchodilators and have published 95% confidence limits of the response as measured by PEFR, FEV_1, and FEF_{25-75}. The latter test showed the greatest percentage of change.

As naloxone (an opiate antagonist) has no effect on the response to cold air challenge, endogenous opiates are thought not to be involved in the response.[3373] It also did not affect the 6 AM dip in function in six asthmatics,[3385] but, for unexplained reasons, flow rates were apparently better on the day after the first naloxone infusion.

A number of studies have been conducted to throw light on the relative importance of H_1 and H_2 receptors in the response to histamine.[537, 554] Both H_1 and H_2 receptors are present in asthmatics,[563] and the histamine response has been thought to be mediated by H_1 rather than H_2 receptors.[1523] In a very detailed and comprehensive study, Eiser and his colleagues[540] concluded (1) that the same pattern of H receptors existed in asthmatics and normal subjects, (2) that histamine-induced constriction was mediated by H_1 and not by H_2 receptors, and (3) that histamine was an important mediator of an immediate airway allergic response.[540] Recent studies with cimetidine (an H_2 blocker) and chlorpheniramine (an H_1 blocker) on modifying the histamine response in asthmatics and normal subjects[3103] have indicated that H_2 receptors mediate bronchodilation in asthmatics but not in healthy subjects. In studies on eight asthmatics, it was shown that chlorpheniramine increased the concentration of histamine required to lower the FEV_1 by 20%.[2615]

The role of prostaglandins in the lung is still poorly understood.[1436, 1469, 1505] In normal subjects, PGE_2 causes initial bronchoconstriction and then maximal bronchodilation in 15 minutes.[3390] If ipratropium bromide is given, the degree of the initial bronchoconstriction is increased. It was concluded that PGE_2 acts directly on bronchial smooth muscle and not via a vagal reflex initiated by airway irritant receptors.

Infusion of prostaglandin intravenously to induce abortion caused a fall of FEV_1 from 2.72 to 2.34 in two patients with a personal or family history of asthma.[1454] Aerosolized $PGPF_{2\alpha}$ produced inconstant effects in 17 asthmatics,[1452] though they have been described as responding to less than one-thousandth of the dose tolerated by normal subjects.[1436] In another comparison between normal and asthmatic subjects, the asthmatics were 8.5 times more sensitive to histamine and 150 times more sensitive to $PGF_{2\alpha}$.[1408] Recent studies on prostaglandins[3090] that made use of indomethacin, an inhibitor of prostaglandin synthesis, showed that this drug produced bronchodilation in normal, but not in asthmatic, subjects. However, it reduced histamine reactivity in the asthmatics but not in the normal subjects. The authors concluded that beta-adrenergic stimulation induced changes that were dependent on prostaglandin production. Experiments with phenylephrine (an $alpha_1$ agonist) indicate that increased $alpha_1$ receptor activity in bronchial smooth muscle is not the primary abnormality responsible for the variability between asthmatics in non-specific airway hyperreactivity.[3372] Experimentally in sheep, histamine produces the same effects by aerosol as by intravenous injection.[3088]

Apart from hyperventilation, exercise (see later section), and irritant gases, such as SO_2 and ozone (see Chapter 6), many other factors and drugs cause increased airflow limitation. Propanolol caused a fall in SGaw, the largest being from 279 to 60.[1544] In eight asthmatics, the fall in SGaw after propanolol was 40% to 56%, with atropine reversing the effect.[1440] It probably acts by unopposed vagal action. Calcium blocking agents such as nifedipine reduced the level of induced bronchoconstriction in dogs[2523] and reduced the effect of antigen challenge in eight grass pollen–sensitive asthmatics.[2485] However, the role of these agents in asthma is complex.*

It seems clear that nocturnal gastroesophageal reflux may worsen asthma at night.[1356] One experimental study apparently showed that in 15 cases of asthma with symptoms of reflux,

---

*See references 2837, 3387, 4175, 4176.

acid perfusion of the lower end of the esophagus lowered the vital capacity by 210 milliliters and increased the SBN_2/L slope.[1371] No reflux occurred into the lung. Cimetidine has been reported as relatively ineffective in such cases, however.[1356] In a study that made use of esophageal pH monitoring in 18 asthmatic children, eight had reflux during sleep, but the relationship of reflux to worsening of their asthma was unclear.[4208] In these subjects, histamine sensitivity increased 90 minutes after a dilute solution of HCl (0.001 N) was drunk. Gastrointestinal reflux should probably be considered as a possible aggravating phenomenon in some asthmatics.[3381]

PULMONARY FUNCTION IN SUBJECTS IN REMISSION OR WITH MILD TO MODERATE AIRFLOW OBSTRUCTION

Level of Perception of Airflow Limitation

In 1971, Cade and Pain[531] studied 56 asthmatics and found, through the use of methacholine, a clear separation between normal and asthmatic subjects. Rubinfeld and Pain more recently studied nine asthmatics in detail and, in a paper entitled "How mild is mild asthma?,"[1539] reported the following data, obtained when the subject first noticed chest tightness:

	Baseline	After Methacholine
TLC (%P)	103.2	109.8
FRC (%P)	107.7	127.6
RV (%P)	141.4	181.3
FEV_1 (%P)	90.6	73.4
SGaw (%P)	75.1	39.6

They note that considerable changes in both airflow and residual volume were present by the time symptoms were noticed. They also studied 82 patients with asthma and noted that 15% of these could not detect a fall of FEV_1 below 50% of the predicted level when airflow limitation was induced with mecholyl.[1517] The "poor perceivers" did not seem distinguishable by other characteristics. The same investigators also noted that a 25% change in airflow was usually not detected by asthmatics, even though a significant elevation of residual volume had also occurred.[1500] However, Burki and his colleagues[1443] reported that asthmatics were better at detecting added loads to inspiration than were normal subjects. Others[4189] have reported similar findings, noting that after bronchodilation the asthmatic's perception returns to normal.

In other studies, no differences between asthmatic and normal subjects have been observed, and some observers have reported reduced load detection when chronic airflow is present.[1403] It has been suggested[3418] that threshold detection may be related to "behavioral styles" in both normal and asthmatic subjects. In this study of 12 normal and 12 asthmatic subjects, there were no differences between the two groups. In another study of 10 asthmatics, tightness of the chest was noted when the FEV_1 was reduced to 72% of its baseline value, and the residual volume was nearly doubled. In this series, the $\dot{V}max_{50\%}TLC$ was reduced to 42% of its control value.[1407]

In a comparison between 19 asthmatics with initial airway obstruction and 11 asthmatics with normal airflows,[3428] 10 of the 19 in the first group felt short of breath, but nine did not; there was no difference in airflow measurements between them. After salbutamol, all improved objectively, but only nine noted subjective improvement. The authors suggested that initial airway obstruction might impair the perception of changing airway tone in some asthmatics. It is possible that those with inaccurate perception are at greater risk.

In one interesting study, 81% of asthmatics found inspiration more difficult during attacks than expiration. Only 19% said that expiration was the problem during attacks; whereas 78% of 56 physicians expected that asthmatics would find expiration more difficult.[1362] This difference may be explained by two factors. First, physicians are influenced by expiratory tests of airflow measurement. Second, physicians do not understand that the patient's perception of a load arises from concentration on respiratory muscles, and most of the work performed by these muscles is during inspiration. Patients are better than physicians at estimating their peak expiratory flow rate.[1508]

Chapman and Rebuck[3426] have also noted that asthmatic patients find inspiration more difficult than expiration. The maximal mouth expiratory pressures measured at TLC and the maximal inspiratory pressures measured at RV were slightly higher in 29 asthmatics, who were between 5 and 25 years old, than they were in a normal control group.[4153]

Pulmonary Function Test Changes

Much attention has been given to the lability and periodicity of airflow limitation in asthmatics. Normal subjects show a slight circadian rhythm effect on expiratory flow rates,[1520] and it has been shown that there is a diurnal rhythm effect that slightly modifies the response to histamine challenge in asthmatics.[3444] The lability of some of these patients is shown by the fact that airway resistance can be modified by suggestion in asthmatics.[1446] Nocturnal and early morning worsening has been well documented[1528, 1537, 1546] and is not influenced by cortisol infusion (which corrects circadian rhythm changes),[1546] by disruption of sleep,[1528] or by the use of slow-release salbutamol or oral theophylline.[1522] Dips of up to a 40% decline in peak expiratory flow rate have been recorded,[1420] and the magnitude of this change does not appear to be related to age, sex, morning level of the peak expiratory flow rate, or duration of asthma.[1420] Airway resistance is highest at 7 AM,[441] and residual volume increases at 6 AM.[1537] It has been suggested that loss of sympathetic tone at night might be responsible for these changes,[1536] but there is no direct evidence for this explanation. These and other changes during sleep were discussed in Chapter 4.

Patients with non-atopic asthma have been said to have a more impressive circadian rhythm than atopic patients. In the latter, nocturnal asthma has been ascribed to low catecholamines at 3 AM.[1375] Chen and Chai[3438] reported that warm humidified air for 8 hours during the night abolished the early morning decrease in PEFR in eight asthmatics and suggested that airway cooling might be important in its genesis. On the basis that 4 hours of recumbency lowers the PEFR, others have suggested that the nocturnal dip might be related to posture.[4246] In REM sleep in asthmatics, there are decreased EMG activity in intercostal muscles, a fall in tidal volume, and an increase in diaphragmatic EMG activity.[1404] A slightly greater fall in oxygen saturation (of about 3.9%) has been noted in asthmatics, as compared with normal subjects,[1404] during REM sleep.

The PEFR has been extensively used for home monitoring by patients. In one study of 69 non-seasonal asthmatics measuring their own PEFR four times daily for 2 weeks, it was shown that those with a higher coefficient of variation were at higher risk of an acute exacerbation.[4233] When the PEFR was monitored daily for 14 days by 27 subjects with mild airway hyperresponsiveness but a normal FEV_1,[4177] only half the subjects showed a variability of PEFR greater than that in normal non-hyperresponsive subjects. In a third study, 246 patients monitored their PEFR four times daily for 2 weeks.[4184] In 38, there was a significant dip in morning PEFR, and in half of these, it increased after bronchodilator therapy was instituted. The authors concluded that the presence of a morning dip was not a risk factor in the long-term prognosis.

By means of comparisons of maximal flow on helium/oxygen and on air, it has been concluded that atropine preferentially dilates larger airways.[1491] Other investigators have reached the same conclusion but found that it only holds in asthmatics without infection, chronic bronchitis, or a smoking history.[1554] Atropine has also been found to lower hyperinflation more than isoproterenol,[1456] from which it was concluded that parasympathetic system–mediated bronchial smooth muscle contraction must be important in asthma.

As noted in Chapter 5, it is unclear whether firm conclusions on the probable site of airway narrowing can be drawn from differential air and helium flow measurements. Possibly, the method used indicates sites of flow limitation. By comparing air and helium flows in 15 asthmatics after terbutaline, Fairshter, Novey, and Wilson[3431] concluded that the first effect was on peripheral airways, but a later effect was on larger airways. In another study, prednisolone in a dose of 40 milligrams IV was followed by improvement in FEV_1, which started 3 hours later and was maximal at 9 to 12 hours.[1409] Effects on both large and small airways were found. Studies on 20 asthmatic children using density-dependent flow measurements led to the conclusion that peripheral airways were mainly involved in five subjects, central airways predominated in four subjects, and both were involved in eight subjects. All the abnormal groups had an increased residual volume, but three of the 20 appeared normal in all tests.[1390]

Changes in Lung Mechanics, Lung Volumes, and Flow Rates

The broad outlines of pulmonary function changes in asthma have been known for many years.[1] However, the data have been considerably refined and extended by recent studies. In Table 9–1, various stages of asthma of increasing

Table 9–1. STAGES IN SPASMODIC ASTHMA

Stage*	Clinical Observations	FEV	FRC and TLC	Gas Distrib.	Regional Distrib. $\dot{V}$	$\dot{Q}$	Arterial Pa_{O_2}	Pa_{CO_2}
I	Complete remission	N	N	N	N	N	N	N
II	Partial remission (asymptomatic)	N or ↓	N or ↑	ABN	ABN	ABN	N or ↓	N
III	Moderate bronchospasm (rhonchi)	↓ or ↓↓	↑	ABN +	ABN +	ABN	↓	N
IV	Severe bronchospasm	↓↓	↑↑	ABN + +	ABN + +	ABN +	↓↓	N
V	Status asthmaticus							
	a. Initial	↓↓	↑↑	ABN + +	ABN + +	ABN + +	↓↓	N
	b. Terminal	↓↓	↑↑	ABN + +	ABN + +	ABN + +	↓↓	↑

*Possible State of Lungs:

  I : Normal, apart from increased bronchial reactivity.
  II : Airway resistance of major bronchi increased: Dynamic compliance is frequency dependent. Small airway blockage?
  III : II + beginning atelectasis: altered lung recoil.
  IV : Obstruction in major bronchi and bronchioles + atelectasis. Beginning mucous plugs.
  V : Extensive mucous plugs; atelectasis; fatigue, severe acidosis, and danger of cardiac arrest.
  N = Normal; ABN = abnormal.

severity are defined. Asymptomatic asthmatics may be found to have abnormalities of function in addition to being hyperreactive to histamine. There has been discussion as to which ventilatory test is most sensitive to detecting change.

Cade and Pain reported that 51 of 57 asthmatics in complete clinical remission showed abnormalities of some tests of function. If spirometry only has been used, one-third of these would have been missed.[1458] The fall of dynamic compliance with frequency may be abnormal in asthmatics when the FEV_1 is still normal.[1543] In another study comparing 18 asymptomatic asthmatics to normal subjects, the following data were obtained[1501]:

	Normal Subjects	Asthmatics
C_{st}	0.29	0.25 (L/cm H_2O)
C_{dyn} (f = 60)	0.28	0.14 (L/cm H_2O)
RL	1.7	2.8 (cm H_2O/L/sec)
C_{dyn} (f = 60) post salbutamol	0.28	0.20 (L/cm H_2O)

In non-smoking asthmatics, C_{dyn}/f (although invasive) is clearly a very sensitive indicator of abnormality.[1385, 1484] However, phase differences between measurements at the mouth and from the plethysmograph may introduce error into this value.[1444] In a study of nine asthmatics before and after induced bronchoconstriction,[3015] it was concluded that the data were consistent with the hypothesis that when a compliant upper airway is coupled with high airway resistance during panting caused by an occluded airway, transmission of changes in

alveolar pressure to the mouth is incomplete. Errors are signaled by the development of a loop between mouth pressure and volume. It is probable that this source of error is not of major significance in asymptomatic patients.

Significant gas compression may occur at 75% VC in mild asthmatics.[1389] PmaxTLC is useful in separating subjects with asthma from those with emphysema, and, as noted in Chapter 7, it is not affected by histamine or isoproterenol.[1219] Measured apparent increases in TLC in asthmatics from body plethysmography have to be interpreted with caution in the light of Stanescu's recent work showing major potential error in this measurement (see Chapter 5). The divergence between helium equilibration (with careful attention to continuing this long enough) and the plethysmographic data are greater the worse the airflow measurements.[1480] The increased TLC, which occurs whatever method of mesurement is used, has been attributed to loss of recoil and to increased inspiratory muscle activity.[1513] Probably, both mechanisms are involved.

In normal subjects challenged with methacholine,[3840] a 20% fall in partial expiratory flow volume was accompanied by an increase in RV from 1.54 to 2.37 liters. The SBN_2/L increased from 0.88% to 2.84% after challenge. The change in RV was thought to account for about 24% of the increased slope. Although the SBN_2/L index may be abnormal in asthmatics with a normal FEV_1,[1] its degree of abnormality is not a sensitive indicator of the extent of regional ventilation changes.[1460] When asthmatics are treated with salbutamol, there is a consistent relationship between the increasing FEV_1 and the decreasing SBN_2/L.[4178] However, in the subjects studied, the VC increased on treatment almost as much as the FEV_1. Other authors have concluded that the FEV_1 is a more sensitive indicator of change after bronchodilator administration than are changes in the SBN_2/L.[1466] Steady-state indices of ventilation distribution are more sensitive to such differences[1, 1481] but may not be superior to flow rate measurements. A detailed study of multibreath N_2 washouts in asthmatics before and after antigen-induced bronchoconstriction[4188] showed poor correlations between changes in ventilation distribution indices and the FEV_1, SRaw, and RV/TLC differences. It has been shown that inequality of time constants does not contribute to the curvilinearity of the expiratory flow curve.[1455] It also has been shown that lung recoil increases when the TLC, which had increased during the asthma episode, returned to normal.[1534]

In some asthmatics, a single deep inspiration is followed by a transient increase in airflow obstruction,[1527] amounting to about a 70% increase in RL.[1453] This transient increase in RL is greater the lower the initial FEV_1.[1401] For this reason, measurements of FEF at 25% VC may be greater if forced expiration is begun at 50% VC after a 5-second breath hold than if a full inspiration to TLC is taken.[1379] In a comparison between 9 normal and 22 asthmatic subjects that made use of the oscillation method of airway resistance measurement,[4240] the data suggested that a faster inspiratory velocity led to more irritant receptor stimulation and that the effect would be minimized if a slower inspiration were taken before the FEV_1 was recorded.

In one group of 16 asthmatics of mean age 46 years, elastic recoil was reduced when the FEV_1 was 72% of predicted and the residual volume was 152% of predicted.[1525] In asthmatics after bronchodilation, P_{st} at low lung volumes has been observed to increase,[4245] probably as a result of reduction in trapped gas volume. Evidence has been published that suggests that a 20 to 60 minute application of negative pressure to the chest wall of normal subjects might lead to an increase in lung distensibility, but the phenomenon was seen only in one of six subjects tested.[3448]

In 16 of 19 symptom-free asthmatics, the CV/VC ratio was elevated or the slope of the alveolar plateau on expiration was abnormal.[1473] In this series, CV was above the level of FRC in some patients, both in sitting and supine positions. However, the CV was found to be less sensitive than the RV/TLC ratio or the MEFV curves in 205 asthmatic children,[1467] a finding others have confirmed.[1188] The FEF_{25-75} is commonly abnormal in asymptomatic adult asthmatics.[1457] In 178 asymptomatic asthmatic children in whom the ventilatory flow rates were all normal, the residual volume was increased in 25%.[1502] Other authors reported that spirometric abnormalities were still present in 24 children even after a year free of symptoms.[1368] Oberger and Engstrom[1412] studied 21 children with severe asthma over a 5-year period and noted that the RV became more elevated as the children grew. They concluded that overinflation could worsen over time, although the FEV_1 did not reflect this.

The FEF_{25-75} should be calculated as an isovolume flow rate; otherwise, it fails to record change correctly when the lung volumes change.[1497] If this is not done, it is an unreliable indicator of change after histamine.[1506] If corrected, it can be a sensitive measurement.[1488, 1504]

There is considerable difference of opinion as to which flow rate measurement is the most sensitive indicator of change. Some authors find the FEV_1 to be as sensitive as other indices.[1499] Others find the $\dot{V}max_{60\%}$ or 70% TLC and $\dot{V}max_{75\%}VC$ to be the best indices of induced bronchoconstriction,[1383] or sometimes the $MEF_{75-90\%}$ is preferred.[1378] The simplest measurement, that of peak flow, has been found satisfactory in following changes in airflow limitation,[343, 345] particularly in children. As the RL has a coefficient of variation of about 19% in children with bronchoconstriction, it is doubtful if its use would add anything to flow rate measurements. Permutt[1495] reviewed the choice of methods for measuring bronchodilator response.

The use of a mouthpiece has been shown to increase resting ventilation in asthmatic subjects.[2994] However, measurements made during resting ventilation have been used to detect airflow obstruction. In 16 asthmatics in whom isoproterenol increased SGaw and VC but did not change FEV_1, the flow during tidal volume breathing increased from 0.61 L/sec to 0.80 L/sec.[1490] The percentage of volume expired to the peak flow point of the tidal volume is correlated with other measurements of airflow limitation.[1357] This value is 50% in normal subjects but fell to between 10% and 30% when the FEV_1 was between 25% and 40% of predicted. However, the measurement is of dubious value, since it is almost certainly influenced to a large extent by the instrumentation used to measure it. Several papers have attempted to identify the site of airflow limitation (or its relief) by the use of air and helium/oxygen during MEFV curve recording. However, it should be noted that it is not clear how valid this approach is (as was pointed out by Knudson and Schroter[3060]).

It is important to note that the coefficient of variation in flow measurements is much greater in reactive subjects than it is in normal ones, as shown by the following data reported by Bonsignore and his colleagues[5412]:

Coefficient of Variation

	$\dot{V}max_{50\%}$ air	$\dot{V}max_{50\%}$ He/O_2	$\Delta \dot{V}max_{50\%}$
Normal subjects	5.3%	7.0%	25%
Reactive subjects	14.0%	17.0%	>45%

Despas and his colleagues[1442] classified asthmatics according to their response, which was measured by flow rates in air and with 80% helium breathing. As noted earlier, it has been suggested that those subjects with a central airway flow limitation pattern are those without infection and who are non-smokers.[1423] Fairshter and Wilson[1398] used this method in 65 asthmatics and concluded that as the airflow limitation became more severe it became more peripheral.

We have recently studied flow curves in 15 asthmatics before and after the use of Berotec or ipratropium bromide.[2921] There were no differences in response to the two agents. The patients were divided into two groups by their response—a group in whom flow was primarily improved (Δ FEV_1/Δ FVC >1), and a group showing volume response (Δ FEV_1/Δ FVC <1). The significance of these differences in response is unclear. No advantage is gained by studying flow rates with SF_6 and helium in asthmatics,[1352] but it has been suggested that boluses of helium and SF_6 may be used to study gas distribution in asthmatics.[3318, 3422]

In quiet breathing, expiratory resistance is always found to exceed inspiratory resistance. However, in a proportion of cases (7/16), inspiratory resistance may exceed expiratory resistance during the early phase of expiration at high breathing frequencies, an effect possibly attributable to changes in the glottis or extrathoracic trachea.[1397] As noted earlier, the general importance of upper airway and laryngeal changes in asthma cannot yet be critically evaluated.

Measurements of Regional Ventilation

A comparison between ventilation distribution measured with ^{133}Xe and deposition of a ^{99m}Tc-labeled pertechnetate aerosol showed that in asthmatics, when the $\dot{V}max_{50\%}$VC improved, central deposition of the aerosol was reduced and peripheral deposition was increased.[1530] Reduced aerosol penetration has been attributed to the presence of mucus plugs.[3400] In asthma, aerosol deposition is very dependent on whether a normal tidal volume or a fast or slow VC is taken.[33] Ruffin and colleagues[44] used a radioactive aerosol to detect the site of deposition of histamine and concluded that "a given dose deposited in large airways was more effective in increasing airway obstruction than the same dose distributed peripherally."

The question of aerosol delivery has become important because aerosol bronchodilators are now so commonly used. It is very important that patients be carefully trained in their use.[57] But even when properly used, only about 3% of the dose reaches alveoli, a further 5.8% reaches conducting airways, and the rest is deposited in the pharynx.[45] A slow deep inspiration with aerosol injection at about 20% VC and a 10-second breath hold at TLC has been found optimal,[1414] but inhalation at 80% TLC, when the airways are more widely dilated, has also been recommended.[502] Three puffs usually produce a maximal effect.[1433] A number of papers have confirmed previous work[1] indicating that zones of regionally reduced ventilation are common in asthma and may be present without measurable airflow limitation.

When data from ^{133}Xe and radioalbumin scans for perfusion were combined in subjects with a mean FEV_1 of 56% of predicted, zones with reduced ventilation commonly also showed reduced perfusion. However, in some instances perfusion appeared unaffected.[1516] Delayed xenon clearance is commonly detected in such studies.[1470, 1509] In one study of eight asthmatic subjects given 4 to 10 milligrams of methacholine intramuscularly,[1503] $\dot{V}max_{60\%}$VC fell from 4.1 to 2.3 L/sec, and $\dot{V}E$ to clear xenon increased from 3.6 to 9.9 liters. All zones of the lung were affected to the same extent. When one of the subjects later had a spontaneous asthma attack, xenon studies showed much more variation in ventilation between zones than was present during the experiment, although the time for half clearance was the same on both occasions. Other studies have shown changes in regional distribution after histamine challenge.[3399]

Andersen and Haghfelt[1421] studied 15 asthmatics with a mean FEV_1 of 80% predicted, 10 of whom had an abnormal SBN_2/L slope before fenoterol was given. After drug administration, the FEV_1 increased from 2.25 to 2.89 (100% of predicted), but the SBN_2/L slope was still abnormal in seven. However, 13 of the 15 still had abnormal zones of regional ventilation as detected by [133]Xe. They noted that the drug generally improved ventilation distribution to the lower zones, with blood flow distribution little changed. Studies of six asthmatics using [81]Kr (13-second half-life), showed grossly abnormal ventilation distribution "with large segmental or even lobar areas of reduced ventilation."[1392] These defects were improved significantly after bronchodilator treatment.

In a recent study of 15 asthmatics, all nonsmokers[3392] in whom PEFR values were slightly lowered, [81]Kr was used for ventilation scanning. Areas of delayed ventilation were detected in all subjects. After isoproterenol administration, which increased PEFR by a mean value of 24%, the regional ventilation defects were unchanged. Defects in perfusion distribution were also noted. Further intensive treatment leading to another increase in PEFR of 29% was followed by improvement in regional ventilation distribution. Bulow, Lindell, and Arborelius[1432] studied 10 asthmatics in remission by having them inhale specific antigens in the right lateral or decubitus positions. Subsequent ^{133}Xe studies showed a reduced ventilation to the right lung when that had received more of the dose. Perfusion was less affected. The phenomenon took 15 minutes to develop fully after inhalation.

It seems clear that regional reductions of ventilation are a feature of asthma, even when ventilatory flow rates are relatively normal. This phenomenon probably accounts for the increased SBN_2/L slope in asthmatics in remission noted 30 years ago.[1] However, the extent of abnormality of ventilation distribution is probably related to the decrement in airflow.[4205]

$\dot{V}/\dot{Q}$ Distribution

As noted in the previous paragraph, regional perfusion may be normal to a zone of reduced ventilation in the lung in asthma or it may be reduced. A widening of $\dot{V}/\dot{Q}$ distribution accounts for the increased physiologic dead space value commonly found.[1542] In 178 asymptomatic asthmatic children, in whom the residual volume was increased in 25%, a reduced arterialized capillary PO_2 was found in 23%.[1502] With increasing severity in children with asthma, the $(A - a) D_{O_2}$ and physiologic VD are both increased when significant symptoms are present.[1487] After isoproterenol is given, an increased $(A - a) D_{O_2}$ has been observed to fall, with little change in RL in symptomatic asthmatics.[1486]

The six inert gas method of quantitating $\dot{V}/\dot{Q}$ has been used to study cases of asthma. Wagner and West summarized this data[1370] collected from seven subjects. One of these, when in remission with an FEF_{25-75} of 2.2 L/sec, had a narrow distribution of $\dot{V}/\dot{Q}$ and a small shunt. In another patient whose FEF_{25-75} was only 0.3 L/sec, a considerable fraction of cardiac output was perfusing zones with $\dot{V}/\dot{Q}$ ratios between 0.01 and 0.1. This pattern was also seen in five other patients. Isoproterenol increased cardiac output by 50%, airflow limitation decreased, pulmonary arterial pressure was unchanged, and the arterial Pa_{O_2} fell by 12 mm Hg. The proportion of blood flow to the low $\dot{V}/\dot{Q}$ regions increased from a mean of 20% to about 40%. The rise in cardiac output with no change in pulmonary artery pressure indicates a fall in pulmonary vascular resistance, presumably attributable to a reduction in resistance in the regions with reduced ventilation. By means of the six inert gas method, a more recent study[4185] of 10 asthmatics with moderately severe symptomatic asthma, whose FEV_1 varied from 22 to 58% of predicted, showed that six had minimal $\dot{V}/\dot{Q}$ abnormality, whereas in four it was increased. The FEV_1 was not different between these two groups. Studies on oxygen breathing and after clemastine (a histamine inhibitor) administration showed that compensatory vasoconstriction was probably common in asthma and led to better $\dot{V}/\dot{Q}$ matching. One of the subjects studied had an unexplained high shunt component. Exercise-induced airflow limitation is followed by a further widening of the $\dot{V}/\dot{Q}$ distribution, as measured by this technique.[3416]

The Bohr isopleth method of analysis[1471] also

showed increased perfusion of the large poorly ventilated region of the lung in asthmatics following use of a bronchodilator; this probably accounts for the observation that use of a bronchodilator is commonly followed by a fall in arterial Po_2. In one series of 25 stable asthmatics of mean age 38 years,[1515] FEV_1 increased from 1.8 to 2.4 liters; $\dot{V}max_{50\%}VC$ increased from 1.3 to 2.1 l/sec; $VD_{physiol}$ increased from 186 to 253 milliliters; and Pa_{O_2} fell from 77 mm Hg to 69 mm Hg. The SBN_2/L was unchanged. However, it is not clear why this phenomenon is seen in some cases but not in others, since the differentiation cannot be made by spirometry or by differences in lung volumes.[1471] In an earlier publication, Wagner[1448] noted that ". . . in some asymptomatic patients with asthma, as many as half of the lung units may lie behind completely closed airways and have very low but finite $\dot{V}A/\dot{Q}$ ratios as a result of collateral ventilation."

No detailed studies of adult asthmatics appear to have been conducted in which the resting Pa_{O_2} was compared with their ventilatory status. However, in a group of 113 asthmatic children, who were studied with an arterialized capillary sample[3445] and during an attack-free period, 70% of them had significant hypoxemia at rest when first tested. A formula was devised that related the Pa_{O_2} to C_{dyn}, total thoracic gas volume, and airflow limitation. The lowered Pa_{O_2} reflects the presence of low $\dot{V}/\dot{Q}$ units and hence indicates that these are commonly present when symptoms are not severe.

Diffusing Capacity

The fact that the diffusing capacity is normal in asthma and it is useful in distinguishing between asthma and emphysema were emphasized in the last edition of this book.[1] It is now known that $DL_{CO}SB$ rises above predicted values in asthmatics as airflow limitation becomes more severe,[253, 1494, 1512] but k_{CO} is commonly unchanged[253] or increases less.[1512] Both return to normal levels as the FEV_1 improves.[1494] This interesting phenomenon has been attributed to two mechanisms:

1. The height of perfusion (Zone 2). This increased by a mean of 4 centimeters in seated asthmatics as compared with normal subjects[1512];
2. The effect of inspiration against a resis-

tance. $DL_{CO}SB$ increased by 18% in 10 normal subjects,[1494] presumably by causing a transient increase in pulmonary capillary blood volume.

Both of these mechanisms may be operative, but it is also possible that the high $DL_{CO}SB$ readings reported in some asthmatics may be artifacts caused by errors in timing in the presence of severe airflow limitation. The $DL_{CO}SB$ in asthmatics is higher if the Ogilvie methodology is used than if the "three equation" computation is employed,[3883] but is not much different from techniques using the Jones or Ferris methods of timing. The observed $DL_{CO}SB$ increases in asthmatics if the breath holding time is prolonged,[3869] a phenomenon not observed in normal individuals. However, this result is only obtained if the "three equation" method of computation introduced by Graham and his colleagues is used.[3869]

In contrast, other studies of the effect of different breath holding times with helium or SF_6 as carrier gases showed that $DL_{CO}SB$ fell with increasing apnea in both normal and asthmatic subjects (in contradistinction to emphysema, in which it rose).[404, 1113] By further analysis, the authors concluded that the ratios of $D/\dot{V}A$ and $VT/\dot{V}A$ in asthma were unequally distributed in parallel units.[404]

In one comparison of $DL_{CO}SB$ and $DL_{CO}SS$ in asthmatics,[1097] the ratio was more than 2.0 in these subjects. As noted in the last edition, very severe airflow limitation in asthma may be accompanied by a lowered steady-state DL_{CO}. Through the use of arterial PCO_2 to compute steady-state DL_{CO} in 10 asthmatics, $DL_{CO}SS$ rose and $DL_{CO}SB$ fell as airflow limitation decreased.[298] It has been noted that $DL_{CO}SB$ does not decline in asthma with duration of the disease.[1457] As noted later, a lowered DL_{CO} in asthma should raise the suspicion of bronchiectasis, concomitant pneumonitis, or complicating aspergillosis.

Tracheal Mucus

Shelhamer and Kaliner[4179] have recently contributed a useful review of respiratory mucus production in asthma, noting evidence that parasympathetic stimulation results in increased secretion of mucous glycoproteins and that many substances, including arachidonic acid, prostaglandins, aspirin, leukotrienes, and histamine, increase secretory activity. Mucociliary function is often, but not universally, found to be impaired in asthmatics.[2945] An important finding has been that asthmatic sputum induces ciliostasis.[2951, 2956] This may be an important mechanism leading to the development of mucus plugs in severe asthma attacks. It has also been shown that leukotrienes increase mucus production.[3374] The physical properties of mucus and mucociliary clearance are discussed in Chapter 3.

As a result of challenge, tracheal mucus velocity was shown to be reduced in six non-smoking asthmatics.[959] A brief report indicated that it might also be reduced when no challenge was administered, but this data was incompletely described.[1510] In another study of 12 asthmatics, however, the tracheal mucus velocity was normal.[1429] Other investigators found a fall in asthmatics in remission or with mild airflow limitation.[94] In another study of eight non-smoking asthmatics in complete remission[4202] on no medication, muciliary clearance measured by a radioaerosol technique was depressed in the asthmatics, compared with parallel studies in eight normal subjects.

These variable results are not surprising in a condition that in other respects is very variable. The fall of mucus velocity on challenge is an important finding: slower transport as asthma worsens could be a significant factor (possibly the major factor) in leading to water loss from mucus and its consequent impaction in small airways—a feature of status asthmaticus. The observation that sputum from asthmatics during an attack of asthma inhibits ciliary function[2951, 2956] may explain reduced mucociliary clearance and mucus plugging phenomena.

COMPARISON BETWEEN CHALLENGE TESTS IN ASTHMATICS

The special sensitivity of asthmatics to SO_2 and to aerosol sulfates is discussed in Chapter 6. In Chapter 5, challenge testing is described. Through the use of histamine, reactivity can be graded as follows, based on the dose required to cause a 20% fall in FEV_1.

- Severely reactive = 0.25 mg/mL or less
- Moderately reactive = 0.25 to 1.0 mg/mL
- Mildly reactive = 1.0 to 8.0 mg/mL
- Normal or non-reactive = >8.0 mg/mL

It is important to note that a significant percentage of "normal" subjects have responses in the range between 0.25 mg/mL and 8.0 mg/mL.[3106] As has been noted, there appears to be no relationship between *in vivo* histamine response and *in vitro* tests of bronchial muscle response after surgical removal of tissue.[4203]

It has been shown in a sheep preparation that histamine increases the flow in bronchial arteries.[4150] Although it may be suspected that histamine response may be affected by bronchial flow, specific understanding is lacking. The demonstration that bronchial flow may be important in exercise-induced airflow limitation is noted in the next section.

The effect of mecholyl is enhanced if two maximal inspirations and expirations are made before the mecholyl is inhaled,[1364] and lung inflation leads to better airflow in those nonreactive to mecholyl than in those reactive.[3084] The response is unaffected by hyperventilation during the test.[3101] It has been shown that both the histamine and mecholyl response are enhanced in asthmatics 40 minutes after inhalation of ultrasonically nebulized water.[4207]

It has been suggested that the slope of the histamine dose response curve is largely determined by the initial airway caliber.[3087] Dehaut and his colleagues[3388] did repeated studies on 18 stable asthmatics and concluded that the $PC20FEV_1$ was the most reproducible of all the indices of response. This value had a 95% confidence limit of ±1.6 times the single two-fold concentration difference and was more reproducible than any of the threshold concentration values. In a paper in the same journal, Cockcroft and his colleagues[3089] compared 27 normal and 41 asthmatic subjects. They showed that the PC20 was the best discriminator of normal and asthmatic subjects and that the threshold measurement might be useful in population studies. The correlation between the two measurements in the asthmatics was close (r = 0.89). Between two separate determinations of the histamine threshold, the r value was 0.91. Between first and subsequent PC20 determinations, the r value was 0.98.[3089]

Others have shown good repeatability in asthmatics in the response to histamine repeated after 2 hours, and reproducibility after an interval of 65 days was also good.[4174] In this study, the confidence limit for the latter interval for PC20 was 2.12 times the twofold concentration. However, in isolated cases there may be considerable short-term variation in response.[4255]

Other studies of survey methods and analytical techniques have been published.*

Ipratropium bromide inhibits the effects of methacholine in both normal and asthmatic subjects but does not change the threshold or slope constants in either group after histamine.[4254] This study led to the interesting suggestion that asthmatics might "lack a normal mechanism that inhibits severe airway narrowing during histamine challenge." Jean-Luc Malo and his colleagues[4197] have studied the response curves after histamine and mecholyl in normal and asthmatic subjects in great detail. They concluded that the PC20 index correlates more closely with clinical status than does the slope of the response curve.

In 15 asthmatics restudied after an interval of a year, the threshold dose to lower the FEV_1 by 20% (PC20) was found to reflect the clinical status of the patient,[560] but it is clear that fluctuations in symptom severity may occur without change in reactivity.[525] Others have found a relationship between the PC20 and the morning PEFR (r = 0.79)[556] and between medication use and PC20.[553] There is some evidence that beclomethasone may reduce airway reactivity,[1555] but it is unaffected by use of salbutamol.[1386] A mean fall of 1% of O_2Hb saturation accompanied a 38% fall in PEFR in 55 reactive adults challenged with histamine.[1427] The largest fall (7%) occurred in two subjects, both of whom had a less than average fall in PEFR, for unexplained reasons. Aerosolized antigens administered to 12 asymptomatic asthmatics caused the expected increases in RV and R_L but no increase in TLC.[1475] The first change noted was a parallel shift in the MEFV curve with no change in slope. $Vmax_{60\%}$ of control TLC was the most sensitive indicator. Induced bronchoconstriction is thought to cause large airway constriction as the initial change,[1459] although other experiments indicate peripheral airway involvement as well in some cases.[527] Some investigators have concluded that both central and peripheral airways are involved in most cases.[533] Subjects with hay fever challenged with mecholyl only show a central airway response.[527] In airflow limitation induced by ragweed antigen in sensitive subjects, the fall in FEV_1 is dose-dependent.[1465] Changes in RV and SBN_2/L were variable and not related to dose. The investigators in this study concluded that reflex spasm involving postganglionic efferent parasympathetic

---

*See references 3093, 3094, 3097, 3099, 3104, 3105, 3196, 3394, 3421.

fibers was not a major component of the response.[1465] The $\dot{V}_{iso}V$ increases after ragweed challenge,[533] and changes can be prevented by giving a slow-reacting anaphylactic antagonist before the challenge is administered.[541] Studies on five atopic asthmatics in which hexamethonium and atropine were administered before histamine and mecholyl challenge[1399] led to the conclusion that in these subjects bronchial hyperreactivity was due "to a change in characteristics of efferent parasympathetic pathway at a site distal to the ganglion, possibly at the smooth muscle. . ."

The change in SGaw after challenge does not offer any advantage over the FEV_1.[4217] However, the differential effects on the two indices in normal and asthmatic subjects probably reflect the fact that a deep inspiration inhibits bronchoconstriction in normal individuals but enhances it in asthmatics. It has been shown that the time required for recovery after increases in R_L are induced by histamine is prolonged with larger doses.[4199] It has also been shown that the response to methacholine and histamine in mild asthmatics is enhanced by the prior administration of prostaglandin (PGD_2).[4152] The authors suggested that there was a postreceptor increase in smooth muscle contractility. This response may be related to the increased reactivity that occurs after inflammation.

Distilled water aerosol produces more coughing and a greater increase in SRaw than does normal saline.[3371] In this detailed study of eight asthmatics, atropine or cromolyn sodium inhibited the SRaw response but did not affect the coughing, whereas lidocaine anesthesia of the upper airway inhibited the cough but not the bronchoconstriction. The water response has been quantified; the volume required to induce a 20% fall in FEV_1 was 9 milliliters or less in 48 of 55 asthmatics. Normal subjects had a less than 10% fall after inhaling 33 milliliters.[3406] Other studies have confirmed these findings,[4213, 4244] and it has also been shown that methacholine response is increased 40 minutes after inhalation of ultrasonically nebulized water.[4207] Although one study indicated that positive ions might accentuate exercise challenge in children,[4243] two other studies of negative and positive ions found no adverse effect.[4218, 4219]

In a large series of 433 atopic patients, Kreukniet and Pijper[567] showed that histamine reactivity was closely related to antigen sensitivity. Others have found a close relationship (r =

-0.91) between wheal diameter on skin tests and the dose of histamine needed to lower the FEV_1 by 29%.[565] In comparisons between normal and asthmatic subjects challenged with mecholyl, wide variations were noted between the dose required to cause a 25% fall in SGaw (bronchial sensitivity) and in the slopes of the dose-response curve (bronchial reactivity).[526] It is not clear whether this differentiation is important in practice. Acetylcholine sensitivity is related to sensitivity to mite allergens[3447] and increases after challenge with them. The study of airway reactivity in asthmatics has added several important new components to our understanding of the syndrome, but it is clear that much remains to be learned. The standardization and increasing use of challenge testing have become useful aspects of the work of the routine pulmonary function laboratory, but a definitive analysis of the contribution of the technique to diagnosis and management has not yet appeared.

CONTROL OF BREATHING

There is conflicting evidence on the respiratory drive in asthmatics. Some investigators have found that as airflow limitation increases, the $P_{0.1}$ increases,[1464] and higher values have been found in asthmatics than in other subjects with chronic airflow obstruction[1492, 1498] or in normal individuals.[1492] However, there is also evidence that in asthmatics the P_{100} slope plotted against change of Pa_{O_2} is depressed,[1493] and a lower dP/dT response has been shown not to be attributable to the increased FRC nor to the airflow obstruction.[1382] In a re-examination of this question, Kelsen, Fleegler, and Altose[1346] found a higher P_{100} response in asthmatics than in normal subjects and showed that it increased with increasing airflow limitation induced by mecholyl. At a Pa_{CO_2} of 55 mm Hg, the P_{100} was 14.6 cm H_2O in asthmatics and 6.3 cm H_2O in normal controls.

In an interesting comparison between 17 asthmatics and six subjects with pneumonia with the same Pa_{CO_2}, dP/dT and inspiratory flow rate (VtT/ti) were increased in the asthmatics during quiet breathing, which showed increased respiratory center output. This phenomenon was not seen in those with pneumonia, although respiratory frequency was increased in both groups. The hyperinflation in those with asthma may be related to the increased drive.

A grossly reduced hypoxic drive is very dangerous in an asthmatic, as shown by the remarkable case of a 17-year-old asthmatic reported by Hudgel and Weil[1363] from Denver. He presented in respiratory failure, severe hypoxemia, cor pulmonale, and polycythemia, with an FEF_{25-75} of 0.74 L/sec and a normal $DL_{CO}SB$. A very depressed hypoxic ventilatory drive was found in three of four healthy members of his family. Operations such as glomectomy not only do not lead to improvement[1483] but would seem to be contraindicated.[1496] Calculation of the optimal breathing frequency in terms of minimal respiratory work in asthmatics shows that it should be lower than in normal individuals. Five subjects had FEV_1/FVC ratios of 35%, 38%, 49%, 50%, and 56% and increased RL values of 6.8 to 21.7 cm H_2O/L/sec. The frequency for minimal work was between five and seven breaths/min in four subjects and 16 breaths/min in one.[1438]

EXERCISE-INDUCED OR HYPERVENTILATION-INDUCED AIRFLOW LIMITATION

In the second edition of this book, the observation that airflow limitation might occur on exercise in some asthmatics was noted. We also described a patient in whom we documented a fall of 60% in FEF_{25-75}, whose function tests were normal at rest, and who had no history of asthma.[1] Others have noted similar cases.[1472] This syndrome, together with airflow limitation induced by cold air hyperventilation, is now known to be common in asthmatics. During the past 15 years, more than 150 papers have appeared in relation to it. In this section, only a brief résumé of this information can be attempted. Several useful reviews of the phenomenon have appeared.* A recent volume on asthma[4247] contains a very useful review by Godfrey of this phenomenon.

The frequency of the phenomenon among asthmatics in different series varies between about 39% and 93%,[1416] and declines in FEV_1, FEF_{25-75}, or PEFR of 30% often occur. The effect is maximal 5 to 20 minutes after exercise. Hyperventilation on dry air may cause a similar fall in FEV_1 to that observed on exercise† and possibly occurs more frequently.[1445] Different

---

*See references 1416, 1529, 4167, 4180, 4204.
†See references 1361, 1374, 1405, 1479.

forms of exercise cause the same degree of airflow limitation if the ventilation is the same.[1548] In occasional patients, bronchodilation has been documented to occur on exercise.[4183] However, maximal exercise is not an adequate screening test for airway hyperreactivity,[3095] and it has been reported that the relationship between mecholyl sensitivity and voluntary isocapnic hyperventilation response is not precise.[3382]

Other studies have suggested that voluntary isocapnic hyperventilation can be used as a screening test.[3446] Some authors have found a close relationship between methacholine response and airflow limitation induced by cold air ($-18°$ C) breathing. In a comparison in 214 asthmatics, the r value between respiratory heat exchange to lower the FEV_1 by 10% (the $PD_{10}RHE$) and PC20 for methacholine was 0.86, and the response was highly reproducible.[3415] The phenomenon is related to histamine reactivity.[1359, 1434] The cold air response is not related to baseline FEV_1.[3244] It has also been shown to be highly repeatable. In studies of 36 asthmatic and 13 normal subjects, the response to cold air provocation—with two estimates at an interval of 2 to 3 weeks—had a least squares regression value of r of 0.93 between the two measurements.[4214] Atopic status was not important. An r value of 0.92 between histamine and cold air response was also documented.

In 1977, Chen and Horton[1381] observed that no airflow limitation occurred if warm and humidified air was breathed. Strauss and his colleagues[1451] confirmed this and concluded that water loss from the airway was the triggering stimulus, a finding others have confirmed.[1422] McFadden[1391] has suggested that heat loss is the trigger, but carefully studied patients have been reported in whom exercise-induced airflow limitation (EIAL) occurred after warm humidified air was breathed.[3404] The question of whether the response is primarily triggered by temperature change or by water loss from the airway has been intensely debated.

Anderson's study of 22 asthmatic children[4173] showed that a response could be elicited on exercise while breathing hot (32 to 40° C) air containing only 3 to 10 mm H_2O/L. It also indicated that water loss and not heat loss was the important mechanism. Other experiments have clearly favored the role of osmotic rather than temperature changes in the genesis of EIAL,[4190, 4224] but some have been equivocal.[4194] Recent data indicate that the prior administration of cromolyn sodium (which inhibits the response) is associated with changes in airway temperature,[4226] and detailed studies of the pattern temperatures of controlled expirations in normal subjects indicate that the respiratory gas-wall heat transfer coefficient is very sensitive to expiratory velocity.[4200]

Detailed temperature measurements in different regions of the airway under different breathing conditions indicate that considerable temperature swings can be recorded in distal airways (subsegmental) with cold air breathing during hyperventilation.[4148] Recent experiments on 10 anesthetized, open-chested dogs have demonstrated that bronchial blood flow is immediately and considerably affected by changes in airway temperature.[4147] It may well be that many of the observed responses (or their attenuation) are to be explained by changes in bronchial blood flow, and this line of enquiry seems promising. We have suggested[4248] that the essential defect may be a failure to control the osmolarity and ion concentration of the fluid lining the airway surface. There may well be a variety of intermediary mechanisms involved, such as reduced beta$_2$-adrenoreceptor activity.[4187]

The observation that nose breathing during exercise prevents or reduces airflow limitation supports either of the hypotheses.[1447] Airflow limitation may also be induced by a cold shower but not a warm one. This response is related to cooling of the airways, since taking cold showers while breathing warm humidified air did not cause airflow limitation.[1489] If a brief spurt of hard exercise is given for 30 seconds before the 6-minute test exercise period, the response is reduced,[1519] suggesting that mediator release is an important component of the phenomenon.[1358, 1413, 1444] Other data are compatible with this theory, but the role of mediator depletion is not yet completely understood.[4206] The interesting observation that a histamine challenge test prior to exercise reduced the response in 29 cases supports this hypothesis.[1526] Some authors have found that cold air inhalation induces "refractoriness" to exercise-induced airflow limitation,[2217] but there is also evidence that "refractoriness" is caused by the exercise rather than by airway cooling.[3420] Response to exercise or hyperventilation is not affected by the order in which the challenges are administered.[3410]

In an interesting comparison between seven atopic and six non-atopic asthmatic subjects on treadmill exercise,[4250] it was shown that both groups had an increase in plasma histamine and in serum high molecular weight neutrophil chemotactic activity as a result of the exercise. These results suggest that release of mast cell mediators is independent of the atopic state.

The technique of cold air eucapnic voluntary hyperventilation testing has been standardized[4191] and shown to differentiate asthmatics from normal individuals. The response to cold air is not only shown by expiratory flow rate measurements. A comparison between nine normal and nine asthmatic subjects showed that in the latter cold air challenge increased the SBN_2/L index from 2.41 to 5.39%.[4211] The change was related to 1/log of the PC20. The initial PC20 of the asthmatics on histamine was 0.47 mg/mL, compared to a value of 22.4 in the normal subjects. Their FEV_1 was 71% of predicted. The response is blocked by salbutamol, isoprenaline, and nifedipine[1348, 1666] and is attenuated by sodium cromoglycate.*

Data on the efficacy of ipratropium bromide are conflicting.[1435, 1541, 4168] Some have found that the response is blocked by atropine sulfate,[527, 1315, 3434] and others report no effect.[1485] Data on the effect of steroids are also conflicting.[1411, 1737] Preliminary data suggest that the response may be modified by verapamil, a calcium antagonist.[4182] Cromolyn and terbutaline have an additive effect.[2702] It has been reported that the exercise-induced response can be modified by hypnosis,[3378] but it is unaffected by negative ions,[3092] lidocaine anesthesia in the airway,[3401, 3402] or acupuncture.[3425] Aerosol salbutamol has been found to be more effective than oral administration in prevention of EIAL.[1461]

The observation that sodium cromoglycate is more effective in a particle size of 2 microns than one of 11 microns[1410] suggests that the small airways are an important site for the exercise-induced effect. However, studies on helium/oxygen mixtures in five asthmatics, in which the $\dot{V}max_{60\%}TLC$ was reduced to 29% of the pre-exercise value,[1450] were interpreted to indicate primarily a large airway response. Other investigators have suggested that a large airway response occurs first and is followed by small airway changes.[1376]

Alpha-blocking agents have been found to block the effect by some investigators but to be ineffective by others.[1369, 1428] Propanolol enhances the effect of hyperventilation and exercise; this effect is inhibited by phentolamine, leading to the conclusion that the vagus and alpha-adrenergic system are involved.[1380] EIAL

has been found to cause an increase in mast cells and in serum neutrophil chemotactic factor,[2676] but isocapnic hyperventilation did not evoke these responses. There is no evidence that acetylcholine is involved in the genesis of the response,[3440] and endogenous opioids are not involved in it.[4164]

Significant hyperinflation of the lung usually accompanies the decline in FEV_1[1406]; in one carefully studied case, the residual volume nearly doubled.[1476] In 19 subjects, the rise in FRC and fall in FEV_1 related significantly (r = −0.43).[1415] In addition, the $(A − a) D_{O_2}$ increases in asthmatics on exercise, in contrast to the decrease in this measurement that occurs in normal individuals.[1419] In six asthmatic boys on hard exercise, the fall in FEV_1 was not accompanied by pulmonary hypertension.[1425] Compared with normal subjects, no changes occur in circulating norepinephrine, in $PGF_{2\alpha}$, or in metabolites.[1430] However, other investigators have reported that plasma catecholamines rise more in asthmatics with EIAL than in those without.[1518] Cyclic AMP rises similarly on exercise in asthmatics and normal subjects.[1550] The observation that clemastine, an H_1 receptor antagonist, inhibited EIAL in 10 adult asthmatics[1521] suggests that these receptors are important in the phenomenon. Changes in blood histamine levels appear variable and inconstant.[3395] It is probable that at least two mechanisms are acting to produce the responses to exercise and hyperventilation.[3396]

Patients with hay fever usually have no response or a minimal change,[1387] and atopic subjects with allergic rhinitis do not develop EIAL.[1373] However, it has been shown that subjects with rhinitis who breathe cold air do have an increase in leukotrienes, as determined from subsequent nasal lavage specimens.[4160]

A remarkable case of acquired EIAL in a nonasthmatic speed skater[1468] serves to emphasize the importance of testing for this phenomenon whenever effort dyspnea is complained of and resting pulmonary function tests and chest x-rays are normal. Another single case report of a 32-year-old woman with a 10-year history of wheezing during exercise, with no atopy and normal baseline spirometry,[4212] showed that both FVC and FEV_1 fell during exercise and that the ratio of expiratory flow rate to inspiratory flow rate went from 0.76 at rest to 1.07 on exercise. Fiberoptic bronchoscopy during the attack showed that an area of corniculate and cuneiform cartilages in the posteroinferior portion of the arytenoepiglottic folds collapsed over

---

*See references 1400, 1402, 1424, 1463, 1533, 2607, 3397, 3420, 4172, 4201.

the laryngeal vestibule, causing upper airway obstruction.

STATUS ASTHMATICUS

In the last edition of this book, we noted that several reports indicated that mortality from asthma was increasing. The international data on mortality experience up to 1972 has been reviewed by Stolley.[1477] It appears that a rise occurred between 1962 and 1966 in the United Kingdom, Ireland, Australia, and New Zealand, but was not reported from Germany, Holland, Belgium, or the United States. It was suggested (but not proved) that the use of pressurized aerosols of isoproterenol in the former countries may have been the cause of the difference.[3407] More recent reports indicate that asthma mortality may be rising in the United Kingdom.[4234, 4235] Sears and his New Zealand colleagues[4256] have noted that asthma mortality in New Zealand still appears to be about double that in the United Kingdom. In a study of fatal cases, they comment that 25% of patients died less than one hour from the apparent onset of the attack and that "in both countries, however, most deaths were associated with poor assessment, underestimation of the severity, and inappropriate treatment (over-reliance on bronchodilators and underuse of systemic corticosteroids), and delays in obtaining help."

A study organized by a research committee in Britain[4242] analyzed 147 cases certified as dying from asthma in the Mersey region in 1979. The panel considered that 89 had probably died of asthma, but there was a net overestimate of 13%. Accuracy was highest in the younger age groups.

Several interesting analyses of mortality have appeared. One report reviewed 1169 consecutive hospital admissions for severe asthma. It was noted that in 458 cases treated in a special unit, only one case of ventricular arrest occurred. Among patients treated on general medical wards, there were nine ventricular arrests, of which three were fatal.[1367] In another series, four of 39 patients, all of whom required mechanical ventilation, died.[1511] All patients who died had very labile asthma. In them, inadequate treatment, underuse of steroids, and overuse of sedatives were identified as characterizing the most severe cases. In this series, the Pa_{CO_2} averaged 77 mm Hg before intubation. Cochrane and Clark[1335] analyzed 19 pa-

tients who died of asthma in London in 1971. They noted that in half these fatalities there had been no physiologic assessment of airflow; seven of the 19 had received no steroids; sedatives had been given to 13 of those who died; and deaths were noted to be frequent in the early hours of the morning on general medical wards. This observation underlines the importance of teaching all medical residents that as the Pa_{CO_2} rises in this condition, the tidal volume falls, and the signs of airway obstruction diminish. When the patient becomes drowsy instead of being restless and agitated, a nurse's note that the patient is "sleeping quietly" may be an indication for immediate intervention.

The question of how rapidly the condition may progress is still difficult to answer. It has been noted that tests of expiratory flow may be normal or better than usual 2 weeks before death, and one patient was found dead in bed having been relatively well and active the day before.[1540] Recently, Stableforth[3407] reported on a 27-year-old woman whose asthma had apparently given no trouble for many months. She became faint and breathless in a supermarket and used an inhaler but died 20 minutes later before an ambulance arrived.

There is little doubt that severe hypoxemia is the usual cause of death, with both mucus plugging in the airways of the lungs and right ventricular hypertrophy being common features.[1540] It has been noted that the adrenals are often small at autopsy. Myocardial changes have also been suspected of being related to death in some patients. In another patient who died, twice daily measurements of PEFR as an outpatient did not prevent a fatal outcome.[1532] Wide diurnal variations in flow rates are a bad sign.* In 10 severely ill asthmatics, the FEV_1 started to improve 1 hour after a single IV dose of 40 milligrams of prednisolone, and the maximal response occurred in 8 hours.[1549] However, in a study of 38 patients with severe disease, McFadden and his colleagues[1514] reported on a comparison between isoproterenol hourly, given to all the subjects, and this regime plus hydrocortisone in a single injection at three different dose levels. There was no evidence that the steroid had a beneficial effect.

One study of the treatment of 10 patients with severe asthma concluded that 20 milligrams of methylprednisone sodium succinate was as effective as 125 milligrams when both were given intravenously every 6 hours for 7

---

*See references 1367, 1372, 1511, 1532.

days of treatment. The initial FEV_1 levels in the two groups compared were 800 milliliters and 600 milliliters, respectively.[3439] The FVC, FEV_1, and PEFR values rose steadily over a 10-day period, with no difference between the two regimes. A recent observation that very high levels of antidiuretic hormone existed in 10 children in status asthmaticus points to the danger of fluid overload in the treatment of this condition.[3398]

The use of mechanical ventilation in 18 patients who required 48 episodes of assisted ventilation between 1973 and 1985 in Edinburgh[4166] (with one patient being ventilated 29 times) was reviewed. The authors stressed that physical exhaustion was the main indication for the need of ventilatory assistance. Apart from one episode of mediastinal emphysema, there were no major complications. The authors noted that "On each occasion, arterial blood gas abnormalities were restored to normal as quickly as possible irrespective of peak inflation pressures." It seems clear that this form of treatment will be required in a small percentage of patients (such as in one young patient recently admitted to our service in whom the arterial pH was 6.8 when first measured). However, not everyone's experience of mechanical ventilation is as favorable as this. One center reported that of 32 severe asthmatics requiring mechanical ventilation on 34 occasions,[4164] three died; pneumothorax occurred in 18%; hypotension in 35%; and gastrointestinal bleeding in 9%. Chest infections occurred in 35%, but this incidence may have been increased by the use of therapeutic bronchial lavage in 19 patients. Other authors have reported a similar mortality experience.

From Lausanne, Switzerland, Darioli and Perret[4249] noted that over a 5-year period 26 of 159 patients with severe asthma required ventilatory assistance. At the time of intubation, 10 were in a coma and five were in respiratory arrest. Mechanical ventilation was required for a mean duration of 2.5 days, and all patients survived. It has been reported that ether administration is useful in moribund patients.[4229]

A recent analysis of emergency room treatment of asthma at one English hospital[4209] (there were no reasons to conclude it to be unrepresentative of many others) revealed that in 152 patients attending over a 12-month period, the blood pressure was five times more likely to be recorded than the peak flow rate; that PEFR values were noted in only 11%; that arterial blood gases were measured in only two patients; and that 47% of the patients presented between midnight on Friday and midnight on Sunday (this figure would have been 29% if attendance was uniformly distributed). The authors commented adversely on failure to record more objective measurements of the severity of airflow obstruction. McFadden[4155] has recently urged a more critical appraisal of therapy in the acute case of asthma. A recent controlled study of the effect of atropine indicated that this drug was not useful.[4157]

Because these patients are usually very sick, relatively few studies of them when acutely ill have been conducted. Recently, however, Hillman, Prentice, and Finucane[4154] reported on the pattern of breathing in eight acutely ill asthmatics aged between 19 and 63 years. FEV_1 values, when they could be first measured, varied from 18% to 36% of predicted. Using magnetometers, they noted a phase lag of the anteroposterior diameter of the rib cage relative to the anteroposterior abdominal motion. This was greatest when the FEV_1 was at its lowest. Fractional inspiratory time was decreased. There was no clear evidence of respiratory muscle fatigue in these patients, though there is little doubt that physical exhaustion may occur.[4249]

In one series of asthmatics, FEV_1 was 20% of predicted on admission to hospital; it rose to 70% of predicted after a week.[1531] In another series of 22 adult patients, the mean admission FEV_1 was 0.6 liters; it had risen to 2.0 liters at discharge from the hospital.[1478] It was noted that the TLC fell as the airflow improved, but the residual volume remained elevated when the patients were free of symptoms. Other authors have noted the importance of the physician realizing that very considerable physiologic abnormalities may be present without the patient appearing acutely ill.[1351]

In a study of 52 patients with severe disease, a slow recovery was noted to be associated with five factors[1349]: patient older than 40; non-atopic asthma; duration of acute attack before admission; poor long-term control; and the use of maintenance oral steroids. The Pa_{O_2} measured at 48 hours after treatment was initiated was a useful predictor of the rate of recovery. Fifteen of 44 patients still had an increased residual volume 5 days after admission, although by that time the PEFR was 80% of predicted.[1349] The recovery period is characterized by great PEFR variability, which is revealed when this is charted several times a day for 3 weeks following a severe attack.[1372]

Evidence relating to lactate increase is conflicting. In one large series of 85 patients with status asthmaticus, no elevation was found.[1431] In another series of 25 patients with severe disease, lactic and pyruvic acid levels and the lactic acid/pyruvic acid ratio were all elevated,[1384] as was the Pa_{CO_2}. In a study of 97 episodes of acute asthma in 47 asthmatic children, the arterial base excess and HCO_3 were significantly lower during the attack than when the subjects were well.[1396] The degree of hypoxemia correlated well with the severity of symptoms and was noted to be present on occasion when the signs of airflow obstruction were relatively slight.[1396]

Increased P waves on the EKG in lead II and lead aVF were noted in 26% of 61 patients with status asthmaticus.[1377] In another series of 10 patients, severe airflow limitation was accompanied by an abnormally vertical frontal plane P-wave axis.[1524]

In the first edition of this book written in 1964, we stressed the importance of monitoring the arterial P_{CO_2} in this condition. By the time the second edition was written in 1970, it had become clear that hypoxemia occurred early and was the most important indicator of severity,[1] and routine arterial oxygen tension measurements were becoming practicable. We stressed that proper management necessitated blood gas measurements. In a 1978 editorial Seaton[1535] wrote: "How many physicians would manage diabetes without measuring the blood and urine sugar levels? Yet these same physicians usually feel able to look after severe asthmatics without ever measuring their peak flow rate or arterial blood gases."

The principles of management of this condition are

1. Frequent monitoring of arterial blood gases.
2. Frequent observation of the chest and abdomen to check the respiratory muscles and the state of the pump.
3. Frequent observation of PEFR or FVC.
4. Ventilatory assistance when respiratory muscle fatigue is developing and the arterial Pa_{CO_2} has started to rise.

PULMONARY FUNCTION TESTS IN THE MANAGEMENT OF ASTHMA

In asthma, pulmonary function testing is useful in the following ways:

1. In differentiating asthma from emphysema in the elderly patient seen for the first time.
2. In assessing the degree of airway reactivity; this may be particularly useful if EIAL is suspected.
3. In employing the DL_{CO} as an indicator of possible aspergillosis, bronchiectasis, eosinophilic pneumonitis, or atelectasis if reduced in the absence of emphysema.
4. In advising on therapy, knowing the severity of EIAL, or documenting marked nocturnal worsening.
5. In following the patient and noting changes in flow rates, lung volumes, and the relationship between symptoms reported and functional status. Also, it may be that patients with a very labile condition are in more danger from sudden very acute and life-threatening exacerbations.
6. In managing severe asthma. Measurements of arterial blood gases and flow rates are essential.

ALLERGIC BRONCHOPULMONARY ASPERGILLOSIS

The first three cases of this syndrome were diagnosed in Britain in 1952. Ricketti and his colleagues[4801] have noted that in acute attacks, reductions may occur in TLC, VC, FEV_1, and $DL_{CO}SB$, with a return to baseline values after steroid therapy. The diagnosis should be suspected if the TLC or the $DL_{CO}SB$ is noted to be lowered in an asthmatic.

PROGNOSIS

The largest series of asthmatics observed for 20 years is a group of 244 asthmatic children.[1355] Half of these appeared to be free of symptoms; 21% had chronic asthma; and three died. From another series of women, which probably included some patients with chronic infective asthma and possibly some with emphysema, it appeared that $DL_{CO}SB$ did not deteriorate with time, although the ratio RV/TLC increased. FEV_1 values as a percentage of predicted fell from 89% between age 25 and 34, 73% between age 55 and 64, and 63% over the age of 65.[1426] Detailed longitudinal studies of carefully defined adult asthmatics have not yet appeared.

The longitudinal data in cases of occupational asthma are reviewed in Chapter 16.

An analysis of mortality among 2547 adult asthmatics attending a national sample of 60 general practices between 1970 and 1976 in Britain[5315] compared them with a matched group of non-asthmatic patients. A significantly excessive mortality rate in the asthma patients (189 deaths versus 112 among the controls) was found. There were 25 asthma deaths in the referent group, compared with no deaths from this cause in the controls.

10 CYSTS AND BULLAE, BRONCHIECTASIS, AND CYSTIC FIBROSIS

CYSTS AND BULLAE

During the past few years, several studies have been published that clarify the indications for surgery and the results to be expected in patients with large bullae and cysts in the lung. It has been suggested that the word "bulla" be used for a space more than 1 centimeter in diameter.[2025] In addition to their occurrence in emphysema, and particularly as part of paraseptal emphysema, bullae may occur as isolated phenomena in otherwise normal lung. These dual etiologic possibilities make management difficult. Certain cases of isolated bullae have a familial occurrence. Three sisters, all with normal alpha$_1$-antitrypsin levels and without Marfan's syndrome, had spontaneous pneumothoraces.[2018] Two of the sisters had large bullae, but there was no generalized emphysema. The sister with the most severe function defect was a non-smoker, and the VC was reduced, the RV increased, the FEV$_1$ was 45% of predicted, and the DL$_{CO}$ was 74% of predicted. The two other siblings had less severe function disturbance.

Fitzgerald and his colleagues[2010] followed 84 cases of surgically resected bullae for a mean of 7.3 years. Local excisions were done in 69 of these, lobectomy in 14, and Monaldi's drainage in four. There were two operative deaths, serious postoperative complications in 10, and minor complications in 13. In 13 patients, there was no improvement in FEV$_1$ postoperatively,

but in 13 it improved by more than 50%. Bronchospirometric studies in 20 patients showed significant improvement in $\dot{V}O_2$ and $\dot{V}E$, usually on the side of the lung resection; postoperative values were nearly normal. These authors[2010] concluded that

1. Patients with chronic productive cough did not do as well as others.
2. Removal of bullae occupying less than one-third of the hemithorax did not result in significant improvement of function.
3. The presence of diffuse emphysema did not preclude surgery.

In another series of 31 subjects treated by Monaldi's drainage (intracavity suction) that was reported by MacArthur and Fountain,[2019] 28 had symptomatic improvement and, in several, VC and FEV$_1$ increased postoperatively. In some of these subjects, the bullae were part of generalized emphysema, but it is difficult to know in how many. Gunstensen and McCormack[2011] reported on 22 subjects, all cigarette smokers, of whom 10 were so breathless that they could not walk 100 yards of flat distance. The FEV$_1$ data ranged from 0.37 to 0.85 in these patients, and the RV was usually elevated. Three of this group had significant improvement in function for more than 2 years. In the 12 less severely ill patients, the FEV$_1$ values ranged from 1.0 to 3.2. Ten of these 12 had improved function for more than 2 years. There were two operative deaths, and four of the total group of 22 were dead within 2 years.

Pride and his colleagues[2008] reported a series of 11 patients, with one postoperative death. Nine had disabling dyspnea, which was treated with resectional surgery. One was not improved by surgery, seven were moderately improved, and one greatly improved. Mean preoperative/ postoperative data were FEV_1 = 1.04/1.24; VC = 2.85/3.02; P_{el} at TLC = 10.9/10.9 cm H_2O; $DL_{CO}SB$ = 14.6/13.8; Pa_{O_2} at rest = 69.3/80.3 mm Hg; and Pa_{O_2} on exercise = 65.3/70.1 mm Hg. The maximal exercise load tolerated for 5 minutes increased from 275 to 350 kpm/min postoperatively. Other investigators have noted improvement in Pa_{O_2} postoperatively. In 18 patients treated surgically,[1997] the most consistent changes were in Pa_{O_2} and FRC, as measured with body plethysmography. The FEV_1 was noted to increase most in those with least impairment preoperatively.

Sackner and Landa[2023] reviewed 16 patients aged between 41 and 75 years, 10 of whom had bullae in the upper lobes. Detailed function studies showed that the VC was generally normal; RV usually increased; $SBN_2\%/L$ was usually abnormal; and FEV_1 ranged from normal to 46% of predicted. $DL_{CO}SB$ (as a percentage of predicted) varied from a low of 14% to 76% of predicted. $DL_{CO}SS$ was also measured and, in several subjects, considerably higher values were recorded than in the $DL_{CO}SB$ data. These authors concluded that differences in ventilatory capacity among the patients could be related to the degree of collapse of intervening lung parenchyma and airways rather than involvement with emphysema.

Roeslin and his colleagues[2033] reported on 18 patients with diffuse emphysema with large bullae who were treated by resection. The mean age was 44 years. Function tests were performed preoperatively and 6 months and 1 year postoperatively. Test values were as follows:

	Pre-operative	6 Months	1 Year
VC	3.14	3.50	4.03
RV (by He)	2.05	1.73	1.71
RV (by BP)	4.88	3.23	—
FEV_1	1.33	1.76	1.85
Pa_{O_2} (rest/exercise) (cm H_2O)	65.2/68.6	71.1/76.3	67.2/70.8
PAP (rest/exercise) (cm H_2O)	17.5/29.8	18.5/27.6	—

In a recent report on 21 patients with bullous disease treated surgically,[2043] four out of six with preoperative hypercapnia improved with surgery. Symptomatic improvement occurred in 14, with improvement in VC and FEV_1 in nine. The single best result led to a postoperative increase of FEV_1 from 0.81 to 2.92.

Pearson and Ogilvie[3459] have reported on 12 patients treated by resection, of whom 11 survived for more than 5 years after the surgery. Nine showed benefit 3 to 6 months after surgery, and several returned to full-time employment. Nine of the patients were restudied 5 years after the resection; all had had a gradual return of dyspnea, and the FEV_1 had declined by a mean value of − 82 mL/year (compared to a predicted value of about − 30 mL/year). Only three had had chronic bronchitis or had smoked after the operation; all but two had bullae occupying half or more of the thorax, and none had preoperative hypercapnia.

There has been interest in the subsequent (postoperative) rate of decline of FEV_1 in these patients. In a series of 11 followed for a minimum of 4 years,[4303] the rate of decline in ex-smokers appeared no different from normal subjects. In those who continued to smoke, it was accelerated; but even in these, the FEV_1 changed only by a mean value of − 34 mL/year, which is not much different from that in smokers without lung disease.

In some individuals, striking functional improvement has followed resectional surgery. In one 45-year-old cigarette smoking woman[2009] with a large bulla in the right upper lobe and compression of the right lower lobe, the preoperative/postoperative data were as follows: VC = 1.4/2.3; FEV_1 = 0.8/2.3; $DL_{CO}SB$ = 2.6/7.9; Pa_{O_2} = 45/63; and Pa_{CO_2} = 41.9/31.3. In another report[2002] on a 52-year-old automobile mechanic unable to work because of dyspnea, who also had a large right upper lobe bulla, the preoperative/postoperative data were FEV_1 = 0.61/1.47; VC = 1.05/2.35; Pa_{O_2} = 35/71; and Pa_{CO_2} = 60/24. The pulmonary arterial pressure changed from 75/40 mm Hg preoperatively to 36/18 mm Hg postoperatively. In a 34-year-old cigarette smoking soldier,[2000] FEV_1 and Pa_{O_2} rose after removal of a right sided bulla, but DL_{CO} did not change. An increase of 2 liters in VC and 1 liter in FEV_1 and considerable improvement in DL_{CO} followed resection in a 31-year-old farmer.[2024] Patients with excessive ventilation of the large bullae are unusual, but in one carefully studied 28-year-old man with a bulla occupying most of the left lung,[2041] regional studies showed good ventilation of the bulla but poor perfusion. The (A − a) D_{O_2}

widened, and the V_D/V_T ratio was much increased. Operation was followed by a reduction in VC, RV, TLC, and FEV_1. His exercise ventilation fell 40%, with considerable decrease in dyspnea; postoperatively, he returned to work as a gardener.

Severe paraseptal emphysema in a 60-year-old man[2035] led to a functionless right lung and severe dyspnea. His course was followed for 7 years before resection, when his FEV_1 fell from 1.49 liters to 0.80 liters (a decline of -98 mL/year). Removal of bullae from the right lung improved the FEV_1 to 1.52 liters; the $DL_{CO}SB$ rose from 9.0 mL/min/mm Hg to 21.0 mL CO/min/mm Hg postoperatively. Regional function studies with ^{133}Xe have been useful in evaluating the ventilation of the bullae and the status of the remaining lung[1995] in these cases. It is likely that CAT scan studies of the lung may prove useful.[4285]

We noted the difficulty of assessing these patients in the second edition of this book.[1] More recent data suggest that the following generalizations can be made:

1. Significant functional improvement may follow removal of cysts or bullae occupying more than a third of the hemithorax.

2. Chronic mucus hypersecretion and generalized emphysema are not contraindications to surgery, although they worsen the prognosis and increase the risk of surgery. When these conditions are present, regional lung function data may be useful in evaluating the integrity of other parts of the lung.

3. A significant reduction in exercise ventilation postoperatively may reduce dyspnea if the bulla is well ventilated and the V_D/V_T ratio and the $(A - a) D_{O_2}$ are increased. However, the FEV_1 may be unimproved.

4. The excessive falls in FEV_1 after successful resection indicate that this disease may be a progressive one. However, such accelerated falls are by no means universal.

We wrote in 1970 that "The physician may be reminded that, however carefully these studies are performed, he will still on occasion be surprised at the degree of improvement that follows resectional surgery in some patients, and in others he will be disappointed that improvement in function and effort tolerance is not greater."[1] This still seems to be relevant.

BRONCHIECTASIS

Immotile Cilia Syndrome: Kartagener's Syndrome

The immotile cilia syndrome includes Kartagener's syndrome but is not limited to it. An excellent review of this syndrome has recently appeared.[3454] Although there are several different dynein defects indentifiable by electron microscopy, the clinical effects are much the same.[3454] The syndrome has complex variants, however, and patients have been described in whom cilia are morphologically abnormal[4270] or in whom they look normal but are immotile.[4269] There is one patient with bronchiectasis and dextrocardia but no ciliary abnormality.[4278] The congenital lack of dynein arms in the cilia leads to very low tracheobronchial clearance rates, which is the primary abnormality.[2027, 2034] This commonly leads to chronic infection and secondary bronchiectasis. These conditions were described in Chapter 1.

In a study of 14 subjects, nine with situs inversus, aged 25 to 40 years, the very slow tracheobronchial clearance rate was documented.[2026] All had rhinitis, sinusitis, and bronchitis. Two had been smokers, five were current smokers, and seven were non-smokers. In the non-smokers, the FEV_1 levels varied between 42% and 89% of predicted and was below 80% of predicted in six. Of the 14 subjects, nine had evidence of obstructive disease on spirometry. In two subjects, the chest x-rays were thought to show emphysema. DL_{CO} levels and blood gases were not reported. In seven patients with this syndrome followed for 4 to 14 years, chronic airflow limitation and increased residual volume remained stable, but there was considerable morbidity from sinusitis, otitis media, chronic cough, and episodes of pneumonia.[2031] On occasion, it may be difficult to exclude this syndrome. In a careful study of seven asthmatic patients, all with severe sinusitis and nasal polyps, cultures of nasal epithelia revealed no structural or functional ciliary defects.[3449]

Young's syndrome is bronchiectasis with obstructive azoospermia and normal testicular function. In 34 men aged between 23 and 53 years with this syndrome,[3460] 19 had severe chronic sinusitis; 12 had chronic bronchitis (three were non-smokers); 10 had bronchiectasis; and three had had a lobectomy. Airflow limitation was moderate in 13 and severe in two. All had a normal DL_{CO} and k_{CO}.

Acquired Bronchiectasis*

As we noted in the last edition of this book, the severity of overall function defect depends on the number of segments involved with disease.[1] With severe generalized cystic bronchiectasis, severe airflow limitation may be present.[2003] There is often some component of reversible airflow limitation, and an increase of FEV_1 of more than 15% may be noted in many subjects.[2020]

In a review of 23 subjects of mean age 36 who were compared with age-matched controls, FEV_1 and PEFR were 67% of predicted; the FVC was 77% of predicted; and, in several, a greater than 15% increase occurred after bronchodilator use.[3461]

A major problem in cystic bronchiectasis is that the sacs are blind, and there is little ventilation through them. Thus, in order for coughing to be effective, equal pressure points must be upstream of the opening of the sacs, otherwise dynamic compression cannot occur. CAT scan studies may sometimes be useful.[4313]

Regional tests of function show reduced ventilation to affected segments.[1] Tests using aerosol inhalation often show abnormal deposition (mainly reduced peripheral filling).[36] Thurlbeck[1507] reported a case of severe peripheral airway disease in a 57-year-old woman in association with bronchiectasis. The reduced MEFV curves, increased residual volume, and reduced dynamic compliance with increased frequency—often starting in childhood[2014]—probably indicate the usual involvement of small airways in this condition. The pattern of reduced dynamic compliance and reduced TLC was found in 31 cases studied in detail,[2012] and the lowering of DL_{CO} correlated with the extent of involvement. Several studies have been reported on the follow-up of subjects treated either medically or with surgical resection. In a 1 to 15 year follow-up of 393 patients, two-thirds of whom had resection and one-third of whom were treated medically, the results suggested that surgery was more valuable than commonly supposed[2015] but no function tests were reported.

Bronchiectasis generally leads to moderately severe airflow limitation associated with a reduced total lung capacity and residual volume (unlike emphysema); DL_{CO} usually is normal in relation to lung volume or is only slightly reduced. It has been suggested that elevation of the RV/TLC ratio is associated with sputum purulence.[4305] In 66 patients with bronchiectasis who were treated surgically and followed up 5 years later,[2021, 2022] 27 were considered to have been cured; 21 had persisting symptoms; and 10 were symptomatic, with evidence of involvement of the remaining lung. In another follow-up study of 116 patients,[2045] 22 had died. The mean follow-up period of the remainder was 14 years. Thirty per cent were better than when first diagnosed, and 11% were worse. Seven per cent were considered to be severely disabled. The rate of decline of FEV_1 was less than -50 mL/year in 43 subjects and more than this in 14. The rate was related to survival.

In one interesting report, it was shown that the results of surgery were related to preoperative airway reactivity, as measured with histamine challenge.[532] In six of eight subjects considered to have a poor postoperative result, airway reactivity was increased as compared with normal. In eight of nine subjects considered to have had a good result from resectional surgery, the test was normal preoperatively. The authors suggested that the presence of increased airway reactivity indicates generalized disease. In the light of this report, it would seem advisable to check airway reactivity before resectional surgery is undertaken.

In a recent study of 50 bronchiectatic adults,[4284] 29 with an FEV_1 >1.5 liters were tested with methacholine. Of these, the majority showed increased reactivity; these subjects had lower baseline FEV_1, VC, and FEF_{25-75}. In the 29 subjects, the $DL_{CO}SB$ and $DL_{CO}SS$ values were about 80% of predicted; the RV was 150% of predicted; and the FEV_1 was 60% of predicted. Other authors note that there is a hyperimmune response in patients with bronchiectasis, but, in contradistinction to cystic fibrosis, there is no increased atopy.[4306] There is often a significant response to bronchodilators.[4306] One case report noted that there were five adults in two families with bronchiectasis, but in none of them were the cilia abnormal.[4277] Severe bronchiectasis following mycoplasma infections has been reported.[4304]

Associated Syndromes

In two siblings aged 13 and 16 years with congenital absence of bronchial cartilage (Williams-Campbell syndrome), the VC was 87% and 40% of predicted; the RV was 205% and

---

*Acquired bronchiectasis as the result of inhalation of corrosive gases is discussed in Chapter 16.

151% of predicted; and the FEF_{25-75} was 25% and 20% of predicted.[1991] Pa_{O_2} was measured in one of the subjects and was 53 mm Hg.

In one patient with ulcerative colitis, autoimmune hemolytic anemia, and Hashimoto's disease, there were pulmonary bullae and bronchiectasis,[2042] but no pulmonary function tests were reported. One unusual case of a patient who developed lung cysts was ascribed to a hamartomatous condition.[3463]

CYSTIC FIBROSIS

During the past 12 years, a significant number of reports in adult patients with cystic fibrosis have appeared, permitting a more detailed account of pulmonary function in this condition. In fact, survival has risen from about 2 years from diagnosis in 1940 to about 20 years in 1980.[4301] Standard sweat tests are negative in other pulmonary diseases.[3234] Boucher and his colleagues[3452] have reviewed the pathophysiology of this condition and noted that respiratory epithelium appears to have three abnormalities:

- increased transepithelial potential difference
- greater reduction in potential difference after amiloride perfusion
- reduced permeability to chloride ion

It is postulated that abnormalities in active ion transport of airway epithelia in cystic fibrosis contribute to the abnormal airway secretions.

Whereas the basic defect in the immotile cilia syndrome is in ciliary function, and hence in tracheobronchial transport, the cilia are normal in cystic fibrosis. Their beat frequency is also normal,[3174] but the nature of the material to be transported is abnormal.[2047] Mucociliary clearance is not invariably reduced in cystic fibrosis,[2027] but it is more commonly slowed.[613] It was reduced to 2.6 mm/min in 14 adult subjects with cystic fibrosis, as compared with a value of 20 mm/min in 20 normal subjects of the same age.[956] Adult subjects with cystic fibrosis often have an upper lobe infiltration, with evidence of atelectasis and bronchiectasis, and chronic staphylococcal infections are common.[2029] Infection with *Aspergillus* occurred in half of the 46 patients with cystic fibrosis in another series;[2044] chronic *Pseudomonas* infection is very common.

In 45 patients, all more than 12 years of age, of mean age 17 years,[2007] three groups could be identified: Group 1, with no physical signs in the chest; Group 2, with physical signs and occasional cough and sputum; and Group 3, with constant cough, sputum and signs. Pulmonary function data were as follows:

Group	Number	FVC (%P)	FEV (%P)
1	3 (initial)	100	94
	3 (5.6 years later)	103	93
2	9 (initial)	82	74
	8 (5.1 years later)	77	67
3	30 (initial)	64	47
	24 (4.1 years later)	62	47

The DL_{CO} was reduced in 10 of 14 patients in Group 3 in whom it was measured.

Other authors have found the FEF_{25-75} to be a more sensitive test of impairment and have confirmed that the DL_{CO} is lowered only when flow rates are abnormal.[3453]

In a report on 75 subjects aged 18 to 47 years (there is also an analysis of 232 subjects in the literature[2006]) hemoptysis occurred in 60% and chest x-rays were abnormal in 98%, with 58% showing evidence of hyperinflation. There was a close relationship between the clinical severity of the condition and abnormalities of VC, FEV_1, RV/TLC, and Pa_{O_2} but the authors noted that the $DL_{CO}SB$ was less abnormal. This observation was also noted in five patients diagnosed after the age of 15.[2005] Their test data showed VC values from 56 to 85% of predicted; RV values from 119 to 219% of predicted; and FEF_{25-75} values from 0.55 L/sec to 1.3 L/sec. DL_{CO} values were greater than 83% of predicted in the four from whom they were recorded. In another series of 40 patients over the age of 25,[2001] elevation of residual volume was noted in most. This does not lead to emphysema, however.[1994]

Recent series of adult cases have included:

1. Sixteen patients between the age of 14 and 32, whose FEV_1 was from 14 to 55% of predicted.[4273] There was evidence from urinary desmosin and plasma elastase activity that proteolytic destruction was occurring in the 11 with chronic infections.

2. Twenty-three male patients aged 16 to 35,[4274] in whom hyperinflation with an RV/TLC ratio above 50% was associated with a reduced maximal inspiratory pressure at the mouth (this may have been influenced by concomitant malnutrition).

3. Four patients aged between 35 and 63 years,[4276] in whom cystic fibrosis was first diagnosed at those ages. Three had finger clubbing, all had grossly reduced FVC and FEV_1 values, and upper zone bronchiectasis was present in all.

4. Twenty adult patients in whom the mean FEV_1 was 27% of predicted and the mean FVC was 47% of predicted.[4257] In this group, steroid administration did not improve lung function.

Using the three equation method of analysis of expired CO, Cotton and colleagues[4271] reported that in 24 cystic fibrosis patients who were compared with controls the DL_{CO} fell as the FEF_{25-75} became more abnormal. This conclusion was at variance with earlier observations.[1494] Possibly, earlier data gave an overestimate of DL_{CO} in these patients.[3883] The measured anatomic dead space is normal in cystic fibrosis,[1998] but $VD_{physiol}$ is usually increased.[2017] Alveolar ventilation is reduced only in severe cases.[3457]

Regional studies that used ^{133}Xe revealed regional ventilatory defects in patients with normal tests of pulmonary function.[1470] The most sensitive index of general ventilatory distribution in 12 children was the measurement of the volume of nitrogen expired during maximal breaths after nitrogen washout to an expired concentration of 2% nitrogen on oxygen breathing.[2038] It has been noted that nitrogen clearance data may be useful in studying small children with this condition.[3027]

Some have found no enhanced airway reactivity to histamine in cystic fibrosis,[2036] but others have found it to be very variable.[4302] One-third of the parents of children with cystic fibrosis have been reported to have a PC20 to methacholine to less than 3 mg/mL.[4309] In a control group, only 4% showed this degree of reactivity.

The presence of significant low $\dot{V}/\dot{Q}$ regions in the lung is shown by the elevated $(A-a) D_{N_2}$ that exists in this condition.[1992] It is clear that peripheral airways are frequently abnormal, either structurally or by mucus blockage. In 46 patients aged between 7 and 26 years, C_{dyn}/f was normal in only seven and fell in those with normal ventilatory function. The MEFV curves changed, and residual volume became elevated with increasing severity. The $\dot{V}max_{50\%}TLC$ was considered to be the most sensitive indicator of abnormality.[1994] In another series of 37 patients aged between 8 and 22 years,[1990] the mean transit times of the FVC curve were studied, and the SD of these was found to correlate with the $MEF_{25\%}VC$. In children with this disease, measurement of the maximal flow rate at FRC divided by the FRC has been found useful.[4308] In 24 patients between 8 and 31 years of age,[1993] the pressure volume curve of the lung studied in 13 of the patients showed "excessive stiffness of the lung near maximal volume, and loss of recoil at lower volumes." The loss of recoil was considered to play a part in the development of gas trapping. Zapletal and his colleagues[2028] confirmed the loss of recoil by finding that in 28 patients P_{st} at 60% TLC was reduced in 60% of them.[2028] The reduced flow rates at low lung volumes were also documented.

Studies of the control of breathing in 14 children with cystic fibrosis[2030] showed that there was no abnormality of neuromuscular drive. By means of the hyperoxic CO_2 test, the slope of the relationship between $\dot{V}E$ and $P_{et}CO_2$ was found to correlate significantly with the FEF_{25-75} expressed as a percentage of vital capacity.[2030] Sleep studies in 20 subjects aged between 9 and 29 years[2032] showed that a fall in oxygen saturation, averaging 7.4% in REM sleep, was common. It was associated with a fall in FRC and was interpreted to indicate increasing airway closure and an increase in low $\dot{V}/\dot{Q}$ regions.

A fall in Pa_{O_2} of between 1 and 23 mm Hg was observed in 33 patients with cystic fibrosis when they went from a sitting to a supine position.[4272] Pa_{CO_2} did not change. The authors felt that this phenomenon contributed to lower Pa_{O_2} values at night and also felt that the changes were not completely explained either by airway closure or by radiologic worsening in the upper lobes. The mean age of their group was 17.7 years; the mean RV was 136% of predicted; and the mean FEV_1 was 72% of predicted.

In later stages of this disease, circulatory factors become important. In six patients aged 24 to 31 years,[4275] all had had a previous episode of right ventricular failure. Their mean resting pulmonary arterial pressure was 31 mm Hg, which increased by 20 mm Hg on exercise but fell on oxygen breathing. In another group of 18 patients[4299] (mean age of 21 years; mean FEV_1 of 61% of predicted) the right ventricular ejection fraction was shown to be abnormal in all of them on incremental exercise. In five subjects the right ventricular response to exercise was abnormal. Nifedipine has been found to lower the pulmonary arterial pressure in this condition without lowering the Pa_{O_2}.[4298]

In 31 subjects of mean age 17 years (21 boys and 10 girls) and with a mean FEV_1 of 58% of predicted,[4300] the mean Pa_{O_2} at rest was 62 mm Hg (ranging from 45 to 75 mm Hg). On exercise, nine were unable to increase their right ventricular ejection fraction more than 5%. These subjects were studied by radionuclide angiography, and the authors concluded that there was no close relationship between pulmonary function and circulatory abnormality.

Some increase in peak flow rate after physiotherapy has been observed,[2037] and improved clearance from large airways, but not from peripheral airways, was shown. Increased sputum clearance has been shown to follow the forced expiration technique of chest physiotherapy.[2040] Other reports have noted improvement in SGaw[2047] and increased sputum clearance after vibration/percussion techniques[2039, 2046] and suggested that coughing is as effective as chest physiotherapy.[4307] However, there is no close relationship between the amount of sputum raised and changes in pulmonary function tests.[4307]

Other studies of physiotherapy[2955] and exercise[3451] indicate that one effect of exercise may be to cause increased coughing and sputum clearance, leading to improved expiratory flow rates. In 17 subjects,[3458] a 14-day hospital admission with intensive physiotherapy led to a significant improvement in VC after 5 days, with reduction in RV and improvement in PEFR.

Progressive bicycle ergometry in 20 patients with cystic fibrosis,[3456] for whom a scoring system of impairment of resting pulmonary function was adopted, showed that exercise impairment was related to the severity of change at rest. Peak work capacity was affected in several patients, and a fall in oxygen saturation was also observed. The mean age of the patients was 16.1 years.

Exercise programs are useful in improving these patients. In a study of 31 subjects, 21 were given an exercise program, and 10 served as controls.[3450] After 3 months of physical conditioning, the exercise group had significantly increased exercise tolerance and maximal $\dot{V}_{O_2}$ and lower heart rates at submaximal exercise loads. Their respiratory muscle endurance also increased, although they had no specific respiratory muscle training. The exercise program consisted of supervised running and was described in detail by the authors.[3450]

In addition to the study just noted,[2007] several interesting longitudinal function studies of this condition have been published. It has been found useful to plot the FEV_1 per centimeter of growth.[2013] In children with no respiratory symptoms, this averaged 29 milliliters. In those with minimal symptoms, it was 17 milliliters.

In those with severe symptoms, the FEV_1 was only 3.1 milliliters. FVC values per centimeter of growth for the three groups were 40 milliliters, 22.5 milliliters, and 10.4 milliliters, respectively. These data originated from studies of 76 children with cystic fibrosis who were observed for 4 to 9 years.[2013] In another series of 132 patients observed for 5 to 7 years,[1989] pulmonary function remained stable or improved in 25%, and 20 of the patients maintained completely normal function. Accelerated rates of decline of FEF_{25-75} and FEV_1 were noted, however, and these were greater in females than in males. The authors concluded that there was not a pattern of "relentless progressive decline for all patients diagnosed as having cystic fibrosis."

An important observation has been the value of respiratory muscle training in reducing the rate of decline of FVC.[1988] Ventilatory muscle endurance was 36% higher in those with cystic fibrosis than in normal subjects, but the faster rate of decline of FVC in girls was probably attributable to the greater athletic training in boys.[1988] In spite of malnutrition, respiratory muscle strength is normal or better than normal in patients with cystic fibrosis,[3462] but training can improve the maximal inspiratory pressure.[3464] It has been shown that the once popular therapy of nightly mist exposure in cystic fibrosis is of no benefit, as indicated by pulmonary function.[1996]

As we noted in the second edition of this book,[1] hypoxemia and hypercapnia with associated pulmonary hypertension develop in patients with severe disease. Right ventricular hypertrophy is related to thickening of the medial muscular layer of the pulmonary arterioles in cystic fibrosis.[2016] Intercurrent infection and cor pulmonale represent the two most important complications that increase the mortality rate in this condition.

More general recognition of the occurrence of adult cases of cystic fibrosis and more effective treatment of the condition in childhood, with much better survival into adult life, serve to emphasize the importance of this disease as a cause of chronic airflow limitation in adults. The concordance between the abnormalities in the lung and the data from function tests is satisfactory, but there is still much to be learned of the reasons for the different natural history in patients with the same basic defect. It seems that cystic fibrosis may be a condition in which lung recoil is lost without the development of morphologic emphysema; the relative preservation of the $D_{L_{CO}}SB$ until severe $\dot{V}/\dot{Q}$ mismatch has occurred is in line with this conclusion (though there is some uncertainty of the reliability of the $D_{L_{CO}}SB$ as ordinarily performed in this condition).

The function test data noted previously would support the view that the increased residual volume in this condition is caused in part by loss of lung recoil and is not to be solely attributed to peripheral airway obstruction. It is also of interest that an increased residual volume seems to be common in patients with cystic fibrosis but is uncommon in persons with acquired bronchiectasis. Pulmonary function tests play a very useful role in the long-term management and supervision of these patients.

11

ALLERGIC ALVEOLITIS OR HYPERSENSITIVITY PNEUMONITIS

INTRODUCTION

It is now known that a wide variety of materials can precipitate allergic alveolitis. Some of these are encountered only in the working environment, and others are the consequence of hobbies or are due to different environmental factors. Pepys,[1572] whose valuable work on the immunologic aspects of this condition uncovered many of these factors, has reviewed the wide spectrum of materials that may cause it. Reynolds[3469] has also recently reviewed the immunologic aspects of these conditions. Another review has dealt with sources of risk in the poultry industry.[4287] The effects on pulmonary function appear to be generally similar irrespective of the etiologic factor. Warren[1589] has made the interesting observation that the syndrome appears to be commoner in non-smokers than in smokers. The pathogenesis of this condition was discussed in Chapter 1.

There is considerable variation in severity. In extreme instances, and very rarely, interference with gas exchange is so severe that an acute respiratory distress syndrome may be produced.[1576] In other individuals, symptoms are mild. In most patients, the acute episode consists of fever, tachypnea, and dyspnea, often with inspiratory rales audible over the lungs. An inspiratory "squawk" has been described as often present in those with extrinsic allergic alveolitis.[3470] This apparently occurs later in inspiration, is shorter in duration, and is higher in frequency than rales or rhonchi heard in

other types of interstitial disease. It is attributed to late opening of airways.

From the clinical point of view, the diagnosis should be suspected from a careful history. However, we have seen cases labeled "viral pneumonia" in which the causative environmental exposure only came to light after very careful investigation. (In one case, someone was exposed to redwood dust while making a canoe in a vocational school class.) A case originally reported in a coffee worker later turned out to be an interstitial fibrosis due to rheumatoid disease.[3471]

Outbreaks in groups of people have been reported in which no causative agent could be identified, even after a thorough investigation for them. Thus, 12 office workers had a febrile illness with chills, fever, muscle aches, and chest tightness after a leak from a cafeteria above the office. The DL_{CO} of those affected differed significantly from that in unaffected workers; the chest x-rays of both groups were normal. Detailed air hygiene studies identified nothing.[4265]

Of great interest has been the recent description of seasonal hypersensitivity pneumonitis in Japan, and many cases have been described.[4286] It seems that this illness may be due to *Trichosporon cutaneum*,[4259] since positive challenge tests to this organism from bird droppings have been reported.[4290] Two severe cases occurred as a result of exposure to *Penicillium chrysogenum* and *Penicillium cyclopium* growing in a leaky central heating system.[4310] No

244

causative agent could be identified in an outbreak in a rayon manufacturing plant.[4288]

The radiologic changes usually consist of a patchy "ground-glass" appearance, often more evident in the lower zones. However, the disease may be present with measurable effects on functions but with an equivocal or normal chest x-ray.

A review of biopsy specimens from 60 patients with farmer's lung[3468] reported the following frequency of observed changes:

Morphologic Change	Frequency (%)
Interstitial infiltrate	100
Pneumonitis	65
Pleural fibrosis	48
Interstitial fibrosis	65
Bronchiolitis obliterans	50
Foam cells	65
Edema	52
Granulomata, with giant cells	50
without giant cells	58
Solitary giant cells	63
Foreign bodies, birefringent	47
non-birefringent	40
Vasculitis	0

These morphologic appearances usually permit a definitive diagnosis to be made, although the clinical, radiologic, and functional characteristics are sufficiently well defined that in the presence of a clear history of exposure to a known precipitating agent lung biopsy is not usually required to confirm the diagnsosis.

The sequence of changes in the lung has been described by investigators at the National Institutes of Health as follows.[1563] An acute inflammatory alveolitis occurs with accumulation of polymorphonuclear leukocytes in the lung. This is followed by more chronic changes, with increasing numbers of mononuclear cells, the appearance of granulomata, and later interstitial fibrosis. Reports on rabbits injected intratracheally with *Micropolyspora faeni*,[3474] and other animal studies,[4280] have shown that a rapid increase in T lymphocytes occurs 24 hours after intratracheal administration of a specific antigen. A rapid change in the population of immune-effector cells occurs before the mononuclear alveolitis develops and is characteristic of the disease. It appears that resolution of pulmonary changes is not dependent on the development of immunologic tolerance.[4292]

Alveolar lavage data in three groups of farmers[3476] are reviewed below. As noted in Chapter 1, lung biopsy specimens often show a bronchiolitis to be present. It is important to distinguish this syndrome from occupational asthma on the one hand,[4289] and non-specific

respiratory changes as a result of exposure to dust, including grain dust, on the other. Those conditions are discussed in Chapter 16. The flu-like illness encountered in workers exposed to a variety of phenol-formaldehyde resins, particularly in the rubber fabrication industry, are also discussed in that chapter. It is possible that alveolitis may be involved in some of those cases, but the precise precipitating agent has not been identified.

PULMONARY FUNCTION CHANGES

Farmer's Lung

Farmer's lung was the first of these conditions to be described in detail, as it was first recognized in 1924.[1] It is caused by exposure to thermophilic actinomycetes, the majority to *M. faeni*. It is still an important cause of illness and incapacity. Two hundred cases were documented in Devon, England, between 1939 and 1971,[1591] and an incidence of 23 cases per 1000 farmers has been found in Somerset.[1586]

A recently reported survey of 428 farmers in different regions of England and Wales[4263] showed that the farmers had lower FEV_1/FVC and FEF_{25-75} values than controls after social class, smoking, and geographic region had been taken into account. These changes were greater in those doing dairy farming and silage work. There was no excess incidence of chronic bronchitis. Large series of cases have been studied in Finland[552] and in Wisconsin.[1565] In one survey of 471 farmers in Utah, 172 had serological tests, chest x-rays, and spirometry. There was a 3% incidence of pulmonary abnormalities, which were considered to be attributable to alveolitis.[1595]

With acute illness, VC and FVC are reduced. The residual volume is not elevated,[1587] and FEV_1 and FEF_{25-75} are usually impaired,[1580, 1587] no doubt reflecting the common occurrence of bronchiolitis. $DL_{CO}SB$ or fractional CO uptake is lowered (usually to a greater degree that can be attributed to reduction of TLC.* Pa_{O_2} is reduced, sometimes at rest,[1584, 4297] but more importantly it falls with exercise, often to very low levels.[2445, 3446, 4297]

C_{stat} is lowered, and C_{dyn}/f falls even in nonsmokers.[1587] Involvement of small airways is also

---

*See references 1566, 1570, 1584, 1587, 1591, 1594, 3477, 4297.

indicated by the considerable volume of trapped gas (730 milliliters versus 320 milliliters in controls) found in 19 patients with farmer's lung.[1566] Severe respiratory failure with dangerous hypoxemia has been described in a 5-year-old child with allergic alveolitis as a result of exposure to moldy hay.[1564] Twelve children with this condition (caused by moldy hay in two children and bird exposure in 10 children) have been described.[4312]

Eleven subjects with extrinsic allergic alveolitis (EAA) (eight dairy farm workers and three mushroom growers) and 23 cases of sarcoidosis (three in Stage 1, 14 in Stage 2, and 6 in Stage 3 of the disease) were compared with 23 normal subjects of similar age. The following data were found[4296]:

	Normal Subjects	Sarcoidosis	EAA
TLC (L)	5.98	5.45	5.46
VC (L)	4.44	3.97	3.80
RV (L)	1.65	1.48	1.55
FEV_1 (L)	3.60	2.72	2.64
FEF_{25-75} (L/sec)	3.91	2.61	2.37
$DL_{CO}SB$	25.8	18.3	15.7

In relation to lung volume, the $DL_{CO}SB$ generally tends to be lower in hypersensitivity pneumonitis than in sarcoidosis.

A recent review of 141 subjects in Wisconsin, of whom 92 (of mean age 54) were restudied,[1565] showed that 20% had significant dyspnea, and 39% had evidence of radiologic change. Pulmonary function test abnormalities were reported as follows:

Test	Abnormalities (%)
VC	12
TLC	12
$DL_{CO}SB$	30
FEV/FVC%	25
FEF_{25-75}	14
$\dot{V}max_{75\%}VC$	19
CV%VC	36
Pa_{O_2} at rest	40

In an interesting series of 82 subjects studied in Finland,[552] 22 were shown to have increased reactivity to histamine during the acute phase of the disease. In 16 of these, the reactivity had reverted to normal after 1 to 2 months. The FEV_1 averaged 76% of predicted in the reactive group and 93.6% of predicted in the non-reactive group in the acute phase. The mean FEF_{25-75} values were 67.5% and 95.5% of predicted, respectively. However, there were no significant differences between the Pa_{O_2} and the $DL_{CO}SB$ between the reactive and non-reactive groups, both values being similarly abnormal.[552]

Follow-up data from Finland of 93 patients followed for 2 years[4267] showed a clear relationship between a lowered $DL_{CO}SB$ and radiologic change. Chronic changes were present in 38 patients, and the authors concluded that steroids did not affect the outcome. The mean age of the patients was 50 years, and 20% were smokers in this series. Three abnormal $DL_{CO}SB$ values were noted in those with a normal chest film. In those with abnormal chest films, the mean value of $DL_{CO}SB$ was 57% of predicted. This index and the FVC and Pa_{O_2} were, in general, noted to change together. Some data suggest that individual sensitivity may have a genetic basis.[4311]

Bronchial lavage studies, as well as pulmonary function tests, have recently been reported in three groups of dairy farmers in Quebec. They were classified as follows:

Group 1: Seven subjects with acute farmer's lung disease

Group 2: Ten asymptomatic farmers with positive serum precipitins to *M. faeni.*

Group 3: Nine normal farmers without serum precipitins.

The lavage data showed that Group 1 had large numbers of cells, with 72% lymphocytes and high IgA and IgG/albumin ratios. Six in Group 2 also had an increase in cells, with 52% lymphocytes. Two in Group 3 had similar findings. Pulmonary function tests in the three groups were as follows:

	Group 1	Group 2	Group 3
Mean age (range)	44 (37–57)	43 (24–58)	43 (25–61)
Male/female	6/1	9/1	8/1
TLC (%P)	85.7	110.4	97.5
FEV_1 (%P)	76.0	104.9	98.4
$DL_{CO}SS(\%P)$	62.4	119.9	111.4

Cormier and his colleagues[4262] have analyzed the interrelationship between radiologic changes, function tests, and findings on bronchoalveolar lavage in 94 Quebec dairy farmers. Very good correlations were found between the increased lymphocytes in BAL fluid, the radiologic changes, and the $DL_{CO}SB$. However, the FEV/FVC ratio did not differ between different groups. Ten of 43 asymptomatic farmers had both radiologic and function test abnormalities.

The same investigators have also noted[4293] that bronchoalveolar lavage in 24 asymptomatic dairy farmers (of whom 13 were seropositive for *M. faeni* and 11 were seronegative) showed that 13 had a high percentage of lymphocytes in their BAL fluid. In most of these, there were no pulmonary function deficits. They conclude that alveolitis can be occurring when all other findings are normal. Other authors have suggested that in hypersensitivity pneumonitis the lymphocyte counts in lavage fluid may be higher than the lymphocytes in lung tissue.[4283]

The Quebec investigators have restudied 27 subjects 2 and 3 years after an acute attack.[4258] All were still on their farms and were asymptomatic. All had normal chest films and no physical signs. There were few changes in function tests, and their $DL_{CO}SB$ had not changed. Nine of 12 still had a lymphocytosis in bronchoalveolar lavage, and the authors concluded that this may persist but may not be associated with significant disease during the same period. In another group of 29 subjects with farmer's lung followed up in England, two had evidence of a chronic restrictive condition.[3472]

It is important to stress that with an intensive educational campaign on the nature of the risk to farmers and the use of simple respirators when some contact with spores cannot be avoided, this disease should be completely preventable.

Positive challenge tests to varieties of *Aspergillus* have been reported in individual subjects.[4297] A recent report[4260] indicated that residual abnormality in farmers after an acute attack of alveolitis may be related to the presence of higher S-GGT (galactosylhydroxylsyl glucosyltransferase) and serum procollagen than in those who recovered fully. The authors concluded that those with residual high values of these enzymes were at risk of developing interstitial fibrosis after an acute attack. It has been shown that ponies with "heaves" develop increased airway response to methacholine after exposure, and their dynamic compliance falls.[4261]

Exposure to Birds

Allergic alveolitis due to exposure to birds, particularly budgerigars, is said to be the commonest form of allergic alveolitis in Britain.[1596] Allergic alveolitis to pigeons was reported in four children aged from 13 to 18 in a Puerto Rican family.[3467] Warren, Tse, and Cherniack studied 14 cases of allergic alveolitis with about equal numbers due to birds and thermophilic actinomycetes.[1594] They were studied 1 week after onset and 4 to 6 weeks later, with the following results expressed as a percentage of predicted values from a control group:

	1 Week	4–6 Weeks
TLC (%)	82	95
FRC (%)	85.7	100.9
RV (%)	89.75	104
FVC (%)	74.9	85
FEV/FVC%	normal	normal
FEF_{25-75}	62%	62%
CO uptake	59%	72%
C_{stat}	reduced	increased
Recoil	increased	reduced

They agreed with Allen and his colleagues[1573]—who had studied nine patients with bird-induced alveolitis—that all cases have initial evidence of small airway involvement. In sequential studies, Allen showed that compliance initially fell with frequency in five out of seven subjects, all non-smokers, and later showed no fall.

Other workers studying bird-sensitive subjects have found lowered arterial oxygen tensions and elevated pulmonary artery pressures (which fell on oxygen breathing), reduced compliance and flow rates, and elevated $(A-a) D_{O_2}$ differences at rest and on exercise.[1569] In 24 proven cases, the lowered $DL_{CO}SB$ was shown to be attributable to a lowered DM, with a normal pulmonary capillary blood volume, V_c.[1568] In this series, FEV_1 and RV were normal, FRC was reduced, and C_{stat}/FRC was lowered. The authors concluded that gas exchange abnormalities were much more significant than mechanical alterations. In seven members of two families affected, VC and F_{CO} fell together.[1585] Some biopsies from the subjects showed moderate interstitial fibrosis and evidence of peribronchiolar changes.[1575] In one of these patients, $DL_{CO}SB$ was still only 42% of predicted 6 months after the acute attack, although the VC had risen from 38% of predicted to 72% of predicted. Pigeons, budgerigars, and even chickens[1574] can all induce the disease.

However, the disease as a result of contact with pigeons appears to be relatively uncommon in relation to exposure, since careful examination of 200 pigeon breeders at a convention turned up no cases. It is important to note that the presence of precipitins is evidence of exposure but is not correlated to hypersensitivity lung changes.[1581] There is also an overlap of IgA and IgG values, which limits the diagnostic value of these tests.[1562] In an interesting comparison between 46 subjects with allergic alveolitis due to birds and 59 sensitized subjects with positive precipitins, Petro and his colleagues[1567] found normal RV values, lowered C_{dyn}/f, increased SBN_2/L slopes, and lowered TL_{CO} values in the affected subjects. In another series, three of nine subjects attributable to budgerigars appeared to have some degree of interstitial fibrosis.[1582]

Hendrick and colleagues[510] studied 144 challenge tests in 31 subjects sensitized to birds. They defined the late response in these subjects and concluded that resting respiratory rate and minute volume, $T_{L_{CO}}$, and lung volumes were too insensitive to be useful indicators; whereas exercise ventilation and frequency, temperature, and circulating neutrophils were more sensitive. Auscultation and chest x-rays were not useful. A fall in FVC was noted in most subjects. In an ingenious follow-up study of six subjects, these authors showed that if the challenge tests were repeated with the subject using a respirator, no response occurred.[559]

A comparison between four symptomatic pigeon breeders and six who were without symptoms[4291] showed that BAL lymphocytes were similar in the two groups, but challenge testing produced significant declines in FVC, FEV_1, and Pa_{O_2} only in the group with symptoms. In another comparison between eight subjects with bird-induced hypersensitivity pneumonitis and 17 subjects with sarcoidosis[4279] (with no differences in FEV_1 between the groups), the author noted that there was a significantly lower ratio of DL to lung volume (70%) in the hypersensitivity pneumonitis subjects than in those with sarcoidosis, in whom it was 92% in inactive cases and 74% in active cases. Antigen challenge in six subjects with disease due to bird exposure[4266] showed that two had an early fall in terminal airflow velocity ($\dot{V}max_{75\%}VC$), followed by later falls in FVC, FEV_1, and RL. In four, only the $\dot{V}max_{75\%}VC$ changed significantly. DL_{CO} did not change, nor did the Pa_{O_2}.

There are several interesting individual cases reported. In one of them,[4295] a 41-year-old woman with a pet bird had severe systemic illness characterized by weight loss, arthralgia, and dyspnea. Lung biopsy showed severe bronchiolitis and patchy alveolitis. The chest film predominantly showed hyperinflation. Her pulmonary function tests were as follows:

	Predicted	Initial	1 Month Later	1 Year Later
FEV_1	2970	1040	1120	1370
FVC	3590	1950	2410	2770
TLC	5380	5490	4940	5580
RV	1810	3340	2840	2730
VC	3590	2150	2100	2850
Raw (kPa/L/sec)	<0.2	0.3	0.34	0.58
SGaw (kPa/L/sec)	1.3–3.6	0.88	0.87	0.51
$DL_{CO}SB^*$	8.76	3.1	2.91	6.21
k_{CO} (kPa)	1.79	0.93	0.80	1.68

*Recorded in units of mMol/60 sec/kPa.

It is not clear whether hypoxemia in this condition is commonly accompanied by pulmonary hypertension, but this has been suggested.[3473]

Other Causes

Severe alveolitis has been recorded in mushroom workers. In two cases, the $DL_{CO}SB$ was only 50% of normal, with FEV_1 45% of predicted.[1593] Resolution occurred in 6 months. This disease can be life-threatening with severe hypoxemia and with the chest x-ray showing extensive miliary mottling.[1576] Many wood dusts may cause alveolitis, challenge tests often being effective in demonstrating the etiology.[1590] In a recent case of extrinsic allergic alveolitis in a Swedish sawmill worker, the causative agent was thought to be molds associated with the wood rather than the wood itself.[3465]

Other etiologic agents causing illnesses of characteristic patterns include pituitary snuff,[1560] swine feed,[1561] *Alternaria* organisms in wood pulp[1559] (two cases were documented in great detail with rest and exercise and challenge studies), and contact with smallpox.[1588] These illnesses have been found in coffee workers[1592] and in workers exposed to sugar cane contaminated with *Aspergillus*.[1571] Also, in workers making Roquefort blue cheese, antibodies to the causative agent (*Penicillium roqueforti*) were found in serum and bronchial lavage fluid. Overexposure to starch and soil repellants in spray cans caused typical illnesses with later positive challenge tests.[520] Some cases of alveolitis have been reported following exposure to porcine pancreatic extract.[4264] Dry tobacco dust exposure (possibly containing *Aspergillus fumigatus* spores) has also been identified as a possible cause of alveolitis.[4294]

Of more general importance is the occurrence of sensitivity reactions to thermophilic actinomycetes or aspergilli in office cooling systems that use water contaminated with these organisms (so-called humidifier fever). In one outbreak, four of 27 exposed office workers were affected.[1578] Challenge tests are useful in establishing the diagnosis,[1583] and the disease may occur through contamination of cool-mist vaporizers.[1558] However, sometimes a specific organism cannot be identified.[4282] In some outbreaks, antibody tests to thermophilic actinomycetes are negative. Although IgG levels are increased, the pattern of function and radiologic change is characteristic.[4281]

Certain drugs, including bleomycin,[1557] furazolidone,[1577] hydrochlorothiazide,[1556] and tetracycline,[1579] have been reported to cause allergic alveolitis. These effects are discussed in Chapter 14.

SUMMARY

Although complete recovery from allergic alveolitis occurs, residual abnormality with dyspnea is not uncommon. Attributability of the illness to the suspected agent may be confirmed by challenge testing after the acute episode is over. The disease has been shown to lead to increased airway reactivity, and ventilatory flow rates are usually reduced. The severity of the alveolitis is indicated by the sensitivity of DL_{CO} measurements, together with exercise Pa_{O_2} recording, to indicate abnormality. The lack of increase of residual volume distinguishes alveolitis from "asthma," but it is not clear why the residual volume is normally decreased rather than increased as it is in that condition. Another unexplained observation is the apparent increased occurrence of alveolitis in non-smokers.[1589]

This disease can cause long-term effects if repeated exposures occur. Farmer's lung can be entirely prevented by an intensive educational program and the wearing of a mask if exposure is likely. It is, in theory, a disease that should no longer be occurring. Families in which severe cases of allergic alveolitis occur as a result of exposure to pet birds should be counseled on the importance of avoiding continued exposure. Pulmonary function testing and evaluation, as others have pointed out, is of the great value, both in diagnosis and in management.[1585]

There is some overlap between occupational asthma and allergic alveolitis, and episodes of bronchiolitis obliterans can cause diagnostic difficulty. One recent report of 94 cases of bronchiolitis in adults noted that in 50, no cause could be identified.[4268] Histologic testing showed polypoid masses of granulation tissue in the lumina of small airways. A cough and a flu-like illness lasted for 3 to 10 weeks, and the chest x-ray showed patchy densities. Seventy-two per cent of the patients had a reduced FVC and TLC, and 86% had a reduced $DL_{CO}SB$. Improvement on steroids occurred, usually with complete functional and radiologic resolution (in 65% of the subjects in this series who were observed for 4 years). The FEF_{25-75} was below 60% of predicted initially in 13 of the subjects. This entity, which seems to combine a bronchiolitis with an alveolitis, is discussed further in Chapter 19.

12

INTER-RELATIONSHIPS BETWEEN CARDIAC AND PULMONARY FUNCTION

INTRODUCTION

The impact of abnormalities in cardiac structure and function on the lungs is subtle and complex; it consists not only of the effects of an elevated left atrial pressure on fluid accumulation and drainage, but also of the impact of cardiac function on inspiratory muscle activity and of chronic hypoxemia on respiratory control. By contrast, the effects of lung disease on the heart are somewhat simpler, although much remains to be learned about the progression of hypoxemia to pulmonary hypertension secondary to lung disease, and about right ventricular failure. A symposium volume entitled The Cardiac Lung published in 1979 should be consulted by anyone interested in the impact of heart disease on pulmonary function. (References 1679 through 1697 are from this volume.)

PULMONARY FUNCTION IN VALVULAR HEART DISEASE

Congenital Heart Disease

In adult patients with atrial septal defects, changes in pulmonary function are related to the degree of pulmonary hypertension. When the resting pulmonary arterial pressure (PAP) is less than 19 mm Hg, lung volumes and expiratory flow rates are usually normal, but the single-breath $DL_{CO}SB$ may be increased.

With pressures between 20 mm Hg and 25 mm Hg, there may be some abnormality of MEFV curves. With pressures greater than 25 mm Hg, some reduction in lung volumes with abnormal MEFV curves and an increased airway resistance will commonly be present. The $DL_{CO}SB$ may be normal.[1637, 1684] Mechanics studies suggest that lung elastic recoil is progressively reduced at low lung volumes as the pressure increases. These changes have been attributed to "competition for space between vessels and airways within the bronchovascular sheaths, with a subsequent compression of small airways."[1637]

Other studies of adults with either ventricular septal defect or atrial septal defect lesions have shown some elevation of residual volume and closing capacity, with mild ventilatory defects and little interference with gas distribution.[1724] $DL_{CO}SB$ is variable,[1655] but some relationship of pulmonary capillary blood volume (V_c) and DM to pulmonary artery pressure has been demonstrated.[1685] Abnormalities of regional ventilation and perfusion distribution have been noted but seem unrelated to any hemodynamic parameter.[1614, 1686] In children, corrective operations have been followed by reduction in the mild pulmonary hyperinflation present preoperatively.[1612]

Adults with tetralogy of Fallot, whether with total correction or treated surgically with shunts, have some reduction of TLC and some non-uniformity of $\dot{V}/\dot{Q}$ distribution.[1658] On exercise, the arterial blood gases were normal in one group of 37 such patients, but maximal $\dot{V}_{O_2}$ was reduced by about 30% as a result of a reduced cardiac output.[1658] Exercise studies of cases of cyanotic congenital heart disease have amplified data from earlier observations.[1] In one group of seven patients, maximal work was about half the normal predicted value, whereas minute volume was the same as in normal subjects doing twice as much work.[1683] The arterial Pa_{O_2} fell from 52 mm Hg at rest to 35 mm Hg on exercise and was unaffected by 100% oxygen breathing. Pa_{CO_2} fell to 24 mm Hg. The authors concluded that carotid chemoreceptor response was normal.[1683]

In a more recent study of eight adults with congenital cyanotic heart disease,[4432] the mean exercise Pa_{O_2} was 27 mm Hg, a drop of 10 mm Hg from the resting value. All had polycythemia. Blood lactate levels increased only slightly. In spite of the very low Pa_{O_2} values, their oxygen uptake doubled on exercise, and the authors noted that mitochondrial oxygen utilization had to be maintained in spite of very low Po_2 values. In four of these patients, heart-lung transplantation was successfully carried out, and their post-transplant Pa_{O_2} was 95.8 mm Hg. Transplantation in six severe Eisenmenger's syndrome patients[4377] with severe pulmonary hypertension has also been successful, with dramatically improved function test data. Studies of children with right to left shunts have noted a reduced ventilatory response to hypoxemia at rest[1671] and improvement after corrective surgery.[1635] A comparison between six patients with chronic airflow limitation and six patients with right to left shunts and equivalent hypoxemia showed that episodes of increased hypoxemia were common in the former group but were not observed in the latter patients.

Tracheobronchial obstruction in infants due to abnormal vascular rings is a well recognized and important condition.[1610] The reverse of Horner's syndrome, which is due to nerve stimulation rather than paralysis (known as the Pourfour du Petit syndrome), has been described as a result of an abnormal aortic arch.[4470]

Mitral Valve Lesions

In mitral stenosis, there is a distinctive change in pulmonary mechanics with increasing pulmonary hypertension. At low lung volumes, elastic recoil is diminished, and at high lung volumes it is increased.[1632] These changes revert toward normal after mitral valve replacement surgery. Preoperatively, the intrapleural pressure at TLC may be reduced, with a shift in the pressure-volume curve.[1604] With increasing severity, there is reduction in vital capacity and increased airway resistance, and the FEF_{25-75} in adults falls with increasing pulmonary hypertension.[1] In a study of 32 patients wtih mitral stenosis, all non-smokers, significant correlations were observed between pulmonary wedge pressure and dynamic compliance and among mean pulmonary arterial pressure, airway resistance, and $MEF_{50\%}$. No significant correlations between hemodynamic measurements and RV or closing volume were found.[1711] In other series, however, a relationship was found between closing capacity and atrial pressure.[1680] Changes in DL_{CO} occur, with an initial increase in V_c[1183] but a reduction in DL_{CO} and DM as the pulmonary hypertension increases.* In subjects with a well preserved working capacity, the DL_{CO} increases normally on exercise.[1701] In 12 patients wtih pure mitral stenosis, a significant correlation was observed between pulmonary vascular resistance on exercise and DL_{CO}.[1707]

Rhodes and colleagues have reported on 26 non-smoking patients aged 23 to 63 with mitral valve disease. Twenty had predominant mitral stenosis, and six had predominant regurgitation.[3495] None had evidence of primary lung disease. The authors showed that the mitral valve pressure gradient significantly negatively correlated with the FEV_1, $FEV_1/FVC\%$, and k_{CO} and positively correlated with residual volume. $DL_{CO}SB$ significantly correlated with pulmonary arteriolar resistance. Reduction in the vital capacity was related to the measured heart size. Initial isotope studies showing increased apical perfusion in patients with mitral stenosis seated upright at rest[1] have been confirmed by more recent measurements. In addition, Dawson and his colleagues[1642] showed that lower zone ventilation is reduced, principally because the initial portion of a full inspiration is poorly distributed to the lung bases, which fill normally as the inspiration is completed. This effect is attributed to a loss of compliance in the lower zones, with probable small airway closure in these regions. Studies in upright and lateral decubitus positions in another series of 10 subjects showed that the ratio of upper zone to lower zone perfusion correlated with pulmonary arterial pressure in both positions.[1648] Changes in perfusion distribution were noted to occur

---

*See references 1, 1616, 1651, 1655, 1706.

Pulmonary Function in Cases of Mitral Valve Disease[4343]

	Number	Age	Predicted Values (%)						R_{tot} (cm $H_2O/L/sec$)
			FVC	FEV_1	RV	$DL_{CO}SB$	PEFR	$\dot{V}max_{50\%}$	
Men	35	32.7	63.5	67.4	134	65	78	60	2.99
Women	44	34.5	67.0	67.8	116	65	77	60	4.02

within 10 minutes of a change in position, which the authors felt probably indicated that edema was not responsible, but local vasoconstriction of dependent vessels might account for the observation.[1648] Other investigators have favored shifts in lung water as the mechanisms inducing changes in perfusion.[1664] The degree of pulmonary venous hypertension can be accurately assessed by measurements of regional function.[1682]

Correction of mitral stenosis by valvotomy is not followed by an increase in vital capacity, and the diffusing capacity is generally unchanged at rest[1616] or is slightly increased on exercise when compared with preoperative values.[1696] However, the major change is a reduction in exercise ventilation, the mechanism of which is unclear.[1616, 1678] Ablett, Reed, and Cotes[1678] noted that exercise tidal volume increases postoperatively in spite of a fall in vital capacity (attributable to the thoracotomy), and respiratory frequency falls. The ventilatory response to CO_2 is slightly reduced or unaffected by valvotomy. The effect of mitral stenosis on increasing the ventilation in relation to $\dot{V}O_2$, which has been known for many years,[1] occurs in patients whose DL_{CO} is normal.[3518] The slope of $\dot{V}O_2$ in relation to heart rate also changes. A report on cases of mitral stenosis from Kuwait provided the following data[4343] (in the table at the top of this page).

The preoperative data showed significant correlations between pulmonary vascular resistance and DL_{CO}, FEV_1, $\dot{V}max_{50\%}$VC, and VC. Postoperative testing showed little change after 50 weeks, but the DL_{CO} level was related to survival. After 2 years, the VC and DL_{CO} had improved and the R_{tot} value had fallen in the survivors.

Aortic Valve Disease

The distinctive change in lung mechanics in mitral stenosis noted previously does not occur

in aortic valve lesions,[1595, 1679] and there is no comparable fall in DL_{CO} with increasing severity.[1651] Some authors have noted a relationship between increasing pulmonary wedge pressures and reduction in vital capacity with an apparent lowering of dynamic compliance.[1723] In other series, this relationship was not significant.[1679] As pulmonary vascular resistance increases in patients with aortic valve disease, there is some increase in upper zone perfusion.[1681] The same series from Kuwait discussed earlier[4343] also provided the data on aortic stenosis (in the table at the bottom of this page).

There was less improvement in this group postoperatively than in the group with mitral stenosis.

CORONARY ARTERY DISEASE

Coronary arterial disease is so dominant as a cause of death in the western world that changes in pulmonary function as a result of it are commonly observed. Because both chronic airflow limitation and coronary artery disease are related to cigarette smoking, these conditions commonly occur together. Therefore, it is not surprising that dyspnea attributable to one of these conditions is not infrequently attributed to the other.

Acute Myocardial Infarction

In patients with very recent myocardial infarction with a normal chest x-ray, VC, FEF_{25-75}, and FEV_1 are reduced. Closing capacity is increased, and TLC is normal or slightly reduced. RV is slightly increased but falls later if congestion increases, and ventilation to dependent parts of the lung is reduced.[1618, 1692] Blood flow is also reduced in dependent parts of the lung.[1630] The arterial oxygen tension falls.[1644] It may be increased transiently by hyperventila-

Pulmonary Function in Cases of Aortic Valve Disease[4343]

	Number	Age	Predicted Values (%)						R_{tot}
			FVC	FEV_1	RV	$DL_{CO}SB$	PEFR	$\dot{V}max_{50\%}$	
Men	44	34.7	73.8	79.1	135	79	92	66	304

tion but returns to its previous level in 3 minutes.[1670] A lowered Pa_{O_2} was found in 86% of 89 patients with acute myocardial infarction.[1690] $DL_{CO}SB$ falls slightly, and the VD/VT ratio increases.[1618] CV/TLC% increases[1654] but may fall if diuretics are used.[1635] In patients with evidence of pulmonary edema or shock, the Pa_{O_2} is reduced to lower levels as the pulmonary diastolic and wedge pressures increase.[1650, 1670] It has been noted that a wedge pressure exceeding 18 mm Hg is usually associated with a fall in ventilatory flow rates.[1712] As noted in the last edition,[1] assisted ventilation may be required in patients with severe left ventricular failure.[4353]

The arterial oxygen tension remains depressed for about a week after an acute infarction, but both it and the $(A - a)\,D_{O_2}$ return to normal in 8 weeks.[1630] The FEF_{25-75} averaged 62% of predicted 3 days post–myocardial infarction in one series,[1689] rising to 88% of predicted 2 weeks later and 98% of predicted at 10 weeks. Other authors have noted that the vital capacity is still reduced up to 4 weeks after the acute episode, but this and ventilatory flow rates are normal at 8 to 10 weeks.[1618, 1643]

McHugh and his colleagues[1716] found that there was a close relationship between radiologic stages of congestion and the pulmonary wedge pressures. The earliest radiologic change was a redistribution of flow to upper vessels with loss of their marginal contour. This was followed by developing perihilar haze, and the third stage involved periacinar rosette formation. Other authors have used more complex radiologic grading based on nine criteria,[1691] and these studies also showed a close correlation between severity of congestion and depression of the arterial oxygen tension.

In 40 patients with coronary artery disease confirmed by angiography and left heart catheterization,[1693] significant relationships were found between left ventricular end-diastolic pressure and TLC/BSA, VC/TLC, and closing capacity as a percentage of TLC. There was also a close relationship between the components of diffusing capacity and this pressure, leading the authors to conclude that "the differential estimation of the CO transfer components . . . is an easy and valuable noninvasive technique, which yields reliable information about the left ventricular dysfunction of patients with coronary heart disease."

In 70 men of mean age 52.3 years who were studied 3 to 5 months after a myocardial infarction,[1694] 23% had a normal left ventricular end-diastolic pressure at rest and on exercise. Eleven per cent had an abnormal pressure on exercise only, and 66% were found to have an elevated pressure, both at rest and on exercise. Exercise ventilation was increased in this group. Although Pa_{O_2} decreased on exercise in nearly half the patients, it was not correlated to any hemodynamic data. Closing volume was not elevated. In another series of patients with similar disease,[1728] elevation of pulmonary arterial pressure on exercise was demonstrated. A similar phenomenon has also been demonstrated through the use of a different method of study that involved the measurement of total pulmonary blood volume.[3514] Exercise in the upright position does not change this volume in normal subjects, but it increased in 27 of 40 patients with coronary artery disease and in every one of the 19 of these who had to stop exercise because of dyspnea. The mean increase was from 550 milliliters to 690 milliliters.

The development of pulmonary hypertension on exercise in men who have apparently made a normal recovery from an acute myocardial infarction is an important observation. It probably accounts for the dyspnea that may be noted by such patients, when resting pulmonary function tests are normal; and it may well complicate the assessment of dyspnea in middle-aged men with evidence of concomitant occupational lung disease (see Chapter 16). It is not clear if it is accompanied by any loss of FVC, since this has not been recorded. If it is, this might explain part of the close relationship between the FEV_1 (lowered due to a loss of FVC) and survival (see Chapter 8). This idea is supported by the work of Wilhelmsen and his colleagues.[1687] In 1967, they used exercise tests to study a random sample of men in Göteborg, Sweden born in 1913. Between 1967 and 1975, 49 men had fatal or non-fatal mycoardial infarcts. They showed that dyspnea and a lower FEV_1 were associated with an increased risk of infarction and that the vital capacities were lower (mean 95.7% predicted) in the dyspneic group than in other subjects (in whom it was 99.1% of predicted). The findings were supported by the studies of Collins, Clark, and Brown[1673] (see later discussion) and by data from Poland[4042] (see Chapter 8). Bloom and his colleagues from Tucson have also suggested that cardiovascular factors may be important in FVC decline.[4493]

Pulmonary Function Following Cardiac Surgery

After aortic and mitral valve replacement operations, the reduction in heart size leads to increases in TLC, FRC, and RV.[1599] Static lung compliance also increases. After aortic valve replacement, the pulmonary pressure volume curve shifts to the left. However, after mitral valve replacement, the postoperative curve crosses the preoperative curve, so that recoil decreases postoperatively at high volumes and increases at low lung volumes.[1598]

There has been considerable interest in pulmonary function changes after coronary artery surgery with cardiopulmonary bypass. Post-perfusion changes in pulmonary function were documented in great detail by Rea and his colleagues.[1731] An increase in resting ventilation and a reduction of Pa_{O_2} (by about 10 mm Hg during air breathing) persisted for several days postoperatively but had returned to normal in 10 days. The $(A - a) D_{O_2}$ had risen by 19 mm Hg 48 hours postoperatively. At this stage there is a considerable increase in the work of breathing, which may be increased by as much as five times.[1735]

The $(A - a) D_{O_2}$ on oxygen rose from 275 mm Hg preoperatively to 342 mm Hg postoperatively in another series[1729] but did not change after coronary artery surgery without bypass. There are pathologic changes in the lung if bypass is prolonged longer than 2 hours[1732] or if homologous blood is used to prime the oxygenator.[1730] The effect of the thoracotomy probably accounts for the lowering of $DL_{CO}SB$ and VC for several months postoperatively, since $DL_{CO}SB/\dot{V}A$ was the same as it had been preoperatively.[1733]

It has been noted that interference with phrenic nerve conduction may follow cooling of the pericardium in bypass surgical procedures[4402, 4405] and may result in diaphragmatic paresis or paralysis (see Chapter 22). Buhlmann and Frick[1736] noted that there was an increased risk of pulmonary problems after cardiac surgery if the FEV_1 was less than 60% of VC or if the VC was less than 70% of predicted. Using length of stay postoperatively in the intensive care unit as a criterion, others have found that this cannot be predicted from preoperative function.[1734] However, the criterion is obviously very indirect.

ACUTE PULMONARY EDEMA AND LEFT VENTRICULAR FAILURE

A full discussion of the physiology of pulmonary edema and pulmonary vascular reactivity cannot be attempted in this volume, but the factors affecting fluid stability in the pulmonary capillaries were noted in Chapter 2. Of clinical importance are the observations that it is the precapillary arterioles that are sensitive to hypoxemia,[1750] and this response may be mediated by histamine.[1751] There is evidence from clinical studies that the magnitude of the response depends on vessel reactivity rather than on the amount of histamine released.[1752]

Pulmonary arterial pressure rises in both normal individuals and patients with chronic airflow limitation when 5% CO_2 is breathed, causing an acute elevation of Pa_{CO_2} by 25 mm Hg.[1753] This effect was not influenced by bicarbonate administration and is therefore thought to be independent of hydrogen ion increase. Experimental studies in dogs have shown that when left atrial pressure increases so that wedge pressure exceeds 25 mm Hg, the closing volume increases, presumably as a result of fluid accumulation around small airways or within small airway walls.[1750]

A detailed review of factors determining fluid flow across the alveoli has been published in the proceedings of a symposium,[3111] but this discussion is beyond the scope of this section. However, it may be noted that recent experimental work has suggested that granulocytes[3489] and release of oxygen radicals,[3488, 4342] platelet activating factor,[3521] and thromboxane[4467] may all be important in alterations of capillary permeability. In experimental studies of edema,[3485] increasing the left atrial pressure leads to increases in extravascular water accompanied by increasing lymph flow from the lung. This reaches a maximum and does not increase further as left atrial pressure and fluid extravasation both increase. It is not clear whether periobronchial edema in dogs reduced the bronchial lumen,[3494] but it has recently been reported that it increases the R_L response to histamine.[4466] The observation in the same experiments that C_{dyn} falls as left atrial pressure increases[4466] indicates probable narrowing of peripheral airways. In oleic acid–induced edema in dogs, the use of positive end-expiratory pressure increases the arterial Pa_{O_2} but does not influence survival.[3497] It probably causes a redistribution of water into extra-alveolar tissues or the cuff space in humans.[3482]

The observation made by Anthonisen and Smith[1725] that respiratory acidosis may occur in some cases of severe pulmonary edema has been confirmed by others.[4380] In one series of 109 patients with pulmonary edema, 55 had severe combined metabolic and respiratory acidosis and Pa_{CO_2} levels of 70 mm Hg.[1609] An interesting observation was that in 12 such patients in whom Pa_{CO_2} elevation was recorded in the acute stage, the ventilatory response to CO_2 was no different from 12 subjects without this finding.[1672] This indicated that non-responsiveness to CO_2 was not a factor in causing the hypercapnia. It has also been noted that patients with hypercapnia did not have more severe pulmonary edema or greater airway obstruction than those without.[1715] Lactic acidosis is a common finding in these cases.[1714] It has been suggested that the effect of a Valsalva maneuver on blood pressure, assessed at the bedside, may be useful in differentiating cardiac edema from respiratory failure, a square-wave response, or an absence of overshoot indicating left ventricular failure.[4355] The differential diagnosis between severe asthma and cardiac failure can, on occasion, cause difficulty.[4355] The clinical differentiation between cardiac edema and edema due to impaired permeability may also be difficult. One study showed that in only 31 of 50 patients was cardiac edema correctly diagnosed.[4324]

In the second edition of this book,[1] we reported observations on pulmonary function in two patients with pulmonary congestion before and after treatment. Recent data from patients with early left ventricular failure and some degree of pulmonary congestion amplify those observations. Collins, Clark, and Brown[1673] studied 72 patients with left-sided heart disease, all non-smokers. Reduction of FVC and FEV_1 to about 75% of predicted values was noted, with elevation in CV/VC%. FEV_1 and FVC both fell further when the patient became supine, but CV/CV% did not change. Although CV/VC% correlated significantly with the degree of dyspnea, it was not closely related to pulmonary wedge pressures or to left ventricular end-diastolic pressures.[1673] Improvement in all respiratory measurements followed inhalation of salbutamol aerosol. Studies of patients with hypertension before and after diazoxide or furosemide administration[1709] showed that these drugs produced a fall in RV and RV/TLC% and significant increases in $Vmax_{50\%}$ and $Vmax_{25\%}$. Furosemide led to a slight increase in vital capacity also. Measurements of $\dot{V}_{iso}V$ on air and helium showed no change. The authors concluded that airflow in small airways had been reduced initially and improved after diuresis. Sorbini and his colleagues[1695] studied 22 cases of congestive heart failure—12 of whom had radiologic evidence of pulmonary congestion

and 10 of whom had evidence of interstitial pulmonary edema—before and after treatment. Comparisons before and after treatment showed that in both groups VC, FEV_1, C_{dyn}, and Pa_{O_2} rose after treatment, and RV/TLC% and CV/VC% fell. A significant correlation was observed between CV (predicted minus observed) and Pa_{O_2} (predicted minus observed). MEFV curves were carefully studied before and after treatment. Those showed considerable increases in peak expiratory flow rate but only minor changes in the middle and end parts of the expiration.

Exercise studies in patients with congestive heart failure, necessarily very limited in scope, indicate that the maximal $\dot{V}O_2$ achievable correlates poorly to indices of resting lung function.[4319] Others have noted that the $(A - a) D_{O_2}$ may increase and that falls in Pa_{O_2} are not often observed, although hypoventilation in relation to oxygen uptake may be present.[4320]

Some observations on normal subjects throw light on the changes during pulmonary congestion. In experiments reported in 1973, 2 liters of saline were rapidly infused into normal subjects.[1669] The following changes were noted:

	Control	Postinfusion
FVC	5.08	4.83
FEV_1	4.03	3.58
CV/VC%	8.4	12.7
C_{stat}	0.283	0.25

In more recent studies,[350] five normal subjects were rapidly infused with 2 liters of normal saline. Mean values (n = 5) before and after infusion were as follows:

	FVC	FEV_1	$MEF_{50\%}$	CV/VC%
Before	5.87	4.85	6.00	3.9
After	5.45	4.40	5.24	11.2

	$V_{iso}V$	$\delta MEF_{50\%}$ (He/O vs air)
Before	9.6	28.7
After	31.2	12.2

Another group of investigators[3486] studying five normal volunteers made measurements before and 20 to 90 minutes after intravenous infusion of 30 mL/kg of warm saline over a 20-minute period. Pulmonary function tests, chest x-rays, and CAT scans of the chest were performed. The data showed a 4.5% decrease in VC, a 14% increase in RV, and a 24% increase in SBN_2/L (which was shown to be a sensitive indicator of change). The azygos vein, observed in chest x-rays and in the CAT scans, increased in size, but apart from this there were no other changes. The authors concluded that tests of small airway function were more sensitive than radiographic techniques in detecting changes under these conditions. Other investigators have reported that $DL_{CO}SB/V_A$ was not changed by saline infusion but was increased by immersion in water up to the neck.[1675]

In normal subjects, extravascular lung water (EVLW), as measured by indicator dilution techniques, increases from a mean of 178 milliliters at rest to 233 milliliters on exercise. This is probably attributable to a redistribution of flow among and within alveolar walls.[1640] EVLW in supine subjects is about 32 milliliters (± 8 mL) per liter of total lung capacity and is not increased by breathing 100% oxygen for up to 12 hours.[1649] It increases in states of shock or sepsis or with fluid overload. In pulmonary edema, it may be 200 milliliters per liter of TLC.[1688] Recent studies in critically ill patients[3519] show that EVLW increases in parallel with the severity of the radiologic appearance of edema in both cardiac and non-cardiac patients. In this series, the normal value in patients with a normal chest x-ray was 5.6, ± 1.8 mL/kg. In the cardiac group with radiologic changes, EVLW was 10.2, ± 3.1 mL/kg, and in the non-cardiac patients it averaged 15.8, ± 4.6 mL/kg.[3519] Others have reported a general relationship between radiologic changes and this measurement.[4436] A recent detailed study of 174 patients with edema of either cardiac or non-cardiac origin[4434] indicated that at any given pulmonary wedge pressure EVLW was greater in non-cardiac edema patients. Clearance of inhaled ^{99m}Tc-labeled DTPA is also more accelerated in non-cardiac than in cardiac types of edema.[4435] In 45 severely ill patients with pulmonary edema,[3506] the $(A - a) D_{O_2}$ was more increased in those with hemodynamic pulmonary edema than in those with capillary damage.

Some studies have indicated that EVLW is increased in the presence of cor pulmonale,[1649] but the reason for this is unclear. Changes in pulmonary function in cirrhosis hepatis and in chronic renal failure are noted in Chapter 19. The etiology of pulmonary edema in brain injury is still not completely understood, as was noted in a recent review of this entity.[4349]

PULMONARY VENO-OCCLUSIVE DISEASE

By 1975, 21 cases of pulmonary veno-occlusive disease had been described.[1611] Some reduction of VC, FEV_1, and Pa_{O_2} may occur, but the $DL_{CO}SB$ is normal[1611] or slightly reduced.[1726] If only one or two lobes are involved, as may occur, spirometry and Pa_{O_2} may be normal.[1613] This condition may give rise to unilateral transradiancy of the lung and hemoptysis.[1720] Diagnostic criteria and clinical features have been discussed in reviews and editorials.[1611, 1622, 1719] It seems unlikely that pulmonary function data can contribute to the diagnosis of this condition (which can be very difficult) during life, except by helping to exclude other conditions. In three cases confirmed by histology,[4441] ventilatory flow rates and subdivisions of lung volume were normal, but the Pa_{O_2} was decreased in all and the $(A - a) D_{O_2}$ was increased. In one, the $DL_{CO}SB$ was reduced. The clinical picture was dominated by cardiomegaly and right ventricular failure.

PULMONARY HYPERTENSION

Pulmonary Embolic Disease and Primary Pulmonary Hypertension*

In studies of autopsy data, there is some evidence that pulmonary hypertension may be commoner in liver cirrhosis.[3487] It also occurs in some collagen diseases, particularly in systemic lupus erythematosus[3478] and polymyositis,[3508] in which it may dominate the clinical picture. Occasionally it occurs in several members of the same family,[4318] in children,[4397] and in adolescents.[4379] We have encountered an apparent case in a 10-year-old boy, in whom the eventual diagnosis was capillary hemangiomatosis (see Chapter 17).

Although pulmonary emboli are very commonly found at autopsy, their clinical recognition is notoriously difficult. Often when these emboli are present at autopsy, they were not suspected during life. In contrast, sometimes when pulmonary emboli were diagnosed during life, they were absent at autopsy. The diagnosis is very difficult when chronic airflow limitation and emphysema are present. Venous thromboses are common in this condition.[3285] In one carefully studied patient,[3507] multiple small emboli caused death, but neither radionuclide scanning nor pulmonary angiography had been useful in diagnosis. The disproportion among the FEV_1, excessive tachypnea, a Pa_{CO_2} of 21

---

*Reviews of this group of conditions have appeared in the last few years,[4350, 4372] one with particular emphasis on therapy.[4473]

mm Hg, and a Pa_{O_2} of 48 mm Hg with right ventricular failure were considered in retrospect to have suggested the diagnosis. Others have noted the fall in both the Pa_{O_2} and the Pa_{CO_2} as suggesting emboli in patients with chronic airflow limitation.[3323] A study of 110 subjects in whom pulmonary embolism was suspected[4468] found that a VD/VT ratio of more than 40% in the presence of a normal spirogram was very suggestive of the presence of embolism. The authors concluded that this measurement was comparable, in terms of specificity and sensitivity, to radioisotope lung scanning. The VD/VT ratio was measured by collecting expired gas while simultaneously determining Pa_{CO_2}. Other studies have attempted to refine the criteria of diagnosis by scanning.[4438] However, a recent study of 51 suspected cases that used both radionuclide ventilation-perfusion scanning and angiography[4406] showed that in nine subjects the methods disagreed. The authors concluded that both methods may give erroneous results. Pulmonary angiography is usually considered the most reliable criterion of a diagnosis of pulmonary embolization.

Comparisons of respiratory function between patients with disease thought to be embolic in origin and patients with primary pulmonary hypertension do not reveal any differences in EKG, symptoms, or radiologic or physical findings.[4375] In one such comparison, comparative pulmonary function data were as follows[4375]:

	Thromboembolic Disease	Primary Pulmonary Hypertension
Number	8	17
Mean age	39	36
FVC (%P)	84	75
FEV_1 (%P)	75	79
TLC (%P)	96	87
RV (%P)	115	114
FRC (%P)	99	94
$DL_{CO}SB$ (%P)	60	59
Pa_{O_2} (mm Hg)	62	65
Hematocrit (%)	44	46

In this series, average survival was 3 years from the onset of symptoms.

In patients with pulmonary embolic disease studied within the first 5 days after the event, the vital capacity is usually reduced, with reductions in both IC and ERV. The FEV_1 is lowered by an equivalent amount, and $DL_{CO}SB$ may be lowered.[1645] The $(A - a) D_{O_2}$ is usually increased,[1601] but this is difficult to interpret. The arterial P_{O_2} is an unreliable indicator of the presence of emboli. The difference between end-tidal P_{CO_2} and arterial P_{CO_2} increases when

emboli are present. This difference may be useful if all measurements in all patients are made with maximal inspirations[285]; this greatly reduces the difference between these two measurements in chronic airflow limitation.

In two patients with massive embolization, studies of $\dot{V}/\dot{Q}$ distribution that used the six inert gas method showed an increase of ventilation in units with a high $\dot{V}/\dot{Q}$. Between 20% and 39% of the cardiac output was perfusing unventilated lung units, thereby constituting a shunt.[3481] The widened $(A - a) D_{O_2}$ was attributed mainly to the increased shunt, and the increased VD/VT ratio was attributed to the increased ventilation of unperfused units. In a recent study, acute pulmonary embolism was demonstrated by angiography in 10 patients. The subjects were between 54 and 78 years old,[4399] and the percentage of vascular obstruction was estimated to be between 30% and 65%. The patients showed slight reductions in VC and a mean Pa_{O_2} of 61.5 mm Hg. The $(A - a) D_{O_2}$ increased in all patients. Using the six inert gas method to quantitate the $\dot{V}/\dot{Q}$ abnormality, the authors concluded (1) that 13% of the $(A - a) D_{O_2}$ was due to a diffusional component; (2) that true shunt and flow in low $\dot{V}/\dot{Q}$ regions was an average of 9% of the cardiac output; and (3) that the fall in mixed venous P_{O_2} accounted for the remainder of the hypoxemia and was to be regarded as the major factor.

In seven patients with chronic pulmonary embolism also studied by the six inert gas method of quantitating $\dot{V}/\dot{Q}$ abnormality, there were no regions of high $\dot{V}/\dot{Q}$ and little gross overall abnormality. In patients with a significantly lowered Pa_{O_2}, this was attributable to a slight $\dot{V}/\dot{Q}$ abnormality, together with a very low mixed venous P_{O_2} that was probably due to a reduced cardiac output. In patients with primary pulmonary hypertension or pulmonary thromboembolic disease studied when stable, there may be a slightly reduced $DL_{CO}SB$, but spirometry is normal.[1603] In other patients with severe disease, venous admixture has been increased,[4439] and shunting only contributed to the hypoxemia when atelectasis was present. It is remarkable that resting oxygen uptake remains normal in spite of very low values of cardiac output in patients with pulmonary hypertension or left ventricular failure.[3479]

Horn and colleagues[3480] reported on studies of eight patients with primary pulmonary hypertension and 17 with chronic thromboembolic disease; all had had right heart catheterization and pulmonary angiography. Five of the eight patients with primary pulmonary hypertension had a severe restrictive ventilatory pattern, with a VC mean of 54% of predicted and a TLC mean of 64.3% of predicted. A similar pattern was found in five of the chronic thromboembolic group.

Others have stressed that the very low mixed venous P_{O_2}, rather than any diffusion limitation or shunt, is the major factor related to widening of the $(A - a) D_{O_2}$ in this condition.[1663, 1698] Pulmonary compliance is normal, and the reductions in VC and TLC are apparently not due to changes in it.[1727]

Ten non-smokers studied in Mexico City had idiopathic pulmonary hypertension,[3520] and their mean pulmonary arterial pressure was 65.7 mm Hg. In the eight subjects with a normal pulmonary elastic recoil pressure, the FEF_{25-75} was decreased, and the closing capacity was increased. The delta $\dot{V}max_{50\%}$ on helium and air was also abnormal in eight subjects. The residual volume was increased in seven. Pulmonary resistance was normal in all. Nine of the 10 subjects had a fall in C_{dyn} with increasing frequency. In two, lung recoil was thought to be increased. The SBN_2/L was increased in only one subject. A biopsy from one subject showed evidence of small airway infiltration. The mean age of the subjects was 25 years (range 16–42); it is possible that the clinical presentation was affected by altitude.

Riedel, Widimsky, and Stanek[1663, 1665] reported on 87 patients with thromboembolic pulmonary hypertension studied at least 2 months after the last episode had occurred. They documented increased resting ventilation and a reduction in FEF_{25-75} with increasing pulmonary arterial pressure. The vital capacity was normal. Pa_{O_2} was slightly lower in the most severe group, and the VD/VT ratio was slightly higher. Using steady-state DL_{CO} with end-tidal sampling, they found that although this was reduced in some patients it bore no relation to the pulmonary arterial pressure. They concluded that it was not useful in the evaluation of this condition. Others have noted lower $DL_{CO}SB$ values in individual patients or in small series,* and some have confirmed the absence of a consistent pattern of abnormality in this index.[1763]

In the interpretation of pulmonary function tests in this condition, it is important to emphasize the lack of a close relationship between DL_{CO} and the severity of vascular change. This discrepancy is probably to be explained by the fact that vessels are commonly seen to be partially recanalized on microscopy. Hence, although flow may be greatly reduced, the alveolar capillaries distal to the lesions are normally filled. The pulmonary capillary blood volume may therefore be normal as a result of retrograde capillary filling. As others have emphasized,[1663] spirometry and diffusion measurements are useful mainly to exclude other conditions.

Pulmonary emboli occur with respiratory failure and in one series[1619] were present in 27% of 66 patients. In these patients, scans were not useful in the diagnosis, and angiograms were required. Schor and his colleagues[1722] carefully compared ^{81}Kr and ^{133}Xe in 44 studies of 41 patients with pulmonary embolism. They concluded that ^{81}Kr offered important advantages over ^{133}Xe in diagnosing emboli because of better spatial resolution, but they found that ^{133}Xe was superior in patients with chronic airflow limitation because it detected areas of low ventilation not visualized with ^{81}Kr. Regional function measurements reveal zones of decreased perfusion with only slight reduction in ventilation,[1645, 4494] but if ^{81}Kr is used, scattered zones of high $\dot{V}/\dot{Q}$ may be found.[1099]

In the second edition of this book, we stressed the importance and invariance of effort dyspnea in this condition,[1] and authors reviewing the clinical aspects of the syndrome have emphasized this feature.[1608, 1636] Excess exercise ventilation commonly occurs and is easier to measure than resting hyperventilation.[1703] It is possible that the increased ventilation, shown by Kan, Ledsome, and Bolter[1756] to follow passive pulmonary arterial distension in dogs, may be related to this phenomenon. Their finding has recently been confirmed by others.[4465] It is important to note that major falls in Pa_{O_2} usually do not occur in these patients, and hypoxemia is probably insufficient to explain the increased ventilation. In one series studied on exercise, the relationship between $\dot{V}E$ and CO_2 appeared (from one of the figures) to be as follows[4321]:

Mean Resting PVR (dyne/sec/cm^{-5})	Minute Volume (L/min/M^2)	$\dot{V}CO_2$ (mL/min/kg)
170	14	10
	22	20
580	18	10
	35	20
1500	22	10 (maximal possible)

A reduction in pulmonary arterial pressure is

---

*See references 1603, 1627, 1646, 1655.

usually followed by improvement in exercise dyspnea.[4473]

Exercise was accompanied by a fall in Pa_{O_2} from 64 mm Hg at rest to 56 mm Hg on exercise in seven recently studied patients.[4344] However, studies of $\dot{V}/\dot{Q}$ inequality do not reveal evidence of incomplete alveolar–end-capillary equilibration.[4344]

There have been few longitudinal studies of this condition, but one series observed 76 patients with thromboembolic disease for between 1 and 15 years.[3510] The pulmonary hypertension appeared to be progressive if it initially exceeded 30 mm Hg. There was some relationship of V_D/V_T ratio to survival, but no relationship of $D_{L_{CO}}$, VC, FEV_1, or Pa_{O_2} to prognosis. This observation is in conformity with the data of Riedel, Widimsky, and Stanek noted earlier. Nineteen patients with pulmonary hypertension were observed for a mean of 8.4 years.[4430] The level of hypertension had increased in 10 of the cases, and this was accompanied by a measurable increase in the diameter of the descending branch of the right pulmonary artery.

Drug Addiction

In drug-addicted patients using intravenous injections, pulmonary abnormalities are commonly present. In one series of 512 patients, 42% had a $D_{L_{CO}}SB$ less than 75% of predicted. In most, this test was the only abnormal function test.[1605] In some of these patients, granulomata and pulmonary hypertension are found.[1606] In four such patients, the $D_{L_{CO}}SB$ was below 51% of that predicted for all. FVC and FEV_1 were lowered in two. In another series of 23 patients,[1625] 13 with normal chest x-rays and normal $D_{L_{CO}}SB$ values had abnormalities on $^{99}TcMAA$ or ^{133}Xe scans. All 10 patients with a lowered $D_{L_{CO}}SB$ had abnormal scans, and 5 of these had hypoxemia at rest. In one patient in whom the $D_{L_{CO}}SB$ was only 32% of predicted, the vital capacity was 4.3 liters. In another study of 22 cases of heroin addiction, the lowest $D_{L_{CO}}SB$ was 50% of predicted, with a VC of 90% predicted and a lowered FEF_{25-75}.[1626]

Six men of mean age 32 years with long histories of intravenous use of crushed suspended pentazocine tablets[3496] had $(A - a) D_{O_2}$ levels at rest and on exercise (rest/exercise) of 24/25; 29/54; 24/11; 26/28; 30/22; and 26/20. In contrast to this variability, the $D_{L_{CO}}SB$ was reduced in all, ranging from 53% to 76% of predicted normal values. Three patients had a normal chest film, but in three the x-rays showed bilateral diffuse reticulonodular infiltrates. In four patients, talc crystals were recovered on bronchoalveolar lavage, and lung biopsies showed that there were birefringent crystals in the granulomata. It seems that the $D_{L_{CO}}SB$ is more commonly and more consistently lowered in these patients than in those with pulmonary thromboembolic disease. The reason for this is not clear.

Fat Embolization

In 1976, Banyai[1621] reviewed the history of early recognition of this condition. Sproule and his colleagues[1615] first documented the severe hypoxemia that may also occur. In one of their three patients with an initial Pa_{O_2} of 25 mm Hg and an $(A - a) D_{O_2}$ of 66 mm Hg, the vital capacity was only 1.6 liters. It rose to 3.3 liters on recovery. The reason for the initial low value was not clear, but it might be explained by severe respiratory muscle fatigue. The condition is probably common in long-bone fractures.[1621] In 17 such patients who were compared with 19 controls, a lower $D_{L_{CO}}SB$ was noted between the third and eighth days after fracture,[1629] probably indicating the presence of fat emboli. Sproule noted the unreliability of clinical cyanosis as an indicator of the presence of fat emboli. It is important that the arterial Pa_{O_2} be measured if the diagnosis is suspected. Guenter and Braun[3509] reported on 54 patients with fat embolism, noting the increased $(A - a) D_{O_2}$ and also the generally favorable prognosis, even in cases requiring assisted ventilation and positive end-expiratory pressure.

Recent experimental studies of fat embolization in sheep have shown that lung lymph flow increases, and Pa_{O_2} falls about 13 mm Hg when pulmonary arterial pressure has doubled.[1641] The volume of pulmonary extravascular water was not increased in these experiments. Since indomethacin blocked the effects, it was suggested that prostaglandins mediated the response.[1641]

Miscellaneous

Two cases involving self-injection with metallic mercury have been reported.[1634, 4437] In one, this lowered TLC and FVC. Both values returned to normal in 20 weeks, and $D_{L_{CO}}SB$ rose from 15.8 to 24.5 in 2 weeks. Improvement in the chest x-ray indicated that metallic mercury was leaving the lung. In the other,[4437] concomitant pulmonary thromboembolism was present. Experimentally, mercury may produce fibrosis around the metallic deposit, but there is no indication of systemic toxicity after it lodges in the lung.

CARDIAC CHANGES SECONDARY TO LUNG DISEASE: COR PULMONALE

Evidence of early pulmonary hypertension well before cor pulmonale develops is discussed in Chapters 7 and 8 and pulmonary hypertension in fully developed chronic obstructive lung disease is detailed in Chapter 8. Additional observations on respiratory failure in chronic airflow limitation can be found in Chapter 23.

"Cor pulmonale" describes the sequence of circulatory changes that may follow chronic lung disease. It has been suggested that it be defined in terms of right ventricular enlargement.[1657] A number of reviews have appeared,[1638, 1653] and Grover[4401] has commented on the control of the pulmonary circulation. Voelkel[4469] has reviewed mechanisms involved in hypoxic pulmonary vasoconstriction. A valuable summary of cardiovascular performance in patients with chronic airflow limitation has also been published.[1700]

Occurrence of cor pulmonale as a percentage of patients with cardiac failure seems to vary from a high of 35% in Sheffield, England to a low of 0.4% in Japan.[1660] It has recently been shown that papain-induced emphysema in dogs is followed by pulmonary hypertension after 6 months.[3264]

In this section, all the studies cited are concerned with patients with chronic airflow limitation. For observations on the pulmonary circulation in interstitial fibrosis, see Chapter 14; in pneumoconiosis, see Chapter 16; in sarcoidosis, see Chapter 15; in scoliosis, see Chapter 21; and in cystic fibrosis, see Chapter 10. In Chapter 2, the physiology of the relationship between pulmonary arterial pressure and hypoxemia is discussed.

The inverse relationship between Pa_{O_2} and mean pulmonary arterial pressure in this condition has been found in many studies,* and oxygen breathing on exercise lowers the pulmonary arterial pressure.[1122] In 136 subjects, an r value of 0.56 was found between Pa_{O_2} and pulmonary arterial pressure at rest.[1249] It has been observed that in persons with chronic

---

*See references 1043, 1115, 1628, 1652, 1702, 1705.

airflow limitation born and living at altitude the pulmonary arterial pressure is no higher than in those at sea level.[3267]

It is common to note that the onset of heart failure occurs when the Pa_{O_2} falls below 60 mm Hg or when the Pa_{CO_2} rises above 50 mm Hg, with the FEV_1 being reduced to about a liter.[1266] As noted in the second edition,[1] the onset of clinical cor pulmonale often occurs at about the age of 57. In one series, 66% of patients died within 2 years of the first episode.[1266] Survival is shortened, the higher the measured pulmonary vascular resistance.[1230] Relatively few studies of the events leading up to clinical edema have been published, but the results of those that have been published are interesting. In one of these,[1656] the increase in peripheral fluid was accompanied by an increase in sodium similar to other types of heart failure. No potassium depletion was noted.

Campbell and colleagues[1674] noted that body weight increased only slightly as peripheral edema and elevation of jugular venous pressure appeared. They suggested that tissue loss was occurring with replacement by edema. Recent studies of plasma renin, aldosterone, and antidiuretic hormone in patients with chronic airflow obstruction in acute respiratory failure[4354] have indicated that the lack of sodium diuresis may be partially due to hyperaldosteronism, and the hyponatremia is caused by inappropriately elevated plasma antidiuretic hormone. In another study, the effect of variation of arterial Pa_{O_2} was varied between 80 mm Hg and 39 mm Hg.[4444] Urinary water excretion was not affected by the hypoxemia. However, the sodium excretion declined, and the systemic blood pressure fell, as did glomerular filtration rate and filtered sodium load. Renal plasma flow and filtration fraction were unchanged. Plasma renin, norepinephrine, aldosterone, and arginine vasopressin levels were unaffected by hypoxemia. The mean FEV_1 of the patients studied was 600 milliliters, and the Pa_{CO_2} varied by only 7 mm Hg between the two sets of observations.

The favorable effect of long-term diuretic therapy[1238] is noted in Chapter 8. We have noted the frequency with which patients with chronic airflow limitation in pulmonary edema are admitted through the emergency department of the hospital. Although there seems no reason to suspect that this is attributable to left ventricular failure, it seems clear that fluid overload may occur in the lung—but the mechanism is obscure. Possibly, this is why diuretics are often found to be helpful. Observations on left ventricular function and pulmonary arterial wedge pressures are noted later. As noted in Chapter 8, studies of renal pathology have shown significant glomerular changes in patients with severe chronic airflow limitation.[3287] Acute exacerbations of respiratory failure are not accompanied by any reduction in cardiac output,[1702] although an increase in pulmonary arterial pressure occurs with the falling Pa_{O_2}.

As noted in Chapter 8, EKG evidence of right ventricular hypertrophy is associated with a lower rate of survival, and clinical cor pulmonale lowers survival, compared with cases with a similar FEV_1.[1022] It has been shown that EKG changes are related to measured right ventricular hypertrophy,[1602] and the authors of this study concluded that six EKG criteria were useful in indicating hypertrophy:

• rightward P vector
• P wave cor pulmonale
• right initial QRS vector
• right terminal QRS vector
• right mean QRS vector
• posterior horizontal QRS vector

Others have suggested that an S/Q_3 pattern and right axis deviation equal to or more than 110 degrees are better indicators than P wave changes.[1623] Others have noted a good correlation between pulmonary arterial pressure and the area of the QRS loop.[3516] Other correlations between EKG criteria and the pulmonary arterial pressure have been published.[1704] Changes on vectorcardiography[1617] are related to pulmonary arterial pressure and hemodynamics on exercise. Results of studies that have used echocardiography are somewhat conflicting. In one study, it was found that estimates of right ventricular wall thickness correlated with Pa_{O_2} and FEV_1.[3503] In another small series, the echocardiographic data correlated with the degree of pulmonary hypertension.[4440] Others have not found the same relationship, however.[4378] In a third study, there appeared to be a clear correlation between the echocardiographic data and estimates of the severity of emphysema.[4381] It has been suggested that the time interval between tricuspid valve closure and pulmonary valve opening rises from a normal value of about 30 milliseconds to 120 milliseconds when the pulmonary diastolic pressure is elevated.[1597] Murphy and colleagues[1251] carried out a careful evaluation of radiologic criteria of cardiac and chamber enlargement in 72 patients with chronic airflow limitation. They

concluded that overall detection of cardiomegaly was satisfactory but that "the inaccuracy and interobserver variability in the detection of enlargement of specific chambers make it evident that the criteria are not valid and that roentgenographic appraisal of cardiac size in these patients is limited to findings of normality or cardiomegaly." Heart chamber sizes were assessed at autopsy. In this series, the mean FEF_{25-75} of the patients during life was less than 0.5 L/sec.[125] Thurlbeck[585] has analyzed the reasons for the conflicting evidence that right ventricular hypertrophy is, or is not, related to the extent of pulmonary emphysema at autopsy. Conflicting data continue to appear.*

Careful measurement of the distance between the bifurcation of the right and left main pulmonary arteries and the mean thoracic diameter can be used to predict an elevated pulmonary arterial pressure. If the ratio between these two lengths multiplied by 100 exceeds 42, pulmonary hypertension can be inferred.[1659] This finding may apparently precede clinical or EKG evidence of cor pulmonale. The transhilar width has also been used to estimate the pulmonary arterial pressure.[3499] Weitzenblum and colleagues[3522] have contributed an editorial summarizing data on clinical methods of estimating the pulmonary arterial pressure in patients with chronic airflow limitation. In spite of the many correlations that have been noted, estimation without measurement is still uncertain in many individuals. The mean diameter of pulmonary vessels measured on angiography is reduced in chronic airflow limitation, and the reduction is related to the increase in TLC.[1721]

Patients with chronic airflow limitation with a small heart size[1710] show a higher TLC, lower $DL_{CO}SB$, and a lower cardiac output, but FEV_1, resting pulmonary arterial pressures, and exercise hemodynamics were not different from those with a normal sized heart. Right ventricular hypertrophy is related to the thickening of the medial muscle layers of the pulmonary arterioles[1599, 1620] (which is also related to smoking history[1624]). Right ventricular hypertrophy may occur in some patients in whom the FEV_1 is still 50% of predicted values.[1326] There is a close correlation ($r = -0.56$) between the degree of hypoxemia and the diameter of right ventricular myocardial fibers.[1631]

Dynamic studies of ventricular function on exercise show that abnormality of the right

---

*See references 1326, 1599, 1633, 1639.

ventricular ejection fraction (RVEF) is common.[1237, 1275, 3491] Some authors have found this to be related to the Pa_{O_2},[3491] but in other series there was no correlation to either FEV_1 or Pa_{O_2}.[1237] In studies of upright exercise in 12 men with severe chronic airflow limitation[4104] whose mean age was 58.5 years, the mean FEV_1 was 33% of predicted and the mean Pa_{O_2} was 77 mm Hg at 58% of maximal $\dot{V}_{O_2}$. There was a significant increase in pulmonary arterial pressure, and the RVEF failed to increase normally. The end-diastolic volume index increased significantly. The results led the authors to suggest that right ventricular dysfunction played an important part in limiting exercise. Others have noted a linear negative correlation between the pulmonary arterial pressure and the right ventricular ejection fraction in similar cases.[4352] Also, a relationship between RVEF and the fall in oxygen saturation on exercise has been found.[4442]

There has been much analysis of left ventricular hypertrophy and dynamics in patients with chronic airflow limitation. In 72 patients, left ventricular hypertrophy was found in 20, of whom 10 had hypertensive or arteriosclerotic heart disease. Two had occult aortic lesions.[1717] The authors concluded that left ventricular hypertrophy was rarely seen without some factor independent of lung disease being present. Its occurrence varies in different series,* and Thurlbeck[585] observed that its percentage occurrence ranged from 15% to 90% in autopsies of patients with chronic airflow obstruction. He concluded that it occurred in between 5% and 15% of patients in whom no explanation could be found.

Left ventricular end-diastolic pressure and stroke volume are most commonly normal.[1661, 1668] In those patients in whom it is elevated, the phenomenon may be attributable to the effect of hypercapnic acidosis on cardiac

*See references 1326, 1599, 1600, 1639.

muscle contractility.[1668] An elevated wedge pressure is not thought to indicate left ventricular dysfunction in patients with severe airflow limitation,[1708] though its elevation is unexplained. It does not appear to be related to the simultaneously measured esophageal pressure.[4044] There may well be an interactive effect between the two ventricles,[4398] and echocardiographic data have recently supported this concept.[4317] Although evidence of pulmonary thromboembolism is commonly found at autopsy in patients with chronic airflow limitation (86% in one series[1647]), the importance of this factor in relation to pulmonary hypertension is not clear.

There are many studies of exercise hemodynamics in patients with chronic airflow limitation. In one of these, which used supine bicycle exercise, Weitzenblum and his colleagues[1043] divided the patients into three groups with increasing severity of pulmonary hypertension (see the table at the bottom of this page).

The normality of the cardiac output in the presence of pulmonary hypertension confirms earlier data.[1] The pulmonary vascular resistance measured on exercise correlates with the predicted percentage of DL_{CO}, with FEV_1,[1292] and with the extent of abnormalities seen on wedge angiography.[1069, 1252] There is a greater difference in swings of pulmonary arterial pressure on exercise (related to inspiration and expiration) in patients with chronic airflow limitation than in normal individuals[1052]; this is probably attributable to the greater swings of intrapleural pressure. The larger swings complicate the measurement in these patients.

Measurements of pulmonary blood volume by differential dye injection methods in patients with chronic airflow limitation show that this volume is generally about the same as in normal individuals when expressed as a percentage of total blood volume (about 6.3%).[1662] In absolute terms, it is slightly lower than in normal persons. In one study, it averaged 343 (± 95)

	Group 1	Group 2	Group 3
Number	23	40	29
Age (year)	54.1	62.6	58.5
PAP, rest (mm Hg)	Normal	Normal	>20
exercise	26.3	44.2	55.4
VC (L)	3.67	2.93	2.94
FEV_1 (L)	1.52	1.19	1.07
Pa_{O_2}, rest/exercise (mm Hg)	67/81	64/69	57/57
Pa_{CO_2}, rest/exercise (mm Hg)	37/34	34/37	38/42
$(A - a) D_{O_2}$, exercise (mm Hg)	34	37	45
$\dot{V}_{O_2}$, exercise (mL/min/M^2)	533	497	487
$\dot{Q}_C$, exercise (L/min/M^2)	6.3	6.0	6.1

milliliters in patients, compared with 469 (± 117) milliliters in normal individuals.[1676] It was not related to an increase in TLC. However, pulmonary blood volume does not increase normally on exercise,[1699] perhaps because of limitation of the pulmonary bed. Although there is no direct shunt on exercise in patients with chronic airflow limitation, there is evidence of an increased shunt component on 100% oxygen breathing.[1245] There have been several observations of the effect of oxygen therapy, both acute and prolonged,[4316, 4041] on cardiac hemodynamics.

In 67 patients studied by cardiac catheterization at rest and on exercise and after 20 minutes of 100% O_2,[4443] the cardiac output was normal in all; the wedge pressure was also normal at rest and on exercise. The pulmonary vascular resistance fell on oxygen, but the change in pulmonary arterial pressure was not striking. Long-term studies indicate that the initial fall in pulmonary vascular resistance on oxygen breathing may be related to survival.[404]

Many studies of the effect of drug therapy on cardiac hemodynamics have appeared. Earlier data showing that digoxin is of no value in these patients have been confirmed. The effects of nifedipine,* hydralazine,[4322, 4346, 4356] felodipine,[4026, 4474] and disodium cromoglycate[4472] have all been studied.

Since the onset of cor pulmonale is such an important adverse prognostic sign, the state of the pulmonary circulation and right ventricle should be evaluated carefully when patients with chronic airflow limitation of moderate severity are first seen. It seems likely that measurement of Pa_{O_2}, careful EKG analysis, and determination of vessel diameters on the chest x-ray will permit a reasonably accurate assessment of pulmonary arterial pressure to be made. But if unusual features seem to be present, measurement of the pulmonary arterial pressure at rest and on exercise may be justified to clarify the status of the lesser circulation. A careful comparison between the measured pulmonary arterial pressure, at rest and on exercise, and Pa_{O_2} should be made. When the pulmonary arterial pressure seems unusually high in relation to the Pa_{O_2}, either thromboemboli may be present or the patient may be an abnormally sensitive responder to a lowered Pa_{O_2} and is, therefore, a candidate for early domiciliary oxygen therapy.

---

*See references 4298, 4323, 4325, 4347, 4495.

INTRAPULMONARY SHUNTS

The comprehensive review by Laros on shunts "in and over the lungs"[1746] summarizes clinical details and methods of investigation of these cases. In patients with arteriovenous fistulae in the lung, a low Pa_{O_2} and normal diffusing capacity and normal spirometry values suggest the diagnosois,[1743] but on occasion the arterial Pa_{O_2} may be as low as 45 mm Hg before the diagnosis is made.[1738]

Occasionally, the diagnosis is confused by coexistent airflow limitation.[1741] In studies of eight patients with arteriovenous fistulae, it was observed that the shunt increased by as much as 25% if a full inspiration was taken and the breath held, presumably because the pulmonary vascular resistance increases under these conditions.[1744] This test was considered clinically useful. Studies on a 23-year-old man with two arteriovenous fistulae in the right middle lobe[4376] showed that the Pa_{O_2} initially rose on exercise to 79.9 mm Hg from a resting value of 73 mm Hg—an effect the authors attributed to the initial fall in pulmonary vascular resistance on exercise. Careful preoperative assessment is required because multiple fistulae are not rare.[1748] One patient with an acquired pulmonary arteriovenous fistula as a result of a bullet wound had a Pa_{O_2} of 47 mm Hg and an FEV_1 of 99% of predicted.[1739]

Pulmonary telangiectasia with multiple capillary sinusoids in the lung is very rare but of special interest because of the unusual combination of pulmonary function test findings. Since our initial report in 1957 of a patient diagnosed during life,[4314] two other similar patients have been reported.[1747, 4403] The second of these was the same age as our patient (19 years), with gross finger clubbing and cyanosis and with splenomegaly. Xenon ventilation scans and technetium perfusion scans were normal, but the outline of the kidneys was noted after the latter test. An intracardiac shunt was excluded by bolus studies. The pulmonary function data were as follows:

	Right Lung	Left Lung
Oxygen uptake	13%	87%
Ventilation	46%	54%

A lung biopsy in this patient showed the characteristic thin-walled telangiectatic vessels lying in the alveolar walls. These patients often have a normal chest x-ray (but an abnormal angiogram), and test values are confusing because a lowered Pa_{O_2}, often with polycythemia, may be accompanied by a normal or lowered diffusing capacity, normal pulmonary mechanical and spirometric findings, and no evidence of an arteriovenous fistula in the lung. Changes of Pa_{O_2} with posture have been described.[1747]

PULMONARY ARTERY ATRESIA AND OBSTRUCTION

Patients with pulmonary artery atresia in which flow is greatly reduced to some part of the lung do not show a comparable reduction in ventilation to the lobe.[1749] Although the bronchial arteries may show enlargement, there is little gas exchange. In one study of 30 patients with obstruction to major pulmonary vessels,[1745] careful measurement of the $A-a$ difference for CO_2 was found to be a useful test. Localized narrowing of pulmonary vessels has been described as part of Takayasu's arterial disease.[1742] In one case in a 27-year-old woman that involved the right pulmonary artery, the VC was 103% of predicted and the $DL_{CO}SB$ was 63% of predicted. Oxygen uptake and ventilation were divided as follows:

	Predicted	Actual	5 Years Later
Hb (g)	15–16	15	18
VC (L)	3.55	2.12	
$DL_{CO}SB$ (%P)	100	36	
Pa_{O_2} (mm Hg)	80	58	44
Pa_{CO_2} (mm Hg)	35–39	30	
O_2Hb (on 100% O_2)	100	100	
Pa_{O_2} (on 100% O_2)	600	357	

In one remarkable study of unilateral pulmonary arterial occlusion at rest and on exercise in 22 normal subjects, exercise ventilation increased 30% on exercise, compared with control values.[1703] A recent case report of a 46-year-old woman with complete obstruction of the right main pulmonary artery by a malignant fibrous histiocytoma[4446] noted that on exercise her arterial Pa_{O_2} fell from 91 mm Hg to 67 mm Hg. Her resting $DL_{CO}SB$ was 14.1, compared with

a predicted value of 23, and her FEV_1 was 82% of predicted. Other cases of obstruction to one main pulmonary artery with some lowering of $DL_{CO}SB$[1607] but relatively little disability have been reported. Anomalous pulmonary venous drainage of the right lung into the inferior vena cava is not associated with interference with pulmonary function.[1740]

SUMMARY

It may be concluded that evidence of the effect of heart disease on pulmonary function, in both acute and chronic conditions, is reasonably consistent and is in concordance with experimental data. The evidence that increased pulmonary arterial pressure may be closely related to dyspnea is very strong, as noted throughout this chapter. When a patient is referred to the pulmonary function laboratory with a complaint of dyspnea, with radiographically normal lung fields, and with normal routine pulmonary function tests, the physician should suspect this diagnosis.

The data summarized in this chapter raise the important question of whether an increasing degree of left ventricular dysfunction or minor degrees of pulmonary hypertension below the level of simple clinical detection, from any cause, may play a role in raising ventilation in relation to oxygen uptake in patients who have some additional disease, such as the early radiologic changes of pneumoconiosis. Further, it is important to consider the possibility that the reason why the FEV_1 has been found to be such a reliable predictor of survival is because the FVC is lowered by a raised left atrial pressure. This is suggested by the literature, but definitive evidence is lacking. Such questions cannot be resolved with precision, yet the physician should be fully aware of pulmonary function data in patients with pulmonary hypertension or with left ventricular failure.

CHAPTER

PULMONARY FUNCTION IN COLLAGEN DISEASES, HEMOSIDEROSIS, AND GOODPASTURE'S SYNDROME

13

INTRODUCTION

The results of pulmonary function tests in collagen diseases, hemosiderosis, and Goodpasture's syndrome depend on the extent and degree of the following changes:

- chronic alveolitis
- vasculitis
- intrapulmonary hemorrhage
- pleural changes and pleural effusions
- associated muscle weakness, including diaphragm paresis

Pulmonary changes as a consequence of drug administration may include alveolitis and vasculitis and hence may mimic these diseases; they are discussed in Chapter 14. Scleroderma and polymyositis in relation to diffuse interstitial fibrosis are also discussed in the next chapter.

Fulmer[3524] states that in the following seven syndromes some degree of vasculitis is invariably found:

- Churg-Strauss syndrome
- "overlap" vasculitis

- Wegener's granulomatosis
- lymphomatoid granulomatosis
- lymphocytic angiitis
- necrotizing sarcoid granulomatosis
- bronchocentric granulomatosis

and may occur in seven other conditions:

- Henoch-Schönlein purpura
- leukocytoclastic vasculitis
- disseminated giant cell arteritis
- Behçet's syndrome
- polyarteritis nodosa
- Takayasu's disease
- essential cryoglobulinemia

A report on 11 patients with collagen vascular disease and 26 with viral pneumonia, all with progressive respiratory insufficiency and abnormal function tests,[3505] noted that endothelial cell cytoplasmic swelling and intracellular tubuloreticular structures were the dominant changes in both groups. The authors concluded that ultrastructural changes were identical in the two groups; that endothelial cell damage was the principal lesion; and that tubuloreticular

265

structures were also seen in peripheral blood lymphocytes in both groups.

PULMONARY CHANGES IN ASSOCIATION WITH RHEUMATOID ARTHRITIS

In the second edition of this book, we noted that up to 1970 no series of cases of rheumatoid arthritis had been systematically surveyed to determine the frequency of pulmonary function abnormalities.[1] Several surveys have now been published. Ninety-nine patients with classic rheumatoid arthritis were compared with 60 controls matched for age, sex, and smoking history.[1793] The FEV_1 and FVC were lower in rheumatoid men and women, but the FEV_1/FVC ratio was normal. The $DL_{CO}SB$ was lower in affected men but not in women with rheumatoid arthritis. More of the rheumatoid patients were reported to show an increased frequency dependence of compliance than the controls.

In 48 patients and controls matched from the same series,[1791] measurement of the components of DL showed no differences in DM but showed lower V_c values in patients with rheumatoid nodules; DL was not much affected. Changes in dynamic compliance were not confirmed. One series of 129 patients has been extensively studied.[387, 1759, 1798] Six had marked pulmonary radiologic changes. Of the 123 remaining, 35% had abnormality of one function test or slight radiologic changes; 28% had reduction in either VC or $DL_{CO}SB$; 7% had reduction in VC and $DL_{CO}SB$; and 2% had radiologic changes plus reduction in VC and $DL_{CO}SB$.[1759] These authors were careful to correct the $DL_{CO}SB$ for anemia. They concluded that DL_{CO}/VA was normal in a higher percentage than $DL_{CO}SB$, but several patients showed lowering of the $DL_{CO}SB$ out of proportion to the lowering of VC. Patients with a normal chest film and definite function test abnormality were documented. In another series of 41 "consecutive" patients with rheumatoid arthritis,[1784] 53% had an abnormal chest film and 41% had an abnormal $DL_{CO}SB$. Needle lung biopsies were abnormal in all those with reduced VC, TLC, $DL_{CO}SB$, and Pa_{O_2}, even in those in whom the chest film was considered normal.

Yousem, Colby, and Carrington[4411] reported on open-lung biopsies in 40 patients with rheumatoid arthritis, of whom seven were thought to have "restrictive" disease; one to have "ob-structive" disease; and nine to have some combination of these findings. Detailed pulmonary function tests were not reported, but pathologically, 13 had pulmonary nodules, six had bronchiolitis obliterans with patchy pneumonitis, five had "usual interstitial pneumonitis"; five had lymphoid hyperplasia, and five had cellular interstitial infiltrates. None had angiitis. The authors stated that "consistent correlations between the results of pulmonary function tests and roentgenologic and histologic findings were not found," but this was not documented in detail.

A second recent study of 24 patients with rheumatoid arthritis, of whom nine had clinical evidence of interstitial lung involvement,[4479] found that bronchoalveolar lavage was abnormal in five with no evidence of lung involvement. Ten were normal, both on lavage and clinically. In this series, the mean FVC was 67% of predicted, and the mean $DL_{CO}SB$ was 74% of predicted in those with clinical evidence of lung involvement; these were normal in the other groups.

The frequency of finding a lowered $DL_{CO}SB$ in this condition varies between 24% and 57% in different series,[1765] but correction for anemia has not been made in all of them. It is possible that the incidence of abnormal DL_{CO} is higher in seropositive than in seronegative patients, as was reported in a comparison between 44 patients in the former category and 40 in the latter.[1801] There was no difference in FRC values. Collins and his colleagues[1755] studied 43 patients of mean age 50 years with rheumatoid arthritis and found the following abnormalities:

	Abnormalities (%)
Pa_{O_2}	15
VC	20
MMEF	65
FVC	26
$FEV_1/FVC\%$	41
Chest x-ray	44

They commented that smokers with rheumatoid arthritis had significantly lower MMEF values than either non-smokers with rheumatoid arthritis or smokers with osteoarthritis. They also stated that PiMS phenotype for alpha$_1$-antitrypsin seemed to be an additional risk factor.

An acute interstitial pneumonitis has been reported in association with a worsening of rheumatoid arthritis (probably the rare "rheumatic pneumonia" that used to be described). In one well studied patient, the Pa_{O_2} rose from 29 mm Hg to 60 mm Hg on recovery, and the VC increased from an initial value of 0.96 liters to 1.67 liters.[1779] A 73-year-old woman with rheumatoid arthritis treated with D-penicillamine developed extensive interstitial pneumonitis with severe hypoxemia but without bronchiolitis.[3523]

Chronic Bronchiolitis

The recognition by Geddes and his colleagues of a syndrome of obliterative bronchiolitis in association with rheumatoid arthritis was a major contribution.[1320] In Table 13–1, the pulmonary function data from Geddes' six cases and one additional case confirmed at autopsy are shown. This disease causes a very severe obstructive defect, with very low values for FEF_{25-75} and FEV_1. There is also reduction of DL_{CO} and Pa_{O_2} initially without hypercapnia.[976, 3367]

In one mild case in a 44-year-old woman on gold therapy, the FEF_{25-75} fell from 3.40 L/sec to 2.69 L/sec, while the FEV_1 was unchanged at 2.80 liters. The bronchiolitis was demonstrated on several transbronchial biopsies.[4386] Patients in whom it was difficult to decide whether their disease was "rheumatoid" in origin have been described in detail. In one of these, a 57-year-old non-smoking woman with no clinical evidence of connective tissue disease,[4332] positive antinuclear and rheumatoid factors were ascribed by the authors to the lung disease. Dyspnea resulted in death from respiratory failure in 2 years. The chest x-ray showed only hyperinflation. The DL_{CO} was 80% of predicted when the FEV_1 had fallen to 19% of predicted. At autopsy, a very severe obliterative bronchiolitis was the only lesion present.[4332] There was no history of any relevant environmental exposure.

As noted in the reported patients, the chest x-ray shows only hyperinflation. This syndrome is additionally important because it illustrates the functional consequences of very severe small airway disease without chronic mucus hypersecretion and without morphologic emphysema (and is briefly discussed in Chapter 7 from this point of view). One case of obliterative bronchiolitis in a 37-year-old woman that was attributed to exposure to cleaning agents[1781] may well have been related instead to her rheumatoid arthritis (noted in the case history). Acute bronchiolitis has been noted in association with an acute worsening of rheumatoid arthritis,[1763] and acute localized necrotizing arteritis also occurs.[1766] Acute bronchiolitis also occurs in the Stevens-Johnson syndrome[3535] and occasionally in systemic lupus erythematosus.[3526] In one case of rheumatoid arthritis in a 55-year-old woman,[3533] bilateral upper lobe shadowing developed, with progressive deterioration of pulmonary function and ending with an FEV_1 of 16% of predicted and a Pa_{O_2} of only 38 mm Hg. At autopsy, there was not only a severe bronchiolitis but, in addition, severe mucosal inflammation of lobar and segmental bronchi

Table 13–1. PULMONARY FUNCTION TEST DATA IN CASES OF BRONCHIOLITIS ASSOCIATED WITH RHEUMATOID ARTHRITIS*

Test	Cases†						Case LH‡
	1	2	3	4	5	6	
TLC	124x	140p	106x	115x	118p	86he	65he
VC or FVC	24	46	47	38	29	49	31
RV	—	309p	—	184	243p	167he	126he
FRC	—	—	—	—	—	—	92he
FEF_{25-75}	—	—	—	8	10	16	11
DL_{CO}	46sb	48sb	—	—	53sb	63sb	64ss
Pa_{O_2} (mm Hg)	54.7	62.2	60.0	60.0	42.0	—	54.0
Pa_{CO_2} (mm Hg)	39.7	36.0	41.2	42.0	48.0	—	41.0

NOTES: x = measured by x-ray planimetry.
     p = measured by body plethysmography.
    he = measured by helium dilution.
    sb = $DL_{CO}SB$.
    ss = $DL_{CO}SS$.
*All data presented as a percentage of predicted.
†Data for cases 1–6 from Geddes, D. M., et al. Progressive airway obliteration in adults and its association with rheumatoid disease. Quart. J. Med. 46:427–444, 1977.
‡Data from Murphy, K. C., et al. Obliterative bronchiolitis in two rheumatoid arthritis patients treated with penicillamine. Arthritis Rheum. 24:557–560, 1981.

throughout the lungs. By 1984, 18 patients with bronchiolitis in association with rheumatoid arthritis had been recorded.[4386]

The use of gold salts in the treatment of rheumatoid arthritis may be followed by pulmonary changes (see Chapter 14). On occasion, it may be difficult to determine whether changes in function are due to the disease or are a consequence of this therapy. This difficulty may be avoided if pulmonary function tests are done routinely before the therapy is initiated.

SJÖGREN'S SYNDROME

In a report from the Mayo Clinic, pulmonary involvement occurred in 31 patients out of a series of 343 persons with this syndrome,[1780] giving an incidence of 9%. Detailed function tests have been reported in a number of small series. In five non-smokers with Sjögren's syndrome, all had an FEF_{25-75} less than 60% of predicted but had normal lung recoil.[1772] Increased residual volume and SBN_2/L slope and a reduced Pa_{O_2} with a normal TLC and static intrapleural pressure indicated probable small airway involvement, as there was no associated chronic bronchitis or asthma. Mononuclear cell infiltration of small airways was found in one biopsy of these patients. There appear to be two forms of pulmonary involvement: xerotrachea causing a troublesome dry cough, but associated with a normal chest x-ray; and diffuse interstitial lung disease.[4370] Pleurisy appears to be rare. A study of 36 patients[4456] revealed six with normal pulmonary function but a dry cough, which was thought to indicate tracheal changes. Nine showed diffuse pulmonary interstitial change, all with a reduced DL_{CO}. Eight had evidence of small airway involvement, as indicated by a reduced $\dot{V}max_{25\%}VC$ with a normal FEV_1 and normal lung volumes and diffusing capacity.

In another group of 17 patients with Sjögren's syndrome, 10 had evidence of pulmonary involvement manifested by recurrent pneumonia, granulomatous infiltration, fibrosing alveolitis, or airway disease.[1771] FEV_1 and $DL_{CO}SB$ were lowered, but the mucociliary clearance rate was noted to be normal. In another series of 20 patients with Sjögren's syndrome, all non-smokers, pulmonary function was normal in 12. The remainder showed evidence of combined restrictive and obstructive changes, with DL_{CO} lowered in three and Pa_{O_2} lowered in five.[1767] In 22 patients with primary Sjögren's syndrome,

12 were thought to have pulmonary involvement.[4370] This syndrome occurs in association with primary biliary cirrhosis, but reduction in DL_{CO} occurred only in patients with cirrhosis who also had Sjögren's syndrome.[1799]

DIFFUSE LUPUS ERYTHEMATOSUS

In the second edition of this book, we presented details of a patient with systemic lupus erythematosus with abnormalities of pulmonary function.[1] At that time there were no data to indicate how commonly the lungs were involved in this condition, but recent series indicate that involvement is not rare. However, some clinical reviews of this condition make scant reference to pulmonary involvement or abnormalities in function.[1790]

In one series of 30 patients,[1786] the VC was less than 80% of predicted in 14 and the $DL_{CO}SB$ was reduced in 24. The authors concluded that the $DL_{CO}SB$ was the most sensitive indicator of abnormality, often being lowered without radiologic change or a respiratory history. In five of their cases, they noted that the inspiratory pressure was abnormally low and suggested that there might be interference with the normal action of the diaphragm. Bilateral diaphragmatic paralysis has been described in this condition.

In another series of 44 patients,[1777] the $DL_{CO}SB$ was often lowered. In 22 patients in another series, all without pulmonary symptoms, reduction in VC and $DL_{CO}SB$ and increases in RV and $(A - a) D_{O_2}$ were common.[1761] Similar findings occurred in another 18 patients, of whom seven had pulmonary symptoms.[1768] Since many of these patients have anemia, it is important that correction for this be applied before the DL_{CO} is reported.

These function test abnormalities are caused by a combination of chronic non-specific interstitial fibrosis (with varying degrees of vasculitis and chronic pleural changes) and diaphragmatic weakness. Thompson and his colleagues[4419] have recently documented the reduced transdiaphragmatic pressures that occur in cases of diffuse lupus erythematosus. They also note that the reduction in TLC may be so marked that the designation "shrinking lung" might well be applied to these cases. Their data[4419] indicate that the reduced diffusing capacity is largely a function of reduced lung volumes, since the "k_{CO}" in their patients was not abnormal. Their series indicated that some improvement in function occurred after albuterol therapy.

In a report[4457] of 18 autopsied cases, visceral pleural thickening was present in all, and interstitial pneumonitis was found in six. There was no specific pulmonary marker of the lung in lupus, and no particular involvement of small airways was noted. Occasionally, there are severe changes in pulmonary arterioles in this condition,[3478] and pulmonary hypertension may dominate the clinical picture. Acute lupus pneumonitis may be accompanied by severe hypoxemia and very low values for VC and $DL_{CO}SB$.[1783]

IDIOPATHIC PULMONARY HEMOSIDEROSIS

Idiopathic pulmonary hemosiderosis is a disease of remissions and exacerbations, and derangements of pulmonary function vary during its course. When the patient has recovered from an acute episode, there may be a slight reduction in VC, but exercise diffusing capacity is little reduced—an observation compatible with the histologic demonstration of normal alveolar septa.[1778] In patients with disease running a course of a few months to death, considerable reduction in VC may occur, with moderate hypoxemia and pulmonary hypertension but with relative preservation of ventilatory flow rates.[1776] The residual volume is reduced, and $DL_{CO}SB$ may be low, if intrapulmonary hemorrhage is not present and the condition has become chronic.[1787] Intrapulmonary hemorrhage in this condition may be detected through the use of CO, as described in the next section.

In children, both restrictive and obstructive syndromes occur.[1775]

GOODPASTURE'S SYNDROME

Episodes of intrapulmonary hemorrhage are a feature of Goodpasture's syndrome, and Greening and Hughes[1762] have recently reported on the use of the diffusing capacity to detect its occurrence. Analyzing patients in a routine laboratory in whom $DL_{CO}SB/\dot{V}A$ occasionally averaged 219% of baseline values, they noted that these included 21 patients with Goodpasture's syndrome, four with polyarteritis nodosa, four with Wegener's granulomatosis, and one with diffuse systemic lupus erythematosus. In an earlier paper, Lipscomb, Patel, and

Hughes[1794] had suggested the use of $DL_{CO}/\dot{V}A$ for this purpose. The combination of hemoptysis, opacities on the chest film, a fall in hemoglobin, and a rise in $DL_{CO}SB/\dot{V}A$ signaled the occurrence of intrapulmonary hemorrhage. Addleman, Logan, and Grossman[4452] have reported sequential studies of $DL_{CO}SB$ in a 25-year-old man with this condition; the value varied from 100% to 150% of predicted and reliably indicated the occurrence of intrapulmonary hemorrhage. In this patient, the DL_{CO} one year after recovery had fallen to 80% of predicted, which the authors interpreted as indicating the development of chronic changes.

The technique of measurement of $DL_{CO}SB/\dot{V}A$ can be performed at the bedside by equilibrating the patient's alveolar gas with a bag containing 10% helium and 0.3% CO; the bag is emptied and filled 10 times in 10 seconds.[344] In 22 tests, this method agreed closely with $DL_{CO}SB$ (r = 0.9923). In stable patients with a chronic form of this condition—and in the absence of intrapulmonary hemorrhage—some reduction in VC, residual volume, and $DL_{CO}SB$ may be seen, together with some hypoxemia.[1787] A review of clinical features of this condition[1789] noted that 37% of patients had rales or rhonchi in the lungs, but it is not clear whether flow limitation is commonly found.

In both hemosiderosis and Goodpasture's syndrome, the major lung function abnormality is generalized airspace disease, creating an effective shunt in regions of zero or nearly zero $\dot{V}/\dot{Q}$ ratios and leading to hypoxemia imposed on anemia and a severe reduction in oxygen delivery. In addition, the work of breathing is increased; lung compliance is decreased as a consequence of a reduction of volume of normally functioning lung.

PULMONARY EOSINOPHILIA SYNDROMES

Tropical Eosinophilia

During the acute stage of this condition, characteristic findings are reduced lung volumes, impaired ventilatory flow rates, and a reduced diffusing capacity (which distinguishes it from the majority of cases of asthma).[1] A 37-year-old Englishman who visited northwest India had a 4-year history of intermittent cough, wheezing, and dyspnea.[353] The chest x-ray showed 2 to 4 millimeter nodules in the middle and lower zones and some generalized haziness.

His FEV_1 was 37% of predicted, and his DL_{CO} was 56% of predicted. The filarial fluorescent antibody titer was very high (1/512), and both FEV_1 and DL_{CO} rose after treatment with diethylcarbamazine.

Recovery may be complete,[1795] but Poh,[1796] in a 2-year follow-up of 15 cases in Singapore, found persistence of a reduced $DL_{CO}SB$ and FEV_1, possibly due to development of mild interstitial fibrosis. Abnormality of function may still be present after complete radiologic clearing has occurred.[1796]

Eosinophilic Pneumonia (Löffler's Syndrome)

In three patients with chronic eosinophilic pneumonia,[1792] all showed reductions in TLC and VC, and two had a reduced $DL_{CO}SB$. The closing volume was increased by steroid administration. A biopsy from one of the patients showed early bronchiolitis obliterans.[1792] The condition seems to be characterized by restrictive or obstructive features or some combination of these.[1788] Rogers and his colleagues[1782] recorded pretreatment and post-treatment function tests in three cases of this syndrome, as follow:

	Pretreatment	Post-treatment
Case 1:		
VC (%P)	78	93
FEF_{25-75} (%P)	27	50
$DL_{CO}SB$ (%P)	57	96
Pa_{O_2} (mm Hg)	68	83
Case 2:		
VC (%P)	83	93
FEF_{25-75} (%P)	34	38
$DL_{CO}SB$ (%P)	48	79
Pa_{O_2} (mm Hg)	65	79
Case 3:		
VC (%P)	69	75
FEF_{25-75} (%P)	67	82
$DL_{CO}SB$ (%P)	50	69
Pa_{O_2} (mm Hg)	66	82

Similar observations have been recorded in other cases.[1769] Familial pulmonary eosinophilia has been described in identical twins, occurring in one at age 25 and in the other at age 29. They had not lived together since the age of 18. In both, there was lowering of the FVC and FEV_1, and the DL_{CO} was 69% of predicted in one and 66% of predicted in the other.[3532]

DIFFUSE LYMPHOID INTERSTITIAL PNEUMONIA

In a patient with diffuse lymphoid interstitial pneumonia who was followed over a 4-year period,[1797] a progressive decline in vital capacity and $DL_{CO}SB$ was documented. In another patient, a fall in exercise Pa_{O_2} of 37 mm Hg was documented at a time when the vital capacity was still 80% of predicted.[1773] These observations may be related to vasculitis. In another case in a 38-year-old man,[4450] the VC was 83% of predicted, the TLC was 63% of predicted, and there was no hypoxemia. In this patient, the chest x-ray was unusual, showing "bizarre central infiltrates."

GRANULOMATOSIS SYNDROMES

Eosinophilic Granuloma

As noted in the second edition of this book,[1] lung volumes may be normal in the early stages of this condition, and there may be no dyspnea. Usually, considerable radiologic change is evident before the diffusing capacity is much reduced. Considerable bronchiolar involvement may lead to evidence of airflow obstruction, as was the case in a 17-year-old patient recorded by us.[1] As more fibrosis develops, the lung volume and compliance are reduced. The late pattern may be similar to other cases of interstitial fibrosis,[1966] except that the course of the disease is often benign, and progressive function deterioration may not occur. Powers, Askin, and Cresson[4338] have recorded 25 years of follow-up of a case, with the autopsy findings. The FVC did not change over the period, but the $DL_{CO}SB$ fell from 31% of predicted to 19% of predicted over the last 3 years of the course and was accompanied by worsening hypoxemia. The characteristic honeycombing was present at autopsy, and the small airways were distorted by infiltrates on the initial lung biopsy.

Wegener's Granulomatosis

In a series of 22 patients with Wegener's syndrome,[1785] airflow obstruction was the commonest abnormality. Reductions of lung volumes were useful in following the course of infiltrative lesions, as was measurement of diffusing capacity. Function tests were found to be useful in the staging of patients and following the course of therapy. In one patient, successful treatment of focal airway lesions was followed by improvement in FEF_{25-75} and FEV_1.[1785] The interpretation of changes in $DL_{CO}SB$ must, however, take into account the possibility of intrapulmonary hemorrhage in this condition, as noted previously.

Bronchocentric Granulomatosis

It has been suggested that bronchocentric granulomatosis is a necrotizing bronchitis caused by hypersensitivity to *Aspergillus*.[1770] Clinical and pathologic reviews have not contained enough data for a conclusion to be reached on pulmonary function in this entity.[1774, 3536, 3538] However, the interpretation may be complicated by the presence of mucoid impaction.[3530]

Allergic Granulomatous Angiitis

In one autopsied case of allergic granulomatous angiitis in a 15-year-old boy, the vital capacity and FEV_1 were reduced to 60% of predicted values, with preservation of a normal diffusing capacity[1760]; the possibility of intrapulmonary hemorrhage influencing these values could not be ruled out.

MISCELLANEOUS

Alpha-Chain Disease

The rare entity of alpha-chain disease is accompanied by pulmonary infiltrates but is without a fibrosing alveolitis. In one case, the $DL_{CO}SB$ was reduced to 36% of predicted values.[1764]

Behçet's Syndrome

Two non-smoking women with Behçet's syndrome had chronic airflow limitation, with a normal chest x-ray and reduced vital capacity and diffusing capacity.[1800] In both patients, there was considerable elevation of residual volume. The report noted that on bronchoscopy there was submucosal inflammation and narrowing of the airway at the level of the fourth and fifth generation. It seems possible that chronic airway disease with bronchiolitis may occur in

this syndrome. It has been suggested that the syndrome might be associated with small airway disease, but definitive evidence is lacking.

Raynaud's Phenomenon

Ploysongsang and Foad[4369] investigated 13 patients with different connective tissue diseases and Raynaud's syndrome. The FEF_{25-75} was below 75% of predicted in five patients, and the $DL_{CO}SB$ was reduced in eight. Their studies led to the conclusion that spasm of the pulmonary vessels may occur in this condition.

Mixed Connective Tissue Disease

Mixed connective tissue disease has features of lupus erythematosus, scleroderma, and polymositis but differs serologically. In 16 collected cases,[4453] C_{st} was reduced by half. Both TLC and DL_{CO} were reduced in most of the cases. The transdiaphragmatic pressure was normal in all 10 patients in whom it was measured. There was no correlation between the pulmonary function abnormalities and the level of the extractable nuclear antigen. The authors concluded that $DL_{CO}SB$ was probably the most sensitive indicator of pulmonary change.

SUMMARY

Pulmonary function tests have been shown to be of value in following the course of collagen diseases, hemosiderosis, and Goodpasture's syndrome and in assessing the results of interventions (which cannot always be reliably deduced from radiologic change). The combination of reduced lung volumes, airflow limitation, a reduced $DL_{CO}SB$, and hypoxemia should always suggest the possibility of one of these diagnoses. However, specific conclusions cannot be drawn from such observations as a lowered DL_{CO}, since this may result either from alveolitis or vasculitis or both. Some degree of airflow limitation is often observed and in nonsmokers may indicate involvement of small airways. Differentiating the effect of diaphragmatic weakness from the effects of pleuritic change and, in turn, differentiating both of these from the effects of interstitial changes in the lung represents a considerable challenge.

14

SYNDROMES OF NON-OCCUPATIONAL DIFFUSE INTERSTITIAL LUNG DISEASE

What I do suggest is that it is always undesirable to make an effort to increase precision for its own sake—especially linguistic precision—since this usually leads to loss of clarity, and to a waste of time and effort on preliminaries which often turn out to be useless, because they are bypassed by the real advance of the subject: one should never try to be more precise than the problem situation demands.

KARL POPPER[1934]

INTRODUCTION

A classification of lung disease into "obstructive" and "restrictive" syndromes is so simplistic that it can lead to error, as is argued in our approach to the interpretation of pulmonary function in Chapter 5.

Carrington[1839] has made the important point that if all syndromes of interstitial fibrosis are classified as necessarily "restrictive," the very important observation that abnormal gas transfer and extensive morphologic changes on lung biopsy may occur with a normal TLC and VC will be lost. Thus, emphasis on "restriction" as a necessary or definitive aspect of function change will deflect attention away from early recognition and diagnosis of disease in which

significant change in function may antedate radiologic change. Apparently, 130 different syndromes of "interstitial" lung disease have now been described.[1929] No attempt is made in this chapter to suggest a particular classification or to adjudicate between various interpretations of similarity or differences between closely related entities. Our emphasis concentrates on defining the usefulness and limitations of function tests in this group of diseases and, where possible, relating function to morphology.

This group of disorders occupies an important position in the history of pulmonary function testing, and the definition of function defect has played a considerable role in improving recognition of an increasingly important group of disorders.[1] Although the general outlines of function defects were clear when we wrote the last edition of this book in 1970, significant additional information is now available. In a review of structure/function correlations, Berend[3359] commented on the relative paucity of correlative data in this group of diseases.

DIFFUSE INTERSTITIAL PNEUMONITIS OR CRYPTOGENIC FIBROSING ALVEOLITIS

Diffuse interstitial pneumonitis is the commonest of the interstitial fibrosis syndromes, and many studies of pulmonary function have now been published.

Morphometric Pathology and Clinical Features

Cassan, Divertie, and Brown[1849] compared stereologic measurements of the lung in nine controls and nine patients with diffuse interstitial fibrosis. The patients with pathologic disease had a mean DL_{CO} of 41% of predicted and TLC of 65% of predicted. They noted the following comparisons:

Mean Thickness of Alveolocapillary Membrane (in microns)

	Normal Subjects	Fibrosis Patients
Arithmetic	1.665 ± 0.128	3.460 ± 0.346
Harmonic	0.829 ± 0.067	1.464 ± 0.187

They concluded that the increases noted were insufficient to account for the associated abnormalities of gas transfer and threw doubt on the validity of the concept of an "alveolar-capillary block" syndrome. There were more striking differences in surface areas, however:

Surface Area (in square meters)

	Normal Subjects	Fibrosis Patients
Alveoli	953 ± 52.8	398 ± 66.5
Capillaries	769 ± 76.9	299 ± 76.6

The mean functional volume of the capillary space in fibrotic lungs was computed to be less than half that in normal lungs.[1849]

The relationship of these syndromes to viral infections is unclear, although experimentally the viral cellular response looks similar to the early stages of this disease.[3543] The pathology of

patients with adult respiratory distress syndrome who survive for more than a few days also looks similar,[3558] and, as noted in Chapter 23, the delayed resolution of some of these cases indicates the development of significant interstitial disease as part of the syndrome.

Immunologic aspects have also been confused,[3469, 3541] but it seems unlikely that DNA antibodies are important.[3562] Cases have been described in sisters,[4449] and Demedts and his colleagues[4407] have described a syndrome with interstitial lung disease, hypocalciuric hypercalcemia, and defective granulocyte function in three siblings. Detailed function test data in one of the patients showed the VC falling from 59.7% of predicted to 47.9% of predicted over 12 years. The DL_{CO} fell from 74% of predicted to 35% of predicted. In a second patient, the DL_{CO} fell from 59% of predicted to 25% of predicted over the same period.

The presence of the distinctive coarse inspiratory rales (often called "Velcro" rales because of their similarity to the noise made by separating the two layers held by this fastener) is the only characteristic physical sign in the lungs.[3470] A careful study of the acoustic nature of the crackles in seven typical cases[4388] correlated these with simultaneous ventilatory flow and esophageal pressure measurements. The authors showed that they occur at the end of the inspiration, with timing closely related to specific lung volumes and pressures. The authors concluded that the crackles were caused by airway opening. A recent paper described digital vasculitis with painful fissures or ulcers of the fingers in this condition[4395]; there was no evidence of an associated pulmonary vasculitis.

As is noted later, it has been shown that considerable alveolar pathology may exist in the lungs in diffuse interstitial pneumonitis and may lead to characteristic functional defect before the chest x-ray has changed in appearance. This feature, together with the inconstancy of such methods as gallium scans,[3540] accounts for the importance of pulmonary function tests in this group of conditions. Recent studies of 10 patients—CAT scans of the lung were used[4330]—indicated that subpleural shadowing was a common feature. Delayed xenon clearance occurred from regions where bullae were visible, and dilated small airways appeared to be visible in some cases. In patients too incapacitated for routine laboratory tests, the diffusing capacity may be followed by a rebreathing method designed for bedside use.[3018]

Pulmonary Function and Hemodynamic Changes

Established Cases

The TLC and VC may both be normal in the presence of histologically proven disease, but as the condition worsens, both fall together.[1874, 1886] Occasionally, the residual volume may be reduced,[1864] but it is more often normal initially, the reduction occurring in TLC and VC.

Studies of lung mechanics generally show an increased maximal P_{st} and a lowered C_{st},[1873] even when related to the reduced lung volume. Dynamic compliance may fall with frequency in this condition.[1870, 1871] Maximal expiratory flow curves show increased flow rates in many cases, especially when the residual volume is reduced. It has been suggested that an increase in the FEF_{25-75} is an early indicator of change.[1911] However, in some patients, including non-smokers, flow rates are reduced in relation to transpulmonary pressure.[1871, 1885, 1891] This has led some authors to state that obstructive changes are often present,[1843] particularly in the small airways.

In one study involving a maximal inspiratory effort against a closed shutter, the relationship between lung volume and transpulmonary pressure appeared normal in 12 patients with diffuse interstitial fibrosis.[1860] In 26 patients, all non-smokers, the increased recoil pressure of the lung led to a lower than normal value for closing volume and closing capacity. The difference between FRC and closing capacity was positive in all.[1907] Tan and Tashkin[1911] compared 32 non-smokers and 22 smokers, all with diffuse interstitial fibrosis. They noted that the ratios FEF_{25-75}/TLC and FEF_{25-75}/FVC were greater than 120% of normal in the non-smokers and that the values were related to elevations in maximal P_{st}. The $DL_{CO}SB$ values were 56% of predicted in this group.

The FEV_1/FVC is commonly increased, especially in early stages of the disease. Morphometric studies of large bronchi in nine patients with diffuse interstitial fibrosis[3556] led Edwards and Carlile to conclude that glandular hyperplasia commonly occurs and is similar to that seen in mucous hypersecretion. Increases in muscle were also observed. Most of their patients had been symptomatic for less than 4 years, and the changes were thought to be a consequence of persistent infection of distal lung parenchyma. In one group of patients, no significant differences in diffusing capacity between those with and without evidence of small airway involvement were found.[1872]

In many of the published series, the DL_{CO} averages about 50% of predicted normal,* and there is no difference between steady-state and single-breath measurements.[1097] The $DL_{CO}SB$ is unaffected by varying the time of breath holding.[1057] The fractional CO uptake is also about 50% of normal.[1906] In a smaller group of patients, the DL measured for oxygen was also about half the normal value.[1899] The ratio $DL/\dot{V}_A$ may reach very low values in this condition.[1902]

Watters and his colleagues[4475] have proposed a composite clinical-radiographic-physiologic scoring system for the evaluation of these patients that uses seven variables. This system correlated well with the severity of the pathologic changes on biopsy, and no individual component of the score correlated better than the score itself in the 26 patients studied. The total pathology score correlated best with the exercise oxygen saturation.

A group from the National Institutes of Health recently reported on bronchoalveolar lavage in 119 patients with diffuse interstitial lung disease, of which 56 had diffuse interstitial fibrosis.[3528] They noted the safety of this procedure, since fewer than 5% had any minor complications. In these patients, the mean DL_{CO} was 59% of predicted, and the TLC was reduced. However, the FEV_1/FVC ratios were all greater than 91% of predicted.

All established cases of this syndrome show evidence of impaired $\dot{V}/\dot{Q}$ distribution. Overall measurements include a widened end-tidal/arterial P_{CO_2} difference,[261] increased V_D/V_T ratio,[261, 1863] and a widened $(A-a)\ D_{O_2}$ at rest.[1863] The six inert gas method indicates that in most, if not all, of these cases when studied at rest, the degree of $\dot{V}/\dot{Q}$ abnormality, combined with the reduction in mixed venous oxygen tension, accounts, for the reduction in arterial Pa_{O_2} observed.[1896, 1930] From these data taken at rest, it might be concluded that the reduced DL_{CO} (however measured) affects only the arterial Pa_{O_2} under exercise conditions in most patients. However, as noted later, this is a difficult point to resolve. In 34 mixed patients, all non-smokers, significant correlations were noted between Pa_{O_2} at rest and DL_{CO} (r = 0.78) and between Pa_{O_2} at rest and C_{dyn}/f (r = 0.66).[1885]

---

*See references 1871, 1874, 1885, 1886, 1893, 1900, 1907, 1925, 3557.

Some impairment of inert gas distribution may be present,[445, 1858, 1891] but it is not usually severe. In 10 patients with interstitial lung disease, including two with diffuse interstitial fibrosis and one with chronic pneumonitis,[4488] the inert gas method showed that the Pa_{O_2} (derived) at rest, was the same as that measured. But on light exercise, the measured Pa_{O_2} fell more than predicted, and the authors concluded that "limitation of diffusion across the alveolar-capillary membrane developed during exercise, contributing approximately 30% to $(A-a) D_{O_2}$."

Studies using Tc-labeled albumin particles have shown that direct shunting is not present in this condition.[4485] There have been few studies of regional function. In 10 patients, McCarthy and Cherniack, using ^{133}Xe, found no abnormalities in regional ventilation but noted a significant reduction in flow to the basal regions in those seated.[1858] Significantly, when arterial PO_2 improved after steroid administration, flow through the lung bases also increased.[1858]

Pulmonary arterial hypertension may be present at rest, and the mixed venous PO_2 was noted to be less than 34 mm Hg, the normal value, in 40% of a group of patients with diffuse interstitial fibrosis.[481] Hypercapnia has been reported in four patients. In one, there was pulmonary hypertension and considerable arteriolar hypertrophy in the lung at autopsy.[1905] This is obviously rarely encountered.

Exercise studies invariably show important abnormalities, most particularly a fall in arterial oxygen tension, often of 20 mm Hg,* and a corresponding increase in $(A-a) D_{O_2}$.[3502, 4337] This increase is greater in this condition than in sarcoidosis.[4337] However, the relationship between exercise $(A-a) D_{O_2}$ and resting function tests (including the $DL_{CO}SB$) is only approximate, except when the $DL_{CO}SB$ is reduced to low levels (below 60%) predicted.[4464]

In studies of 23 biopsied cases, Fulmer and his colleagues[1872] concluded that the measured fall in Pa_{O_2} per liter of oxygen uptake on exercise was the best index of gas exchange abnormality in this condition, but the correlation with severity (as judged from biopsy material) was not close. Pa_{O_2} on 100% oxygen also falls on exercise.[1875] As one would expect, the pulmonary arterial pressure rises as the Pa_{O_2} falls on exercise.[1881] In a recent study of 31 patients with

*See references 1833, 1870, 1875, 1876, 1896, 1899, 1900, 1925, 3502.

diffuse interstitial fibrosis, Pa_{O_2} fell from a mean of 67.8 mm Hg at rest to 56.0 mm Hg on exercise, and the $(A-a) D_{O_2}$ rose from 39 mm Hg to 51.7 mm Hg.[3502] The VC, as a percentage of predicted, was not correlated with the pulmonary arterial pressure. The correlation between Pa_{O_2} and pulmonary arterial pressure $(r = -0.51)$ led the authors to suggest that part of the pulmonary hypertension in this condition is due to alveolar hypoxemia. The mixed venous PO_2 may fall to very low levels on exercise[1896] and may become a significant factor in relation to the arterial hypoxemia.

The control of breathing has been studied, both at rest and on exercise. $P_{0.1}$, frequency, and the ratio V_T/T_i are generally elevated.[1894] There is a significant negative correlation between FRC as a percentage of predicted and $P_{0.1}$ values.[1894] V_T and T_i are both reduced, and T_i/T_{tot} and $\dot{V}_E$ are generally not different from normal, the pattern being similar to that observed in elastic loading.[1894] The increased $P_{0.1}$ also correlates with increased lung elastance,[1890] and the relationship between increased elastance and increased respiratory frequency is close $(r = 0.81$ in 12 patients).[1890] In 1982, Renzi, Milic-Emili, and Grassino[3572] reported on studies on six patients with diffuse interstitial fibrosis and six patients with sarcoidosis. The increased frequency of breathing and $P_{0.1}$ both correlated positively with lung elastance, whereas V_T decreased significantly with increasing elastance. They suggested that inspiratory muscle drive was increased as a function of elastic load in those with diffuse interstitial fibrosis and that signals from the rib cage were probably responsible for this change. Elastic but not resistive load detection may be increased in these patients.[4420] These changes are small, however, and others have found no difference from normal subjects in load detection.[4055]

DiMarco and his colleagues[3548] studied 16 patients, finding that both $\dot{V}_E$ and $P_{0.1}$ at a Pa_{CO_2} of 55 mm Hg were elevated but the responses were not different from normal. They concluded that both vagal and chest wall mechanoreceptors contributed to the responses. Burdon, Killian, and Jones[3560] studied 41 patients with a mean VC of 62% of predicted. Their maximal power output was 53% of predicted, and O_2Hb fell by more than 5% on exercise in 13 of the 31 patients. Both T_i and T_i/T_{tot} were shorter in patients than in a control group. The authors concluded that exercise was limited by reduced ventilatory capacity, despite the adoption of a short T_i and a high inspiratory flow rate.

Aldrich, Arora, and Rochester[3307] have recently compared respiratory muscle function in eight normal subjects, eight patients with diffuse interstitial fibrosis, and 16 patients with chronic airflow limitation. In those with diffuse interstitial fibrosis, differences in respiratory muscle strength estimated from maximal static inspiratory and expiratory mouth pressures accounted for 83% of the variance in maximal voluntary ventilation, and differences in SGaw explained none. Studies of proportional rib cage movement in seven with diffuse interstitial fibrosis[3561] showed that there was reduced motion of the upper thoracic cage and proportionately greater expansion of the lower thoracic cage. The k_{CO}, FEV_1, and RV were all reduced in the patients studied. Difficulty in interpreting function test changes may be caused by coexistent pulmonary interstitial change and respiratory muscle weakness; this is discussed later. A significant fall in $\dot{V}E$ on 100% oxygen breathing is considered to indicate the presence of a significant hypoxic reflex drive.[1893]

In a reported study of 16 patients with interstitial lung disease of mixed origin breathing air and oxygen on exercise (including seven patients with occupational lung disease),[3477] maximal exercise performance when breathing air was 61% of predicted. Exercise time improved with oxygen breathing, and this improvement correlated significantly with the fall in O_2Hb during air breathing. The patients were a mixed group, and five had diffuse interstitial fibrosis. Jones and Rebuck[1880] noted a relationship between the tidal volume on maximal exercise and the vital capacity in six patients, as expressed by the following equation:

$$\text{maximal } V_T = 0.65 VC - 0.64$$

Early Function Test Changes

Although a few isolated patients in whom function test abnormality antedated definite radiologic change had appeared in the literature,[1906] it was not until 1978 when Epler and his colleagues[1866] published a review of 44 patients with a normal chest film (as determined by several radiologists) and significant function test impairment that the importance of this combination of findings could be appreciated. Seventeen of Epler's subjects had chronic interstitial pneumonitis of non-occupational origin. The earliest function test changes in this

condition are therefore of great importance. They are:

1. A fall in Pa_{O_2} on exercise with a widening of $(A-a) D_{O_2}$.
2. A lowered $DL_{CO}SB$ or DL_{CO}, which may be found with a normal resting Pa_{O_2} and normal spirometry findings.
3. A lowered static or dynamic compliance.

In one study in which both the DL_{CO} and lung mechanics were measured in 34 patients, all non-smokers, the DL_{CO} had the greater percentage change from predicted of all indices.[1885] Other data confirm this finding.[1901] However, as noted earlier, widening of the exercise $(A-a) D_{O_2}$ may be found when the resting $DL_{CO}SB$ is within the predicted limits.

It has been claimed[1911] that the finding of an increase of the ratio of FEF_{25-75} to TLC should lead to a measurement of diffusing capacity, particularly if the x-ray is normal, since this may indicate early interstitial change. It should be noted that functional abnormalities are more severe in this syndrome than in sarcoidosis for patients with a similar degree of radiologic change.[1909] This is to be explained by the fact that almost all alveolar walls are often involved in diffuse interstitial fibrosis, whereas in sarcoidosis the primary change is that of discrete granulomata without generalized alveolar wall pathology.

Lowering of Arterial Pa_{O_2}

As we noted in the previous edition,[1] the concept of an "alveolar-capillary block" syndrome characterized by a significant alveolar–end-capillary oxygen difference had been questioned. The finding that the abnormalities in $\dot{V}/\dot{Q}$ distribution, as measured by the six inert gas method, accounted for most of the lowered Pa_{O_2} at rest has led to further controversy, since the Bohr integral analysis method clearly indicates the probability of significant diffusion limitation. For readers interested in following this controversy, the following guideposts may be helpful:*

1. All patients with established diffuse interstitial fibrosis have evidence of abnormal $\dot{V}/\dot{Q}$ distribution, which, together with the lowered

---

*Considerable discussion of this problem can be found in references 332, 1279, 1863, 1882, 1887–1889, 1896, 1899.

mixed venous oxygen tension, no doubt contributes significantly to a widened $(A-a) D_{O_2}$.

2. It is clear that on exercise the lowered DL_{CO} may commonly contribute to the lowered Pa_{O_2}, as shown by the six gas method.[1896] Neither shunts nor $\dot{V}/\dot{Q}$ distribution accounts fully for the measured hypoxemia in a number of patients.[4488]

3. A complex study by Cohen and Overfield[1862] (sometimes quoted as providing definitive evidence of a diffusion defect) is difficult to interpret, since one of the two patients had only a slightly lowered DL_{CO}.

4. Significant evidence of a diffusion component to the widened $(A-a) D_{O_2}$ without a major $\dot{V}/\dot{Q}$ component has been secured in some patients.* The lowered DL_{CO} correlates closely with the reduced maximal oxygen uptake on exercise in these patients.[1870, 1931]

5. There may be an increase in the shunt component on oxygen breathing.[1875]

6. The gross reduction in capillary bed area[1849] and the redirection of flow from the bases (noted previously) lead to the suggestion that these factors lower the observed DL_{CO} significantly. This is in addition to lowered values caused by non-uniformity of $DL/\dot{Q}_c$ ratios or thickening of the alveolar wall. The sensitivity of the DL_{CO} in this condition no doubt resides in the fact that all these factors lower it, but precise quantitation of each component is not possible.

Summary

The question of whether the lowered DL_{CO} caused by alveolocapillary wall thickening (morphometrically present) contributes to the lowered Pa_{O_2} at rest or on exercise is an interesting one, but it should not divert attention from the (practically) far more important observation that changes in DL_{CO} and in arterial P_{O_2} on exercise antedate significant radiologic change in this condition. The pattern of progressive function defect is well established in these cases, and careful (and repeated) tests of function are not only important in indicating the need for biopsy in the presence of symptoms and a normal chest film, but also are important in following progress and response to treatment. The usefulness of tests of function used intelligently in these

conditions is not diminished by the reported lack of close correlation between function defect and morphologic severity (as judged from biopsies and noted by Fulmer and his colleagues[1872]). It has been suggested that the polymorphonuclear cells in bronchial lavages increase in this condition as the arterial P_{CO_2} falls[3579] and that the latter non-invasive index can be used as an indicator of severity.

Prognosis

Several studies have been published on factors related to prognosis. In one follow-up of 96 patients,[1815] deterioration was not related to the extent of radiographic change or to rheumatoid or antinuclear factors. Deterioration was related to steroid response, degree of dyspnea and hypoxemia, and abnormality of vital capacity. Rapidly fatal cases (with death within 7 months of the first symptoms and which are similar to the original cases collected by Hamman and Rich[1807]) do occur,[1] but these are not as common as cases with a much longer course. In one series of 220 patients, a Pa_{O_2} below 60 mm Hg was a bad prognostic sign, but the FVC was not related to prognosis.[1804] Responders to steroids do not differ from non-responders in respect to FEV_1, FVC, DL_{CO}, Pa_{O_2}[1803] or DL_{CO}/V_A.[1895] However, in one study responders had an initially more abnormal FVC.[1895] In another study of 50 patients studied twice, the DL_{CO} was noted to decline more rapidly than the VC as the disease progressed.[1927]

In a recent study of 100 consecutive patients followed for at least 3 years and all treated with steroids,[3557] early objective functional improvement occurred in 30%. Factors favorable to survival were youth, shorter duration of symptoms, less severe chest x-ray changes, and less impairment of DL_{CO}. There was significantly better survival in those with a DL_{CO} >45% of predicted. Prognosis was not related to a more cellular histologic appearance, but early steroid response was a favorable indicator.

Improvement in function has been documented to follow the use of immunosuppressive drugs in some cases[1832] or to follow prednisone and azathioprine therapy.[1824, 3574] In some carefully studied patients, remarkable improvement has been noted, with the DL_{CO} doubling, the VC improving by 1.7 liters, and the Pa_{O_2} increasing from an original value of 35 mm Hg to 86 mm Hg.[1851] In some patients, changes in function move in different directions, with the

---

*See references 1279, 1830, 1852, 1863, 1899.

DL_{CO} improving but the arterial P_{O_2} falling.[1845] It has been suggested that prognosis is better in patients with desquamative interstitial pneumonitis (DIP) than in those with usual pneumonitis (UIP) and that there is a longer period of survival in the former condition.[1865] However, the function tests do not appear to be different in the two conditions.

In one series of 56 patients observed for periods up to 19 years,[1886] four variables were predictive of non-survival:

• a mean pulmonary arterial pressure of >30 mm Hg
• a VC of <60% of predicted
• a $DL_{CO}SB$ of <40% of predicted (if greater than this, 90% survived 6 years, and if less, 50% survived 6 years)
• age at onset greater than 30 years

The mean initial $DL_{CO}SB$ of the patients followed was 35% of predicted. A score system was proposed based on these variables to permit assessment of prognosis.[1886]

There is no doubt that pulmonary function tests are very useful in following these patients and in assessing the rate of decline or response to treatment. However, in structural terms, changes in function tests are not easy to interpret.[1034, 1874]

SCLERODERMA

Several observations have been reported in patients with systemic sclerosis that distinguish the thoracic involvement in this condition from the usual pattern in other types of interstitial fibrosis:

1. A 73-year-old woman has been reported in whom the lung parenchyma and the DL_{CO} were normal, but death occurred during respiratory failure as a result of respiratory muscle involvement.[1818]

2. Elastic recoil pressure may be less negative than in other types of interstitial fibrosis, even when the loss of VC is comparable. This is probably due to atrophy of respiratory muscles.[1904]

3. Lowered static compliance is the principal mechanical defect.[4447] This is not closely related to the extent of the radiographic change and is not related to RV levels. Involvement of pulmonary vasculature may be more severe. Pulmonary hypertension may occur early. A radiologic assessment of pulmonary arterial vessel size in upper and lower zones in 20 patients with scleroderma[1883] showed a probable redistribution of flow from bases to apices similar to that reported in patients with interstitial fibrosis, as noted earlier in this chapter. This is not thought to be due to more basal disease but to loss of capillary bed at the bases. A "syndrome of malignant pulmonary hypertension" has been described in scleroderma.[1825]

4. Exposure to cold causes a decrease in DL_{CO} in patients with Raynaud's syndrome without scleroderma. In patients with scleroderma with Raynaud's phenomenon, the DL_{CO} does not change.[3577, 4396]

5. Only one patient in 24 studied had a fall of Pa_{O_2} on exercise.[4447] The ratio of VD/VT does not fall on exercise in this condition, probably due to the fact that additional capillaries cannot be recruited as the cardiac output increases.[1897]

6. Tests of small airway function are usually normal in non-smokers with this condition.[1823]

7. A significant increase in alveolar clearance of inhaled aerosols was found in 10 patients with systemic sclerosis,[1810, 1903] suggesting that there may be a widening of interepithelial junctions.

8. There does not appear to be any correlation between the age of the patient, the duration of the disease, and the degree of pulmonary involvement.[661] Bagg and Hughes[1808] observed nine patients with this condition for a mean period of 10 years by means of pulmonary function tests. The results show that even when initial changes are severe little progression may occur. This led the authors to stress that pronounced early involvement of the lungs in systemic sclerosis does not necessarily imply a poor prognosis. In three of their patients, little change in $DL_{CO}SB$ occurred over the period of observation. In another patient, the $DL_{CO}SB$ declined from 80% of predicted to 64% of predicted, and the VC increased from 2.6 liters to 2.9 liters over the same period. In four patients, both DL_{CO} and VC declined together.

An entity called the "CREST" syndrome, which may be related to systemic sclerosis, is characterized by calcinosis, Raynaud's syndrome, esophageal dysfunction, sclerodactyly, and telangiectasia. Severe pulmonary hypertension occurs in this condition.[1932] In 10 patients there was said to be no pulmonary fibrosis, but the $DL_{CO}SB$ was reduced to less than 52% of predicted in six patients, apparently in conjunction with a normal chest film.

Serial studies of bronchoalveolar lavage fluid in 13 patients with scleroderma indicated that there was an active inflammatory response in all.[4409] Steroids did not affect either the gallium scan or the percentage of neutrophils in the BAL fluid. Mean data in this series showed VC of 59% of predicted, $DL_{CO}SB$ of 52% of predicted, mean Pa_{O_2} of 69 mm Hg, and a normal FEV_1/FVC ratio. Individual cases in which steroids affected the number of neutrophils and may have improved function[4389] have been reported. In this patient, steroids did not improve the k_{CO}, however.[4389]

POLYMYOSITIS, DERMATOMYOSITIS, AND INTERSTITIAL FIBROSIS

In 1970, only a few cases of polymyositis, dermatomyositis, and interstitial fibrosis had been published.[1] In 1974, Frazier and Miller[1848] reviewed 213 patients and performed pulmonary function tests in nine. As other authors have pointed out,[1827] the pulmonary involvement sometimes becomes evident before there is obvious evidence of muscle disease. Hence, the diagnosis should be suggested when the FEF_{25-75} is unexpectedly low in a patient with interstitial fibrosis in whom there is radiologic change and lowered $DL_{CO}SB$. It may be very difficult to determine how much of the functional abnormality ("restriction") is due to muscle weakness and how much is due to the interstitial lung disease. In general, the FEV_1 is decreased out of proportion to the FEF_{25-75} in muscular disease, and the reverse occurs in airway obstruction. Often pulmonary function tests are no different from those of patients with interstitial fibrosis.[1817, 1861]

In one case in a 59-year-old man, pulmonary interstitial changes with hypoxemia improved on steroids. Eighteen months later, muscular weakness developed, and a biopsy revealed polymyositis.[4463] Over the next 2 years, the DL_{CO} improved but remained impaired. Another case was complicated by diaphragmatic paresis.[4335] Initially the transdiaphragmatic pressure difference was 15 cm H_2O, and this rose to 25 cm H_2O after a course of steroids.

A case of dermatomyositis in a 58-year-old man with a 6-week history of joint swelling in his hands, skin rashes, and an abnormal chest film ran a very rapid course, with death during hypoxic respiratory failure 4 months after the first symptom.[3563] Another patient responded to treatment with azathioprine.[3574]

MISCELLANEOUS VARIANTS

Familial Disease

Four cases of the Hermansky-Pudlak syndrome with fibrosing alveolitis have been described in one family,[1822] and cases occur with oculocutaneous albinism.[1831] Other cases have also been reported.[4491]

Two remarkable cases of diffuse interstitial fibrosis have been noted in monozygotic twin brothers, aged 51, who had not shared the same environment.[1834] The histologic findings were identical, and pulmonary function tests were as follows:

	Predicted	Case 1	Case 2
TLC, liters	7.2	5.3	5.1
VC, liters	5.4	3.9	3.9
RV, liters	2.2	1.4	1.2
FEV_1, liters	3.9	3.1	3.0
Pa_{O_2}, rest, mm Hg	80	84	76
exercise, mm Hg	—	71	46
$DL_{CO}SS$, mL CO/min/ mm Hg	22	10	12

Coexistence of diffuse interstitial fibrosis and alveolar cell carcinoma has been reported in one family.[1922] Cases have also been reported in sisters.[4449]

Other Associated Syndromes

Diffuse interstitial fibrosis has been reported in association with infectious mononucleosis,[1914] with a return to normal of abnormal chest x-rays, $DL_{CO}SB$, and VC. It also occurs in association with von Recklinghausen's disease,[1850] with hepatitis B infection,[1821] and following mycoplasmal pneumonia.[1804] The serious epidemic from ingestion of contaminated cooking oil (denatured rapeseed oil) in Spain[1919] led to a complex syndrome of respiratory failure attributable to interstitial pulmonary changes, severe pulmonary arteriolar lesions,[3559] and severe muscle weakness. Twenty thousand people were affected by this, and the condition had a mortality rate of 1.7%.[4392] In 19% of the patients, moderate hypoxemia persisted, although the chest x-ray cleared. Fourteen patients with persistently lowered $DL_{CO}SB$ values were presumed to have chronic changes after the acute effects had cleared.[4459] The chemical nature of the toxic agent has not yet been reported.

It is unclear whether celiac disease may be associated with diffuse interstitial fibrosis[1913] or whether this may be caused by sulfasalazine used in treatment of the condition.[3578]

In two non-smoking women, diffuse interstitial fibrosis was followed by the development of chronic obstructive pulmonary disease. These patients were well documented with pulmonary function tests, and the gradual shift of pressure volume curves from a pattern characteristic of fibrosis to one of loss of compliance is of particular interest.[1836] Alveolar proteinosis may progess to interstitial fibrosis.[1847, 3565]

Differentiation of idiopathic diffuse interstitial fibrosis from asbestosis may be difficult and may require electron microscopy studies.[1868] Indeed, it is important to be highly suspicious whenever a diffuse interstitial lung disease occurs in an employee in industry.[3568, 3580]

A few cases of a progressive pulmonary fibrosis particularly involving the upper lobes have been described. These were without evident etiology and were associated with severe progressive weight loss.[1812] It is not clear whether there is anything characteristic about changes in function in these rare cases.

DRUG-INDUCED PULMONARY DISEASE AND TOXIC SYNDROMES

A recent review listed 25 drugs that have been reported to cause interstitial fibrosis.[3524] Cooper, White, and Matthay[4489] have published a very useful review of non-cytotoxic drugs that may cause pulmonary changes. In addition, many experimental studies of interstitial fibrosis have appeared,[3573] and the response to bleomycin and other such drugs has been extensively studied. These suggest that this drug is chemokinetic for neutrophils but not for lymphocytes.[3539] Its effects are reduced by low temperatures[3544] and are enhanced by hyperoxia[3552, 3553]; they are not potentiated by x-irradiation.[3571] Studies of lung strips from bleomycin-treated rats[3567] generated more force in response to acetylcholine, epinephrine, and potassium than did control strips, and it was concluded that both actin and myosin are increased in the fibrotic strips. Sequential studies in dogs indicated that total cells and the per-

centage of polymorphonuclear cells both increased in lavage fluid before the x-ray appearances or lung compliance changed.[3569] Other experimental studies may be consulted by those especially interested in this field.*

Interstitial pneumonitis of varying degrees of severity, and with characteristic pulmonary function test changes of hypoxemia, lowered DL_{CO}, and lowered VC, has been reported as a result of administration of sulfasalazine,[1814, 3578] cyclophosphamide,[1811, 1856, 4366] bleomycin,† vincristine,[1820] phenylhydantoin,[1846, 3564] azathioprine (also used in treatment of dermatomyositis),[3555] procarbazine,[3554, 4329] cephalosporin,[4390] carbamazepine,[1933] carmustine,[1838] melphalan,[1835] gold salts,‡ hydralazine,[1928] mitomycin,[1923] tocainide,[1921] pindolol,[1918] practolol,[1917] phenylbutazone,[1915] furazolidine,[1577] nitrofurantoin,§ D-penicillamine,[3523] and amiodarone.‖ Drugs such as Naproxen,[3583] tolazamide,[3582] salazopyrin,[4462] and bleomycin[4454] may cause pulmonary infiltrates and eosinophilia. Bromocriptine, used in the treatment of Parkinson's disease, has been reported to cause pleuritis, but it is not clear whether an associated interstitial fibrosis occurs.

In a 10-year period between 1966 and 1976, 447 cases of nitrofurantoin toxicity were reported to the Swedish Adverse Drug Committee.[1892] This report notes the presence of changes in pulmonary function but makes no recommendation on prevention. Detailed studies of 66 patients with nitrofurantoin toxicity showed that acute effects with a drop in DL_{CO} might occur 8 days or so after starting, subacute changes after 1 month might appear, or chronic changes with interstitial fibrosis might develop after several months.[1879] Lower zones of the lungs might be more heavily involved due to higher flow through these regions. In other reported cases, including one fatal case in which the VC fell to 33% of predicted,[1877] recognition came very late. In a patient being given bleomycin and in whom the DL_{CO} was measured weekly while the drug was administered, the DL_{CO} fell from 30 to 15 over 3 weeks, and the FVC fell from 3.2 to 2.5 liters. Neither the chest x-ray nor the Pa_{O_2} changed.[1859] The au-

---

*See references 3542, 3546, 3549, 3550, 3566, 3570, 3576, 4334, 4358, 4362, 4363, 4365, 4408, 4413, 4414, 4482.

†See references 1557, 1819, 1826, 1855, 1859, 1860, 3547, 4454.

‡See references 1867, 1884, 1898, 1912, 1916, 4384.

§See references 1828, 1841, 1853, 1869, 1879, 1892.

‖See references 4326, 4383, 4393, 4455, 4484.

thors of this paper stated "baseline and frequent subsequent serial determinations of DL_{CO} and FVC are imperative in all patients receiving bleomycin."[1859]

Eighteen patients with testicular non-seminomatous germ cell tumors were treated with bleomycin, vinblastine, and chlorophenothane. Pulmonary function tests were performed serially over a 4-month period. Although DL_{CO} did not change significantly, the measured pulmonary capillary blood volume (V_c) fell from 75% of predicted to 64% of predicted, which the authors interpreted to mean early vascular damage in the lung.[3547]

A more recent series of 39 patients with disseminated testicular non-seminomatous tumors treated with bleomycin[4364] showed that eight (20%) developed pneumonitis. It was found that low creatinine clearance in combination with a fall in VC and no increase in pulmonary capillary blood volume (V_c) all pointed to an increased risk. The DL_{CO} was poorly predictive in this series. Another study of 77 patients noted that the $DL_{CO}SB$, after correction for hemoglobin, fell 35% in 15 of 18 patients who had no clinical or radiologic evidence of toxicity.[4448] These authors recommended routine use of $DL_{CO}SB$ measurements and discontinuation of bleomycin if this value fell more than 35%, even if no other signs were present. In three patients, the FVC was found a satisfactory indicator of the course of pulmonary changes.[4458]

This brief review of the available information shows that function test changes may antedate radiologic change or severe symptoms and certainly reinforces the view that serial pulmonary function tests should be used routinely to follow many of these patients. In most instances, a weekly check of function is sufficient. However, in a few reported patients, the reaction has been so swift and occurred after such small drug doses that even this might not be adequate forewarning of an adverse effect.[1556, 1908]

The extreme danger of ingestion of paraquat has become well recognized and fatal cases have been carefully described.[1813, 1829] Experimental studies have clarified the sequence of changes in the lung that follow ingestion* and also indicate that oxygen administration with paraquat is more lethal than the drug alone.[1857] This factor greatly complicates management in the presence of hypoxemia. It is important to recognize the common occurrence of an initial

asymptomatic period.[1829] It is not clear what effects low doses of this material may have, but sequential changes of function in a non-fatal case showed the DL_{CO} falling from an initial value of 22.6 to 14.0 and subsequently rising to its predicted value of 29.0 in a 47-year-old man.[1816] Another patient who survived has been reported.[4331] A survey of nine workers using paraquat showed that in six the $DL_{CO}SB$ was lowered.[1809] A lung biopsy in one showed the presence of medial hypertrophy of the pulmonary arteries.

RADIATION

Little has been added to the description of pulmonary function test changes in radiation pneumonitis noted in the previous edition.[1] Characteristically, a fall in diffusing capacity and in lung compliance occurs, together with an irritative unproductive cough, between 3 and 16 weeks after cessation of exposure.

A comprehensive and useful review article[1924] brings this information up to date and might only be faulted because the author assumes that only the chest film can be used in early detection, although he recognizes that pulmonary function test changes occur early.

Some interesting data have been published on the effects of radiation in children. One survey of 48 children treated with radiation for Wilms's tumors with pulmonary metastases[1926] showed reduced lung volumes and dynamic compliance but normal static pressures and DL_{CO} values. The authors thought the radiation might have interfered with chest wall growth. The DL_{CO} was 72% of predicted on the basis of height, but 112% on the basis of lung volume. One infant was treated with radiation at the age of 7 months for a neuroblastoma. By the age of 14, there was grossly reduced perfusion of the left lung without evidence of pulmonary fibrosis, and the DL_{CO} was only 50% of predicted. Considerable pulmonary hypertension was present,[1920] probably indicating irreversible damage to the pulmonary vasculature.

SUMMARY

Pulmonary function tests have played and will continue to play an important role in clinical diagnosis and management of patients with chronic interstitial fibrosis. There is little doubt that they should be much more widely used in

---

*See references 1840, 3570, 3576, 4333, 4340.

the early detection of pulmonary changes due to drug administration. Patients in whom interstitial pulmonary changes, muscle weakness, and atrophy occur are challenging clinical problems. Careful mechanics studies are indicated in patients with a discrepancy between dyspnea and other findings or when the FEF_{25-75}/TLC ratio is reduced rather than increased. When effort dyspnea is present with a normal chest film, with or without the finding of a few inspiratory rales, the normality of the lung can be assured only if there is no fall in arterial Po_2 on exercise and the diffusing capacity is normal.

It is important that early recognition be stressed, since it seems possible that early treatment may improve the prognosis significantly.[1910] Massive doses of intermittent intravenous corticosteroids (2 grams methylprednisone IV once a week) have recently been used to suppress the neutrophil component of the alveolitis of interstitial fibrosis.[3545] What the long-term effect on function is of this regime is not yet known. Immediate drug withdrawal is, of course, mandatory as soon as pulmonary function is adversely affected by any one of the drugs known to lead to interstitial pneumonitis.

Sarcoidosis

INTRODUCTION*

A recent estimate of incidence concluded that in the United States the incidence of sarcoidosis is about 11 per 100,000 per year. In Europe, the incidence ranges between 2 to 32 per 100,000 per year. Peak incidence is between the ages of 20 and 34.[4341]

There is little doubt that it is the variability of distribution of granulomata in the lung in sarcoidosis, together with the fact that they may evolve or possibly resolve, that makes the interpretation of changes in function particularly difficult in this condition. The usual and earliest change is discrete granulomata of varying size occurring in relation to lymphatics—peribronchiolar, subpleural, and along lobular septae—scattered throughout the interstitium of the lung and lying in alveolar walls but not in alveolar lumina. Divertie, Cassan, and Brown[1953] quantitated various components of the lung in seven patients with sarcoidosis. The mean age was 40 years, with a mean TLC of 65% of predicted and a $DL_{CO}SB$ of 63% predicted. The authors obtained the following measurements:

	Normal	Sarcoidosis
Alveolocapillary tissue	21.2%	13.9%
Intercapillary tissue	15.9%	57.6%
Alveolocapillary/intercapillary ratio	1.33	0.24
Alveolocapillary thickness (microns)		
arithmetic mean	1.665	3.299
harmonic mean	0.829	1.321

They concluded that "the bulk of additional

---

*Detailed reviews of epidemiology, clinical manifestations, and pathology, together with four important papers on pulmonary function, will be found in the 750-page Volume 278 of the Annals of the New York Academy of Science report on the Tenth International Conference on sarcoidosis in 1976.

tissue was deposited preferentially between septal capillaries and not in alveolocapillary membranes." In other electron microscopy studies, a normal alveolocapillary barrier is seen in many areas, but the capillaries are displaced.[1960]

There may be exceptions to this typical picture, and these different presentations are very important in analyzing the ways in which this disease may affect pulmonary function:

- lesions may occur intrabronchially[1948, 1983, 1984]
- small and medium-sized arteries may be particularly involved[1942, 1946]
- peribronchiolar fibrosis may be extensive[1945]
- the larynx may be involved[1956, 1961, 1979]
- the pleura, very rarely, may be involved[1959, 4328]
- sarcoidosis followed by a "vanishing lung" syndrome with extensive emphysema is occasionally seen[1981]
- large solitary granulomata that mimic a lung cancer have been described[1954]

Although the alveoli are usually empty, a syndrome of alveolar filling has been described,[4394] and the earliest changes may be a non-granulomatous interstitial pneumonitis.[1949] Bronchial lavage data indicate that the alveolitis of active sarcoidosis is characterized by large numbers of T-lymphocytes in the lung[1987] elevation of the IgG/albumin% ratio,[3592] and an increase in angiotensin-I converting enzyme.[5264] Reynolds[3469] has contrasted the immunologic changes found in sarcoidosis and in diffuse interstitial fibrosis.[3469]

In describing this disease, it is useful to classify it into the following stages[1]:

Stage I: Hilar adenopathy alone, with no radiologic evidence of parenchymal involvement.

Stage II: Hilar adenopathy and mottling or reticular lung change.

Stage III: Pulmonary parenchymal changes and no adenopathy.

Stage IV: Parenchymal changes known to have been present for 2 or more years (pulmonary fibrosis).*

Patients with "active" and untreated sarcoidosis show evidence of elevated levels of angiotension converting enzyme[1974-1976, 1978] and serum lysozyme activity.[1972] Although these tests are positive in 75% of patients with untreated sarcoidosis,[1986] they are not specific for the condition.[1974] Alpha$_1$-antitrypsin levels are also elevated.[1957] These tests are poor predictors of the intensity of alveolitis, as judged by measurements of T-lymphocytes on lavage or gallium-67 (^{67}Ga) scanning.[1985]

PULMONARY FUNCTION

Data up to 1970[1] had indicated that the following were the main pulmonary function findings in sarcoidosis:

1. Pulmonary function might be normal in the presence of radiologic changes or hilar adenopathy in Stage I patients.

2. Lung volumes and diffusing capacity decreased to varying degrees. These changes were present in some Stage I patients and were still present after radiologic clearing in others. The diffusing capacity might or might not be lower than normal in relation to the reduced lung volume.

3. Pulmonary compliance decreased, but this was sometimes normal when related to the reduced lung volume.

4. The arterial oxygen tension was usually normal at rest but sometimes fell on exercise.

5. The fibrotic stage of sarcoidosis, which occurred in only a few per cent of patients, was accompanied by serious loss of volume; hypoxemia was often present.

During the past 12 years, at least 70 studies of function in sarcoidosis have been published, and much more detailed information is available, although some of it is contradictory. A

---

*DeRemee[3587] has recently reviewed the radiologic staging of sarcoidosis.

study of 130 patients in all stages showed that there was no consistent relationship between DL_{CO}, compliance, and duration of the disease.[1941] Four patients without parenchymal radiologic change had dyspnea and a lowered compliance. In this series, 26 patients had a DL_{CO} less than 80% of predicted, but only six had a Pa_{O_2} less than 75 mm Hg. In another series of 29 patients, the vital capacity was less than 80% of predicted and correlated significantly with the static compliance.[1941] In the series reported by Epler and his colleagues,[1866] there were six patients with sarcoidosis with normal chest films, abnormal tests of function, and positive lung biopsies.

Several reports show that small airway changes may be present. In studies of 11 smokers and seven non-smokers, six of the non-smokers had an elevated CV/VC%. In four of these, C_{dyn}/f fell significantly.[1943] The $MEF_{50\%}$ is often abnormal, and the SBN_2/L index is also abnormal in about half the patients studied.[1940] Low values of FEF_{25-75} are not explained by smoking.[1952] In another series of 16 patients, 15 were not smoking at the time, and six were lifetime non-smokers. In 12, the reduction in airflow exceeded the reduction in vital capacity. There was no hyperinflation, however, although the SBN_2/L test was abnormal in 10 of the patients.[1958]

Careful studies of lung mechanics in 21 patients, six of whom were smokers, showed that the $FEF_{50\%}VC$ was reduced in nine.[1970] In four patients, this was due to reduced peripheral airway conductance. In three, it was due to loss of elastic recoil. In two others, both of these factors contributed.

In 14 patients in another study, the disease had been present for less than 6 months. Reductions in lung volumes, DL_{CO}, and C_{st} were noted in most, but C_{st} was normal when related to lung volume. These authors recorded DL_{CO} values of less than 65% of predicted in several patients in whom the TLC was more than 90% of predicted.[1973] They concluded that "in early sarcoidosis, surviving ventilated alveoli retain normal elastic properties, and there is no airway obstruction."

In another series of 25 patients in Stage I or II that included 17 non-smokers, VC and FEV/FVC% were within predicted limits. Half of these had an increased SBN_2/L gradient, and almost the same number had a reduced MEFV at low lung volumes.[1940] C_{st} was noted to be normal in some of these patients.

Lamberto and his colleagues[4451] studied 24

patients with disease of less than 2 years duration. The subjects were between 31 and 36 years old, and 22 were non-smokers. No patient was receiving steroids. These were compared with nine patients with disease of longer duration. They noted that DL_{CO} was reduced in the group with disease of longer duration, but it was also significantly reduced in several members of the other group. TLC, FEV/FVC, and RV/TLC data were not abnormal and were no different between the groups. $Vmax_{25\%}VC$ delta He/O_2, and $\dot{V}_{25\%}VC$ were abnormal in both groups and were significantly lower in the group with long-term disease. The SBN_2/L was abnormal only in a few patients. The ratio of C_{dyn}/C_{st} was abnormal in 75% of the patients. C_{dyn} (measured at 15 and 60 breaths/min) was reduced in both groups and was also worse in those with long-term disease. The authors wrote: "We conclude that patients with sarcoidosis are probably affected by intrinsic small airway disease, but an increase in elastic recoil often conceals its consequences." This comment was based on the observation that there was an increased P_{st} in a few patients.

Another series studied 39 patients with Stage I and 20 patients with Stage II disease,[4367] all non-smokers. C_{dyn} fell with increasing breathing frequency in 40% of Stage I patients and in 50% of Stage II patients. CV/VC% was increased in most, and the RV was increased in 37% of Stage I and 35% of Stage II patients. C_{st} and P_{max} were normal in both groups.

Yernault and Gibson[3584] have noted that if the pressure-volume curve in sarcoidosis patients is expressed in terms of the absolute TLC, the curve is shifted. If it is plotted against the percentage of the actual TLC, it is normal. These findings indicate loss of alveoli but normal compliance in the remainder. The residual volume is the last volume to be affected. Hence, the ratio of RV to TLC increases initially.[3584] The lowered DL_{CO} in Stage II patients appears to be due to a lowered DM component.[1966]

In Stage IV sarcoidosis, DL_{CO} correlates negatively with the pulmonary artery pressure,[1944] and the arterial saturation may fall on exercise.[3586] By this stage of the disease, the FEV_1 is commonly lowered, perhaps partially because of bronchial distortion. However, it must be remembered that significant ventilatory obstruction may result from sarcoidosis of the larynx, which may occur without parenchymal change, and improvement in the MEFV curve may follow treatment.[1979] However, chronic laryngeal scarring may be present.[1961]

Studies of regional lung function in sarcoidosis that use isotopes show that abnormalities are common. Alterations in regional ventilation or perfusion were documented to be present in 24 patients in a series of 26 with different stages of disease.[1971] In 20 non-smoking patients, all in Stage I or II, regional abnormalities of ventilation were found in 16 of 36 zones studied.[1969] The presence of these abnormalities correlated significantly with a reduction of the DL_{CO}/FRC ratio, compared with normal values for this measurement.

Saumon and colleagues[1936] studied 77 patients with sarcoidosis by measurement of DM and V_c. They used the $DL_{CO}SB$ method and obtained at least six DL_{CO} determinations at increasing inspired oxygen tensions. They gathered the following data:

	Normal Subjects	Stages of Sarcoidosis			
		I	II	III	IV
Number	52	19	49	9	20
VC (%P)		110	100	77	77
SB argon test		6.6	7.9	16.3	14.7
$DL_{CO}BSA$	17.3	14.2	14.1	9.0	8.2
SD ($\pm$)	3.06	3.39	3.98	3.58	2.48
DM/BSA	37.4	31.4	31.4	20.0	24.0
SD	9.99	4.72	12.3	9.64	9.64
V_c/BSA	43.3	42.8	40.4	25.7	19.4
SD	9.72	12.4	13.1	8.47	7.49

The single-breath argon test was an index of gas distribution derived from inspiration of a single argon bolus.

The authors found that DL_{CO} was reduced in Stage I. DM was similar in Stages I and II, but some Stage II patients showed a reduced V_c. Significant reduction in DM and particularly in V_c occurs in Stage III, probably indicating obliteration of the capillary network. This obliteration is more marked in the stage of established fibrosis (Stage IV).[1936]

Miller and his colleagues[1937] studied pulmonary function in 25 patients with Stage I and 19 with Stage II disease. They reported a significantly lower VC in Stage II patients, and a lower FEF_{25-75} in non-smokers in Stage II, as compared with Stage I. $DL_{CO}SB$ was significantly lower in Stage II patients, and hypoxemia on exercise was more frequent.

Exercise studies have given somewhat varied results, probably influenced by the status of the patients included. In one series of 40 patients,[1939] significant falls (of about 20 mm Hg) in arterial oxygen tension on exercise (as compared with resting values) were recorded in four subjects. In 106 patients with varied disease undergoing exercise evaluation,[4464] there were 32 cases of sarcoidosis. Ear oximetry was used to record a fall of more than 4% in oxygen saturation, and this was generally related to a $DL_{CO}SB$ of less than 50% of predicted. The widening of arterial $(A - a) D_{O_2}$ on exercise bears a general relationship to the resting VC, TLC, and $DL_{CO}SB$ in sarcoidosis.[4337] In mild cases, there may be no increase of $(A - a) D_{O_2}$ observed.[4371] A number of authors have noted that although the $(A - a) D_{O_2}$ may be increased in sarcoidosis, it is much less abnormal than in patients with diffuse interstitial fibrosis[1876, 1966] and in patients with extrinsic allergic alveolitis.[4296]

In rare cases of sarcoidosis, the main site of the lesions may be in pulmonary vessels, leading to cor pulmonale.[1942] In one such patient with multiple concentric pulmonary artery stenoses, severe dyspnea, and pulmonary hypertension, regional studies showed severe reduction in ventilation to the left lung and the right upper lobe.[1946] Milder cases may be more common. In five patients with sarcoidosis—all of whom had reduced exercise diffusing capacity—studies of lung tissue suggested that considerable displacement of capillaries might explain the findings.[1960]

Although bronchial lavage is not a "routine" measurement,[3591] detailed studies have been reported in which the intensity of the alveolitis in sarcoidosis was assessed by cell content of lavage and by ^{67}Ga scanning.[3593] It is not possible to review all of these studies in detail.*

It has been suggested that a combination of lavage and gallium scanning involving an "in vitro" measurement of macrophages 48 hours after ^{67}Ga is administered might be a useful technique.[4361] In some series, the relationship between alveolitis and radiologic changes has been poor.[4385] There has also been discussion as to whether gallium scanning or lavage is indicated in the management of sarcoidosis.[4336, 4387]

Comparisons between function test status, radiology, and the degree of alveolitis (as judged by lavage) have yielded somewhat contradictory results. In some series, there is a loose relationship between changes in VC and $DL_{CO}SB$ and the intensity of alveolitis.[3593] However, it was concluded that function test criteria could not predict progression. Other authors have noted no relationship between pulmonary function and lavage data[4423] and have concluded that

lymphocyte surface markers are not good predictors of clinical outcome.

In another series of 35 patients with sarcoidosis, all non-smokers and all with recent disease, a group of French investigators[3589] reported that there was a strong correlation between $DL_{CO}/\dot{V}A$ adjusted for age and the IgG/albumin ratio in lavage fluid $(r = -0.72)$ and also between $DL_{CO}/\dot{V}A$ and the percentage of lymphocytes in the fluid $(r = -0.42)$. Other indices of function were not related to the lavage results. Their article contains an interesting discussion of the mechanisms of lowering of DL_{CO} in this disease.

In 19 patients with sarcoidosis and six controls, standardized methods were used for lavage (BAL). Nine of the sarcoidosis patients had more than 8×10^6 helper T-cells and were considered to have a high intensity alveolitis. Only the Pa_{O_2} at maximal exercise discriminated between these patients and the others.[4418] Lin, Haslam, and Turner-Warwick[4425] studied 33 consecutive untreated patients with sarcoidosis. Twenty-nine had had an abnormal chest x-ray for 1 year or more, and 20 for 2 years or more. Only 24% of the group had dyspnea. Twenty of 33 were found to have increased lymphocytes on BAL, but only in eight did the percentage exceed 28%. Fourteen had an excess of neutrophils. There was a significant correlation between the percentage of neutrophils and the radiology score, and there were significant inverse relationships to VC and $DL_{CO}SB$. All patients with high lymphocyte counts had lower radiologic scores. The variation in pulmonary function tests was noted. Individual patients had a VC of 100% predicted and a $DL_{CO}SB$ of 50% of predicted, or, conversely, a VC of 62% of predicted and a $DL_{CO}SB$ of 79% of predicted.

Bechtel and colleagues[544] studied airway reactivity in 20 patients with sarcoidosis using methacholine challenge. Half of the patients had an increased response, and the authors concluded that this was related to five factors: (1) greater airway obstruction; (2) lower vital capacity; (3) lower DL_{CO}; (4) more symptoms, especially wheezing and cough; and (5) longer disease duration. Different results were reported in 17 non-smokers who were not treated with steroids and who were tested shortly after diagnosis.[4422] These had normal spirometric values and no increase in methacholine reactivity could be demonstrated.

Studies of pulmonary permeability that used ^{99m}Tc DTPA in 14 patients with untreated sarcoidosis[4410] showed increased clearance rates,

---

*See references 4439, 4359, 4360, 4416, 4424, 4426, 4476–4478, 4481, 4483, 4492.

compared with controls, in eight of the subjects. There was positive correlation between faster clearance and albumin concentration in BAL fluid. No pulmonary function tests were reported. Other studies have given similar data.[4391]

From data based on 250 patients observed over the past 6 years and studied at a clinic for sarcoidosis in Milan,[4478] mild to moderate pulmonary hypertension was found to exist in many Stage II and Stage III patients. Measurement of a "total perfusion score" by perfusion lung scans correlated well with the pulmonary arterial pressure. A 10% or more reduction in VC or in DL_{CO} was thought to represent clinical activity in these patients, and steroid treatment was recommended if this occurred.

It is probable that pulmonary hypertension on exercise occurs in all Stage III patients[4368] and is accompanied by a fall in Pa_{O_2}. When it occurs in Stage II patients, it may indicate granulomatous involvement of arterioles.[4368] Using non-invasive radionuclide measurements[4374] in 14 cases of sarcoidosis, 7 mild and 7 severe, Baughman and his colleagues reported the following data:

Mild Disease (n = 7)

	TLC (%P)	$DL_{CO}SB$ (%P)	Pa_{O_2} (mm Hg) Rest	Pa_{O_2} (mm Hg) Exer-cise	RVEF% Rest	RVEF% Exer-cise
Mean	73 (7.0)*	57 (23.1)	82 (8)	74 (12.9)	57	54
Most abnormal	64	27	70	52	44	42

Severe Disease (n = 7)

	TLC (%P)	$DL_{CO}SB$ (%P)	Pa_{O_2} (mm Hg) Rest	Pa_{O_2} (mm Hg) Exer-cise	RVEF% Rest	RVEF% Exer-cise
Mean	44 (9.1)	32 (5.6)	72 (17)	57 (39)	43	25
Most abnormal	29	26	55	39	14	8†

*Numbers in parentheses refer to SD of data.
†This patient had evidence of RV failure.

There was a significant correlation between TLC, DL_{CO}, and the right ventricular ejection fraction (RVEF).

Endobronchial Sarcoidosis

Endobronchial sarcoidosis may occur without parenchymal change. Hadfield and colleagues[1984] have recorded four patients with this

syndrome with multiple narrowings and occlusions of bronchi. In one 32-year-old non-smoking man, the FEV_1 was only 2.1 liters, and the flow loop suggested small airway obstruction. $DL_{CO}/\dot{V}A$ was normal. Excellent bronchograms accompany the clinical data in these cases. In another report, an athletic 25-year-old man, who had been a light smoker but who had stopped a year before the onset of the disease, presented with dyspnea. The chest x-ray showed hilar adenopathy and reticulation. The bronchograms were abnormal and sarcoid tissue was obtained on bronchoscopy.[1965] Tests of function were as follows:

	Predicted	Initial	After Prednisone
FEV_1	5.05	1.91	2.7
FVC	5.28	4.32	6.0
FEV_1/FVC	80.5	44.0	45.00
$\dot{V}max_{50\%}$	4.4	0.77	1.30
FRC	3.99	5.03	4.87
RV	2.02	3.91	3.95
TLC	7.30	8.46	9.2
$DL_{CO}SB$	35.0	35.0	40.0
$DL_{CO}SS$, rest	24.5	15.1	16.7
exercise		26.6	43.0
P_{st} at TLC	40–50 (cm H_2O)	40.0 (cm H_2O)	32.0 (cm H_2O)
SGaw	0.13–0.36	0.03	0.07

These data are of considerable interest and indicate the possibility of significant elevation of residual volume. The discrepancy between the $DL_{CO}SB$ and $DL_{CO}SS$ might be explained by much more severe $\dot{V}/\dot{Q}$ abnormality during tidal breathing than when a maximal inspiration was taken. Other cases of bronchiolar sarcoidosis may be characterized by wheezing, stridor, and repetitive infections.[1983]

In one series of 99 patients with sarcoidosis, 8% had significant bronchial stenoses, and the clinical presentation resembled that in other patients with chronic airflow limitation.[1948] In two patients with sarcoidosis and extensive peribronchiolar fibrosis,[1945] the FEV_1 was 27% of predicted in one and 55% of predicted in the other. FEF_{25-75} values were 48% and 14% of predicted. In one of these patients, the DL_{CO} was only slightly reduced at 84% of predicted; it was not recorded in the other patient.

INTERPRETATION OF FUNCTION TESTS: STRUCTURE/FUNCTION

In 1976, Carrington and his colleagues[1935] reported on a comparison between pulmonary function tests and radiologic appearances in 48 patients with sarcoidosis and 13 patients with berylliosis, in whom detailed examinations of the histologic features had been performed. The best correlation was between steady-state exercise DL_{CO} and an index of interstitial cellular infiltration. A multiple index based on $FEV_1/FVC\%$, DL_{CO}, $(A - a) D_{O_2}$, and exercise $\dot{V}E$ also correlated with interstitial change. Radiologic abnormality correlated poorly with the histologic findings. Comparisons with other patients with interstitial pneumonitis showed better $DL_{CO}SB$ at rest in sarcoidosis patients, but little difference in steady-state exercising DL_{CO} or in $(A - a) D_{O_2}$ on exercise between the two groups. However, there was considerable variation in all these relationships.

In 1979, Huang and his colleagues[1980] published correlative studies on 81 patients with sarcoidosis. They used function and radiologic data and lung biopsy examination. In general, function test defects reflected severity. Eleven individuals with normal function showed minimal changes on biopsy and no fibrosis. Those with abnormalities in several tests of function showed more extensive morphologic changes. However, the tests did not distinguish between apparently moderate and severe histologic changes, and they could not differentiate between alveolitis, granulomata, or fibrosis. The reduction in Pa_{O_2} on exercise appeared the most sensitive test but did not differentiate between histologic categories.

Reviewing all this data, Keogh and Crystal[1833] concluded that defects of function bore a general relationship to severity of involvement but that specific interpretations were not possible. Other authors[1844, 1947] have concluded that tests of function are important in evaluating and in following the course of the disease.[3589]

FUNCTION TESTS IN RELATION TO TREATMENT

In 1974, Mitchell and Scadding[1964] published a detailed review of sarcoidosis that omitted all mention of pulmonary function in the condition. This led to a correspondence on the use of function tests in managing treatment. DeRemee and Anderson[1962] stated that, in their experience, leaving treatment of patients with abnormal function but without significant symptoms until symptoms developed was to leave it until too late. Mitchell and Scadding[1963] replied that

there was no evidence that steroids reduced the incidence of disabling fibrosis and that a controlled trial was needed. Other correspondents have discussed the same issue.[1950, 1951]

Colp and her colleagues[1938] reported on a follow-up study of 120 patients with sarcoidosis. Untreated patients were followed for an average period of 2 years and 8 months. Of 67 patients in this category whose VC was originally greater than 65% of predicted, only three improved. Seventeen worsened, and the remainder were unchanged. $DL_{CO}SB$ remained the same or worsened in most of the untreated patients and improved in nine with good initial function and four with poor initial function. In treated patients, most had either no change or some improvement in both vital capacity and diffusing capacity. In this group of 53 patients 36 had an improved VC, and 42 had an improved $DL_{CO}SB$. In only one patient did both these indices worsen. In patients with poor function initially, there was little difference in final DL_{CO} figures between the treated and untreated groups. The authors stressed that this was not a controlled trial, but their data indicated some benefit, in functional terms, from treatment.

Hillerdal and colleagues[4341] reported on a 15-year study of 214 men and 291 women with sarcoidosis. Fifty per cent of Stage I patients had normal chest films 15 months after disease detection. In Stage II patients, 50% had normal chest films after 3 years. In Stage III, only 33% had normal chest films after 5 years.

Selroos and Sellergren[1977] have reported on 39 patients with Stage II disease of less than 5 years' duration. The subjects were randomly allocated to 7 months of prednisolone treatment or to no treatment and were compared at the end of that time and later. The authors obtained the following data:

	Start	7 Months Later*	2 Years Later	4 Years Later
FVC (%P)				
No treatment	84.9	82.4	87.4	85.6
Steroids	83.4	87.9	82.0	85.7
$DL_{CO}SB$ (%P)				
No treatment	76.4	74.7	78.9	77.7
Steroids	77.4	85.2	77.2	79.2

*Treatment ended at 7 months, and the authors concluded that the data indicated the importance of continuing it for a much longer period if significant benefit in the long term was to be obtained.

In another study of 25 patients, follow-up data showed no favorable effect in terms of function tests or radiologic changes between those treated with steroids and those not given steroids. After 10 to 15 years, the mean function tests were not different in the two groups.[3585] A recent study reported no difference in outcome between one group receiving daily steroids and another group observed for 6 months receiving them on alternate days.[4460] All of these were Stage II patients, and all had a TLC or $DL_{CO}SB$ <80% predicted.

In smaller groups, some evidence has been obtained that steroids improve DL_{CO} and $(A - a) D_{O_2}$ but do not affect abnormal small airway tests.[1982] In one unusual case in which a patient's alveoli were filled with mononuclear cells, marked improvement followed steroid therapy.[1955] The FVC rose from 1.76 to 2.69. TLC increased from 2.54 to 3.91, but the $DL_{CO}SB$ dropped from 13.8 to 7.9 as the chest x-ray improved.

Ten patients with biopsy proven sarcoid, who had had no treatment for 6 months or at all, were followed after steroids were given. It was concluded that steroids reduced the percentage of lymphocytes in BAL fluid, lowered the ^{67}Ga index, and increased the VC and $DL_{CO}SB$ in all but two of the patients.[4461] The authors concluded that suppression of the alveolitis was more impressive than improvement in function, and that the initial function defect had not been very severe. Others have noted that improvement in the FVC following steroid administration correlated with the percentage of pretreatment lymphocytes in BAL fluid.[4412] In this series of 21 patients, $DL_{CO}SB$ did not improve after steroids were given. Others have found that improvement in the VC following treatment is often more significant than changes in DL_{CO}.[4486] Steroids did not affect function in 12 patients with Stage III sarcoidosis.[4490] Positron tomography was used to measure regional lung density in studies of seven patients with sarcoidosis. In two of these subjects, steroid treatment was followed by a reduction in regional lung density[4327] and improvement in function test data.

A follow-up study of 192 biopsy proven cases of sarcoidosis showed that 89% of these patients were not "socially disabled" as a result of the disease and 78% were free of symptoms.[1967] No function test data were reported. Two hundred fifty patients followed for 7.4 years had a survival rate lower than that of the general population.[1968] Abnormal spirometry values were said to be a predictor of mortality, but detailed data were not given.

SUMMARY

The interpretation of pulmonary function tests in sarcoidosis represents a considerable challenge. We suggest the following guidelines:

1. Relative normality indicates an early stage of the disease without significant fibrosis. If the only lesions are space-occupying granulomata, the vital capacity and $DL_{CO}SB$ will fall together. C_{st} is reduced in proportion to the reduction in lung volume (i.e., the shape of the static pressure-volume curve is normal).

2. In some cases of early disease, there may be significant changes in tests influenced by small airways. These occur independently of changes in VC or $DL_{CO}SB$. This reduction suggests that small airways are being compromised by adjacent granulomata or that significant endobronchial sarcoidosis exists. Lowered flow rates with a relatively normal DL_{CO} should suggest the possibility of significant endobronchial lesions and should be regarded as an indication of the need for further investigation.

3. The exercise $(A - a) D_{O_2}$ may be the most sensitive indicator of abnormality, as it is in the interstitial fibrosis syndromes.

4. A lowering of DL_{CO} disproportionate to the reduction in vital capacity should suggest the possibility of abnormal $DL/\dot{Q}_c$ distribution, which is probably attributable to vascular abnormalities caused by granulomata in close proximity to small vessels. Capillary distortion and obliteration will be indicated by a lowered pulmonary capillary blood volume.

5. Reductions in pulmonary function cannot be interpreted in terms of severity of alveolitis, nor can distinctions be drawn between different aspects of the manifestations of sarcoidosis, except in the general terms noted previously. However, disease of longer standing and greater fibrosis are both associated with worsening of function.

Although much new information has been added since 1970,[1] there are still uncertainties in the interpretation of tests of function in this condition. On balance, we consider that longitudinal tests of function do contribute to the management of sarcoidosis. (Indeed, data we have reviewed in this chapter clearly indicate this to be the case.) However, "hard" evidence of the benefits of early treatment (and hence of the importance of initiating treatment when function is deranged rather than when symptoms are complained of) has not yet been published. Until it is, many chest physicians will be unwilling to withhold long-term steroid therapy if significant deterioration of pulmonary function is known to be occurring, even when symptoms and radiologic status have not suggested progression of the disease.

OCCUPATIONAL LUNG DISEASES

16

Et quam artem exerceat? (What is his job?)
BERNARDINO RAMAZZINI[2451]

Longe praestantius est preservare quam curare, sicut satius est tempestatem praevidere ac illam effugere quam ab ipsa evadere.
(It is much better to prevent than to cure, and so much easier to foresee future harm and avoid it rather than have to get rid of it after having fallen prey.)
BERNARDINO RAMAZZINI (FROM A TALK GIVEN IN THE YEAR 1711)[2448]

Prevention is so much better than healing.
REVD. THOMAS ADAMS (1612–1653)[4692]

INTRODUCTION

At the time the second edition of this book was published, relatively little attention had been given to problems of occupational lung disease. Over the past 12 years, hundreds of papers have appeared documenting different patterns of function test change in a spectrum of disease that has been rapidly expanding. As this chapter reveals, however, there are still many difficult and unresolved questions, but the essential contribution made by studies of lung function no longer requires the emphasis we thought necessary in 1970.[1]

Several excellent texts on occupational lung disease[2452, 2470, 4651] describe in detail the syndromes briefly presented in this chapter. One recent volume on methodology in relation to

occupational disease contains chapters on exercise testing,[2460] epidemiology,[2461] worker surveys,[2462] and statistical analyses.[2463] A recent review article discusses the use of pulmonary function tests in the industrial setting,[4655] and others have described the use of spirometry in the field[2459, 3711] and the use of the DL_{CO} in industrial surveys.[3718] These issues were noted in Chapter 5.

The following discussion is intended to provide a background for the general chest physician whose contact with occupational lung disease is episodic and who wishes to know whether the pattern of function test derangement in any given cases is similar to, or different from, other cases described in the very extensive literature. One of the major problems in contemporary occupational lung disease is the interaction between the effects of cigarette smoking and the effects of exposure to dangerous materials. Although smoking is unrelated to the risk of mesothelioma or to the occurrence of occupational asthma, in such diseases as coal worker's pneumoconiosis, byssinosis, and silicosis, this interaction is of great importance—but difficult to resolve in epidemiologic studies. In the individual patient, it presents the physician with an insoluble problem.

Every chest physician encounters patients who have been exposed to hazardous materials. In a survey in Tucson, Arizona, Lebowitz[2253] found that more than half of the surveyed population had some form of exposure to a potentially harmful substance, and of the population of 1132 individuals surveyed, 4% had been exposed to silica, 5% to asbestos, 12.8% to sawdust, 9.9% to smoke, 15% to organic solvents, and 3.9% to radiation. These are remarkable observations. The slow development of concern about occupational disease in general, which began with Ramazzini more than 150 years ago, has been documented by several authors. Vilma Hunt contributed an excellent review entitled "The Emergence of the Worker's Right to know Health Risks,"[2251] and Lee[2206] traced the development of occupational medicine and hygiene in Victorian England.

A recently uncovered quotation from Samuel Johnson (1706–1784) may represent the first statement of ethical responsibility in relation to hazardous work: "No man has a right to any good without partaking of the evil by which that good is necessarily produced; no man has a right to security by another's danger, nor to plenty by another's labour, but as he gives something of his own which he who meets the danger or undergoes the labour considers as equivalent. . . ."[2469]

Recent reconsiderations of ethical and organizational problems in relation to occupational disease have analysed these questions.* In this volume, no detailed consideration of the complex problems of measuring actual worker exposure to a wide variety of dusts and chemicals can be attempted; but it may be noted that personal dosimetry, when practicable, tends to show higher values than environmental monitoring.[2152] Nor can any comprehensive review of lung defenses and clearance mechanisms be given. Several excellent contributions have been made to this field in the past few years.†

---

*See references 2137, 2229, 2435, 3595, 3639, 3654, 3697, 3711, 3721, 4506, 4508, 4598.

†See references 2286, 2303, 2305, 2363, 2365, 2535.

In cases of pneumoconiosis, the radiologic appearances are often classified according to the system proposed by the International Labour Office (ILO).[2101] In this classification, the numbers 1, 2, and 3 are given to progressive grades of profusion of small opacities, and they are further classified as

- "p" type with a diameter less than 1.5 mm
- "m" or "q" type with diameters between 1.5 and 3.0 mm
- "n" or "r" type with diameters between 3 and 10 mm

Opacities are also described as "irregular." Progressive massive fibrosis is often designated as type B or C or as "complicated" pneumoconiosis.

Every part of the respiratory tract may be involved in different syndromes of occupational lung disease. Some years ago, we drew attention to the probability that small airways might be a target zone for the deposition of inhaled particles or as the first site of action of certain inhaled gases.[2148] Recent work by Churg and Wright has produced evidence that pathologic changes may be found in this region in persons exposed to a variety of dusts.[2454] This completes the list of affected zones that earlier had been dominated by mucus hypersecretion, alveolitis, and alveolar fibrosis.

PNEUMOCONIOSES DUE TO METAL AND MINERAL DUSTS

Iron, Tin, Barium, and Borax

Exposure to iron oxide (magnetite) or to other forms of iron generally leads to radiologic change without significant function impairment,[2169] as we noted in the previous edition.[1] Bronchitis was noted to be common in one group of underground iron ore miners but was thought to be possibly attributable to diesel fumes; FEV_1 values were not low.[2141] An exception to this generality are the iron ore miners of the Lorraine region of France, in whom extensive generalized pulmonary changes have been described and in whom this condition may lead to cor pulmonale[2379]; there also appears to be a considerably increased mortality by age 69. A recent study of 1109 iron mine workers showed that 210 had a positive methacholine test,[4567] as judged by a more than 10% fall in FEV_1, and 5 years later, cough, sputum, and chronic bronchitis were more common in this group. Their mean FEV_1 fell from 99% of predicted initially to 91% 5 years later. The questionnaire data showed the variability of criteria of "chronic bronchitis" on repeat inquiry in such a population, 14.6% of those negative on the first inquiry being positive on the second, and 54% of those positive on the first occasion being negative on the second. A more recent report on the same population[4649] showed that most of the accelerated FEV_1 decline was in smokers, whose mean FEV_1 fell from 108% of predicted to 99% of predicted 5 years later.

In Cornish tin miners, there is a high incidence of silicosis and an increased risk of lung cancer attributed to radon daughters,[3680] but the tin itself is not blamed for disease. No new reports have appeared on stannosis, or tin oxide inhalation, which also is generally unaccompanied by function defect.[1] Barium is also benign, possibly because of its insolubility. In one survey of miners of barites, there were radiologic changes but no respiratory symptoms[2495] and the mean vital capacities and FEV_1 values were normal. In five cases followed for 5 years after leaving the mine, the chest x-ray slowly cleared.

A recent survey of 629 borax workers showed no radiologic changes and normal FEV_1 levels.[4684]

Coal Worker's Pneumoconiosis

Over the past 13 years, a great deal of new information on this condition has appeared. The first major review of coal worker's pneumoconiosis in the United States showed that about one-third of working miners had radiologic evidence of the condition.[2115]

In Great Britain, surveys of as many as 30,000 working miners have been published.[2095] Useful reviews by Higgins[2060, 2381] and by Morgan and Lapp[2299] in 1975 deal with many of the difficult questions raised by this complex disease. Factors relating to the prevalence of coal worker's pneumoconiosis in different coal fields are poorly understood. In Great Britain, the variation is apparently not explained by differences in dust composition nor by intensity of exposure,[2116] though it is clear that the differences are real.[2051] Nor is it clear why rates are almost 10 times higher in eastern Pennsylvania anthracite miners than in bituminous coal miners in Colorado.[2085] It is been suggested that silica content may be important in determining rate of progression of the disease.[2434] In Britain, it has been reported that in the lungs of miners who work in "high-rank" collieries there is coal but little silica, whereas in the lungs of those who worked in "low-rank" collieries there is a higher fraction of noncoal minerals and silicotic nodules are sometimes found.[3596] Underground exposure to oxides of nitrogen or diesel fumes does not seem to be important.[4569, 4638] Underground coal miners in Utah show remarkably little function defect by comparison with other groups.[2112] As one might expect, the disease is rare in surface coal miners, and in the few cases reported there was a history of previous underground experience.[2068]

There is a fair correlation between dust exposure and radiologic category,[2054] but it is important to note that classification of radiologic stage may vary between one study and another, as there have been shown to be considerable differences between observers in classifying chest films according to the ILO classification,* and systematic differences between readers in the United States and in Britain have been reported.[2090] In one study of 106 applicants for benefits for this condition, in more than half the cases there was disagreement about the presence or absence of radiologic pneumoconiosis.[2170]

Across the whole spectrum of the disease, from the earliest stages of simple pneumoconiosis to the entity of progressive massive fibrosis, the FEV_1 is correlated with the degree of dyspnea.[2115] However, the FEV_1 is still commonly within normal limits when the earliest radiographic evidence of change is present.[2084, 2086] Although there is some correlation between FEV_1 decline and advancing radiologic category, it is not close. In one series, the FEV_1 averaged 3.46 L in 141 miners with normal x-rays, 3.49 in 31 men in category one, and 3.07 in 18 men with progressive massive fibrosis.[2104] Higgins concluded that "Since there is a clear correlation between the x-ray category of pneumoconiosis and the weight of dust found in the lungs at autopsy, these findings indicate that chronic obstructive lung disease is not closely related to long-term dust exposure."[2060] One study investigated 25 miners with simple pneumoconiosis radiologically but with a normal FEV_1. Their average age was 55 years, and they all were non-smokers or had not smoked for 10 years. Of the 25 miners, 17 had a fall in C_{dyn} with increasing frequency, and 10 of these had chronic mucus hypersecretion.[2086] The residual volume was not elevated. It is likely that when

---

*See references 2054, 2094, 2096, 2101.

the FEV_1 is lower than predicted, the RV is commonly increased,* and it may be elevated in some miners whose x-ray is normal.[2081] It appears to be related to obstruction and smoking history in general,[2089] rather than to radiologic category.[2077] In another group of 24 miners in whom RL was not elevated, CV%VC and CC%TLC were significantly increased,[2063] as was RL measured at low lung volumes.

Elevation of residual volume and a reduced C_{dyn}/f commonly occur together.[2109] These findings have been interpreted to indicate that small airway function is compromised early in this condition.

In a recent report on 36 non-smoking, non-bronchitic South Wales miners,[3659] there was a significant loss of lung recoil, with some reduction in ventilatory flow rates, and an increased residual volume. In other series,[3629] the residual volume was rarely raised except with complicated pneumoconiosis.

As noted in the second edition, in simple pneumoconiosis there is some evidence of abnormal gas exchange. This appears to be particularly true of cases showing the "p" (pinhead opacities up to 1.5 mm in diameter) type of change radiographically. In a comparison between two small groups of miners of the same age, the "p" type had a lower DL_{CO}, lower K_{CO}, a larger VD/VT ratio, and an increased exercise ventilation compared with the "m" type.[2099] The $(A-a) D_{O_2}$ on exercise was closely related to the DL_{CO}. There is also some evidence that the presence of irregular opacities (ILO classification) is associated with more impairment of FEV_1 and may possibly indicate the presence of emphysema.[2114] In one recent study, it was attributed to the coexistence of emphysema and interstitial fibrosis.[3622] Irregular opacities occur in about 20% of miners with pneumoconiosis.[3636]

In studies of 1886 coal miners in Germany,[2081] reductions in vital capacity and elevations of residual volume were noted in miners with normal chest films. Impairment of gas distribution, demonstrated by a prolonged mixing index, was found in most men over the age of 40, and Pa_{O_2} on exercise was reduced and $(A-a) D_{O_2}$ elevated on exercise in all age groups and in all dust-exposed men whether with pneumoconiosis on x-ray or not. C_{dyn}/f was lower in miners than in a control group. With 30 years of exposure but without radiologic change, the FEV_1 was 20% lower than in control groups, and the $(A-a) D_{O_2}$ was 80% higher. This series

as well as others[2052, 2075] confirmed the generally poorer function in the presence of the "p" type of change radiographically. Smidt, Worth, and Bielert[2406] in a major study of 3652 coal workers also found the worst defects of function, both in terms of vital capacity and gas exchange, in men with "p" type radiographs. There does not appear to be any detectable difference in mortality rates, however.[2098]

The interpretation of the significance of interrelationships in coal worker's pneumoconiosis is complicated by three factors: the distinction between chronic mucus hypersecretion and its effects, and the effects of dust deposition; the influence of the confounding variable of cigarette smoking; and the question of whether the dust leads to development of emphysema. Much of the data appear to be contradictory, but the questions are of sufficient importance that an evaluation of the present status of these questions must be attempted.

Muir and colleagues in 1977[2113] summarized British experience on the first of these questions by noting that "results are compatible with a simple model in which dust exposure in the mining industry may cause pneumoconiosis, bronchitis, or both," and they noted that there was no evidence that mucus hypersecretion offered any protection against the development of simple pneumoconiosis. In the survey of 30,000 British coal miners already referred to,[2095] there appeared to be two separate groups—those with chronic mucus hypersecretion and those with complaints of breathlessness and chest wheezing. All symptoms increased with increasing age and smoking.

Non-smoking coal miners certainly develop bronchitis,[2111, 2430] and their FEV_1 is lower than in those without bronchitis.[2111] Ex-miners have more chronic bronchitis and lower FEV_1 values than control groups when age and smoking are taken into acount.[2100] Comparisons between 4479 smoking miners and 1687 non-smoking miners in West Virginia[2097] showed that the mean FEV_1 was lower and RV and TLC higher in the smoking miners. From the same laboratory, Morgan and colleagues[2103] excluded all men with significant bronchitis and all cigarette smokers and found evidence of slight elevation of residual volume and increased VD/VT ratio. Also from the same region, Kibelstis and colleagues[2091] studied 8555 miners and found more bronchitis in smoking than non-smoking miners, concluding that "the effect of smoking was five times greater than that of coal dust." In this larger series, there was no evidence that

---

*See references 2081, 2084, 2103, 2108.

residual volume was increased in the non-smoking group.[2089]

Hankinson, Reger, and Morgan in 1977[2087] selected four groups of 428 age- and height-matched men from a sample of 9000 working miners in West Virginia and reported the following data:

Comparison of X-ray Findings

CXR Category	Non-Smokers (number of subjects)		Smokers (number of subjects)	
	WITHOUT CHRONIC BRONCHITIS	WITH CHRONIC BRONCHITIS	WITHOUT CHRONIC BRONCHITIS	WITH CHRONIC BRONCHITIS
0	385	371	371	356
1	35	45	47	54
2	8	12	10	15
3	0	0	0	3

Comparison of Mean Pulmonary Function Test Values

	Non-Smokers		Smokers	
	WITHOUT CHRONIC BRONCHITIS	WITH CHRONIC BRONCHITIS	WITHOUT CHRONIC BRONCHITIS	WITH CHRONIC BRONCHITIS
FEV_1	3.77	3.60	3.49	3.34
$\dot{V}max_{50\%}VC$	4.4	4.21	3.72	3.43
TLC*	7.09	7.03	7.30	7.41
RV	2.20	2.32	2.54	2.75

*Measured by planimetry of chest x-ray.

They noted the decrease in flow rates at low lung volumes in non-smokers and the increased TLC in smokers without symptoms of chronic bronchitis.

Dechoux and colleagues from the Lorraine[3662] noted that in 655 coal miners about to retire at the age of 50 after 30 years underground, the FEV_1 was lowered in 20% of non-smokers and 35% of smokers without evidence of radiologic change. The $DL_{CO}SS$ was found to be related to radiologic category, falling from a mean value of 17.8 in those with normal x-rays to a mean of 13.9 in those with complicated pneumoconiosis. In a quantitative study of the bronchi from 94 coal miners age 67 years,[3621] smoking was found to be significantly correlated with mean and maximal mucus gland/wall ratios, and coal mine dust was significantly related to the maximal gland/wall ratio. The gland dimensions were not related to the amount of dust in the lung or to the degree of pneumoconiosis.

A recent study of 20 anthracite coal miners, 17 of whom had mucus hypersecretion, compared with 10 normals[3719] illustrates the separation of bronchitic symptoms from other changes. Fourteen of the miners were non-smokers, and 6 were ex-smokers, none of whom had smoked in the 10 years before the study.

Their mean age was 66.5 years. There were no significant differences between the miners and the control group in lung volumes, DL_{CO}, or compliance, either static or dynamic. Dust exposure had presumably been light in this group.

Cowie, Lloyd, and Soutar[4721] have recently reported a more sophisticated approach to the analysis of lung function in 458 coal miners using principal component analysis. Their criteria for clinical definition were as follows:

Group	Number	FEV_1 (%P)	FEV_1/ FVC (%P)	TL_{CO} (%P)
A	27	<80	<90	<80
B	27	<80	<90	>80
C	12	<80	>90	<80
D	30	<80	>90	>80

where A = airflow obstruction with low gas transfer; B = airflow obstruction with preserved gas transfer; C = restrictive defect with low gas transfer; D = restrictive defect with preserved gas transfer.

This method of analysis results in a set of linear combinations of the original variables, each of which explains a percentage of the total variation in the data. Comparisons with criteria of normality based on predicted values indicated that this method selected more young men with unusual lung function than the conventional comparison. The authors considered that this approach "unifies the analysis of results of multiple tests, and may also provide insight into associations between the results of one test and others and into the various functional patterns of abnormality which the lung may express."[4721]

Detailed mechanics studies in 20 miners, of whom 17 were non-smokers,[2073] showed that the pressure/volume curves were shifted to the right. The authors concluded that in three of the miners, regional inhomogeneity of elastic recoil due to focal emphysema probably accounted for the observed fall in C_{dyn} with increasing frequency.

Other authors have noted that reduced diaphragm excursion during life is correlated with the degree of emphysema at autopsy.[2107] Studies of perfusion distribution using ^{99m}Tc-MAA in 37 miners and ex-miners showed that all 14 with complicated coal worker's pneumoconiosis had avascular zones in relation to conglomerate masses and bullae.[2093] In 24 of these cases, the DL_{CO} was less than 70% of the predicted value.

Studies using ^{133}Xe in 10 miners with normal chest films and in 15 with simple coal worker's pneumoconiosis, in all of whom the FEV_1/FVC ratio was normal,[2072] showed reduced ventilation in upper zones in those with pneumoconiosis. TL_{CO} values were lower in this group, and mean FEV_1 values were 3.68 in those with normal films and 3.23 in those with pneumoconiosis. Studies of aerosol deposition have suggested that abnormalities in small airways of miners lead to a higher than normal rate of deposition in smokers, but cases of simple coal worker's pneumoconiosis did not show any additional differences.[2088] More recent aerosol deposition studies have indicated, however, that the "p" type of pneumoconiosis may be associated with decreased rates of disappearance with breath holding,[2056] possibly indicating larger peripheral air spaces.

The question of whether emphysema occurs as a complication of coal worker's pneumoconiosis, and the influence of cigarette smoking, was raised by Ryder and colleagues,[2110] who compared 247 autopsy specimens on miners with a control group and noted that the mean emphysema score derived by point counting was twice as high in the miners' group as in the control group. The FEV_1 was closely related to the extent of emphysema present. This study was later questioned on the basis of possible sampling bias.[2080] Lyons and colleagues recently published data from 139 autopsies on miners, 19 of whom were non-smokers[2071]; 95 had pneumoconiosis, and 44 had early progressive massive fibrosis. The FEV_1 levels were slightly less abnormal in the non-smokers, but the difference was not significant. They concluded that the amounts of emphysema in smokers and non-smokers were similar and that centrilobular emphysema was the most common type in both groups. They showed a lung from a 66-year-old lifelong non-smoking miner with very extensive centrilobular emphysema involving at least 60% of all lobules.

In a recent autopsy study on the lungs of 886 coal workers from New South Wales, Australia,[3665] quantitative morphometric studies led to the following conclusions, among others:

1. The severity of emphysema had a significant positive regression on years of work at the coal face independently of age at death.

2. The severity of emphysema was related to the severity of radiologic change, particularly in the non-smoking and non-bronchitic group.

3. There were significant relationships between emphysema, bronchial gland ratio, and pneumoconiosis.

4. Smoking was not correlated with the severity of emphysema or the gland/wall ratio.

5. The FEV_1 was significantly negatively correlated with bronchitis, emphysema, and pneumoconiosis.

Cockcroft and colleagues from Wales[3663] recently reviewed the lungs of 39 coal workers who died of ischemic heart disease and compared them with 48 controls (non-miners) who also died of ischemic heart disease. There was a significantly greater score of centrilobular emphysema in the miners. Reviewing this and other data in a recent editorial,[3623] Seaton concluded that the reasons for progression of the disease remain obscure, but that there was a clear relationship between coal dust exposure and FEV_1 decline, attributable to more emphysema. These conclusions were disputed in subsequent correspondence,[3625] and the discussion was interesting,[3626] but the objections were well answered by Seaton.[3627] Kennedy has suggested that exposure to underground fumes may be important,[3624] but there is little evidence that this may be occurring, as noted earlier.

Other autopsy data on 215 coal miners, 115 with simple or no pneumoconiosis and 100 with progressive massive fibrosis,[3629] showed that right ventricular hypertrophy was rare without advanced pneumoconiosis. It was related to emphysema and to airways disease (but not closely) and was predominant in smokers, though when progressive massive fibrosis was present, it also occured in non-smokers.

More recent autopsy comparisons between coal workers and non–coal workers all aged 50 to 70 years and dying of ischemic heart disease[4499] have shown beyond much doubt that 22 years of work at the coal face (the mean for the miners) is associated with higher scores for centrilobular emphysema than occur in the controls. This conclusion has been supported by autopsy data on 450 coal miners, in whom it was also shown that the degree of emphysema was related to increasing amounts of dust retained in the lungs.[4525] A recent review of this question[4605] pointed out the implications for compensation policy.

There have been several studies of the interrelationship between radiologic and function tests status, and hemodynamic changes.

A recent study of 26 coal miners, all with a normal airway resistance, divided them into three groups[4722]:

- Gp C: Normal chest x-ray; TL_{CO} 77.6 %P; k_{CO} 83.6 %P; VC 91.9 %P; (n = 8)
- Gp S1: Micronodular silicosis; TL_{CO} 79.2 %P; k_{CO} 80.3 %P; VC 89.1 %P; (n = 10)
- Gp S2: Complicated silicosis; TL_{CO} 71.1 %P; k_{CO} 80.6 %P; VC 67.7 %P; (n = 8)

At rest, blood gases and pulmonary arterial pressure were normal, but values for pulmonary artery pressure were slightly higher in groups S1 and S2 compared with group C. However, on exercise, pulmonary hypertension occurred in half of the cases in group S2. The increased pulmonary vascular resistance was correlated with loss of VC and FEV_1. There was no fall in Pa_{O_2} on exercise, but values were 6 mm Hg lower in group S2.

In another study of 47 symptomatic coal miners, the following data were obtained[2092]:

	Group A No Airway Obstruction	Group B Airway Obstruction
Number	23	24
FEV_1	3.15	1.83
$\dot{V}_D/\dot{V}_T$ (at rest)	41%	51%
$(A-a) D_{O_2}$ (rest mm Hg)	27	27
PAP increased at rest	1	7

These data confirm the probability that pulmonary hypertension is related to FEV_1 in this condition.

Kremer[2062] also found a relationship between FEV_1 and resting pulmonary arterial pressure. He reported that if the FEV_1 was less than 1.0 L, there was a 1-year mortality of 40% and a 5-year mortality of 80%. In a group with a similar FEV_1 but also with a resting pulmonary arterial pressure of more than 30 mm Hg, there was a 70% 1-year mortality.[2062]

Exercise data generally show an increased $\dot{V}_E$ in relation to oxygen uptake.[2072, 2082] Recent data of great interest suggest that diaphragmatic fatigue may limit exercise capability in men with pneumoconiosis.[2070, 2074] This is an important finding, since if it is confirmed, it may explain the poor relationship between exercise endurance and the FEV_1. An interesting comparison between cases of chronic airflow limitation of non-occupational origin and coal worker's pneumoconiosis[2079] showed that the relationship between Pa_{O_2} and pulmonary arterial pressure was not different between the two groups, the pressure rising when the Pa_{O_2} fell below 70 mm Hg. It has been shown that the risk of developing progressive massive fibrosis increases with a rising category of simple pneumoconiosis.[2053]

Caplan's syndrome complicating coal worker's pneumoconiosis does not seem to be associated with any characteristic function defect.[2083, 2105]

Longitudinal studies of decline of FEV_1 in this condition have provided different estimates. Musk and colleagues[2069] studied 125 miners after an interval of 9 years and found a rate of FEV_1 decline of -23 mL/year, which is no different from non-smoking normals (see Chapter 5). Muir reported rates of FEV_1 decline of between -35 mL/year and -40 mL/year in non-smoking miners, and of -39 mL/year and -44 mL/year in smokers with and without respiratory symptoms and with different radiologic categories.[2078] These declines were computed from cross-sectional data.

Love and Miller[2067] recently reported longitudinal data on 1677 coal miners studied after an interval of 11 years in Great Britain. Their data show the following FEV_1 declines in mL/year:

	Age			
	<39	40–49	>50	ALL
Non-smokers	-32.7	-39.0	-38.2	-37.2
(Number)	(57)	(90)	(68)	(215)
Current smokers	-42.7	-47.2	-53.6	-46.3
(Number)	(245)	(506)	(358)	(1109)

Values in intermittent and ex-smokers were intermediate between these two groups. Their data clearly showed that faster declines in FEV_1 occurred with higher dust exposures in all categories of smoking. Lyons and colleagues reported FEV_1 declines of -70 mL/year in category "p" cases, and in non-smokers and ex-smokers with category B and C complicated pneumoconiosis, rates of -105 mL/year.[2050] By contrast, Hildick-Smith[2049] recently studied 107 coal miners over the age of 65 from Kent, England, and found that 72 of the 95 men tested had a normal FEV_1. This result may have been influenced by survivor sample bias, though it suggests that in this coalfield accelerated rates of decline of FEV_1 must be uncommon. In another study by Lyons and Campbell,[2106] serial FEV_1 data over 15 years in 215 miners and ex-miners showed that the most accelerated rates of decline occurred in men with category B progressive massive fibrosis. Faster than normal rates were also observed in men with simple pneumoconiosis in this series. In 675 Nigerian underground miners, an average rate of FEV_1 decline of -34 mL/year was reported.[2055]

We have recently completed a study of 139 non-smoking and 254 smoking miners from the Lorraine coal field in France, who were followed for 18 years.[2117] The rates of FEV_1 and FVC decline were as follows:

		Decline		Age	
	Number	FVC (mL/ year)	FEV₁ (mL/year)	(at start)	Period (years)
Non-smokers					
Deceased	101	−69.7	−68.9	50.9	17.3
Alive	38	−40.5	−47.7	49.1	18.7
Smokers					
Deceased	110	−81.0	−78.4	49.8	15.3
Alive	144	−59.1	−63.7	46.6	17.7

The rates of decline were noted to be the same before and after retirement when further exposure ceased. It seems likely that in these groups it is the accelerated rate of decline of FVC that is responsible for the decline in FEV_1.

Attfield[4640] recently reported on longitudinal FEV_1 decline in 1440 United States miners studied over 9 years. Their ages ranged from 20 to 49 years.

	Age			
	<39	40–49	>50	All
Non-smokers (n = 211)				
FEV₁ decline (mL/year)	−39	−46	−49	−44
Mean FEV₁ (liters)	4.21	3.53	3.50	3.81
Ex-smokers (n = 199)				
FEV₁ decline (mL/year)	−32	−42	−50	−44
Mean FEV₁ (liters)	4.05	3.65	3.27	3.56
Smokers (n = 431)				
FEV₁ decline (mL/year)	−45	−54	−64	−52
Mean FEV₁ (liters)	3.92	3.67	3.08	3.54

A careful regression analysis on this population was possible using approximate dust exposure data. There is little doubt that heavier dust exposure leads to faster rates of decline.

An 11-year follow-up of 4059 men from 24 collieries[4647] indicated that the rate of fall of FVC (which varied from −70 mL/year to −30 mL/year) depended on the initial level of FVC, which averaged 4.0 L in this sample of men with a mean age of 47 years.

A study of 1261 United States coal miners over a 9-year interval indicated that the level of pneumoconiosis is being reduced by application of the 2-mg/m³ dust standard[4609]; however, it has been observed that dust levels are underreported by mine owners in the United States.[4611]

MacLaren and Soutar[4682] have reported on 17,738 working miners in the United Kingdom examined between 1953 and 1958 and re-examined between 1974 and 1980. Of these, 4526 had left the industry. They reported that the incidence of progressive massive fibrosis was 27 per 1000 in those still in the industry but was 94 per 1000 in those who had left it. Cumulative dust exposure, category of simple pneumoconiosis, and age each were found to influence the risk of developing this lesion in a subgroup of 1902 of the men. Exposure to mixed dusts might also be an added risk factor.[4570]

Hurley and Soutar[4691] have also shown that more severe FEV_1 declines occurred in 199 men who had left the coal industry before normal retirement age and who had bronchitic symptoms than in those remaining in it over a 20-year period. In this study, smoking history and dust exposure were accurately known, and the FEV_1 loss could be related to both. These studies indicate the importance of selection bias in both cross-sectional and longitudinal studies in this industry.

It is the combination of a variety of pathologic changes in this condition that makes the interpretation of function defect difficult. Both alveolar destruction and chronic mucus hypersecretion may lead to overinflation, but space-occupying large fibrotic lesions lead to restriction. Until severe lung destruction has occurred, because remaining alveoli are still normal, the DL_{CO} may remain relatively normal. The faster than normal FEV_1 decline may be attributed to developing emphysema, or possibly to the effect of loss of recoil due to aging in further compromising small airway function that is already jeopardized by selective dust collection at this location.

Reports of single cases of progressive massive fibrosis with remarkable preservation of function,[2061] together with studies of non-smoking miners without symptoms,[2103] have led some reviewers to conclude that coal dust alone is generally harmless. Brooks in a recent review[2066] concluded the following:

The problems arise when differentiating spirometric changes due to cigarette smoking from those due to occupational exposures. In general, significant obstructive airways disease does not occur as the result of chronic inhalation of mineral dusts. Now the term significant airway obstruction must be clarified. If there is airway obstruction, for example, FEV_1/FVC of less than 55 per cent, it is probably not due to the dust, but rather to some other cause, such as chronic bronchitis or emphysema from cigarette smoking, or reversible airways obstructive disease of occupational or nonoccupational origin. Small changes in FEV_1 and FEV_1/FVC per cent can occur in industrial bronchitis from dusts, but the changes are small and disability does not occur.

By contrast, we think it important to stress that defects of function are induced by dust loading of the lungs, and these may have long-term effects greater than one would assume from finding a well-preserved FEV_1 in the presence of simple coal worker's pneumoconiosis at age 45. Accelerated declines in FEV_1 and FVC continuing after exposure has ceased, greater in smokers but greater in nonsmoking miners than in nonexposed nonsmokers,[2117] may fairly be attributed to the presence of mineral dust. They may well indicate developing emphysema. Furthermore, it has also been shown that some persons with coal worker's pneumoconiosis may occasionally develop severe lesions after a relatively short period of exposure to coal dust.[2102]

It is possible that coal dust in the lungs leads to an intensification of the adverse effects of cigarette smoke. There is no reason to assume that adverse changes in a smoking coal miner would have occurred if he had smoked as heavily but not been exposed to coal, though a number of those who discuss this problem seem to start from this position.

However, mortality rates for miners and ex-miners with simple pneumoconiosis are not much different from those of the general population.[4539, 4681]

Sadoul[2118] has stressed the importance of deploying a number of tests in studying individuals with pneumoconiosis, and there is some hazard that too much reliance may be placed on a single measurement of FEV_1 in this condition. Exercise testing may, on occasion, show a fall in oxygen saturation,[4464] which would be unsuspected unless the requisite tests were performed. Smidt, Worth, and Bielert, from the laboratory in Moers, Germany, that has published many studies on coal worker's pneumoconiosis concluded that both Pa_{O_2} and $(A-a) D_{O_2}$ should be measured in any complete evaluation of function in this condition.[2406] Longitudinal data that they published[2406] on vital capacity in 265 coal miners indicated the variability of these observations, and this factor diminishes their value. Exercise evaluation of disability is discussed later in this chapter.

Silica

Silica is the most abundant material in the earth's crust. Churg[3599] recently reported that silica can be found in most, if not all, of the lungs of the general population and, with talc and asbestos fibers, constitutes the major component of the 13 different mineral species that can ordinarily be identified. It is likely that it is to be found particularly around small airways.[2454]

Leonardo da Vinci made a cryptic note of the hazards of dust (probably silica from marble quarries) in his notebook, as illustrated in Figure 16–1. However, we still do not have a quantitative "dose-response" curve for silica.

A useful review of silicosis by Ziskind, Jones, and Weill appeared in 1976.[2300] Respiratory disease in British foundry workers was the subject of a British government report in 1971.[2203]

Acute Silicosis

Silica in very finely divided form, to which sandblasters may be exposed, is extremely dangerous. It causes an acute form of silicosis with diffuse change throughout the lung and commonly presents initially as an attack of pneumonia. We presented a case of this condition in the previous edition of this book,[1] in whom the vital capacity declined from 2.9 liters to 1.1 liters over a period of 18 months—a decline of −1200 mL/year. Twenty-two cases of this syndrome in 83 sandblasters in New Orleans have been described and their working conditions analyzed.[2341] Their average age was 44, and the severity of their condition varied, but 8 died from respiratory failure.[2512] When surveyed, the VCs varied from 47% of predicted to normal, and the $DL_{CO}SB$ values were between 36% of predicted and normal. In another report on the same group,[2348] 14 had nodular silicosis, 10 had large opacities, and 31 had major distortions of lung architecture. In the latter two groups, VC and FEV_1 values were reduced, and the mean DL_{CO} values of the groups were below 80% of predicted. Acute silicosis has been described in four tombstone sandblasters, with an average of 35 months exposure.[2304] In one of these cases, the VC fell from 3.13 liters to 1.82 liters over a 13-month period, a rate of decline of −1190 mL/year. The $DL_{CO}SB$ fell from 16.0 (54% predicted) to 13.8 (47% of predicted) over the same period, but the Pa_{O_2} changed only 2 mm Hg, from 80 mm Hg to 78 mm Hg.

A group of United States and British authors have reported on the rate of decline of FEV_1 in New Orleans sandblasters.[5101] Sixty-one men with silicosis were followed longitudinally for up to 7 years. Dust estimates were based on "extensive measurements of airborne dust and protective equipment used." Sixty-three per cent had chest x-ray evidence of disease progression. Declines in pulmonary function tests were associated with average concentration of silica dust exposure, with those in the lowest category having normal rates of decline. Initial levels of function were as follows:

	Radiologic Category	
	Simple	Complicated
Number	31	52
FVC (%P)	87	78
FEV_1 (%P)	83	67
FEF_{25-75} (%P)	70	44
RV (%P)	116	131
TLC (%P)	95	94
$DL_{CO}SB$ (%P)	104	84

The following data on longitudinal decline were reported:

	Comparison of Mean Annual Change in Function	
	No Radiologic Progression	Radiologic Progression
Number	21	38
FVC (mL/year)	−21	−116
FEV_1/FVC (mL/year)	−55	−109
FEV_1/FVC	−0.960	−1.209
RV (mL/year)	−46	−9
TLC (mL/year)	−63	−102
DL_{CO} (mL/min/mm Hg)	−0.946	−0.755

There was evidence of disease progression radiologically in 50% of those with exposure to dust levels of less than 1.25 mg/m³. In those with dust levels above 3.0 mg/m³, all showed radiologic progression. Mean age of all groups was 42 years, and mean exposure was about 11 years. Eighty per cent were smokers, but no differential rates of decline for smokers and non-smokers were reported. The authors of this important study noted that sandblasting with silica was banned in the United Kingdom in 1949 and in the European Economic Community in 1966, but it is still permitted in North America.

Quartz milling is also a very dangerous occupation, and acute silicosis occurred in a 58-year-old man employed in this work.[2497] His vital capacity fell from 2.65 liters to 2.0 liters over the course of a year, and the DL_{CO} fell from 11.0 to 7.0 mL/min/mm Hg. It goes without saying that these cases should never occur; it is the responsibility of chest physicians to ensure that the extreme hazard of finely divided silica is understood and that regulations for protection against it are rigorously enforced. That this can be done successfully was shown by one survey of 32 men with more than 25 years service as sandblasters, in all of whom the vital capacities and FEV_1 data were normal.[2160]

Chronic Silicosis

Exposure to silica dust occurs in a wide variety of occupations. The majority of cases of silicosis are seen in hard-rock drillers, particularly those working underground, and in foundry workers and steelworkers. In 126 stonecutters working in a quarry, 49 had radiologic evidence of silicosis, and dyspnea and reductions of FVC were noted in half of these.[2493] Cases also occur in workers in more unexpected occupations, including people who make slate pencils,[2261] furniture makers,[2265] people who work with bentonite clay,[2288] those who make silica flour (tripoli) used as an abrasive,[2374] and even those who make dental prostheses[2393, 4694] and work with jade.[4683]

Churg and colleagues[4623] recently studied in detail the state of the small airways in 53 persons who had been either hard-rock miners or who had worked in asbestos, construction, or shipyard industries. They described "mineral dust airways disease" in 13 of the 53 workers, compared with 1 in 121 controls without occupational dust exposure. The lesion was associated with lower values of VC, FEV_1, FEV_1/FVC ratio, and FEF_{25-75}; also SBN_2/L values were higher in the exposed group. The mean DL_{CO} values were 76% predicted in the group with airway disease and 96% of predicted in the controls. Pathologically, there was significant fibrosis of the walls of both respiratory and membranous bronchioles. The smoking history was not different between those with and without the lesion.

Kennedy and colleagues[4637] studied resected specimens and confirmed the bronchiolar changes in men exposed to mineral dusts or fumes, but this change was not associated with specific lung function changes, though the mean $Vmax_{50\%}VC$ was lower and the SBN_2/L was higher in the exposed group.

This form of silicosis is usually more evident radiologically in the upper lobes. Interpretation of pulmonary function is complicated by the fact that subsequent contraction of these leads to overinflation of the lower lobes, and gross distortions of architecture occur in the later stages.

There is a general relationship between function defect and radiologic change, as was shown in an analysis of 97 cases of silicosis[2392]:

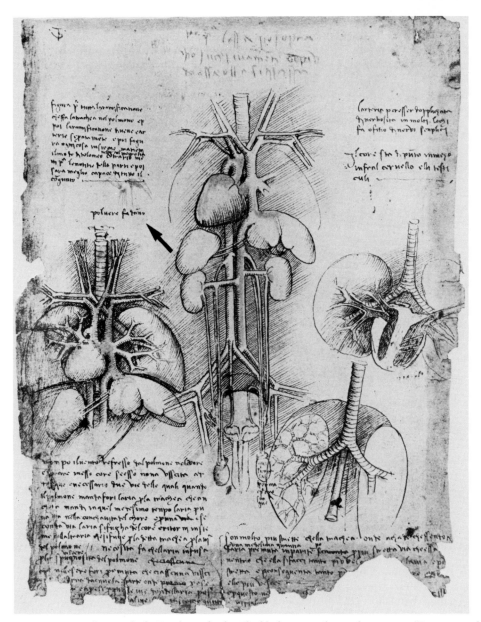

Figure 16–1. From one of Leonardo da Vinci's notebooks. The black arrow refers to the sentence "Dust causes damage." (Courtesy of Her Majesty, Queen Elizabeth II, from the Da Vinci drawings at Windsor Castle.)

Number	CXR (by ILO grade)	Mean Age	VC (%P)	FEV$_1$ (%P)	DL$_{CO}$SS (mL/min/ mm Hg)
39	0/1:1/0:1/1	53.2	88.2	87.7	17.4
26	1/2:2/1:2/2	53.2	80.3	75.4	13.4
32	2/3:3/2:3/3 or B and C	57.9	73.6	64.5	13.6

All those who have studied the condition have noted that individual discrepancies between function data and radiologic category are common. DL$_{CO}$SB and DL$_{CO}$SS data are similar in this condition.[453]

A fall in dynamic compliance and later in static compliance may predate much change in VC or FEV$_1$.[1] Teculescu and Stanescu[2344] studied 47 cases, mostly in drillers, all with radiologic change, all non-smokers, none with radiologic evidence of emphysema nor with a history of heart disease, and all without sputum. The FEV$_1$/FVC was above predicted normal in this group, whose mean exposure was 10.7 years. Eighteen had retired, 10 with conglomerate silicosis. They found that the DL$_{CO}$SB was normal in all except 5 with advanced disease. In three of the five, the lowered $D_{L_{CO}}$ was attributable to the lowered TLC, and in only two was there a defect of gas exchange independent of the change in lung volume. They concluded that gas exchange defects were rare in this form of silicosis.

However, a recent survey of 144 cases from Finland gives a somewhat different perspective.[4688] Forty-six per cent of these had phlegm, and 87% were dyspneic. The data reported were as follows:

	CXR Profusion Category		
	Category 1	Category 2	Category 3
Number	55	68	12
Dyspnea grade (%)			
1	20	10	8
2 or more	80	90	92
3 or more	40	46	83
4 or more	7	12	33
5	0	0	8

Note: 1 = No dyspnea; 2 = hurrying on slight hill; 3 = walking on flat surface with others of same age; 4 = having to stop when walking on level surface; 5 = shortening of breath on dressing or moving.

The pulmonary function test data were as follows:

CXR Category	VC <80%P	FEV$_1$ <80%P	$D_{L_{CO}}$ <80%P
1	48%	35%	44%
2	44%	33%	44%
3	50%	50%	75%

VC, FEV$_1$, and $D_{L_{CO}}$SB all were very significantly different from a referent population. The authors concluded that "$D_{L_{CO}}$ proved to be a rather sensitive lung function parameter for advanced simple silicosis."

In a study of 14 steelworkers,[2198] 4 had silicosis with ILO category 2/3 changes radiologically. They had been exposed to mixed dusts. The $D_{L_{CO}}$ values were normal, but accelerated rates of decline of VC and FEV$_1$ were noted over a 2-year interval. A cross-sectional sample of 1973 white South African gold miners between ages 45 and 54 years[2312] was analyzed to compare those with radiologic evidence of silicosis (S) and those without (N). The incidence of chronic bronchitis was the same in both groups. The following data were obtained.

	Radiologic Silicosis	Normal Chest Radiographs
Number	122	1708
Non-smokers	9.8%	12.3%
Ex-smokers	28%	23.5%
Current smokers	63.1%	64.2%
FEV$_1$	2.98	3.15
FEF$_{25-75}$	2.40	2.80

The FVC values were the same in the two groups. The authors concluded that "chronic obstructive lung disease may well be more important than silicosis as an occupational cause of morbidity in gold miners." Progression to progressive massive fibrosis is very rare in this population.

In an interesting comparison between 22 foundry workers, age 40, with 30 coal miners, 30 welders, and 30 unexposed controls, all of the same age,[2346] the foundry workers had significantly lower vital capacities, increased RV values, increased physiologic dead space values (by 42 mL), and lower exercise Pa$_{O_2}$ values (by 7 mm Hg) than the other groups. Their exercise ventilation, at a $\dot{V}_{O_2}$ of 1.5 L/min, was 42.8 L/min, compared with 37.9, 37.0, and 34.8 L/min for the other three groups. No $D_{L_{CO}}$ nor mechanics data were reported, but the authors concluded that the foundry workers had significantly worse function than the other three groups. Increase in physiologic dead space and exercise ventilation in silicosis has been noted by others.[2349] Other authors have noted that gas distribution is impaired in cases of silicosis[2347] but more abnormal in smokers than nonsmokers,[2391] and some early derangement of $\dot{V}/\dot{Q}$ distribution may be common. A decreased TLC and increased static pressure at all lung volumes have been recorded in non-smoking men with silicosis without bronchitis,[2356] and reductions in flow rates at 50% and 75% of VC were related to the altered lung volumes and not abnormal when corrected.

In another study of 77 men, all with silicosis, between the ages of 39 and 70 years, 37 were from iron foundries, 15 from steelworks, 9 from a quartz mill, and 16 from drilling.[2375] The VC was abnormal in only a few men, but helium mixing times and arterial Pa$_{O_2}$ values were abnormal in most, and exercise ventilation was commonly increased. These authors pointed out the possibility that complicating left heart disease might be related to the increased exercise ventilation (a problem discussed below). They divided the sample into those with and without evidence of left-sided heart disease and showed that there was still an elevation of exercise $\dot{V}_E$ in men with no evidence of it, but much greater elevation in the 18 men with evidence of left-sided disease. The VC data and arterial Pa$_{O_2}$ values were not different in the two groups.[2375]

As noted in Chapter 5, the studies of Finnish foundry workers are among the most thorough in any occupationally exposed group.[2917]

A comparison of data from 78 foundry workers

in Vancouver with data from 372 railway repair yard workers[4669] showed that respiratory symptoms were more common in the foundary workers, but these had been exposed to MDI and formaldehyde as well as to silica. Of the foundry workers, 4.8% had radiologic evidence of pneumoconiosis. In Brisbane, respiratory symptoms in a group of foundry workers were ascribed to formaldehyde exposure.[4670]

Workers in Nevada producing silica flour (also known as tripoli), in which 30% of the particles are less than 1 μm in size, had a high incidence of silicosis, and more than 100 men of the 1000 employed since 1900 were believed to have died from silicosis.[2374] A survey of 61 currently employed workers showed that 11% had progressive massive fibrosis, with reduced FVC and FEV_1 values. Of 40 men exposed to amorphous silica vapor,[2370] 11 had nodular or reticular x-ray changes; but in only one case was there significant function defect, both the FEV_1 and DL_{CO} being abnormally low. A lung biopsy showed pulmonary fibrosis. Makers of dental prostheses are exposed to cobalt and molybdenum as well as to silica. Five cases of silicosis in these workers were found,[2393] and in one a VC decline of −200 mL/year was noted, accompanied by a fall of F_{CO} from 0.48 to 0.38 over a 3-year period. The authors raised the question of the importance of the cobalt in inducing these changes.

Reductions in FEV_1 and FVC were found in two of four shale miners with radiologic silicosis.[2410] A recent survey of 725 slate workers compared with 530 men from the same area but not so employed[4538] showed that 33% of the slate workers had evidence of pneumoconiosis, and 10% had category 2 disease or higher. FVC and FEV_1 declines were related to radiologic category.

Brick workers are also at risk. Two workers in a refractory brick factory[4532] had bilateral radiologic densities, and lung biopsy showed silicon carbides and tungsten carbide in the lungs. In one of the cases, arterial Pa_{O_2} fell from 88 mm Hg at rest to 65 mm Hg on exercise, although his $DL_{CO}SB$ was normal; his VC was 77% of predicted. Cases of silicosis from a similar factory in Egypt have been reported but not documented in detail.[4545]

In some occupations, such as that of glass etching, it may be difficult to determine the role of silica in the pneumoconiosis produced.[4603]

Although it has been stated for years that silicosis commonly progresses after exposure

ceases (and this is probably always true of acute silicosis), the rate of progression or its frequency in chronic forms was not precisely defined until a recent report from Hong Kong was published.[4606] Eighty-one cases of silicosis from two granite quarries were studied. Seventy-three were followed for 2 to 10 years (mean 7.2 years), with a mean of 3.5 serial readings on each man. Sixty-two of the cases were no longer exposed to dust when the follow-up began. Twenty-four of 53 cases with simple silicosis and 11 of 20 with complicated disease showed evidence of radiologic progression during follow-up.

Baseline Characteristics

	Simple Silicosis	Complicated Silicosis
Number	58	23
Age	52.9	54.8
Smoking history	14	4
Past smokers	7	5
Current	37	14
Current (packs/year)	25.4	23.9
Dust cumulative mg/m³ × year	11.0	12.7
Exposure years	23.7	22.5
Av silica mg/m³	0.46	0.57
FEV_1 (liters)	2.406	2.118
%P	94.0	83.6
n <75 %P	10	6
FVC (liters)	3.097	2.796
%P	96.5	86.7
n <75 %P	7	6

The report contained the following data on decline of function in relation to radiologic progression:

	Simple		Complicated	
	No Progress	Progress	No Progress	Progress
Number	29	24	9	11
Initial FEV_1	2.47	2.43	2.17	2.26
FVC	3.18	3.09	2.75	2.99
Age (years)	51.9	53.1	54.9	52.6
Smoking history	8	6	2	2
Past smoker	4	3	2	3
Current	17	15	5	6
FEV_1 (mL/year)	−64	−97	−65	−100
adjusted*	−64	−96	−66	−102
FVC (mL/year)	−59	−95	−66	−104
adjusted*	−59	−94	−73	−103

*Adjusted for age at follow-up, smoking, and lung function on initial examination.

A decline of −182 mL/year over 5 years was noted in the only tool grinder in the group. There may have been a history of complicating tuberculosis in a few of the cases. The authors noted a general relationship between radiologic progression and FEV_1 and FVC decline. The rate of decline was not related to smoking but was related to history of tuberculosis, average dust exposure, and most strongly to radiologic progression in multiple regression analysis. From the data in this important study, the fact of progression of disease in about half of all the cases appears to have been established.

Before this study was published, one brief report from Sweden[3127] noted progression of radiologic change in all but about 10% of a sample of quartz workers followed for 10 years. Pham and colleagues[2355] documented a faster fall in all aspects of pulmonary function over a 5-year period in 196 steelworkers compared with 186 workers in a clean atmosphere. Recent data from Italy on 90 men with recognized silicosis followed for 9 years, of mean age 60.7 years, and with a mean smoking history of 21.9 pack/years, in whom a numerical chest x-ray score was used, gave the following values:

	1974	1983	mL/year
Smokers (%)	72.2	38.9	
VC (liters)	3.73	3.42	−34
	± 0.63	± 0.68	
FEV$_1$ (liters)	2.77	2.40	−41
	± 0.58	± 0.63	
CXR score	4.34	6.07	
	± 1.54	± 1.35	

These rates of decline are not much different from those in non-exposed smokers. The authors noted no relationship between changing VC and changing radiologic score. Other studies have not found an unusually fast rate of decline in those exposed to silica,[4583] but the Hong Kong data described above would seem to invalidate this as a general conclusion.

It is to be assumed that differences between follow-up studies of men with silicosis are probably due to differences in dust loading of the lungs.

As one would expect, survival in silicosis is related to hypoxemia and pulmonary arterial hypertension. In 60 cases followed for not less than 12 years, the following equation predicted survival[2357]:

$$\text{Survival (years)} = 9.967 - 0.478 \text{ PAP (mm Hg)} + 0.145 \text{ FEV}_1/\text{FVC}$$

Right ventricular hypertrophy is common in this condition,[2405] and complicating pulmonary emphysema is often observed, though with what frequency in non-smoking cases of silicosis is not clear.[2405] However, a recent report on the use of CAT scan in cases of silicosis indicates that this method can be used to quantitate the coexisting degree of emphysema[4718] and in a small group of cases the degree of emphysema so quantitated was found to be closely related to the $DL_{CO}SB$. A report of rapid progression in a group of Vermont granite workers[2306] was later shown to be an artifact attributable to instrumental and methodologic error.[2376] However, recent data from bronchoalveolar lavage indicate that alveolitis may be common in these exposed workers.[4631]

Silicon Carbide

Silicon carbide is produced by heating petroleum coke and silica sand to 2000 degrees centigrade in an electric furnace for 36 hours. A detailed study of 171 men involved in this work[4562] showed that the FVC level and the chest film changes were related to exposure levels to respirable particulates. A 10% difference in FEV$_1$ separated the least exposed group from the most exposed group in the non-smokers, but a bigger difference was demonstrated in relation to concomitant levels of sulfur dioxide exposure.

Kaolin

Kaolin consists of a group of clay materials with various names (kaolinite, nacrite, dickite) consisting of a two-layer crystal in which silicon-oxygen and aluminum-hydroxyl sheets alternate; the approximate composition is $Al_2O_3 \cdot 2SiO_2 \cdot Al_2O_3 \cdot 2SiO_2 \cdot 2H_2O$.[3670] In a survey of Cornish china clay workers,[3632] 17.9% of 1676 men had category 1 radiologic change and 4.7% were in categories 2 and 3. Smoking was unrelated to radiologic change. Pulmonary function was not very abnormal, and a follow-up study in non-smokers suggested that the excess FEV$_1$ fall amounted to about 500 milliliters between the ages of 20 and 65.[3632] In 459 kaolin workers in the United States, spirometry was different in men with large opacities,[3690] and in another study[3691] of 65 current and former workers in a kaolin mine, in which the dust was kaolinite, there were significant reductions in FVC and FEV$_1$. In an editorial on these two studies,[3669] Morgan questioned the control of smoking versus non-smoking groups and pointed out the need for longitudinal studies.

A more recent study of the 62 Cornish china clay workers exposed to kaolinite[4709] showed that many had nodular and interstitial fibrosis; pulmonary function test data were not reported. Similar findings with some lowering of FVC and FEV_1 were reported from a kaolin mine in Georgia in the United States,[4516] and five cases of complicated pneumoconiosis from kaolinite, with autopsy findings, have also been reported.[4548] Diatomite (silicon dioxide in opaline or amorphous form), when heat treated, forms cristobalite, which can lead to disabling pneumoconiosis,[4512] but no detailed studies of pulmonary function have been reported.

Talc

Twenty-seven cases of talc pneumoconiosis with reticulonodular radiologic changes have been reported.[2394] Talc particles were demonstrated on biopsy of some of these cases. In others,[3496] talc has been demonstrated in the sputum or in bronchial washings. In this condition, the reported VC and FEV_1 values have not been much reduced, but complete gas exchange studies have not been included in the literature.

In the rubber tire industry, talc exposure has been linked to declines in FEV_1,[2369] but other dusts may have been present also.[2471] However, in one study of 80 exposed workers compared with 189 unexposed, the FEV_1 was lowered if exposure had exceeded 10 years.[2369] The chest x-rays were not abnormal, but the authors concluded that each year of talc exposure lowered the FEV_1 by 26 milliliters. They suggested that a dust level of 25 mg/m^3 as a time-weighted average would probably be a safe exposure level.

There is no doubt that talc may cause a severe pneumoconiosis, and this occurred in a man who spent 10 years cleaning ventilators in a factory where talc was used in molding and packaging rubber goods.[2243] His VC was less than 50% of predicted. C_{dyn}/f was grossly reduced, and the MVV was 60% of predicted. Hypoxemia and pulmonary hypertension were detectable at rest, and the lung biopsy revealed talc (identified by x-ray diffraction) in lung tissue; it constituted 50% of the lung residue. The case we reported (see case 42 in reference 1) and others[2246] represent lesser degrees of the condition. Mining of talc ore may also lead to radiologic changes and an accelerated decline of FEV_1.[2425] It may be difficult to distinguish talc granulomas from sarcoidosis.[3496]

Carbon and Graphite

Activated carbon is a steam-derived product of lignite, a variety of soft coal. Inhalation of this dust led to radiographic changes in about 10% of one group of exposed workers[2528] but produced no symptoms or function test change. Graphite, or "black lead," is an allotropic form of carbon, and it can cause a severe pneumoconiosis. In seven exposed workers, FEV_1 and FVC annual decrements of -80 mL/year and -90 mL/year were observed over a 10-year period.[2196] In a survey of 344 exposed workers in Ceylon, 22% had radiographic changes, and clubbed fingers were noted in about the same number.[2199] No pulmonary function test results were reported. There are 605 cases of graphite pneumoconiosis reported in the literature.[4724] In reviewing these data, Handa recently concluded that many of these cases were due to exposures to mixed dusts.[4724]

Mica

Mica consists of a group of phyllosilicate materials with a sheet-like structure. The molecules contain aluminum and silica, as well as iron, magnesium, lithium, and calcium.[3670] In a recent report, two men exposed to this material developed pneumoconiosis, with progressive dyspnea and linear and nodular radiographic changes.[3658] In one of them, age 61 in 1981, sequential changes in function were as follows:

Date	FVC	FEV_1	$D_{L_{CO}}$ (%P)
1958	3.8	—	—
1967	3.9	3.1	57
1977	3.3	2.5	55
1981	2.7	2.0	—
	(P = 4.0)	(P = 2.8)	

In the second case in a 54-year-old man, the FEV_1 fell at a rate of -97 mL/year between 1957 and 1976.

A literature review in 1985 concluded that 66 cases of mica pneumoconiosis had been reported up to that date.[4687] Although Parkes[3744] doubted that mica caused pneumoconiosis, it seems likely that if the dose is high enough, it can do so, as it can cause fibrosis experimentally.

Summary

Silica is not only the most common of the earth's minerals, but the danger of silica dust in the lungs has been known for as long as humans have been exposed to it. The recent data on progression of the disease after exposure has ceased have added an important new dimension to its understanding. As we noted recently,[4498] the correct assessment of individual cases may prove difficult and can only be established by careful autopsy examination.

Asbestos

The fascinating historical background of asbestos, which we noted in 1970,[1] has been well described by Lee and Selikoff.[2475] Asbestos, in different forms, affects the local population in Turkey,[4714] Greece,[4662] Finland,[4500] and Corsica,[4715] most recently described. During the past 12 years, asbestos has been the object of intensive inquiry. This has in part been stimulated by the recognition of its ability to induce pleural mesothelioma after relatively brief contact and a latent period as long as 60 years.[2442] Its role in the genesis of lung cancer has become one of the major questions in environmental medicine, with reviews[2322] of possible public hazard resulting from city exposures or from low-level exposures within buildings in which asbestos was sprayed during construction 30 years ago.

Becklake contributed an excellent review of information on all aspects of asbestos up to 1975.[2513] Reviews of safety standards,[2440, 2534, 2450] discussions of the reasons for the long delay in United States recognition of the carcinogenicity of asbestos,[2316] and a report to the European Economic Community on public hazards of asbestos exposure[2447] all have resulted from the growing recognition of the dangers associated with its use. Enterline[3723] has reviewed the epidemiologic basis for an exposure standard. There has also been much controversy on the problem of risk estimates for very low-level exposures. The Report of a Royal Commission on Asbestos in Ontario,[3642] which contains an excellent analysis of the evidence relating to carcinogenicity from different types of fiber, and a National Academy of Sciences Report from the United States[3601] have provided important syntheses of the data. The risk estimates in the latter report have subsequently been revised.[4496] A detailed review of the cancer risk is beyond the scope of this volume, but reviews of exposed workers in Canada and elsewhere reinforce the risks of even short periods of exposure, and the long latency period.* Hughes and Weill's risk estimates for low-dose exposure are the most recent.[4693]

Problems of attributability in the United Kingdom have recently been discussed.[4523] Brodeur's remarkable account of the history of claims against the asbestos industry in the United States[4497] traces the sequence of events that led the Johns-Manville Company to file for bankruptcy. At that time there were about 26,000 outstanding claims in the United States, about a third of which were for cancer related to asbestos exposure. That serious overexposures to asbestos could result in Britain, where there is a well-developed system of factory inspections and where information on the hazards of asbestos was generally available, was documented as recently as 1978.[2473] I have recently commented on the dilemma of whether continued production of asbestos is justified.[4719]

Recent experimental work has confirmed that chrysotile asbestos instilled into the lung induces an intense alveolitis[3630, 3652] with a peribronchiolitis.[3610] In studies of sheep following instillation, changes in vital capacity and static compliance and reductions in Pa_{O_2} and $DL/\dot{V}A$ ratio have been documented.[3630] The deposition of fibers in the rat lung after inhalation has been documented in detail and particularly well illustrated by Brody and colleagues.[2941, 3751] Other experimental data are available.†

Advances in detection and analyses of different types of asbestos in lung tissue[2409, 2423, 2530] have been important in defining tentative dose-response relationships.‡ Concentrations of asbestos fibers vary in different sites in the lung.[3605, 3729] Higher values in the upper lobes than in the lower have been reported by some investigators.[3661] Churg and colleagues have documented aggregation of fibers around small airways[2454, 4577, 4677] in a comparison between nine chrysotile miners with small airway aggregation but no interstitial fibrosis and nine miners matched for age, smoking history, and duration of exposure but with no histologic evidence of small airways disease. He found greater numbers of fibers in those with the airway lesions[3608] but concluded that factors other than the degree of loading were probably important in determining the airway changes. Asbestos fibers can be recovered from the lung by bronchoalveolar lavage,[3611, 4701] and cell ratios have been reported to be different in asbestos-exposed workers.[4634] Lung permeability as studied with ^{99m}Tc-labeled DTPA is increased in fully developed asbesto-

---

*See references 3633, 3634, 3643–3645, 3649, 3656, 3681, 3684.

†See references 4529, 4535, 4547, 4572, 4574, 4624, 4629, 4695.

‡See references 6502, 7315, 7912, 8271, 8272.

sis,[4660, 4725] and this acceleration seems to involve all zones of the lung.[4617] The BAL albumin/serum albumin ratio is also elevated.[4660]

A positive gallium scan, indicating active alveolitis, may occur in humans, it has been shown to follow intratracheal instillation of asbestos in sheep.[3602]

Asbestos exposure may cause the following effects:

1. Pleural thickening and pleural plaques.
2. Interstitial fibrosis ("asbestosis").
3. Peribronchiolitis, with or without interstitial changes.
4. Pleural mesothelioma.
5. An increased risk of lung cancer, particularly when combined with cigarette smoking.

As we pointed out in the second edition,[1] asbestos fibers are found in the lungs of most city dwellers. A recent comparison of their presence in the lungs in inhabitants of Southampton, England, and Wellington, New Zealand,[3650] found them in 83% of men and 74% of women in the English city and in 78% of men and 63% of women in Wellington. There has recently been a collaborative study between seven different centers in quantitating asbestos fibers in the lungs.[4689] These useful techniques have recently been reviewed.[4707, 4708]

The formation of pleural plaques is associated with asbestos exposure, and in Sweden, where this condition has been extensively studied,[2353, 2411] the frequency of occurrence has been clearly related to increasing use.[2361] In some surveys, these are detected in as many as a third of exposed workers[2358]; 13% of insulation workers in the United States, 5% of United Kingdom dockyard workers,[4543] and 14% of Swedish dockyard workers had pleural plaques.[2360] A recent survey of 5000 marine engineers found that 12% had pleural abnormalities.[4513] In the United States, 339 male shipyard workers were surveyed and 28% had parenchymal disease, 37% had pleural disease only, and 35% had both.[4654]

The detection of plaques is not easy radiologically, and autopsy comparisons show that false-positive x-rays are about as common as false negatives in which they are found at autopsy but were not visible radiologically.[2360] In another study of 434 autopsies, 5.8% had pleural plaques, but only in a third of these were they visible radiologically.[4591] In this series, there was an association between pleural plaques and laryngeal cancer rate. The evidence on the general relationship of plaques to lung cancer

is conflicting.[4590] Plaques can be much better visualized by use of a CAT scan of the thorax than on conventional x-rays.[4571]

A recent study from Philadelphia[3609] analyzed 824 radiographs from consecutive hospital admissions screened by two radiologists. The maximal width of pleural thickening was measured and carefully classified. Bilateral pleural thickening was found in 52 cases, 19 of whom were men aged 35 to 60 and 23 of whom were older than 60 years. Of the 52 cases, 25% had a definite history of asbestos exposure, 19% had probable exposure, and 23% had possible exposure—for a total of 67% of the group. McMillan and Rossiter[3682] reassessed 155 men of a group of 201 with asbestos exposure with pleural abnormalities 10 years after they were first x-rayed. They found that 10.3% had radiographic changes in lung parenchyma, and 4.5% satisfied all the criteria for parenchymal involvement. This rate was substantially higher than in men with no pleural abnormality and was unrelated to age, smoking history, occupation, duration of exposure, or type of pleural abnormality when first seen.

In a recent study of pulmonary function in 45 men with pleural plaques but without evidence of pulmonary fibrosis, Fridriksson and colleagues[2364] found evidence of significant reductions in TLC, VC, RV, FEV_1, C_{st}, and TL_{CO} in the exposed group, with increases in SBN_2/L and CV/VC% indices. Exposure levels were correlated with C_{st}/TLC but not with the other changes. There was no evidence of differences between smokers and non-smokers.

In a study of construction workers exposed to asbestos, Hillerdal[2353] compared three groups: Group A had a history of exposure, pleural plaques, but no evidence of interstitial change; group B had the same exposure history, but no plaques and no interstitial change; and group C had no exposure and no plaques. Pulmonary function data were as follows:

	Group A	Group B	Group C
Number	55	52	55
Age (years)	57	53	54
FVC	4.25	4.41	4.66
FEV_1	3.11	3.27	3.54
FEV_1/FVC%	73.2	74.1	75.9
$MEF_{50\%}$(L/sec)	3.55	4.09	4.34
CV (liters)	1.33	1.18	1.08
DL_{CO}SB (mL/min/mm Hg)	25.6	26.3	29.4

Static pressure/volume curves were not different between the three groups, and differences appeared to be somewhat greater in the indices between exposed and non-exposed non-smokers than between exposed and non-exposed smokers. In another series of 42 cases of pleural plaques,[2345] work capacity was considered to be affected if pulmonary mechanics were abnormal, but 6 of these cases had slight evidence of interstitial change on their x-ray. Exercise limitation in one asbestos worker with pleural disease but a normal diffusing capacity was caused by the fact that the tidal volume was limited to 1 liter,[4530] and we have observed the same phenomenon in an asbestos-exposed steelworker with an active pleuritis.

Asbestos causes pleural "pseudotumours" with lung atelectasis caused by invagination of lung by fibrotic pleura*; 306 cases were seen at the Karolinska Institute in Stockholm between 1954 and 1976.[4657] It is not clear whether all of these had been exposed to asbestos. Diffuse pleural involvement may also occur,[4519] occasionally with a "shrinking pleuritis."[4620, 4643] The sedimentation rate is elevated in these cases.[4522] We have recently observed such a case, without interstitial pulmonary asbestosis on lung biopsy, in which the FVC fell by 500 mL over a 2-year period as the lesion was developing. Miller, Teirstein, and Selikoff have recently documented severe ventilatory impairment as a result of asbestos pleurisy,[2453] but it is not clear how often this occurs.

Hemorrhagic pleural effusions may occur without malignant change in asbestos workers.[2414]

These data do not show definitively that pleural plaques alone interfere with function, since it is not possible to exclude the presence of some interstitial change in the lung without radiologic evidence of it. As noted below, function defect may be present in asbestosis with a normal chest x-ray, and there is no reason why this situation may not occur in cases with pleural plaques.

The diagnosis of pulmonary asbestosis is generally considered to be indicated by some combination of the following factors when there is a history of exposure:

- Radiologic change
- Coarse basal rales
- Clubbing of the fingers
- Evidence of TLC and VC reduction and lowered $DL_{CO}SB$ or changes in lung recoil pressure

In one survey of 270 asbestos workers, sound

*See references 2449, 3672, 3724, 4580, 4587.

amplification and recording techniques were used to detect basal rales. Comparison with a control non-exposed group revealed that 32.2% of the asbestos workers had rales, compared with an incidence of 4.5% in controls.[2407] Rales occurred in late inspiration and were most common in the midaxillary line. They were well detected by trained technicians whose skills were compared with sound recordings in a survey of 386 asbestos workers.[4531]

In a friction component factory, rales were heard twice as commonly in 79 asbestos-exposed workers as in others not exposed,[2385] and their VCs were slightly but significantly reduced. Two men were described as having "slight" radiologic change. DL_{CO} data were not recorded.

Other studies have shown that the detection of rales is not a reliable indicator except in the presence of radiographic change or function defect.[13] Clubbing of the fingers is also an unreliable indicator,[2244] and there is considerable interobserver variability in reading chest films of exposed workers.[2278, 2419] Repeat questionnaire data on symptoms in asbestos workers show poor repeatability, although estimates of exposures are reliably duplicated.[2351] It is these factors that accentuate the importance of function tests in this condition.

There is little doubt that cigarette smoking not only increases the risk of lung cancer in exposed workers but also increases the risk of pulmonary parenchymal change.[6549] In Hawaii, Fournier-Massey found few abnormalities among 741 former asbestos-exposed workers who were contacted, and 83% had been non-smokers.[4600] Surveys of shipyard workers exposed to asbestos compared with those not exposed have shown lower FVC and FEV_1 values in those exposed.[2318] The incidence of pulmonary parenchymal change varies in different surveys of different industries; it was 3% in a survey of United Kingdom dockyards.[4504]

In one survey of 175 asbestos workers with radiologic changes compared with 139 workers with asbestos exposure but without radiologic change, the mean VC values were 400 mL lower, and the mean $DL_{CO}SB$ 4.0 mL/min/mm Hg lower in those with radiologic changes.[2283] Eleven cases of asbestosis were included in Epler's study of abnormal function tests and confirmed lung biopsy changes in cases with a chest film considered normal by a panel of four radiologists.[1866]

Jodoin and colleagues reported studies on 24 workers with exposures varying between 6 months and 24 years, all with normal chest films.[2289] They found evidence of lowered VCs, and the 13 men with the heaviest exposures had a 30% increase in static recoil of the lung. The diffusing capacities both at rest and on exercise were not different, however. They concluded that TLC and C_{st} both were lower in the more heavily dust-exposed group and that these indices reflected change earlier than $DL_{CO}SB$. A stratified random sample of 1069 asbestos workers in Quebec[2343] also produced evidence that the DL_{CO} was not depressed if the chest x-ray was normal. Another study of 983 currently working asbestos miners in Quebec[4663] indicated that asbestos dust exposure led to airway abnormalities and defined the interaction with smoking.

It may be noted that there is evidence from cancer data of differences between workers exposed in producing asbestos and those employed in textile and other industries using the product,[4673] being very low in the friction products industry.[4563, 4674] Differences may also exist in the pattern of function test change between different types of exposure in different industries.

A cross-sectional study of 377 railroad workers intermittently exposed to asbestos[4627] found that 22.9% had pleural plaques; 1.9% had evidence of interstitial disease; only 18 had an abnormal $DL_{CO}SB$. A later analysis of these data[4699] illustrated the problem of normal criteria, since if the percentage of predicted values was used, 71 would have been considered to have "restrictive" disease; but if the 95% confidence limit criterion was used, only 41 would have been considered to be abnormal.

In a major study in Italy, Zedda and colleagues[2396] reported on 724 men exposed to asbestos dust. These men were divided into five groups as follows:

Group	Exposure	CXR by ILO Category	Number	Age (years)
A	<10 years	Normal or equivocal	161	44.0
B	>10 years	Normal or equivocal	228	49.7
C	>10 years	1/0 or 1/1	215	51.3
D	>10 years	1/2–2/1 or 2/2	107	54.3
E	>10 years	2/3–3/2 or 3/3	13	53.0

Length of exposures were about the same in groups B, C, D, and E. Pulmonary function data were as follows:

Group	VC (%P)	RV/ TLC%	$DL_{CO}SS$ (mL/min/ mm Hg) Rest	F_{CO} Rest	$DL_{CO}SS$ Exercise (mL/min/mm Hg) 50 Watts	100 Watts
A	−9.9	28.4	20.0	0.52	36.1	44.1
B	−14.5	28.8	17.7	0.48	32.9	39.5
C	−17.2	33.8	16.6	0.48	32.3	37.3
D	−24.4	36.9	12.8	0.45	25.6	29.4
E	−35.4	39.5	9.8	0.34	17.0	24.1

The FEV_1 values followed VC declines. They found evidence of function test abnormality in several workers before definitive x-ray changes were present and noted the generally good relationship between degree of radiologic change and function test abnormality. Early restrictive disease was present in many of those studied. These results were generally confirmed in a smaller study of 20 workers with radiologic change compared with 10 exposed workers with negative or doubtful chest films.[2390] By comparison with 20 unexposed controls, both of the asbestos groups had lowered DL_{CO} values, and in both exposed groups, the Pa_{O_2} fell on exercise (by a mean of about 5 mm Hg), and the $(A-a) D_{O_2}$ rose by about 10 mm Hg on exercise. Other surveys have found slightly lower mean FVC and FEV_1 mean values in asbestos-exposed workers.[4594]

In 40 asbestos workers employed in secondary industries, flow rates at low lung volumes were often found to be abnormal, but only 2 of the subjects were non-smokers.[2403] Chronic bronchitis has been reported to be more common in non-smoking asbestos workers than in non-exposed workers,[2259] but for the same level of asbestos exposure, radiologic changes and the presence of rales are related to smoking history.[2352] Becklake and colleagues recently reported a follow-up of 722 Quebec miners between 1968 and 1974.[3720] FEF_{25-75} fell significantly in all groups, with faster declines than normal being noted. There was also some evidence that stature affects the development of asbestosis, since a comparison between 44 men with exposure and interstitial lung change with 88 men with comparable exposure but no lung changes[3603] revealed that the affected men had shorter intrathoracic tracheal lengths and narrower transthoracic diameters than the others, and in addition were shorter in stature. In these men, both the FVC and DL_{CO} were closely related to the calculated cumulative exposure, as shown by the following data:

Deficit compared to non-exposed men (% decrease)	Cumulative Exposure (mpcf/year*)				
	<10	10–99	100–199	200–399	400–799	800+
FVC	0	−4	−9	−11	−14	−15
DL_{CO}	0	−3	−6	−5	−9	−11

*Millions per cubic foot/years.

Liddell and McDonald reported on 4559 Quebec asbestos miners[4542] and noted a close association between FVC decrement and duration of exposure. Radiologic progression occurred after withdrawal from exposure. A longitudinal study of 181 asbestos cement workers in Ontario[4526] also showed radiologic progression after exposure ceased, and faster progression with higher exposures. Similar follow-up data on 280 former employees at the crocidolite mine in Wittenoom in western Australia[4702] showed that although none had radiographic changes at the end of their exposure, all except 37 had radiographic changes at the end of 10 years.

Cohen, Adasczik, and Cohen recently reported on studies in 610 claimants for asbestos-related disease, 575 men and 35 women, in whom the smoking history was known. All had been exposed in a single workplace.[4581] MEFV curves and SBN_2/L data were recorded:

	Duration of Exposure					
	<15 Years		15–30 Years		>30 Years	
	S	NS	S	NS	S	NS
FVC						
Predicted	4.18	3.97	4.04	3.78	3.86	3.86
Actual	3.32	3.25	3.18	3.06	3.00	3.08
FEV_1						
Predicted	3.34	3.18	3.11	2.90	2.91	2.89
Actual	2.78	2.77	2.57	2.58	2.33	2.48
CC						
Predicted	36.5	38.8	48.4	45.9	45.9	46.9
Actual	48.9	51.5	55.5	61.4	59.2	64.5
SBN_2/L						
Predicted	1.28	1.16	1.26	1.28	1.34	1.30
Actual	3.71	3.01	4.35	3.80	5.05	4.25

The data in non-smokers clearly indicate small-airway disease and hence provide a clinical counterpart to the observations by Churg noted earlier in this chapter that fiber aggregation occurs around small airways in asbestos-exposed workers.

Similar evidence was collected in 97 non-smoking male insulators,[4665] and the authors suggested that in some cases, parenchyma stiffening might "protect" the FEF_{25-75}, since they found a disproportionate decline in the terminal part of the expiratory flow curve (FEF_{75-85}).

Studies of regional ventilation in 12 men exposed to asbestos showed minor abnormalities in ventilation distribution,[3671] but it seems unlikely that this method of examination would contribute much to the understanding of the disease.

Striking individual cases have been reported. In the wife of one asbestos worker, pleural plaques were present and the FVC was 73% of predicted; $DL_{CO}SB$ was 68% of predicted, and $DL_{CO}SS$ was less than 50% of predicted on exercise.[2404] In a 47-year-old man whose only exposure was at the age of 31 for 9 months to Cape blue asbestos, then used in making cigarette filters,[2395] the VC was 1.9, $DL_{CO}SB$ was 55% predicted, $DL_{CO}SS$ was also 55% of predicted, and there were basal rales, finger clubbing, and diffuse basal shadows on the chest x-ray. The diagnosis of asbestosis was proved by lung biopsy. In this man, the resting Pa_{O_2} was still 82 mm Hg when he had serious disability. The difficulty of establishing the diagnosis was illustrated by a case of diffuse interstitial pneumonitis in a 63-year-old man who had no occupational history of asbestos exposure and whose lung volumes were normal.[1868] Light microscopy examination of the lung showed no particles, but on electron microscopy many uncoated chrysotile fibers were visible, all less than 0.5 microns long. The total asbestos load was calculated to be at least 0.45 grams, three to four times the load found in unexposed New York residents. His hobby had been furniture finishing, and this constituted his likely exposure.

Exercise studies in cases of asbestosis are usually described together with other interstitial conditions. The increased $(A-a)$ D_{O_2} on exercise or a drop in arterial Pa_{O_2} is probably the most sensitive parameter.[4371] A comparison between 73 non-smoking asbestos exposed workers and 73 smokers also asbestos exposed, using incremental cycle exercise,[4632] found a mean level of resting $DL_{CO}SB$ of 113% in the nonsmokers; 15 of the 73 had a maximal $\dot{V}O_2$ of less than 80% of predicted. Of the 33 smokers who could not exceed 80% of the predicted maximal $\dot{V}O_2$, 16 were judged to have heart disease. The non-smokers presumably had minimal parenchymal or small airway disease. In six asbestos-exposed workers, the ratio VD/VT was elevated during exercise[4690]; but when the subjects were coached to breathe more slowly and deeply, a normal value was recorded.

Some studies of longitudinal change have been reported. Lee and Selikoff[2399] reproduced data from a few cases reported, but not discussed in detail, in a symposium at the New York Academy of Sciences in 1965. This shows that in one case, the VC dropped from about 120% predicted in 1956 to 62% predicted in 1964, a decline of about -330 mL/year. Average falls seemed to be about -220 mL/year in the group as a whole. No detailed clinical data accompany the graph from which these numbers have been read.

Sixty-five exposed workers and 30 controls studied at an interval of 7 years[4593] revealed an annual rate of FVC decline of -52.5 mL/year in the asbestos workers with more than 15 years of exposure, and of -24.3 mL/year in those with less than this duration. The control group declined at a rate of -6 mL/year compared with an overall rate of -48 mL/year for all the asbestos workers. The smoking history was taken into account.

A Swedish study of 75 former asbestos cement workers[4678] found that 32% had pleural plaques but none had interstitial disease. The follow-up data expressed as a percentage of the initial lung volumes were as follows:

Mean 4-Year Decrements

| | Exposure (in years) | | | | |
	<14	15–22	>23	All	Referents
Number	28	23	24	75	56
FVC	−4.5%	−7.3%	−8.2%	−6.6%	−4.5%
FEV$_1$	−4.6%	−8.2%	−8.7%	−7.0%	−5.6%

The problem of assessing disability in asbestos-exposed workers is discussed below.

Aluminum

Studies of workers in the pot rooms of aluminum plants, who are exposed to a variety of gases and dusts, generally show some evidence of fluorosis.[2121] There is contradictory evidence whether they have an increased incidence of chronic obstructive pulmonary disease, some studies indicating increased respiratory symptoms,[2239] an increased mortality for emphysema,[2174] and a slight increase in obstructive disease compared with control populations,[2252] and at least one other study showing no evidence of difference between pot-room workers and others.[2132] A significant fall in FEV$_1$ over a work shift has been reported in aluminum pot-room workers using the AluSwiss process,[2239] and this was prevented by atropine. Others have also noted significant shift declines.[4521]

Our own recent studies[2466] of workers at a large smelter in Kitimat have indicated some excess of chronic respiratory symptoms, and function test change in 797 pot-room workers compared with 713 workers in the casting area or in office work at the same plant. The difference in FEV$_1$ was about 100 mL, and in FEF$_{25-75}$ about 0.2 L/sec between high-exposure workers and controls, and cough and wheezing were more common. No significant work shift changes in FEV$_1$ were found; so in this study, the existence of so-called pot-room asthma could not be confirmed.

A cross-sectional study of 1141 men at a plant in Arkansas[4636] showed that among those who had never smoked, the FEV$_1$ decreased in relation to increased duration and density of exposure. The decrement amounted to about 400 mL after 20 years of exposure. FVC data were not reported.

Increased mecholyl airway reactivity has been found in men exposed to aluminum fluoride.[2362]

A 44-year-old man working for 6 years as an aluminum rail grinder in a very dusty environment[4550] had alveolar proteinosis, but the lung tissue was loaded with aluminum particles. Aluminum polishing with abrasives can also lead to pulmonary changes, and in one 61-year-old man with radiologic infiltrates and clubbed fingers, the biopsy showed numerous dust-laden macrophages containing metallic aluminum and corundum particles.[4713] This man's DL$_{CO}$SB had been observed to fall from 51% of predicted in 1978 to 36% of predicted 5 years later. Over the same period, the FVC declined from 99% predicted to 81% predicted.

Beryllium

Beryllium is of considerable historical interest, since the granulomas that it causes in the lungs were described as being associated with severe abnormalities of gas exchange in pioneer studies more than 30 years ago.[1] In the previous edition, we noted that the hazards of exposure were now sufficiently well recognized and that few new cases occurred; but it is clear that it is a continuing hazard, since 76 new cases were added to a beryllium registry between the years 1966 and 1974.[2254] These have mostly occurred in relation to beryllium production, but a few have been recorded after exposure in the ceramics and electronics industries. A recent review noted that as a result of stringent control, although beryllium production in the United States has risen since 1940, very few new cases now occur.[4503] It is recognized, however, that some cases occur in persons who have had very light exposure.

The x-ray usually shows a mixed pattern of fibrosis and granulomatous infiltration. Of the 76 new cases referred to above,[2254] 31% had interstitial function defects, 16% principally had a reduction in lung volumes, 14% had obstructive defects, and only 6% were found to have normal pulmonary function. In a survey of 214 workers in a beryllium plant in 1973, 31 had radiologic changes and 11 were hypoxemic at rest.[2514] In five hypoxemic cases, the Pa_{O_2} values were 54, 66, 67, 68, and 73 mm Hg, and $DL_{CO}SS$ values as a percent of predicted were 14%, 33%, 41%, 50%, and 69%. This report noted results of lung biopsy studies in two cases,[2514] and the authors stressed the importance of continuing and careful surveillance of any workers exposed to beryllium. It is clear that removal from exposure can result in improvement in lung function, and in 11 workers studied in 1971 and again in 1974, improvements in arterial Pa_{O_2}, $(A-a)\ D_{O_2}$, and FVC were noted to have occurred.[2314]

A longitudinal study of men exposed to beryllium but without clinical or radiologic evidence of disease[3657] found normal rates of FVC and FEV_1 decline.

A new beryllium lymphocyte transformation test has been shown to be valuable in the surveillance of exposed workers.

Cobalt, Tungsten, Mercury, Zinc, Cadmium, Vanadium, Arsenic, Chromates, Nickel, Manganese, Vitallium, Uranium Hexafluoride, and Titanium Tetrachloride

Workers in some specialized industries are commonly exposed to both tungsten carbide and cobalt, and it is difficult to be sure of specific effects. A recent editorial on hard metal disease was subtitled "A Continuing Enigma."[4588] A recent survey of two tungsten carbide production plants involving 290 subjects[4589] uncovered 11 with interstitial infiltrates. Pulmonary function data on seven of these showed four with a lowered FEV_1, four with mild hypoxemia, and three with a lowered $DL_{CO}SB$, but the $DL_{CO}SS$ was 80% of predicted or lower in all. The authors refer to a German survey of 331 tungsten carbide workers, of

whom 18% had radiologic evidence of infiltrates.

These metals may cause an allergic alveolitis or reversible bronchospasm, and resolution may follow removal from exposure,[2507] although some reduction of FEV_1 and FVC values may persist. More severe exposure, particularly to tungsten carbide, may cause an interstitial pneumonitis, which can lead to reduction of DL_{CO} to 35% of predicted values[2130] and may prove fatal. In one case with patchy pneumonitis and basal atelectasis, x-ray diffraction studies of lung tissue were strongly positive for tungsten carbide[2131] and there was patchy alveolar wall thickening and small irregular crystals in alveolar septae.

A recent study from England of five cases of hard metal disease has increased our knowledge of this condition.[3752] In five cases, multinucleate macrophages recovered in bronchial lavage were characteristic. In case 1, electron probe analysis of lung biopsy material showed abundant tungsten and no cobalt. The FVC in this man fell from 5100 milliliters in 1977 to 2370 milliliters in 1980; it increased to 2960 milliliters in 1981. The k_{CO} was at the lower level of normal throughout. A second case had some cobalt as well as tungsten. In a third man, titanium and tungsten were present; the FVC was reduced in this case. The other cases were predominantly asthma, with positive bronchial provocation tests and an FEV_1 fall to 42% of control values 10 hours after exposure to hard metal powder. Cobalt may cause interstitial disease in welders and was responsible for interstitial lung disease in five diamond polishers.[4534] Lung biopsies were performed in four of these men, whose lung function test results are shown below:

	Cases				
	1	*2*	*3*	*4*	*5*
Sex	F	M	M	M	F
Age	17	21	27	23	28
TLC (%P)	51	42	57	90	69
VC (%P)	20	31	26	90	56
$DL_{CO}SB$ (%P)	13	39	44	76	83

Case 1 improved after steroids and withdrawal from exposure, with DL_{CO} doubling and VC increasing. Case 4 was considered to be primarily an alveolitis, but other cases showed severe chronic pneumonitis and interstitial fibrosis changes. Exposure had been only to cobalt. In three other diamond workers,[4661] cobalt caused an occupational asthma syndrome, with positive challenge tests demonstrated. The DL_{CO} was normal in all of these cases.

Vanadium pentoxide is dangerous material. One hundred boilermakers were exposed to this fume during conversion of a power plant from oil to coal in Massachusetts.[4511] Although chest films were normal in many with upper respiratory tract symptoms, the mean FEF_{25-75} was only 57% of predicted in the 24 workers in whom it was measured. Wheezing was commonly noted, and mild hypoxemia was documented. No detailed follow-up data have been reported on this group.

Seventeen men exposed to 15.3% vanadium dust while cleaning out the bottom ash from the boiler of an oil-fired generating station[4541] were noted to have falls of 500 milliliters in FVC within 24 hours of the first exposure. The values were still depressed 8 days later but returned to normal at the end of 4 weeks. Respirators had been worn, but they were believed to have been leaking. No abnormalities were detected in 75 employees making vanadium pentoxide from magnetite.[4546]

Inhaled mercury vapor causes a severe pneumonitis in high concentration. Four such cases with severe function test abnormalities were described.[2477] The chest x-ray showed irregular patchy opacities in both lower zones, which cleared within a week. In one of the men, the FEV_1 recovered over a 10-day period from an initial value of 48% of predicted to 102% of predicted, and the DL_{CO} improved from 65% of predicted to 95% of predicted over the same interval. Four other cases have occurred[2186] in men working in a confined space; function data were not reported, however. An episode of overexposure to mercury vapor[4656] led to a severe acute pneumonitis; the DL_{CO} was only 57% of predicted 11 months later and was only 45% of predicted after the chest x-ray had returned to normal. Urinary mercury levels reached 1900 μg/L. In a bizarre episode of exposure of four adults and three children to mercury vapor caused by heating a mercury-gold amalgam,[4579] the victims developed fever and leukocytosis, in addition to acute respiratory symptoms and depression of FEV_1 and DL_{CO}.

As we noted in the previous edition,[1] acute exposure to zinc chloride may cause a severe interstitial fibrosis of the lungs. Since then, no further cases appear to have been reported.

Cadmium exposure was reported to represent a special risk in relation to development of emphysema, and inhalation of fumes of cadmium oxide may cause an acute pneumonitis.[1] An acute cadmium pneumonitis in a welder, followed up for 17 years,[3692] ran a slow course.

After apparent recovery, a progressive pulmonary fibrosis developed some years later, and finger clubbing was noticed 9 years after the acute exposure. The DL_{CO}, first measured 12 years after exposure, was 53% of predicted and was the same 5 years later. The author stressed the importance of careful and long-continued follow-up after a severe acute episode. A well-documented case with excellent longitudinal data of cadmium pneumonitis in a 34-year-old welder showed slow resolution over a period of 4 years after the acute event.[4592]

Evidence in relation to chronic effects is contradictory, one survey of 29 exposed men finding slight evidence of interstitial fibrosis radiologically in about a third,[2301] with evidence of lowering of FVC and PA_{O_2} values but with no evidence of obstructive defects. Teculescu and Stanescu[2387] studied 11 workers exposed to cadmium oxide for 7 to 11 years and reported both FEV_1 and DL_{CO} values to be normal, with no evidence of loss of vascular pattern on the chest x-ray. A poster presented at a recent American Thoracic Society meeting showed data from the United Kingdom that clearly indicated an increased risk of emphysema in cadmium-exposed workers, but these data have not yet been fully reported.

Although arsenic exposure is associated with an increased incidence of lung cancer,[2123, 3732] chronic respiratory effects attributable to it have not to our knowledge been reported.

Chromates are also associated with increased respiratory tract cancers,[2529] but there is no note of increased chronic respiratory tract disease. Nickel exposure is associated with respiratory cancers,[2223, 2231] and exposure to nickel salts may induce bronchospasm. This was shown in a study of 24 men with normal chest x-rays but with a complaint of wheezing.[2439] Challenge with nickel sulfate produced a fall of 40% in FEV_1, but no fever and no fall in DL_{CO}. There was no note of whether methacholine or histamine reactivity was affected.

Although manganese oxide produces toxic effects in mice,[2282] in humans it apparently causes psychoses before it produces effects on the lungs.[2187]

Vitallium, used in dental prostheses, caused diffuse pulmonary fibrosis in a 49-year-old man and a 30-year-old woman, both dental technicians.[4694] In the man, the vital capacity fell from 5.2 L to 4.3 L over a 3-year period, and the DL_{CO} was not initially abnormal. Although chromium, cobalt, and molybdenum with some asbestos fibers were present in the lung biopsy, the changes were thought to have been caused by Vitallium.

Uranium hexafluoride is contained in a number of materials such as floor sealants, spray paint, metal coat remover, and others. In 10 cases this produced an asthma syndrome, with increased methacholine reactivity.[4658] Bronchial mucosa biopsies showed chronic inflammation and edema.

An engineer accidentally sprayed with titanium tetrachloride in an industrial accident[4551] had severe respiratory failure and was respirator dependent for 5 weeks. Fleshy polypoid lesions had developed in major bronchi, occluding them at segmental and subsegmental levels. Slow improvement occurred after a year on steroids.

Studies of pulmonary function in welders, who may be exposed to many of these metals, and others, are noted below.

BYSSINOSIS, SISAL WORKER'S DISEASE, AND DISEASES CAUSED BY WOOL, COCONUT FIBERS, AND KAPOK

We noted in 1970 that byssinosis provided "a classic example of the use of respiratory function tests to clarify a clinical entity, the accurate description of which was otherwise entirely dependent on the subjective complaint of dyspnea, since usually the chest x-ray is normal."[1] Corn[2533] has provided a fascinating review of the extraordinary history of recognition of respiratory disease in textile workers. A recent supplement to *Chest*, volume 79 of 1981, contained a comprehensive review of many aspects of this condition.[3697-3717]

A recent review by Lee and Stretton[4704] contained the following quotation from the novel *North and South*, published in 1854, by British novelist Elizabeth Gaskell:

"Fluff"? said Margaret inquiringly.
"Fluff", repeated Bessy. "Little bits, as fly off fro' the cotton, when they're carding it, and fill the air till it looks all fine white dust. They say it winds round the lungs, and tightens them up. Anyhow, there's many a one as works in a carding-room, that falls into a waste, coughing and spitting blood, because they're just poisoned by the fluff."

There have been a number of experimental studies to determine the causative agent.* A

*See references 4555, 4557, 4558, 4566, 4671.

recent review concluded that the evidence indicated the possible involvement of histamine, 5-HT, platelet activating factor, and metabolites of arachidonic acid[4703] or prostaglandin $PGF_{2\alpha}$.[3612] Endotoxins, which some studies had suggested might play a role,[4626] are not believed to be the primary offending agents. Polyphenol, isolated from cotton bracts, is also not thought to be primarily responsible.[4584]

In a recent experimental study,[4576] 226 healthy non-asthmatic subjects inhaled cotton dust at levels of 1.02 mg/m³. FEV_1 decrements were related to atopic status, as measured by skin testing, but also occurred in non-atopic subjects. A purified extract of cotton bracts has been shown to induce airflow limitation in healthy normal subjects.[3703] In another study, 22 healthy normal subjects breathed cotton bract extract.[4652] Partial MEFV curves were measured; 12 responded with a fall in $MEF_{40\%}VC$ of >20%. The mean methacholine threshold in the responders was 26.8 mg/mL, compared with 55.6 mg/mL in the non-responders. Metaproterenol increased the $MEF_{40\%}VC$ by 41% in the responders and by 24% in the non-responders. All the baseline FEV_1 data were normal. The FEV_1 fell from a mean of 3.44 L to a mean of 3.11 L after exposure in the responders.

The disease first came to light by virtue of complaints of episodic shortness of breath.

The first demonstration of a decline in FEV_1 over a work shift, by Schilling, McKerrow and Gilson,[1] has been amply confirmed by recent studies. Monday shift declines of −126 mL in "non-byssinotics" and of −458 milliliters in workers with "grade 2 byssinosis," with the falls related to fine dust contamination, have been documented.[2125, 2149] In another survey, shift FEV falls averaged −254 milliters. In three grades of byssinosis of increasing severity, the $\dot{V}max_{50\%}$ shift falls were 3.3 to 2.4, 3.8 to 3.0, and 4.4 to 3.3 in the less-severe category.[2212] Shift declines of >15% in FEF_{25-75} and >10% in FEV_1 led another group of authors to conclude that flow measurements were more sensitive.[2220] If a bronchodilator is used, shift declines are much reduced,[2216] in one study, from a mean of −156 milliliters to a mean of −23 milliliters.[2230] It is also diminished by antihistamines.[2383]

In a recent Ontario study of shift decline,[4501] there were close relationships between dust level and observed FEV_1 shift change, and between dust, symptoms, and FEV_1 level. In one mill, 8% of workers had a greater than 10%

fall in FEV_1. It was concluded that a dust level of no more than 0.2 mg/m^3 will protect workers against shift FEV_1 changes (and possibly, by inference, from long-term effects).

No changes in DL_{CO} occur over a shift, nor does the total lung capacity change,[2241] but the residual volume increases.[2383] Most of the decline occurs in the first hour,[2354] and it seems likely that small airways are affected first, as Field and Owen in Australia noted that the $\dot{V}max_{50\%}VC$ fell first.[2354] The relationship of different dust levels to FEV_1 decline has been carefully studied.[3708]

Chronic byssinosis is characterized by irreversible chronic airflow limitation. It has proved difficult to define, and a recent committee of the National Academy of Sciences[2444] wrestled with the problem of accurate definition. Jones[4585] discussed the problem in a recent editorial.

Cotton dust exposure in non-smokers causes mucous gland hyperplasia and goblet cell metaplasia, but not emphysema.[2372, 4726] There may be some hypertrophy of bronchial smooth muscle.[2494] There is no evidence of extrinsic alveolitis.[2494] The autopsy findings have been described as resembling those seen in "asthmatic bronchitis," and there are no cotton fibers in the lungs.[3706]

Respiratory symptoms, particularly of chronic mucus hypersecretion and wheezing, are common.[2354] Comparisons between cotton-exposed workers, both smokers and non-smokers, and non-exposed controls consistently show more respiratory symptoms and more objective evidence of chronic obstruction in the cotton workers.[4524, 4533] However, data on 153 women with byssinosis[4705] showed no evidence of abnormality in DL_{CO} in spite of FEV_1 decrements—findings that confirmed the absence of morphologic emphysema or alveolitis noted histologically in these cases.

In one survey of 80 workers, 50 were considered to have byssinosis.[2200] FEV_1 values averaged 3.1 in the least severe category and 1.5 in those most affected.

In a recent survey of an Italian cotton mill,[3660] of 352 workers, 17.9% were considered to have byssinosis. In New South Wales, Australia, only 12 of 493 surveyed workers had byssinosis, although dust levels were high.[2161] This low incidence might be explained by lack of air pollution or, more probably, by climatic factors, though a self-selection process might also be operating. In a survey in Yugoslavia, 28% of operatives had byssinosis,[2194] and in the United States, 63 of 500 surveyed operatives were considered to have the disease.[2285] In this study, FEV_1 data were as follows:

Mean FEV_1 Values

Shop Location	Without Byssinosis	With Byssinosis
Carders	3.0	2.4
Weavers	3.1	2.2
Spinners	3.1	2.3

Of 135 men and 236 women in an urban cotton mill, in whom work shift FEV_1 changes averaged −340 milliliters, and FVC changes were −420 milliters,[2354] 25% of the men and 13% of the women had a productive cough. Effort dyspnea was much less common, being present in only 2%. In this study, 55% of the men and 28% of the women were smokers.

Byssinosis was found in 21% of the most heavily exposed workers in a survey of 506 men in a textile plant in Alexandria.[4601] Shift declines were more frequent than byssinosis and occurred in about a third of workers in the most dusty areas.

The interaction between smoking and cotton dust exposure in determining the outcome in this disease is a very difficult problem,[2444] though there is no doubt that chronic disease may occur in non-smokers. There is evidence that longitudinal declines of FEV_1 are accelerated in cotton workers, with faster declines in smokers.[2119, 2136, 2511] In a recently reported 5-year prospective study of 1241 textile workers in India,[2373] Kamat and colleagues noted the following data:

Annual Declines

	FVC (mL/year)	FEV_1 (mL/year)
Asymptomatic	−112	−76
Non-specific	−118	−88
Specific	−144	−114
"Mixed"	−151	−124

In one group with more than 6 years of service, the FEV_1 decline averaged −214 mL/year. There was a close relationship between dust load and rate of FEV_1 decline. Smoking was very light in this population, and its role was considered small in relation to cotton dust. Byssinosis was considered to be present in 14% of workers in carding rooms and 10% in other areas. In these workers, dyspnea occurred in 56%, chest tightness in 54%, wheezing in 29%, and cough in 36%. Although these data lack control observations of FEV_1 decline in Indian workers of comparable economic status but unexposed to cotton dust, they clearly indicate the adverse effect of this dust in the absence of a major smoking effect. FEV_1 declines of -53.3 mL/year in hemp workers in Spain have been recorded.[2436] Merchant and colleagues reported that workers with byssinosis had more chronic bronchitis and more dyspnea than matched controls, and that by the age of 50 to 70 years, the mean FEV_1 was 80% of predicted normal in non-smokers.[2438]

Beck and colleagues recently reported on a 6-year follow-up of 383 cotton textile workers in the United States[3676] compared with controls of similar ages. Higher attack rate of respiratory symptoms, after standardization for smoking, occurred in their textile workers, and the incidence of chronic bronchitis in them was much higher. The FEV_1 was declining at an annual rate of -42 mL/year in the textile workers compared with a decline of -25 mL/year in the control population, with similar data in men and women. The authors concluded that "chronic lung disease is not only irreversible but may progress even after exposure to cotton dust has ended." Subsequent correspondence in the journal questioned some of the conclusions drawn from this data, but the study represents the most complete longitudinal data from the United States. In another report on the same study, the authors showed that smoking differences could not account for the data, and there was a relationship between early retirement from the mills and FEV_1 decrement.[3700] In Britain, there is no evidence that survival is adversely affected by byssinosis,[3699] but FEV_1 follow-up data have not been published.

The pioneer work of the late Arend Bouhuys in drawing attention to this important condition and in clarifying its mechanism is well known. He showed that positive challenge tests using an extract of hemp dust and producing falls in FEF_{25-75} and increases in residual volume occurred in sensitized workers,[2159] and hemp dust exposure in workers retired from the industry could cause a fall in Pa_{O_2} without a change in FEV_1.[2291] Sisal extract apparently releases histamine from human lung tissue[2207]; however, healthy subjects sensitive to cotton bract extracts do not show any increased reactivity to histamine, and hence the responders are not to be thought of as "subclinical asthmatics."[2377] This is surprising, since it has been shown that blood histamine levels are elevated after the Monday work shift.[3705] It has recently been suggested that the "Monday morning" effect may be due to sudden release of histamine accumulated in the lungs during the weekend.[4565]

Subjects with byssinosis have no increase in IgE levels.[3660]

Bouhuys and colleagues in 1977[2384] concluded that as many as 35,000 United States men and women "may suffer from disabling lung function loss, owing to chronic lung disease, as a result of their work in cotton textile mills." By contrast, the National Academy of Science Committee[2444] had difficulty in concluding that there was any clearly defined entity; possibly they overemphasized the importance of distinct morphologic criteria. Workers in cottonseed mills have a small FEV_1 shift decline and a low incidence of byssinosis.[2498] However, a recent survey of 255 workers in four cottonseed crushing mills[4536] found shift declines of 100 milliliters in FEV_1 and 0.28 L/sec in FEF_{25-75}.

Jute workers are not afflicted with the condition.[2200] A survey of 252 wool workers of average age 36 with 11 years of exposure[2525] showed that FEV_1 shift declines of -120 milliliters occurred in non-smokers and of -90 milliliters in smokers. Lower preshift $MEF_{50\%}VC$ values were recorded in those exposed for more than 10 years. Coconut fiber exposure does not produce respiratory symptoms.[2218] Kapok, which comes from the fruit of *Ceiba pentandra*, a tree grown in Ceylon, produces "mill fever" and possibly chronic bronchitis, but typical byssinosis does not occur.[2227] Cork, on the other hand, has been associated with three syndromes[2490]: asthma, extrinsic alveolitis, and chronic bronchitis with bronchiectasis. In 13 of 63 workers, positive challenge tests to cork dust were found.[2490]

Summary

The pulmonary function data clearly indicate that chronic byssinosis is a real entity, even though not morphologically definable. It thus resembles asthma and, like asthma, does not lead to emphysema. The data clearly indicate the adverse effects on function that cotton dust may produce. However, in the absence of a specific morphology, precise definition is not possible. This accounts for the uneasiness with which prestigious committees have regarded this entity. In the light of the function test data, this hesitancy would seem to be misplaced.

BAGASSOSIS

The literature on bagassosis, which indicated some reductions in lung volumes and defects in gas transfer,[1] has been enlarged by a study from Trinidad, which showed evidence of reductions in vital capacity, FEV_1, and DL_{CO} in affected men.[2189] The residual volume was normal. A provocation test produced fever and malaise 6 hours after exposure to the dust, with the FEV_1 falling from 2.76 to 2.34 liters. After an acute episode, the chest x-ray cleared after about 8 weeks.[2189] No further lung biopsy material has been described in addition to the two noted in the previous edition,[1] which showed interstitital infiltrates and granulomas. Experimental data have shown that bagasse fiber has an adverse effect on macrophage function.[2280]

Another recent paper from Spain[3745] describes work shift changes in a group of workers with bagassosis as high as a 28% decline in FVC. After improvement in the condition, both C_{st} and $DL_{CO}SB$ rose, but the FEF_{25-75} was still abnormal. In one case, a biopsy showed lymphocytic and plasmocytic infiltration, with granulomas and obliterative bronchiolitis.

OCCUPATIONAL ALLERGIC ALVEOLITIS AND ASTHMA: CHRONIC EFFECTS

A wide variety of agents produce

- Reversible airflow limitation
- Induced non-specific (or specific) airway reactivity
- Airflow limitation accompanied by allergic alveolitis
- Long-term effects, possibly unresolved allergic alveolitis or changes leading to chronic mucous hypersecretion and emphysema

In some instances, the agent only produces the first of these effects. In others, high doses produce severe alveolitis, and lower doses produce reversible airflow limitation—but abnormally fast rates of FEV_1 decline are observed, suggesting long-term effects. In others, increased airway reactivity induced by the agent, together with mucus hypersecretion, dominates the long-term consequences of exposure. These factors complicate the description of the effects of the large number of agents associated with "occupational asthma." The use of the word *asthma* in this context may wrongly suggest that all effects are to be attributed to inherited characteristics in the exposed workers. In a recent editorial, Newman Taylor[2506] noted that the number of agents to which exposure at work

has been reported to cause asthma now exceeds 200. All of these are not discussed in this section, but the function test defects described in all those noted in his table of main agents causing occupational asthma are described below. The work on occupational asthma over the past 20 years has led to an impressive body of knowledge. An editorial written in 1982 was entitled "Occupational Asthma: Coming of Age."[3639] An indication of how this field of knowledge has developed is the fact that a recent comprehensive review by Chan-Yeung and Lam[4698] contained 257 references.

The many conditions that may cause occupational asthma, apart from contact with flour, recognized by Ramazzini,[2451] have only been defined over the past two decades. Apart from the useful editorials noted above,[2506] there have also been published a book with emphasis on grain dust exposure,[2470] symposia proceedings,* the Amberson lecture by Pepys,[1572] and an editorial on asthma inducers.[561] Challenge testing with occupational agents has been reviewed by Hendrick.[4613] It is discussed in detail in Chapter 5.

An important general point is that the diagnosis may be easily missed in isolated cases, because asthmatic symptoms may begin at night and not occur at the workplace, and also because chronic bronchitis and cough are prominent in some cases and may mask the underlying reactivity.

Toluene Diisocyanate, Diphenylmethane Diisocyanate, 1,5-Naphthylene Diisocyanate, N-Methylmorpholine, and Hexamethylene Diisocyanate

These chemicals, which are widely used, are important causes of occupational asthma. In very high doses in accidental exposures, toluene diisocyanate (TDI) can cause a fatal acute pneumonitis[2145] or an acute bronchitis with an FEV_1 decline and hypoxemia.[2255] In one case,[2255] arterial Pa_{O_2} was 58 mm Hg acutely and rose to 91 mm Hg over the next 4 days.

Recent experimental studies using guinea pigs suggest that TDI may have a direct effect on tracheal smooth muscle.[4528] Other guinea pig experiments showed that TDI caused a 15-fold increase in polymorphonuclear neutrophils in

---

*See references 2359, 3465, 3734, 3735.

the lamina propria of the trachea,[4635] followed by an eosinophil flux, as well as an increased acetylcholine response.

Other data[3613] suggest that mechanisms other than direct beta-adrenergic blockade are likely to be important.

A 35-year-old worker exposed to prepolymerized isocyanate developed a very severe life-threatening reaction.[3733] Allergy to both TDI and diphenylmethane diisocyanate (MDI) were shown in a RAST test.

Sensitivity develops after chronic exposure to low levels of these compounds. A recent development has been the recognition that specific antibodies are formed.[2455] This may lead to techniques important in prevention of chronic effects. Specific IgE antibodies have also been detected to MDI, and positive challenge tests occur in foundry workers exposed to the material.[2465] MDI is somewhat safer than TDI[2491] but may cause an allergic alveolitis. In one exposed worker, a challenge test with MDI was followed by a significant fall in FEV_1 and $D_{L_{CO}}$ and by fever.[3641] In this man and in two others with a history of pneumonitis, both specific IgG antibody and total antibody binding of MDI-HSA were elevated. In another worker, MDI caused an acute alveolitis with hypoxemia and fever.[4515] Challenge caused a fall in $D_{L_{CO}}$, as well as FEV_1. Other cases have been reported with positive challenges to MDI, and IgG antibodies to MDI have been demonstrated in serum and in bronchoalveolar lavage fluid.[4622] A recent report from France indicated that pulmonary function levels were depressed in relation to exposure to MDI.[4720]

TDI also may cause an allergic alveolitis, and in one worker, a challenge test was followed by a fall of FEV_1 to 40% of the control value; in Pa_{O_2} from 78 mm Hg to 56 mm Hg; and in $D_{L_{CO}}SB$ from 34 to 26.[2315] In one worker exposed to TDI, recovery from occupational asthma took longer than 70 days.[2504] Work shift declines in FEV_1 were found to be proportional to exposure in one study of 111 exposed workers[2153]:

TDI Concentration (ppm)	Work Shift Change in FEV_1
0.002	− 78 mL
0.005	− 106 mL
0.006–0.013	− 180 mL

Although one worker was reported to be very sensitive to TDI but to have normal non-specific airway reactivity,[2181] a more usual finding is that airway reactivity to methacholine or histamine is increased.[2274, 2310, 2465] This was clearly shown in studies of 254 exposed workers,[4697] of whom 64 were found to have an increased methacholine response.

Sequential studies in a TDI-sensitized patient[4552] showed that methacholine sensitivity regressed after exposure ended. However, other studies on six workers led to the conclusion that in single cases a normal methacholine response does not indicate that TDI sensitivity (and symptomatology) may not be present.[4712] In detailed studies on five cases of TDI sensitivity,[4650] a late asthmatic reaction was prevented by prednisone. The data suggested that inflammatory mediators were involved in the TDI response.

In 114 subjects with TDI-induced asthma,[4711] bronchial provocation showed that 24 had an immediate response, 50 had a late response, and 40 had a dual response to TDI. Those with a dual response were most reactive to methacholine. Of those with a dual reaction, 22% had chronic bronchitis. It was noted that there were few smokers among the late reactors.

A comparison between 180 asymptomatic men with possible TDI exposures with 61 TDI workers with symptoms showed that the latter group had a mean FEV_1 267 milliliters lower and mean FVC 269 milliliters lower compared with predicted values.[2219] Longitudinal declines of FEV_1 (measured over a 2-year period only, however) of − 103 mL/year in the highest exposure group of 63 TDI workers have been reported,[2228] with a significant association between shift FEV_1 fall and chronic decrement. The authors of this study concluded that exposure to more than 0.003 ppm of TDI was unsafe, and there has been much discussion of what threshold value should be established.[2317] An increase in airway resistance has been reported after exposures to concentrations between 0.006 and 0.02 ppm,[2402] and 37 workers reacted to concentrations below 0.005 ppm.[2431]

Diem and colleagues[3607] recently reported on 277 workers in a new TDI plant followed prospectively over a 5-year period. Personal TDI monitors were used in more than 2000 sample analyses. FEV_1 declines were shown to be related to level of exposure, and the effect of exposure in non-smokers with high exposures resulted in an FEV_1 annual decline of 38 milliliters more than in non-smokers with lighter exposures. The conclusions from this study were disputed in subsequent correspondence.[3614]

A comparison between 95 isocyanate workers

and 37 controls in Ontario[4514] showed that the FEV_1 and FEF_{25-75} values in the exposed group were about 5% lower after adjustment for smoking history. Significant shift declines were also recorded, with a mean fall of 52 mL in FEV_1 on Mondays. In this study, personal samplers were used. Only one sample was greater than 20 ppb, and fewer than 5% of samples were greater than 5 ppb.

There is some evidence that TDI exerts its first effect on small airway function,[2274] but this has not been studied in detail.

The importance of TDI was clearly shown in a study of 47 men exposed to a polyurethane material with and without TDI as an activator.[2398] Immediate effects occured on challenge with TDI, but not with the polyurethane.

The physician should be aware that TDI may be contained in many industrial materials. Twenty-one cases of occupational exposure occurred in a steel coating plant after the process was changed.[4676] The new material liberated TDI. Steelworkers are also exposed intermittently.[4669]

Significant FEV_1 decrements have been reported in exposed workers in Nigeria.[2282]

Isocyanate asthma occurred after exposure to 1,5-naphthylene diisocyanate also,[2305] and in this case, a challenge test to TDI was negative.

Exposure to amines evolved during polyurethane foam production may be important in addition to isocyanate exposure. N-Methylmorpholine occurs in concentrations higher than 10 ppm, and this substance was believed to have been responsible for causing increased airway reactivity in a group of workers.[3664]

Hexamethylene diisocyanate (HDI) has been shown to lead to an increase in histamine reactivity, which persisted for 18 months after exposure ended.[4612]

Wood Dusts

Several wood dusts are capable of causing allergic alveolitis or occupational asthma. Cases have been reported as a result of exposure to ramin (*Gonystylus bancanas*)[2496]; California redwood,[2302] in one case of which challenge testing produced falls in FEV_1 from 3.8 to 2.6 over 8 hours and DL_{CO} from 32 to 28 mL/min/mm Hg; and African zebrawood (*Microberlinia*).[2313]

The most extensively studied wood is western red cedar (*Thuja plicata*). Occupational asthma from this wood was first recognized in Australia by Gandevia and Milne in 1970.[2185] Six cases

were described, and challenge testing produced falls in FEV_1 from 3.8 to 1.0. They also noted that "delayed responses occurring after 4 to 6 hours and also at night to bronchial provocation tests provided an effective diagnostic aid in our series." These observations have been extended and confirmed by us in Vancouver. We reported positive bronchial challenges in 18 of 22 cases[2293] and showed that the response to plicatic acid, which the wood contains, was similar. The methacholine response is also abnormal and remains abnormal after exposure ends.[2284] Histamine reactivity remained abnormal for 16 days after challenge in another study.[717] In a 55-year-old cedar worker, non-atopic changes in FEV_1, closing capacity, and SBN_2/L were documented 2 days after exposure,[566] and histamine reactivity remained abnormal for 2 days after all pulmonary function test results returned to normal. These changes are discussed in Chapter 5.

The group in British Columbia have recently summarized their follow-up experience with 125 cedar workers, 50 of whom remained at work and the remainder who ceased exposure.[2456] All of the 50 who stayed at work continued to have asthmatic attacks requiring regular medication. Their pulmonary function deteriorated, and their methacholine reactivity increased. Of those who left the industry, half lost their symptoms and half did not. Those who remained symptomatic had had longer exposure and a longer duration of symptoms. At the time of diagnosis, their lung function was more abnormal and their methacholine reactivity greater than in those whose symptoms disappeared, and dual asthmatic reactions were more common in them. Smoking, race, and the presence of eosinophilia were not related to the occurrence of the syndrome, and it was evident that the enhanced reactivity was acquired as a result of exposure and did not antedate it. These observations on prognosis have recently been summarized in an editorial.[4641]

Brooks and colleagues[3739] have reported studies on 74 shake mill workers exposed to western red cedar compared with 58 planer mill operators exposed to other wood dusts. By comparison with clerical workers, both groups of woodworkers had about twice the incidence of chronic bronchitis. Occupational asthma was only found in the group exposed to cedar, who were working in a dust level of about 6.8 mg/m^3.

A recent comparison between 652 cedar mill workers and 440 male office workers in Vancouver[4554] showed that the cedar mill workers had a higher prevalence of respiratory symptoms after adjustment for age and smoking; lower FVC, FEV_1, and FEF_{25-75} mean values; and a positive methacholine challenge test in 19.4%, compared with 11.6% positive in the office workers. The prevalence of atopy was not different between the two groups. It was of interest that the prevalence of increased methacholine reactivity rose in the cedar workers with years of exposure, whereas it fell in the office workers with increasing years of employment.

Western red cedar exposure represents the inducer of occupational asthma on which we have the best longitudinal data to this point. It is, of course, not certain that the conclusions will apply to occupational asthma from other agents, but the data illustrate the importance of early diagnosis and removal from contact with the agent if disability is to be avoided. The symptoms of this type of asthma, with the percentage of patients in whom they occur, are cough (87%), sputum production (46%), wheezing (89%), chest tightness (89%), dyspnea (96%), and rhinitis (40%). Before the syndrome was identified, some of these cases were considered to have bronchitis, since in some cases the productive cough appeared to be the dominant symptom.

In a recent report on two carpenters,[3738] both had a dual asthmatic response to cedar urea formaldehyde but none to spruce or western red cedar. Both had increased histamine airway reactivity, and in both, rhinitis was a prominent symptom.

Tea and Coffee

Tea packers have excessive FEV_1 declines during work shifts,[2418, 3679] and 125 tea blenders had a high incidence of chronic bronchitis (24%) and asthma (6.4%) with very light cigarette smoking. A variety of tea known as "dog-rose" appeared to cause most symptoms in a recent study, in which an 8% mean shift fall in $\dot{V}max_{50\%}$ was documented.[4560] This study also indicated that chronic symptoms may be caused in these workers.

Monday work shift declines similar to those in the cotton textile industry also occur in coffee workers,[2237] possibly predominantly indicating small airway dysfunction. In a recent review of 45 coffee workers,[2417] skin tests were positive in 40% of those emptying bags. Most of these workers had a productive cough. The

$MEF_{25\%}VC$ declined 18% over a work shift, and the $MEF_{50\%}VC$ declined 8%. Characteristic occupational asthma occurred in nine coffee workers, of whom four had positive challenge tests to green coffee allergen.[4675]

Exposure to green coffee beans seems to be the important factor in producing FEV_1 declines.[3685] An erroneous attribution of interstitial pneumonitis to coffee, later realized to be due to concomitant rheumatoid disease,[3471] has already been noted.

Tobacco Dust

Workers with tobacco (unsmoked), all nonsmokers, had wheezing but normal FEV_1 values.[2526] But in one high-exposure group, FEV_1 work shift declines of -489 milliliters over a work shift were noted.

Grain Dust and Flour: Thermophilic Actinomycetes

Apart from allergic alveolitis in agricultural workers (farmer's lung; see Chapter 11), chronic respiratory disease in grain elevator workers and others in contact with grain dust has been extensively studied. The book edited by Dosman and Cotton[2470] provides a comprehensive review of these data up to 1980. The microflora of grain dusts is very complex, as it includes many bacteria, yeasts, and actinomyces, more than a dozen spore types, and many fungi. Thirty different species of bacteria and yeasts were recovered from the air of Canadian grain elevators.[2470]

Those exposed to this environment have increased respiratory symptoms[2509] and an increased non-specific airway reactivity[2269, 2307] and may show evidence of lowered FEV_1 values or low flow rates on terminal expiration. FEV_1 values are lower in workers with positive challenge tests to grain dusts.[2269]

Shift declines in FEV_1, prevented by wearing masks, have been shown to be related to dust levels in grain elevator workers.[3647] Personal monitors have been used to measure dust levels in these workers, and decrements of FEV_1 are closely related to the dust level encountered.[3615] The acute response is blocked by disodium cromoglycate and seems to be particularly related to the dust from durum wheat. Challenges with dust from mites in the grain were negative.[3737]

Grain elevator workers with positive skin tests to grain do not appear to have an excess of respiratory symptoms or lower FEV_1 levels.[4502] A comparison between 310 grain handlers and 237 city hall workers[4553] showed that both symptoms and the occurrence of rhonchi were higher in the grain handlers, with about a fourfold increase in risk. The effects of smoking and grain dust were additive. Atopic status does not seem to be different between grain handlers and control groups.[4628]

There is evidence of "worker selection" in this industry, in that those who join the industry and notice early symptoms probably leave it.[2386, 4561] It is clear that this condition is aggravated by cigarette smoking,[2470] but it is not yet possible to arrive at some general assessment of the burden of increased respiratory disease associated with grain dust exposure. It appears to cause symptoms rather similar to those observed in cotton workers (whose disease is also difficult to define).

Earlier data indicating no accelerated rate of FEV_1 decline in grain handlers[2172] have been superseded by our data from a 6-year follow-up of 267 grain elevator operators from Vancouver.[4586, 4727] These observations may be summarized as follows:

Annual Rates of Decline

Age Groups (years)	Number	FEV_1 (mL) loss	±	FVC (mL) loss	±	FEF_{25-75} (mL/sec) loss	±
Non-smokers							
<30	28	−24.5	115	−16.3	114	−48.7	203
30–49	29	−26.9	56	−11.3	72	−91.4	108
>50	12	−45.1	40	−9.3	73	−124.0	59
Ex-smokers							
<30	9	−1.1	31	−5.4	23	−20.0	130
30–49	47	−21.8	50	−14.2	52	−87.9	101
>50	28	−31.2	43	−10.5	49	−113.8	101
Smokers							
<30	30	−16.9	53	−2.3	53	−77.7	112
30–49	65	−34.9	58	−19.6	64	−126.2	112
>50	18	−70.1	52	−47.0	95	−125.3	45

It is shown that acute changes in lung function over the course of one workweek during the initial study were correlated with subsequent decline in FEV_1, as was bronchial hyperreactivity, but this was measured after declines were noted (hence not prospective). Differences in rate of decline were noted as between groups in whom the methacholine PD20 was greater than or less than 8 mg/mL. Differences between smokers and non-smokers did not reach statistical significance, nor were positive skin reac-

tions, symptom occurrence, or initial lung function level related to rate of decline.

Studies of six men handling barley[4672] showed shift declines of up to 800 mL in FEV_1. After 2 hours of exposure, recovery took up to 72 hours. Five volunteers exposed in a silo to 31 mg/m³ of dust for 5 hours showed progressive falls in FVC and FEV_1 and changes in the shape of flow/volume curves.

There are several individual cases of interest in the literature. One farmer reacted positively to challenge by dust from his own fields that did not contain aspergillus, showing falls in FEV_1, fever, malaise, and radiographic changes.[1590] The agent could not be identified. In another non-smoking farmer with grain dust sensitivity, a positive bronchial provocation test to a grain mite (*Glycophagus destructor*) produced a fall of FEV_1 from 3.3 to 1.0 liters, and a fall in DL_{CO} from 32 to less than 20 mL/min/mm Hg.[2527] A farmer's wife had a severe allergic alveolitis after contact with infected oats, and a lung biopsy showed multiple granulomata.[1584]

Thermophilic actinomycetes contaminating air-conditioning systems have caused allergic alveolitis,[1578] but asthmatic attacks do not seem to have been a feature (see Chapter 1).

Mold antigens are responsible for the alveolitis that occasionally occurs in malt workers.[2214]

Baker's asthma has been a well-recognized entity for more than 200 years. Eighteen cases were studied with placebo drugs and bronchodilators, and the bronchodilator was shown to normalize airway resistance in 5 minutes.[2522] Detailed challenges with rye and wheat flour to 85 baker's apprentices, 29 healthy bakers, and 38 bakers with occupational asthma[2276] showed increases in airway resistance in the symptomatic group, who also had enhanced responses to acetylcholine. An Australian comparison between 176 bakers and 24 bread slicers[4575] showed that the bakers had a greater prevalence of wheeze and dyspnea. Airway reactivity was increased in 41% of the bakers and in 21% of the slicers, and in bakers with work-related asthma, 75% had increased airway reactivity to methacholine. Symptoms were more common in oven handlers rather than in general bakers or dough handlers, and the mean baseline FEV_1 was 500 milliliters lower in the oven handlers than in other groups.

A recent detailed study of a symptomatic baker shows how difficult it can be to make a definitive diagnosis in some cases.[2464]

Mushroom Workers, Swine Barn Workers, Animal Protein Exposure, and Poultry Workers

Mushroom workers may develop a severe alveolitis, with marked reductions in FEV_1, DL_{CO}, and Pa_{O_2} in the acute stage.[1593] Occupational asthma has not been documented. Swine barn workers with positive precipitins to the feed are said to have excessive dyspnea,[1561] but FEV_1 values have not been reported. Laboratory workers exposed to rat proteins may develop sensitivity to them, as shown by challenge testing.[2311]

Risks in the poultry industry have been defined.[4287] Increased shift declines of FEV_1 have been described in hog farmers in Iowa.[4595] A study from Israel[4717] indicates significant occupational asthma in animal house workers.

Detergent Enzymes and Papain

Exposures to detergent enzymes cause acute falls in FEV_1,[2142] but one survey found normal DL_{CO} values and FEV_1 values not much different between exposed workers and clerical staff.[2163] In another survey of 98 workers, half complained of asthmatic symptoms, particularly at night.[522] These were not related to smoking or atopy, and no differences were found between FEV_1, FVC, or DL_{CO} values between symptomatic and asymptomatic groups.

Proteolytic enzymes are potentially dangerous, and biphasic responses to challenge by maxatase, an enzyme prepared from *Bacillus subtilis*, occurred in five workers.[2290] An interesting follow-up of 62 workers previously exposed to enzymes,[2298] with six readers of the chest x-rays, cataloged four changes:

- a—thickened bronchial walls
- b—attenuation of midzone vessels
- c—hyperinflation
- d—abnormal peripheral markings

The FEV_1 values were lowered in relation to b, c, and d; RV/TLC% was elevated in relation to a and d; DL_{CO} was lowered in relation to b; and compliance and recoil pressure measurements were not related to any. Exposure to proteolytic enzymes has been reported to be accompanied by a loss of recoil,[2226] a very important finding if confirmed.

Fourteen employees of a pharmaceutical company handling porcine pancreatic extract[4264] had significant illness, with two developing an acute alveolitis; three had mild radiologic interstitial change; and seven had emphysema. Hyperreactivity to the extract was shown by skin testing and bronchial provocation. Pancreatic alpha$_1$-amylase was the causative allergen. Thirteen of the employees had evidence of airflow obstruction or bronchial hyperreactivity or an increased $(A-a)$ D_{O_2}. It is obviously very dangerous material.

Solder Flux

An interesting series of papers documented the occurrence of occupational asthma in a large percentage of workers exposed to solder flux in an electronics factory in England,[2500–2503] and cases have also occurred in the industry manufacturing this material.[2413] The recognition that many workers had asthma from their work exposure and that asthma had been a major cause of workers leaving this employment took several years. Detailed function test studies were required to prove the association beyond doubt.

A survey of 104 electronics workers in the United States using two types of solder flux (rosin core, colophony; or aqua core, phosphorous hexate) showed small shift FEV_1 deficits with no differences between those using the two types of solder. All had normal FEV_1 levels before starting work on Mondays. Another survey of 1611 employees in this industry showed little evidence of increased respiratory symptoms, though these were increased in previously exposed workers.[4573] A recent follow-up of 39 electronics workers[2412] over a 4-year period showed that enhanced histamine reactivity returned to normal in 10 of 20 cases, but only two were free of symptoms, the remainder complaining of bronchospasm provoked by exercise, infections, and non-specific irritants. The data support the conclusion from studies of the western red cedar workers that the nonspecific histamine reactivity was a result of the occupational asthma, not the cause.

Miscellaneous Chemicals, Plastics, and Metals

Polytetrafluoroethylene (PTFE) may cause an acute pneumonitis, probably through workers' contamination of cigarettes while on the job.[2126] Tetrachlorophthalic anhydride (TCPA) causes occupational asthma with no IgE antibody,[2166] and exposure is followed by a slow decline of FEV_1 over an 8-hour period. In five cases, the $\dot{V}max_{50\%}VC$ fell to 25% of the control value over a 4-hour period.

PVC dust may cause a pneumoconiosis,[2279, 2499] with small radiologic opacities and falls in FEV_1 and FVC closely related to dust exposure. A study of 818 workers led to a calculation that the loss of FEV_1 was 4.1 mL per unit of dust exposure calculated as years $\times$ mg/mm^3 concentration.[2499] Other studies have not found differences.[4537, 4568] More recent data on 28 men showed that small rounded opacities on the chest film were common, but FEV_1 values were not abnormal.[3694] Whether this material actually causes disease is disputed, however.[3747] Increased respiratory symptoms have been reported,[3749] but not found in other surveys.[4537, 4568]

Vinyl chloride exposure for more than 10 years led to small linear reticular changes, with rounded opacities in some.[2258] FEV_1/FVC values were lowered in relation to exposure, but other tests were not reported.

Teflon polymer causes a fume fever with a flu-like illness, but apparently without long-term effects.[2154] Surveys of workers exposed to nylon and Orlon dusts have not included FEV_1 data.[2492] Bakelite[2294] has been reported to cause a pulmonary granuloma. Initial studies of workers exposed to fiberglass did not indicate any chronic adverse effects,[2143, 2209, 2257] but the period of exposure was generally short. More recently, studies of 1028 men in seven different plants showed clear evidence of radiologic change, the severity of which was related to the level of exposure to fibers less than 1 micron in diameter.[3620] Although the FEV_1 values were not lower, there was evidence that FEF_{25-75} and DL_{CO} values were lower in men with radiologic changes. Symptoms were minimal, however. A European collaborative study on fiberglass exposure involving 25,146 workers[4578] is not reassuring, as an increased risk of lung cancer was found.

This material will obviously have to be closely watched, since fibrous glass dust has been shown to cause a focal bronchiolitis in baboons.[3607] Fiberglass batt makers are also exposed to formaldehyde, and this may be related to work shift FEV_1 declines.[4664] Styrene exposure occurs in builders of fiberglass boats,[4540] but this appears to cause mental symptoms before any respiratory symptoms occur in most workers, although respiratory sensitivity to it does occur.[4510]

Meat packers may be exposed to fumes from a hot wire used for cutting plastic in packaging the meat. Occupational asthma in a 58-year-old worker, whose FEV_1 fell from 2.35 to 0.95 1 minute after exposure,[2171] showed that this syndrome could occur. Recent survey data support this,[4685] but there does not appear to be a long-term hazard,[2408] and recent studies have been negative.[3740]

There has been great concern and controversy over the possibility that urea-formaldehyde foam installed in houses might lead to asthma and other adverse health effects. Exposure to high concentrations of formaldehyde in hospital workers was believed to have caused occupational asthma in a nurse and a pathologist.[2443] A fall in FEV_1 on challenge was demonstrated; however, there is little information on how frequent this syndrome may be. A single case in a 47-year-old farmer's wife seemed to be attributable to sensitivity to some component of the house insulating material (to which a challenge test was positive) rather than to formaldehyde.[3736] Levels of formaldehyde in factories have been carefully measured,[3726] as it is a widely used material. There is no evidence of increased mortality in those exposed.[3646]

Dimethyl ethanolamine is used in certain paint sprays. In one worker, challenge by the paint produced a 30% fall in FEV_1, but it fell 60% with challenge with pure dimethyl ethanolamine, which the paint contained as a solvent.[524] Increased histamine reactivity in this man continued for 6 months after exposure ceased.

Ethylene diamine is used in color photograph processing. It was shown to cause a late asthmatic reaction in one exposed worker.[2531] Diazonium salts used in dye-coupling reactions have been shown to cause falls in PEFR on challenge.[2416]

Two workers exposed to persulfate dust had increases in airway resistance 8 hours after exposure, accompanied by a fall in DL_{CO}.[2400] Hair bleaches contain persulfates. Four of 23 employees in a large hair salon were found to have occupational asthma and, on challenge testing, sensitivity to these chemicals.[4706]

Of 151 workers exposed to azodicarbonamide dust, 18.5% had late onset asthma.[2415] Thirteen were considered to have enhanced and prolonged increased airways reactivity after exposure.

Chloramine-T is used in breweries, and dyspnea has been alleged in exposed workers, but no challenge tests were reported.[2441]

Platinum salts have long been known to be capable of inducing asthma, but detailed surveys of exposed workers do not seem to have been reported. Asthma was shown to have been induced in a metal polisher by a positive challenge test.[2544] Nickel can also induce sensitivity.[4556]

Exposure to oil mists,[4666] formaldehyde,[4507, 4615, 4670] acrylates used in solvent manufacture,[4619] piperazine used in chemical manufacture,[4604] tetrazine,[4518] freon,[4520] hexachlorophene (in a children's nurse),[4728] and cimetidine (during manufacture)[4596] have all been shown, by positive challenge testing, to be capable of inducing airflow limitation and symptoms.

GASES AND VAPORS

Sulfur Dioxide

As we noted in the previous edition,[1] inhalation of high concentrations of sulfuric acid or sulfur oxides may cause a chemical bronchiectasis with severe reduction of pulmonary function. Two additional reports have appeared since 1970.

One involved a healthy, non-smoking 25-year-old man who inhaled a high concentration of SO_2 for about 15 minutes after an industrial accident.[2401] The chest film showed patchy infiltrates but cleared in 5 days. There was severe cough and wheezing, with sputum production, and assisted ventilation was required initially. Over the next 20 months, the VC increased from 2.18 to 3.58 L (predicted 4.32); but the FEF_{25-75} only changed from 0.48 to 0.56 L/sec. The residual volume remained twice the normal value at 2.18 L. There was some reduction of $DL_{CO}SS$, but the $DL_{CO}SB$ was normal.

Another report involved the accidental exposure of seven men to high levels of SO_2 after a pyrite dust explosion.[3616] After the acute episode, they were followed for 4 years. After 3 months, no further decrement in function occurred, but six had severe chronic airflow limitation, and interstitial fibrosis was thought to be present in the seventh. Pre-exposure lung function tests were available, and in the group of six men, the FEF_{25-75} fell from a pre-exposure mean value of 115% of predicted to 25% of predicted a week after the exposure. Four years later it only averaged 40% of predicted. In four of the men, there was evidence of acquired increased airway reactivity as a result of the exposure.

One summary of 24 cases of SO_2 inhalation does not permit detailed analysis of the effects of this gas on pulmonary function.[2388]

SO_2 is one of the most important air pollutants (see Chapter 6). Apart from community studies of the relationship between SO_2 levels, respiratory symptoms, and function, there are some studies of smelter workers and pulp and paper employees that may indicate a chronic effect from low-level exposure. These are reviewed below. However, interpretation is difficult since in these environments exposure is commonly to a number of different gases.

Oxides of Nitrogen

Henderson and Haggard[2120] noted the delayed effect of inhalation of oxides of nitrogen, commenting that

The nitrous fumes are by no means the most toxic of the irritant gases, but they are among the most insidious. The inflammation of the lungs gives rise to little pain, but is out of all proportion to the irritation of the upper respiratory tract. These fumes, therefore, give little warning; a man may, without serious discomfort, breathe an atmosphere containing a concentration of nitrous fumes sufficient to cause death some hours later.

Exposure to high concentrations may occur when welding is performed in confined spaces, or after explosives have been used underground, or occasionally from exposure to silage gas. Four cases, two from the first of these, one from the third, and the fourth from a leak at a chemical plant,[2489] showed that the very acute stage was characterized by a severe ventilatory defect and hypoxemia and that recovery, usually to near normal values, occurred slowly but did occur in all the cases. In one case, a second phase of abnormality with a lowering of DL_{CO} occurred 17 days after the exposure. All cases had a considerable polymorphonuclear leukocytosis. In five other new cases, recovery was also complete,[2250] and the authors raise the question of whether the chronic bronchiolitis earlier described after oxide of nitrogen inhalation might not have been due to some other gas present in those cases in whom this was observed. In four episodes of NO_2 inhalation in three cases, all from silage gas, Pa_{O_2} levels in the acute phase were 38, 51, 52, and 65 mm Hg.[2248] Complete radiologic clearing occurred in all cases, and recovery was thought to be complete, although in one of these cases the FEF_{25-75} was not reported to have risen above

1.8 L/sec. These authors also raise the question whether the long-term sequelae earlier reported from underground exposures might not have been due to some other inhaled material, since chronic bronchiolitis seems unusual in silage gas exposures, when oxides of nitrogen were present in relatively pure form.

A remarkable episode was reported in a 21-year-old gardener exposed to silage gas. He developed respiratory failure 3 weeks after exposure, after the initial fever, cough, and nausea had disappeared.[2397] A needle lung biopsy showed the presence of interstitial pneumonitis distal to bronchiolitis obliterans. The changes of function (from worst value to best value) were FVC from 2.5 to 5.1; FEV_1 from 2.5 to 4.3; RV 1.3 and unchanged; $DL_{CO}SS$ exercise from 25 to 30 mL/min/mm Hg; and $DL_{CO}SB$ from 26 to 37 mL/min/mm Hg. Steroids were given and were thought to have assisted recovery.

An interesting pattern of function test change was reported in a non-smoker who inhaled nitric acid fumes at work. Dyspnea developed 6 hours later, and the chest film showed soft and confluent densities. Over the next 13 weeks, the Pa_{O_2} returned to normal, as did the $DL_{CO}SS$, but small airway change was considered to be maximal some weeks after the episode and then to improve. The FEF_{25-75} was still 0.5 L/sec below the predicted value 10 weeks after the episode.[2275]

Chronic exposure to low levels of NO_2 occurs as a result of community exposure (see Chapter 6). There has recently been great interest in whether cooking with gas (as compared with electric), which results in higher NO_2 levels in the home, is or is not associated with an increase in respiratory infections in children, and both positive and negative findings have been reported.

Another environment in which long-term exposure to oxides of nitrogen occurs (but in combination with other constituents of automobile exhaust) is in automobile tunnels. Ayres and colleagues[2326] produced suggestive evidence that this led to small airway dysfunction, as indicated by an increased closing volume and by an increased airway resistance. Five hundred fifty employees of the Triborough Bridge and Tunnel Authority in New York City were studied, and it was of interest that half of the non-smoking workers were found to have carboxyhemoglobin levels in excess of 3%—indicating chronic exposure to automobile exhaust. Pham and colleagues[2378] found evidence that respiratory function was significantly more impaired in underground iron ore miners in mines where

nitrate fuel was used as an explosive, compared with other miners not exposed to oxides of nitrogen.

A recent study of miners found no evidence that exposure to diesel fumes underground had a measurable adverse effect.[3686]

Oxides of nitrogen are a common and dangerous constituent of smoke in fires; data relevant to this are discussed below.

Ammonia

An experimental study in which 20 cats were exposed to 1000 ppm of ammonia for 10 minutes and then studied in detail[4614] showed that the lung reaction was biphasic. Initial resolution was followed by secondary effects, still apparent 35 days later.

Exposure of six volunteers for 6 weeks to concentrations of ammonia of 25, 50, and 100 ppm led to mild irritation of the eyes, nose, and throat but no changes in FEV_1. The authors concluded that those levels were easily tolerated.[2133] Acute exposures to high concentrations occur in industrial accidents or transportation accidents. In seven cases acutely exposed to a high concentration,[2205] one patient died and the other six were followed for 5 years. The autopsy on the fatal case showed intense edema. Symptoms were severe searing pain in the mouth and throat, blood-stained mucus, edema of exposed membranes, and pulmonary edema. Improvement occurred in 48 hours. Radiologic changes were not striking and not persistent in those who recovered. All tests of function, including the DL_{CO}, were back to normal after 1 year except in one case, in whom the FEV_1 improved slowly from 1.30 at 1 year, to 2.86 at 2 years, to 3.60 at 5 years after the episode.[2205] In another near-fatal case,[2144] there was only a mild residual cough 6 months later. Severe exposure to ammonia following a tank car derailment[2247] led to severe bronchiectasis. Function tests in two cases in whom bronchograms showed moderate (case 2) and severe (case 1) changes, with predicted values in brackets, were as follows:

	Case 1	Case 2
Age (years)	22	20
TLC	4.5 (4.3)	5.5 (4.9)
FRC	3.3 (2.2)	3.3 (2.9)
VC	1.9 (3.1)	3.6 (3.4)
RV	2.6 (1.2)	1.9 (1.5)
SBN_2/L	5.0 (<1.5)	2.0 (<1.5)
FEV_1	1.2 (2.7)	2.9 (3.0)
FEF_{25-75} (L/sec)	1.1 (4.7)	3.9 (5.0)
C_{st}	0.14 (0.1–0.3)	0.2 (0.1–0.3)
C_{dyn}/f	not recorded	48% (>80%)
V_D/V_T%	43 (30)	54 (30)
$DL_{CO}SB$	18 (22)	22 (24)
Pa_{O_2} (mm Hg)	66 (>75)	85 (>75)

These data were interpreted to indicate severe generalized airway involvement in case 1 and probable peripheral airway dysfunction in case 2, with no considerable chronic pneumonitis in either. Ammonia inhalation can also cause tracheal and bronchial strictures.[2260] In a 28-year-old non-smoker exposed to a high concentration, the sequelae were reduced perfusion to the posterior part of the left lung, with bronchial changes within it, in addition to two tracheal strictures. This case serves to emphasize the importance of careful follow-up studies on such patients, since his chest film showed no abnormality. Fourteen cases occurred after a leak in a ship's refrigeration system.[2272] Nine of these had transient radiologic change, but improvement occurred over 7 days. In five, both the x-ray and the Pa_{O_2} were normal; in one the Pa_{O_2} was 48 mm Hg initially with a normal x-ray, and it rose to 80 mm Hg within the next 7 days.

A committee of the National Academy of Sciences in the United States recently published a useful review of the consequences of exposure to ammonia.[5371] They recommended a maximal 1-hour exposure level of 100 ppm.

Chlorine

In the previous edition of this book, we noted that persistent abnormal function could follow acute chlorine exposure.[1] This chemical is so widely used and transported that accidental exposure has unfortunately been common. Within 10 minutes, seven workers exposed to a high concentration had severe symptoms, which lasted for up to 8 days.[2124] One man had radiologic changes of congestion and edema. In another, severe hypoxemia persisted for 4 days. After 8 weeks, one man had an FEV_1 of 48% of predicted, and in another it was 57% of predicted. DL_{CO} data were not abnormal. The author stated that "all patients recovered completely" but did not record the restitution of all function test data to normality.[2124] In another study of 139 workers at risk with an average chlorine concentration of less than 1 ppm, 55 had had accidental higher exposures.[2129] Mean FEF_{25-75} values were recorded as follows:

	Smokers		Non-Smokers	
	No Cl	+ Cl	No Cl	+ Cl
Number	56	46	25	12
FEV_{25-75} (L/sec)	4.13	3.57	4.36	4.10

These data indicate some evidence of a long-term effect in both smokers and non-smokers.

Twelve patients studied 7 years after an acute accidental exposure had no evidence of abnormalities in flow rates, mechanics, diffusing capacity, or arterial gas tensions.[2482] In an unusual report of two sisters acutely exposed to chlorine, one was treated with steroids and one not.[2264] The sister that received steroids had normal pulmonary function after 1 year, but the sister who did not receive steroids had persistent gas exchange abnormalities over a 55-month period, with an elevated $(A-a) D_{O_2}$, a fall in Pa_{O_2} on exercise, and a $DL_{CO}SS$ "still abnormal" (but no value quoted) at the end of that period. Although this report cannot be taken to prove the value of steroid administration, it emphasizes the possibility of residual effects in the presence of a normal chest film. Kaufman and Burkons reported the effects of accidental exposure of five chlorine workers and 13 non-workers following a leak in a storage tank in Cleveland. The cases were studied within 24 and 48 hours, and serially over the following 14 months.[2319] Airway obstruction and persisting hypoxemia generally cleared within 3 months, but the plant workers showed persistent reduction in ventilatory flow rates 14 months later. Twelve cases of chlorine exposure were noted in the report referred to above, but although both DL_{CO} and C_{dyn} were said to be lowered, exact data were not reported.[2388] Precise details are difficult to derive from another report,[2484] but both of these lead to the conclusion that long-term sequelae may follow chlorine exposure.

The only report of experimental chlorine exposure in normals that we have been able to trace[2545] indicated that in eight normal subjects exposed to 1.0 ppm of chlorine for 4 hours, the FEV_1 had fallen significantly. After 4 additional hours of exposure, the mean fall from the initial value was 800 mL.

Phosgene

Exposure to phosgene gas is followed by the development of pulmonary edema, often after a latent period of several hours.[1] No new cases have been reported over the past 12 years, as far as we know.

Ozone

The effects of oxone, a very irritant gas, were discussed in Chapter 6. Accidental high exposure, which may occur in plants using ozone for water purification or where ultraviolet light sterilization is used,[2157] causes pulmonary edema. It is not known whether recovery from such an episode is followed by restitution of normal lung function or not.[1]

Recent occupational exposures have been described in flight attendants, whose symptoms were very characteristic.[850] A bizarre episode in Hong Kong in an electric motor factory[4680] involved acute illness in 191 employees, following introduction of a new process. Levels of up to 1.6 ppm of ozone were recorded; 125 cases had to be admitted to the hospital with cough, severe dyspnea, and fever. Eleven per cent had crepitations, and 8% were hypoxemic. The authors considered that the effects were due to a combination of ozone and acid chloride aerosol, which was also present.

Hydrogen Sulfide

In high concentration, hydrogen sulfide gas is an acute central nervous system poison. Communities in proximity to plants treating natural gas may be exposed to low levels over a considerable period of time. This has been reported to cause general symptoms of malaise, headache, nausea, and eye irritation, but chronic respiratory effects have not been documented.

Hydrocarbons, Gasoline, Kerosene, and Oil Mists

The acute danger of gasoline fumes was noted in the previous edition.[1] Benzol is also acutely toxic.[2138] In several specialized industries, workers are exposed to oil mists. Pulmonary function studies of such employees did not reveal evidence of adverse effects,[2140] though in one case in a steel-rolling mill, pulmonary granulomas might have resulted from such exposure.[2256] In underground mines, workers may be exposed to diesel fumes, as noted above; but although these may be related to lung cancer incidence,[2180] there is no clear evidence that they cause increased chronic respiratory disease. Coke oven workers are exposed to polycyclic hydrocarbons, and they are at a considerably increased risk of lung cancer.[2468] There is evidence that this exposure leads to increased bronchitis and a lowered FEV_1, with the effect being greater in cigarette-smoking workers exposed to these fumes.[2193]

Kerosene may cause a chronic paraffin pneumonitis, and one case had severe respiratory impairment; autopsy findings were reported.[2486] Acutely, it may denature pulmonary surfactant and cause patchy atelectasis and edema.

Miscellaneous Substances

Chloromethyl Ether. Chloromethyl ether exposure is associated with an increased lung cancer risk, and in a study of 103 exposed workers, of whom 72 had been exposed for some years,[2483] lowered expiratory flow rates were associated with length of exposure. FEF_{25-75} values were reported, and these were less than 60% of predicted in one-third of the exposed men, compared with the same abnormality in only 3% of unexposed workers.

Trimellitic Anhydride. Trimellitic anhydride is formed from trimellitic acid, which is 1,2,4-benzenetricarboxylic acid, used in the preparation of adhesives, dyes, inks, and resins. Seven young men developed acute pulmonary hemorrhage and edema from inhaling this chemical, with acute reductions in VC, DL_{CO} and Pa_{O_2}.[2511] Follow-up studies indicated that complete recovery occurred. It is believed that acute alveolar wall injury occurs, with hypertrophy of type II cells. Recent longitudinal data of workers exposed to this substance[3689] indicated that respiratory symptoms were common and that high levels of IgE antibody could be demonstrated in those with rhinitis or asthma. No detailed pulmonary function tests were reported. McGrath and colleagues[4509] recently summarized the various syndromes that this substance may cause and mention adverse long-term effects but do not give details.

Hydrogen Selenide. Hydrogen selenide is used in the preparation of semiconductor materials. A non-smoker exposed to this dangerous material developed a severe cough and had a pneumomediastinum and subcutaneous emphysema,[2273] but the chest x-ray did not show any interstitial change. Acutely, the arterial Pa_{O_2} was 69 mm Hg, and the following function test changes were noted:

	Predicted	Day 1	Day 5	Day 30	3 years later
FVC	4.65	2.00	2.50	3.80	4.20
FEV_1	3.86	0.90	1.50	3.20	3.20
TLC	6.14	3.33	—	4.91	5.04
$V_{50\%}$TLC (L/sec)	5.98	0.40	1.00	3.80	3.00

Aerosols. Aerosols have been noted to affect

pulmonary function in high concentrations, particularly those containing starch and soil repellents.[530] Hair sprays have similar effects.[2309] A recent case attributable to hair spray occurred in a 66-year-old woman who developed diffuse interstitial fibrosis.[3575] NMR analysis of lung tissue identified the presence of the laquering agent (8-copolymer-maleic anhydride-butylic alcohol) in the lung tissue. Her TLC was 52% of predicted; P_{st} was -51 cm H_2O; and $DL_{CO}SB$ was 47% of predicted. Freon, which may be the carrier gas, is without effect on the lung.[2309]

Complex Mixtures. A few reports of effects of complex mixtures have appeared. In one remarkable case from Alberta,[2245] exposure to chlorine, hydrogen sulfide, and methane in an oil rig worker led to diffuse parenchymal lung disease with pulmonary infiltrates. After this, the lung slowly became hyperinflated and emphysema developed, with disrupted alveoli and hemosiderin-laden macrophages on lung biopsy. The pattern of function test changes was as follows:

	Predicted	Sept. 1972	March 1983
VC	5.0	5.1	4.1*
FEV$_1$	4.1	2.9	1.4
FEF$_{25-75}$	5.3	1.4	0.5
RV	2.3	2.6	4.9
TLC	7.3	7.7	9.0
P$_{st}$max	>20	34	11
Coefficient of retraction	3–5	4.4	1.2
Pa$_{O_2}$ (mm Hg)	>75	48	38

*This would represent a decline of -91 mL/year.

This man had smoked a pack of cigarettes a day for 25 years and had a normal alpha$_1$-antitrypsin level.

Exposure to mixtures of mustard gas, lewisite, phosgene, and hydrogen cyanide in Japan led to a high incidence of chronic respiratory tract symptoms, with considerable sputum production and lowered values for FEV$_1$ and $DL_{CO}SB$.[2287]

Alkyl Benzene Sulfonate. Alkyl benzene sulfonate[4621] used in a detergent factory produced significant shift falls in FEV$_1$ and respiratory tract symptoms. It was not clear whether there were any long-term adverse effects.

SMOKE INHALATION AND BURN EFFECTS

In fires, firefighters and victims are exposed to a wide variety of substances in addition to the smoke. Of these, oxides of nitrogen and carbon monoxide are commonly encountered, but the list of toxic chemicals produced in fires is a long one.[2262] A number of reports have dealt with the effects of smoke inhalation on firefighters and others.[2270] In observations of 39 firefighters,[2236] 137 observations showed a mean FEV decline of 50 mL after an episode of firefighting, with decreases in excess of 100 milliliters recorded on about a third of the occasions. In another 30 firefighters, there were no differences in FEV$_1$ after a severe episode and 2 to 18 months later. Transient exposure to dense smoke containing polyvinyl chloride and other irritants[2262] led to transient hypoxemia in 19 of 21 firefighters studied; 2 to 10 hours after the exposure, their mean Pa$_{O_2}$ was 64 ± 7 mm Hg, and 20 hours later it was 88 ± 7 mm Hg. One month after this exposure, there was no evidence of ventilatory impairment.[2263]

Studies of 54 firefighters, 32 smokers and 22 non-smokers,[2271] showed evidence of small airway changes in the non-smokers with more than 25 years at the job; in one man trapped in a fire, whose carboxyhemoglobin was measured at 42%, severe ventilatory defect persisted for 2½ years after the fire, and he developed saccular bronchiectasis with a normal $DL_{CO}SB$. In this study, the cigarette-smoking firefighters were not different from the smoking population as a whole.[2271] Detailed studies have been reported on 1768 Boston firefighters.[2292, 2295, 2296] Exposures were followed by increased mucus secretion and depression of ventilatory data. The data showed that "the firefighter incurred an increased risk of disease due to his occupation and cigarette smoking." A 5-year longitudinal study of 168 Boston firefighters (FF) compared with 2280 men enrolled in a study of aging in the same city[3687] revealed the following comparative data:

	Number	Annual Declines FVC (mL)	(SE) (±)	FEV$_1$ (mL)	(SE) (±)
Never smokers					
FF	50	-76.9	10.7	-81.2	19.2
Controls	447	-71.3	4.1	-64.1	3.9
Former smokers					
FF	47	-86.7	9.4	-68.2	8.7
Controls	484	-77.1	3.9	-62.8	3.7
Current smokers					
FF	71	-109.9	11.2	-77.9	8.5
Controls	543	-76.8	3.8	-65.2	3.2

The reasons for the fast rate of decline in the control group of non-smokers were not clear; but in all groups, the firefighters had a faster rate than the controls. Another longitudinal study of 1006 London firefighters[4667] had apparently shown accelerated declines of FVC over a period of a year. This was ascribed to faulty instrumentation, but it might have been because the interval was too short for reliable longitudinal data. This may be a difficult population to study longitudinally (like asthmatics), as on a single follow-up visit data may be influenced by a transient decline.

It has recently been reported that lung permeability may be increased in fire-fighters.[4679]

A 25-year-old non-smoker fighting a fire in a plastics factory[3742] had severe bronchiolitis on lung biopsy. At the time he was first tested, his FEF_{25-75} was 14% of predicted, and FEV_1 16% of predicted. The residual volume was twice normal. The DL_{CO}/VA ratio was normal, but his Pa_{O_2} was 53 mm Hg. Eleven people were involved in a factory explosion in which the smoke contained hydrogen chloride, phosphorus oxychloride and pentachloride, oxalyl chloride, and oxalic acid.[2267] Of these, nine had respiratory effects, which cleared rapidly in six. In one case, however, the tests were not normal for 4 weeks; in another, for 10 weeks. In one case, tests were still abnormal 2 years later, when dyspnea was still present, and there were rales in the lungs. The DL_{CO} was reduced on exercise (though normal at rest), the VC was 80% of predicted, and the residual volume was elevated.

A 26-year-old non-smoker who had no previous respiratory symptoms and who was caught in an apartment fire[2268] showed the following pattern of changes:

	Number of Weeks After Prednisone Treatment		
	12	24	32
FEV_1 (%P)	20	28	34
FVC (%P)	35	47	54
RV (liters)	4.3	3.3	4.9
TLC (liters)	6.3	6.4	8.2
$DL_{CO}SB$ (mL/CO/min/mm Hg)	16.6	21.3	28.7
Pa_{O_2} (mm Hg)	64	82	84

It seems clear that residual airway damage was present, probably without much associated alveolar pathology.

Exposure to aluminum fluoride or sulfate has led to occupational asthma in a group of workers in Sweden.[4644]

Burn Effects

A recent report on 42 burn patients[5411] stressed the importance of upper airway lesions.

Eighteen of the cases had abnormal inspiratory flow curves consistent with extrathoracic obstruction, and 12 had abnormal expiratory flow curves. These were related to structural changes observed during nasopharyngoscopy, and the authors concluded that flow curves were useful in the detection of upper airway lesions in these cases. In some cases, laryngeal edema may be so severe that a tracheostomy is required.[5408]

Pruitt and colleagues reporting on 697 cases[5409] noted that the occurrence of pulmonary complications was reduced from 33% to 24% by the use of topical chemotherapy. Pulmonary edema up to 5 days after admission occurred in 7%, and atelectasis in 3%. In 3.6% of all admissions, pneumonia was the primary cause of death.

Whitener and colleagues[5410] studied 28 cases in detail, dividing them into groups with smoke inhalation alone, with surface burns alone, or with both. All cases were studied at 9 hours, 22 hours, 58 hours, 11.5 days, and 5 months after the episode. In the smoke inhalation cases, the FEF_{25-75} was reduced to 25% of the predicted value at 22 hours, and it had only risen to 60% of predicted a month later. Those with both surface burns and smoke inhalation had the most severe defects of function, with early development of a restrictive defect in spite of a normal pulmonary capillary wedge pressure. The management of these cases may be complicated by the additional consequences of acute exposure to carbon monoxide. This may lead to significant metabolic acidosis due to lactic acid accumulation and may be detected by a widening of the anion gap (as noted in Chapter 23).

SPECIAL WORKING ENVIRONMENTS

In several working environments, exposures are multiple, and the data cannot be described under headings related to only one agent.

Welding

Welders are exposed to a wide variety of gases, including ozone, and to the fumes of many metals. Zinc fume fever is commonly recognized by them, but vanadium, manganese, and many other substances are encountered, particularly if scrap metal is being cut. A survey of 209 arc welders and comparison with 109 controls[2122] showed evidence of differences from controls in FEV_1 of 200 milliliters in smokers and 350 milliliters in non-smokers. Another review of 119 welders and 90 controls[2371] matched for age, height, and smoking history showed that there were significantly more respiratory symptoms in the welders and a slight elevation in both closing volume and closing capacity. The authors suggested that the effects were due to deposition of small particles in small airways. The particle sizes commonly encountered were very small, between 0.01 microns and 1 micron. In the previous edition of this book, we recorded data on a welder who had 15 years of exposure and in whom a micronodular pattern of radiologic change was accompanied by significant lowering of FEF_{25-75} but normal exercise diffusing capacity.[1] In another cross-sectional study of 30 controls, 30 welders, 30 coal miners, and 22 foundry workers, the foundry workers were the most abnormal. The welders had a slight increase in exercise ventilation and a slight increase in physiologic VD, probably indicating $\dot{V}/\dot{Q}$ abnormality of mild degree.[2346] In one longitudinal study comparison over a 6-year interval between 29 welders, 22 men with coal worker's pneumoconiosis, and 13 men with silicosis, the rate of decline of FEV_1 was lower in the welders than the coal workers and not increased above normal.[2349]

A recent detailed study of 83 stainless steel welders and 29 mild steel welders[3722] indicated that decrements in flow rates and possibly in DL_{CO} occurred in relation to length of exposure to manual metal-arc welding, which is a relatively high-fume process. The authors thought that this type of welding might result in small airway changes.

Other comparisons between arc welders and controls from the same plant but not welding show a high level of respiratory symptoms in both groups, but no major function test differences between them.[3746]

A comparison between 258 welders and age-matched controls[4517] showed no differences in pulmonary function, but more respiratory symptoms and work absences for respiratory infections in the welders. In a subset of 186 of the welders, however, there were significant differences in the lower part of the MEFV curves between the welders and controls with the same smoking history. Non-smoking welders were not abnormal in this respect.

A comparison between 64 aluminum welders, 46 stainless steel welders, and 149 railroad track welders in Sweden,[4686] all with more than 2 years exposure, compared with a referent group of non-welding railroad and industrial workers, showed that respiratory symptoms were more common in the welders. In aluminum welders, the symptoms appeared to be related to ozone exposure; in other groups, possibly to chromium exposure.

The data therefore indicate that as a whole welders are not more severely impaired than other groups, though respiratory symptoms are more common. However, it is very important that the physician should be aware that severe lung damage may on occasion follow exposures, as shown by individual case reports.

In one 51-year-old man with 16 years of exposure,[2389] the VC was 73% of predicted, and $DL_{CO}SB$ only 38% of predicted normal. The lung biopsy showed an alveolitis with fibrosis and many intraluminal histiocytes. The same report[2389] also described a significantly lowered DL_{CO} (43% of predicted) and a fall in Pa_{O_2} from rest to exercise from 82 mm Hg to 67 mm Hg in another welder. The smoking history of these men was not noted, but there was no sputum, although in the second case, the FEV_1 was only 66% of predicted. Detailed analysis of the metal content of the lung in a 55-year-old welder who was exposed for 18 years and whose x-ray showed extensive interstitial fibrosis revealed a high content of cobalt, iron, chromium, and nickel.[2340]

The occurrence of severe disease in an aluminum welder working in the confined spaces of boat hulls[3748] has already been noted.

Cement Industry

There have been a number of studies of cement workers, some[2350] indicating no differences from other workers and others indicating an excess of respiratory tract symptoms.[2324] In one comparison between 39 non-smoking cement workers and 23 non-smoking controls, the cement workers had significantly lower FEF_{25-75} values,[2342] indicating either a loss of recoil or small airway dysfunction. The FEV_1/FVC ratio was also noted to be lower in cement workers in one study.[2325] A detailed comparison between 301 cement factory workers, 649 blue collar workers, 218 white collar workers, and 102 farmers[4729] found no evidence of worse pulmonary function in the cement workers.

Longitudinal studies of cement workers have been inconclusive, but the standard mortality ratio for respiratory disease is not increased.[4564] Asbestos-cement pipe manufacture may involve concomitant asbestos exposure.

Rubber Industry

A detailed series of studies of rubber plant workers by physicians in the occupational health program at the Harvard School of Public Health[2366–2369] showed that FEV_1 values were significantly lowered in workers in the curing plant, and shift decrements of 115 milliliters in FEV_1 were noted. In the processing area, chronic cough and decrements in FEV_1 were related to length of exposure.

Rubber workers are also exposed to talc (see previous section) in the curing process, and this may relate to respiratory impairment and disability in these workers.[2471] In 1975, doPico and colleagues[2536] described a remarkable epidemic of an influenza-like illness in 210 rubber workers after the introduction of a new thermosetting resin into the process. Pneumonic infiltrates on chest x-ray occurred in a quarter of the cases, and abnormal diffusing capacities and ventilatory data were found in more than a third of the workers tested. Lung biopsy showed focal interstitial fibrosis and a chronic inflammatory reaction. In one case, resolution did not occur, and there was permanent disability. The chemical agent responsible was not identified.

Pulp and Paper Industry

Workers in the pulp and paper industry are exposed to sulfur dioxide and chlorine, usually episodically. Studies do not show evidence of chronic differences in function,[2478] and a recent study of a large plant in British Columbia in which gas concentrations were relatively low showed little evidence of chronic impairment.[2382] A 10-year follow-up of 659 workers found an average rate of decline of FEV_1 of -37 mL/year in non-smokers, rising to -49 mL/year in smokers in this industry.[2380] Ferris, Puleo, and Chen[2238] noted FEV_1 declines within the expected range in another 10-year follow-up of pulp and paper workers, with no evidence of excessive mortality or morbidity. It therefore appears that in general the levels of exposure in this industry do not lead to excessive rates of FEV_1 decline, though of course individual workers may be adversely affected by episodic

exposures to high concentrations of chlorine or sulfur dioxide.[1]

Enarson and colleagues[4639] recently reported that 392 pulp mill workers had more wheezing, chest tightness, and missed work due to respiratory tract illness than occurred in 310 rail yard workers. Lower FEV_1 values were found in those working in the bleach plant of the mill, and pulp mill maintenance workers had lower FVC values than comparable rail yard workers.

A survey of a population of 2374 individuals living near a sulfite pulp factory in Sweden[4646] found no evidence of an increase in chronic bronchitis compared with other populations. Employment at the factory did carry an increased risk, however.

Inorganic Chemicals

Sodium sulfate exposure does not affect the FEV_1.[2168] However, workers exposed to high levels of copper sulfate in agricultural spraying in Portugal show a diffuse interstitial fibrosis with characteristic granulomas in the lungs.[2297] Detailed pulmonary function test surveys of these workers have not been reported.

Printing Industry

An unusual episode of work-related wheezing, chest tightness, and breathlessness in 35 printers led to two hourly records of PEFR being kept for 2 weeks.[5102] Fifteen of the workers had consistent work-related decreases. This asthma was later shown to be due to something (not identified) in a humidifier in the plant and was not attributable to materials they were handling.

Glassblowing

Glassblowers complain of excess coughing and wheezing, but there is little evidence of excessive decline of vital capacity or FEV_1.[2175]

Brass Instruments

Chest physicians and respiratory physiologists who play brass instruments will be encouraged to note that larger vital capacities, residual volumes, total lung capacities, and expiratory flow rates were found in 45 young men who played brass instruments,[2320] with very high-peak intraoral pressures. They will be less encouraged to read that cardiac arrhythmias during instrument playing were commonly noted in these musicians, premature atrial and ventricular contractions occurring predominantly in inspiration.

High-Pressure Environments

Although deep-sea diving is associated with a high mortality, the increased work of breathing results in a higher than predicted FVC and FEV_1, each being increased about 20% over predicted values in 404 North Sea divers.[2225] Caisson disease still occurs.[2139] An episode involving several workers was reported from Egypt.[2192]

A first longitudinal study of divers[7872] showed that in 224 men so employed, the mean fall in FVC was -68.5 mL/year over a 3.5-year interval. Fifty-seven non-smokers in the group had an average fall of -69.4 mL/year. The significance of these high values (more than three times what would have been predicted) is unclear. Physiologic aspects of diving were considered in Chapter 2.

CHRONIC BRONCHITIS AND OCCUPATIONAL LUNG DISEASE

From the previous sections, it is apparent that symptoms of chronic mucus hypersecretion are common in a variety of occupational settings. Epidemiologic studies reveal that these symptoms occur in a higher fraction of coal miners, textile workers, or workers exposed to wood dust or grain dust (to take a few examples) than in control populations. *Industrial bronchitis* is a term often used to refer to this syndrome.

Becklake has recently reviewed the data relating occupational exposures to chronic respiratory tract disease.[4659] She concluded that the answer to the question, "Can the exposures which men and women encounter in the course of their daily work eventually lead to chronic airflow limitation?" was affirmative. She continued, "There is no reason to suppose that the answer to the second part of the question, 'Can it be of a degree sufficiently severe to disable them for their occupation?' is not also in the affirmative." The review contained 83 references.

Smidt and Worth organized a major study of more than 13,000 workers from different regions of Germany, grouped as follows[2539]:

Number of Workers	Industry
3050	Ceramic, asbestos
3008	Foundry
2230	Coal mine; cement
1724	Foundry
1500	Machine factory
1450	Coal mine
985	Cement

The workers were divided into three types on the basis of symptoms and into three categories of function defect based on (1) airway resistance data, (2) FEV_1/FVC as per cent of predicted, and (3) resting Pa_{O_2} also expressed as per cent of predicted. The authors concluded from their analysis that the adverse effect of dust was evident in both smokers and non-smokers; that smoking more than 10 g of tobacco per day had a greater effect than the dust on symptoms and function defect; and that age had an important effect on both symptoms and function independent of dust exposure and smoking. Dust-exposed men between the ages of 20 and 35 years had a similar excess of bronchitis as moderate smokers. Single influences were additive. They also concluded that "it is not safe to state that smoking is more hazardous with respect to chronic bronchitis than occupational dust exposure, particularly in coal miners."[2539] Smidt[2540] also presented another analysis of the same data, with similar conclusions. Morgan[2234] noted that the British Medical Research Council in 1966 issued a Report of a Select Committee, which concluded that "occupationally induced bronchitis did not play a significant part in the aetiology of airways obstructed in dust-exposed men." His review of the data led him to the conclusion that although dust exposure caused chronic bronchitis, "unlike bronchitis induced by cigarette smoke, the predominant effect of industrial bronchitis is on large rather than small airways and the condition is not accompanied by emphysema." A comment by Brooks[2066] in which he indicated that dust alone rarely caused significant airway obstruction was noted previously.

Reviewing all the information in this chapter on this question, it seems to us that the data at the present time hardly permit a definitive conclusion. That chronic mucus hypersecretion, however caused, does not inevitably lead to emphysema has been stressed in Chapter 7. That dust exposure without tobacco smoke may lead to emphysema in some individuals cannot be ruled out, although it may be true that dust exposure without smoking less commonly leads to emphysema than does smoking without dust exposure. However, to teach that dust exposure alone does not cause significant functional impairment invites the kind of error of attributability that we have documented.[4498]

What seems to be needed is more data of every kind. In its absence, the question of defining precisely the role of dusts in the genesis of chronic mucus hypersecretion, small airway changes, and alveolar destruction seems impossible.

Evaluation of Dyspnea and Disability in Occupational Lung Disease

Most chest physicians at one time or another become involved in questions of assessment of disability and attributability, and they commonly find themselves enmeshed in complex arguments with little firm ground on which to stand. The following notes are intended for general guidance but do not constitute a comprehensive coverage of these complex issues.

Assessment of Functional Impairment

In most jurisdictions, some measurement of function impairment is required in cases of pulmonary disease thought to have been caused by occupation. The extent to which they are used and the thoroughness with which they are performed vary greatly between countries. To our knowledge, the assessment of function at this time seems most thorough in the European Economic Community, where exercise testing is routinely performed; very variable in North America as a whole; and not relied on in any rigorous way in Britain. Cotes[2335] wrote that "lung function tests are of great use in environmental medicine and for medical diagnosis and treatment; they can probably also make a useful contribution to assessment." He also indicated that in his view[2334] steady-state diffusing capacity measurements, FEF_{25-75}, and measurements of changes in dynamic compliance with frequency all were either obsolete, or superseded, or of limited usefulness. By contrast with this rather lukewarm endorsement of function testing, it seems to us that in most occupational cases, function testing is a necessity. We agree that the FEV_1 and FVC and $DL_{CO}SB$ tests are obligatory and are first choices. In some cases,

more difficult tests including measurements of gas exchange on exercise and of maximal exercise capability and even studies of lung mechanics may be required. In difficult cases, measurements that the individual cannot influence may be of special significance.

Table 16–1 is a suggested categorization of dyspnea severity, with the approximate correlated levels of FEV_1 as indicated by Cotes[2335] in brackets.

Table 16–2 is an abbreviated form of the table of assessment recommended by a Canadian Task Force on pneumoconiosis[2446] based on resting measurements of FEV_1 and $DL_{CO}SB$.

We cannot attempt here to present a complete review of exercise testing. In sections on chronic airflow limitation, diffuse interstitial fibrosis, and elsewhere in this chapter, we have indicated the results of exercise studies in a variety of conditions. Jones and Campbell's excellent text on clinical exercise testing[2445] sets out in detail a precise protocol for exercise tests of increasing complexity and provides invaluable guidance on their interpretation. In the assessment of disability, as opposed to their use in differential diagnosis, the following comments seem to us to be important:

1. Submaximal exercise testing is the preferred mode, with a standardized incremental protocol. However, there are still considerable variations in methods used.[2336]

2. It seems clear that exercise capability cannot be accurately predicted from resting data, though severe airflow limitation is accompanied by reduced maximal oxygen uptake, and dys-

Table 16–1. CLASSIFICATION OF DYSPNEA

Activity Level	Dyspnea Grade	Approximate FEV_1 (liters)
Can hurry on level ground and walk uphill	0–1	3.1
Can walk at normal pace on level ground	2	2.6
Can walk unlimited distance at slow pace	3	2.1
Can walk about 400 meters	4	1.6
Can walk 100 meters, sing, or climb 8 stairs	5	1.1
Can converse, walk 10 meters, bathe with help	6	0.7
Can dress and sit out of bed with help	7	0.5
Needs help with feeding	8	<0.3

Modified with permission from Bull. Physiopathol. Respir., vol. 11, Cotes, J. E. Assessment of disablement due to impaired respiratory function. Copyright 1975, Pergamon Press plc.

Table 16–2. CLASSIFICATION OF IMPAIRMENT

Function Test Data	Grades of Dsypnea (see Table 16–1)									
	0–1		2–3		3–4		5–6		>6	
	O	R	O	R	O	R	O	R	O	R
FVC (%P)	N	N	N	>60	^	40–60	^	<40	^	<20
FEV$_1$ (%P)	N	N	>60	^	40–60	^	<40	^	<20	
DL$_{CO}$ (%P)	N	N	>75	<75	>50	<60	<60	<40	<50	<40
V̇max$_{O_2}$ (mL/min/kg)	>25	>25	<25	<25	<15	<15	<7	<7	<7	<7
Rest Pa$_{O_2}$ (mm Hg)	N	N	N	N‡	>60	>60‡	>60	>60‡	<50	<50
Rest Pa$_{CO_2}$ (mm Hg)	N	N	N	N	<45	<45	40–50	<40	40–60	<40

Key: O = Obstructive syndromes; R = Restrictive syndromes.
  N = Normal.
  ‡ = Often falls on exercise.
  ^ = Too variable to specify.
Modified with permission from Ostiguy, G. L. Summary of task force report on occupational respiratory disease (pneumoconiosis). Can. Med. Assoc. J. 121:414–421, 1979.

pnea occurs as the requirement for ventilation approaches capacity.[2537] Others have noted that dyspnea on exercise occurs when tidal volume per centimeter of esophageal pressure change falls below 0.08,[2496] though this method of measurement could not be generally applied.

Epler and colleagues documented the fact that clinical and radiologic data were inadequate in defining impairment[2477] and made a valuable critical assessment of different criteria of disability in relation to function test change. A study of 277 cases of industrial lung disease[2474] showed the considerable scatter between level of dyspnea and ventilatory measurements at rest. It seems probable that two factors are responsible for this poor correlation. First, exercise may be limited by the impending onset of respiratory muscle fatigue,[2070, 2516] and this is only loosely related to ventilatory data. Second, a significant number of middle-aged men may well have exercise pulmonary hypertension (with consequent dyspnea) as a result of left ventricular inadequacy—a point stressed in Chapter 12 and based on studies of men who were not in heart failure and who had made a normal recovery from a myocardial infarct a few months before.[1728]

3. The research group in Nancy has recently studied maximal oxygen uptake capability in 43 cases of silicosis requesting compensation, measuring this parameter on two separate days.[2522] They found a very close correlation between the maximal V$_{O_2}$ on the two occasions, the "r" value being 0.972. Such repeatability could not occur by intent.

4. Cotes[2335] found a different relationship between FEV$_1$ and alleged dyspnea in coal workers seen for compensation, on the one hand, and those studied for research purposes, on the other. Morgan[2188] quoted these data in an editorial rather less censorious than its title (Disability or Disinclination?) would indicate and suggested that such disparity probably commonly occurred. By contrast, Rubinfeld and Pain recently repeated this study in Melbourne[2520] and did not find evidence of disparity between FEV$_1$ and dyspnea level as between compensation claimants and a population of hospital patients. It is clear that conclusions of this kind cannot be generalized between populations, let alone assumed to be operative in every individual case, without serious risk of error. The mechanism of dyspnea is still poorly defined,* but its assessment in experimental subjects can be successfully graded by the use of a serial visual analogue scale.[2339] The distance walked can also be used as a test of dyspnea level, and in one study of 44 cases of chronic airflow limitation and 18 cases with diffuse interstitial fibrosis,[2521] this was noted to be better correlated with the FVC than with the FEV$_1$. These tests were successfully used to show that oxygen breathing relieved dyspnea in cases of chronic airflow limitation even when there was no initial hypoxemia (see Chapter 8[1004]).

In view of these data, it seems evident to us that factors causing excessive dyspnea in cases of industrial lung disease are very complex. Excessive exercise ventilation occasioned by a widened $(A-a)$ D$_{O_2}$, early onset of respiratory

*See references 2337, 2338, 2524, 2537.

muscle fatigue on account of increased respiratory work and decreased efficiency due to an increased residual volume, and precipitated by hypoxemia—these interacting factors probably explain a lower exercise capability in relation to a simple measurement like the FEV_1 in some cases compared with others. Disinclination may be present, but it cannot be assumed unless the other factors have been ruled out. In addition, we think that in many individuals, excess exercise ventilation may be amplified by pulmonary hypertension consequent on unrecognized left ventricular inadequacy.

Smidt and Worth[2515] summarized their experience of ergometric measurements in more than 3000 subjects in 1976 and concluded that "an increased specific ventilation besides an increase of airway resistance is an important measure for an increased work of breathing, which is sensitized as dyspnea. However, pulmonary dyspnea may be caused also by pulmonary hypertension, so that in a single patient we have to apply all necessary methods to understand the causes of his dyspnea." Their work underlines the importance of measurements of gas exchange during exercise in disability assessment.

Worker's Compensation Evaluation

Discussions of Worker's Compensation legislation and administration in different jurisdictions provide examples of different social and political traditions applied to similar problems. Policy in Britain,[2277, 2517, 2519] West Germany,[2311] and the United States[2330, 2333, 2476] and general discussions of the problems* may be consulted by those interested in these questions. In one analysis of general safety improvement over the past 50 years, it was noted that home fatalities in the United States fell from 22 per 100,000 per year in 1930, to 13 per 100,000 per year in 1970.[2134] The authors concluded that general factors, as well as the possible influence of Worker's Compensation legislation, should be credited with a decrease in on-the-job fatalities over the same period.

Questions of attributability that the chest physician confronts are very complex. An editorial in the British Medical Journal in 1981 noted[2518]

In clinical practice, patients disabled by chronic bronchitis who have never been smokers are extremely rare. Talk of occupational bronchitis, as

though occupation were the sole cause of the potentially disabling or fatal disease, in an individual, is misleading. Claims that exposure to dust does not contribute to the disease are, however, equally false, since there is good evidence in the coal industry of relations between measured dust exposure and symptoms, impairment of lung function, and mortality from chronic bronchitis. To disentangle the relative effects of dust and cigarettes in causing the disease is difficult epidemiologically and impossible in the individual exposed to both; nevertheless, both have played their part—at least in the past.

An editorial in 1970 in the same journal[2017] addressing the same question stated

Assessing the degree of a miner's disability is difficult; allotting the proportion of this disability between pneumoconiosis, chronic bronchitis, and emphysema is more difficult; but deciding what share of the chronic bronchitis or the emphysema or both together is due to mining, and what is due to the rest of the miner's environment is an almost impossible undertaking. Yet this is what equitable compensation of the miner requires.

In these questions, the chest physician should, in our view, keep in mind the following generalities:

1. The imprecision of the relationship between impairment and dyspnea, but the necessity for objective assessment of impairment.

2. Decisions of compensation policy are social decisions, and the medical profession may participate in these but must not claim sole competent input into them. We have commented elsewhere[2195] on the "statistics of equity" that underlie such social decisions.

3. The chest physician can summarize the probable relationship between occupational exposure, radiologic change, and function defect in individual cases. Such opinions are no more than opinions, and though they may be influenced by pulmonary function data or radiologic findings, the physician should not speak as if talking with a "scientific authority" that the scientific base of the data would hardly support.

4. The importance of autopsy data in cases in which compensation has been refused during life should be known to the physician and emphasized to claimants and their families. The responsibility of physicians to their patients in this situation extends beyond the life span of the patients.

5. Death of industrial workers may be accelerated but not caused directly by their condi-

---

*See references 2195, 2331, 2332, 2538.

tion. In one study over a 7-year period of coal miners and slate workers receiving industrial compensation in Britain,[2135] 10% of the deaths of the miners and 40% of the deaths of the slate workers were considered to have been accelerated by their disease. We have noted the continued accelerated decline of FEV_1 after retirement from the industry in French coal miners. The same phenomenon has been documented to occur in cases of silicosis. This means that careful follow-up is mandatory. Single payments at one point in time to those who have been adversely affected by dust are probably inequitable.

Interactions of Causative Agents

Occupational lung disease provides many examples of the effect of multiple factors on disease causation. The strongest interaction is between cigarette smoking and dusts encountered in the workplace. Saracci,[2541] in an interesting essay on this question, has pointed out the problem of defining how much disease can be attributed to which factor. He illustrated the point by reference to the interaction of smoking and asbestos exposure in causing excess lung cancer. These data, which are based on very large numbers of subjects, are summarized as follows:

Exposure Group	Death Rate (1)	Excess Rate (2)	% Excess Rate Removable by Eliminating	
			Smoking (3)	Asbestos (4)
A− S−	11.3	0.0	—	—
A+ S−	58.4	47.1	—	100.0
A− S+	122.6	111.3	100.0	—
A+ S+	601.6	590.3	92.0	81.2

The excess rate is expressed per 100,000 person-years. The excess rate in those exposed only to asbestos is 47.1, but it is 590.3, or 12.5 times greater, in the group exposed to both agents. Saracci notes,

Should the analysis stop here, the conclusion would almost automatically follow that in a situation as that portrayed by the death rates in column (1), smoking is by far the dominant factor and its removal is, correspondingly, by far more effective as a preventive measure than asbestos removal. That things are not so simple is indicated by the figures in columns (3) and (4). If smoking is removed, the excess rate will go down from 590.3 to 47.1, i.e., some 543 lives will be saved (per 100,000 person-years) or 92% of the excess rate will be removed. If, on the other hand, asbestos is removed, the excess rate will go down from 590.3 to 111.3, i.e., 479 lives will be saved, or 81.2% of the excess rate will be removed. This means that removal of smoking is more effective than removal of asbestos, but only 1.14 times (543/479) and not 12.5 times as it superficially appeared.

This analysis is important. Its principles apply to all interactions that are multiplicative. It is not known, however, to what extent this applies to other interactions such as between air pollution and smoking, or cotton dust and smoking. Unfortunately we do not have such precise data for many of these situations as we have for asbestos and smoking. Nor is mortality necessarily the correct end point, making quantitation very difficult.

The definition of risk in precise mathematical terms has become an important field of study; an excellent example of recent methods applied to a serious health concern is the detailed calculation of risk of environmental exposure to asbestos, published by the National Academy of Science,[3601] though the risk estimates of cancer have since had to be revised.[4496]

Relative risks and absolute risks are computed as follows:

	Dead	Alive	Total
Exposed	a	b	a + b
Not exposed	c	d	c + d
Total	a + c	b + d	n

If P1 = a/a + b, and PO = c/c + d, relative risk = P1/PO and, absolute risk = P1 − PO.

This example would apply to a cohort study. If a case-control study of a rare disease is being conducted, the odds ratio (a × d/c × b) gives a better index of the relative risk.

MALIGNANT DISEASE: LUNG RESECTION

EFFECT OF RESECTIONAL SURGERY AND THORACOTOMY ON PULMONARY FUNCTION

Thoracotomy without lung resection has a measurable effect on lung function. Observations on 14 such patients showed that the Pa_{O_2} fell an average of 28% in the immediate postoperative period, but it slowly rose after 48 hours.[2553] All of these patients had a normal preoperative value, and the FEV_1 values varied from 1.35 to 3.2 liters. The maximal cough pressure was measured in 24 patients after thoracotomy with lung resections and was found to be reduced by half for a week after the surgical procedure.[967] Pain was considered to be the most important inhibitor.

Lobectomy

Lobectomy is followed by expected reductions in total lung capacity and vital capacity. In one series,[2547] these fell from 7.1 to 6.2 liters and from 4.1 to 3.7 liters, respectively. The maximal negative intraesophageal pressure rises slightly after lobectomy. In another series in which 37 patients had preoperative and postoperative measurements of pulmonary artery pressure,[2596] the intraesophageal pressure increased after lobectomy from a mean of 29.9 mm Hg to a mean of 35.7 mm Hg. In 227

lobectomies and 169 pneumonectomies in Oslo,[2584] the 30-day postoperative mortality rate was 3% after lobectomy and 11% after pneumonectomy.

Pneumonectomy

After pneumonectomy,* regional measurements of ventilation and perfusion distribution in the remaining lung are unchanged from that measured in the same lung preoperatively.[2550] In patients whose FEV/FVC ratio was >70% preoperatively, pneumonectomy was followed by a 25.8% fall in FEV_1, but a small increase in DL_{CO} and in Pa_{O_2} were noted.[2551] In patients whose FEV/FVC ratio was <70% preoperatively, FEV_1 fell 28.6%, and DL_{CO} fell 8.4%. Studies of diaphragm excursion after pneumonectomy, compared with vital capacity measurements, suggested that the increased tidal volume on exercise must have been attained by use of muscles other than the diaphragm.[2580] Function appears to be good after a surgical procedure to move the diaphragm upward after resectional surgery.[2555] Pneumonectomy is followed by an increase in pulmonary arterial pressure. Resting pulmonary arterial pressure increased from a mean of 32.3 mm Hg to a

---

*An excellent account of undergoing a pneumonectomy, written by an exceptionally articulate patient,[4793] should be read by all those caring for such individuals.

mean of 37.2 mm Hg after pneumonectomy in one series of patients.[2596]

Several interesting individual cases have been reported in the last few years. In one patient with severe pleural and parenchymal disease from old tuberculosis, pneumonectomy was followed by an increase in Pa_{O_2} from 50 mm Hg to 81 mm Hg, but the vital capacity increased only from 1.16 to 1.42 liters.[2575] Pneumonectomy in a 61-year-old man was followed by an unexpectedly low arterial tension of 40 mm Hg when sitting,[137] with marked postural changes. This was due to a patent foramen ovale. After that was successfully closed, normal arterial tensions were measured.

There have been two longitudinal studies of pulmonary function change after pneumonectomy.[2581, 4771] In one,[2581] the following data were reported. After pneumonectomy for tuberculosis, 78 patients of mean age 49 years were observed for 22 years. The average VC decline was only −10.3 mL/year. In 56 postpneumonectomies, mostly for lung cancer, the patients were of average age 61 and were observed for 11 years. The VC fall was −20 mL/year. In a comparison group, 81 patients with chronic obstructive pulmonary disease of mean age 54 were observed for 12 years. The VC decline was −29 mL/year.

In the other study,[4771] 123 pneumonectomy patients were studied in 1955 and 20 years later. VC had declined only at the rate of −4 mL/year, and the FEV_1 rate of decline was −5 mL/year. In the same group, the RV increased by +12 mL/year.

From these studies, it may be inferred that pneumonectomy does not cause a faster than expected rate of decline of vital capacity in the remaining lung. Pneumonectomy is no contraindication to pregnancy, and there were no obstetrical difficulties in 196 deliveries after pneumonectomy.[2598]

ESTIMATION OF POSTOPERATIVE FUNCTION FROM PREOPERATIVE MEASUREMENTS

During the past few years, considerable attention has been devoted to refining the preoperative assessment of patients before resectional surgery. Three editorials have addressed this question.[2554, 2565, 2602] In one series of 85 patients with lung cancer, all were studied preoperatively with ^{133}Xe ventilation scans and ^{99m}Tc-MAA perfusion scans.[2556] After lobectomy, the closest prediction of FEV_1 was given by multiplying the preoperative FEV_1 by the number of segments resected and dividing by the total segments. Close predictions were also given by the estimated regional function of the lobe to be resected. The best estimate was obtained when the regional function was predicted from the preoperative perfusion fraction. In this case, the relationship between preoperative predicted FEV_1 and postoperative measured FEV_1 was close (r = 0.95), both for lobectomy and pneumonectomy patients.

Others have also reported that a combination of preoperative FEV_1 and perfusion data is useful in predicting postoperative function.[4805] However, in a recent series of 36 patients, preoperative perfusion data was not considered useful in the evaluation.[4862] In another series, the preoperative FEV_1 was considered the most important measurement, and values below 2 liters were considered likely to be followed by difficulty.[2559] However, other authors consider that simple reliance on conventional tests is not adequate, and their series shows the importance of regional data in some patients.[2563] In one series of 13 patients with a mean FEV_1 of 1.9 liters and DL_{CO} of 14.0, all with moderately severe chronic airflow limitation, both regional perfusion measurements and preoperative function tests were used in the evaluation.[2568] Calculation of postoperative FEV_1 by multiplying the preoperative value by [1.22 − 0.048 × V], where V was the percentage ventilation of the lung to be resected, was successfully applied to 27 patients.[2564]

In another series of 33 patients, all with an FEV_1 of less than 2 liters, operations were carried out if the postoperative FEV_1 predicted from the perfusion scan and the preoperative FEV_1 were greater than 800 milliliters. In all these patients, successful resections were performed.[2566]

Regional ventilation measurements with ^{133}Xe in 44 lobectomy and 47 pneumonectomy patients were used to predict the postoperative FEV_1,[2569] with a subsequent r value between the predicted value and actual value of 0.83. In another series of 100 patients who were evaluated preoperatively with ^{133}Xe measurements, an r value of 0.83 was found between preoperative predicted FEV_1 and postoperatively measured values.[2596] Other authors report similar data, with successful resections in some patients with a preoperative FEV_1 as low as 1.3 liters.[2582]

In 23 patients older than 65 years, whose FEV_1 averaged 1.94 preoperatively, postoperative function was satisfactory.[2590] However, resection of more than one lobe if the FEV_1 is less than 1 liter is not advisable.[2591] Both differential function measurements and measurements of diffusing capacity are useful in evaluating these patients.[2591]

In attempting to predict postoperative function, either the ventilation or perfusion regional data can be successfully used, and a table for calculation of functional segments of lung from the measured perfusion fractions has been published.[2591] When bronchospirometric data was used, measurement of differential ventilation between the two lungs preoperatively was used to predict probable postoperative vital capacity.[2579]

In a series of papers based on over 200 patients,* Lockwood concluded that right pneumonectomy involved a higher risk than left. Adverse risk factors were an FEF_{25-75} below 1.2 L/sec, an RV >2.08 liters, a TLC >6.13 liters, and a delayed helium equilibration time. However, the prediction value of these indices seems inferior to that based on careful regional measurements. A "lateral position" test for measuring the increase in FRC when the patient moves from a supine to a lateral decubitus position has also been recommended for preoperative evaluation[2558, 2567, 4802] but is unlikely to be precise enough.

Exercise data have been used in preoperative evaluations, and a V_D/V_T ratio of greater than 43% on exercise was noted in patients with postoperative insufficiency.[2549] In 75 patients subjected to a graded exercise test,[2562] there were no postoperative respiratory problems in any who completed the test. In eight of 14 who could not complete it, there was respiratory insufficiency and dyspnea. The test consisted of treadmill walking for 4 minutes at 2 mph on a flat surface; for 2 minutes at 2.5 mph flat; for 2 minutes at 3 mph flat; and for 2 minutes at 3 mph on a 5 degree grade.[2562] Measurement of perfusion distribution by means of ^{133}Xe during seated exercise was also used to predict the postoperative FEV_1 (r = 0.95).[2588]

Colman and his colleagues[2604] have evaluated the use of exercise tests in 59 candidates for lung resection. Routine tests of function and a measurement of the maximal $\dot{V}O_2$ on exercise, together with a clinical assessment of dyspnea on climbing two flights of stairs in 15 seconds,

were compared with the incidence of postoperative complications. They concluded that the FEV_1 and FVC were related to the incidence of complications, whereas the measured maximal $\dot{V}O_2$ was not useful in predicting the occurrence of complications. The commonest complication was pneumonia, which occurred in 11 patients, followed by atelectasis in six and arrhythmias in five. Respiratory failure was noted to have occurred in three patients, but no details were given. The 12-minute walking test was not useful in preoperative assessment in a small series of 22 patients,[4794] but in another series of the same size[4785] the occurrence of postoperative complications was reported to be related to the preoperative maximal $\dot{V}O_2$.

Brundler, Chen, and Perruchoud[4840] reported on 637 consecutive patients with lung cancer undergoing right heart catheterization. Ninety-five had precapillary hypertension, 44 at rest and 51 on exercise only. In contrast, 276 patients had pulmonary hypertension secondary to abnormal left ventricular function, 67 at rest and 209 on exercise only. Discriminant analysis using the FEV_1, Pa_{O_2}, $DL_{CO}SS$ on exercise, and RV/TLC% yielded a qualitative prediction of precapillary pulmonary hypertension with a sensitivity of 95% and a specificity of 50%. The authors concluded that patients with a negligible risk of having an increased pulmonary arterial pressure could be identified by these noninvasive measurements.

Hirschler-Schulte, Hylkema, and Meyer[4833] have reported that 16 (4.4%) of 365 patients surgically treated for bronchial cancer required postoperative mechanical ventilation. Their FEV_1 values varied preoperatively from 36% of predicted to 60% of predicted. Four of the 16 patients were not recognized to be high-risk cases. In the remainder, a moderately increased risk had been recognized, but respiratory failure was related to largely unpredictable intraoperative or postoperative events.

The FEV_1 is undoubtedly useful as the first test to be done. If it is below about 60% of predicted, it may be advisable to recommend a more thorough evaluation. When it is reduced to 40% of predicted (after bronchodilator administration), regional ventilation and perfusion tests and an exercise evaluation should be undertaken before a pneumonectomy is performed. Macklem and his colleagues[2855] have reported a patient with severe dyspnea after pneumonectomy, probably ascribable to undiagnosed generalized small airway disease without a major reduction in FEV_1.

---

*See references 2593, 2594, 2599, 2601.

Recent studies from Sweden on the careful evaluation of the quality of survival after different forms of treatment for lung cancer in a large series of patients[2548, 2552] provide a necessary corrective for complacency.

PULMONARY FUNCTION IN SPECIFIC SYNDROMES OF MALIGNANT DISEASE OF THE LUNG

Positive Sputum Cytology and Normal Chest Films

Lindell and his colleagues[2587] reported on six consecutive patients with a normal chest x-ray and positive sputum cytology. Regional ventilation distribution was studied with ^{133}Xe. All six showed abnormalities outside the normal variation. In all six, cancers were located from these zones of decreased ventilation. Two of these were inoperable, and four were successfully resected. All patients had histories of hemoptysis.

Bronchial Adenoma, Alveolar Cell Carcinoma, Lymphangitic Carcinoma, and Lymphoma

Several interesting cases of intrabronchial obstruction, subsequently relieved by surgery, have appeared. One patient[2557] presented with a unilateral hyperlucent lung. There was gross reduction of perfusion to the left lung, of which the main bronchus was partially obstructed. The following function test data were reported:

	Predicted	Preoperative	Postoperative
VC	3.88	2.18	3.28
RV	1.73	0.84	1.28
TLC	5.61	3.03	4.57
$DL_{CO}SB$	29.2	20.6	28.9

Six months after the bronchial obstruction had been relieved, there was still very little flow to the left lung. A year after the surgery, it had returned to normal. A similar slow return of perfusion to the affected lung was also noted after removal of an intrabronchial carcinoid in the left upper lobe of another patient.[2577] Pulmonary function tests were as follows:

	Predicted	Pre-operative	After 14 Months
VC	3.6	2.02	3.59
RV, N_2 washout	1.4	0.61	1.36
body plethysmography		2.21	1.50
TLC, N_2 washout	5.0	2.63	4.95
FRC, N_2 washout	2.3	1.10	2.50
FEF_{25-75}	2.4	2.0	4.1
Pa_{O_2}, air	>80	86	91
DL_{CO}, exercise	26.0	13.0	19.0
C_{dyn}	0.23	0.13	0.21

A preoperative angiogram showed marked tapering of the left pulmonary artery. Normal perfusion returned after a year. Other cases illustrate the reduction in perfusion that follows lobar obstruction.[2585]

Although large clinical series of cases of alveolar cell carcinoma[2560] and lymphangitic carcinoma[2561] have been published, there is no note of accompanying pulmonary function data. Hence, it is not possible to state whether or not these conditions are associated with a characteristic pattern of function defect. As we have noted,[1] an early loss of diffusing capacity and a fall in compliance may characterize lymphangitic carcinoma. These defects are seen in extensive alveolar cell carcinoma, along with a lowered arterial oxygen tension.[1] In one case of alveolar cell carcinoma in a 64-year-old man,[2576] an arterial Pa_{O_2} of 21 mm Hg was recorded, probably due to veno-arterial shunting within the tumor.

It has recently been shown that poorly differentiated lymphoma of a centroblastic centrocytic type can involve the mucosae of major bronchi. In a 43-year-old woman[4872] who smoked 15 cigarettes/day, there was increasing dyspnea. The chest x-ray showed features consistent with emphysema. The FEV_1 at 2.1 liters was initially 77% of predicted, but it fell to 1.3 liters. The TL_{CO} was 45% of predicted. The flow volume loop suggested central obstruction, and at bronchoscopy, the mucosae of both main bronchi was thrown into folds, with the lumina narrowed to about one quarter of their normal diameter. Palliative radiotherapy was given, and the FEV_1 improved to 3.1 liters.

Fibroleiomyomatosis

Fibroleiomyomatosis consists of diffuse tumors arising from smooth muscle and connective tissue of the walls of airways or in the lung periphery, with solitary, multiple, or diffuse nodules of differing size and locations. In a 33-year-old man with this condition[2600] who had smoked 15 cigarettes/day for 15 years, there was no sputum, and the condition was diagnosed on biopsy of the lung. Function test data were as follows:

	Predicted	Measured
TLC	6.23	7.6
VC	4.67	4.5
RV	1.56	3.2
FEV_1	4.12	2.0
$\dot{V}max_{50\%}$	5.16	0.8
R_L	—	4.3
C_{st}	—	0.29
P_{st} (at 70% TLC)	—	2.5
$DL_{CO}SB$	32.1	8.2
Pa_{O_2}, rest	>80	69.3
exercise	>80	46.3
Pa_{CO_2}, rest	<42	40.3
exercise	<42	39.2
PAP, rest	<16	24.0
exercise	<20	37.0

This disease evidently is associated with a gross reduction in lung recoil, with no "restriction," but there are severe ventilatory flow abnormalities and gas exchange impairment.

Lymphangiomyomatosis

In the last edition of this book, we described a case of pulmonary lymphangiomyomatosis in a 37-year-old woman.[1] We noted the unusual pattern of function defect, which included a loss of recoil, severe ventilatory abnormality, and marked reduction in diffusing capacity. In 1977, Carrington and his colleagues[2578] wrote an excellent review of this interesting entity, adding six new cases to those already in the literature (but not noting our case). The condition most commonly occurs in women of childbearing age, is not associated with smoking (and is therefore an important diagnosis to consider in non-smokers with chronic airflow limitation), and the chest x-ray shows a reticular pattern with cyst-like spaces. Pneumothoraces and chylothoraces occur. The pattern of function test derangement is sufficiently distinctive to suggest this diagnosis, since it is quite unlike that seen in diffuse interstitial fibrosis syndrome: the lung volume increases, and the recoil pressure is reduced rather than increased. $DL_{CO}SB$ values as low as 3.5 mL/min/mm Hg have been recorded, and the total lung capacity is not reduced, even when such low values are seen. In 1980, Bradley and colleagues[2589] noted that six cases had

been seen at the Mayo Clinic between 1937 and 1979, all in young women. They noted that 65 cases had been reported (66 with our case) and added six new cases to these. They confirmed the pattern of function test changes previously described.

The importance of diagnosing this condition has been enhanced by the recent report of a case in a 29-year-old woman whose DL_{CO} was less than 50% of the predicted value and who improved after progesterone therapy.[4799] It has been suggested that this condition may be linked to tuberous sclerosis.[4838]

Pulmonary Capillary Hemangiomatosis

Wagenvoort and colleagues[4804] reported the first case of pulmonary capillary hemangiomatosis in 1978 in a 71-year-old woman, but no function test data were included in the report. Magee and his colleagues[4831] have reported this rare condition in a 35-year-old woman. Severe pulmonary hypertension was present, and death occurred 5 years after the onset of symptoms. The FVC was lowered by one liter, the DL_{CO} and C_{st} were both slightly reduced, and the resting Pa_{O_2} was 77 mm Hg. The pressure/volume curve showed decreased elastic recoil at low lung volumes and increased recoil at higher volumes. This condition is believed to be a malignant change, with proliferation of capillaries within the walls of arterioles and venules and with only mild interstitial fibrosis.

In 1983, Whittaker and colleagues[4803] reported a case in a 22-year-old man who had recurrent hemoptyses and dyspnea that progressed over 4 years. There were coarse inspiratory crackles over both lung fields, and the chest x-ray showed a diffuse reticular pattern. The TLC was 3.3 liters (the predicted was 5.7), and there was no airway obstruction. The TL_{CO} was said to be elevated, with a value of 120% of predicted. Death occurred from a pulmonary hemorrhage, and the autopsy showed sheets of thin-walled vessels invading the lung, with secondary veno-occlusive disease.

We have encountered a case in a 10-year-old boy. He initially presented with dyspnea, a normal chest x-ray, and clinical evidence of pulmonary hypertension. His pulmonary function test data were as follows:

	Predicted	Observed
Vital capacity	3.5	4.2
TLC	4.5	6.7
Residual volume	1.0	2.5
$DL_{CO}SS$	17.2	4.4

All of these measurements were made on several occasions. The diagnosis was not definitive from an initial lung biopsy, but it was revealed by histologic examination after autopsy. He survived for 4 years after the initial complaint of dyspnea.

Metastatic Carcinoma

Pulmonary function tests in nine patients with metastatic lung carcinomata showed reductions in vital capacity and FEV_1 in most and a lowered $DL_{CO}SB$ in all.[2595] The authors concluded that there was generally more airflow obstruction and a lower $DL_{CO}SB$ than is seen in patients with diffuse interstitial fibrosis, in relation to the radiologic extent of involvement.

Small-Cell Carcinoma

Studies of regional pulmonary function have been successfully used by Bake and his colleagues[2586] to follow the course of these patients while being treated with chemotherapy.

LUNG TRANSPLANTATION

A perspective on lung transplantation concluded that continued attempts at this procedure were justified in centers equipped with major diagnostic and support facilities.[2570] Rejection of the transplant has not yet been completely surmounted, however. Even in a patient with acute silicosis who lived for 10 months after the procedure, the DL_{CO} never rose above 30% of predicted, and the FEV_1 slowly fell.[2574]

In our case of acute silicosis in a 29-year-old man who received a lung transplant[1] and died 7 days after surgery, necrosis of the bronchial anastomosis was present. This has been noted in another patient[2571] and has been attributed to intense immunosuppressive therapy.

Seven episodes of rejection occurred in a single lung transplant in a patient with emphysema who lived for 3 months after the operation.[2603] In this patient, the transplanted lung

had better ventilation than the remaining diseased lung. Two unsuccessful lung transplant operations in men aged 37 to 39 with very severe emphysema were reported.[2572] Possibly, successful surgery can only be undertaken when both lungs can be replaced.[2573] Preliminary reports of combined heart-lung transplants have noted that there are now a number of such patients who have survived for many months, although obliterative bronchiolitis was an important complication in five of 14 such cases.[4800] Pulmonary function data in these cases were as follows:

	FEV$_1$		FEV$_{25-75}$ (L/sec)		Months After Surgery	
Case	Best	Final	Best	Final	Best	Final
1	2.9	0.8	3.7	0.3	4	24
2	3.7	0.8	4.4	0.4	5	14
3	3.3	2.5	2.2	0.6	2	8
4	3.0	1.0	3.6	0.4	6	14
5	3.2	2.3	3.8	1.0	6	30

Recurrent lung infections occurred in all patients. Ten of the 14 patients reported were leading relatively normal lives.

The ideal candidate for this complex procedure is a young patient with severe primary pulmonary hypertension. However, a few cases of advanced emphysema have also been successfully treated.

In one report of seven patients with combined heart and lung transplantation,[5248] six were well 4 to 33 months after transplantation. There was one case each of diffuse interstitial fibrosis, cystic fibrosis, sarcoidosis, histiocytosis X, and bronchiectasis, and two cases of emphysema. In the six cases, the FEV_1 after recovery was greater than 75% of the recipient's normal predicted value. Similar good results are beginning to be reported after lung transplantation alone.

SUMMARY

There is little doubt that pulmonary function tests can play a useful part in decisions on the feasibility of resectional surgery. It is evident that in some centers, this evaluation is carried out with great thoroughness. In others, the evaluation is more empirical. The importance of regional studies of ventilation and perfusion in some patients has been clearly demonstrated, and there seems little doubt that these investigative facilities should be routinely available in centers undertaking a major load of resectional surgery. Most physicians have encountered patients in whom postoperative function was better than one would have predicted, and others in whom unexpected respiratory failure occurred.

Lung transplantation, at centers properly equipped to handle such patients, is beginning to offer a reasonable chance of success in selected cases, and recent results have been far more encouraging.

18

ACUTE AND CHRONIC INFECTIONS

INTRODUCTION

In 1964, in the first edition of this book, we drew attention to the studies by Bervan of pulmonary function changes resulting from viral pneumonia. By the second edition, 7 years later, few additional studies had been reported. Over the past 12 years, a great deal of new information has become available. In part, these studies have been stimulated by the speculation (suspicion) that repetitive episodes of chest infection in children may be associated with later chronic airflow limitation.[2741, 2794]

ACUTE UPPER RESPIRATORY INFECTIONS

Acute rhinovirus infections in children are associated with a wheezing bronchitis.[2611] These are probably associated with exacerbations of asthma in asthmatic children, although such infections apparently account for only about 10% of such episodes.[1553] There are 14 different rhinovirus serotypes, and apparently all are associated with wheezing.[2750] In another study of 243 routine visits of 19 asthmatics, it was concluded that infections could occur without worsening of asthma.[1345] In 84 exacerbations of wheezing, viral infections were identified as the cause in eight patients. This was compared with checks for viral infections during the 243 routine visits, when an incidence of only 3.3% was recorded.

A study of "respiratory illnesses," in 26 normal individuals[2843] showed that FVC, FEV_1, PEFR, and $\dot{V}max_{50\%}VC$ all fell during acute infections, with generally larger falls in cigarette smokers. The FEV_1 fall averaged 110 milliliters, and PEFR fell by 0.37 L/sec. In 12 adults studied on the third to fifth days of an upper respiratory tract infection,[2666] there were no abnormalities of forced expiratory flow curves. However, four had a drop in C_{dyn} at increasing respiratory frequencies, suggesting small airway involvement. These changes were still present 4 weeks after the infection but had returned to normal by 14 weeks. In another study, lowered C_{dyn}/f values returned to normal in 2 weeks,[2744] and the closing volume was unaffected.

Collier and his colleagues[2735] studied 55 children between 2 and a half and 11 years of age over a 2-year period. The authors performed spirometry and lung volume measurements every 3 months during upper respiratory tract infections, and every 4 weeks thereafter. They found that the FEV_1 declined about 140 milliliters during such episodes, and FVC, PEFR, and $MEF_{50\%}VC$ values all fell. The functional residual capacity was unchanged. They suggested that lower respiratory tract involvement usually accompanied an upper respiratory tract infection in children. Others have reported lower PEFR values in children with upper respiratory tract infections.[2788] In nine children with adenovirus infection,[4777] only one had normal function test values. Hyperinflation, reduced C_{dyn}, and even hypoxemia persisted for several months.

Population studies have provided rather different information. Vedal and his colleagues[3964] surveyed 4000 elementary school children from rural western Pennsylvania. They found

FEF_{25-75} values to be lower in those with "asthma" or with a persistent wheeze. These values were not lower in children who had had chest illnesses before the age of 2 years. However, a prior history of croup or bronchiolitis was associated with increased airway reactivity to cold air in a population-based cohort of 194 children aged 12 to 16 years of age in East Boston.[4049]

Cate and colleagues[2707] observed 18 healthy young adults during an upper respiratory infection. Ten were non-smokers, six smoked pipes, and only one smoked cigarettes. Eight of the 24 illnesses studied were due to rhinovirus infections. They found that $DL_{CO}SS$ fell in 12 of 14 attacks (by a mean of 4.3 mL CO/min/mm Hg), which they felt was probably attributable to $\dot{V}/\dot{Q}$ changes resulting from bronchiolitis. Similar data have been recorded in uncomplicated influenza, as noted later. In another study of rhinovirus infections in healthy normal individuals, an increased closing volume was found only in smokers.[2825] This was accompanied by reduced flow at low lung volumes at 80% helium breathing. The adverse function test changes lasted about 30 days.

In a comparison between 11 controls and 16 subjects with upper respiratory tract infections, Empey and his colleagues[2748] compared the effects of 10 breaths of 1.6% histamine diphosphate. In the controls, this produced a 30% increase in R_L. In those with infections, R_L increased 218%. Saline was without effect, and the baseline R_L values were the same in the two groups. Subjects with colds had a lower citric acid aerosol cough threshold. These workers concluded that an upper respiratory tract infection is accompanied by airway epithelial damage, which exposes and sensitizes receptors in the airway, much as ozone exposure does. They also concluded that the induced bronchoconstriction is mediated by a vagal reflex.

In a prospective study of 44 non-smoking asthmatics and 30 normal subjects,[4791] 15 had an upper respiratory infection within the next 4 months. No changes in pulmonary function tests occurred, but there was a slight increase in airway reactivity in both groups. This did not achieve statistical significance, however.

Documented cases of increased airway reactivity in non-atopic normal individuals, such as that in a long distance skater,[1468] may well be attributable to repetitive trivial infections, but the frequency of this phenomenon and its importance in the general spectrum of chronic adult respiratory disease is difficult to assess.

Studies of children with chronic hyperinflation and chronic bronchitis have suggested viral infections in their etiology.[4820]

Live attentuated influenza A virus instilled into the nose of six asthmatics produced a significant increase in histamine reactivity[2772] but did not affect baseline levels of SGaw. Acute coryzal upper respiratory infections in 24 young adults were not followed by any increased airway reactivity on a cold air challenge.[4873] In another study, 13 non-smoking normal adults with an upper respiratory infection were observed during acute disease and then at 1, 3, and 6 week intervals.[2792] In nine of them, histamine reactivity was acutely increased, but had fallen by the end of 6 weeks. The acute reactivity was blocked by atropine. There is good evidence that airway reactivity in children is increased after an attack of croup. In 96 children who had had croup an average of 8.5 years before, mean flow rates were slightly lower than in controls, and 35% had increased airway reactivity.[2793] In another study of 17 children, 14 had increased reactivity after an attack of croup.[2808]

As noted in Chapter 6, elevated levels of SO_2 and particulate pollution (and possibly exposure to NO_2 in the home as a result of the use of gas for cooking) may be associated with an increased risk of bronchitis in pre-adolescent children.[4860] In England, infant mortality from respiratory disease in the years 1921 to 1925 was compared with adult bronchitis mortality in the years 1959 to 1978, on a regional basis.[4867] The findings suggested that the later bronchitis might have had more to do with increased childhood illness than with an air pollution effect in adult life.

ACUTE PULMONARY INFECTIONS

Acute Viral Infections: Influenza and Viral Pneumonia

No detailed review of the extensive experimental work on virus infections can be attempted here, but such infections impair the intracellular killing mechanisms of macrophages and lead to a higher mortality rate in mice with subsequent bacterial challenge.[2767] The epithelial desquamation following virus infections has been elegantly illustrated.[2841] Repair begins in 5 days and is generally complete in about 2 weeks, following acute viral infections induced in mice. It has also been shown that mice with viral infections have an increased susceptibility to the effects of 100% oxygen.[2850] These and other pathologic changes are noted in Chapter 1.

Acute viral infections were found to be responsible for 31 of 49 exacerbations of chronic bronchitis in patients with chronic mucus hypersecretion[2641]; influenza and para-influenza were the main agents. Adult respiratory virus infections are followed by increased airway reactivity, which returns to normal after about 5 weeks.[2689]

Live attenuated flu vaccine given intranasally to 15 volunteers[2753] caused symptoms in 3 days. The $FEF_{25\%}VC$ (low lung volume) changed significantly at 3 days. FEF_{25-75} fell at 7 days, but closing volume was unaffected. The FEF measured at 25% of VC was found to be a sensitive index of change in this study. All tests returned to normal a few days later. Intramuscular injection of killed influenza virus in 19 asthmatics[4836] resulted in a fourfold increase in hemagglutinin antibodies in nine of the patients. All had an increased histamine reactivity 48 hours later. This increased reactivity was not accompanied by more severe symptoms, a fall in PEFR, or an increase in bronchodilator usage. Studies of 29 children who had an average of four attacks of bronchitis per year[2816] showed that increases in R_L and C_{dyn}/f were common. Most of the patients were between 1 and 7 years old. Airway reactivity increased in 12 of the 17 in whom it was measured. Regional ventilation distribution abnormalities measured with inhaled ^{133}Xe were present in seven of nine in whom this was studied. Most of the tests were done 6 weeks after the last acute attack of bronchitis.[2816]

A remarkable prospective study of 10,989 school children in Sydney, Australia[656] showed that the $\dot{V}max_{50\%}$ was lowered in those with a history of bronchitis and/or asthma during the surveillance period. The FEV_1 was relatively insensitive, compared with the $\dot{V}max_{50\%}VC$. Studies of 39 college students with documented influenza A infection[2728] showed that density-dependent flow rates fell in 36 of the subjects. A comparison between placebo and amantidine therapy suggested that amantidine accelerated a return of these values to normal. Airway reactivity was also increased, and this effect lasted for 7 weeks. Airway reactivity to a sodium nitrite aerosol was also increased in 11 subjects after uncomplicated influenza[2634] and returned to normal after 3 weeks.

In another study of 13 non-smoking adults[2749] affected by influenza A infections, airway resistance was followed by the forced oscillation method. Although spirometric measurements were generally unchanged, 10 were abnormal on the oscillation test; seven of these were still abnormal 3 weeks later. At 5 weeks after the acute infection, two subjects still showed abnormal test values. Non-uniformity of airway time constants was postulated as the probable mechanism.[2749]

Johanson, Pierce, and Sanford[2851] studied 10 subjects during and after an attack of influenza A. They found an average fall of 400 milliliters in FVC and FEV_1, which returned to normal at the end of 2 weeks. The FEF_{25-75} fell by 0.6 L/sec during the acute illness. A rise in the $(A-a) D_{O2}$ was also documented, in some patients by as much as 30 mm Hg. In most patients, the elevated values returned to normal 6 weeks after the acute attack.

Flow rates on breathing helium steadily improved over the 7 weeks following an attack of influenza A in 21 subjects.[2689] In a 20-month study of 20 cases of acute viral infections, Horner and Gray[2708] documented a fall in $DL_{CO}SS$, which was greater in women than in men. This value rose to >90% within 10 to 12 weeks after the attack in most subjects. In four it did not return to normal for several months (confirming Bervan's original observations). Influenzal pneumonia may be very severe and may lead to acute respiratory failure.[886, 2852] Very slow resolution and improvement in function after severe attacks have been well documented. In two such cases, the VC was still reduced 3 years later,[2737] and chronic inflammatory changes with bronchiolitis were found on lung biopsy. Much attention has been given to respiratory syncytial virus (RSV) infections in children. These are an important cause of morbidity. In a large study in England, hospital admission rates per capita were more than twice as high in industrial areas, compared with rural areas.[752] It is possible that these infections are related to increased NO_2 levels in homes with gas cooking, compared with homes with electric cooking.[745] As noted in Chapter 6, the question of whether urban NO_2 levels might account for the difference in incidence is not yet resolved.

Residual pulmonary function deficits in children who have had bronchiolitis have been described,[2636] although sample selection may have influenced these results. One study compared 100 RSV and 100 non-RSV cases with 200 matched controls. The patients with pulmonary function deficits were seen an average of 7 years after the acute episode.[2822] It was found that the prevalence of cough, wheezing, nasal discharge, and hearing difficulties were greater in the RSV group. "Bronchitis" and "asthma" were also more common. The FEF_{25-75} averaged 91.8% of predicted in the index cases and 102.3% of predicted in the controls.[2822] The authors of this study were careful to point out that they did not know whether the index group were more sensitive to respiratory illness from the beginning, or whether subsequent illnesses were related to the original infection. Other follow-up data have yielded similar results.[2821]

There is obviously still much to be learned of the etiologic factors affecting episodes of respiratory disease in children. In one study in Britain of 2228 children, a higher incidence of respiratory illnesses was shown to occur in South Wales, which was not thought to be attributable to air pollution.[2838] Whether it is associated with higher rainfall, and if so why, is not known. There were no differences in pulmonary function between children from different regions in this study,[2838] although falls in FEV_1 with episodes of infection were documented.[2834] Respiratory syncytial virus infections may be severe enough to cause respiratory failure, and elevation of Pa_{CO_2} has been used to classify severity.[2819] In 84 severe cases, values between 60 and 80 mm Hg were recorded in nine. Eleven children needed ventilatory assistance, and one died in this series.[2819] Respiratory syncytial virus infections in 26 8-year-old children[2823] suggested that atopy did not predispose to these infections, and the induced exercise airflow limitation that occurred did not correlate with either eosinophil counts or IgE levels.

An acute attack of influenza or rhinovirus infection in 13 normal subjects was shown to lead to a marked slowing of tracheal mucus velocity.[4839] As has been noted in Chapter 16, respiratory illness caused by industrial exposures may mimic viral respiratory infections.[2536]

Mycoplasmal Pneumonia

Severe mycoplasmal pneumonia may be followed by slow recovery. In one 50-year-old woman, the VC was 2.6 liters 15 weeks after the illness, rising to 3.0 a year later.[2621] The TLC rose a liter over the same period, and DL_{CO} increased from 55% of predicted to 107% of predicted. In a 31-year-old woman with very severe mycoplasmal pneumonia, death occurred on the fifteenth day. At autopsy, severe fibrosis was developing.[2607]

In milder cases, the FEV_1 is initially reduced, and the $SBN_2\%/L$ and $(A-a)$ D_{O_2} differences are both increased.[2606] Mycoplasmal pneumonia in a 27-year-old cigarette smoker,[2711] in whom the Pa_{O_2} was initially only 39 mm Hg, slowly resolved. Neither the VC nor the FEV_1 had returned to predicted values, although the Pa_{O_2} was 78 mm Hg, 4 months later. Other studies[2606] have shown that persistent small airway flow limitation may follow this disease.

An important sequela of the bronchiolitis of mycoplasmal pneumonia may be the later development of a hyperlucent lung. This was documented in an 11-year-old girl following a severe attack of mycoplasmal pneumonia.[2734]

Bacterial Pneumonia

Experimentally, the infectivity and mortality from bacterial aerosols in mice are both increased if the animal is exposed beforehand to ozone, oxides of nitrogen, or sulfate aerosols.[722, 732, 2635] It is not known whether current ambient levels of these substances have any influence on human disease. Somewhat paradoxically, there is evidence in animal experiments that pre-exposure to tobacco smoke may enhance the macrophage response to bacterial challenge.[2768] Experiments of mice have also indicated that pneumococcal elastase inhibitors may play a role in minimizing lung injury during pneumococcal pneumonia.[4792, 4818] In experimentally induced lobar inflammation in cats, it was shown that the increased respiratory frequency depended on an intact vagus on the affected side.[2774]

In the acute stage, the Pa_{O_2} is commonly lower in cases of bacterial pneumonia than in viral pneumonia.[2756] Regional ventilation studies were abnormal after the chest x-ray had cleared in four of nine cases of bacterial pneumonia.[2756] This phenomenon was noted in the second edition of this book.[1] The data that suggest a fall in lung compliance greater than can be accounted for by the radiologic extent of the pneumonia, also noted in that edition, have not been extended by any further observations.

In acute bacterial pneumonia, the acute hypoxemia is attributable to a large shunt component, perfusion presumably still occurring through consolidated lung.[266] In a recent study, 11 cases of severe bacterial pneumonia were studied by use of the six inert gas method.[4817]

During ventilation via an endotracheal tube, between 2% and 43% of perfusion was distributed to low $\dot{V}/\dot{Q}$ units. Thirty minutes of oxygen ventilation resulted in a fall in $\dot{Q}v_A/\dot{Q}T$ from 31% to 25%, and the shunt fraction did not increase. The authors concluded that in these cases, hypoxic vasoconstriction, while present, was not at a fully effective level.

Slow recovery from Legionnaire's pneumonia was reported in a 30-year-old woman.[2682] Eight months after the acute disease had resolved, the DL_{CO} was only 34% of predicted. The FEV_1 was 77% of predicted, with residual abnormalities on the chest x-ray.

It is clear that worsening of patients with chronic airflow limitation is associated with increased frequency of *Streptococcus pneumoniae* in the sputum.[2746]

Pulmonary Infections in the Acquired Immunodeficiency Syndrome

Severe pulmonary infections occur in at least 50% of those with the acquired immunodeficiency syndrome (AIDS), often with cytomegalovirus or *Pneumocystis*.[5103] A fall in DL_{CO} has been noted to be a predictor of these infections,[4835, 4837, 4863] sometimes changing before the chest radiograph has become abnormal. The exercise $(A-a)$ O_2 difference has also been found useful in screening for pulmonary abnormality.[5103] Hypoxemia may antedate significant radiologic change and may be an early indicator of abnormality. The hypoxemia later may become severe.[4787] Acute tuberculosis may also be a complication in AIDS patients.[4816]

ACUTE MILIARY TUBERCULOSIS

Patients with acute miliary tuberculosis and acute respiratory distress are still reported. In one, the Pa_{O_2} fell to 20 mm Hg on 60% oxygen breathing before death, and the diagnosis was made at autopsy.[2699] Other severe cases have also been noted.[2693, 2832]

CHRONIC INFECTIONS

Tuberculosis

In a study of 30 patients with chronic tuberculosis, reductions in TLC, VC, and RV, all proportional to their normal values, were found.[2759] Where the RV/TLC ratio was increased, chronic bronchitis was invariably present. Tests of airway reactivity in 12 patients with tuberculosis showed a normal response, both to histamine and charcoal dust.[2760] Evidence of airway obstruction relieved by bronchodilators is occasionally encountered.[2759] A study of 112 patients with chronic tuberculosis showed that 87% had impaired ventilatory capability, 23 of 73 were hypoxemic at rest, and 44% had resting elevation of pulmonary arterial pressure.[2804] On exercise, pulmonary hypertension may be revealed in those in whom it was normal at rest.[2804] In another study, separate measurement of DL_{CO} in each lung in 20 patients[2807] showed that this closely correlated with flow and oxygen uptake in that lung. In the most comprehensive study of chronic tuberculosis so far attempted, Lopez-Majano[2809] compared patients with far advanced disease with patients with moderate and minimal disease. He noted a good correlation between decreases in VC and DL_{CO} and documented the importance of restriction. Improvement in function was observed after treatment in a number of patients.

A report of 18 patients with "destroyed lung" due to very extensive tuberculosis, 10 of whom were under the age of 40, indicated that the affected lung often contributed less than 10% to ventilation and oxygen uptake.[2762] Excellent results can follow pneumonectomy in such patients,[2575] even in persons over the age of 60. Reports of 12 patients with tuberculosis, studied while in different body positions and by means of ^{133}Xe,[2717] showed that both ventilation and perfusion of affected zones were relatively normal, but their volume was reduced. Shifts of perfusion with changes in body position were less than in normal subjects, probably as a result of the presence of pulmonary hypertension. A comparison among lesions caused by *Mycobacterium tuberculosis* with those due to *M. kansasii* and *M. intracellulare* suggested that the latter two organisms might cause greater impairment of function than *M. tuberculosis*.[2747]

Blastomycosis

Blastomycosis in generalized form gives rise to scattered pulmonary infiltrations. Of 16 patients, all smokers, 11 had signs of obstructive disease. The FEV_1 values varied between 42% and 69% of predicted.[2668] All patients had elevated residual volumes, and hypoxemia was present in a few. The pathologic studies indicated that bronchiolitis and bronchiolar lesions were probably common in this condition. Detailed clinical classifications, without notes of pulmonary function defect, have been published.[2645]

Histoplasmosis

A report of acute pulmonary histoplasmosis in four young men[2643] showed reduced diffusing capacities in two and a reduction in exercising arterial P_{O_2}. In another patient, TLC, VC, and C_{st} were all reduced. The condition may be so severe as to present as an acute respiratory distress syndrome.[2701, 4786] In five patients with chronic disease, normal lung mechanics were reported.[2703]

In addition to intrapulmonary lesions, this condition can cause a severe fibrosing mediastinitis. In such cases, pulmonary hypertension may become a prominent feature, but no pulmonary function details have been recorded.[2655]

Trichinosis

A remarkable case of acute trichinosis in a 51-year-old butcher deserves notice because the acute bronchitis of this condition was later complicated by severe respiratory muscle weakness due to muscle involvement.[2721] The diagnosis was made on muscle biopsy.

ASPERGILLOSIS AND ASTHMA

Allergic bronchopulmonary aspergillosis in asthmatics is noted in Chapter 9. Detailed studies of atopic asthma complications showed that an unexpectedly low DL_{CO} in a known asthmatic should suggest the possibility of *Aspergillus* infection.[2618] During exacerbations of allergic bronchopulmonary aspergillosis, falls into TLC, FEV_1, VC, and $DL_{CO}SB$ are observed,[2647] with values returning toward normal on treatment with steroids. A reduction in these parameters not responsive to treatment suggests the possibility of either chronic bronchiectasis or chronic pneumonitis or both. However, it has recently been noted that abnormalities in pulmonary function tests may not clearly define the extent of lung damage induced in this syndrome,[4801] although acute attacks are associated with a deterioration in function.

ACUTE MALARIA

In 16 patients with *Plasmodium falciparum* malaria studied between the second and fifth day after onset,[2719] 13 had a normal chest x-ray and normal function tests. Three had evidence of pulmonary infiltrates with hypoxemia, an increased $(A-a) D_{O_2}$ shunt component, and a decreased C_{st}. Improvement had occurred by the ninth day of treatment.

MISCELLANEOUS INFECTIONS

Smallpox handler's lung, which may show extensive punctate calcified lesions radiographically, was characterized by normal pulmonary function in five nurses in whom it occurred.[2615] Varicella pneumonia can be so severe as to be life-threatening. In one such patient, PEEP ventilation was found to be essential for adequate oxygenation, since it reduced the shunting through unventilated atelectatic regions.[2678] In a patient with herpes zoster infection involving C4 and C5 segments, unilateral diaphragmatic paralysis accompanied the infection.[2679]

Changes in lung function in the acute stage of *Pneumocystis carinii* pneumonia in 23 children showed that VC, FEV_1, and DL_{CO} were reduced to about 65% of predicted values.[2786] These were largely back to normal after a month, although the DL_{CO} continued to improve for a further 2 months. As noted previously, pneumocystic infections are common complications of AIDS patients, as well as others who are immunologically compromised. Pneumocystic infections are associated with an early fall in DL_{CO}, and hypoxemia may antedate radiologic changes.

CHAPTER

19

MISCELLANEOUS CONDITIONS

CENTRAL AIRWAY OBSTRUCTION SYNDROMES AND BRONCHIOLITIS

Laryngeal Paralysis and Tracheal Stenoses

Proctor's review of the physiology of the upper airway and the larynx[2303, 2742] and the exhaustive listing of all known congenital and genetic lung disorders by Landing[2853] will be found useful. The function of the posterior cricoarytenoid muscle is complex and is probably only partly understood.[273, 2824] Its phasic activity, with contraction on inspiration, can be observed in normal subjects during voluntary hyperventilation,[2785] and may be present on normal resting breathing in those with chronic airflow limitation. The role of the larynx in relation to airflow limitation in asthma is not yet clear,[1387] as noted in Chapter 9. Upper airway obstruction during sleep is discussed in Chapter 4.

During the past 10 years, several studies of persons with upper airway obstruction have been published. A comparison among 11 patients with upper airway obstruction, 15 normal subjects, and 20 patients with chronic airflow limitation caused by diffuse lung disease[2696] showed that four measurements were useful in distinguishing those with central obstruction. These were

1. A forced inspiratory flow rate equal to or less than 100 L/min.
2. A ratio of $FEF_{50\%}VC$ to $FIF_{50\%}VC$ equal to or greater than 1.0.
3. A ratio of FEV_1 (in milliliter) to PEFR (in L/min) equal to or greater than 10.0.

4. A ratio of FEV_1 to $FEV_{0.5}$ equal to or greater than 1.5.

In patients with bilateral vocal cord paralysis, inspiratory and expiratory flow rates are greatly reduced, and tracheostomy is often required.[2683] It may complicate patients with general paralysis due to the Guillain-Barré syndrome.[4808] Surgical procedures on the larynx in patients with bilateral vocal cord paralysis lead to improvement in expiratory flow rates.[4842] Unilateral vocal cord paralysis also leads to a high ratio of $\dot{V}E_{50}/\dot{V}I_{50}$.[2614] Inspection of the expiratory and inspiratory flow curves shows suggestive flattening. These curves can be reproduced by normal subjects breathing through added resistance.[2718]

Attention has been drawn to the syndrome of unexplained laryngeal wheezing. This was apparently first described in 1842 and may be confused with irreversible airflow obstruction.[4779] These episodes can be severe, and in one 23-year-old non-smoking woman,[4815] the Pa_{O_2} fell to 40 mm Hg during an attack. A tracheostomy had to be performed, and a vocal cord abnormality of unknown origin was diagnosed. In a 32-year-old woman[4810] whose baseline function tests were normal, an area of the corniculate and cuneiform cartilages in the posteroinferior portion of the aryepiglottic folds collapsed over the laryngeal vestibule during increased ventilation. This caused the FEV_1 to fall from 4.28 liters to 3.60 liters. The differential diagnosis from exercise-induced airflow limitation would be difficult in such a case.

Tracheal stenosis is also an important cause of upper airway obstruction. Miller and Hyatt[2709] studied 16 patients with tracheal stenosis, 14 patients with obstructive neoplasms,

350

and 13 patients with bilateral vocal cord paralysis. With fixed narrowing, equal decreases in inspiratory and expiratory flow loops were seen. Intrathoracic lesions distorted the expiratory loop, and extrathoracic obstruction distorted the inspiratory loop. The ratio of $\dot{V}$max expiration to $\dot{V}$max inspiration at mid-VC was a useful index. In patients with fixed obstruction this index averaged 0.85. With extrathoracic obstruction it was 2.2, and with variable intrathoracic obstruction it was 0.32. This differentiation has also been noted by others.[2660, 2716] In some cases, however, main bronchial stenoses could not be distinguished from laryngeal stenoses by flow/volume curve analyses.[2705]

Hoffstein and Zamel[4788] measured airway cross-sectional area using an acoustic reflection method in six patients with tracheal stenosis. The subjects were between 15 and 70 years old. This important study provided the following data:

	Patients						
	1	2	3	4	5	6	Mean
Age	67	59	15	70	32	80	
$\dot{V}$max$_{50\%}$ (L/sec), expiratory	3.1	3.0	4.5	3.4	7.1	2.4	3.9
inspiratory	5.8	2.7	1.6	3.9	6.5	2.7	3.9
Expiratory/inspiratory ratio	0.5	1.1	2.8	0.9	1.1	0.9	1.2
LSS (cm), Ac	4.0	4.9	5.0	5.0	5.0	5.3	4.9
XR	3.5	5.0	5.0	5.5	4.5	5.5	4.8
MGMS (cm), Ac	7.1	6.5	6.0	5.0	5.5	4.0	5.7
XR	7.0	7.0	6.0	4.0	5.8	3.5	5.6
MCSA (cm^2) Ac	1.9	1.8	1.2	2.1	1.6	1.8	1.7
XR	1.4	1.2	0.8	1.5	1.0	1.3	1.2

LSS = Length of stenotic segment; Ac = acoustic method; XR = by radiology; MGMS = distance between midglottis and middle of stenotic segment; MCSA = minimal cross-sectional area of stenotic segment.

It is of interest that patient 3 had the most severe stenosis, with a minimal tomographic diameter of 4 millimeters and a clearly abnormal inspiratory flow volume curve. However, the forced expiratory $\dot{V}$max$_{50\%}$VC was 4.5 L/sec. The acoustic method has a tendency to overestimate the minimal cross-sectional area of the stenotic segment, as measured radiologically.

In normal subjects, the ratio of FEV_1 to PEFR was <10 (mean, 7.3), but it was >10 (mean, 14) in patients with upper airway obstruction with orifices of 6 millimeters or less.[337] However, in another series of 16 patients with upper airway obstruction,[2673] the ratio of FEV_1 to PEFR was found to be of limited value. The authors of this study found that the inspiratory flow loops were useful in following progress and

noted that the position of the neck was important when flow curves were being recorded. In another study of 21 cases of tracheal stenosis,[2801] four patients with flow/volume loops failed to demonstrate abnormality, although stenoses could be seen radiologically.

Tracheal obstructions can result in significant falls in arterial oxygen tension on exercise. In seven patients, the resting/exercise Pa_{O_2} values were 83/73; 97/94; 73/65; 94/88; 95/76; 84/72; and 101/80. These studies showed that respiratory failure is a hazard if the orifice is less than 8 millimeters in diameter.[2752] The fall in Pa_{O_2} on exercise documented in this paper might well cause diagnostic difficulty.

Upper airway obstruction can be identified by the improved flow with 80% helium, even in patients with chronic obstructive airway disease.[2731] We noted an increase in FEF_{25-75} from 1.18 to 1.78 L/sec on 80% helium breathing in one patient with tracheal stenosis.[1] Sometimes central obstruction leads to an increase in residual volume.[26, 39, 2761] Gas distribution indices and normal diffusing capacities are useful in excluding generalized lung disease.[2639, 2743] Several of these cases have been misdiagnosed as asthma.[2673] Other causes of significant airflow limitation have included fibrosarcoma of the trachea[2628]; carcinoid intratracheal tumor (which led to an FEV_1 of 1.2 liters in a 36-year-old man initially diagnosed as having asthma[4796]); sarcoid lesions in the larynx or trachea;* tuberculosis[4869]; cartilaginous ring dislocation[2715]; and the rare syndrome of tracheopathica osteoplastica.[2675] In small infants, vascular ring abnormalities lead to obstruction of the trachea at the carina.[2676]

External pressure from a large goiter may also cause airflow obstruction.[4845] In one carefully studied patient with variable extrathoracic obstruction, both laryngoscopy and bronchoscopy findings were normal. The cause could not be determined but was thought possibly to be patient with stenosis functional origin.[2796] In another study of a patient with a stenosis caused by a previous tracheostomy, it was noted that the extrathoracic stenosis increased when the arms were raised. The FIF fell 37%, compared with when the arms were lowered.[4807]

All these cases serve to illustrate the importance of a close study of the pattern of the expiratory airflow curve in patients with dyspnea.[4814, 4843, 4868]

_____

*See references 1901, 1979, 2702, 4850.

Relapsing Polychondritis

Krell, Staats, and Hyatt[4861] have reported on five patients with this syndrome; four were white, and one was black. All except Patient 2 were non-smokers:

	Patient				
	1	*2†*	*3*	*4*	*5*
Age	55	46	48	44	32
TLC*	80	94	72	102	89
VC*	107	60	92	117	85
RV/TLC*	65	122	51	67	105
FEV/FVC*	120	57	46	112	80
MVV*	105	16	44	103	47
$D_{L_{CO}}SS*$	—	—	91	—	90
MEF/MIF ratio	0.89	0.40	0.26	0.98	0.99
C_{st}	—	0.56	0.17	0.41	0.29
R_L	—	8.4	11	1.0	5.8

*Data as a percentage of predicted.
†Smoker.

Patients 1, 2, and 4 had normal chest x-rays and tomograms of the airways. Narrowing of the trachea or mainstem bronchi were seen in Patient 3 and Patient 5. The authors stressed the importance of spirometry in the diagnosis. Other single cases,[4826] one in a physician,[4856] indicate how difficult this disease may be to diagnose.

Bronchial Obstruction

Injuries may lead to isolated bronchial obstruction,[2854] and improvement in flow rates may follow surgical repair. In one such case, perfusion of the right lung continued, although the right bronchus was occluded. This led to a Pa_{O_2} of only 37 mm Hg and an $(A - a) D_{O_2}$ of 63.6 mm Hg.[2642] Pneumonectomy restored these values to normal. Isolated bronchial stenoses in sarcoidosis are noted in Chapter 15.[2637] In some cases, the etiology may be obscure.[2690] Bronchial adenomata in a main bronchus may lead to an FEV_1 of only 46% of predicted and slight hypoxemia.[1411] Other cases are noted in Chapter 17.

The rare syndrome of tracheobronchiomegaly (Mounier-Kuhn syndrome) causes collapse of the affected bronchus on expiration and a major difference between inspiratory and expiratory flow rates.[2660]

Non-occupational, Non-rheumatoid Chronic Obliterative Bronchiolitis

In 1971, Macklem and his colleagues drew attention to the syndrome of "chronic obstruc-tive disease of small airways,"[2855] in which inflammation of small airways and bronchioles without concomitant emphysema is the main lesion. Three of the patients had some degree of bronchiectasis. One had had chronic chest illness since two episodes of pneumonia, and one had sarcoid infiltration of small airways. Two had a syndrome of chronic obliterative bronchiolitis without associated rheumatoid arthritis being present. In every case, there was evidence that the small airways were the main site of the pathologic process and the severe airflow limitation. Cases similar to the final two cases in this series have been described by others.

In 1981, Turton, Williams, and Green published an interesting study[2839] in which they reviewed all cases of severe airflow obstruction over a 3-year period. They excluded all smokers and ex-smokers, and all cases of chronic bronchitis, asthma, and emphysema. Ten patients with obliterative bronchiolitis remained, of whom five had rheumatoid arthritis (see Chapter 13). In these and in the five without rheumatoid arthritis, k_{CO} values were normal, residual volumes were slightly increased, and TLC values were normal. The flow/volume curves indicated the presence of volume-dependent airway obstruction.

In 1983, Epler and Colby[3741] wrote an editorial entitled "The spectrum of bronchiolitis obliterans," reviewing the data up to that time. More recently, the same authors have described a syndrome they call "Bronchiolitis obliterans organizing pneumonia" (quickly christened "BOOP"),[4268] in which they report 50 cases of bronchiolitis obliterans without an identified cause. Polypoid masses of granulation tissue were found in the lumina of small airways. Usually there had been a flu-like illness for between 3 and 10 weeks, rales were heard in 68% of the patients, and the chest x-ray showed scattered densities. Seventy-two per cent of the patients had a reduced FVC, and 86% had a reduced $D_{L_{CO}}SB$. The FEF_{25-75} was below 60% of predicted in 13 of the patients. No measurements of SBN_2/L or C_{dyn} were reported. Complete clinical and physiologic recovery after steroid administration occurred in 65% of the patients. It is not clear whether this condition is completely distinct from other entities, nor what the etiologic factors are.

Other investigators have reported cases of severe bronchiolitis in adults that have been proved on biopsy but were without evident cause. In four such adults,[4849] there was a rapid onset of severe dyspnea; a severely reduced FEV$_1$ and FEF$_{25-75}$, without a bronchodilator response; overinflation but no interstitial lung disease on the chest x-ray; no large airway involvement (no bronchitis or bronchiectasis); and normal serum alpha$_1$-antitrypsin levels. The diffusing capacity was normal in these patients, but bronchoalveolar lavage showed high neutrophil percentages (which fell from 53% of total cells to 8% of total cells after steroid administration). It seems clear that acute inflammation is an important part of this syndrome and may be distinguished from "BOOP" by the lack of infiltrates on the chest film.

A single case in a 40-year-old engineer, a non-smoker who had had no dusty occupation, also illustrates this condition.[2771] He had had pneumonia at the age of 7, developed a dry cough at about age 24 and a productive cough at age 38, and had had occasional episodes of low grade fever and hemoptysis. The chest x-ray showed linear opacities and mottling over both lungs, and basal rales were present. Bronchoscopy was normal. Pulmonary function tests showed:

	Predicted	Observed
TLC	7.0	7.7
VC	5.6	4.4
RV	2.0	2.6
FEV$_1$	4.3	3.3
$\dot{V}$max$_{50\%}$VC	5.5	4.3
$\dot{V}$max$_{25\%}$VC	2.0	0.8
SBN$_{2\%}$/L	1.1	4.0
DL$_{CO}$SB	37.0	31.0
DL$_{CO}$/$\dot{V}$A	3.4	3.5
Pa$_{O_2}$, rest	80.2	72.2
exercise: 40 watts	80.2	66.9
160 watts	80.2	60.9

The very low airflow during the terminal part of the expiratory flow curve was a striking feature. The lung biopsy from this man showed normal alveolar walls, but considerable peribronchiolar inflammation and fibrosis in various stages of progression. There was no vasculitis.

In another single fatal case, a 57-year-old non-smoking woman with no evidence of connective tissue disease[4332] had an FEV$_1$ of only 19% of predicted and a normal k$_{CO}$. The chest x-ray showed overinflation only. Death occurred with severe hypoxemia after 2 years. The cases described by Rubin and Bruderman[2638] in 1973 might also be this same entity.

These cases of bronchiolitis represent a considerable diagnostic challenge, since many other conditions have to be carefully excluded before the diagnosis can be made. Although probably not common, they do represent an important subcategory not easily distinguished from other far more common syndromes of chronic airflow limitation. Experimental studies using nitric or sulfuric acid in dogs confirm the general specificity of tests of small airways in relation to acute small airway changes[3141, 4790] (see Chapter 1).

As noted in Chapter 17, bronchiolitis may be an important complication of heart-lung transplant operations. As documented later, it may also occur following bone marrow transplant procedures. Occasionally, bronchiolitis dominates the findings in cases of allergic alveolitis (see Chapter 11).

Microlithiasis Alveolaris

Up to 1970, about a hundred cases of this hereditary disease had been published.[1] Apart from some reduction in lung volumes, there has usually been little disability, and other tests of function have been normal. A case has been described in an 80-year-old woman. The TLC was normal, but the diffusing capacity was much reduced.[2631] Another case has been described in a 5-year-old girl.[2720] In a 16-year-old boy with this disease, all function tests were normal, including the DL$_{CO}$.[2803] In a boy who was 13 when first diagnosed,[4830] studies when he was aged 21 showed that his VC fell from 48% of predicted to 32% of predicted over this period. His FEV$_1$ fell from 51% of predicted to 39% of predicted. At the end of the period, his Pa$_{O_2}$ was only 44 mm Hg, and the EKG showed evidence of right ventricular hypertrophy. No measurements of DL$_{CO}$ were reported. It is clear from this patient that this condition can lead to serious disability.

Alveolar Proteinosis

As we have noted,[1] this condition may occur with little interference with function. However, more severe cases have been reported, and the literature now contains observations made over longer periods of time than before. Gee and Fick have reviewed the use of bronchoalveolar lavage in this condition,[2608] as have Claypool, Rogers, and Matuschak.[4806]

In one report,[2856] 14 patients were followed for up to 8 years. In addition to radiologic abnormalities, 13 had an increased serum lactate dehydrogenase. Improvements in all aspects of function, including diffusing capacity and resting and exercise Pa_{O_2}, followed lavage treatments. Data illustrating the fluctuations in function on one patient were as follows:

	TLC	FVC	FEV_1	Pa_{O_2} Rest	Pa_{O_2} Exercise	$D_{L_{CO}}$ (mL/min/mm Hg)
Before Lavage	5.22	4.02	3.04	60	50	20
After Lavage	5.32	4.21	3.26	70	75	24
5 Months	6.26	4.79	3.61	69	90	34
8 Months	5.78	4.74	3.50	68	87	40
16 Months	5.39	4.33	3.24	63	71	37
33 Months	5.47	4.35	3.06	71	62	24
46 Months	5.22	4.36	3.23	68	53	24

These data suggest that a complete assessment would have to include gas exchange or diffusing capacity information, since the considerable changes in these were accompanied by relatively small reductions in volumes or FEV_1.

Other studies indicate that the effects of lavage on function are variable and somewhat unpredictable.[2626, 2680, 2723] The use of trypsin aerosol was followed by striking improvement in function in two patients.[2652, 2710] In some patients, the VC and $D_{L_{CO}}$ may be reduced to 40% of predicted values, and moderately severe hypoxemia may be present.[2645, 4809] It has been shown that the lowered Pa_{O_2} is mostly attributable to an increased shunt component.[2730] One patient with severe alveolar proteinosis had a sarcoid reaction of the lymph nodes.[2810] In another, a gradual transition to a diffuse interstitial fibrosis occurred over a 13-year period, with a final Pa_{O_2} of only 39 mm Hg.[1847] This condition has been reported in four siblings.[4772]

ENDOCRINE DISORDERS

Thyrotoxicosis and Myxedema

In the second edition of this book,[1] we noted that dyspnea is the commonest symptom of thyrotoxicosis and commented that it was probably related to excess exercise ventilation, a lowered pulmonary compliance, and muscular weakness. Freedman[2612] studied pulmonary mechanics in detail in six patients with thyrotoxicosis and three patients with myxedema before and after treatment. He found that VC rose in three of the six thyrotoxic patients, and static compliance rose in four of them. He could find no evidence of muscular weakness contributing

to the respiratory manifestations of this condition and suggested that the mechanics data supported the theory that pulmonary vascular engorgement was responsible for most of the changes. He thought the increase in VC that occurred after treatment of myxedema might be explained by improvement in muscle force.

Seven patients with thyrotoxicosis were studied by switching from air to oxygen for 20 seconds. The $\dot{V}E$ fell in all patients by a significant average decrement of 21% below control values.[2784] This response was unaffected by propranolol, and the authors concluded that there is an increased hypoxic drive to ventilation in thyrotoxicosis. Their patients all had a normal VC, but the mean FEV_1 was slightly below the predicted value. After treatment, the change in $\dot{V}E$ on 100% oxygen was reduced to 11.7%.

It has been reported that thyrotoxicosis is associated with deterioration in patients with asthma,[4773] and that an inverse relationship exists between the level of thyroid function and airway beta-adrenergic responsiveness. However, thyrotoxicosis induced by triiodothyronine administration was not accompanied by any change in airway reactivity.[4857]

The lowered $D_{L_{CO}}$ in thyrotoxicosis is probably related to the lowered stroke volume in the presence of tachycardia. The hypoxic ventilatory response is considerably depressed in myxedema and rises after treatment.[2724] The CO_2 response is also depressed. In a case of myxedema coma and respiratory failure, the delta $\dot{V}E/Pa_{CO_2}$ rose from 0.45 to 2.00 after treatment.[2714]

Patients with myxedema are at an increased risk of developing sleep apnea (see Chapter 4). In studies of nine patients with myxedema whose mean age was 49 years,[4795] five had hypersomnolence. In these five, there were an increased number of apneic episodes during sleep. Two of the five had severe sleep apnea, but the mechanism was not clear. In a 56-year-old man with hypothyroidism, episodes of apnea during sleep were eliminated after treatment with medroxyprogesterone acetate. The delta $\dot{V}E/Pa_{CO_2}$ and $P_{0.1}$ increased.[2787]

Acromegaly and Hypopituitarism

As noted in Chapter 4, patients with acromegaly have a greatly increased risk of obstructive sleep apnea as a result of hypertrophy of soft tissues around the upper airway.[2644] In 11 patients with acromegaly, five were found to have sleep apnea,[2820] and central obstructive and mixed types were seen. Sometimes the problem is compounded by the presence both of acromegaly and of chronic obstructive lung disease.[4870] It is of great interest that patients with acromegaly develop increased lung volumes. In one series of 20 patients,[2617] six men had a mean TLC that was 112% of predicted; the DL_{CO} was 96% of predicted. In 30 patients, TLC was 115% of predicted in men and 112% of predicted in women. TLC values were noted to be higher in smokers.[2672] This change was noted only in patients whose disease had been recognized for more than 8 years. In addition, eight patients had evidence of small airway narrowing. In some patients, reduction in maximal inspiratory flow velocity at 50% of VC were interpreted to indicate probable extrathoracic airway narrowing. In another series of nine men and seven women, the following data were obtained:

	TLC (%P)	VC (%P)	RV (%P)	DL_{CO} (%P)	$DL_{CO}/$ TLC (%P)
Men	121	122	110	132	108
Women	111	116	100	107	101

The data were considered to be consistent either with an increased number of alveoli or with an increase in the size of existing alveoli.

In a group of 11 patients with acromegaly, eight were treated by pituitary irradiation. The mean TLC was not increased before treatment, but eight of 10 had slight hypoxemia. This was attributed to defects of perfusion seen on lung scans, but of unknown cause.[2798]

Fewer cases of hypopituitarism have been studied. In one comparison between six patients with acromegaly and eight patients with hypopituitarism, those with hypopituitarism were found to have TLC values only 76.7% of predicted.[2671] Studies of lung mechanics showed that this was not due to neuromuscular deficit or to abnormal chest wall mechanics. P_{st} values at TLC were higher in patients with hypopituitarism than in those with acromegaly. The authors concluded that growth hormone influences lung volume in adults and is necessary to maintain a normal lung volume. It is not known whether significant reductions in TLC take 8 years to develop, in parallel with the time span needed in acromegaly for the TLC to increase.

Acute Pancreatitis

In acute pancreatitis, there is commonly significant hypoxemia.[2828] As noted in Chapter 23,

the condition may lead to acute respiratory distress syndrome. In 14 patients, the mean Pa_{O_2} was 64.6 mm Hg, the lowest observed value being 36.8 mm Hg.[2670] In this series, five patients had pleural effusions, and there were no consistent spirometric changes; the DL_{CO} was reduced in three. The hypoxemia was attributed to an increased shunt component. In 22 patients with uncomplicated acute pancreatitis, all with normal x-rays,[2692] four had mild hypoxemia, and DL_{CO}/VA values were reduced to 68% of predicted. The mean VC was 3.55, compared with a mean predicted value of 4.76. In 20 patients, the Pa_{O_2} varied between 44 mm Hg and 56 mm Hg, and the chest x-rays showed a diffuse infiltration in several.[2828] Autopsy studies revealed a diffuse non-specific pneumonitis with no evidence of bacterial infection.[2828]

Experiments inducing acute pancreatitis in sheep have indicated that this condition increases pulmonary vascular permeability to proteins,[2791, 4781] with an increase in extravascular lung water of about 25%. This seems compatible with clinically observed changes.

Diabetes Mellitus

Morphologic changes in the lung of adult diabetics, including thickening of endothelium, have been documented,[2844] but there do not appear to be any carefully controlled observations on pulmonary function to indicate whether these have any functional consequence.

An initial report that there was a significant loss of lung recoil in 11 patients with juvenile diabetes[2751] and reduced TLC was not confirmed by other workers[2745] who found that TLC was reduced but recoil was normal. The diffusing capacity was normal in both series. In another study, no distinctive changes in juvenile diabetics were found.[2738] As there are known connective tissue changes in this disease, further data should be obtained to resolve the question of alterations in lung recoil.[2732] Changes in diabetic ketoacidosis are noted later.

In a comparison study, 11 patients with insulin-dependent diabetes and normal joints and 12 with severe joint movement limitation[4789] were matched for age, sex, and glycemic control. The FEV_1 and FVC were both significantly lower in those with joint limitation; there was no evidence of airflow obstruction, since the FEF_{25-75} was normal. It was not clear whether there were changes in the chest wall or whether lung compliance may have been abnormal.

It has been suggested that autonomic dysfunction may be present in some diabetics. Douglas and his colleagues[5104] studied 11 patients with diabetic neuropathy, all with a normal FEV_1. Changes on administration of ipratropium bromide suggested that there was reduced airway vagal tone. In other studies, a normal ventilatory response to hypoxia was found and was taken to indicate that peripheral chemoreceptors are intact. However, Montserrat and his colleagues[4841] studied 20 diabetics with autonomic neuropathy, 20 diabetics without the syndrome, and 20 controls. They found that the $\dot{V}E$ response to hypoxia was lower in the diabetics and lower in those with autonomic neuropathy than in those without. The response was evaluated by noting the ventilatory response to five breaths of nitrogen. The hypercapnic response was also depressed. In another report,[4774] 52 diabetics were compared with 65 controls. Twenty-five per cent of the diabetics had impaired sensitivity to hypoxia or hypercapnia, and 7% had abnormal respiration on exercise. These findings bore no relation to complications of diabetes and were not predictable from routine pulmonary function tests.

HEMATOLOGIC DISORDERS

Anemia: Polycythemia and Other Abnormal Hemoglobin Syndromes

The correction of DL_{CO} for anemia should be a routine procedure in the function test laboratory. Otherwise, its depression may lead to an erroneous interpretation. Several formulae have been proposed for this, but the differences between them are small. The DL_{CO} falls by 7% for each 1 g/100 ml fall in hemoglobin.[306] In another study of 23 patients before and after changes in hematocrit, the DL_{CO} changed by 6.5% for each 1 g/100 mL change in hemoglobin.[443] In a third study of 13 patients, DL_{CO} changed 6.3% for the same hemoglobin change.[467] In 1978, Clark, Woods, and Hughes[411] found that the ratio between the components of DL, DM/V_c, was unchanged in anemia and that the corrected DL_{CO} was calculated from:

$$DL_{CO} \text{ (observed)} \times (10.2 + Hb)/(1.7 \times Hb)$$

with Hb expressed in g/100 mL.

Petermann[4852] has proposed the following formula to calculate a corrected $DL_{CO}SB$:

$$(\text{Actual } DL_{CO}SB \times 100)/Hb\ (\%) = \text{Corrected } DL_{CO}SB$$

A formula has also been published to correct calculations of V_c and DM for differences in hemoglobin.[380]

DM falls with a reduced concentration of Hb in capillary blood.[443] The observed value of V_c in anemia and polycythemia falls with increasing apnea times in the single-breath test,[467] but the mechanism is not clear.

Anemia is not accompanied by any differences in other aspects of pulmonary function at rest. On exercise, however, ventilation is higher than in normal subjects. In a study of 22 Jamaicans whose Hb was equal to or less than 8 g/100 mL,[2776] excess exercise ventilation was accompanied by excess lactic acidemia. The heart rate was not increased. The ratio of $\dot{V}E/\dot{V}O_2$ was 27.2 in controls and 40.0 in patients with anemia. Observed increases in $(A - a)\ D_{O_2}$ and the VD/VT ratio were also noted. Anemia lowers the maximal exercise capacity, with a higher cardiac output at a given level of oxygen uptake.[4780]

In studies of 15 patients with very severe anemia,[2815] Hb concentrations varied between 1.4 and 4.0 g/100 mL. Central CO_2 responsiveness was normal, as judged by response to CO_2 in a hyperoxic mixture. But the hypoxia response, mediated through peripheral chemoreceptors, was markedly depressed. However, the tests were not conducted under steady-state conditions.

The polycythemia secondary to hypoxemia in patients with chronic airflow limitation has been studied[2763, 2777] and has been shown to be closely related to the level of COHb,[2831] that is, it is affected by current cigarette smoking.[2835] No further studies of cases of primary polycythemia have appeared. Earlier observations[1] suggested that DL_{CO} was lowered in these patients when the hemoglobin was restored to normal, possibly as a result of the presence of pulmonary thromboses. Studies of high-affinity hemoglobin (Hb Andrew-Minneapolis)[2754] showed that there was no fall in O_2Hb at a PA_{O_2} of 40 mm Hg and the $\dot{V}E$ response to hypoxia was normal. No observations of DL_{CO} were recorded—it would be interesting to know if this was higher than predicted. Four brothers with abnormal hemoglobin (Hb Malmö) had complex abnormalities of function.[2757] The chest x-rays showed a reticular pattern, with dilated central pulmonary arteries and sparse peripheral vessels. Two of the brothers had restrictive changes, and one had obstructive abnormalities. The Pa_{O_2} fell on exercise in all four, with rest/exercise values of 79/66; 56/44; 67/57; and 87/70. In the patient with a 56/44 ratio, there was probably a right to left shunt. DL_{CO} was impaired in one of the patients.

In an unusual study of 20 normal subjects, 20 patients with emphysema, and 20 patients with anemia, all of whom breathed 0.03% CO for 45 minutes, the rise in COHb was observed. In the normal subjects, it increased 4.27%. In emphysema patients, it increased 3.48% (81% of the normal subjects), in anemia patients, it rose 5.75%.[2775] The effect of COHb on the Hb/O_2 dissociation curve (the Haldane effect) was recently re-examined.[4858]

Sickle Cell Anemia

Studies of patients with sickle cell anemia have given somewhat varied results. Twelve affected children, compared with 12 matched normal controls,[2847] showed no differences in $DL_{CO}SB$. Mild hypoxemia and increased shunts were seen in children with anemia. Lung volumes and ventilatory flow rates were not different. In adult patients, VC and TLC are reduced. In 16 affected men and nine affected women, the average hemoglobin value was 7 g/100 mL. DL_{CO} values after correction for anemia averaged 21.8 (P = 33.1) in the men and 16.7 (P = 23.5) in the women.[2632] FEV_1 values were normal. $DL_{CO}/\dot{V}A$ values (k_{CO}) were also depressed. In 61 patients with this disease,[2765] VC was reduced in about half, and there was slight hypoxemia at rest. Studies using 100% oxygen breathing suggested that an increased shunt effect was present. In crises of this condition, the Pa_{O_2} falls further, and there is alveolar hypoventilation.[2765] It seems probable that the functional status in this condition is affected by the presence of pulmonary thromboses, since in 36 autopsies thromboemboli were present in the lungs of two-thirds of the cases.[2722] Because lowered TLC values are found in some children with this condition, it has been suggested that there may be a reduced growth of air spaces in the lung relative to the vascular bed.[2802]

Bone marrow replacement may be followed by the development of obliterative bronchiolitis.* In one of the reported cases,[4782] the

---

*See references 4776, 4782, 4846, 4848.

FEF_{25-75} fell from 4.0 L/sec to 1 L/sec. Bone marrow replacement may also be complicated by interstitial pneumonitis[4828] or pulmonary vascular abnormalities.[4846] In an existing series of 625 patients, pulmonary complications developed in more than half.[4846]

Miscellaneous Disorders

Hypogammaglobulinemia. In 55 patients with hypogammaglobulinemia, bronchograms were performed on 21. All of these showed cylindrical bronchiectasis.[2613] Five others had no evidence of pulmonary disease, and four were found to have thymomas.

Macroglobulinemia. Pulmonary infiltrations are common in patients with Waldenstrom's macroglobulinemia and may be the major presenting sign.[2664] Pulmonary function tests in five patients with lung involvement showed gross reductions in VC, grossly lowered DL_{CO} values (3.4 mL/min/mm Hg in one patient), and hypoxemia.[2700]

Cryoglobulinemia. Abnormal chest x-rays were present in 18 of 23 patients with essential mixed cryoglobulinemia.[2650] Vital capacity, TLC, and FEV_1 values were all noted to be normal, but defects were recorded in terminal flow velocity, with very abnormal values of FEF_{75-85} and $\dot{V}max_{75\%}VC$. The $(A - a) D_{O_2}$ was elevated in nine patients. No DL_{CO} measurements were recorded in this series, but some patients had abnormal lung perfusion scans.

Immunoglobulin A Deficiency. Immunoglobulin A deficiency with hepatitis was associated with fibrosing alveolitis. Radiologic changes and a grossly lowered DL_{CO} (48% of predicted) and Pa_{O_2} (50 mm Hg) were seen in one patient.[2651] The lung biopsy showed generalized intra-alveolar cellularity. Autoimmune hemolytic anemia is occasionally associated with a fibrosing alveolitis.[2622]

Angioimmunoblastic Lymphadenopathy. A case of angioimmunoblastic lymphadenopathy with dysproteinemia, considered to be a nonneoplastic proliferation of the B-lymphocyte system, has been reported.[2833] This patient had a reduced VC and FEV_1 with mild hypoxemia, probably caused by interstitial pneumonia. Other bizarre cases of lymphocytic illness with pneumonitis have been reported.[1773, 2656]

Hyperlipidemia

Six patients with hypercholesterolemia with triglyceride values between 814 and 7567 mg%

and cholesterol values between 238 and 638 mg% had a lowered $DL_{CO}SS$ on exercise.[2758] In six family members with lower triglyceride values (118 to 430 mg%) but similar cholesterol levels (312 to 585 mg%), the DL_{CO} was lowered in three.[2758] In another series of 43 hyperlipidemia patients, all with normal hemoglobin values, the $DL_{CO}SS$ was lowered by about 5 units in every subject.[2766] A close correlation was noted between DL_{CO} values and triglyceride levels (r = −0.86). The Pa_{O_2} was lowered by about 8 mm Hg at rest but rose to normal values on exercise. Xenon-133 studies showed abnormalities of perfusion distribution in the lungs of some patients.

Chronic Eosinophilia

Pulmonary function changes in chronic eosinophila are noted in Chapter 13.

Histiocytosis X and Malignant Histiocytosis

Primary pulmonary histiocytosis X may cause respiratory failure. In two such patients,[2685] the reticulonodular radiographic pattern was accompanied by hyperinflation, and there was a severe obstructive defect, with an FEV_1 of only 0.5 liters. The residual volume was 3.4 liters (P = 0.8), and the SBN_2/L test was grossly abnormal. Severe hypoxemia was seen on one hospital admission, but DL_{CO} values were not recorded. This disease has been recorded in a father and his son, 62 and 42 years old, respectively.[2712] Abundant histiocytes and moderate interstitial pneumonitis were present in the lungs of both. Severe abnormalities of pulmonary function were present, and the son had a $DL_{CO}SS$ value of 24% of predicted. The Pa_{O_2} at rest was 64 mm Hg, falling to 59 mm Hg on exercise. The RV was increased (113% of predicted), and the FEV_1 was 83% of predicted.[2712]

In a large series of 78 cases, this syndrome[2857] occurred four times more often in males than in females. Some were asymptomatic but most had dyspnea, cough, or malaise, and some had a history of pneumothoraces. The reticular and micronodular lesions were mostly in the midzones and bases, but apparently the costophrenic angles were spared. The VC was decreased in 59% of the patients. The RV/TLC ratio increased in 61%, the FEV_1/FVC ratio decreased in 21%, and the DL_{CO} decreased in

74%. Test results were entirely normal in 15% of the patients. The authors of this study[2857] made the interesting observation that RV/TLC and DL_{CO} changes were related to radiologic cyst formation and followed radiologic changes fairly closely.

A classification of radiologic changes in this condition has been proposed.[2842] One case has been reported[2858] in which it was suggested that the condition might be caused by a neoplastic proliferation of pulmonary macrophages.

Acute and Chronic Leukemia

A study of 47 episodes of pulmonary infiltration in 43 patients showed that 55% had local consolidations on the chest film, 13% developed cavitary disease, and 32% had a diffuse interstitial infiltrative pattern.[2659] Although it was noted that several patients had a Pa_{O_2} of less than 50 mm Hg, no detailed function tests were reported in this series. In acute leukemia, acute respiratory failure may be the first manifestation of the condition,[2684] with severe hypoxemia caused by intense infiltration of the alveolar septae by blast cells. In such patients, ventilatory support may be needed to permit survival until a remission can be induced. In the second edition of this book,[1] we noted that pulmonary infiltrations and associated function test defects were probably commoner in leukemia than reports would indicate. This view has been supported by a study of 139 adults with leukemia, 98 of whom had patchy lung infiltrates—43 local and 55 diffuse.[2681] In this series, no function tests were reported.

In Chapter 14, which deals with drug-induced changes in the lung, we noted the occasional difficulty of distinguishing between drug effects and lesions attributable to the disease itself. This problem was illustrated by a patient with lymphadenoma and pulmonary infiltrates who was treated with bleomycin.[2725] The same problem may be encountered in patients with leukemia.

Pulmonary Amyloidosis

Severe cases of diffuse pulmonary amyloidosis continue to be reported.[2669] Some patients show radiologic changes but a normal DL_{CO}.[2695] Others have gross reduction in VC but relative preservation of DL_{CO}.[2799] In some patients, both VC and DL_{CO} are reduced.[2633, 4822] Sometimes these decrease to very low levels, as in a 58-year-old woman in whom the $D_{L_{CO}}$ was only 13% of predicted values and k_{CO} was 0.7 (compared with a predicted value of 4.0).[2629] In this patient, who had associated myelomatosis, the TLC was remarkably preserved at 108% of predicted values. A similar very low F_{CO} (0.23, compared with the predicted 0.45), with normal lung volumes and ventilatory flow rates, was noted in a 61-year-old man with amyloid infiltration of alveolar walls proved by biopsy.[2625] According to the published reports, the disease may run a very slow course. In one 51-year-old man with diffuse nodular infiltrates, ventilatory flow rates were normal and the Pa_{O_2} was 64 mm Hg 7 years after the condition had been diagnosed.[4797]

We have recently seen a biopsy-proven case in a 57-year-old man with marked radiologic changes, a reduction in TLC of 1.4 liters, and a normal FEF_{25-75}. His single-breath and steady-state diffusing capacities were 6.2 and 6.0, respectively. It may be that this condition is characterized by a greater diffusion reduction than one would predict from the loss of lung volume, but more data on this rare condition are needed before this conclusion can be firmly reached.

A 51-year-old man survived 6 years with pulmonary infiltrative amyloidosis,[2648] during which time the VC declined at an average rate of -470 mL/year. In another case, hemoptysis was the presenting symptom.[4825] A form of this disease that may give rise to airway obstruction and present diagnostic difficulty is localized amyloidosis of the lower respiratory tract.[2727] Tracheobronchial amyloidosis in a 40-year-old woman[4829] lowered the FEV_1 to 64% of predicted. In a 47-year-old man, it was reduced to 56% of predicted. In each patient some improvement followed CO_2 laser treatment. Others have also noted airflow obstruction in this rare condition.[4827]

Thrombotic Thrombocytopenic Purpura, Leukopenia, and Hemophilia

Bleeding into the lung, which may lead to respiratory failure, is not uncommon in thrombotic thrombocytopenic purpura and is signaled by a rise in respiratory rate.[2654] Mechanical ventilation may be required. As in other diseases that cause intrapulmonary hemorrhage

(noted in Chapter 13), a rise in $D_{L_{CO}}$ may be recorded after such episodes.

It has recently been shown that intense leukopenia can give rise to an adult respiratory distress syndrome of acute respiratory failure.[7242] Studies of cases of hemophilia being treated by infusion of factor VIII concentrates[4854] showed that careful filtration prevented any measurable adverse pulmonary effects.

PULMONARY FUNCTION IN LIVER DISEASE: PULMONARY TELANGIECTASIA

During the past decade, considerable attention has been devoted to the cause of hypoxemia in patients with chronic liver disease. It has become clear that several mechanisms may be involved:

1. Ruff and his colleagues[2849] showed that closing volume was increased in many of these patients. They also found that there was significant airway closure in dependent parts of the lung, which led to low $\dot{V}/\dot{Q}$ regions and hypoxemia.

2. Patients with ascites were compared with subjects without ascites. In the former group, it was common to find Pa_{O_2} lower in recumbency than when the patient was sitting.[2624] In this series, there was no consistent relationship between closing capacity and hypoxemia.

3. The $D_{L_{CO}}$ is commonly lowered (after correction for anemia), as was shown in studies of 170 patients with chronic liver disease of mixed etiology.[2630] The $(A - a) D_{O_2}$ is elevated.

4. In some cirrhotic patients with finger clubbing, Pa_{O_2} falls on exercise,[127] the $D_{L_{CO}}$ is lowered (67% of predicted), and FEV_1 and SBN_2/L are both normal. In such cases, there are probably shunts within the lung. One severely cirrhotic patient had a $D_{L_{CO}}$ of 50% of predicted and a $(A - a) D_{O_2}$ of 60 mm Hg. At autopsy, there were spider nevi on the pleural surface and many precapillary arteriovenous anastomoses with thickened capillary walls.[2616] In this patient, high radiation counts over the kidney were seen immediately after a lung scan, showing that significant shunting was present. Similar findings have been reported in a 35-year-old man,[2691] also with a lowered $D_{L_{CO}}$ and an increased shunt component. In others, vas-

cular abnormalities in the lung are so prominent that the disease resembles pulmonary telangiectasia[2795] (see later discussion).

In another case in a 49-year-old man[2806] $DL_{CO}SB$ and $DL_{CO}SS$ were 66% of predicted and Pa_{O_2} was 49 mm Hg. The pulmonary angiogram showed dilatations but no intrapulmonary shunts. These authors noted that arterial desaturation in liver disease was first noted in 1935, and they suggested that there was "recruitment of pre-existing non-functioning shunts at the pre-capillary level within the lung parenchyma."

Other authors have been unable to demonstrate an increase in ventilated slow space in these patients, as would be expected if an increased closing volume was important. They concluded that vascular changes within the lung are probably more important.[2811] They also noted a lowered DM component and suggested that there was an increased flow through abnormal shortened pulmonary capillaries.[2812]

5. In 17 patients with encephalopathy, consistent elevations in both closing capacity and residual volume were noted,[2817] and the $(A - a) D_{O_2}$ averaged more than twice the predicted value.

6. It is possible that in some cases, there is also a shunt through portacaval/pulmonary anastomoses of portal venous blood into pulmonary veins via collateral channels connecting portal, mediastinal, and pulmonary venous beds.[1746] In some patients there is secondary pulmonary hypertension.[2846]

7. A very interesting observation is that the pulmonary vasoconstrictive response to hypoxemia is lost in this condition. This was shown to be the case in 10 patients with alcoholic cirrhosis breathing 10% oxygen.[2736] This phenomenon clearly indicates that abnormality of the pulmonary vasculature is common. It has been suggested that the rarity of systemic hypertension in liver disease may be attributable to pulmonary shunts preventing the conversion of angiotensin-I to angiotensin-II.[2658]

8. In overt liver failure, there is increased sensitivity of the peripheral chemoreceptors to hypoxemia.[2782] the delta $\dot{V}E/P_{CO_2}$ response is diminished,[2781, 2782] leading to the paradox of increased resting $\dot{V}E$ and reduced CO_2 response. In such cases, a lowered Pa_{O_2} is found with a lowered Pa_{CO_2}.

9. In view of the many possibilities of abnor-

mality in pulmonary telangiectasia, it is perhaps not surprising that no significant differences in blood gases were found between patients with relatively good and those with relatively poor liver function.[2790]

10. In patients with primary biliary cirrhosis, reduction in DL_{CO} was found only in those with concomitant Sjögren's syndrome.[2837] It was suggested that liver disease alone is not accompanied by the changes seen in other types of cirrhosis.

In Chapter 12, the syndrome of pulmonary telangiectasia is discussed. Some of the instances of liver cirrhosis in the literature[2691] appear very similar to this syndrome.

ALCOHOL INGESTION

In 12 normal subjects, acute ingestion of alcohol was followed by a decline in both DL_{CO} and $DL_{CO}/\dot{V}A$ 90 minutes later.[2686] In these studies, the CO was measured by gas chromatography, which avoids the possible error that alcohol in the breath may produce by interfering with the CO meter reading.[983] Acute sensitivity to ethanol, with bronchoconstriction, has been documented.[2729] Of considerable interest is the observation that alcohol ingestion (to a blood level of 80 to 100 mg/100mL) in 10 healthy normal persons depressed the citric acid cough threshold.[966] It also depressed the delta $\dot{V}E/P_{O_2}$ response after 20 minutes. The P_{CO_2} response is depressed 50 minutes later.[2779] This, together with the increase in pharyngeal resistance that occurs following alcohol ingestion,[4823] may explain why alcohol ingestion worsens sleep apnea.

The question of whether heavy alcohol intake predisposes to the progression of chronic airflow limitation is not resolved. This was originally suggested[2662] and supported by a study of 44 former alcoholics. In four non-smoking women, FEF_{25-75} values were 35%, 55%, 65%, and 72% of predicted values.[2694] $DL_{CO}SB$ values were normal. In 30 acute alcoholics, 15 had mild airway obstruction, and the DL_{CO} was reduced to a mean of 19.3 (P = 31).[2706] However, the possible interference of alcohol in the breath on the CO meter was not excluded in these studies. In other studies, after correction for smoking and socioeconomic status, no effect of alcohol ingestion on the FEV_1 was detectable.[2789, 2797] From these data, it was concluded that alcohol ingestion, *per se*, is not a significant risk factor in the development of chronic airflow limitation. This conclusion is supported by a recent study of 27 chronic alcoholics, in whom no function defects were demonstrable in the non-smokers or in the ex-smokers.[4865]

PULMONARY FUNCTION IN CHRONIC RENAL FAILURE

Lee, Stretton, and Barnes studied 55 patients with chronic renal failure, all without radiologic or clinical evidence of lung disease[2627] and with DL_{CO} data corrected for anemia. The mean data were as follows:

	Number	Mean	Predicted	p
FEV_1, men	29	3.05	3.75	0.001
women	26	2.20	2.50	0.001
VC, men	29	3.86	4.63	0.001
women	26	2.75	2.95	0.001
FEV/FVC, men	29	78%	76%	ns
women	26	81%	82%	ns
DL_{CO} (mL/min/ mm Hg), men	29	19.2	31.5	0.001
women	26	14.5	25.1	0.001
DM, men	13	31.6	62.8	0.001
women	7	19.8	41.8	0.001
V_c (mL), men	13	62.8	76.8	0.05
women	7	63.4	59.4	ns

DL_{CO} was closely related to blood urea and creatinine clearance data.

In three non-smokers and three smokers studied before and after dialysis, VC increased, RV fell, and FEF_{25-75} increased after the procedure. There was also a decrease in closing capacity.[2663] The $(A - a) D_{O_2}$ was not much affected, and changes in the reduced diffusing capacity were inconsistent. Regional studies showed that before dialysis, $\dot{V}E$ and $\dot{Q}_c$ were both diminished at the lung bases and both improved after dialysis.

Other authors have noted overinflation and air trapping in chronic renal failure, with a normal RL and elevated RV.[2697] Dialysis usually produces a significant increase in the difference between expiratory reserve volume and closing volume, often with a decrease in $(A - a) D_{O_2}$.[2764, 2770] All of these findings indicate that there is an increase in peribronchial fluid before dialysis, with premature airway closure caused by fluid overload. The fall in body weight after dialysis correlates with the fall in closing volume.[2780] The persistently reduced DL_{CO}, present even after dialysis, has been noted by most of those who have studied this condition.[2818] Its cause is not clear. The slope

of the delta $\dot{V}E/PCO_2$ relationship has been said to be normal in these patients, but others have found that it and the $P_{0.1}$ measurement are lowered before dialysis and increase after dialysis is completed.[4798] The Pa_{CO_2} is linearly related to the HCO_3^- level. If this rises, it leads to relative hypoventilation and a fall in Pa_{O_2}.[2778]

Serial studies on 13 patients undergoing continuous ambulatory peritoneal dialysis[4812] noted that both FVC and FEV_1 fell by equal amounts (about 10%) during induction, with no change in Pa_{O_2}. The mean DL_{CO} values were below 60% of predicted and were unaffected (the reason for these low values was not explained). Other investigators, using the six inert gas method to quantitate $\dot{V}/\dot{Q}$ change,[4784] have concluded that hemodialysis improved the $\dot{V}/\dot{Q}$ relationships, although the Pa_{O_2} declined as the ventilation fell. There was no evidence of a diffusion defect in the patients studied.

A recent editorial pointed out that there were over 10,000 patients on chronic dialysis in the United States.[4811] It has been found that unless microembolic filters are used, the $(A - a) D_{O_2}$ may increase after dialysis.[2698]

Intrapulmonary calcification occasionally occurs in these patients, and the material in the lung has been shown to be $(CaMg)_3(PO_4)$. In nine such patients, significant decreases in VC, DL_{CO}, and Pa_{O_2} were present in all.[2830] Acute respiratory failure occasionally occurs.[2609]

MISCELLANEOUS

Intestinal Diseases

Ulcerative colitis is associated with bronchial disease. In one series of 10 patients, all non-smokers, all had a productive cough. Six had abnormal chest x-rays, but four had some increased pulmonary markings. The FEV_1 was abnormal in the four with radiologic changes, and DL_{CO} was below 74% of predicted in the same four patients.[2605] Bronchial epithelial biopsies showed submucosal inflammatory changes. In one patient, colectomy was followed by the development of pulmonary bullous disease and bronchiectasis.[2042]

Data on 18 patients with Crohn's disease with normal chest x-rays and no pulmonary symptoms showed that the FVC was less than 80% of predicted in four and that the $DL_{CO}SB$ was less than 80% of predicted in eleven.[4847] Bronchoalveolar lavage revealed that there was a lymphocytic alveolitis in six patients. Fourteen of the 18 patients had taken no sulfasalazine (which can cause pneumonitis) for 3 months before the study.

Gaucher's disease has been noted to cause death in respiratory failure, with massive infiltration of alveolar wlls by abnormal cells.[2657] In one patient, the VC was reduced to 30% of the predicted value.

Whipple's disease may cause foamy macrophages in the lung[2635] with bilateral basal infiltrations on the x-ray, but pulmonary function tests have not been recorded. Oculocutaneous albinism (Hermansky-Pudlak syndrome) occurs with inflammatory bowel disease and associated pulmonary fibrosis.[2649] In five patients with this rare syndrome, all had a DL_{CO} less than 56% of predicted, with similar reductions in VC. Lung biopsies revealed ceroid-like material in pulmonary macrophages, with other changes in the interstitium.

There has been some controversy as to whether celiac disease is sometimes accompanied by pulmonary changes. A study of 24 patients with this condition[2840] indicated that fine reticular shadowing occurred on the chest x-ray in several patients, with a normal FEV_1 and lowered DL_{CO}. However, the specificity of these findings is unclear.[1913] In one case of celiac disease, pulmonary hemosiderosis was also found to be present.[4813]

Gastrointestinal reflux was found to be present in 65% of patients with chronic airflow obstruction, but there was no evidence that this was aggravating their pulmonary disease.[4783] The possible importance of reflux of acid from the stomach into the lower esophagus in asthmatics led to experimental acid infusions. It was noted that this was followed by a fall of 210 milliliters in VC and an increased SBN_2/L.[1371] It was postulated that there might be a neural esophagobronchial reflex mechanism to explain the findings. It has been suggested that this might be related to night-time symptoms in asthmatics, but the use of cimetidine did not lead to any change in function.[1356] Studies of pulmonary function in patients with hiatus hernia do not reveal any differences from normal subjects without this condition.[2688, 2813, 2814]

An intriguing observation was made that there was an increase in hydrogen gas detectable in alveolar gas samples in carbohydrate malabsorption syndrome patients given lactulose.[2783]

Recently, the acute effects of glucose in hypocaloric and hypercaloric amounts were studied. The glucose was given to four normal volunteers and four acutely ill patients for 6 days. The $\dot{V}CO_2$ increased by 18% in the normal subjects and 7% in the others. $\dot{V}O_2$ did not change and the RQ rose. The $\dot{V}E/Pa_{CO_2}$ curve did not change. The authors[4851] concluded that the $\dot{V}O_2$ increases with total parenteral nutrition, and the CO_2 sensitivity also rises. These effects must be due to the protein infusion, since they could not be demonstrated with glucose alone.

Metabolic Acidosis and Alkalosis

In three patients, severe hypokalemic metabolic alkalosis with dehydration and azotemia led to a rise in Pa_{CO_2} of more than 60 mm Hg.[2667] In such a situation, rapid reduction of Pa_{CO_2} by ventilation can be dangerous. In another patient in whom the Pa_{CO_2} was 75 mm Hg, the alveolar hypoventilation led to hypoxemia and a Pa_{O_2} of 50 mm Hg.[2665] On voluntary hyperventilation, the Pa_{CO_2} fell to 28 mm Hg, and the pH rose to more than 7.8 units. Hypoventilation leading to hypoxemia has been recorded in this condition on several occasions.[2713, 2829]

In 159 cases of diabetic ketoacidosis,[2773] the relationship between hydrogen ion $[H^+]$ (in nmol/L) and Pa_{CO_2} (in mm Hg) was given by:

$$Pa_{CO_2} = -224.2 + 2140/H^+ + 0.163[H^+]$$

The r value was 0.79. There is also a linear relationship between Pa_{CO_2} and HCO_3^- (in mmol/L)

$$Pa_{CO_2} = 1.30(HCO_3) + 9.8$$

The authors of this study noted that maximal resting ventilation was observed for pH values between 6.90 and 6.95. When HCO_3 is increasing or decreasing from a previous high level, it takes between 11 and 24 hours for a new steady state to be reached between Pa_{CO_2} and HCO_3.[2836]

Fabry's Disease

Fabry's disease is also known as angiokeratoma corporis diffusum universale. In seven patients, two of whom were non-smokers, there was significant airflow obstruction.[2646] Three had significant hyperinflation. Airway epithelial cells have increased deposits of sphingolipid in this condition, and this is believed to be responsible for changes in MEFV curves and delayed ^{133}Xe clearance. In this series, the changes were more marked in the smokers, suggesting that smoking, in addition to the pathologic changes, produced more functional impairment.

Marfan's Syndrome

Marfan's syndrome, a connective tissue disorder, is associated with a considerable loss of elastic recoil and an increased frequency of spontaneous pneumothorax.[1] In two patients, one a 29-year-old smoker of 10 cigarettes/day (case 1) and the other a 30-year-old non-smoker (case 2), pulmonary function data were as follows[2623]:

	Case 1	Case 2
TLC*	123	124
FRC	121	118
RV	121	139
FVC	127	121
$DL_{co}SB$	66	75
k_{co} ($DL_{co}/\dot{V}A$)	48	56

*All values given as a percentage of predicted.

Studies of pulmonary mechanics demonstrated the considerable loss of recoil in both cases.

A definitive review of no fewer than 100 cases of this syndrome[4775] confirmed that spontaneous pneumothoraces and bullae, together with bronchiectasis and recurrent respiratory infections, were common features. Apical pulmonary fibrosis was also observed. Four men between 30 and 46 years old showed skeletal and cardiac manifestations, and three had abnormally low values for FVC, FEV_1, and DL_{co}.

Down's Syndrome

In Down's syndrome, the alveoli are hypoplastic, and alveolar elastic fibers are deficient.[4824] The consequential changes in pulmonary function do not appear to have been defined.

Tuberous Sclerosis

Thirty-one patients with tuberous sclerosis and pulmonary involvement had been recorded in the literature up to 1971.[2674] Dyspnea was a prominent symptom, and the chest x-ray showed fine reticulation proceeding to cystic changes. Spontaneous pneumothoraces are common. No detailed function tests in this condition have been reported, but it is probable that the pattern of function disorder resembles that seen in pulmonary lymphangiomyomatosis (see Chapter 17).

20 PNEUMOTHORAX, FIBROTHORAX, PLEURAL EFFUSION, AND ATELECTASIS

INTRODUCTION

The function of the pleural linings of the lung is often taken for granted. However, interference with the normal pleura, which is designed to enable one layer to slide over the other with very low (but calculable) frictional forces, causes major functional abnormalities. Hills[4832] has contributed a valuable review of the forces acting on the pleura, and Herbert[4864] has summarized the pathophysiologic aspects of pleural disease.[4864] Brandi[4871] appears to have been the first investigator to calculate the probable work required in overcoming frictional forces in the normal pleura, and Stamenovic[4859] has investigated the mechanical characteristics of pleural strips.

The effects of pleural plaques and of aggressive pleuritis, which occasionally occurs in asbestos-exposed patients, on pulmonary function is described in Chapter 16. In Chapter 5, a patient with asbestos pleuritis (rounded atelectasis) is discussed (see Case 10).

PNEUMOTHORAX

The effect of a pneumothorax is to abolish the vertical gradient normally present in pleural pressure. Anthonisen[2740] found that this led to the abolition of the vertical gradient of ventilation distribution in the affected lung, with probable airway closure occurring in the collapsed lung at low lung volumes. Nitrogen clearance

364

does not seem to be much reduced, unless the degree of lung collapse exceeds 50%. The ventilation per unit of lung volume of the collapsed lung is the same as that for the inflated lung.

Studies of lung function after re-expansion following spontaneous pneumothorax in 21 healthy subjects aged 16 to 38[2769] showed that four had some evidence of emphysema. A raised residual volume and lowered $DL_{CO}SB$ was found in many of the others with normal mechanical properties of lung function. The authors concluded that these results probably indicated the presence of "disseminated blebs with high ventilation/capillary blood flow ratio." Others have also found a reduced DL_{CO}. In many of these patients, DL_{CO} and k_{CO} ($DL_{CO}/\dot{V}A$) reductions are accompanied by evidence of loss of elastic recoil.[2805]

A comparison of pulmonary function after re-expansion among 15 patients conservatively treated, 23 treated by drainage tube, and nine who had a thoracotomy and local repair[2755] showed no major differences in function between the first two categories, but slightly lower VC was found in those treated by operation. In this total series of 47 patients, 20 of 30 studied had a delayed nitrogen clearance after complete re-expansion had occurred. It has been shown that active vasoconstriction occurs in the affected lung and that a reticulocytosis accompanies spontaneous pneumothoraces.[1]

Induction of experimental pneumothorax in dogs leads to an immediate increase in respiratory rate, a shift in ventilation from the affected side to the normal lung, and a fall in Pa_{O_2} from 85 mm Hg to 51 mm Hg.[2677] Complete restitution of function occurred after re-expansion. Earlier studies had indicated that changes in arterial oxygenation were much more marked in anesthetized dogs than when a pneumothorax was induced without anesthesia.[1]

PLEURAL EFFUSIONS

In studies of six subjects with small pleural effusions, (by means of ^{133}Xe), Anthonisen and Martin found that boluses inspired from residual volume were equally distributed between the affected and unaffected sides.[2739] However, regional washouts were prolonged from the affected side, probably as a result of a reduction in dynamic pressure swings by the presence of the effusion. Studies of pulmonary function before and after removal of between 600 and 1800 milliliters of fluid from the pleural cavity[188] showed that small increases in FRC and TLC occurred. Pa_{O_2} rose by 6 mm Hg. RV and VC were not affected, however. The effect of thoracentesis on lung volumes is noted in detail in Chapter 4.

PLEURITIS, PLEURAL THICKENING, AND FIBROTHORAX

Studies of "unilateral pleuritis" in 11 cases (by means of $^{133}Xe^{2827}$) showed that ventilation was reduced more than perfusion on the affected side. In these cases, VC was reduced to 58% of predicted, and the authors concluded that "unilateral pleuritis thus appears to affect the mechanical function of both lungs."

The severity of function defects in association with severe pleural disease and a fibrothorax was documented in the previous edition.[1] Reports of marked improvement in function after surgery continue to appear.[2575, 2800, 2826] A vital capacity of less than 70% of predicted was found to be a useful criterion for decortication in a series consisting of 66 cases of pleural disease caused by tuberculosis and three post-traumatic cases of fibrothorax.[2800] The grossly compromised pulmonary function that follows the now obsolete operation of thoracoplasty was noted in the second edition.

Recurrent pleurisy commonly occurs in diffuse lupus erythematosus. As noted in Chapter 13, there is evidence that diaphragmatic function may be compromised in this disease, possibly as a result of chronic pleural thickening.

IDIOPATHIC MEDIASTINAL FIBROSIS

Although three of five patients with this syndrome were successfully treated by venous graft surgery,[4866] there was no note of preoperative or postoperative function tests.

CHAPTER

21 DISORDERS OF THE CHEST WALL

This chapter is concerned with "structural" defects of the thoracic cage. The effects of neuromuscular disorders and diaphragmatic paralysis are discussed in the next chapter.

In 1979, Bergofsky[4898] reviewed the factors leading to respiratory failure in conditions involving defects of the thoracic cage. He suggested five principal mechanisms:

1. $\dot{V}/\dot{Q}$ inhomogeneity—airway closure caused by compressed lung.
2. Inability to cough.
3. Defect in respiratory control in conjunction with increased work of breathing.
4. Excess load on certain groups of respiratory muscles.
5. Excess blood volume and fluid retention aggravating the work of breathing.

The new understanding of the respiratory muscles and the possibility of their fatigue (reviewed in the next chapter) would lead one to suppose that this might be an additional important cause of ventilatory failure. In general, the degree of resting hypoxemia determines the level of pulmonary hypertension and, hence, the risk of cor pulmonale.

IDIOPATHIC SCOLIOSIS

Idiopathic scoliosis usually begins in adolescence. Studies in children show normal thoracic mobility, but the VC, FEV_1, and DL_{CO} are usually reduced.[4899] Studies of 48 subjects—39 girls and 9 boys of average age 14—showed that the corrective Harrington operation does not immediately produce improved function but this improves as normal growth occurs.[4902] Oth-

ers have also noted that spinal fusion does not improve function.[4884] Kafer[4889] has considered whether such measurements as arm span or tibia length should be used for predicted values of pulmonary function tests, but the latter index is inaccurate. Her review of this condition (with 114 references) surveyed the data up to 1977.[2958] When the spinal curvature is less than 30 degrees in adolescents, there are usually no symptoms, although the FVC may be reduced.[4904] The FVC correlates with the maximal inspiratory and expiratory pressures more closely than with the degree of curvature at this stage.

In 22 subjects, whose mean angle of curvature was 66 degrees, $DL_{CO}SB$ was 17% lower than in controls, but the $DL/\dot{V}A$ ratio was the same.[4900] In this series, the FEF_{25-75} averaged 75% of predicted, and gas distribution indices were normal. Kafer[4890] studied 55 patients of mean age 25 years and a TLC of 70% of predicted. She noted that the residual volume was reduced. Correlation coefficients between the angle of scoliosis and the degree of abnormality in TLC or VC were shown to be highly significant. In the same series,[4889] 50 patients with a mean scoliosis angle of 80 degrees were studied. The Pa_{O_2} was also related to the VC and the angle of deformity. The coefficient of variation of various parameters was not much different from normal; for the Pa_{O_2}, it was 3.6%.[4887]

In older subjects (and in 14 patients of mean age 28 years[4901]), as the angle of scoliosis increases with age, both VC and FEV_1 fall. RV/TLC increases, as does the resting respiratory rate, and hypoxemia and hypercapnia precede the development of cor pulmonale. Comparisons between patients aged 17 with those aged 40 show that exercise hypoxemia is commoner in the older group,[4895] even though the vital capacities may not be much different. In the last edition, we noted that regional studies of these patients that used ^{133}Xe had been reported.[1] More recent data on 10 patients[4897] showed that ventilation is more severely impaired in the region of maximum convexity than in the opposite lung. Perfusion distribution is less affected. The widened $(A - a) D_{O_2}$ is attributed to this $\dot{V}/\dot{Q}$ imbalance. In the patients studied, the mean FVC was only 48% of predicted, and the $(A - a) D_{O_2}$, at 33.7 mm Hg, was twice the normal value. Others have found less regional differences in ventilation, without a clear relationship to convexity.[4877] It has been suggested that early $\dot{V}/\dot{Q}$ disturbance occurs only when the scoliosis affects the higher level of the cervical vertebrae (T1 through T5).[4876]

With greater angles of curvature in patients with more severe disease, airway closure may occur in parts of the lung at respiratory levels above the FRC.[4874] The low TLC seen in some patients may be caused by defective mechanical coupling between the respiratory muscles and the chest cage, since the Harrington operation has been found to lead to an increase in PI_{max} in 15 patients studied before and a year after the operation.[4907] Exercise studies show that pulmonary arterial pressure increases linearly with increasing $\dot{V}O_2$.[4883] Oxygen breathing did not affect the pulmonary pressure at rest, but during exercise it caused it to fall by a mean of 5.2 mm Hg. There is a close relationship between Pa_{O_2} and pulmonary arterial pressure in these patients.[4880] In mild cases, the maximal $\dot{V}O_2$ may be little reduced,[4885] but later exercise is limited by ventilation.[4882]

Some very severe cases of this condition have been documented. In one infant, it developed before the age of 1 year[4903]; death from cardiopulmonary failure occurred at age 36; and postmortem morphometry of the lung showed that it was about the size of the lung of a 5-year-old child. The FVC was 600 milliliters. At rest, the pulmonary arterial pressure was 140/440 mm Hg.

KYPHOSCOLIOSIS

The commonest cause of this condition is childhood poliomyelitis.

In 12 patients, resting Pa_{O_2} was a mean of 70.0 mm Hg; this fell on exercise to a mean of 47.7 mm Hg.[4892] Pulmonary hypertension closely followed the degree of hypoxemia. In advanced cases, nocturnal ventilation by means of a specially built cuirass may be helpful,[4905] and restitution of the blood gases to normal has been reported as a result of this treatment. In such patients, the VC is usually less than one liter and the TLC is less than 2 liters.[4906] A short period of high inflation pressure has also been suggested, since this was followed by some improvement in six patients.[4910]

Often the PI_{max} is reduced to low levels. Nine patients with severe disease were of mean age 48. Their mean TLC was 44% of predicted, and the mean Pa_{O_2} was 66 mm Hg.[4908] The transdiaphragmatic pressure was also lower than in normal subjects, and it correlated with the blood gas changes. The investigators concluded that impairment of respiratory muscle function was closely related to the development of ventilatory failure. The marked abnormalities in blood gases upon change in body position[4769] in a patient with very severe kyphoscoliosis are noted in Chapter 4.

Rom and Miller[4881] have pointed out that some patients with severe disease survive for many years. They found 10 patients, all with curvatures greater than 100 degrees, who had survived into their seventh decade; their mean age was 69.3 years. In three whose TLC values were 26%, 55%, and 70% of predicted, Pa_{O_2} levels varied between 59 mm Hg and 77 mm Hg. The highest Pa_{O_2} was 57 mm Hg.

ANKYLOSING SPONDYLITIS

As noted in the last edition,[1] ankylosing spondylitis causes some reduction in TLC and VC. Ventilatory capability is well maintained because of unimpaired diaphragmatic action. Thoracic wall compliance is reduced. More recent studies have noted that the residual volume may be increased[4878] and have documented the increased diaphragmatic excursion.[4911] In a study of 25 patients,[4896] it was computed that their diaphragmatic contribution was 84% during quiet breathing, compared with 68% in a normal control group. As was also noted in the last edition,[1] this dependence on diaphragm function means that respiratory depressants and upper abdominal incisions represent a special risk.

Regional lung function using ^{133}Xe[4879] studies have noted some reduction of ventilation at the lung apices. This is of interest in view of the association of apical fibrosis with ankylosing spondylitis. In the nine patients investigated in this study, the VC was 65% of predicted, and the DL_{CO} was 80% of predicted.

It is known that upper lobe fibrosis may occur in this condition, associated with the presence of the HLA-B27 antigen.[4894] The affected areas may develop cavitary changes. The VC was reduced to between 0.9 and 1.9 liters in five of seven patients between 35 and 70 years old.[4886] Secondary aspergillosis may occur as a complication. Reductions in VC and TLC in the presence of apical fibrosis have been documented in other series.[4894] Although apical fibrosis is strongly associated with ankylosing spondylitis, it may occur alone.[4893]

In a study of exercise in ankylosing spondylitis, six patients with a mean maximal chest expansion of 1.4 cm[4909] were compared with six normal subjects of the same age and sex. The following data were reported:

	Controls	Ankylosing Spondylitis
Age	47.2	47.8
Weight (kg)	84.3	83.2
Height (cm)	187	180
FVC	5.62	3.81
FEV_1	4.43	3.16
TL_{CO} (mL/min/mm Hg)	—	28.8
$\dot{V}max_{O_2}$ (L/min)	2.78	2.15
Work (maximal)	225	175
$\dot{V}E_{max}$ (L/min)	109.8	92.9
Maximal respiratory rate/min	34.8	40.8
VT_{max} (L)	3.02	2.26

The authors concluded that exercise performance was decreased. Because maximal voluntary ventilation exceeded the exercise ventilation by 15 L/min, the exercise was not limited by ventilation. However, they might have been limited by incipient diaphragmatic fatigue.

There is little $\dot{V}/\dot{Q}$ disturbance in this condition, and blood gases are normal.[1] There is consequently little risk of cor pulmonale.

PIGEON CHEST DEFORMITY

As noted in the last edition, this deformity is associated with little interference in pulmonary function.[1] There do not appear to have been any additional studies of the condition.

MYOSITIS OSSIFICANS PROGRESSIVA

Studies of a 15-year-old girl with rare myositis ossificans progressiva[4888] led to the conclusions that the severe reduction in TLC, which was 66% of predicted, was due to thoracic wall changes and that no interstitial lung disease was present.

POST-THORACOPLASTY DEFORMITY

As noted in the last edition,[1] patients who had thoracoplasty operations for tuberculosis, with the resulting severe deformity, may develop respiratory failure. Ten such patients have been described, all of them successfully treated with long-term negative pressure ventilation.[4912]

THE RESPIRATORY MUSCLES AND THEIR DISORDERS

INTRODUCTION

It has been recognized since ancient times that breathing is a rhythmic contraction of muscles, although the purpose of the resultant air movement remained obscure. The mechanism of breathing became clearer after the early years of the twentieth century, but the past two decades have witnessed a remarkable resurgence of interest in the muscles of respiration. Many new insights have been gained. Principles learned from the study of skeletal muscles in general have been applied to the respiratory muscles, and some differences, for example between the diaphragm and other skeletal muscles, have been identified.[5075] The diaphragm indeed has some metabolic similarities to heart muscle. This is not surprising since, unlike other skeletal muscles, the muscles of inspiration contract phasically under non-voluntary control (for the most part) throughout our lives. Any condition that impairs the normal function of these muscles is important, since respiratory failure is the potential consequence. This chapter outlines current understanding of the muscles of breathing and of the many diseases that may interfere with their normal function.

THE NEUROMUSCULAR PUMP

The muscles of breathing are customarily divided into inspiratory and expiratory muscles. During quiet breathing, inspiratory muscles are active, and expiration is mostly passive. The diaphragm produces the major fraction of the tidal volume, but it requires the co-ordinated activity of other respiratory muscles for efficient function. Muscles that dilate the upper airway are important in preventing collapse of the soft tissues in this region during inspiration. In addition, the parasternal intercostal muscles (intercartilagenous, internal intercostal muscles) prevent collapse of the anterior rib cage during diaphragmatic contraction.[4913] Augmented breathing during exercise is associated with the recruitment of additional inspiratory muscles. Similarly, the expiratory muscles become phasically active as ventilation increases to speed up the respiratory cycle.

Inspiratory Muscles

In addition to those muscles of inspiration just mentioned, it is now known that the scalene muscles are phasically active in humans during quiet breathing.[4914] These neck muscles appear to be important because only when they are active can the parasternal muscles elevate the rib cage.[4915] Thus, the diaphragm, the intercostal muscles (particularly the parasternals), and the scalene muscles may be considered primary muscles of inspiration.[4916] Diseases that impair their function may be expected to impair normal ventilation. Other muscles of inspiration, the accessory muscles, include the sternomastoid, trapezius, serrati, pectorals, levator scapulae, and the costal levators. These muscles are active during augmented breathing or when the primary muscles have failed and recruitment of the accessories is needed to prevent respiratory failure. An extreme clinical example of such a situation is seen in the high quadriplegic patient who is able to use only the neck accessory muscles to maintain ventilation.[4917]

The diaphragm is a thin curved muscle with its insertion on the ribs and its origin in the central tendon. Its motor innervation is via the phrenic nerve, which arises from the cervical segments C3 through C5. The diaphragm consists of two main parts, costal and crural.[4918] The lateral walls of the diaphragm are adherent to the rib cage and therefore run parallel to it. The fibers curve medially to join the central tendon and form the dome of the diaphragm. Contraction and shortening of the diaphragm causes the upper margin of the adherent part of the diaphragm to progressively "peel away" from the rib cage as the dome descends. This downward piston-like movement of the diaphragm increases abdominal pressure. The increase in abdominal pressure acts as a fulcrum to allow elevation of the rib cage by force applied on the rib cage insertions of the diaphragm (insertional action) and also acts to distend the lower rib cage in the area below the diaphragmatic dome (appositional action).[4919] When lung volume is near TLC at full inspiration, the muscle fibers of the diaphragm are approximately perpendicular to the rib cage. In other words, there is no appositional component and no fulcrum, so that subsequent contraction leads to inward motion of the rib cage at the insertional ring. In patients with chronic airflow limitation who are very hyperinflated, this paradoxical motion of the rib cage may be noted during tidal breathing (Hoover's sign). The normal downward descent of the diaphragm is best seen when the subject is supine, and it is indicated by the outward movement of the anterior abdominal wall. Absent contraction is signaled by an inward, paradoxical movement of the abdominal wall during inspiration.

The intercostal muscles are thin flat muscles located between the ribs. Their sequential activation in a descending or ascending manner promotes inspiration or expiration. That is, although both of these muscles have an elevating action on the rib cage at low lung volumes when activated in a co-ordinated manner, either an elevation or a depression of the ribs ensues.[5249] Phasic inspiratory and expiratory activity has been recorded from the appropriate intercostal muscles in humans. The internal intercostals (excluding the parasternals) exhibit expiratory activity, whereas the external intercostals and the parasternals exhibit activity in inspiration. The degree to which these muscles contribute to ventilation is unknown. With disease, however, some indications can be deduced. In bilateral diaphragmatic paralysis, contraction of the inspiratory intercostal muscles expands the rib cage along both anteroposterior and lateral diameters. Paralysis of several intercostal nerves, as occurs in poliomyelitis, results in decreased movement of the affected part of the rib cage. Accordingly, the intercostal muscles must have a significant inspiratory action.

Expiratory Muscles

The muscles of expiration consist of two groups, the abdominal muscles and the rib cage muscles. The transversus abdominis, the rectus abdominis, and the obliques are the major abdominal muscles. The expiratory muscles of the rib cage include the internal intercostals (interosseous portion) and the transversus thoracis. The expiratory muscles are generally recruited during high levels of ventilation, particularly when the tidal volume increases to include some fraction of the resting expiratory reserve volume.[5414] In patients with severe airflow obstruction, these muscles may be recruited during resting expiration, and they are of major importance in the act of coughing. In addition to this phasic activity, tonic expiratory activity of the abdominal muscles is now known to be important in regulating diaphragm length, particularly when the subject moves from the supine to the upright position.[5415] Without increased tone in the abdominal musculature during such a change in position, the diaphragm would be shortened and would become less effective as a pressure generator. Quadriplegics moving from the supine to the erect position can significantly improve their vital capacity if an abdominal tensor is used to replace the lost activity of the abdominal muscles.[4917] The expiratory muscles, accordingly, should not be regarded as purely antagonistic muscles since they can serve to improve the function of the inspiratory muscles, especially of the diaphragm.

INTRINSIC PROPERTIES OF THE RESPIRATORY MUSCLES

As is the case with other striated muscles, the respiratory muscles are composed of muscle fibers, the contractile elements of which are sarcomeres. The amount of force these fibers can develop is determined by the degree of overlap of the actin and myosin filaments within the sarcomere. The length-tension relationship is believed to be the expression of this interaction.[4920] The diaphragm[4921] and parasternal intercostals[4922] demonstrate such properties *in vitro*. Predictably, the force output also decreases *in vivo*, since diaphragm length decreases with increasing lung volume. This has been shown to be true in both the canine[4923] and human[4924, 4996] diaphragm. Accordingly, reduced pressure output as an index of force occurs with reduced diaphragm length or with increased lung volume. Similarly, the inspiratory intercostal muscles produce less force as lung volume increases. However, parasternal intercostal muscle length is less reduced (possibly by only 10%) as lung volume increases to TLC—at least in dogs.[4925] Therefore, it is likely that the inspiratory intercostals may be more effective than the diaphragm at higher lung volumes.

The response of a muscle fiber to a single electric shock (the twitch) is determined by the fiber type. Slow twitch oxidative fibers (SO) develop tension more slowly during the twitch (100 to 200 milliseconds). These are the "red fibers," with a high mitochondrial content and high oxidative capacity. These fibers are capable of sustained activity and are predominantly recruited during low levels of repetitive activity. In contrast, fast twitch glycolytic white fibers (FG) have fewer capillaries and rely on anaerobic glycolysis. These fibers are recruited during high intensity tasks and are "fatigue-sensitive," as opposed to the "fatigue-resistant" slow twitch (SO) fibers. There is also an additional group of fast twitch fatigue-resistant fibers that are both oxidative and glycolytic; these are known as fast twitch oxidative and glycolytic fibers (FOG).

Skeletal muscles are composed of differing proportions of these fiber types. Slow twitch oxidative fibers predominate in postural muscles such as the soleus. Fast twitch glycolytic fibers predominate in muscles such as the ankle dorsiflexor, the tibialis anticus. The diaphragm is composed of all three fiber types in the following proportions: SO, 55%; FOG, 21%; and FG, 24%.[4926, 4927] In contrast, the diaphragm of the newborn infant only contains 10% SO fibers,[4928] which would predispose the muscle to fatigue. In general, the diaphragm has greater oxidative capacity and larger blood flow

in relation to volume than do limb muscles.[4930] Accordingly, it is more fatigue-resistant. The intercostal muscles have between 5% and 15% more FG fibers than the diaphragm.[4933]

METABOLISM OF RESPIRATORY MUSCLES

The diaphragm has an excellent blood supply,[4929] receiving abundant collaterals from the intercostal, inferior phrenic, internal mammary, and pericardiophrenic arteries. There is no definite evidence that blood flow limitation impairs contractile force under normal circumstances.[4930] The diaphragm derives its energy from carbohydrate oxidation (glucose and lactate) and lipid metabolism, predominantly free fatty acids. It has a remarkable capacity to resist net anaerobic metabolism and has a greater oxidative capacity than limb muscles.[4930] These features, in combination with the abundant blood supply, are similar to the features of the heart and provide the potential for prolonged endurance work.[4930] However, the presence of disease can significantly alter these capabilities. For example, in chronic hyperinflation with associated decreased cardiac output, hypoxemia, malnutrition (combined with a greatly increased work of breathing and increased ventilatory demand), the diaphragm must operate under conditions very different from those in healthy normal subjects. In such circumstances, the endurance capability of the diaphragm and other inspiratory muscles may well be compromised. When the limits of endurance are reached, the force output of both skeletal and respiratory muscles will be reduced. This reduction in force is termed "fatigue." Fatigue of the respiratory muscles has been described in humans[4931] and, specifically, in patients undergoing weaning from assisted ventilation.[4932]

SPECIFIC TESTS OF RESPIRATORY NEUROMUSCULAR FUNCTION

Respiratory Muscle Force

During the past few years, the measurement of maximal inspiratory pressure (MIP) and maximal expiratory pressure (MEP) has been used to evaluate respiratory muscle function. Normal values are noted in Chapter 5. In performing the MIP maneuver, the subject inspires from residual volume against an occluded, non-compliant mouthpiece. A small leak (1 millimeter in diameter) is introduced to prevent glottic closure and the development of pressure above the glottis by the cheek muscles. The pressure should be a sustained plateau for at least 1 second. Air leaks around the mouth must be prevented. Measurements are made at RV for MIP and at TLC for MEP because the pressure generated varies sharply with lung volume.[4940] Correction for lung volume becomes particularly relevant when measuring MIP and MEP in patients with chronic airflow obstruction.

Comparisons should be made only with normal values obtained by an identical technique to that being used. Normal values have been defined for adults,[3827, 4944, 4945] adolescents,[3829] and children.[3827, 3828] There is variation in these values, with the highest values for adults being reported by Ringqvist and his colleagues.[4945] In their study, military conscripts repeated the maneuver 20 times. On some occasions, the subjects developed nose bleeds or conjunctival hemorrhages. Black and Hyatt[4944] studied 120 adults, 60 men and 60 women, and took the two best values from each subject. They reported slightly lower values than Ringqvist and noted a coefficient of variation of 9% for both MIP and MEP. A similar coefficient has been reported from other series.[3827, 3828] An improvement in MIP and MEP with repeated testing, i.e., a learning effect, has been noted in one study.[3828] After the age of 55, the value declines.[4944] Wilson and his colleagues[3827] have reported lower values than those found by others.

Diaphragmatic Strength

Diaphragmatic weakness can be assessed by several methods. Recording the pressure above and below the diaphragm gives transdiaphragmatic pressure (P_{di}). This measurement, when obtained during a maximal maneuver, has been found to be very variable. Although P_{di} is the algebraic sum of the change in gastric and pleural pressures during the maneuver, normal subjects can inspire with varying amounts of rib cage or diaphragmatic contraction. Accordingly, the P_{di} may be reduced as a result of pronounced rib cage recruitment during the maneuver.[4949] Hence, the range of P_{di} reported varies from 18 to 137 cm H_2O.[4949] However,

if subjects are trained with visual feedback to co-ordinate the abdominal muscles and diaphragm, a reproducible (and consistently higher) value can be obtained.[4950] Using this technique, the coefficient of variation of the measured P_{di} was found to be 19%. It has been reported that a maneuver involving a sniff[4951] requires little instruction and gives a better defined lower limit than the P_{di} without feedback (range 82 to 204 cm H_2O, with a coefficient of variation of 7.2%). This test may be useful in following the course of a patient with suspected diaphragmatic weakness.

If diaphragmatic paralysis or weakness is suspected, phrenic nerve conduction time can be measured.[4952] The recording electrodes are placed on the rib cage over the diaphragm, and the phrenic nerve is stimulated in the neck. The normal mean conduction time is 7.7 ± 0.8 milliseconds.[4952] Diaphragm function can also be assessed fluoroscopically.[4953] Decreased excursion alone is non-specific, as this can be caused by subphrenic disease, pulmonary fibrosis, or atelectasis. However, decreased excursion associated with paradoxical motion during a sniff is highly specific. A lateral radiographic view is recommended during the sniff to rule out paradox of just the anterior portion of the diaphragm. False-negative findings during spontaneous breathing can be caused by abdominal muscle contraction during expiration, producing downward movement of the diaphragm when the abdominal muscles relax at the beginning of inspiration.

Respiratory Muscle Endurance

In addition to respiratory muscle force, respiratory muscle endurance can also be measured. The maximum voluntary ventilation can normally be sustained for about 30 seconds. As ventilation drops, an asymptote is reached at 15 minutes. This is defined as the maximal sustainable ventilation.[4955] The maximal sustainable ventilation is therefore an index of respiratory muscle endurance. However, since ventilation does not reflect the load placed on the muscles in patients with lung disease, the application of the method is limited. More recently, inspiratory threshold loading has been used to produce a measurable load.[4954] The resulting sustainable inspiratory pressure follows a parabolic relationship over time similar to that of ventilation. Recent modifications have expanded on this technique.[4957] These measurements have practical value for research studies in which interventions are being made and the tests repeated by the same subject. Normal values for assessing respiratory muscle endurance in the general population are currently not available.

PULMONARY FUNCTION STUDIES AND RESPIRATORY MUSCLE WEAKNESS

The disease process resulting in respiratory muscle weakness may or may not be evident at the time of presentation. However, the tests of respiratory muscle strength already described can be used to assess whether the respiratory muscles are affected in a neuromuscular disease. The vital capacity may be used as an indicator of respiratory muscle weakness, and it is useful when there is no intrinsic lung disease (as indicated by a normal chest film) or no evidence of rib cage restriction. Normally, a small fraction of the maximal strength of the respiratory muscles is required to inflate the lung. Because of the curvilinear shape of the pressure/volume curve of the respiratory system, proportionally more loss of pressure is required before a similar proportional loss of vital capacity occurs (see Fig. 22–1). Hence, a 50% reduction in maximum inspiratory pressure leads to only a 15% reduction in vital capacity. Thus the MIP may be reduced before the vital capacity is altered. However, the vital capacity has been noted to be lowered below the value predicted (see theoretical curve in Fig. 22–1) in most studies of patients with respiratory muscle weakness.[3023, 4934, 4935] In Figure 22–1, the measured relationship between vital capacity and respiratory muscle strength in 25 patients with respiratory muscle weakness is shown. The authors of the study from which this illustration is taken noted that specific lung compliance was reduced, that is, the compliance curve of the lung was shifted to the right and did not simply terminate at an earlier point as a result of muscle weakness. Other studies support this finding.[4935] The mechanism of this loss of compliance is thought to be a loss of gas exchanging units caused by atelectasis. This atelectasis may be detectable radiographically in some patients. In association with the reduction of FRC often found in these patients, DeTroyer and his colleagues[4934] found a reduced static recoil pressure of the lung; this suggested a reduction in outward chest recoil. In patients

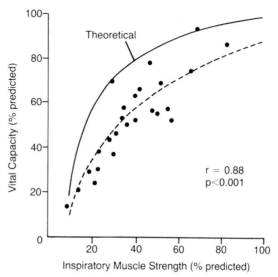

Figure 22–1. The solid curve indicates the theoretical effect of respiratory muscle weakness on vital capacity constructed by assuming (1) that the relaxation PV characteristic of the chest wall is normal and (2) that the inspiratory and expiratory muscles are involved uniformly. The dashed curve is the logarithmic regression calculated from the data obtained in the 25 patients with various neuromuscular diseases (*closed circles*). (Reprinted with permission from DeTroyer, A., Borenstein, S., and Cordier, R. Analysis of lung volume restriction in patients with respiratory muscle weakness. Thorax 35, 607, 1980.)

with chronic respiratory muscle weakness, the chest wall could conceivably become stiffer and hence lose recoil. In acute muscle weakness, reduced tonic inspiratory muscle activity in the intercostals may reduce chest wall recoil as well.[4936] Therefore, a reduction in vital capacity beyond that predicted by the normal pressure/volume curve may be explained by a combination of reduced lung compliance and reduced elastic recoil of the chest wall. The vital capacity is, accordingly, a useful index for monitoring the course of respiratory muscle weakness.

The subdivisions of lung volume are also altered by respiratory muscle weakness. A reduction in the FRC as a result of respiratory muscle weakness is not an invariable finding. In some studies, it has not been found.[4937–4939] Residual volume has been noted to be increased in some series,[4933, 4937–4939] but in others it was unchanged.[4935, 4941, 4942] Total lung capacity, inspiratory capacity, and expiratory reserve volume are usually reduced.[4943] Although lung volumes, particularly the vital capacity, are useful in following the course of the disease, maximal inspiratory and expiratory pressures may be demonstrably abnormal before changes in lung volumes are apparent.[4947]

SYNDROMES OF RESPIRATORY MUSCLE WEAKNESS

Respiratory Muscle Fatigue

Fatigue is defined as the inability of a muscle to maintain a given force. The duration that any given force can be maintained is termed endurance. The endurance of the respiratory muscles and limb muscles is determined by the amount of force developed.[5067, 5074] The greater the force of contraction, the shorter the endurance. Bellemare and Grassino showed that endurance is also dependent on the fraction of the breathing cycle that is spent on inspiration, i.e., the duty cycle.[5074] Hence, the longer the duty cycle, the shorter the endurance. The location of fatigue may be at the muscle level (peripheral fatigue) or at higher levels (central fatigue), such as at the neuromuscular junction. In general, fatigue results when the demand for energy exceeds the supply. As already noted, the diaphragm is normally well adapted to resist fatigue, but there may well be clinical situations in which a combination of adverse factors can lead to it.

The clinical manifestations of inspiratory muscle fatigue include tachypnea, paradoxical abdominal motion and respiratory alternans (variations between normal expansion and abdominal paradox), hypercapnia, and, as a preterminal event, bradypnea.[5075] There are a number of diagnostic tests available to identify fatigue in the respiratory muscles. In the experimental setting, a reduced high/low ratio on the electromyograph (EMG) and a reduced rate of relaxation, together with a rightward shift of the force frequency curve, may be demonstrated.[5075] Normal values are not available, so the subject must act as his or her own control. Thus, patients on ventilators can be rested; then, during weaning, these parameters can be followed and compared with previous values. From this, the onset of fatigue can be deduced. Some patients with chronic airflow limitation have been shown to develop a reduced high/low ratio of their diaphragmatic EMG during exercise, suggesting that respiratory muscle fatigue may limit their maximal workload.[5076] A simple test to diagnose fatigue is not available as yet, and this has limited our knowledge of the prevalence of respiratory muscle fatigue in clinical conditions.

Another example of fatigue is encountered with the start of electrophrenic stimulation in quadriplegic patients with deconditioned diaphragms. Quadriplegic patients who have been mechanically ventilated develop a disuse atrophy of their diaphragm (deconditioning); this becomes immediately evident when electrophrenic stimulation is started and it is found that the P_{di} can only be sustained for a brief period.[5077, 5078] In such patients ventilation cannot be maintained by phrenic stimulation until the diaphragm has been retrained by intermittent stimulation. Disuse atrophy has been shown to result in a reduction of the number of skeletal muscle fibers—in addition to a reduction in their mean diameter—resulting in a loss of force-generating capacity.[5014, 5416]

It is clear from the results of electrophrenic stimulation that the respiratory muscles can be trained to increase their endurance and strength. Training can be performed at home. Patients can use an inspiratory loading device, can perform repeated MVV maneuvers, or can adopt a general exercise program. The results of such attempts in patients with chronic airflow limitation are reviewed in Chapter 8.

NEUROMUSCULAR DISEASES

A diminution in respiratory muscle force can be the end result of dysfunction at many levels. Overall, the term neuromuscular disease applies, and this embraces disease at four levels:

1. The spinal cord, as in amyotrophic lateral sclerosis or poliomyelitis.
2. The peripheral nerve, as in the Guillain-Barré syndrome.
3. The neuromuscular junction, as in myasthenia gravis.
4. Failure of the contractile elements, as in the myopathies.

In Table 22–1, the diagnostic abnormalities that differentiate these diseases are shown.

DISEASES OF THE SPINAL CORD

There is little information about the respiratory muscles and the spinal muscular atrophies. Weakness in these conditions is generally more marked proximally, and the prognosis is related to respiratory muscle weakness and later respiratory failure. In amyotrophic lateral sclerosis, there is a progressive disorder of motor neurons in the brain stem and spinal cord. Typically, the disease presents in the fifth or sixth decade, with weakness of the hands; muscle atrophy

Table 22–1. ELECTRODIAGNOSTIC FINDINGS IN ACUTE GENERALIZED WEAKNESS

Syndrome	EMG	Motor Nerve Conduction		Sensory Nerve Conduction		Repetitive Stimulation
		Amplitude	Velocity	Amplitude	Latency	
Motor neuron disorders	Sparse recruitment pattern; rapid firing	Normal	Normal	Normal	Normal	Normal
Polyneuropathy	Sparse recruitment pattern; rapid firing	May be reduced	May be reduced	May be reduced	May be prolonged	Normal
Disorders of neuromuscular transmission	Recruitment full for effort; MUPs* small, brief in weak muscle	Reduced in weak muscles	Normal	Normal	Normal	Abnormal decrement or increment (may be normal)
Myopathy	Recruitment full for effort; MUPs* small, brief in weak muscles	Reduced in weak muscles	Normal	Normal	Normal	Normal

*MUPs: Motor unit potentials.
Reprinted with permission from Layzer, R. B. Neuromuscular Manifestations of Systemic Disease. F. A. Davis, Philadelphia, 1984, p. 6.

and hyperreflexia predominate. More rarely, progressive muscular atrophy occurs, presenting with weakness and atrophy but without evidence of corticospinal tract dysfunction. Progression is rapid, with death in respiratory failure in 2 to 5 years. In one study of 27 patients with amyotrophic lateral sclerosis,[4939] two subgroups could be identified based on the shape of the flow/volume curve. One of these groups showed a curve of characteristic shape consisting of a sharp drop in flow rate at low lung volumes. This group had larger residual volumes, lower vital capacities, and lower maximal expiratory pressures, findings suggesting predominant expiratory muscle weakness. The other subgroup had a normal flow/volume curve and no evidence of expiratory muscle weakness or a reduction in vital capacity. Since the inspiratory pressures were similar in both groups, reduced expiratory muscle strength was the major factor reducing the vital capacity. In this condition, respiratory failure usually occurs when the disease is well established, and a falling vital capacity is a poor prognostic sign.[4958] However, there have been several reports of respiratory failure as a presenting symptom in amyotrophic lateral sclerosis.[4948, 4959, 4962]

Other studies have identified a group of patients with amyotrophic lateral sclerosis who presented with predominant diaphragmatic weakness[4961] or paralysis.[4960, 4963] Bulbar involvement, which can result in death from aspiration pneumonia, can be manifested by a peculiar flow/volume curve that may be caused by glottal closure during expiration.[4958] Performance of

expiratory flow maneuvers with an oral airway in place has been suggested as a means of separating abnormal curves attributable to muscle weakness from those that may be caused by bulbar involvement.[4964]

Poliomyelitis, an infectious disease of the anterior horn cell, is rarely encountered today following the introduction of vaccines. Paralyzed muscles recover to a varying degree over the 2 years subsequent to the acute attack. Respiratory muscle weakness is more common in older age groups, and its degree is reflected in the vital capacity, the expiratory reserve volume, and, particularly, the inspiratory capacity.[4937] Patients in whom the VC has fallen below 30% of the predicted value usually require assisted ventilation.[4965] Intercostal muscles are affected in the upper and lower rib cage, and involvement can be unilateral or bilateral. The diaphragm can be similarly involved, either unilaterally or totally.[4966] The compliance of the respiratory system has been found to be reduced in these patients, even with a relatively short duration of paralysis of 6 to 18 months and in patients maintained on negative pressure ventilators.[4938] The FRC has been measured with divergent results, some finding a decrease[4967] and others no change.[4937] Although MIP and MEP were not recorded in these studies, these pressures may be predicted to be good indicators of respiratory muscle involvement in this disease.

Patients who contract poliomyelitis when older are at increased risk of developing respiratory failure after the convalescent period.

Lane and his colleagues[4968] studied 55 patients who had had poliomyelitis at least 15 years before. None had required initial ventilatory assistance, but several presented in later life with hypersomnolence, fatigue, and dyspnea. This phenomenon has been termed post-polio progression. In this group, whose mean age was 37 years, the vital capacity was between 20% and 40% of the predicted value. A high proportion had unilateral or bilateral diaphragmatic paralysis (13/32) or kyphoscoliosis (12/41), and some were obese or had chronic airflow obstruction. In many, the generalized muscle weakness had developed insidiously and may have been caused by progressive muscular atrophy occurring in segments contralateral to the areas initially involved by the acute disease.[4969]

Spinal cord lesions produce variable effects on respiratory muscle strength, depending on the level of the lesion. In 40 such patients, Fugl-Meyer[4971] documented the effect on respiration. The vital capacity is more affected the higher the lesion and is reduced by two factors, an increase in residual volume and a decrease in inspiratory capacity. The reduction in inspiratory capacity is related to the reduced MIP, but there may also be increased chest wall stiffness,[4970] together with reduced lung compliance.[4972] In a subgroup of quadriplegic patients, phasic inspiratory intercostal activity is seen. In them, lung volumes, FRC, and TLC may all be relatively preserved.[4972] These patients did not have inspiratory paradoxical inward movement of the upper rib cage, which limits the inspiratory capacity and may lead to regional atelectasis. Loss of inspiratory intercostal activity therefore contributes to the reduced compliance and TLC. Paraplegics with thoracic lesions have similar changes in TLC, probably reflecting similar pathophysiology. The increase in residual volume seen after spinal cord trauma is also related to the level of the lesion, the expiratory reserve volume being less reduced the lower the lesion in the cord. The increased RV is, not unexpectedly, paralleled by a reduction in MEP, which in turn reflects the loss of expiratory muscle mass.

The effect of changes in body position in quadriplegic patients is shown in Figure 22–2. As the patient goes from the supine toward the sitting position, the RV increases and the VC decreases. The RV increase is due to loss of abdominal muscle tone and the resultant hydrostatic pull that shortens the diaphragm. As noted previously, this effect can be reduced by use of an abdominal binder. Positional changes

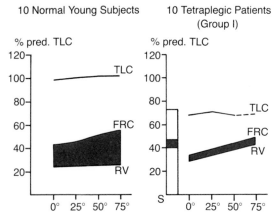

Figure 22–2. Mean total lung capacity (TLC) and its subdivisions in 10 normal young subjects and 10 tetraplegic patients at different body positions. Values expressed as per cent of predicted TLC. (Four tetraplegic patients could not be tilted to the 75° position.) For the tetraplegic patients mean values at the sitting position (S) are included. *FRC*, functional residual capacity; *RV*, residual volume. 0°, supine position; 25°, 50°, and 75°, different head-up tilted positions. (Reprinted with permission from Fugl-Meyer, A.R. Effects of respiratory paralysis in tetraplegic and paraplegic patients. Scand. J. Rehab. Med. 3, 145, 1971.)

in residual volume also occur in patients with upper thoracic lesions in which expiratory muscle function is impaired. Patients with lesions above the level of C3 have no expiratory muscle activity, and residual volume and FRC are equal.[4917] The neck accessory muscles in such a patient are capable of inflating the upper rib cage and in association with glossopharyngeal breathing can support ventilation for finite periods of time. These patients benefit from an abdominal binder when upright. The binder probably reduces the pull of the abdominal contents on the rib cage and thus assists the neck accessory muscles.

HEMIPLEGIA

Acute hemiplegia has been shown to reduce chest movement[5006] and electrical activity[5024] in inspiratory muscles ipsilateral to the paralyzed side. However, the extent of this weakness, and whether it could lead to respiratory complications, is unclear.

DISEASES OF THE PERIPHERAL NERVES: DIAPHRAGMATIC PARALYSIS

Neuropathies may be hereditary or acquired. Diaphragmatic paralysis is in the latter category. When phrenic nerve activity is lost bilaterally, there are significant and characteristic effects on ventilation. The breathing pattern is more rapid and shallow than usual, and there is significant dyspnea when the patient lies flat (orthopnea). Although there is usually some complaint of dyspnea on walking, it is not severe. The combination of definite orthopnea but moderately good effort tolerance should always raise the possibility of the diagnosis. Inspection of the anterior abdominal wall with the patient supine reveals paradoxical inward motion during inspiration. There is a striking fall in the supine vital capacity compared with the upright vital capacity. In normal subjects, the VC decreases by less than 20% in moving from the upright to the supine position.[5417] In patients with diaphragmatic paralysis, the TLC, FRC, and VC are all reduced when the patients are supine, the VC by more than 30%.[5417] The P_{di} measured during spontaneous breathing is either absent[4988] or greatly reduced. Fluoroscopy and the measurement of phrenic nerve conduction time serve to confirm the diagnosis.

Hypoventilation with hypercapnic respiratory failure can develop,[4974, 4975] but this does not occur in all patients with bilateral diaphragmatic paralysis. However, it may be out of proportion to the degree of muscle weakness.[5062] Hypoventilation may worsen at night, during REM sleep, when the activity of rib cage muscles is reduced. The genesis of the hypoventilation is not entirely clear, but the shortened inspiratory time and the resultant increased dead space ventilation may contribute.[5062] Other conditions, including myopathies, with mild to moderate respiratory muscle weakness, may also lead to hypoventilation out of proportion to the degree of muscle weakness.[5083] The mechanism of this hypoventilation is unclear. Hypoxemia may be a feature of bilateral diaphragmatic paralysis. The alveolar-arterial O_2 difference increases when the subject is supine, and the Pa_{O_2} falls.

Bilateral diaphragmatic paralysis is much less common than unilateral paralysis. It results from high cervical cord lesions, invasive lesions in the mediastinum, polyneuropathies, poliomyelitis, surgery involving cardiac hypothermia,[4981] or trauma.[4990] In several reported cases no cause could be identified.[4979, 4992]

Unilateral diaphragmatic paralysis is usually not clinically detectable by paradoxical abdominal wall motion.[4989] The reductions in lung volume are less than with bilateral paralysis, there being no change in FRC and the VC falling by about 25%.[4980, 4991] In some patients, there may be a small fall in Pa_{O_2}.[4978] The MIP is usually not reduced unless some other condition is present.[4991] Patients appear to compensate for unilateral paralysis by recruiting the rib cage muscles and the opposite hemidiaphragm.[4983, 4991] The commonest cause of unilateral paralysis is invasive mediastinal lesions,[4984] but it also may result from trauma or following surgical dissection. Less common causes include herpes zoster,[4987] neuralgic amyotrophy,[5000] injection of tetanus antitoxin,[4993] and diphtheria.[4994]

Diaphragmatic paresis, as opposed to paralysis, has been reported in multiple sclerosis[5001] and after neck surgery[4999] or upper abdominal surgery.[4997] The mechanism of the paresis after abdominal surgery may be a reflex, arising from the upper abdomen, so that diaphragmatic activation is suppressed in relation to rib cage activation.[4998]

Guillain-Barré syndrome, an acute polyneuropathy of unknown etiology, often profoundly affects the respiratory muscles. Gracey and his colleagues[5002] reviewed 72 patients observed in the hospital. Twenty-one required admission to a respiratory intensive care unit, and 13 of these needed mechanical ventilation for a mean period of 58 days. In other series, between 10% and 28% have required mechanical ventilation.[4995] Frequent monitoring of MIP, MEP, and vital capacity are obviously needed in such cases. The complications are those associated with prolonged intubation. Mortality is generally less than 5% and is caused by management complications,[5002] not the disease *per se*.

DISEASE AT THE NEUROMUSCULAR JUNCTION

The commonest disease of the neuromuscular junction is myasthenia gravis (MG), an autoimmune disorder affecting the acetylcholine receptors of skeletal muscle. In 20% of patients, symptoms are confined to the eyes ("ocular MG"). The remainder have generalized MG. Ocular MG may progress to generalized MG. If it does so, this usually occurs within 2 years of onset. Muscle weakness distribution, in order of frequency, is extraocular, bulbar, neck, limb girdle, distal limbs, and trunk.[5003] Antibodies to acetylcholine are present in 90% of patients, but there is little correlation between disease activity and antibody titer. The disease has a significant mortality, which is related to respiratory muscle or bulbar involvement. Thyroid disease can exacerbate the muscle weakness.[5005] Treatment is with anticholinesterase drugs, thymectomy, corticosteroids, and, recently, plasmapheresis.[5005]

Concern over possible bronchoconstriction occurring as a result of medication with anticholinesterase compounds has not been substantiated.[4943] Patients given these medications show increases in vital capacity, airflow, and respiratory muscle force with no evidence of a decrease in airway conductance. Chest wall recoil has been shown to increase when these patients are given anticholinesterase compounds, suggesting that the initial chest wall recoil, and the FRC, were determined to some extent by tonic muscle tone.[4943]

Hypercapnic respiratory failure occurs in MG in some well defined circumstances. A "myasthenic crisis" is usually precipitated by a reduction in anticholinesterase medications or by infections, emotional stress, surgical operations, or the inadvertent use of drugs that exacerbate the condition. Initiation of steroid therapy may worsen the disease for a brief period before improvement occurs. Such therapy should be started in the hospital, where the patient can be closely monitored for respiratory muscle weakness. A "cholinergic crisis" is produced by an excess of anticholinesterase medication resulting in a depolarizing blockade. Gracey and his colleagues[5002] reviewed 28 cases of MG requiring mechanical ventilatory assistance. Most of these were secondary to surgery, particularly thymectomy. Bulbar involvement represents a particular risk,[5007] and such cases may require plasmapheresis before surgery. Plasmapheresis may be particularly useful when the usual treatable causes have been rectified.[5008, 5009]

Botulism is caused by the ingestion of *Clostridium botulinum* toxin, which leads to neuromuscular paralysis. This poisoning has become rare as food canning has improved, but sporadic cases still occur. It can also develop from contaminated wounds.[5013] The toxin interferes with release of acetylcholine at the neuromuscular junction.[5010, 5011] The resultant paralysis affects extraocular, bulbar, and limb muscles. Bulbar involvement is expressed by dysphonia, dysarthria, and difficulty in swallowing. Involvement of respiratory muscles can occur early or late in the disease. It may be insidious, and its onset may be missed unless the patient is specifically watched for its development. Provided respiratory failure is treated, recovery in all cases eventually occurs, but there may be some residual weakness.[5011]

DISEASES OF THE MUSCLES

The myopathies form the largest group of neuromuscular diseases; most of them have been shown to cause alveolar hypoventilation.[5014]

Braun, Arora, and Rochester[3023] reviewed 53 patients with proximal myopathies. In half, the MIP and MEP were less than 50% of the normal predicted value. When these values were below 50% of predicted, the Pa_{CO_2} increased linearly. When the maximal pressures were 30% of predicted, it increased sharply. Fifty-three per cent of these patients developed respiratory complications, such as pneumonia or atelectasis.

Studies of pulmonary function in patients with Duchenne's muscular dystrophy usually show the features of respiratory muscle weakness.[5015] Residual volume increases, and the MEP decreases in association with reduced inspiratory capacity, total lung capacity, and MIP. There is usually little difference between VC values when the patient is upright or supine, suggesting that the diaphragm is relatively spared. It has been noted, however, that there is not a close relationship between abnormalities of pulmonary function and general muscle status.[5017] Kilburn and his colleagues[5016] reported considerable respiratory insufficiency when mild or moderate muscular dystrophy was apparent in other muscle groups. There is a correlation between abdominal muscle performance and VC, MVV, and expiratory flow rates, which indicates the importance of abdominal muscle strength in these aspects of function.[5017] Chest wall deformities, including scoliosis and "drooping of the ribs," are noted during progression of the disease. These deformities probably account for some of the increased stiffness and loss of recoil of the chest wall observed in these patients.[5017] As respiratory muscle function deteriorates, respiratory failure occurs and can worsen rapidly if respiratory infections are not promptly treated. Once chronic hypoventilation develops, the prognosis is much less favorable.[5014, 5015] Nocturnal ventilation at this stage has been shown to prolong survival.[5018–5020]

Myotonic dystrophy is an inherited myopathy. The myotonia is due to a reduction in the rate of muscle relaxation secondary to a defect in the muscle membrane. These patients can present in adult life with weakness and hypercapnic respiratory failure. This myopathy has been associated with a central defect in chemosensitivity,[4941, 5021] but studies of respiratory drive have indicated that reduced response to CO_2 may be the result of muscle weakness alone.[5022] Others[198, 5023, 5026] have found reduced CO_2 responsiveness in those with mild muscle weakness. In some patients, there does appear to be an imperfect relationship between muscle weakness and CO_2 response.

Respiratory muscle dysfunction in myotonia congenita (Thomsen's disease) has been well described.[5027] Routine pulmonary function tests and tests of respiratory muscle strength are normal. However, patients described breathlessness associated with chest tightness on exertion. Electromyographic studies show a delayed rate of relaxation of respiratory muscles, and the sensation of dyspnea may be attributed to this. It is of interest that the dyspnea resolves if a warm-up period is allowed, a feature seen in limb muscles in this condition.

Acid maltase deficiency (Pompe's disease) is an inherited glycogen storage disease that usually presents in childhood. However, it can present in adults with respiratory failure.[5028, 5029] Patients have been noted who presented initially with marked orthopnea, probably indicating predominant diaphragm involvement.[5030] A recent case report[5035] indicated that improvement in respiratory muscle strength could follow the use of a high protein diet in this condition, and training of the respiratory muscles may also be of benefit.

In cases of slowly progressive muscle weakness, it should not be assumed that the cause is muscular dystrophy. Myopathies secondary to inflammatory or metabolic disease or endocrine conditions or myopathies caused by drug use should be excluded.

GENERALIZED NEUROMUSCULAR DEFECTS

Impairment of the respiratory muscles due to spasm of the laryngeal and intercostal muscles is the major cause of death in tetanus. The toxin released by *Clostridium tetani* acts at the nerve, the neuromuscular junction, and also on the muscle itself. Trismus is the first sign, followed by severe muscle spasms. Progression is rapid, and the mortality used to be at least 50%. This has been reduced to 10% with intensive care monitoring, tracheotomy, administration of diazepam, or assisted ventilation following paralysis with muscle relaxants in severe cases. In one report of 100 severe cases,[5031] 97 required paralysis to control muscle spasms, for

a mean duration of 21 days. Deaths in this series were mainly attributable to bronchopneumonia or to cardiac arrest during tracheal suctioning. Prolonged delayed recovery has been reported, but it is more usually fairly rapid and complete. Mild cases of tetanus are associated with reduction in vital capacity.[5033] Diaphragmatic dysfunction is a prominent feature.[5032] However, there are no data on the use of current techniques in assessing diaphragm function in this disease.

NUTRITIONAL AND ELECTROLYTE DEPLETION

Significant weight loss is a feature of some patients with chronic airflow limitation. As noted in Chapter 8, Openbrier and colleagues[3342] documented loss of body weight probably associated with the degree of emphysema. Animal studies have shown that malnutrition results in a reduction in the cross-sectional area of muscle fibers and affects all striated muscles, including the diaphragm. This is greater in fast twitch than in slow twitch fibers.[4946] The weight of the diaphragm[1294] is reduced in patients with chronic airflow limitation; and MIP, MEP, and the maximal voluntary ventilation are reduced in malnourished patients in conjunction with reduced diaphragmatic mass.[5064] Thus, there is supportive evidence implicating nutritional depletion as a factor compromising respiratory muscle strength in patients with chronic airflow limitation.

Electrolyte disturbance can compromise muscle function. It is generally recognized that severe hypokalemia can lead to flaccid paralysis and hypercapnic respiratory failure. However, to what degree lesser reductions in potassium can affect respiratory muscle strength is unknown. Hypophosphatemia can precipitate respiratory failure,[5065] and repletion improves diaphragmatic strength.[5068, 5069] Table 22–2 summarizes the electrolyte and acid-base disturbances that have been associated with impaired respiratory muscle strength.

RESPIRATORY MUSCLE FUNCTION IN THE PRESENCE OF LUNG DISEASE

Chronic Airflow Limitation

Several factors reduce the effectiveness of the ventilatory muscles in this condition. Hyperin-

Table 22–2. ELECTROLYTE AND ACID-BASE DISTURBANCES ASSOCIATED WITH REDUCED RESPIRATORY MUSCLE STRENGTH

Disturbance	Reference
Hypokalemia	
Hypomagnesemia	5070
Hypophosphatemia	5065
Hypocalcemia	5072
Hypercapnia	5071
Metabolic acidosis	5073

flation shortens the inspiratory muscles. This may result in the muscle's contracting at a suboptimal part on the length-tension curve and hence, less force is developed for a given intensity of neural activation. However, chronically shortened muscles tend to adapt by reducing the number of sarcomeres arranged end to end and hence can re-establish a new length that optimizes contraction.[5037] The effectiveness of the action of the diaphragm in inflating the rib cage may also be compromised as the diaphragm becomes more perpendicular to the rib cage. When the diaphragm is perpendicular to the rib cage, diaphragmatic shortening deflates the lower rib cage (Hoover's sign). The MIP is generally reduced in these cases. However, when corrected for the increase in lung volume, the pressures developed are generally in the normal range,[4052, 5034] although the MIP was reduced in a subgroup with severe chronic airflow limitation and weight loss. The maximal P_{di} is usually reduced as well,[5036] but data on P_{di} corrected for the change in lung volume and the consequent decrease in diaphragm length are not available. Such patients may be found to have reduced diaphragmatic area and weight at autopsy (see Chapter 8).

Since the inspiratory intercostal and scalene muscles are less affected by hyperinflation,[5042, 5043] their function is less impeded than that of the diaphragm. Patients with chronic airflow limitation tend to breathe more with these rib cage muscles. The resulting exaggerated rib cage expansion, in association with a reduced descent of the diaphragm, can lead to paradoxical inward movement of the abdominal wall during inspiration.[5044] Clinical examination of such patients may reveal palpable activity of the scalene muscles and visible contraction of the sternomastoids, even during quiet breathing. The abdominal muscles are often recruited during resting ventilation in these patients. Contraction of these muscles cannot improve airflow during expiration if airway collapse has

occurred, but they will assist the diaphragm to return to a longer (and hence more optimal) length during the next inspiration. Posture can have a similar effect.[144] Some patients experience relief from dyspnea by leaning forward. They may be benefiting from the weight of the abdominal contents optimizing diaphragm length and hence reducing the neural activation required to produce a given diaphragmatic pressure. The supine position may also relieve dyspnea through a similar mechanism.[144, 2976, 2977]

Acute Hyperinflation

The inspiratory muscles are compromised in the acute hyperinflation that occurs in severe asthma, and the accessory and expiratory muscles can be seen to be activated during resting ventilation. Part of the hyperinflation has been shown by Martin and his colleagues[5046, 5047] to be produced by tonic activity of the inspiratory muscles during expiration—a mechanism that may help to prevent airway closure. Patients with recurrent attacks of asthma undergo a training effect, such that the endurance of their expiratory muscles may be increased.[5051] But a subgroup of asthmatics, who may be obese and steroid-dependent, have been found to have reduced muscle strength.[5048] It is suspected that the steroids may play a dominant role in this weakness. Tests of respiratory muscle strength may be indicated in such patients. It is possible that a reduction in vital capacity might be an indication to taper rather than to increase steroid dosage.

RESPIRATORY MUSCLES IN CONNECTIVE TISSUE DISEASES AND LUNG FIBROSIS

The lung recoil pressure is increased in pulmonary fibrosis, and the pressure recorded at the mouth measures the muscle and lung recoil pressure together. When an esophageal balloon is used for measurements of MIP and MEP to circumvent this problem, respiratory muscle strength is shown to be normal.[1806] But in mitral stenosis, it has been shown to be reduced.[5053] Whether this is a "detraining," effect or is related to a reduced cardiac output or to malnutrition is unclear.

As noted in Chapter 13, chronic pleuritis is common in diffuse lupus erythematosus, but the diaphragm may also be involved. Gibson,

Edmonds, and Hughes[1786] noted that 13 of 30 consecutive patients with systemic lupus erythematosus had a TLC of less than 80% of predicted. The patients with the lowest lung volumes had a past history of pleurisy. Seven patients had a lowered MIP. In four, the maximal P_{di} values were reduced. None had complete diaphragmatic paralysis. Others[5058] have also documented reduced MIP and MEP data in patients with this disease, and diaphragmatic weakness has been documented in a few cases.

As noted in Chapter 14, the diagnosis is complicated in polymyositis by the concurrence of interstitial lung disease and respiratory muscle weakness. The diaphragm can be predominantly affected in this condition.[4335] Respiratory muscle involvement in scleroderma is discussed in Chapter 14. The combination of peripheral neuropathy affecting the respiratory muscles and an interstitial pneumonitis in persons poisoned by toxic oil in Spain is also noted in Chapter 14.

SUMMARY

The recent renewed interest in the respiratory muscles led by the work of Rochester, Macklem, DeTroyer, and their colleagues has alerted all chest physicians to the great importance of the "pump" in a wide variety of clinical circumstances. It is clear that much remains to be learned, particularly the general importance of fatigue, and the relationship between dyspnea and imminent fatigue; the frequency with which the diaphragm is involved in different diseases; and even the precise mode of action of the respiratory muscles. The diaphragm is clearly a complex muscle, both in terms of its structure and its activation. These issues and many others will no doubt be addressed in the future.

23

SYNDROMES OF RESPIRATORY FAILURE

INTRODUCTION

The recognition of a condition generally classified as "adult respiratory distress syndrome" (ARDS) has led to a large body of work aimed at clarifying the cause and sequence of changes that occur in the lung. Modes of treatment have also generated considerable research, motivated in part by the recognition that prognosis of this condition has not improved in recent years. In this volume, neither of these aspects of the group of diseases can be considered; rather, the relationship between the stages of the syndrome and pulmonary function is covered. In addition, some aspects of acute respiratory failure in patients with chronic airflow limitation, not covered in earlier chapters, are reviewed.

ADULT RESPIRATORY DISTRESS SYNDROME

Reviewing the syndrome of "shock lungs," or respiratory distress syndrome after trauma, Wardle[4734] noted that Moore and his associates, in a monograph published in 1969,[4752] described four phases in the development of the condition:

Phase 1. Traumatic shock; blood or plasma infusion; hyperventilation and hypocapnia.

Phase 2. Early respiratory distress; V/Q imbalance; hypoxemia and hypocapnia.

Phase 3. Increasing hypoxia necessitating mechanical ventilation.

Phase 4. Terminal hypoxia and developing hypercapnia.

In Harrison's *Principles of Internal Medicine,*

tenth edition, Roland Ingram[4753] summarized the conditions now known to lead to this syndrome as follows:

1. Diffuse pulmonary infections: viral, bacterial, fungal, *Pneumocystis.*

2. Aspiration: Mendelson's syndrome, near drowning.

3. Irritant gases or fumes: Cl_2, O_3, NO_2, high concentrations of oxygen or smoke (see Chapter 16).

4. Narcotic overdoses: heroin, methadone, morphine.

5. Non-narcotic drugs: nitrofurantoin (see Chapter 14).

6. Immunologic response to host antigens: Goodpasture's syndrome, systemic lupus erythematosus (see Chapter 13).

7. Effects of non-thoracic trauma with hypotension: "shock lung."

8. Systemic reactions to processes initiated outside the lung (gram-negative septicemia, hemorrhagic pancreatitis, amniotic fluid embolism, fat embolism) (see Chapter 12).

9. Postcardiopulmonary bypass: "pump lung" or "postperfusion lung."

Adult respiratory distress syndrome has also been observed concomitantly with acute miliary tuberculosis,[2699, 2832] acute histoplasmosis,[2701] and following anaphylactoid shock.[4757]

In 1971, Petty and Ashbaugh[4770] drew attention to the syndrome by christening it the "Adult Respiratory Distress Syndrome." Others have suggested that the common mechanism may be non-cardiac pulmonary edema and call it by that name. In addition to Wardle's review, which contained 126 literature references to "shock lung" alone,[4734] there have been many review articles on different aspects of the condition. A review of a conference on ARDS was published in 1985.[4819]

SEQUENCE OF CHANGES IN THE LUNG AND IN PULMONARY FUNCTION IN ARDS

Bachofen and Weibel in 1977 studied nine fatal ARDS cases following septicemia[5413] and suggested that changes occurred in the following sequence:

1. Widespread interstitial and alveolar edema with preservation of the capillary endothelium and no large endothelial gaps.
2. Local destruction of squamous epithelium and proliferation of Type II cells.
3. Cuboidal transformation of epithelium and fibrotic alterations to the interstitium.

The illustrations to this paper clearly indicate the interstitial thickening that occurs as an end result of this condition. They later published the following morphometric data from three fatal cases[1101]:

	Normal	Cases
Epithelial thickness	0.74	2.94: 3.14: 3.79 (microns)
Endothelial thickness	0.52	0.82: 1.26: 1.40 (microns)
Interstitial thickness	1.39	3.53: 8.31: 9.12 (microns)

The capillary volume per unit of tissue was less than half normal. None of these cases had had more than 40% oxygen. The increase in lung collagen that occurs in these cases has been quantitated[1037] and amounts to a doubling or trebling of the normal content. In one case, established diffuse interstitial fibrosis was present at autopsy 22 days after severe trauma and ARDS.[2909]

Changes in pulmonary function are generally consistent with these findings. As ARDS develops, the first change is widening of the $(A-a)$ O_2 difference. As the condition worsens, this may exceed 200 mm Hg. Arterial P_{O_2} values of less than 50 mm Hg while the patient is breathing 100% oxygen have been recorded.[3970] In 88 patients with aspiration pneumonitis, the lowest Pa_{O_2} recorded during air breathing was 31 mm

Hg.[4345] In 50 consecutive patients with acute pancreatitis,[2838] the Pa_{O_2} during air breathing varied between 44 mm Hg and 56 mm Hg. When there are mixed alveolar and interstitial opacities on the chest x-ray, static compliance is usually reduced, and the pressure/volume curve shows considerable hysteresis.[5050] An early report noted no increase in extravascular lung water in ARDS.[5052] More recent observations that made use of the thermal green dye method found consistent increases in patients with non-cardiac edema. For a given level of wedge pressure, extravascular lung water was higher in these patients than in those with pulmonary edema secondary to cardiac failure.[5084] The association between a rising extravascular lung water and a falling Pa_{O_2} has been observed in experimental preparations.[5087]

The six inert gas method of quantitating $\dot{V}/\dot{Q}$ distribution has been used to study the effect of positive and expiratory pressure in 16 patients with ARDS.[5088] It was found that PEEP raised the Pa_{O_2} by reducing the shunt component and reducing the perfusion of poorly ventilated zones. In a few, PEEP led to an increase in ventilation to low $\dot{V}/\dot{Q}$ units. Similar findings were reported in another 8 patients.[5060] Dantzker and his colleagues[5061] studied 16 patients with ARDS by this method and concluded that there was a bimodal distribution of $\dot{V}/\dot{Q}$ ratios, with 52% of the cardiac output going to units with a normal $\dot{V}/\dot{Q}$ ratio. The remainder went either to shunts or to units with a very low $\dot{V}/\dot{Q}$ ratio. A close correlation was noted between the calculated and measured Pa_{O_2}. This finding is surprising, since illustrations of this condition[944] indicate that diffusion impairment must exist, both because of reduction in the capillary bed and because of the documented interstitial thickening.

Severe viral infections may be followed by ARDS[1280, 2661] and it may be difficult to know whether the clinical condition is directly due to the infection or to ARDS complications.

With head injuries, an increased $(A-a)$ D_{O_2} is commonly observed.[2962] In five such patients,[2965] all with normal chest X-rays, the six inert gas method was used to quantitate the $\dot{V}/\dot{Q}$ distribution. Schumaker and his colleagues[2965] found that 41% of the cardiac output was distributed to the low $\dot{V}/\dot{Q}$ region or shunt. This decreased to 21%, with no change in the shunt, when assisted ventilation was instituted. They concluded that head injury led to hypoxemia through a failure of the normal $\dot{V}/\dot{Q}$ regulatory mechanism. All the patients had a normal chest film and normal Pa_{CO_2} when studied.

PULMONARY FUNCTION AFTER RECOVERY FROM ARDS

It is not yet clear what determines survival in established cases of this syndrome, but there is evidence that infection in the lung worsens the prognosis.[4729, 4730] It is clear that the recovery process is slow in many cases. Yernault and his colleagues[2998] in 1975 reported on seven patients who had recovered. They noted a lowered $DL_{CO}SB$ but a normal static compliance. In 1977, they reported on four additional patients.[3116] In two of these, after 16 and 19 months, the DL_{CO} and k_{CO} were still abnormal, but the FEV_1 was normal. In two others, after 40 months, the DL_{CO} and k_{CO} were still depressed. In one, the static compliance was still reduced. In this patient, the Pa_{O_2} and the chest x-ray were both normal. In one patient with ARDS following a septic abortion,[3188] the following data were recorded:

	Months After Acute ARDS			Predicted
	1	3	5	
FVC	1.85	3.45	3.72	3.15
FEV_1	1.72	3.07	3.18	2.73
$DL_{CO}SB$	11.0	17.0	21.0	23.0
k_{CO}	2.92	3.38	3.51	4.71
Pa_{O_2} (mm Hg)	80.0	—	92.0	85.0

These data show that although the Pa_{O_2} had returned to normal within a month the other four measurements were all abnormal. Also, the DL_{CO} and the k_{CO} were still reduced after the FEV_1 had returned to a normal value.

A 19-year-old boy who survived near drowning[3245] went on to develop ARDS. Assisted ventilation with PEEP and a high oxygen pressure was required for 2 days to maintain his Pa_{O_2}. There were persistent infiltrates on the chest film, and a lung biopsy showed that interstitial fibrosis was present. The chest x-ray cleared over a 10-day period. His function test data were as follows:

	Days After Near Drowning		
	12	19	103
VC (%P)	40	28	82
FEV_1 (%P)	34	28	78
TLC (%P)	50	39	83
RV (%P)	85	83	100
FRC (%P)	66	61	87
$DL_{CO}SB$ (%P)	27	20	62
Pa_{O_2} (mm Hg)	62	54	88

The deterioration in all aspects of function between the twelfth and nineteenth days after the event is apparent. The DL_{CO} was still depressed after 103 days. A similarly slow recovery of DL_{CO} was observed in another person after near drowning.[3251]

It is clear that slow recovery of the DL_{CO} and slow restitution of the $(A-a) D_{O_2}$ is commonly observed. Nine survivors of ARDS, all with normal spirometry findings and chest-x-rays, were studied with exercise and noted to be limited by tachycardia.[3294] In two, there was a 10 mm Hg fall in Pa_{O_2} on exercise. Measurements of D_M and V_c (pulmonary capillary blood volume) showed that V_c varied between 36% and 65% of the predicted value, indicating a significant loss of capillary bed.

Six patients with disease of varied etiology, all under the age of 37 years,[3366] were observed for up to 16 months after recovery. In three, the $DL_{CO}SB$ and the $(A-a) D_{O_2}$ were still abnormal, although clinical recovery was complete. In the many instances in which high oxygen pressures have had to be used, some of the observed consequences may have been due to this factor. However, the characteristic pathologic changes occur even when no oxygen above 40% has been used (as noted by Bachofen and Weibel[5413]).

In another series of 10 patients,[3581] residual abnormality of the FEF_{25-75} was observed. Organizing exudate in the bronchioles in one of these patients was thought to be possibly a consequence of the administration of oxygen at high pressure. In three of nine survivors of ARDS studied for several years,[3673] the persistence of a restrictive pattern was noted, and in three of them there was exercise-induced airflow limitation with a positive methacholine challenge test. It is not clear how frequently this occurs in survivors.

In two of eight patients studied after recovery with regional measurements and ^{133}Xe,[3753] reduced ventilation and perfusion of one lung, as compared with the other, was observed. Slow resolution, with a rise in F_{CO} from 48% of predicted to 92% of predicted over a 4-month period, was noted in a patient with Mendelson's syndrome.[3767] Over the same period, the VC increased from 1.8 liters to 3.9 liters.

In one study of 86 survivors of blunt chest injury,[3803] all had a normal FVC and FEV_1, but 27% claimed that they had persistent cough. Twenty-one per cent complained of persistent wheezing. About the same number also complained of dyspnea. The symptoms were noted to be commoner in smokers than non-smokers. These patients had not suffered the generalized changes of ARDS. Hence, the pattern of extensive alveolar damage was not present.

Pulmonary function during and after survival in ARDS is closely related to the observed pattern of pathologic changes. The syndrome therefore provides one of the more striking structure/function correlations.

RESPIRATORY FAILURE IN CHRONIC OBSTRUCTIVE LUNG DISEASE

Factors associated with respiratory failure in patients with severe chronic airflow limitation are noted in Chapter 8. Pulmonary hypertension (cor pulmonale) is discussed in Chapter 12. This section contains additional observations.

Domiciliary oxygen has been increasingly used in the management of chronic obstructive pulmonary disease.* In 1976, Lertzmann and Cherniack[4054] reviewed the problem of rehabilitation in these patients, and Anthonisen[4149] has recently published a comprehensive review of oxygen therapy. It is now clear that continuous oxygen therapy (1) leads to improvement in neuropsychiatric tests[422]; (2) relieves the vicious circle of hypoxemia, depression, lack of appetite, and deconditioning due to lack of physical activity[3337]; (3) reduces hospital admissions[4222]; and (4) probably postpones the onset of overt right ventricular failure. For those able to maintain a reasonable level of intellectual activity and to put up with the inconvenience of the therapy, these are, without doubt, major benefits.

Flenley and his colleagues studied 10 severely hypoxemic patients at rest and on exercise and noted that the administration of 30% oxygen on exercise led to an increase in mean Pa_{O_2} from 41.9 mm Hg on air to 65.6 mm Hg on oxygen, with only a 1 mm Hg increase in Pa_{CO_2}.[1336] The overall benefit of oxygen is not easy to quantitate in these patients. Degaute and his colleagues,[4236] studying 35 patients, showed that oxygen delivery significantly rose in 15. There was also an increase in mixed venous oxygen pressure. In 20, there was a fall in cardiac output that offset the increased arterial Pa_{O_2}, leading to no significant improvement in oxygen delivery.

Cases of chronic airflow obstruction in right ventricular failure have also been intensively studied. The rate of respiratory work and the respiratory work per liter of ventilation are increased.[4046] At end expiration, alveolar pressure is commonly between 6 to 13 cm H_2O (an effect the authors described as "intrinsic PEEP"[4046]). Detailed studies on one subject with a maximal recoil pressure of only 6.5 cm H_2O[3266] showed that inspiratory work was seven times the normal value, most of it being elastic work on the chest wall. Patients with chronic hypoxemia have a lower $P_{0.1}$, a smaller tidal volume, and a faster respiratory rate than comparable subjects not in respiratory failure.[4400] Severe hypoxemia in these patients may be accompanied by a lactic acidosis; this may be detected by measurement of the "anion gap,"[2726] which may be computed by subtracting the chloride (Cl) and bicarbonate (HCO_3) ions from the sodium (Na) component, a difference that is normally less than 15 mEq/L.

Inducing bronchoconstriction with mecholyl leads to increased airflow resistance, hyperinflation, and a decrease in respiratory muscle performance.[4415] In 12 patients so studied, Pa_{CO_2} increased, although $\dot{V}E$ also rose. Tidal volume fell and the frequency of respiration increased. In 14 patients with severe chronic airflow limitation, airway anesthesia led to a 6% decline in $\dot{V}E$; expiratory time increased 10%, and respiratory frequency slowed.[3301] $P_{0.1}$ increased after airway anesthesia, an effect attributed to the fall in Pa_{O_2} by 6 mm Hg and the rise in Pa_{CO_2} by 8 mm Hg. These studies are unlikely to be repeated because mechanical assistance was needed in all the patients. Comparisons between air and 24% oxygen breathing in 40 patients in an intensive care unit[4429] showed that the rise in Pa_{O_2} (from a mean of 40.4 mm Hg to a mean of 57.3 mm Hg) was mainly attributable to better oxygenation of the 81% of the cardiac output that was traversing low $\dot{V}/\dot{Q}$ units. The initial Pa_{O_2} value was mainly determined by the fractional perfusion of the poorly ventilated regions of the lung. Oxygen administration in patients in respiratory failure appears to cause a greater increase in Pa_{CO_2} than in those not experiencing an acute episode.[4433] The increased Pa_{CO_2} is attributable to an initial fall in $\dot{V}E$, but Pa_{CO_2} continues to rise because of an increase in $\dot{V}/\dot{Q}$ inequality.[4599]

There have been some reports of survival following episodes of acute respiratory failure. Following acute episodes of respiratory failure,[4607] 100 consecutive patients in a British series were observed for 4 years after discharge from the hospital. Thirty per cent survived 4 years. Asmundsson and Kilburn from the United States[4608] observed 146 patients after acute episodes of respiratory failure for between

---

*See references 3983, 3959, 4002, 4010.

5 and 8 years. Thirty per cent survived 2 years, and 16% survived 5 years. Bronchitis without emphysema was considered a favorable feature in terms of survival. In another series of 111 patients whose Pa_{O_2} averaged 36 mm Hg and Pa_{CO_2} averaged 67 mm Hg on admission,[4642] 28% who left the hospital alive survived 5 years. In most of these series, domiciliary oxygen has been used after the acute episode. This may account for better survival, as compared with earlier reported series in which 66% of the patients died within 2 years of the first episode of respiratory failure.[4723]

Keller, Ragaz, and Borer[4041] recently reported on 87 patients on long-term domiciliary oxygen therapy who were observed for 3 years. Their mean age was 62.9 years. Initial mean values were a Pa_{O_2} of 46.4 mm Hg; VC of 57.6% of predicted; and FEV_1 32.6% of predicted. Fourteen hours of oxygen were administered each day. In this group, 23.7% died in the first year, 37.4% after 2 years, and 45% after 3 years. In the early death group, the mean PAP had been 40 mm Hg. In the survivors, it was 29.4 mm Hg. Severe airway obstruction and hypoxemia were not related to early death in these patients, but the response of the pulmonary vascular resistance to oxygen breathing was a factor.

REFERENCES*

1. Bates, D. V., Macklem, P. T., and Christie, R. V. Respiratory Function in Disease. 2nd ed. W. B. Saunders, Philadelphia, 1971.
2. Sakula, A. R T H Laennec 1781–1826, his life and work: a bicentenary appreciation. Thorax 36: 81–90, 1981.
3. Bishop, P. J. Reception of the stethoscope and Laennec's book. Thorax 36: 487–492, 1981.
4. Murphy, R. L. Auscultation of the lung: past lessons, future possibilities. Thorax 36: 99–107, 1981.
5. McFadden, J. P., Price, R. C., Eastwood, H. D., and Briggs, R. S. Raised respiratory rate in elderly patients: a valuable physical sign. Br. Med. J. 284: 626–627, 1982.
6. Kraman, S. S. Does laryngeal noise contribute to the vesicular lung sound? Am. Rev. Respir. Dis. 124: 292–294, 1981.
7. Kraman, S. S. Determination of the site of production of respiratory sounds by subtraction phonopneumography. Am. Rev. Respir. Dis. 122: 303–309, 1980.
8. Leblanc, P., Macklem, P. T., and Ross, W. R. D. Breath sounds and distribution of pulmonary ventilation. Am. Rev. Respir. Dis. 102: 10–16, 1970.
9. Ploy-Song-Sang, Y., Macklem, P. T., and Ross, W. D. Distribution of regional ventilation measured by breath sounds. Am. Rev. Respir. Dis. 117: 657–664, 1978.
10. Bunin, N. J. and Loudon, R. G. Lung sound terminology in case reports. Chest 76: 690–692, 1979.
11. Nath, A. R. and Capel, L. H. Inspiratory crackles and mechanical events of breathing. Thorax 29: 695–698, 1974.
12. Forgacs, P. Breath sounds (editorial). Thorax 33: 681–683, 1978.
13. Epler, G. R., Carrington, C. B., and Gaensler, E. A. Crackles (rales) in the interstitial pulmonary diseases. Chest 73: 333–339, 1978.
14. Grassi, C., Marinone, G., Morandini, G. C., Pernice, A., and Puglisi, M. Normal and pathological respiratory sounds analysed by means of a new phonopneumographic apparatus. Respiration 33: 315–324, 1976.
15. Shirai, F., Kudoh, S., Shibuya, A., Sada, K., and Mikami, R. Crackles in asbestos workers: auscultation and lung sound analysis. Br. J. Dis. Chest 75: 386–396, 1981.
16. Forgacs, P. The functional basis of pulmonary sounds. Chest 73: 399–405, 1978.
17. Bohadana, A. B., Peslin, R., and Uffholtz, H. Breath sounds in the clinical assessment of airflow obstruction. Thorax 33: 345–351, 1978.
18. Pardee, N. E., Martin, C. J., and Morgan, E. H. A test of the practical value of estimating breath sound intensity. Chest 70: 341–344, 1976.
19. Forgacs, P., Nathoo, A. R., and Richardson, H. D. Breath sounds. Thorax 26: 288–295, 1971.
20. Pardee, N. E., Winterbauer, R. H., Morgan, E. H., Allen, J. D., and Olsen, D. E. Combinations of four physical signs as indicators of ventilatory abnormality in obstructive syndromes. Chest 77: 354–358, 1980.
21. Ploy-Song-Sang, Y., Pare, J. A. P., and Macklem, P. T. Lung sounds in patients with emphysema. Am. Rev. Respir. Dis. 124: 45–49, 1981.
22. Cohen, B. M. Color presentation of breath sounds. Respiration 29: 234–246, 1972.
23. Brain, J. D. and Valberg, P. A. Deposition of aerosol in the respiratory tract. Am. Rev. Respir. Dis. 120: 1325–1373, 1979.
24. Environmental Factors in Respiratory Disease. Fogarty Center International Proceedings. No. 11. Edited by D. H. K. Lee. Sponsored by NIEHS and Fogarty Center. Academic Press, New York and London, 1972.
25. Gomm, S. A., Keaney, N. P., Winsey, N. J. P., and Stretton, T. B. Effect of an extension tube on the bronchodilator efficacy of terbutaline delivered from a metered dose inhaler. Thorax 35: 552–556, 1980.
26. Pavia, D., Bateman, J. R. M., Sheahan, N. F., and Clarke, S. W. Effect of ipratropium bromide on mucociliary clearance and pulmonary function in reversible airways obstruction. Thorax 34: 501–507, 1979.
27. Pavia, D., Thomson, M. L., Clarke, S. W., and Shannon, H. S. Effect of lung function and mode of inhalation on penetration of aerosol into the human lung. Thorax 32: 194–197, 1977.
28. Schlesinger, R. B. and Lippmann, M. Particle deposition in the trachea: in vivo and in hollow casts. Thorax 31: 678–684, 1976.
29. Lapp, N. L., Hankinson, J. L., Amandus, H., and Palmes, E. D. Variability in the size of airspaces in normal human lungs as estimated by aerosols. Thorax 30: 293–299, 1975.
30. Morgan, A., Evans, J. C., Evans, R. J., Hounam, R. F., Holmes, A., and Doyle, S. G. Studies of the deposition of inhaled fibrous material in the respiratory tract of the rat and its subsequent clearance using radioactive tracer techniques. ii. Deposition of the UCICC standard reference samples of asbestos. Environ. Res. 10: 196–207, 1975.
31. Pflug, A. E., Cheney, F. W. Jr., and Butler, J. The effects of an ultrasonic aerosol on pulmonary mechanics and arterial blood gases in patients with chronic bronchitis. Am. Rev. Respir. Dis. 101: 710–714, 1970.
32. Riley, D. J., Liu, R. T., and Edelman, N. Enhanced responses to aerosolized bronchodilator therapy in asthma using respiratory maneuvers. Chest 76: 501–507, 1979.
33. Newhouse, M. T. and Ruffin, R. E. Deposition and fate of aerosolized drugs. Chest 73(Suppl.): 936–943, June 1978.
34. Asmundsson, T., Johnson, R. F., Kilburn, K. H., and Goodrich, J. K. Efficiency of nebulizers for depositing saline in human lung. Am. Rev. Respir. Dis. 108: 506–512, 1973.
35. Jakab, G. J. and Green, G. M. Effects of pneumonia on intrapulmonary distribution of inhaled particles. Am. Rev. Respir. Dis. 107: 619–673, 1973.
36. Lourenco, R. V., Loddenkemper, R., and Carton, R. W. Patterns of distribution and clearance of aerosols in patients with bronchiectasis. Am. Rev. Respir. Dis. 106: 857–866, 1972.
37. Michel, F. B., Marty, J. P., Quet, L., and Cour, P. Penetration of inhaled pollen into the respiratory tract. Am. Rev. Respir. Dis. 115: 609–616, 1977.
38. Dolovich, M. B., Killian, D., Wolff, R. K., Obminski, G., and Newhouse, M. T. Pulmonary aerosol deposition in chronic bronchitis: intermittent positive pressure breathing versus quiet breathing. Am. Rev. Respir. Dis. 115: 397–402, 1977.
39. Love, R. G. and Muir, D. C. F. Aerosol deposition and

*This bibliography is available on two diskettes (MICROSOFT WORD format) from the author.

airway obstruction. Am. Rev. Respir. Dis. 114: 891–897, 1976.

40. Bohning, D. E., Albert, R. E., Lippmann, M., and Foster, W. M. Tracheobronchial particle deposition and clearance. Arch. Environ. Health 30: 457–462, 1975.

41. Thomson, M. L. and Pavia, D. Particle penetration and clearance in the human lung. Arch. Environ. Health 29: 214–219, 1974.

42. Brain, J. D. and Valberg, P. A. Models for lung retention based on ICRP Task Group Report. Arch. Environ. Health 28: 1–11, 1974.

43. Hiller, C., Mazumder, M., Wilson, D., and Bone, R. Aerodynamic size distribution of metered-dose bronchodilator aerosols. Am. Rev. Respir. Dis. 118: 311–317, 1978.

44. Ruffin, R. E., Dolovich, M. B., Wolff, R. K., and Newhouse, M. T. The effects of preferential deposition of histamine in the human airway. Am. Rev. Respir. Dis. 117: 485–492, 1978.

45. Newman, S. P., Pavia, D., Moren, F., Sheahan, N. F., and Clarke, S. W. Deposition of pressurised aerosols in the human respiratory tract. Thorax 36: 52–55, 1981.

46. Valberg, P. A. and Brain, J. D. Generation and use of three types of iron-oxide aerosol. Am. Rev. Respir. Dis. 120: 1013–1024, 1979.

47. Smaldone, G. C., Itoh, H., Swift, D. L., and Wagner, H. N. Jr. Effect of flow-limiting segments and cough on particle deposition and mucociliary clearance in the lung. Am. Rev. Respir. Dis. 120: 747–758, 1979.

48. Greening, A. P., Miniati, M., and Fazio, F. Regional deposition of aerosols in health and in airways obstruction: a comparison with krypton-81M ventilation scanning. Bull. Eur. Physiopathol. Respir. 16: 287–298, 1980.

49. Stahlhofen, W. Experimentally determined regional deposition of aerosol particles in the human respiratory tract. Bull. Eur. Physiopathol. Respir. 16: 145P–147P, 1980.

50. Agnew, J. E., Pavia, D., and Clarke, S. W. Airways penetration of inhaled radioaerosol: an index to small airways function? Eur. J. Respir. Dis. 62: 239–255, 1981.

51. Pavia, D., Thomson, M., and Shannon, H. S. Aerosol inhalation and depth of deposition in the human lung. Arch. Environ. Health 32: 131–137, 1977.

52. Hahn, F. F. and Hobbs, C. H. The effect of enzyme-induced pulmonary emphysema in Syrian hamsters on the deposition and long-term retention of inhaled particles. Arch. Environ. Health 34: 203–211, 1979.

53. Newman, S. P., Moren, F., Pavia, D., Little, F., and Clarke, S. W. Deposition of pressurized suspension aerosols inhaled through extension devices. Am. Rev. Respir. Dis. 124: 317–320, 1981.

54. Ryan, G., Dolovich, M. B., Roberts, R. S., Frith, P. A., Juniper, E. F., Hargreave, F. E., and Newhouse, M. T. Standardization of inhalation provocation tests: two techniques of aerosol generation and inhalation compared. Am. Rev. Respir. Dis. 123: 195–199, 1981.

55. Brody, A. R., Hill, L. H., Adkins, B. Jr., and O'Connor, R. W. Chrysotile asbestos inhalation in rats: deposition pattern and reaction of alveolar epithelium and pulmonary macrophages. Am. Rev. Respir. Dis. 123: 670–679, 1981.

56. Braun, J. M., Gongora, G., Gongora, R., Roy, M., Bedu, M., du Perron, M. C., Jammet, H., and Drutel, P. Dépositions tracheo-bronchique et pulmonaire mesurées par traceurs radioactifs. Poumon Coeur 35: 355–360, 1979.

57. Gayrard, P. and Orehek, J. Mauvaise utilisation des aerosoldoseurs par les asthmatiques. Respiration 40: 47–52, 1980.

58. Poppius, H. Inhalation of a terbutaline spray through an extended mouthpiece. Respiration 40: 278–283, 1980.

59. Colebatch, H. J. H., Greaves, I. A., and Ng, C. K. Y. Exponential analysis of elastic recoil and aging in healthy males and females. J. Appl. Physiol.: Respir. Environ. Exercise Physiol. 47: 683–691, 1979.

60. Berend, N., Skoog, C., Waskiewicz, L., and Thurlbeck, W. M. Maximum volumes in excised human lungs: effects of age, emphysema, and formalin inflation. Thorax 35: 859–864, 1980.

61. Hurwitz, S., Allen, J., Liben, A., and Becklake, M. R. Lung function in young adults: evidence for differences in the

chronological age at which various functions start to decline. Thorax 35: 615–619, 1980.

62. Schoenberg, J. B., Beck, G. J., and Bouhuys, A. Growth and decay of pulmonary function in healthy blacks and whites. Respir. Physiol. 33: 367–393, 1978.

63. Milne, J. S. Longitudinal respiratory studies in older people. Thorax 33: 547–554, 1978.

64. Yager, J., Chen, T-M., and Dulfano, M. J. Measurement of frequency of ciliary beats of human respiratory epithelium. Chest 73: 627–633, 1978.

65. Gelb, A. F. and Zamel, N. Effect of aging on lung mechanics in healthy nonsmokers. Chest 68: 538–541, 1975.

66. Cantwell, J. D. and Watt, E. W. Extreme cardiopulmonary fitness in old age. Chest 65: 357–359, 1974.

67. Schmidt, C. D., Dickman, M. L., Gardner, R. M., and Brough, F. K. Spirometric standards for healthy elderly men and women. Am. Rev. Respir. Dis. 108: 933–939, 1973.

68. Kronenberg, R. S., Drage, C. W., Ponto, R. A., and Williams, L. E. The effect of age on the distribution of ventilation and perfusion in the lung. Am. Rev. Respir. Dis. 108: 576–586, 1973.

69. Cherniack, R. M. and Raber, M. B. Normal standards for ventilatory function using an automated wedge spirometer. Am. Rev. Respir. Dis. 106: 38–46, 1972.

70. Chiang, S. T., Wang, B. C., Chi, Y. L., and Hsieh, Y. C. Ventilatory components of lungs in relation to sex and age. Am. Rev. Respir. Dis. 104: 175–181, 1971.

71. Martin, C. J., Chihara, S., and Chang, D. B. A comparative study of the mechanical properties in aging alveolar wall. Am. Rev. Respir. Dis. 115: 981–988, 1977.

72. Pump, K. K. Emphysema and its relation to age. Am. Rev. Respir. Dis. 114: 5–13, 1976.

73. Georges, R., Saumon, G., and Loiseau, A. The relationship of age to pulmonary membrane conductance and capillary blood volume. Am. Rev. Respir. Dis. 117: 1069–1078, 1978.

74. Kronenberg, R. S. and Drage, C. W. Attenuation of the ventilatory and heart rate responses to hypoxia and hypercapnia with aging in normal men. J. Clin. Invest. 52: 1812–1819, 1973.

75. Bottiger, L. E. Regular decline in physical working capacity with age. Br. Med. J. 3: 270–271, 1978.

76. Kronenberg, R. S., L'heureux, P., Ponto, R. A., Drage, C. W., and Loken, M. K. The effect of aging on lung perfusion. Ann. Intern. Med. 76: 413–421, 1972.

77. Thurlbeck, W. M. The effect of age on the lung. Aging—its chemistry. Third Arnold O. Beckman Conference in Clinical Chemistry Proceedings. Edited by Albert A. Dietz. American Association for Clinical Chemistry, Washington, D.C., 1979.

78. Sugihara, T., Martin, C. J., and Hildebrandt, J. Length-tension properties of alveolar wall in man. J. Appl. Physiol. 30: 874–878, 1971.

79. Niewohner, D. E., Kleinerman, J., and Liotta, L. Elastic behaviour of post-mortem human lungs: effects of aging in mild emphysema. J. Appl. Physiol. 36: 943–949, 1975.

80. Knudson, R. J., Clark, D. F., Kennedy, T. C., and Knudson, D. E. Effect of aging alone on mechanical properties of normal adult human lung. J. Appl. Physiol. 43: 1054–1062, 1977.

81. Holland, J., Milic-Emili, J., Macklem, P. T., and Bates, D. V. Regional distribution of pulmonary ventilation and perfusion in elderly subjects. J. Clin. Invest. 47: 81–92, 1968.

82. Fleetham, J. Cough and the elderly. Personal communication, 1987.

83. Tautulier, M., Bourret, M., and Deyrieux, F. Les pressions arterielles pulmonaires chez l'homme normal. Effets de l'age et de l'exercise musculaire. Bull. Physiopathol. Respir. 8: 1295–1321, 1972.

84. Pasquis, P., Cevear, A. M., Denis, P., Hellot, M. F., Pietrini, C., and Lefrancois, R. Normal values of TL_{co} measured in steady state. Bull. Physiopathol. Respir. 9: 553–568, 1973.

85. Oxhoj, H., Bake, B., and Wilhelmsen, L. Closing volume in 50- and 60-year-old men. Scand. J. Respir. Dis. 85(Suppl.): 259–265, 1974.

86. Amaducci, S., Mandelli, V., Morpurgo, M., and Rampulla, C. Aging, cigarette smoking, and respiratory function. Bull. Eur. Physiopathol. Respir. 13: 523–532, 1977.

87. Yernault, J. C., Baran, D., and Englert, M. Effect of growth and aging on the static mechanical lung properties. Bull. Eur. Physiopathol. Respir. 13: 777–788, 1977.

88. Jammes, Y., Auran, Y., Gouvernet, J., Delpierre, S., and Grimaud, C. The ventilatory pattern of conscious man according to age and morphology. Bull. Eur. Physiopathol. Respir. 15: 527–540, 1979.

89. Kauffmann, F., Querleux, E., Drouet, D., Lellouch, J., and Brille, D. Evolution du VEMS en 12 ans et tabagisme chez 556 travailleurs de la région Parisienne. Bull. Eur. Physiopathol. Respir. 15: 723–737, 1979.

90. Bigler, A. H., Renzetti, A. D. Jr., Watanabe, S., Begin, R., and Clark, J. Regional lung expansion and vertical pleural pressure gradients in normal human subjects. Bull. Eur. Physiopathol. Respir. 15: 773–788, 1979.

91. Holtz, B., Bake, B., and Winstedt, P. Effect of inspired volume on airway closure in relation to age. Scand. J. Respir. Dis. 60: 119–127, 1979.

92. Derks, C. M. Ventilation-perfusion distribution in young and old volunteers during mild exercise. Bull. Eur. Physiopathol. Respir. 16: 145–154, 1980.

93. Demedts, M. Regional distribution of lung volumes and of gas inspired at residual volume: influence of age, body weight and posture. Bull. Eur. Physiopathol. Respir. 16: 271–285, 1980.

94. Pavia, D., Bateman, J. R. M., and Clarke, S. W. Deposition and clearance of inhaled particles. Bull. Eur. Physiopathol. Respir. 16: 335–366, 1980.

95. Andreotti, L., Cammelli, D., Bussotti, A., and Arcangeli, P. Biochemical measurement of lung connective tissue. Bull. Eur. Physiopathol. Respir. 16(Suppl.): 83–89, 1980.

96. Davies, C. T. M. The oxygen transporting system in relation to age. Clin. Sci. 42: 1–13, 1972.

97. Adams, W. C., McHenry, M. M., and Bernauer, E. M. Multistage treadmill walking performance and associated cardiorespiratory response of middle-aged men. Clin. Sci. 42: 355–370, 1972.

98. Milne, J. S. and Williamson, J. Respiratory function tests in older people. Clin. Sci. 42: 371–381, 1972.

99. Tweeddale, P. M., Leggett, R. J. E., and Flenley, D. C. Effect of age on oxygen-binding in normal human subjects. Clin. Sci. 51: 185–188, 1976.

100. Peterson, D. D., Pack, A. I., Silage, D. A., and Fishman, A. P. Effects of aging on ventilatory and occlusion pressure responses to hypoxia and hypercapnia. Am. Rev. Respir. Dis. 124: 387–391, 1981.

101. Zeilhofer, R. Totale Dehnbarkheit von Lunge und Thorax bei Gesunden. Respiration 31: 318–331, 1974.

102. Mastrangelo, D., Chau, N., and Pham, Q. T. Les differents modes d'expression du test au monoxyde de carbone en regime stable: discussion et proposition de valeurs de reference pour les études epidemiologiques. Respiration 39: 28–38, 1980.

103. Islam, M. S. Mechanism of controlling residual volume and emptying rate of the lung in young and elderly healthy subjects. Respiration 40: 1–8, 1980.

104. Robinson, N. E. and Gillespie, J. R. Morphologic features of the lungs of aging beagle dogs. Am. Rev. Respir. Dis. 108: 1192–1199, 1973.

105. Davis, C., Campbell, E. J. M., Openshaw, P., Pride, N. B., and Woodroof, G. Importance of airway closure in limiting maximal expiration in normal man. J. Appl. Physiol.: Respir. Environ. Exercise Physiol. 48: 695–701, 1980.

106. Dhainaut, J-F., Bons, J., Bricard, C., and Monsallier, J-F. Improved oxygenation in patients with extensive unilateral pneumonia using the lateral decubitus position. Thorax 35: 792–793, 1980.

107. Seaton, D., Lapp, N. L., and Morgan, W. K. C. Effect of body position on gas exchange after thoracotomy. Thorax 34: 518–522, 1979.

108. Clague, H. W. and Hall, D. R. Effect of posture on lung volume: airway closure and gas exchange in hemidiaphragmatic paralysis. Thorax 34: 523–526, 1979.

109. Chevrolet, J. C., Martin, J. G., Flood, R., Martin, R. R., and Engel, L. A. Topographical ventilation and perfusion distribution during IPPB in the lateral posture. Am. Rev. Respir. Dis. 118: 847–854, 1978.

110. Hyland, R. H., Krastins, I. R. B., Aspin, N., Mansell, A., and Zamel, N. Effect of body position on carbon monoxide diffusing capacity in asymptomatic smokers and nonsmokers. Am. Rev. Respir. Dis. 117: 1045–1053, 1978.

111. Michaelson, E. D., Sackner, M. A., and Johnson, R. L. Jr. Vertical distributions of pulmonary diffusing capacity and capillary blood flow in man. J. Clin. Invest. 52: 359–369, 1973.

112. Burki, N. K. The effects of changes in functional residual capacity with posture on mouth occlusion pressure and ventilatory pattern. Am. Rev. Respir. Dis. 116: 895–900, 1977.

113. Douglas, W. W., Rehder, K., Beynen, F. M., Sessler, A. D., and Marsh, H. M. Improved oxygenation in patients with acute respiratory failure: the prone position. Am. Rev. Respir. Dis. 115: 559–566, 1977.

114. Rea, H. H., Withy, S. J., Seelye, E. R., and Harris, E. A. The effects of posture on venous admixture and respiratory dead space in health. Am. Rev. Respir. Dis. 115: 571–580, 1977.

115. Zack, M. B., Pontoppidan, H., and Kazemi, H. The effect of lateral positions on gas exchange in pulmonary disease. Am. Rev. Respir. Dis. 110: 49–55, 1974.

116. Hamosh, P. and Luchsinger, P. C. Lung mechanics and gas exchange in the squatting position. Am. Rev. Respir. Dis. 102: 112–115, 1970.

117. Begin, R. Platypnea after pneumonectomy. N. Engl. J. Med. 293: 342–343, 1975.

118. Khan, F. and Parekh, A. Reversible platypnea and orthodeoxia following recovery from adult respiratory distress syndrome. Chest 75: 526–528, 1979.

119. Walkup, R. H., Vossel, L. F., Griffin, J. P., and Proctor, R. J. Prediction of postoperative pulmonary function with the lateral position test. Chest 77: 24–27, 1980.

120. West, J. B. Regional differences in the lung. Chest 74: 426–437, 1978.

121. Pierson, D. J., Dick, N. P., and Petty, T. L. A comparison of spirometric values with subjects in standing and sitting positions. Chest 70: 17–20, 1976.

122. Marion, J. M., Alderson, P. O., Lefrak, S. S., Senior, R. M., and Jacobs, M. H. Unilateral lung function. Chest 69: 5–9, 1976.

123. Hazlett, D. R. and Watson, R. L. Lateral position test: a simple, inexpensive, yet accurate method of studying the separate functions of the lungs. Chest 59: 276–279, 1971.

124. Sarlin, R. F., Schillaci, R. F., Georges, T. N., and Wilcox, J. R. Focal increased lung perfusion and intrapulmonary veno-arterial shunting in bronchiolo-alveolar cell carcinoma. Am. J. Med. 68: 618–623, 1980.

125. Teculescu, D. B. and Stanescu, D. C. Lung diffusing capacity. Normal values in male smokers and non-smokers using the breath-holding technique. Scand. J. Respir. Dis. 51: 137–149, 1970.

126. Trimble, C., Smith, D. E., Cook, T. I., and Trummer, M. J. The effect of supine bedrest upon alveolar-arterial oxygen gradients and intrapulmonary shunting in normal man. J. Thorac. Cardiovasc. Surg. 63: 873–879, 1972.

127. Kennedy, T. C. and Knudson, R. J. Exercise-aggravated hypoxemia and orthodeoxia in cirrhosis. Chest 72: 305–309, 1977.

128. Sandham, J. D., Shaw, D. T., and Guenter, C. A. Acute supine respiratory failure due to bilateral diaphragmatic paralysis. Chest 72: 96–98, 1977.

129. Laval, P., Feliciano, J. M., Fondarai, J., Kleisbauer, J. P., and Poirier, R. Variations de la capacité respiratoire fonctionelle et des resistances des voies aeriennes chêz les sujets normeaux en position assisé puis couchée. Bull. Physiopathol. Respir. 7: 743–764, 1971.

130. Cumming, G., Abraham, A. S., Horsfield, K., and Prowse, K. Regional hypoxia and dependent airway closure. Scand. J. Respir. Dis. 51: 37–41, 1970.

131. Sundstrom, G. Influence of ventilation, exercise, and body position on techniques for determining steady state diffusing capacity. Scand. J. Respir. Dis. 92(Suppl.): 1–74, 1975.

132. Lilja, B. and Arborelius, M. Jr. Factors affecting pulmonary blood flow in the lateral decubitus position. Scand. J. Respir. Dis. 85(Suppl.): 28–32, 1974.

133. Schaanning, J. and Refsum, H. E. Influence of posture on

pulmonary gas exchange and heart rate in chronic obstructive lung disease. Scand. J. Respir. Dis. 57: 12–16, 1976.

134. Prefaut, C., Monnier, L., Ramonatxo, M., Chardon, G., and Mirouze, J. Influence de la posture et de la fermeture des voies aeriennes sur les échanges respiratoires du sujet obèse. Bull. Eur. Physiopathol. Respir. 14: 249–263, 1978.

135. Marcq, M. and Minette, A. Nongravitational terminal nitrogen rise in smokers. Bull. Eur. Physiopathol. Respir. 16: 607–621, 1980.

136. McClean, P. A., Duguid, N. J., Griffin, P. M., Newth, C. J. L., and Zamel, N. Changes in exhaled pulmonary diffusing capacity at rest and exercise in individuals with impaired positional diffusion. Bull. Eur. Physiopathol. Respir. 17: 179–186, 1981.

137. Roos, C. M., Romijn, K. H., Braat, M. C. P., and van Leeuwen, A. M. Posture-dependent dyspnoea and cyanosis after pneumonectomy. Eur. J. Respir. Dis. 62: 377–382, 1981.

138. Minh, V., Chun, D., Dolan, G. F., Lee, H. M., and Vasquez, P. Mixed venous oxygenation, exercise, body posture, and V/Q ratio in chronic obstructive pulmonary disease. Am. Rev. Respir. Dis. 124: 226–231, 1981.

139. Rehder, K., Knopp, T. J., Brusasco, V., and Didier, E. P. Inspiratory flow and intrapulmonary gas distribution. Am. Rev. Respir. Dis. 124: 392–396, 1981.

140. Lilja, B. The distribution of pulmonary blood flow in man during oxygen breathing and breath-holding. Scand. J. Clin. Lab. Invest. 26: 105–112, 1970.

141. Lilja, B. Pulmonary blood flow distribution at different lung volumes and body positions. Scand. J. Clin. Lab. Invest. 29: 351–358, 1972.

142. Lilja, B. Regional lung function and central haemodynamics in man during two hours of sitting. Scand. J. Clin. Lab. Invest. 30: 5–9, 1972.

143. Lilja, B. Regional lung function and central haemodynamics during hypoxia, hyperoxia, and breath-holding. Scand. J. Clin. Lab. Invest. 30: 11–15, 1972.

144. Sharp, J. T., Moisan, W. S. D. T., Foster, J., and Machnach, W. Postural relief of dyspnea in severe chronic obstructive pulmonary disease. Am. Rev. Respir. Dis. 122: 201–211, 1980.

145. Jay, S. J., Stonehill, R. B., Kiblawi, S. O., and Norton, J. Variability of the lateral position test in normal subjects. Am. Rev. Respir. Dis. 121: 165–168, 1980.

146. Parot, S., Chaudun, E., and Jacquemin, E. The origin of postural variations of human lung volumes as explained by the effects of age. Respiration 27: 254–260, 1970.

147. Jebavy, P., Widimsky, J., Hurych, J., and Stanek, V. Relationship between orthostatic changes of pulmonary diffusing capacity and haemodynamics of lesser circulation. Respiration 28: 101–113, 1971.

148. Arborelius, M. Jr., Granqvist, U., Lilja, B., and Zauner, C. W. Regional lung function and central haemodynamics in the right lateral body position during hypoxia and hyperoxia. Respiration 31: 193–200, 1974.

149. Arborelius, M. Jr., Lilja, B., and Zauner, C. W. The relative effect of hypoxia and gravity on pulmonary blood flow. Respiration 31: 369–380, 1974.

150. Hedenstierna, G., Bindslev, L., and Santesson, J. Pressure-volume and airway closure relationships in each lung in anaesthetized man. Clin. Physiol. 1: 479–493, 1981.

151. Russell, W. J. Position of patient and respiratory function in immediate postoperative period. Br. Med. J. 283: 1079–1080, 1981.

152. Bates, D. V. Impact of radioactive gas studies of the lung on surgery and postoperative care. Bull. Am. Coll. Surg. 54: 355–357, 1969.

153. Kronenberg, R. S., Drage, C. W., and Stevenson, J. E. Acute respiratory failure and obesity with normal ventilatory response to carbon dioxide and absent hypoxic ventilatory drive. Am. J. Med. 62: 772–776, 1977.

154. Zwillich, C. W., Sutton, F. D., Pierson, D. J., Creagh, E. M., and Weil, J. V. Decreased hypoxic ventilatory drive in the obesity-hypoventilation syndrome. Am. J. Med. 59: 349–353, 1975.

155. Kronenberg, R. S., Gabel, R. A., and Severinghaus, J. W. Normal chemoreceptor function in obesity before and after

156. Rochester, D. and Enson, Y. Current concepts in the pathogenesis of the obesity-hypoventilation syndrome. Am. J. Med. 57: 402–420, 1974.

157. Kryger, M., Quesney, L. F., Holder, D., Gloor, P., and MacLeod, P. The sleep deprivation syndrome of the obese patient. Am. J. Med. 56: 531–539, 1974.

158. Miller, A. and Granada, M. In-hospital mortality in the Pickwickian syndrome. Am. J. Med. 56: 144–150, 1974.

159. Licht, J. R., Smith, W. R., and Glauser, F. L. Tonsillar hypertrophy in an adult with obesity-hypoventilation. Chest 70: 672–674, 1976.

160. Luce, J. M. Respiratory complications of obesity. Chest 78: 626–631, 1980.

161. Barrera, F., Hillyer, P., Ascanio, G., and Bechtel, J. The distribution of ventilation, diffusion, and blood flow in obese patients with normal and abnormal blood gases. Am. Rev. Respir. Dis. 108: 819–830, 1973.

162. Emirgil, E. and Sobol, B. J. The effects of weight reduction on pulmonary function and the sensitivity of the respiratory center in obesity. Am. Rev. Respir. Dis. 108: 831–842, 1973.

163. Comroe, J. H. Jr. Retrospectroscope: Frankenstein, Pickwick, and Ondine. Am. Rev. Respir. Dis. 111: 689–692, 1975.

164. Meunier-Carus, J., Lampert, E., Lonsdorfer, J., Kurtz, D., and Micheletti, G. La fonction respiratoire et cardiaque droit des obèses selon leur type. Bull. Physiopathol. Respir. 8: 915–935, 1972.

165. Gunella, G. Evolution des conceptions pathogeniques sur le syndrome de Pickwick. Bull. Physiopathol. Respir. 8: 981–1003, 1972.

166. Reichel, G. Lung volumes, mechanics of breathing and changes in arterial blood gases in obese patients and in Pickwickian syndrome. Bull. Physiopathol. Respir. 8: 1011–1020, 1972.

167. Tassinari, C. A., Bernardina, B. D., Cirignotta, F., and Ambrosetto, G. Apnoeic periods and the respiratory related arousal patterns during sleep in the Pickwickian syndrome. A polygraphic study. Bull. Physiopathol. Respir. 8: 1087–1102, 1972.

168. Carroll, D. Nosology of "Pickwickian" syndrome. Bull. Physiopathol. Respir. 8: 1241–1247, 1972.

169. Gunella, G. Interpretation pathogenique des troubles du sommeil et de la respiration dans le syndrome de Pickwick et dans l'hypoventilation alveolaire primaire. Bull. Physiopathol. Respir. 8: 1257–1276, 1972.

170. Duron, B., Quichaud, J., and Fullana, N. Nouvelles recherches sur le mecanisme des apnées du syndrome de Pickwick. Bull. Physiopathol. Respir. 8: 1277–1288, 1972.

171. Jacobsen, E., Dano, P., and Skovsted, P. Respiratory function before and after weight loss following intestinal shunt operation for obesity. Scand. J. Respir. Dis. 55: 332–339, 1974.

172. Rorvik, S. and Bo, G. Lung volumes and arterial blood gases in obesity. Scand. J. Respir. Dis. 95(Suppl.): 60–64, 1976.

173. Sixt, R., Bake, B., and Kral, J. Closing volume and gas exchange in obese patients before and after intestinal bypass operation. Scand. J. Respir. Dis. 95(Suppl.): 65–67, 1976.

174. Blondal, T. and Torebjork, E. Hypersomnia and periodic breathing. Scand. J. Respir. Dis. 58: 273–278, 1977.

175. Partridge, M. R., Ciofetta, G., and Hughes, J. M. B. Topography of ventilation-perfusion ratios in obesity. Bull. Eur. Physiopathol. Respir. 14: 765–773, 1978.

176. Freyschuss, U. and Melcher, A. Exercise energy expenditure in extreme obesity: influence of ergometry type and weight loss. Scand. J. Clin. Lab. Invest. 38: 753–759, 1978.

177. Chiang, S. T., Lee, P. Y., and Liu, S. Y. Pulmonary function in a typical case of Pickwickian syndrome. Respiration 39: 105–113, 1980.

178. Walsh, R. E., Michaelson, E. D., Harkleroad, L. E., Zigelboim, A., and Sackner, M. A. Upper airway obstruction in obese patients with sleep disturbance and somnolence. Ann. Intern. Med. 76: 185–192, 1972.

179. Farebrother, M. J. B., McHardy, G. J. R., and Munro, J. F. Relation between pulmonary gas exchange and closing

ileal bypass surgery to force weight reduction. Am. J. Med. 59: 349–353, 1975.

volume before and after substantial weight loss in obese subjects. Br. Med. J. 3: 391–393, 1971.

180. Douglas, F. G. and Chong, P. Y. Influence of obesity on peripheral airways patency. J. Appl. Physiol. 33: 559–563, 1972.

181. Holley, H. S., Milic-Emili, J., Becklake, M. R., and Bates, D. V. Regional distribution of pulmonary ventilation and perfusion in obesity. J. Clin. Invest. 46: 475–481, 1967.

182. Gastaut, H., Tassinari, C. A., and Duron, B. Polygraphic study of the episodic diurnal and nocturnal (hypnic and respiratory) manifestations of the Pickwick syndrome. Brain Res. 1: 167–186, 1966.

183. Gazioglu, K., Kaltreider, N. L., Rosen, M., and Yu, P. N. G. Pulmonary function during pregnancy in normal women and in patients with cardiopulmonary disease. Thorax 25: 445–450, 1970.

184. Salisbury, B. G., Metzger, L. F., Altose, M. D., Stanley, N. N., and Cherniack, N. S. Effect of fiberoptic bronchoscopy on respiratory performance in patients with chronic airways obstruction. Thorax 30: 441–446, 1975.

185. Garrard, G. S., Littler, W. A., and Redman, C. W. G. Closing volume during normal pregnancy. Thorax 33: 488–492, 1978.

186. Farmer, W. C., Glenn, W. W. L., and Gee, J. B. L. Alveolar hypoventilation syndrome. Am. J. Med. 39–49, 1978.

187. Man, G. C. W., Jones, R. L., Macdonald, G. F., and King, E. G. Primary alveolar hypoventilation managed by negative-pressure ventilators. Chest 76: 219–221, 1979.

188. Brown, N. E., Zamel, N., and Aberman, A. Changes in pulmonary mechanics and gas exchange following thoracentesis. Chest 74: 540–542, 1978.

189. Montenegro, H. D., Chester, E. H., and Jones, P. K. Cardiac arrhythmias during routine tests of pulmonary function in patients with chronic obstruction of airways. Chest 73: 133–139, 1978.

190. Child, J. S., Wolfe, J. D., Tashkin, D., and Nakano, F. Fatal lung scan in a case of pulmonary hypertension due to obliterative pulmonary vascular disease. Chest 67: 308–310, 1975.

191. Collins, D. D., Scoggin, C. H., Zwillich, C. W., and Weil, J. V. Hereditary aspects of decreased hypoxic response. J. Clin. Invest. 78: 105–110, 1978.

192. Kafer, E. R. and Leigh, J. Recurrent respiratory failure associated with the absence of ventilatory response to hypercapnia and hypoxemia. Am. Rev. Respir. Dis. 106: 100–108, 1972.

193. Gimeno, F., Berg, W. C., Sluiter, H. J., and Tammeling, G. J. Spirometry-induced bronchial obstruction. Am. Rev. Respir. Dis. 105: 68–74, 1972.

194. Naughton, J., Block, R., and Welch, M. Central alveolar hypoventilation. Am. Rev. Respir. Dis. 103: 557–565, 1971.

195. Moore, G. C., Zwillich, C. W., Battaglia, J. D., Cotton, E. K., and Weil, J. V. Respiratory failure associated with familial depression of ventilatory response to hypoxia and hypercapnia. N. Engl. J. Med. 295: 861–865, 1976.

196. Rose, G. Environmental factors and disease: the man made environment. Br. Med. J. 294: 963–965, 1987.

197. Nattie, E. E., Bartlett, D. Jr., and Rozycki, A. A. Central alveolar hypoventilation in a child: an evaluation using a whole body plethysmograph. Am. Rev. Respir. Dis. 112: 259–265, 1975.

198. Bellamy, D., Davis, J. M. N., Hickey, B. P., Benatar, S. R., and Clark, T. J. H. A case of primary alveolar hypoventilation associated with proximal myopathy. Am. Rev. Respir. Dis. 112: 867–873, 1975.

199. Hyland, R. H., Jones, N. L., Powles, A. C. P., Lenkie, S. C. M., Vanderlinden, R. G., and Epstein, S. W. Primary alveolar hypoventilation treated with nocturnal electrophrenic respiration. Am. Rev. Respir. Dis. 117: 165–172, 1978.

200. Bubis, M. J. and Anthonisen, N. R. Primary alveolar hypoventilation treated by nocturnal administration of O_2. Am. Rev. Respir. Dis. 118: 947–953, 1978.

201. Bevan, D. R., Holdcroft, A., Loh, L., MacGregor, W. G., O'Sullivan, J. C., and Sykes, M. K. Closing volume and pregnancy. Br. Med. J. 1: 13–15, 1974.

202. Moskowitz, M. A., Fisher, J. N., Simpser, M. D., and Strieder, D. J. Periodic apnea, exercise hypoventilation, and hypothalamic dysfunction. Ann. Intern. Med. 84: 171–173, 1976.

203. Weiss, S. T., Weinberger, S. E., Weiss, J. W., and Johnson, T. S. Normal pregnancy and delivery in a woman with severe underlying lung disease. Thorax 36: 878–879, 1981.

204. Forbes, A. R. and Gamsu, G. Lung mucociliary clearance after anesthesia with spontaneous and controlled ventilation. Am. Rev. Resp. Dis. 120: 857–862, 1979.

205. Morgan, E. J., Baidwan, B., Petty, T. L., and Zwillich, C. W. The effects of unanaesthetized arterial puncture on P_{CO_2} and pH. Am. Rev. Resp. Dis. 120: 795–798, 1979.

206. Hunt, C. E., Inwood, R. J., and Shannon, D. C. Respiratory and nonrespiratory effects of doxapram in congenital central hypoventilation syndrome. Am. Rev. Resp. Dis. 119: 263–269, 1979.

207. Guilleminault, C., Eldridge, F., and Dement, W. C. Insomnia, narcolepsy, and sleep apneas. Bull. Physiopathol. Respir. 8: 1127–1138, 1972.

208. Fruhmann, G. Hypersomnia with primary hypoventilation syndrome and following cor pulmonale (Ondine's curse syndrome). Bull. Physiopathol. Respir. 8: 1173–1179, 1972.

209. Vachon, L., Fitzgerald, M. X., Solliday, N. H., Gould, I. A., and Gaensler, E. A. Single-dose effect of marihuana smoke. N. Engl. J. Med. 288: 985–989, 1973.

210. Gunella, G. Interpretation pathogenique des troubles du sommeil et de la respiration dans le syndrome de Pickwick et dans l'hypoventilation alveolaire primaire. Bull. Physiopathol. Respir. 8: 1257–1276, 1972.

211. Folgering, H., Kuyper, F., and Kille, J. F. Primary alveolar hypoventilation (Ondine's curse syndrome) in an infant without external arcuate nucleus. Bull. Eur. Physiopathol. Respir. 15: 659–665, 1979.

212. Walkove, N., Altose, M. D., Kelsen, S. G., and Cherniack, N. S. Respiratory control abnormalities in alveolar hypoventilation. Am. Rev. Respir. Dis. 122: 163–167, 1980.

213. Barlow, P. B., Bartlett, D. Jr., Hauri, P., Hellekson, C., Nattie, E. E., Remmers, J. E., and Schmidt-Nowara, W. W. Idiopathic hypoventilation syndrome: importance of preventing nocturnal hypoxemia and hypercapnia. Am. Rev. Respir. Dis. 121: 141–145, 1980.

214. Giroud, M., Flandrois, R., Calamai, M., Buffat, J. J., Quiviger, P., Mouret, J. R., and Fisher, C. L'hypoventilation alveolaire primaire "malediction d'Ondine." Poumon Coeur 30: 101–108, 1974.

215. Solliday, N. H., Gaensler, E. A., Schwaber, J. R., and Parker, T. F. Impaired central chemoreceptor function and chronic hypoventilation many years following poliomyelitis. Respiration 31: 177–192, 1974.

216. Phillipson, E. A. Pickwickian, obesity-hypoventilation, or fee-fi-fo-fum syndrome (editorial). Am. Rev. Respir. Dis. 121: 781–782, 1980.

217. Patakas, D., Louridas, G., and Stavropoulos, K. Respiratory drive in idiopathic alveolar hypoventilation. Respiration 36: 135–137, 1978.

218. Milne, J. A., Mills, R. J., Coutts, J. R. T., Macnaughton, M. C., Moran, F., and Pack, A. I. The effect of human pregnancy on the pulmonary transfer factor for carbon monoxide as measured by the single breath method. Clin. Sci. 53: 271–276, 1977.

219. Weinberger, S. E., Weiss, S. T., Cohen, W. R., Weiss, J. W., and Johnson, T. S. Pregnancy and the lung. Am. Rev. Respir. Dis. 121: 559–581, 1980.

220. Laros, K. D. The postpneumonectomy mother. Respiration 39: 185–187, 1980.

221. Bjure, J., Ekstrom-Jodal, B., and Elgefors, B. Pulmonary gas exchange after radioisotope scanning of the lungs. Scand. J. Respir. Dis. 51: 242–248, 1970.

222. Kokkola, K. Respiratory gas exchange after bronchography. Scand. J. Respir. Dis. 53: 114–119, 1972.

223. Rootwelt, K. and Vale, J. R. Pulmonary gas exchange after intravenous injection of ^{99m}Tc-sulphur-colloid albumin macroaggregates for lung perfusion scintigraphy. Scand. J Clin. Lab. Invest. 30: 17–21, 1972.

224. Silvestri, R. C., Huseby, J. S., Rughani, I., Thorning, D., and Culver, B. H. Respiratory distress syndrome from lymphangiography contrast medium. Am. Rev. Respir. Dis. 122: 543–549, 1980.

225. Gelb, A. W., Southorn, P., and Rehder, K. Effect of general anesthesia on respiratory function. Lung 159: 187–198, 1981.

226. Goff, A. M. and Gaensler, E. A. Respiratory distress syndrome following lymphangiography. Respiration 28: 89–97, 1971.

227. Lode, H., Hutteman, U., and von Wolff, C. Der einfluss endoskopischer abdomineller Untersauchungen auf die Atmung. Respiration 29: 61–73, 1972.

228. Randazzo, G. P. and Wilson, A. F. Cardiopulmonary changes during flexible fiberoptic bronchoscopy. Respiration 33: 143–149, 1976.

229. Karotsky, M. S., Kothari, G. A., Fourre, J. A., and Khan, A. U. Effect of thoracentesis on arterial oxygen tension. Respiration 36: 96–103, 1978.

230. Clark, E. H., Woods, R. L., and Hughes, J. M. B. Effect of blood transfusion on the carbon monoxide transfer factor of the lung in man. Clin. Sci. Mol. Med. 54: 627–631, 1978.

231. Crapo, R. O. and Morris, A. H. Standardized single breath normal values for carbon monoxide diffusing capacity. Am. Rev. Respir. Dis. 123: 185–189, 1981.

232. Frans, A., Gerin-Portier, N., Veriter, C., and Brasseur, L. Pulmonary gas exchange in asymptomatic smokers and non-smokers. Scand. J. Respir. Dis. 56: 233–244, 1975.

233. Pierce, R. J., Brown, D. J., and Denison, D. M. Radiographic, scintigraphic, and gas-dilution estimates of individual lung and lobar volumes in man. Thorax 35: 773–780, 1980.

234. Jordanoglou, J., Tatsis, G., Vesmemes, M., Charalampakis, S., and Hadjistavrou, C. Partial effective times of the forced expiratory spirogram in health and mild airways obstruction. Thorax 35: 375–378, 1980.

235. Macdonald, J. B. and Cole, T. J. The flow-volume loop: reproducibility of air and helium-based tests in normal subjects. Thorax 35: 64–69, 1980.

236. Pierce, R. J., Brown, D. J., Holmes, M., Cumming, G., and Denison, D. M. Estimation of lung volumes from chest radiographs using shape information. Thorax 34: 726–734, 1979.

237. Oldham, P. D. Percent of predicted as the limit of normal in pulmonary function testing: a statistically valid approach (letter to editor). Thorax 34: 569, 1979.

238. Ching, B. and Horsfall, P. A. L. Lung volumes in normal Cantonese subjects: preliminary studies. Thorax 32: 352–355, 1977.

239. Jordanoglou, J., Koursouba, E., Lalenis, C., Gotsis, T., Kontos, J., and Gardikas, C. Effective time of the forced expiratory spirogram in health and airways obstruction. Thorax 34: 187–193, 1979.

240. Liang, A., Macfie, A. E., Harris, E. A., and Whitlock, R. M. L. Transit-time analysis of the forced expiratory spirogram during clinical remission in juvenile asthma. Thorax 34: 194–199, 1979.

241. Pride, N. B. Analysis of forced expiration—a return to the recording spirometer? (editorial). Thorax 34: 144–149, 1979.

242. Sobol, B. J. and Sobol, P. G. Per cent of predicted as the limit of normal in pulmonary function testing: a statistically valid approach (editorial). Thorax 34: 1–3, 1979.

243. Lord, P. W. and Edwards, J. M. Variation in airways resistance when defined over different ranges of airflows. Thorax 33: 401–405, 1978.

244. Williams, D. E., Miller, R. D., and Taylor, W. F. Pulmonary function studies in healthy Pakistani adults. Thorax 33: 243–249, 1978.

245. Pack, A. I., McKusker, R., and Moran, F. A computer system for processing data from routine pulmonary function tests. Thorax 32: 333–341, 1977.

246. Cochrane, G. M., Prieto, F., and Clark, T. J. H. Intrasubject variability of maximal expiratory flow volume curves. Thorax 32: 171–176, 1977.

247. Lord, P. W. and Brooks, A. G. F. A comparison of manual and automated methods of measuring airway resistance and thoracic gas volume. Thorax 32: 60–66, 1977.

248. Lord, P. W., Brooks, A. G. F., and Edwards, J. M. Variation between observers in the estimation of airway resistance and thoracic gas volume. Thorax 32: 67–70, 1977.

249. Macdonald, J. B., Cole, T. J., and Seaton, A. Forced expiratory time—its reliability as a lung function test. Thorax 30: 554–559, 1975.

250. Stanley, N. N., Cunningham, E. L., Altose, M. D., Kelsen, S. G., Levinson, R. S., and Cherniack, N. S. Evaluation of breath holding in hypercapnia as a simple clinical test of respiratory chemosensitivity. Thorax 30: 337–343, 1975.

251. Bhoomkar, A., Davies, S., Geary, M., and Hills, E. A. Comparison of peak flow gauge and peak flow meter. Thorax 30: 225–227, 1975.

252. Stebbings, J. H. Jr. Fractional carbon monoxide uptake in an employed population. Thorax 29: 505–510, 1974.

253. Haydu, S. P. Single breath transfer factor measured concurrently by two methods in asthmatic and normal subjects. Thorax 29: 232–236, 1974.

254. Lapp, N. L., Amandus, H. E., Hall, R., and Morgan, W. K. C. Lung volumes and flow rates in black and white subjects. Thorax 29: 185–188, 1974.

255. Malik, M. A., Moss, E., and Lee, W. R. Prediction values for the ventilatory capacity in male West Pakistani workers in the United Kingdom. Thorax 27: 611–619, 1972.

256. Fletcher, E. C. A nomogram for the transfer factor for carbon monoxide in the lungs. Thorax 27: 382–385, 1972.

257. Reger, R. B., Young, A., and Morgan, W. K. C. An accurate and rapid radiographic method of determining total lung capacity. Thorax 27: 163–168, 1972.

258. Dugdale, A. E., Bolton, J. M., and Ganendran, A. Respiratory function among Malaysian aboriginals. Thorax 26: 740–743, 1971.

259. Elebute, E. A. and Femi-Pearse, D. Peak flow rate in Nigeria: anthropometric determinants and usefulness in assessment of ventilatory function. Thorax 26: 597–601, 1971.

260. Salorinne, Y. Single-breath pulmonary diffusing capacity. Reference values and application in connective tissue diseases and in various lung diseases. Scand. J. Respir. Dis. 96(Suppl.): 1976.

261. Poppius, H., Korhonen, O., Viljanen, A. A., and Kreus, K-E. Arterial to end-tidal CO_2 difference in respiratory disease. Scand. J. Resp. Dis. 56: 254–262, 1975.

262. Schlesinger, Z., Goldbourt, U., Medalie, J. H., Oron, D., Neufeld, H. N., and Riss, E. Pulmonary ventilatory function values for healthy men aged 45 years and over. Chest 63: 520–524, 1973.

263. Gaensler, E. A. and Smith, A. A. Attachment for automated single breath diffusing capacity measurement. Chest 63: 136–145, 1973.

264. Guisan, M., Tisi, G. M., Ashburn, W. L., and Moser, K. M. Washout of [133]xenon gas from the lungs: comparison with nitrogen washout. Chest 62: 146–151, 1972.

265. McCarthy, D. S., Spencer, R., Greene, R., and Milic-Emili, J. Measurement of "closing volume" as a simple and sensitive test for early detection of small airway disease. Am. J. Med. 52: 747–762, 1972.

266. Davidson, F. F., Glazier, J. B., and Murray, J. F. The components of the alveolar-arterial oxygen tension difference in normal subjects and in patients with pneumonia and obstructive lung disease. Am. J. Med. 52: 754–762, 1972.

267. Harris, T. R., Pratt, P. C., and Kilburn, K. H. Total lung capacity measured by roentgenograms. Am. J. Med. 50: 756–763, 1971.

268. Brody, A. W., Navin, J. J., Stoughton, R. R., and Barta, F. Standards and significance for three tests of the distribution of ventilation. Am. J. Med. 48: 424–433, 1970.

269. Harris, E. A., Seelye, E. R., and Whitlock, R. M. L. Revised standards for normal resting dead-space volume and venous admixture in men and women. Clin. Sci. Mol. Med. 55: 125–128, 1978.

270. Bradley, C. A., Harris, E. A., Seelye, E. R., and Whitlock, R. M. L. Gas exchange during exercise in healthy people. 1. The physiological dead-space volume. Clin. Sci. Mol. Med. 51: 323–333, 1976.

271. Harris, E. A., Kenyon, A. M., Nisbet, H. D., Seelye, E. R., and Whitlock, R. M. L. The normal alveolar-arterial oxygen-tension gradient in man. Clin. Sci. Mol. Med. 46: 89–104, 1974.

272. Ray, J. F. R. III, Thompson, S., Moallem, S., Sanoudos, G. M., Yost, L., Goodall, C. W., and Clauss, R. H. Nomogram for estimating pulmonary arteriovenous shunt during ventilation with room air. J. Thorac. Cardiovasc. Surg. 64: 611–617, 1972.

273. Lanese, R. R., Keller, M. D., Foley, M. F., and Underwood, E. H. Differences in pulmonary function tests among whites, blacks, and American Indians in a textile company. J. Occup. Med. 20: 39–44, 1978.

274. Levison, H., Featherby, E. A., and Weng, T-R. Arterial blood gases, alveolar-arterial oxygen difference, and physiologic dead space in children and young adults. Am. Rev. Respir. Dis. 101: 972–974, 1970.

275. Miller, J. M., Ali, M. K., and Howe, C. D. Clinical determination of regional pulmonary function during normal breathing using ^{133}xenon. Am. Rev. Respir. Dis. 101: 218–229, 1970.

276. Dosman, J. A., Cotton, D. J., Graham, B. L., Hall, D., Li, R., Froh, F., and Barnett, G. D. Sensitivity of variables derived from the single breath nitrogen test in smokers. Chest 77(Suppl): 286–289, 1980.

277. Charan, N. B., Hildebrandt, J., Butler, J., and Saxon, R. Measurement of alveolar gas compression to detect mild airway obstruction. Chest 77(Suppl): 290, 1980.

278. Nathan, S. P., Lebowitz, M. D., and Knudson, R. J. Spirometric testing. Chest 76: 384–388, 1979.

279. Heldt, G. P. and Peters, R. M. A simplified method to determine functional residual capacity during mechanical ventilation. Chest 74: 492–496, 1978.

280. Rebuck, A. S. Measurement of ventilatory response to CO_2 by rebreathing. Chest 70(Suppl): 118–121, 1976.

281. Severinghaus, J., Ozanne, G., and Massuda, Y. Measurement of the ventilatory response to hypoxia. Chest 70(Suppl): 121–124, 1976.

282. Weil, J. V. and Zwillich, C. W. Assessment of the ventilatory response to hypoxia. Chest 70(Suppl): 124–128, 1976.

283. McClelland, K. and Mittman, C. A simplified method for measuring helium closing volume. Chest 67: 110–111, 1975.

284. Marmorstein, B. L. and Cianciulli, F. D. Planimetric measurement of total lung capacity in asthma. Chest 66: 378–381, 1974.

285. Hatle, L. and Rokseth, R. The arterial to end-expiratory carbon dioxide tension gradient in acute pulmonary embolism and other cardiopulmonary diseases. Chest 66: 352–357, 1974.

286. Sobol, B. J. Setting the limits of normal for pulmonary function: a problem and a paradox. Chest 65: 240–241, 1974.

287. Yokoyama, T. and Mitsufuji, M. Statistical representation of the ventilatory capacity of 2,247 healthy Japanese adults. Chest 61: 655–661, 1972.

288. Snider, G. L. Interpretation of the arterial oxygen and carbon dioxide partial pressures. Chest 63: 801–806, 1974.

289. Gilbert, R. and Keighley, J. F. The arterial/alveolar oxygen tension ratio. An index of gas exchange applicable to varying inspired oxygen concentrations. Am. Rev. Respir. Dis. 109: 142–145, 1974.

290. Hoeppner, V. H., Cooper, D. M., Zamel, N., Bryan, A. C., and Levison, H. Relationship between elastic recoil and closing volume in smokers and nonsmokers. Am. Rev. Respir. Dis. 109: 81–86, 1974.

291. Brody, A. W., Herrera, H. R., Shehan, J., Campbell, J. C., Zarlengo, M., Blessum, W. T., and Johnson, J. R. The residual volume. Am. Rev. Respir. Dis. 109: 87–97, 1974.

292. Brody, A. W., Johnson, J. R., Townley, R. G., Herrera, H. R., Snider, D., and Campbell, J. C. The residual volume. Am. Rev. Respir. Dis. 109: 98–105, 1974.

293. Adler, J. J. A simplified method for evaluating the ventilatory response to carbon dioxide. Am. Rev. Respir. Dis. 108: 1449–1450, 1973.

294. Buist, A. S. and Ross, B. B. Quantitative analysis of the alveolar plateau in the diagnosis of early airway obstruction. Am. Rev. Respir. Dis. 108: 1078–1087, 1973.

295. Teculescu, D. B. Lung volume changes in asthma measured concurrently by two methods (letter to the editor). Am. Rev. Respir. Dis. 108: 391, 1973.

296. Higgins, M. W. and Keller, J. B. Seven measures of ventilatory lung function. Am. Rev. Respir. Dis. 108: 258–272, 1973.

297. Gullot, R. F. A comparison of two methods of evaluating total thoracic compliance. Am. Rev. Respir. Dis. 108: 62–68, 1973.

298. Ohman, J. L. Jr., Schmidt-Nowara, W., Lawrence, M., Kazemi, H., and Lowell, F. C. The diffusing capacity in asthma. Am. Rev. Respir. Dis. 107: 932–939, 1973.

299. Strachova, Z. and Plum, F. Reproducibility of the rebreathing carbon dioxide response test using an improved method. Am. Rev. Respir. Dis. 107: 864–869, 1973.

300. Kuperman, A. S. and Riker, J. B. The predicted normal maximal midexpiratory flow. Am. Rev. Respir. Dis. 107: 231–238, 1973.

301. Hyatt, R. E. and Black, L. F. The flow-volume curve. Am. Rev. Respir. Dis. 107: 191–199, 1973.

302. Woolcock, A. J., Colman, M. H., and Blackburn, C. R. B. Factors affecting normal values for ventilatory lung function. Am. Rev. Respir. Dis. 106: 692–709, 1972.

303. Van Ganse, W. F., Ferris, B. G. Jr., and Cotes, J. E. Cigarette smoking and pulmonary diffusing capacity (transfer factor). Am. Rev. Respir. Dis. 105: 30–41, 1972.

304. Sackner, M. A., Raskin, M. M., Julien, P. J., and Avery, W. G. Effect of lung volume on steady state pulmonary membrane diffusing capacity and capillary blood volume. Am. Rev. Respir. Dis. 104: 408–417, 1971.

305. Allen, G. W. and Sabin, S. Comparison of direct and indirect measurement of airway resistance. Am. Rev. Respir. Dis. 104: 61–71, 1971.

306. Dinakara, P., Blumenthal, W. S., Johnston, R. F., Kauffman, L. A., and Solnick, P. B. The effect of anemia on pulmonary diffusing capacity with derivation of a correction equation. Am. Rev. Respir. Dis. 102: 965–969, 1970.

307. Miller, G. J., Ashcroft, M. T., Swan, A. V., and Beadnell, H. M. S. G. Ethnic variation in forced expiratory volume and forced vital capacity of African and Indian adults in Guyana. Am. Rev. Respir. Dis. 102: 979–981, 1970.

308. Hathirat, S., Renzetti, A. D. Jr., and Mitchell, M. Intrapulmonary gas distribution. A comparison of the helium mixing time and nitrogen single breath test in normal and diseased subjects. Am. Rev. Respir. Dis. 102: 750–759, 1970.

309. Hathirat, S., Renzetti, A. D. Jr., and Mitchell, M. Measurement of the total lung capacity by helium dilution in a constant volume system. Am. Rev. Respir. Dis. 102: 760–770, 1970.

310. Brody, A. W., Blessum, W. T., Wagner, J. R., and Weaver, M. J. The inelastic saclike component versus the slow time constant component of the distribution of ventilation by stage of respiratory dysfunction. Am. Rev. Respir. Dis. 102: 526–542, 1970.

311. Milic-Emili, J. Clinical methods for assessing the ventilatory response to carbon dioxide and hypoxia. N. Engl. J. Med. 293: 864–865, 1975.

312. Buist, S. The single-breath nitrogen test. N. Engl. J. Med. 293: 438–440, 1975.

313. Marshall, R. A rebreathing method for measuring carbon monoxide diffusing capacity. Am. Rev. Respir. Dis. 115: 537–539, 1977.

314. Conference Reports. Workshop on assessment of respiratory control in humans: II. Analyses of ventilatory responses. Am. Rev. Respir. Dis. 115: 363–365, 1977.

315. Conference Report. Workshop on assessment of respiratory control in humans. 1. Methods of measurement of ventilatory responses to hypoxia and hypercapnia. Am. Rev. Respir. Dis. 115: 177–181, 1977.

316. Tager, I., Speizer, F. E., Rosner, B., and Prang, G. A comparison between the three largest and three last of five forced expiratory maneuvers in a population study. Am. Rev. Respir. Dis. 114: 1201–1203, 1976.

317. Knudson, R. J., Burrows, B., and Lebowitz, M. D. The maximal expiratory flow-volume curve: its use in the detection of ventilatory abnormalities in a population study. Am. Rev. Respir. Dis. 114: 871–879, 1976.

318. Irsigler, G. B. Carbon dioxide response lines in young adults: the limits of the normal response. Am. Rev. Respir. Dis. 114: 529–536, 1976.

319. Guy, H. J., Gaines, R. A., Hill, P. M., Wagner, P. D., and West, J. B. Computerized, noninvasive tests of lung function. Am. Rev. Respir. Dis. 113: 737–744, 1976.

320. Knudson, R. J., Slatin, R. C., Lebowitz, M. D., and Burrows, B. The maximal expiratory flow-volume curve. Am. Rev. Respir. Dis. 113: 587–600, 1976.

321. Craven, N., Sidwall, G., West, P., McCarthy, D. S., and Cherniack, R. M. Computer analysis of the single-breath

nitrogen washout curve. Am. Rev. Respir. Dis. 113: 445–449, 1976.

322. Barrett, W. A., Clayton, P. D., Lambson, C. R., and Morris, A. H. Computerized roentgenographic determination of total lung capacity. Am. Rev. Respir. Dis. 113: 239–244, 1976.

323. de Hamel, F. A. and Glass, W. J. Observations on Maori-European lung function differences. Aust. N.Z. J. Med. 5: 44–48, 1975.

324. Hensley, M. J. and Read, D. J. C. A test of the ventilatory response to hypoxia and hypercapnia for clinical use. Aust. N.Z. J. Med. 7: 362–367, 1977.

325. Morris, J. F., Koski, A., and Breese, J. D. Normal values and evaluation of forced end-expiratory flow. Am. Rev. Respir. Dis. 111: 755–762, 1975.

326. Kryger, M., Aldrich, F., Reeves, J. T., and Grover, R. F. Diagnosis of airflow obstruction at high altitude. Am. Rev. Respir. Dis. 117: 1055–1058, 1978.

327. Stebbings, J. H. and Tietjen, G. L. Means or maxima in lung function testing? (letter to editor). Am. Rev. Respir. Dis. 117: 399–400, 1978.

328. Habib, M. P. and Engel, L. A. Influence of the panting technique on the plethysmographic measurement of thoracic gas volume. Am. Rev. Respir. Dis. 117: 265–271, 1978.

329. Frankel, D. Z. N., Mahutte, C. K., and Rebuck, A. S. A noninvasive method for measuring the P_{CO_2} of mixed venous blood. Am. Rev. Respir. Dis. 117: 63–69, 1978.

330. Wagner, P. D., Laravuso, R. B., Uhl, R., and West, J. B. Continuous distributions of ventilation-perfusion ratios in normal subjects breathing air and 100 per cent O_2. J. Clin. Invest. 54: 54–68, 1974.

331. Comroe, J. H. Jr. Retrospectroscope. Man-Cans. Am. Rev. Respir. Dis. 116: 1091–1099, 1977.

332. West, J. B. Ventilation-perfusion relationships. Am. Rev. Respir. Dis. 116: 919–943, 1977.

333. Comroe, J. H. Jr. Retrospectroscope. Man-Cans. Am. Rev. Respir. Dis. 116: 945–950, 1977.

334. von Nieding, G., Lollgen, H., Smidt, U., and Linde, H. Simultaneous washout of helium and sulfur hexafluoride in healthy subjects and patients with chronic bronchitis, bronchial asthma, and emphysema. Am. Rev. Respir. Dis. 116: 649–660, 1977.

335. Read, D., Nickolls, P., and Hensley, M. Instability of the carbon dioxide stimulus under the "mixed venous isocapnic" conditions advocated for testing the ventilatory response to hypoxia. Am. Rev. Respir. Dis. 116: 336–339, 1977.

336. Mustafa, K. Y. Spirometric lung function tests in normal men of African ethnic origin. Am. Rev. Respir. Dis. 116: 209–213, 1977.

337. Empey, D. W. Assessment of upper airways obstruction. Br. Med. J. 3: 503–505, 1972.

338. Gregg, I. and Nunn, A. J. Peak expiratory flow in normal subjects. Br. Med. J. 3: 282–284, 1973.

339. Cumming, G. and Guyatt, A. R. Alveolar gas mixing efficiency in the human lung. Clin. Sci. 62: 541–547, 1982.

340. Hetzel, M. R. The pulmonary clock (editorial). Thorax 36: 481–486, 1981.

341. Miller, A., Thornton, J. C., Smith, H. Jr., and Morris, J. F. Spirometric "abnormality" in a normal male reference population. Am. J. Indust. Med. 1: 55–68, 1980.

342. Godfrey, S., Konig, P., and Andrea, T. Measurement of lung function in the asthma clinic (letter to editor). Lancet ii: 205–206, 1973.

343. Campbell, I. A., Smith, I., Johnson, A., Prescott, R. J. Anderson, C., and Campbell, J. Peak-flow meter versus peak-flow gauge. Lancet ii: 199, 1974.

344. Clark, E. H., Jones, H. A., and Hughes, J. M. B. Bedside rebreathing technique for measuring carbon monoxide uptake by the lung. Lancet i: 791–793, 1978.

345. van der Lende, R., Jansen-Koster, E. J., Knijpstra, S., Reig, P. R., and Barkmeyer-Degenhart, P. Peak flow meter versus peak flow gauge. Lancet ii: 950–951, 1974.

346. Murray, A. B., Hardwick, D. F., Pirie, G. E., Fraser, B. M. Assessing severity of asthma with Wright peak flow meter (letter to editor). Lancet i: 708, 1977.

347. Kelman, G. R. Theoretical basis of alveolar sampling. Br. J. Indust. Med. 39: 259–264, 1982.

348. Miller, M. R. and Pincock, A. C. Repeatability of the

349. Chowienczyk, P. J., Rees, P. J., and Clark, T. J. H. Automated system for the measurement of airways resistance, lung volumes, and flow-volume loops. Thorax 36: 944–949, 1981.

350. Cormier, Y., Mitzner, W., and Menkes, H. Reverse nitrogen gradients in the study of phase III and cardiogenic oscillations of the single-breath nitrogen test. Am. Rev. Respir. Dis. 120: 15–20, 1979.

351. Peslin, R., Bohadana, A., Hannhart, B., and Jardin, P. Comparison of various methods for reading maximal expiratory flow-volume curves. Am. Rev. Respir. Dis. 119: 271–277, 1979.

352. Stanescu, D. C., Rodenstein, D., Caubergs, M., and Van De Woestijne, K. P. Failure of body plethysmography in bronchial asthma. J. Appl. Physiol.: Respir. Environ. Exercise Physiol. 52: 939–948, 1982.

353. Pare, P. D., Brooks, L. A., Bates, J., Lawson, L. M., Nelems, J. M. B., Wright, J. L., and Hogg, J. C. Exponential analysis of the lung pressure-volume curve as a predictor of pulmonary emphysema. Am. Rev. Respir. Dis. 126: 54–61, 1982.

354. Bohadana, A. B., Peslin, R., Hannhart, B., and Teculescu, D. Influence of panting frequency on plethysmographic measurements of thoracic gas volume. J. Appl. Physiol.: Respir. Environ. Exercise Physiol. 52: 739–747, 1982.

355. Whitelaw, W. A., Derenne, J. P., and Milic-Emili, J. Occlusion pressure as a measure of respiratory centre output in conscious man. Respir. Physiol. 23: 181–199, 1975.

356. Rodenstein, D. O. and Stanescu, D. C. Reassessment of lung volume measurement by helium dilution and by body plethysmography in chronic air-flow obstruction. Am. Rev. Respir. Dis. 126: 1040–1044, 1982.

357. Kvale, P. A., Davis, J., and Schroter, R. C. Effect of gas density and ventilatory pattern on steady-state CO uptake by the lung. Respir. Physiol. 24: 385–398, 1975.

358. Newth, C. J. L., Cotton, D. J., and Nadel, J. A. Pulmonary diffusing capacity measured at multiple intervals during a single exhalation in man. J. Appl. Physiol.: Respir. Environ. Exercise Physiol. 43: 617–625, 1977.

359. Amrein, R., Keller, R., Joos, H., and Herzog, H. Valeurs théoriques nouvelles de l'exploration de la fonction ventilatoire du poumon. Bull. Physiopathol. Respir. 6: 317–349, 1970.

360. Smidt, U. and Muysers, K. A simplified oscillation method with electronic signal handling for the determination of airway impedance. Bull. Physiopathol. Respir. 7: 281–290, 1971.

361. Teculescu, D. B. Validity, variability and reproducibility of single-breath total lung capacity determinations in normal subjects. Bull. Physiopathol. Respir. 7: 645–658, 1971.

362. Drutel, P., Timsit, G., du Perron, M. C., Hennetier, C., Legrand, M., and Vanroux, R. Réparation normale des valeurs bronchospirometriques chez 50 hommes de plus de 50 ans. Bull. Physiopathol. Respir. 7: 925–932, 1971.

363. Kreukniet, J. Relation between rebreathing CO-diffusing capacity of the lung and unequal ventilation. Scand. J. Respir. Dis. 51: 49–54, 1970.

364. Van Ganse, W., Comhaire, F., and van der Straeten, M. Residual volume determined by single breath dilution of helium at various apnoea times. Scand. J. Respir. Dis. 51: 73–81, 1970.

365. Van Ganse, W., Comhaire, F., and van der Straeten, M. Alveolar volume and transfer factor determined by single breath dilution of a test gas at various apnoea times. Scand. J. Respir. Dis. 51: 82–92, 1970.

366. Vale, J. R. Pulmonary gas exchange and venous-arterial shunt in normal subjects breathing oxygen, at rest and during exercise. Scand. J. Respir. Dis. 51: 305–315, 1970.

367. Saidel, G. M., Militano, T. C., and Chester, E. H. A theoretical basis for assessing pulmonary membrane transport. Continuous CO monitoring during a single breath manoeuvre. Bull. Physiopathol. Respir. 9: 481–496, 1973.

368. Davis, J., Kvale, P. A., Schroter, R. C., and Sudlow, M. F. Effect of gas density on the uptake of CO during steady state breathing. Bull. Physiopathol. Respir. 9: 510, 1973.

369. Rutland, J., Griffin, W., and Cole, P. Human ciliary beat

moments of the truncated forced expiratory spirogram. Thorax 37: 205–211, 1982.

frequency in epithelium from intrathoracic and extrathoracic airways. Am. Rev. Respir. Dis. 125: 100–105, 1982.

370. Stanescu, D., Frans, A., and Brasseur, L. Echanges respiratoires et transfert de gaz dans la bronchite chronique et l'emphysème. Bull. Physiopathol. Respir. 9: 1045–1068, 1973.

371. Cotes, J. E. Genetic component of lung function. Bull. Physiopathol. Respir. 10: 109–117, 1974.

372. Hatzfeld, C. and Nury, A-M. Les méthodes de rincage d'un gaz traceur pour l'étude de la mixique pulmonaire. Bull. Physiopathol. Respir. 10: 177–215, 1974.

373. Yernault, J. C. and Englert, M. Static mechanical lung properties in young adults. Bull. Physiopathol. Respir. 10: 435–450, 1974.

374. Frans, A. and Brasseur, L. La mésure de la capacité de diffusion de la membrane alveolo-capillaire (DM) et du volume capillaire pulmonaire (Vc) chez 65 volontaires normaux de sexe masculin. Le Transfert de l'Oxyde de Carbone. Soc. Eur. Physiopathol. Respir. Masson et Cie, Paris, 1969.

375. Rouch, Y. Influence de la fréquence ventilatoire sur les ductances pulmonaires. Le Transfert de l'Oxyde de Carbone. Soc. Eur. Physiopathol. Respir. Masson et Cie, Paris, 1969.

376. Rode, A. and Shephard, R. J. Pulmonary function of Canadian Eskimos. Scand. J. Respir. Dis. 54: 191–205, 1973.

377. Connolly, T., Bake, B., Wood, L., and Milic-Emili, J. Regional distribution of a ^{133}Xe labelled gas volume inspired at constant flow rates. Scand. J. Respir. Dis. 56: 150–159, 1975.

378. Frans, A., Stanescu, D. C., Veriter, C. V., Clerbaux, T., and Brasseur, L. Smoking and pulmonary diffusing capacity Scand. J. Respir. Dis. 56: 165–183, 1975.

379. Yager, J. A., Ellman, H., and Dulfano, M. J. Human ciliary beat frequency at three levels of the tracheobronchial tree. Am. Rev. Respir. Dis. 121: 661–665, 1980.

380. Simecek, C. Formulae for calculation of membrane diffusion component and pulmonary capillary blood volume. Bull. Physiopathol. Respir. 11: 349–351, 1975.

381. Rasmussen, F. V. and Andersen, L. H. Intra- and interobserver variation on the measurement of closing volume and quantitative analysis of the alveolar plateau of the single-breath nitrogen washout. Bull. Physiopathol. Respir. 11: 27P–32P, 1975.

382. Secker-Walker, R. H., Alderson, P. O., and Hill, R. L. Regional ventilation in chronic obstructive pulmonary disease. Bull. Physiopathol. Respir. 11: 143P–145P, 1975.

383. Pasquis, P., Denis, P., Hellot, M. F., and Lefrancois, R. Compliance pulmonaire dynamique. Valeurs de référence. Bull. Physiopathol. Respir. 12: 659–668, 1976.

384. Castillon Du Perron, M., Korobaeff, M., and Drutel, P. Valeur et réproducibilité des mésures de TL_{co} et de ses composantes chez le sujet sain. Bull. Eur. Physiopathol. Respir. 12: 443–451, 1976.

385. Adaro, F., Meyer, M., and Sikand, R. S. Rebreathing and single breath pulmonary CO diffusing capacity in man at rest and exercise studied by $C^{18}O$ isotope. Bull. Eur. Physiopathol. Respir. 12: 747–756, 1976.

386. Chinn, D. J. and Lee, W. R. Within- and between-subject variability of indices from the closing volume and flow volume traces. Bull. Eur. Physiopathol. Respir. 13: 789–802, 1977.

387. Salorinne, Y. Single-breath pulmonary diffusing capacity. Scand. J. Respir. Dis. (Suppl)96: 1976.

388. Whitaker, C. J., Chinn, D. J., and Lee, W. R. The statistical reliability of indices derived from the closing volume and flow volume traces. Bull. Physiopathol. Respir. 14: 237–247, 1978.

389. Piiper, J., Meyer, M., and Scheid, P. Pulmonary diffusing capacity for O_2 and CO at rest and during exercise. Advantages of rebreathing techniques using stable isotopes. Bull. Eur. Physiopathol. Respir. 15: 145–150, 1979.

390. Poh, S. C. The effects of opium smoking in cigarette smokers. Am. Rev. Respir. Dis. 106: 239–245, 1972.

391. Flenley, D. C. Methods and results of assessing the hypoxic ventilatory drive in patients and normal subjects. Bull. Eur. Physiopathol. Respir. 15(Suppl): 23–24, 1979.

392. Prefaut, C., Tcheriatchoukine, J., Guerrero, A. J., Moutou, H., and Chardon, G. Débit maximum expiratoire 25–75 per

393. Rhodes, C. G., Macarthur, C. G. C., Swinburne, A. J., and Heather, J. D. Influence of pulmonary recirculation and the chest wall upon measurements of regional ventilation, perfusion, and water volume. Bull. Eur. Physiopathol. Respir. 16: 383–394, 1980.

394. Ronchetti, R., Jones, H. A., Rhodes, C. G., Herring, A., Eiser, N. M., Benci, S., and Hughes, J. M. B. Clearance of radioactive nitrogen and xenon from the lungs of anaesthetized dogs and human subjects. Bull. Eur. Physiopathol. Respir. 16: 395–409, 1980.

395. Colomer, P. R., Presas, F. M., Llombart, R. Ll., Lopez-Merino, V., and Sanchon, B. R. Application du modèle exponentiel à l'étude des courbes pression-volume en pathologie respiratoire. Bull. Eur. Physiopathol. Respir. 16: 443–458, 1980.

396. Derks, C. M. Mésure de la distribution des rapports ventilation/perfusion par la méthode des gaz inertes. Bull. Eur. Physiopathol. Respir. 16: 555–577, 1980.

397. Demedts, M. and van de Woestijne, K. P. Which technique for total lung capacity measurement? Bull. Eur. Physiopathol. Respir. 16: 705–709, 1980.

398. Pride, N. B., Osmanliev, D. P., and Davies, E. E. Does transit time analysis make the forced expiratory spirogram a "sensitive" test? Bull. Eur. Physiopathol. Respir. 16: 169P–172P, 1980.

399. Douglas, R. B. The maximum midexpiratory flow (letter to the editor). Bull. Eur. Physiopathol. Respir. 283P–285P, 1980.

400. Scheid, P. Mathematical models for intrapulmonary gas mixing. In: Piiper, J. and Scheid, P. (eds.). Progress in Respiration Research, Vol. 16. S. Karger, Basel, 1981.

401. Smidt, U. and Worth, H. Gas mixing in patients. In: Piiper, J. and Scheid, P. (eds.). Progress in Respiration Research, Vol. 16. S. Karger, Basel, 1981.

402. Meyer, M. Pulmonary diffusing capacity for O_2 and CO in man at rest and during exercise by rebreathing stable isotopes. In: Piiper, J. and Scheid, P. (eds.). Progress in Respiration Research, Vol. 16. S. Karger, Basel, 1981.

403. Hughes, J. M. B., Clarke, E. H., Ewan, P. W., Greening, A. P., Jones, H. A., Lipscomb, D. J., Middleton, H. C., Pande, J. N., and Rhodes, C. G. Overall and regional DL_{CO}: studies in normal and abnormal lungs. In: Piiper, J. and Scheid, P. (eds.). Progress in Respiration Research, Vol. 16. S. Karger, Basel, 1981.

404. Magnussen, H. Single breath diffusion capacity for carbon monoxide in bronchial asthma and emphysema. In: Piiper, J. and Scheid, P. (eds.). Progress in Respiration Research, Vol. 16. S. Karger, Basel, 1981.

405. Bohadana, A. B., Jansen Da Silva, J. M., Hannhart, B., and Peslin, R. The unreliability of indirect lung compliance in healthy subjects and patients with chronic lung disorders. Bull. Eur. Physiopathol. Respir. 17: 879–889, 1981.

406. Cotes, J. E., Dabbs, J. M., Elwood, P. C., Hall, A. M., McDonald, A., and Saunders, M. J. Iron-deficiency anaemia: its effect on transfer factor for the lung (diffusing capacity) and ventilation and cardiac frequency during submaximal exercise. Clin. Sci. 42: 325–335, 1972.

407. Godfrey, S. and Wolf, E. An evaluation of rebreathing methods for measuring mixed venous PCO_2 during exercise. Clin. Sci. 42: 345–353, 1972.

408. Harris, E. A., Hunter, M. E., Seelye, E. R., Vedder, M., and Whitlock, R. M. L. Prediction of the physiological dead-space in resting normal subjects. Clin. Sci. 45: 375–386, 1973.

409. Burki, N. K. and Dent, M. C. The forced expiratory time as a measure of small airway resistance. Clin. Sci. 51: 53–58, 1976.

410. Al-Dulymi, R. and Hainsworth, R. A new open-circuit method for estimating carbon dioxide tension in mixed venous blood. Clin. Sci. 52: 377–382, 1977.

411. Clark, E. H., Woods, R. L., and Hughes, J. M. B. Effect of blood transfusion on the carbon monoxide transfer factor in man. Clin. Sci. 54: 627–631, 1978.

412. Higenbottam, T. and Clark, T. J. H. A method for standard-

izing airway resistance for variations in lung volume. Clin. Sci. 57: 397–400, 1979.

413. Higenbottam, T. and Clark, T. J. H. Practical importance of a preceding full inhalation or exhalation upon the measurement of airway resistance. Clin. Sci. 58: 249–253, 1980.

414. Li, K-Y. R., Tan, L. T-K., Chong, P., and Dosman, J. A. Between-technician variation in the measurement of spirometry with air and helium. Am. Rev. Respir. Dis. 124: 196–198, 1981.

415. Block, A. J., Bush, C. M., White, C., Boysen, P. G., Wynne, J. W., and Taasan, V. C. A radiographic method for measuring steady-state functional residual capacity in the supine patient. A method suitable for sleep studies. Am. Rev. Respir. Dis. 124: 330–332, 1981.

416. Cutillo, A., Perondi, M. R., Turiel, M., Egger, M. J., Watanabe, S., and Renzetti, A. D. Jr. Reproducibility of multibreath nitrogen washout measurements. Am. Rev. Respir. Dis. 124: 505–507, 1981.

417. Schoene, R. B., Pierson, D. J., and Butler, J. Constancy of functional residual capacity in the supine position during hypoxia and hyperoxic hypercapnia. Am. Rev. Respir. Dis. 124: 508–510, 1981.

418. Korhonen, O. Xenon 133 radiospirometry with moving detectors. Scand. J. Clin. Lab. Invest. 27: 113–122, 1971.

419. Sackner, M. A., Greeneltch, D., Heiman, M. S., Epstein, S., and Atkins, N. Diffusing capacity, membrane diffusing capacity, capillary blood volume, pulmonary tissue volume, and cardiac output measured by a rebreathing technique. Am. Rev. Respir. Dis. 111: 157–165, 1975.

420. Skoogh, B-E. Normal airways conductance at different lung volumes. Scand. J. Clin. Lab. Invest. 31: 429–441, 1973.

421. Schaanning, C. G. and Gulsvik, A. Accuracy and precision of helium dilution technique and body plethysmography. Scand. J. Clin. Lab. Invest. 32: 271–277, 1973.

422. Arvidsson, E. and Dano, G. Evaluation of the peak expiratory flow rate. Scand. J. Clin. Lab. Invest. 32: 279–284, 1973.

423. Cormier, Y. F. and Belanger, J. The influence of active gas exchange on the slope of phase III at rest and after exercise. Am. Rev. Respir. Dis. 123: 213–216, 1981.

424. Christopherson, S. K. and Hlastala, M. P. Pulmonary gas exchange during altered density gas breathing. J. Appl. Physiol.: Respir. Environ. Exercise Physiol. 52: 221–225, 1982.

425. Quanjer, P-H., Dalhuijsen, A., and Van Zomeren, B. C. Standardised lung function testing. Interim Report, EECS Working Party, Luxembourg, June, 1981.

426. Ringqvist, T. and Ringqvist, I. Respiratory forces and variations of static lung volumes in healthy subjects. Scand. J. Clin. Lab. Invest. 33: 269–276, 1974.

427. Sundstrom, G. Ventilation rate and end-tidal steady state pulmonary diffusing capacity (DL_{coss2}) at rest. Scand. J. Clin. Lab. Invest. 33: 379–386, 1974.

428. Kauppinen-Walin, K., Sovijarvi, A. A., Muittari, A., and Uusitalo, A. Determination of functional residual capacity with Xenon 133 radiospirometry: comparison with body plethysmography and helium spirometry. Effect of body position. Scand. J. Clin. Lab. Invest. 40: 347–354, 1980.

429. Crapo, R. O., Morris, A. H., and Gardner, R. M. Reference spirometric values using techniques and equipment that meet ATS recommendations. Am. Rev. Respir. Dis. 123: 659–664, 1981.

430. Von Westernhagen, F. and Smidt, U. The significance of the difference between slow inspiratory and forced vital capacity. Lung 154: 289–297, 1978.

431. Gilbert, R., Auchincloss, J. H. Jr., and Bleb, S. Measurement of maximum inspiratory pressure during routine spirometry. Lung 155: 23–32, 1978.

432. Sorensen, J. B., Morris, A. H., Crapo, R. O., and Gardner, R. M. Selection of the best spirometric values for interpretation. Am. Rev. Respir. Dis. 122: 802–805, 1980.

433. Douglas, R. B. The maximal expiratory flow-volume curve, normal standards, variability, and effects of age. Am. Rev. Respir. Dis. 122: 990, 1980.

434. Gardner, R. M., Hankinson, J. L., and West, B. J. Evaluating commercially available spirometers. Am. Rev. Respir. Dis. 121: 73–82, 1980.

435. Petusevsky, M. L., Lyons, L. D., Smith, A. A., Epler, G.

R., and Gaensler, E. A. Calibration of time derivatives of forced vital capacity by explosive decompression. Am. Rev. Respir. Dis. 121: 343–350, 1980.

436. Matthys, H., Keller, R., and Herzog, H. Plethysmographic assessment of trapped air in man. Respiration 27: 447–461, 1970.

437. Schmidt, W. and Schnabel, K. H. Methodische Verbesserungen des Verfahrens zur Verteilungsanalyse von Ventilation, Perfusion und O_2-diffusionskapazitat der Lunge. Respiration 27: 15–23, 1970.

438. Glindmeyer, H. W. III, Anderson, S. T., Kern, R. G., and Hughes, J. A portable, adjustable forced vital capacity simulator for routine spirometric calibration. Am. Rev. Respir. Dis. 121: 599–603, 1980.

439. Beeckman, P., Demedts, M., and Vanclooster, R. Radiographic evaluation of lung dimensions in different postures. Bull. Eur. Physiopath. Respir. 18: 557–564, 1982.

440. Lopez-Majano, V. Reproducibility of the carbon monoxide diffusion capacity method. Respiration 28: 114–119, 1971.

441. Zedda, S. and Sartorelli, E. Variability of plethysmographic measurements of airway resistance during the day in normal subjects and in patients with bronchial asthma and chronic bronchitis. Respiration 28: 158–166, 1971.

442. Thews, G., Schmidt, W., and Schnabel, K. H. Analysis of distribution inhomogeneities of ventilation, perfusion and O_2 diffusing capacity in the human lung. Respiration 28: 197–215, 1971.

443. Hilpert, P. Die Anderung der Diffusionskapazitat der Lunge fur CO durch die Hamoglobinkonzentration des Blutes. Respiration 28: 518–525, 1971.

444. Schmidt, K. Zur Frage der Haufigkeitsverteilung der ventilations-perfusions relation in der gesunden und kranken Lunge. Respiration 29: 330–343, 1972.

445. Fleming, G. M., Chester, E. H., Saniie, J., and Saidel, G. M. Ventilation inhomogeneity using multibreath nitrogen washout: comparison of moment ratios and other indexes. Am. Rev. Respir. Dis. 121: 789–794, 1980.

446. Colebatch, H. J. H. and Greaves, I. A. Exponential analysis of lung elastic behaviour (letter to editor). Am. Rev. Respir. Dis. 121: 898, 1980.

447. Joshi, R. C., Madan, R. N., and Eggleston, F. C. Clinical spirometry in normal North Indian males. Respiration 30: 39–47, 1973.

448. Jebavy, P. and Widimsky, J. Lung-transfer factor at maximal effort in healthy men. Respiration 30: 297–310, 1973.

449. Riepl, G. and Hilpert, P. Der Einfluss funktioneller Inhomogenitaten auf die Single-Breath-CO-Diffusionsskapazitat ($DL_{co}SB$). Respiration 31: 60–70, 1970.

450. Heise, M., Koppe, H., and Schmidt, K. Mathematical treatment of inert gas clearance curve as a method for studying regional inhomogeneity of alveolar ventilation in the lung. Respiration 31: 310–317, 1974.

451. Rossman, C. M., Lee, R. M. K. W., Forrest, J. B., and Newhouse, M. T. Nasal ciliary ultrastructure and function in patients with primary ciliary dyskinesia compared with that in normal subjects and in subjects with various respiratory diseases. Am. Rev. Respir. Dis. 129: 161–167, 1984.

452. Demedts, M., De Roo, M., Vandercruys, A., Kiebooms, L., Drieskens, L., and Cosemans, J. L'exploration fonctionelle des poumons par le ^{133}Xe à l'aide de la gamma camera. Respiration 31: 484–502, 1974.

453. Lollgen, H., Smidt, U., von Nieding, G., and Krekeler, H. Vergleichende Bestimmung des Transferfaktors fur Kohlenmonoxyd mit der Single-Breath und der Steady-State-Methode. Respiration 31: 503–514, 1974.

454. Secker-Walker, R. H., Alderson, P. O., Wilhelm, J., Hill, R. L., and Markham, J. Regional ventilation-perfusion relationships. Respiration 32: 265–276, 1975.

455. Paiva, M. Two new pulmonary function indexes suggested by a simple mathematical model. Respiration 32: 389–403, 1975.

456. Worth, H. Pulmonary diffusing capacity for CO during breathing of inert gas mixtures with differing physical properties. Respiration 32: 436–444, 1975.

457. Borngen, U. Normalwerte der ventilatorischen Atemarbeit. Respiration 33: 22–35, 1976.

458. Islam, M. S. Differential diagnosis of ventilatory disorders

with the help of volume/flow diagram. Respiration 33: 104–111, 1976.

459. Thews, G. and Schmidt, W. Partitioning of the alveolar-arterial O₂ pressure difference under normal, hypoxic and hyperoxic conditions. Respiration 33: 245–255, 1976.

460. Rampulla, C., Marconi, C., Buelcke, G., and Amaducci, S. Correlations between lung-transfer factor, ventilation, and cardiac output during exercise. Respiration 33: 405–415, 1976.

461. Pivoteau, C. and Dechoux, J. Méthode non sanglante d'estimation du gradient alvéolo-artériel et de la pression artérielle de CO₂. Respiration 33: 455–467, 1976.

462. Breant, J. and Fleury, M. F. Les deux composantes de l'échange global du monoxyde de carbone: prise de CO et ductance. Poumon Coeur 36: 13–24, 1980.

463. Breant, J. and Fleury, M. F. La prise de monoxyde de carbone au cours de l'exercice chez le sujet sain et chez le malade. Poumon Coeur 36: 315–326, 1980.

464. Talvik, R. Nomogram for estimating standard PaO₂ and alveolar-arterial gradient for oxygen during ventilation with room air. Respiration 34: 118–120, 1977.

465. Jebavy, P., Hurych, J., and Widimsky, J. Relation of pulmonary diffusing capacity to ventilation and haemodynamics in healthy subjects. Respiration 34: 152–161, 1977.

466. Devos, P., Demedts, M., Vandercruys, A., Cosemans, J., and De Roo, M. Comparison of ¹³³Xe washout curves after bolus inhalation, perfusion, and equilibration. Respiration 35: 115–121, 1978.

467. Riepl, G. Effect of abnormal hemoglobin concentration in human blood on membrane diffusing capacity of the lung and on pulmonary capillary blood volume. Respiration 36: 10–18, 1978.

468. Hantos, Z., Galoczy, G., Daroczy, B., and Dombos, K. Computation of the equivalent airway resistance. Respiration 36: 64–72, 1978.

469. Pande, J. N. and Guleria, J. S. Comparison of single breath and steady state methods for the measurement of pulmonary diffusing capacity for carbon monoxide in non-homogeneous lungs. Respiration 36: 117–126, 1978.

470. Pande, J. N. Indirect assessment of lung compliance in chronic lung diseases. Respiration 36: 201–206, 1978.

471. Wiessmann, K. J. and Steinijans, V. W. Computation of the average in- and expiratory airway resistance. Respiration 37: 15–22, 1979.

472. Vermaak, J. C., Bunn, A. E., and De Kock, M. A. A new lung function index. Respiration 37: 61–65, 1979.

473. Dull, W. L. and Secker-Walker, R. H. Helium-oxygen flow curves in young healthy adults. Respiration 38: 18–26, 1979.

474. Lavietes, M. H., Clifford, E., Silverstein, D., Stier, F., and Reichman, L. B. Relationship of static respiratory muscle pressure and maximum voluntary ventilation in normal subjects. Respiration 38: 121–126, 1979.

475. Bradley, J., Bye, C., Hayden, S. P., and Hughes, D. T. D. Normal values of transfer factor and transfer coefficients in healthy males and females. Respiration 38: 221–226, 1979.

476. Todisco, T., Grassi, V., Dottorini, M., and Sorbini, C. A. Reference values for flow-volume curves during forced vital capacity breathing in male children and young adults. Respiration 39: 1–7, 1980.

477. Barnikol, W. K. R. and Diether, K. Dependence of the anatomical dead space on the tidal volume and on the endexpiratory lung volume. Respiration 39: 8–19, 1980.

478. Tashkin, D. P., Shapiro, B. J., and Frank, I. M. Acute pulmonary physiologic effects of smoked marihuana and oral Δ⁹-tetrahydrocannabinol in healthy young men. N. Engl. J. Med. 289: 336–341, 1973.

479. Bres, M. On-line computation of dead space and nitrogen clearance curve. Respiration 39: 213–218, 1980.

480. Lamedica, G., Brusasco, V., Tiano, A., and Ramoino, R. Analysis of nitrogen multibreath washout curves through a statistical approach. Respiration 39: 333–343, 1980.

481. Radwan, L. and Daum, S. Evaluation of mixed venous oxygenation on the basis of arterial oxygen tension in chronic lung diseases. Respiration 40: 194–200, 1980.

482. Petro, W., von Nieding, G., Boll, W., and Smidt, U. Determination of respiratory resistance by an oscillation method. Respiration 42: 243–251, 1981.

483. Hedenstierna, G., Jorfeldt, L., and Bygdeman, S. Flow-volume curves in healthy non-smokers and in smokers. Clin. Physiol. 1: 339–348, 1981.

484. Milic-Emili, J. Recent advances in clinical assessment of control of breathing. Lung 160: 1–17, 1982.

485. Drouet, D., Kauffmann, F., Brille, D., and Lellouch, J. Valeurs spirographiques de référence. Modèles mathématiques et utilisation pratique. Bull. Eur. Physiopathol. Respir. 16: 745–767, 1980.

486. Teculescu, D. B., Pino, J., and Peslin, R. Composite flow-volume curves matched at total lung capacity in the study of density dependence of maximal expiratory flows. Lung 159: 127–136, 1981.

487. Stanescu, D. Predicted values for closing volumes using a modified single breath nitrogen test (letter to editor). Am. Rev. Respir. Dis. 109: 685, 1974.

488. Belanger, J. and Cormier, Y. L'influence d'apnées sequentielles sur le plateau alvéolaire. Bull. Eur. Physiopathol. Respir. 17: 65–74, 1981.

489. Fridriksson, H. V., Malmberg, P., Hedenstrom, H., and Hillerdal, G. Reference values for respiratory function in males: prediction formulas with tobacco smoking parameters. Clin. Physiol. 1: 349–364, 1981.

490. Horsfield, K., Barer, D. H., and Cumming, G. Centrilobular emphysema studied with a mathematical model. Scand. J. Respir. Dis. 54: 53–64, 1973.

491. Smidt, U. and Worth, H. Gas mixing in patients. Prog. Respir. Res. 16: 86–92, 1981.

492. Knudson, R. J., Mead, J., Goldman, M. D., Schwaber, J. R., and Wohl, M. E. The failure of indirect indices of elastic lung recoil. Am. Rev. Respir. Dis. 107: 70–82, 1973.

493. Reichel, G. and Islam, M. S. Measurement of static lung and thorax compliance in health and pulmonary diseases. Respiration 29: 507–515, 1972.

494. Finley, T. N., Engelman, E. P., Packer, B., Aronow, A., and Cosentino, A. M. Use of the RC time constant for CO in the measurement of diffusing capacity. Am. Rev. Respir. Dis. 109: 682–684, 1974.

495. Mohsenifar, Z. and Tashkin, D. P. Effect of carboxyhemoglobin on the single breath diffusing capacity: derivation of an empirical correction factor. Respiration 37: 185–191, 1979.

496. Toulou, P. and Walsh, P. M. Measurement of alveolar carbon dioxide tension at maximal expiration as an estimate of arterial carbon dioxide tension in patients with airway obstruction. Am. Rev. Respir. Dis. 102: 921–926, 1970.

497. Hertle, F. H., Georg, R., and Lange, H-J. Die arteriellen Blutgaspartialdrucke und ihre Beziehungen zu alter und anthropometrischen Grossen. Respiration 28: 1–30, 1971.

498. Pepys, J. and Hutchcroft, B. J. Bronchial provocation tests in etiologic diagnosis and analysis of asthma. Am. Rev. Respir. Dis. 112: 829–859, 1975.

499. Hansen, P. and Penny, R. Immune mechanisms and diagnosis of pigeon breeder's disease. Med. J. Austral. 1: 984–987, 1974.

500. Report of subcommittee on bronchial inhalation challenges. Guidelines for bronchial inhalation challenges with pharmacologic and antigenic agents. Am. Thor. Soc. News. 6: 11–19, 1980.

501. Ryan, G., Dolovich, M. B., Eng, P., Obminski, G., Cockcroft, D. W., Jennifer, E., Hargreave, F. E., and Newhouse, M. T. Standardization of inhalation provocation test: influence of nebulizer output, particle size, and method of inhalation. J. Allergy Clin. Immunol. 67: 156–161, 1981.

502. Riley, D. J., Weitz, B. W., and Edelman, N. H. The responses of asthmatic subjects to isoproterenol inhaled at different lung volumes. Am. Rev. Respir. Dis. 114: 509–515, 1976.

503. Rosenthal, R. R. (ed.). Workshop proceedings on bronchoprovocation techniques for the evaluation of asthma. J. Allergy Clin. Immunol. 64: 560–692, 1979.

504. Lam, S., Wong, R., and Chan-Yeung, M. Non-specific bronchial reactivity in occupational asthma. J. Allergy Clin. Immunol. 63: 28–34, 1979.

505. Cockcroft, D. W., Killain, D. N., Mellon, J. J. A., and Hargreave, F. E. Bronchial reactivity to inhaled histamine: a method and clinical survey. Clin. Allergy 7: 235–243, 1977.

506. Chai, H., Farr, R. S., Froehlich, L. A., Mathison, D. A.,

McLean, J. A., Rosenthal, R. R., Sheffer, A. L., Spector, S. L., and Townley, R. G. Standardization of bronchial inhalation challenge procedures. J. Allergy Clin. Immunol. 56: 323–327, 1975.

507. Spector, S. L. and Farr, R. S. Bronchial inhalation procedures in asthmatics. Med. Clin. North Am. 58: 71–84, 1974.

508. Hazucha, M., Silverman, F., Parent, C., Field, S., and Bates, D. V. Pulmonary function in man after short-term exposure to ozone. Arch. Environ. Health 27: 183–188, 1973.

509. Bouhuys, A. and Van De Woestijne, K. P. Respiratory mechanics and dust exposure in byssinosis. J. Clin. Invest. 49: 106–118, 1970.

510. Hendrick, D. J., Marshall, R., Faux, J. A., and Krall, J. M. Positive "alveolar" responses to antigen inhalation provocation tests: their validity and recognition. Thorax 35: 415–427, 1980.

511. Burge, P. S., O'Brien, I. M., and Harries, M. G. Peak flow rate records in the diagnosis of occupational asthma due to colophony. Thorax 34: 308–316, 1979.

512. Burge, P. S., O'Brien, I. M., and Harries, M. G. Peak flow rate records in the diagnosis of occupational asthma due to isocyanates. Thorax 34: 317–323, 1979.

513. Benson, M. K. Bronchial responsiveness to inhaled histamine and isoprenaline in patients with airway obstruction. Thorax 33: 211–213, 1978.

514. Orehek, J. and Gayrard, P. Les tests de provocation bronchique non-spécifiques dans l'asthme. Bull. Eur. Physiopathol. Resp. 12: 565–598, 1976.

515. Hendrick, D. J. and Lane, D. J. Occupational formalin asthma. Br. J. Ind. Med. 34: 11–18, 1977.

516. Gandevia, B. and Milne, J. Occupational asthma and rhinitis due to Western red cedar (Thuja plicata), with special reference to bronchial reactivity. Br. J. Ind. Med. 27: 235–244, 1970.

517. Juniper, E. F., Frith, P. A., Dunnett, C., Cockcroft, D. W., and Hargreave, F. E. Reproducibility and comparison of responses to inhaled histamine and methacholine. Thorax 33: 705–710, 1978.

518. Smith, A. B., Brooks, S. M., Blanchard, J., Bernstein, I. L., and Gallagher, J. Absence of airway hyperreactivity to methacholine in a worker sensitized to toluene diisocyanate (TDI). J. Occup. Med. 22: 327–331, 1980.

519. Pain, M. C. F. and Symons, H. S. Bronchial reactivity in occupational asthma. Med. J. Austral. 1: 522–524, 1972.

520. doPico, G. A., Layton, C. R. Jr., Clayton, J. W., and Rankin, J. Acute pulmonary reaction to spray starch with soil repellant. Am. Rev. Respir. Dis. 108: 1212–1215, 1973.

521. Halprin, G. M., Buckley, C. E. III., Zitt, M. J., and McMahon, S. M. Changes in arteriovenous complement activity induced by inhalation challenge. Am. Rev. Respir. Dis. 108: 343–352, 1973.

522. Mitchell, C. A. and Gandevia, B. Respiratory symptoms and skin reactivity in workers exposed to proteolytic enzymes in the detergent industry. Am. Rev. Respir. Dis. 104: 1–12, 1971.

523. Pepys, J. Inhalation challenge tests in asthma. N. Engl. J. Med. 293: 758–759, 1975.

524. Vallieres, M., Cockcroft, D. W., Taylor, D. M., Dolovich, J., and Hargreave, F. E. Dimethyl ethanolamine-induced asthma. Am. Rev. Respir. Dis. 115: 867–871, 1977.

525. Rubinfeld, A. R. and Pain, M. C. F. Relationship between bronchial reactivity, airway caliber, and severity of asthma. Am. Rev. Respir. Dis. 115: 381–387, 1977.

526. Orehek, J., Gayrard, P., Smith, A. P., Grimaud, C., and Charpin, J. Airway responses to carbachol in normal and asthmatic subjects. Am. Rev. Respir. Dis. 115: 937–943, 1977.

527. Fish, J. E., Rosenthal, R. R., Batra, G., Menkes, H., Summer, W., Permutt, S., and Norman, P. Airway responses to methacholine in allergic and nonallergic subjects. Am. Rev. Respir. Dis. 113: 579–586, 1976.

528. Hamilton, R. D., Crockett, A. J., Ruffin, R. E., and Alpers, J. H. Bronchial reactivity in Western red cedar induced asthma. Aust. N. Z. J. Med. 9: 417–419, 1979.

529. Blake, J. R. and Winet, H. On the mechanics of mucociliary transport. Biorheology 17: 125–134, 1980.

530. Fink, J. N. and Schlueter, D. P. Bathtub refinisher's lung:
an unusual response to toluene diisocyanate. Am. Rev. Respir. Dis. 118: 955–959, 1978.

531. Cade, J. F. and Pain, M. C. F. Bronchial reactivity. Its measurement and clinical significance. Aust. N.Z. J. Med. 1: 22–25, 1971.

532. Holmgren, A. and Ripe, E. Airway conductance after inhalation of microaerosols of histamine chloride in healthy subjects and in patients with bronchiectasis before and after operation. Scand. J. Respir. Dis. 54: 215–222, 1973.

533. Ahmed, T., Mezey, R. J., Fernandez, R. J., and Wanner, A. Peripheral airway function in antigen-induced bronchoconstriction. Bull. Eur. Physiopathol. Respir. 16: 721–731, 1980.

534. Orehek, J., Kabondo, P., Charpin, J., and Grimaud, C. Mésure spirometrique de la réponse bronchique au carbachol dans l'asthma. Bull. Eur. Physiopathol. Respir. 14: 493–502, 1978.

535. Simonsson, B. G. Clinical implications of bronchial hyperreactivity. Meeting on Bronchial Hyperreactivity Syndrome Proceedings. Eur. J. Respir. Dis. 61(Suppl.): 7–18, 1980.

536. Kivity, S. and Souhrada, J. F. A new diagnostic test to assess airway reactivity in asthmatics. Bull. Eur. Physiopathol. Respir. 17: 243–254, 1981.

537. Michoud, M. C., Lelorier, J., and Amyot, R. Factors modulating the interindividual variability of airway responsiveness to histamine. The influence of H1 and H2 receptors. Bull. Eur. Physiopathol. Respir. 17: 807–821, 1981.

538. Eiser, N. M., Macrae, K. D., and Guz, A. Evaluation and expression of bronchial provocation tests. Bull. Eur. Physiopathol. Respir. 17: 427–440, 1981.

539. Eiser, N. M., Mills, J., McCrae, K. D., Snashall, P. D., and Guz, A. Histamine receptors in normal human bronchi. Clin. Sci. 58: 537–544, 1980.

540. Eiser, N. M., Mills, J., Snashall, P. D., and Guz, A. The role of histamine receptors in asthma. Clin. Sci. 60: 363–370, 1981.

541. Ahmed, T., Greenblatt, D. W., Birch, S., Marchette, B., and Wanner, A. Abnormal mucociliary transport in allergic patients with antigen-induced bronchospasm: role of slow reacting substance of anaphylaxis. Am. Rev. Respir. Dis. 124: 110–114, 1981.

542. Dimeo, M. J., Glenn, M. G., Holtzmann, M. J., Sheller, J. R., Nadel, J. A., and Boushey, H. A. Threshold concentration of ozone causing an increase in bronchial reactivity in humans and adaptation with repeated exposures. Am. Rev. Respir. Dis. 124: 245–248, 1981.

543. Sheppard, D., Nadel, J. A., and Boushey, H. A. Inhibition of sulfur dioxide-induced bronchoconstriction by disodium cromoglycate in asthmatic subjects. Am. Rev. Respir. Dis. 124: 257–259, 1981.

544. Bechtel, J. J., Starr, T. III, Dantzker, D. R., and Bower, J. S. Airway hyperreactivity in patients with sarcoidosis. Am. Rev. Respir. Dis. 124: 759–761, 1981.

545. Schachter, E. N., Brown, S., Zuskin, E., Buck, M., Kolack, B., and Bouhuys, A. Airway reactivity in cotton bract-induced bronchospasm. Am. Rev. Respir. Dis. 123: 273–276, 1981.

546. Zuskin, E., Valic, F., and Bouhuys, A. Byssinosis and airway responses due to exposure to textile dust. Lung 154: 17–24, 1976.

547. Aquilina, A. T., Hall, W. J., Douglas, R. G. Jr., and Utell, M. J. Airway reactivity in subjects with viral upper respiratory tract infections: the effects of exercise and cold air. Am. Rev. Respir. Dis. 122: 3–10, 1980.

548. Lam, S. and Chan-Yeung, M. Ethylenediamine-induced asthma. Am. Rev. Respir. Dis. 121: 151–155, 1980.

549. Boushey, H. A., Holtzmann, M. J., Sheller, J. R., and Nadel, J. A. State of the art: bronchial hyperreactivity. Am. Rev. Respir. Dis. 121: 389–413, 1980.

550. Jorde, W. E., von Nieding, G., Krekeler, H., and Worth, G. Inhalativer Provokationstest und protektive Wirkung von Orciprenalin bei allergischem Asthma bronchiale. Respiration 28: 360–365, 1971.

551. Woitowitz, H-J. and Woitowitz, R. H. Clinical experience with a new beta-sympathicomimetic substance in the provoked attack in occupational asthma. Respiration 29: 549–555, 1972.

552. Monkare, S., Haahtela, T., Ikonen, M., and Laitinen, L. A.

Bronchial hyperreactivity to inhaled histamine in patients with farmer's lung. Lung 159: 145–151, 1981.

553. Juniper, E. F., Frith, P. A., and Hargreave, F. E. Airway responsiveness to histamine and methacholine: relationship to minimum treatment to control symptoms of asthma. Thorax 36: 575–579, 1981.

554. Nogrady, S. G. and Bevan, C. H_2 receptor blockade and bronchial hyperreactivity to histamine in asthma. Thorax 36: 268–271, 1981.

555. Tattersfield, A. E. Measurement of bronchial reactivity: a question of interpretation (editorial). Thorax 36: 561–565, 1981.

556. Ryan, G., Latimer, K. M., Dolovich, J., and Hargreave, F. E. Bronchial responsiveness to histamine: relationship to diurnal variation of peak flow rate, improvement after bronchodilator, and airway calibre. Thorax 37: 423–429, 1982.

557. Harries, M. G., Parkes, P. E. G., Lessof, M. H., and Orr, T. S. C. Role of bronchial irritant receptors in asthma. Lancet i: 5–7, 1981.

558. Cockcroft, D. W. and Berscheid, B. A. Effect of pH on bronchial response to inhaled histamine. Thorax 37: 133–136, 1982.

559. Hendrick, D. J., Marshall, R., Faux, J. A., and Krall, J. M. Protective value of dust respirators in extrinsic allergic alveolitis: clinical assessment using inhalation provocation tests. Thorax 36: 917–921, 1981.

560. Beaupre, A. and Malo, J. L. Histamine dose-response curves in asthma: relevance of the distinction between PC20 and reactivity in characterising clinical state. Thorax 36: 731–736, 1981.

561. Dolovich, J. and Hargreave, F. The asthma syndrome: inciters, inducers, and host characteristics (editorial). Thorax 36: 641–644, 1981.

562. Cade, J. F. and Pain, M. C. F. Role of bronchial reactivity in aetiology of asthma. Lancet ii: 186–188, 1971.

563. Nathan, R. A., Segall, N., Glover, G. C., and Schocket, A. L. The effects of H1 and H2 antihistamines on histamine inhalation challenges in asthmatic patients. Am. Rev. Respir. Dis. 120: 1251–1258, 1979.

564. Martelli, N. A. Bronchial and intravenous provocation tests with indomethacin in aspirin-sensitive asthmatics. Am. Rev. Respir. Dis. 120: 1073–1079, 1979.

565. Cockcroft, D. W., Ruffin, R. E., Frith, P. A., Cartier, A., Juniper, E. F., Dolovich, J., and Hargreave, F. E. Determinants of allergen-induced asthma: dose of allergen, circulating IgE antibody concentration, and bronchial responsiveness to inhaled histamine. Am. Rev. Respir. Dis. 120: 1053–1058, 1979.

566. Cockcroft, D. W., Cotton, D. J., and Mink, J. T. Nonspecific bronchial hyperreactivity after exposure to western red cedar. Am. Rev. Respir. Dis. 119: 505–513, 1979.

567. Kreukniet, J. and Pijper, M. M. Response to inhaled histamine and to inhaled allergens in atopic patients. Respiration 30: 345–359, 1973.

568. Haluszka, J. and Scislicki, A. Bronchial lability in children suffering from some diseases of the bronchi. Respiration 32: 217–226, 1975.

569. Zedda, S., Cirla, A., Aresini, G., and Sala, C. Occupational type test for the etiological diagnosis of asthma due to toluene-di-isocyanate. Respiration 33: 14–21, 1976.

570. Buist, A. S. and Ross, B. B. Predicted values for closing volumes using a modified single breath nitrogen test. Am. Rev. Respir. Dis. 107: 744–752, 1973.

571. Burki, N. K., Barker, D. B., and Nicholson, D. P. Variability of the closing volume measurement in normal subjects. Am. Rev. Respir. Dis. 112: 209–212, 1975.

572. Ducic, S., Swift, J., Martin, R. R., and Macklem, P. T. Appraisal of a new test: between-technician variation in the measurement of closing volume. Am. Rev. Respir. Dis. 112: 621–627, 1975.

573. Knudson, R. J. and Lebowitz, M. D. Maximal midexpiratory flow (FEF25–75 per cent): normal limits and assessment of sensitivity (letter to editor). Am. Rev. Respir. Dis. 117: 609–610, 1978.

574. Little, J. W., Hall, W. J., Douglas, R. G. Jr., Mudholkar, G. S., Speers, D. M., and Patel, K. Airway hyperreactivity and peripheral airway dysfunction in influenza A infection. Am. Rev. Respir. Dis. 118: 295–303, 1978.

575. Martin, R. R., Lemelin, C., Zutter, M., and Anthonisen, N. R. Measurement of "closing volume": application and limitations. Bull. Physiopathol. Respir. 9: 979–995, 1973.

576. Sudlow, M. F., Costello, J. F., Flenley, D. C., and Millar, J. Reproducibility and correlation of tests of "small airways disease." Bull. Physiopathol. Respir. 11: 16P–20P, 1975.

577. Marcq, M. and Minette, A. Diurnal variation and reproducibility of the N2 closing volume test in healthy subjects. Bull. Eur. Physiopathol. Respir. 12: 757–770, 1976.

578. McCarthy, D. S., Craig, D. B., and Cherniack, R. M. Intraindividual variability in maximal expiratory flow-volume and closing volume in asymptomatic subjects. Am. Rev. Respir. Dis. 112: 407–411, 1975.

579. Bake, B., Oxhoj, H., Sixt, R., and Winstedt, P. Effect of the slope of the alveolar plateau on determination of closing volume. Scand. J. Respir. Dis. 59: 82–90, 1978.

580. Green, M. and Travis, D. M. A simplified closing-volume method suitable for field use. Lancet ii: 1138–1139, 1972.

581. Dosman, J. A., Chong, P., and Cotton, D. J. Detection of peripheral airways obstruction in smokers using air vs helium spirometry. Bull. Eur. Physiopathol. Respir. 14: 137–143, 1978.

582. Peslin, R., Hannhart, B., and Pino, J. Impédance mécanique thoraco-pulmonaire chez les sujets fumeurs et non-fumeurs. Bull. Eur. Physiopathol. Respir. 17: 93–105, 1981.

583. Jansen, J. M., Peslin, R., Bohadana, A. B., and Racineux, J. L. Usefulness of forced expiration slope ratios for detecting mild airway abnormalities. Am. Rev. Respir. Dis. 122: 221–230, 1980.

584. The lung in the transition between health and disease. In: Macklem, P. T. and Permutt, S. (eds.). Lung Biology in Health and Disease, Vol. 12. Marcel Dekker, New York and Basel, 1979.

585. Thurlbeck, W. M. T. Chronic Airflow Obstruction in Lung Disease. W. B. Saunders, Philadelphia, 1976.

586. Taylor, D. R., Reid, W. D., Paré, P. D., and Fleetham, J. A. Cigarette smoke inhalation patterns and bronchial reactivity. Thorax 43: 65–70, 1988.

587. Small Airways in Health and Disease. Proceedings of a symposium. Copenhagen, March 29–30, 1979. Excerpta Medica, Amsterdam, 1979.

588. Dosman, J., Bode, F., Urbanetti, J., Martin, R., and Macklem, P. T. The use of a helium-oxygen mixture during maximum expiratory flow to demonstrate obstruction in small airways in smokers. J. Clin. Invest. 55: 1090–1099, 1975.

589. Frans, A., Stanescu, D. C., Veriter, C., Clerbaux, T., and Brasseur, L. Smoking and pulmonary diffusing capacity. Scand. J. Respir. Dis. 56: 165–183, 1975.

590. Frans, A., Gerin-Portier, N., Veriter, C., and Brasseur, L. Pulmonary gas exchange in asymptomatic smokers and non-smokers. Scand. J. Respir. Dis. 56: 233–244, 1975.

591. Engel, L. A., Grassino, A., and Anthonisen, N. R. Demonstration of airway closure in man. J. Appl. Physiol. 38: 1117–1125, 1975.

592. Vulterini, S., Bianco, M. R., Pellicciotti, L., and Sidoti, A. M. Lung mechanics in subjects showing increased residual volume without bronchial obstruction. Thorax 35: 461–466, 1980.

593. Higenbottam, T., Feyeraband, C., and Clark, T. J. H. Cigarette smoke inhalation and the acute airway response. Thorax 35: 246–254, 1980.

594. Ashutosh, K. and Keighley, J. Passive expiration as a test of lung function. Thorax 33: 740–746, 1978.

595. Prieto, F., English, M. J., Cochrane, G. M., Clark, T. J. H., and Rigden, B. G. Spirometry in healthy men: a correlation with smoking and with mild symptoms. Thorax 33: 322–327, 1978.

596. Sobol, B. J., Van Voorhies, L., and Emirgil, C. Detection of acute effects of cigarette smoking on airway dynamics: a critical and comparative study of pulmonary function tests. Thorax 32: 312–316, 1977.

597. Saric, M., Lucic-Palaic, S., and Horton, R. J. M. Chronic nonspecific lung disease and alcohol consumption. Environ. Res. 14: 14–21, 1977.

598. Niewohner, D. E., Knoke, J. D., and Kleinerman, J. Pe-

ripheral airways as a determinant of ventilatory function in the human lung. J. Clin. Invest. 60: 139–151, 1977.

599. Niewohner, D. E., Kleinerman, J., and Rice, D. B. Pathologic changes in the peripheral airways of young cigarette smokers. N. Engl. J. Med. 291: 755–758, 1974.

600. Larsson, C., Dirksen, H., Sundstrom, G., and Eriksson, S. Lung function studies in asymptomatic individuals with moderately (Pi SZ) and severely (Pi Z) reduced levels of alpha₁ anti-trypsin. Scand. J. Respir. Dis. 57: 267–280, 1976.

601. McFadden, E. R. and Linden, D. A. A reduction in maximum mid-expiratory flow rate. Am. J. Med. 52: 725–737, 1972.

602. McFadden, E. R., Kiker, R., Holmes, B., and deGroot, W. J. Small airway disease. Am. J. Med. 57: 171–182, 1974.

603. Bode, F. R., Dosman, J., Martin, R. R., and Macklem, P. T. Reversibility of pulmonary function abnormalities in smokers. Am. J. Med. 59: 43–52, 1975.

604. Hales, C. A. and Westphal, D. Hypoxemia following the administration of sublingual nitroglycerin. Am. J. Med. 65: 911–918, 1978.

605. Kuperman, A. S. and Riker, J. B. The variable effect of smoking on pulmonary function. Chest 63: 655–660, 1973.

606. Chiang, S. T. and Wang, B. C. Acute effects of cigarette smoking on pulmonary function. Am. Rev. Respir. Dis. 101: 860–868, 1970.

607. Guyatt, A. R., Berry, G., Alpers, J. H., Bramley, A. C., and Fletcher, C. M. Relationship of airway conductance and its immediate change on smoking to smoking habits and symptoms of chronic bronchitis. Am. Rev. Respir. Dis. 101: 44–54, 1970.

608. Woolf, C. R. and Zamel, N. The respiratory effects of regular cigarette smoking in women. Chest 78: 707–713, 1980.

609. Hogg, J. C. Structure and function of small airways. Chest 77(Suppl): 279–282, 1980.

610. Knudson, R. J., Armet, D. B., and Lebowitz, M. D. Re-evaluation of tests of small airways function. Chest 77(Suppl.): 284–286, 1980.

611. Pride, N. B., Tattersall, S. F., Benson, M. K., Hunter, D., Mansell, A., Fletcher, C. M., and Peto, R. Peripheral lung function and spirometry in male smokers and exsmokers. Chest 77(Suppl.): 289, 1980.

612. Buist, S. and Nagy, J. A longitudinal study of smokers and nonsmokers. Chest 77(Suppl.): 259, 1980.

613. Sackner, M. A. Effect of respiratory drugs on mucociliary clearance. Chest 73(Suppl.): 958–964, 1978.

614. Hamosh, P. and Da Silva, A. M. T. The effect on expiratory flow rates of smoking three cigarettes in rapid succession. Chest 72: 610–613, 1977.

615. DaSilva, A. M. T. and Hamosh, P. Airway response to short-term inhalation of tobacco smoke. Chest 71: 139–141, 1977.

616. Woolf, C. R. Clinical findings, sputum examinations, and pulmonary function tests related to the smoking habit of 500 women. Chest 66: 652–659, 1974.

617. Buist, A. S. Early detection of airways obstruction by the closing volume technique. Chest 64: 495–499, 1973.

618. Lim, T. P. K. Airway obstruction among high school students. Am. Rev. Respir. Dis. 108: 985–988, 1973.

619. Grimes, C. A. and Hanes, B. Influence of cigarette smoking on the spirometric evaluation of employees of a large insurance company. Am. Rev. Respir. Dis. 108: 273–282, 1973.

620. Zamel, N., Kass, I., and Fleischli, G. J. Relative sensitivity of maximal expiratory flow-volume curves using spirometer versus body plethysmograph to detect mild airway obstruction. Am. Rev. Respir. Dis. 107: 861–863, 1973.

621. Buist, A. S., Van Fleet, D. L., and Ross, B. B. A comparison of conventional spirometric tests and the test of closing volume in an emphysema screening clinic. Am. Rev. Respir. Dis. 107: 735–743, 1973.

622. Verdugo, P., Johnson, N., and Tam, P. Beta-adrenergic stimulation of respiratory ciliary activity. J. Appl. Physiol. 48: 868–871, 1980.

623. Krumholz, R. A. and Hedrick, E. C. Pulmonary function differences in normal smoking and nonsmoking, middle-aged, white-collar workers. Am. Rev. Respir. Dis. 107: 225–230, 1973.

624. Weissbecker, L., Creamer, R. M., and Carpenter, R. D. Cigarette smoke and tracheal mucus transport rate. Am. Rev. Resp. Dis. 104: 182–187, 1971.

625. Cosio, M., Ghezzo, H., Hogg, J. C., Corbin, R., Loveland, M., Dosman, J., and Macklem, P. T. The relations between structural changes in small airways and pulmonary-function tests. N. Engl. J. Med. 298: 1277–1281, 1978.

626. Thurlbeck, W. M. Small airways: physiology meets pathology (editorial). N. Engl. J. Med. 298: 1310–1311, 1978.

627. Webster, P. M., Zamel, N., Bryan, A. C., and Kruger, K. Volume dependence of instantaneous time constants derived from the maximal expiratory flow-volume curve. Am. Rev. Respir. Dis. 115: 805–810, 1977.

628. Knudson, R. J., Lebowitz, M. D., Burton, A. P., and Knudson, D. E. The closing volume test: evaluation of nitrogen and bolus methods in a random population. Am. Rev. Respir. Dis. 115: 423–434, 1977.

629. Burrows, B., Knudson, R. J., Cline, M. G., and Lebowitz, M. D. Quantitative relationships between cigarette smoking and ventilatory function. Am. Rev. Respir. Dis. 115: 195–205, 1977.

630. Kjeldgaard, J. M., Hyde, R. W., Speers, D. M., and Reichert, W. W. Frequency dependence of total respiratory resistance in early airway disease. Am. Rev. Respir. Dis. 114: 501–508, 1976.

631. McCarthy, D. S., Craig, D. B., and Cherniack, R. M. Effect of modification of the smoking habit on lung function. Am. Rev. Respir. Dis. 114: 103–113, 1976.

632. Buist, A. S., Sexton, G. J., Nagy, J. M., and Ross, B. B. The effect of smoking cessation and modification on lung function. Am. Rev. Respir. Dis. 114: 115–122, 1976.

633. McCarthy, D. S., Craig, D. B., and Cherniack, R. M. The effect of acute, intensive cigarette smoking on maximal expiratory flows and the single-breath nitrogen washout trace. Am. Rev. Respir. Dis. 113: 301–304, 1976.

634. Armstrong, J. G. and Woolcock, A. J. Lung function in asymptomatic cigarette smokers—the single breath nitrogen test. Austral. N.Z. J. Med. 6: 123–126, 1976.

635. Gelb, A. F., Molony, P. A., Klein, E., and Aronstam, P. S. Sensitivity of volume of isoflow in the detection of mild airway obstruction. Am. Rev. Respir. Dis. 112: 401–405, 1975.

636. Malo, J. L. and Leblanc, P. Functional abnormalities in young asymptomatic smokers with special reference to flow volume curves breathing various gases. Am. Rev. Respir. Dis. 111: 623–629, 1975.

637. Seltzer, C. C., Siegelaub, A. B., Friedman, G. D., and Collen, M. F. Differences in pulmonary function related to smoking habits and race. Am. Rev. Respir. Dis. 110: 598–608, 1974.

638. Hutcheon, M., Griffin, P., Levison, H., and Zamel, N. Volume of isoflow: a new test in detection of mild abnormalities of lung mechanics. Am. Rev. Respir. Dis. 110: 458–465, 1974.

639. Marcq, M. and Minette, A. Lung function changes in smokers with normal conventional spirometry. Am. Rev. Respir. Dis. 114: 723–738, 1976.

640. Thomson, M. L. and Pavia, D. Long-term tobacco smoking and mucociliary clearance. Arch. Environ. Health 26: 86–89, 1973.

641. Camner, P., Philipson, K., and Arvidsson, T. Withdrawal of cigarette smoking. Arch. Environ. Health 26: 90–92, 1973.

642. Tattersall, S. F., Benson, M. K., Hunter, D., Mansell, A., Pride, N. B., and Fletcher, C. M. The use of tests of peripheral lung function for predicting future disability from airflow obstruction in middle-aged smokers. Am. Rev. Respir. Dis. 118: 1035–1050, 1978.

643. Enjeti, S., Hazelwood, B., Permutt, S., Menkes, H., and Terry, P. Pulmonary function in young smokers: male-female differences. Am. Rev. Respir. Dis. 118: 667–676, 1978.

644. Seaton, D. and Ogilvie, C. M. Regional lung function in asymptomatic cigarette smokers. Am. Rev. Respir. Dis. 118: 265–270, 1978.

645. Goodman, R. M., Yergin, B. M., Landa, J. F., Golinvaux, M. H., and Sackner, M. A. Relationship of smoking history and pulmonary function tests to tracheal mucous velocity in nonsmokers, young smokers, ex-smokers, and patients with chronic bronchitis. Am. Rev. Respir. Dis. 117: 205–214, 1978.

646. Manfreda, J., Nelson, N., and Cherniack, R. M. Prevalence

of respiratory abnormalities in a rural and an urban community. Am. Rev. Respir. Dis. 117: 215–226, 1978.

647. Knudson, R. J. and Lebowitz, M. D. Comparison of flow-volume and closing volume variables in a random population. Am. Rev. Respir. Dis. 116: 1039–1045, 1977.

648. Herning, R. I., Jones, R. T., Bachman, J., and Mines, A. H. Puff volume increases when low-nicotine cigarettes are smoked. Br. Med. J. 283: 187–189, 1981.

649. Ashley, F., Kannel, W. B., Sorlie, P. D., and Masson, R. Pulmonary function: relation to aging, cigarette habit, and mortality. Ann. Intern. Med. 82: 739–745, 1975.

650. Costello, J. F., Douglas, N. J., Sudlow, M. F., and Flenley, D. C. Acute effects of smoking tobacco and a tobacco substitute on lung function in man. Lancet ii: 678–680, 1975.

651. Rees, P. J., Chowienczyk, P. J., and Clark, T. J. H. Immediate response to cigarette smoke. Thorax 37: 417–422, 1982.

652. Hayes, D. A., Pimmel, R. L., Fullton, J. M., and Bromberg, P. A. Detection of respiratory mechanical dysfunction by forced random noise impedance parameters. Am. Rev. Respir. Dis. 120: 1095–1100, 1979.

653. Buist, A. S., Nagy, J. M., and Sexton, G. J. The effect of smoking cessation on pulmonary function: a 30-month follow-up of two smoking cessation clinics. Am. Rev. Respir. Dis. 120: 953–957, 1979.

654. Corbin, R. P., Loveland, M., Martin, R. R., and Macklem, P. T. A four-year follow-up study of lung mechanics in smokers. Am. Rev. Respir. Dis. 120: 293–304, 1979.

655. Buist, A. S., Ghezzo, H., Anthonisen, N. R., Cherniack, R. M., Ducic, S., Macklem, P. T., Manfreda, J., Martin, R. R., McCarthy, D., and Ross, B. B. Relationship between the single-breath N2 test and age, sex, and smoking habit in three North American cities. Am. Rev. Respir. Dis. 120: 305–318, 1979.

656. Woolcock, A. J., Leeder, S. R., Peat, J. K., and Blackburn, C. R. B. The influence of lower respiratory illness in infancy and childhood and subsequent cigarette smoking on lung function in Sydney schoolchildren. Am. Rev. Respir. Dis. 120: 5–14, 1979.

657. Webster, P. M., Lorimer, E. G., Man, S. F. P., Woolf, C. R., and Zamel, N. Pulmonary function in identical twins: comparison of nonsmokers and smokers. Am. Rev. Respir. Dis. 119: 223–228, 1979.

658. Zamel, N., Leroux, M., and Ramcharan, V. Decrease in lung recoil pressure after cessation of smoking. Am. Rev. Respir. Dis. 119: 205–211, 1979.

659. Seely, J. E., Zuskin, E., and Bouhuys, A. Cigarette smoking: objective evidence for lung damage in teen-agers. Science 172: 741–743, 1971.

660. Ingram, R. H. Jr. and O'Cain, C. F. Frequency dependence of compliance in apparently healthy smokers versus nonsmokers. Bull. Physiopathol. Respir. 7: 195–210, 1971.

661. Brundin, A. Pulmonary fibrosis in scleroderma and dermatomyositis. Scand. J. Respir. Dis. 51: 160–170, 1970.

662. Huettemann, U. and Criee, C. D. Cigarette smoking: increase of lung compliance as an early factor to influence the relationship of maximum expiratory flow to lung volume. Bull. Physiopathol. Respir. 9: 1251–1252, 1973.

663. Stanescu, D. C., Veriter, C., Frans, A., and Brasseur, L. Maximal expiratory flow rates and "closing volume" in asymptomatic healthy smokers. Bull. Physiopathol. Respir. 9: 1300, 1973.

664. Trinquet, G., Clauzel, A-M., Saindelle, A., and Meyer, A. Influence de la fumée de cigarette et de l'un des ses constituents, sur le transfert de l'oxyde de carbone en etat stable. In: Le Transfert de l'Oxyde de Carbone. Soc. Eur. Physiopathol. Respir. Masson et Cie, Paris, 1969.

665. Gayrard, P., Orehek, J., Grimaud, C., and Charpin, J. Bronchoconstriction due a l'inhalation de fumée de tabac: effets comparées chez le sujet normal et l'asthmatique. Bull. Physiopathol. Respir. 10: 451–461, 1974.

666. Stanescu, D. C., Veriter, C., Frans, A., and Brasseur, L. Maximal expiratory flow rates and "closing volume" in asymptomatic healthy smokers. Scand. J. Respir. Dis. 54: 264–271, 1973.

667. Frans, A., Gerin-Portier, N., Veriter, C., and Brasseur, L. Pulmonary gas exchange in asymptomatic smokers and non smokers. Scand. J. Respir. Dis. 56: 233–244, 1975.

668. Benson, M. K. and Mansell, A. Tests of uneven ventilation: differences between smokers and non-smokers. Bull. Physiopathol. Respir. 11: 33P–36P, 1975.

669. McDermott, M., Gilson, J. C., and Ridley, N. Closing volume and the single breath nitrogen index in a Danish population—a ten-year follow-up. Bull. Physiopathol. Respir. 11: 41P–45P, 1975.

670. McKusick, K. A., Wagner, H. N. Jr., Soin, J. S., Benjamin, J. J., Cooper, M., and Ball, W. C. Jr. Measurement of regional lung function in the early detection of chronic obstructive pulmonary disease. In: Regional lung function and closing volume. Scand. J. Respir. Dis. 85(Suppl.): 51–63, 1974.

671. Closing volume: physiology, methodology, epidemiology and clinical investigation. Scand. J. Respir. Dis. 95(Suppl.): 1–116, 1976.

672. Benson, M. K. The closing volume as a screening test in smokers. Physiology, methodology, epidemiology and clinical investigation. Scand. J. Respir. Dis. 95(Suppl.): 84–90, 1976.

673. Oxhoj, H., Bake, B., and Wilhelmsen, L. Nitrogen closing volume test in 50 and 60 year old men. Physiology, methodology and clinical investigation. Scand. J. Respir. Dis. 95(Suppl.): 97–101, 1976.

674. Buist, A. S. and Nagy, J. M. Relationship between smoking and the single breath nitrogen washout. Physiology, methodology, epidemiology and clinical investigation. Scand. J. Respir. Dis. 95(Suppl.): 108–116, 1976.

675. Kristufek, P., Virsik, K., Bajan, A., Badalik, L., and Dreviankova, V. Early detection of airway abnormalities in a selected group of population. Bull. Eur. Physiopathol. Respir. 12: 467–475, 1976.

676. Oxhoj, H., Bake, B., and Wilhelmsen, L. Ability of spirometry, flow-volume curves and the nitrogen closing volume test to detect smokers. Scand. J. Respir. Dis. 58: 80–96, 1977.

677. Bake, B., Oxhoj, H., Sixt, R., and Wilhelmsen, L. Ventilatory lung function following two years of tobacco abstinence. Scand. J. Respir. Dis. 58: 311–318, 1977.

678. Mercke, U., Hakansson, C. H., and Toremalm, N. G. The influence of temperature on mucociliary activity. Acta. Otolaryngol. 78: 444–450, 1974.

679. Krzyzanowski, M. Changes in ventilatory capacity in an adult population during a five year period. Bull. Eur. Physiopathol. Respir. 16: 155–170, 1980.

680. Huhti, E. and Ikkala, J. A 10-year follow-up study of respiratory symptoms and ventilatory function in a middle-aged rural population. Eur. J. Respir. Dis. 61: 33–45, 1980.

681. Peslin, R., Hannhart, B., and Pino, J. Impédance mécanique thoraco-pulmonaire chez les sujets fumeurs et non-fumeurs. Bull. Eur. Physiopathol. Respir. 17: 93–105, 1981.

682. Sterk, P. J., Quanjer, P. H., van Zomeren, B. C., Wise, M. E., and van der Lende, R. The single breath nitrogen test in epidemiological surveys: an appraisal. Bull. Eur. Physiopathol. Respir. 17: 381–397, 1981.

683. Sterk, P. J., Quanjer, P. H., van Zomeren, B. C., Wise, M. E., and van der Lende, R. Toward identifying the susceptible smoker. Bull. Eur. Physiopathol. Respir. 17: 399–410, 1981.

684. Kujala, P. Smoking, respiratory symptoms and ventilatory capacity in young men. Eur. J. Respir. Dis. 62(Suppl.): 55, 1981.

685. Martin, R. R., Anthonisen, N. R., and Zutter, M. Flow dependence of the intrapulmonary distribution of inspired boluses of ^{133}Xe in smokers and non-smokers. Clin. Sci. 43: 319–329, 1972.

686. Rees, P. J. and Clark, T. J. H. Pattern of breathing during cigarette smoking. Clin. Sci. 61: 85–90, 1981.

687. Nemery, B., Moavero, N. E., Brasseur, L., and Stanescu, D. C. Significance of small airway tests in middle-aged smokers. Am. Rev. Respir. Dis. 124: 232–238, 1981.

688. Martin, R. R., Lindsay, D., Despas, P., Bruce, D., Leroux, M., Anthonisen, N. R., and Macklem, P. T. The early detection of airway obstruction. Am. Rev. Respir. Dis. 111: 119–125, 1975.

689. Beck, G. J., Doyle, C. A., and Schachter, E. N. Smoking and lung function. Am. Rev. Respir. Dis. 123: 149–155, 1981.

690. Ingemann-Hansen, T., and Halkjaer-Kristensen, J. Cigarette

smoking and maximal oxygen consumption rate in humans. Scand. J. Lab. Clin. Invest. 37: 143–148, 1977.

691. Cosio, M. G., Hale, K. A., and Niewohner, D. E. Morphologic and morphometric effects of prolonged cigarette smoking on the small airways. Am. Rev. Respir. Dis. 122: 265–271, 1980.

692. Hale, K. A., Niewohner, D. E., and Cosio, M. G. Morphologic changes in the muscular pulmonary arteries: relationship to cigarette smoking, airway disease, and emphysema. Am. Rev. Respir. Dis. 122: 273–278, 1980.

693. Gerrard, J. W., Cockcroft, D. W., Mink, J. T., Cotton, D. J., Poonawala, R., and Dosman, J. A. Increased nonspecific bronchial reactivity in cigarette smokers with normal lung function. Am. Rev. Respir. Dis. 122: 577–581, 1980.

694. Azen, S. P., Linn, W. S., Hackney, J. D., Jones, M. P., and Schoentgen, S. A comparison of eight lung function indices in smoking and non-smoking office workers. Lung 154: 213–221, 1977.

695. Teculescu, D. B., Pino, J., and Sadoul, P. Cigarette smoking and density-dependence of maximal expiratory flow in asymptomatic men. Am. Rev. Respir. Dis. 122: 651–656, 1980.

696. Harrison, G. N., Mohler, J. L., Lewis, L. A., and Speir, W. A. Jr. Peripheral airway function in healthy young cigarette smokers. Lung 156: 205–215, 1979.

697. Toomes, H., Vogt-Moikopf, I., Heller, W. D., and Ostertag, H. Measurement of mucociliary clearance in smokers and nonsmokers using a bronchoscopic video-technical method. Lung 159: 27–34, 1981.

698. Da Silva, A. M. T. and Hamosh, P. The immediate effect on lung function of smoking filtered and nonfiltered cigarettes. Am. Rev. Respir. Dis. 122: 794–797, 1980.

699. Milne, J. S. and Williamson, J. The relationship of respiratory symptoms and smoking in older people. Respiration 29: 206–213, 1972.

700. Teculescu, D. B. and Manicatide, M. Smoking and blood oxygen tension in healthy middle-aged males. Respiration 33: 54–63, 1976.

701. Vezzoli, F., Calienno, A., and Longhini, E. Small airways disease: a trial of an easy functional discrimination of preclinical emphysema. Respiration 37: 282–290, 1979.

702. Fairshter, R. D. and Wilson, A. F. Relative sensitivities and specificities of tests for small airways obstruction. Respiration 37: 301–308, 1979.

703. Kieft, K. H., Steinijans, V. W., and Wiessmann, K. J. Normal ranges of the mean in- and ex-piratory airways resistance and gas-dynamic breathing efficiency. Respiration 40: 13–21, 1980.

704. Bosisio, E., Grisetti, G. C., Panzuti, F., and Sergi, M. Pulmonary diffusing capacity and its components (DM & Vc) in young, healthy smokers. Respiration 40: 307–310, 1980.

705. Da Silva, A. M. T. and Hamosh, P. Airways response to inhaled tobacco smoke: time course, dose dependence and effect of volume history. Respiration 41: 96–105, 1981.

706. Marrazini, L., Vezzoli, F., and Longhini, E. Respiratory function 8 years after a diagnosis of peripheral airways disease. Respiration 42: 88–97, 1981.

707. Huttemann, U., Oswald, P., Lode, H., and Huckauf, H. Uber den Einfluss langjahrigen Zigarettenrauchens auf die lungenfunktion jugenlicher Normalpersonen. Respiration 29: 270–287, 1972.

708. Da Costa, J. L., Tock, E. P. C., and Boey, H. K. Lung disease with chronic obstruction in opium smokers in Singapore. Thorax 26: 555–571, 1971.

709. Zwillich, C. W., Doekel, R., Hammill, S., and Weil, J. V. The effects of smoked marihuana on metabolism and respiratory control. Am. Rev. Respir. Dis. 118: 885–891, 1978.

710. Tashkin, D. P., Shapiro, B. J., Lee, Y. E., and Harper, C. E. Effects of smoked marihuana in experimentally induced asthma. Am. Rev. Respir. Dis. 112: 377–386, 1975.

711. Bates, D. V. A Citizen's Guide to Air Pollution. McGill-Queen's University Press, Montreal and London, 1972.

712. Stern, A. C. (ed.). Air Pollution. 3rd. ed. Academic Press, New York, 1977.

713. Bates, D. V. and Sizto, R. Relationship between air pollutant levels and hospital admissions in Southern Ontario. Can. J. Public. Health 74: 117–122, 1983.

714. Hesterberg, T. W. and Last, J. A. Ozone-induced acute pulmonary fibrosis in rats. Am. Rev. Respir. Dis. 123: 47–52, 1981.

715. Holland, W. W., et al. Health effects of particulate pollution: reappraising the evidence. Am. J. Epidemiol. 110: 527–659, 1979.

716. Holtzmann, M. J., Cunningham, J. H., Sheller, J. R., Irsigler, G. B., Nadel, J. A., and Boushey, H. A. Effect of ozone on bronchial reactivity in atopic and non atopic subjects. Am. Rev. Respir. Dis. 120: 1059–1067, 1979.

717. Hamilton, L. D. Health effects of electricity generation. First International Conference on Health Effects of Energy Production Proceedings. Sponsored by Atomic Energy of Canada Ltd., Chalk River Ontario. September 1979.

718. Heidorn, K. C. Sulfate and nitrate in total suspended particulate in Ontario. J. Air Pollution Control Assn. 28: 803–806, 1978.

719. Guidotti, T. L. The higher oxides of nitrogen: inhalation toxicology. Environ. Res. 15: 443–472, 1978.

720. Haagen-Smit, A. J. Chemistry and physiology of Los Angeles smog. Ind. Eng. Chem. 44: 1342–1346, 1952.

721. Goldstein, I. F. and Dulburg, E. M. Air pollution and asthma: search for a relationship. J. Air Pollution Control Assn. 31: 370–376, 1981.

722. Gardner, D. E., Miller, F. J., Illing, J. W., and Kirtz, J. M. Increased infectivity with exposure to ozone and sulfuric acid. Toxicol. Letters 1: 59–64, 1977.

723. Fletcher, C. M., Peto, R., Tinker, C., and Speizer, F. The Natural History of Chronic Bronchitis and Emphysema. Oxford, Oxford University Press, 1976.

724. Folinsbee, L. J., Silverman, F., and Shephard, R. J. Decrease of maximum work performance following ozone exposure. J. Appl. Physiol.:Respir. Environ. Exercise Physiol. 42: 531–536, 1977.

725. Folinsbee, L. J., Bedi, J. F., and Horvath, S. M. Respiratory responses in humans repeatedly exposed to low concentrations of ozone. Am. Rev. Respir. Dis. 121: 431–440, 1980.

726. Folinsbee, L. J., Horvath, S. M., Raven, P. B., Bedi, J. F., Morton, A. R., Drinkwater, B. L., Bolduaan, N. W., and Gliner, J. A. Influence of exercise and heat stress on pulmonary function during ozone exposure. J. Appl. Physiol. 43: 409–413, 1977.

727. Folinsbee, L. J., Horvath, S. M., Bedi, J. F., and Delehunt, J. C. Effect of 0.62 ppm NO_2 on cardiopulmonary function in young male nonsmokers. Environ. Res. 15: 199–205, 1978.

728. Ferris, B. G. Jr., Higgins, I. T. T., Higgins, M. W., and Peters, J. M. Chronic nonspecific respiratory disease in Berlin, New Hampshire, 1961 to 1967: a follow up study. Am. Rev. Respir. Dis. 107: 110–122, 1973.

729. Ferris, B. G. Jr. Health effects of exposure to low levels of regulated air pollutants. J. Air Poll. Control Assn. 28: 482–497, 1978.

730. Fenters, J. D., Bradof, J. N., Aranyi, C., Ketels, K., Ehrlich, R., and Gardner, D. E. Health effects of long term inhalation of sulfuric acid mist-carbon particle mixtures. Environ. Res. 19: 244–257, 1979.

731. Ehrlich, R., Findlay, J. C., Fenters, J. D., and Gardner, D. E. Health effects of short-term inhalation of nitrogen dioxide and ozone mixtures. Environ. Res. 14: 223–231, 1977.

732. Ehrlich, R., Findlay, J. C., and Gardner, D. E. Susceptibility to bacterial pneumonia of animals exposed to sulfates. Toxicol. Lett. 1: 325–330, 1978.

733. DeLucia, A. J. and Adams, W. C. Effects of O_3 inhalation during exercise on pulmonary function and blood biochemistry. J. Appl. Physiol. 43: 75–81, 1977.

734. Cohen, A. A., Bromberg, S., Buechley, R. W., Heiderscheit, L. T., and Shy, C. M. Asthma and air pollution from a coal-fueled power plant. Am. J. Publ. Health 62: 1181–1188, 1972.

735. Chow, C. K., Plopper, C. G., Chiu, M., and Dungworth, D. L. Dietary vitamin E and pulmonary, biochemical and morphological alteration in rats exposed to 0.1 ppm O_3. Environ. Res. 24: 315–324, 1981.

736. Chow, C. K., Plopper, C. G., and Dungworth, D. L. Influence of dietary vitamin E on the lungs of ozone-exposed rats. A correlated biochemical and histological study. Environ. Res. 20: 309–317, 1979.

737. Buechley, R. W., Riggan, W. B., Hasselblad, V., and

VanBruggen, J. B. SO$_2$ levels and perturbations in mortality. Arch. Environ. Health 27: 134–137, 1973.

738. Boushey, H. A., Holtzmann, M. J., Sheller, J. R., and Nadel, J. A. Bronchial hyperreactivity. Am. Rev. Respir. Dis. 121: 389–413, 1980.

739. Becklake, M. R., Soucie, J., Gibbs, G. W., and Ghezzo, H. Respiratory health status of children in three Quebec urban communities: an epidemiological study. Bull. Eur. Physiopathol. Respir. 14: 205–221, 1978.

740. Air Quality Criteria for Ozone and Other Photochemical Oxidants. Washington, D.C., Office of Research and Development, US Environmental Protection Agency, April, 1978.

741. Apling, A. J., Sullivan, E. J., Williams, M. L., Ball, D. J., Bernard, R. E., Derwent, R. G., Eggleton, R. E. J., Hampton, L., and Waller, R. E. Ozone concentrations in southeast England during the summer of 1976. Nature 269: 569–573, 1977.

742. Lawther, P. J., Waller, R. E., and Henderson, M. Air pollution and exacerbations of bronchitis. Thorax 25: 525–539, 1970.

743. Whittemore, A. S. and Korn, E. L. Asthma and air pollution in the Los Angeles area. Am. J. Publ. Health 70: 687–696, 1980.

744. Watanabe, S., Frank, R., and Yokoyama, E. Acute effects of ozone on lungs of cats. Am. Rev. Respir. Dis. 108: 1141–1151, 1973.

745. Speizer, F. E., Ferris, B. G. Jr., Bishop, Y. M. M., and Spengler, J. Respiratory disease rates and pulmonary function in children associated with NO$_2$ exposure. Am. Rev. Respir. Dis. 121: 3–10, 1980.

746. Sterling, T. D., Phair, J. J., Pollack, S. V., Schumsky, D. A., and deGroot, I. Urban morbidity and air pollution. Arch. Environ. Health 13: 158–170, 1966.

747. Schoettlin, C. E. and Landau, E. Air pollution and asthmatic attacks in the Los Angeles area. Publ. Health Reports 76: 545–548, 1961.

748. Shenfeld, L., Yap, D., and Kurtz, J. Long range transport of ozone into and across Southern Ontario, Canada. Long Range Transport of Photochemical Oxidants Conference, Oslo, Sept. 12–14, 1978.

749. Sheppard, D., Saisho, A., Nadel, J. A., and Boushey, H. A. Exercise increases SO$_2$ induced bronchoconstriction in asthmatic subjects. Am. Rev. Respir. Dis. 123: 486–491, 1981.

750. Sheppard, D., Wong, W. S., Uehara, C. F., Nadel, J. A., and Boushey, H. A. Lower threshold and greater bronchomotor responsiveness of asthmatic subjects to sulfur dioxide. Am. Rev. Respir. Dis. 122: 873–878, 1980.

751. Silverman, F., Folinsbee, L. J., Barnard, J., and Shephard, R. J. Pulmonary function changes in ozone—interaction of concentration and ventilation. J. Appl. Physiol. 41: 859–864, 1976.

752. Respiratory syncytial virus infection: admissions to hospitals in industrial, urban, and rural areas. Report to the MRC Subcommittee on Respiratory Syncytial Virus Vaccines. Br. Med. J. 2: 796–798, 1978.

753. Richters, A. and Kuraitis, K. Inhalation of NO$_2$ and blood borne cancer cell spread to the lungs. Arch. Environ. Health 36: 36–39, 1981.

754. Hayes, J. A. Racial, occupational, and environmental factors in relation to emphysema in Jamaica. Chest 57: 136–140, 1970.

755. Cross, C. E., De Lucia, A. J., Reddy, A. K., Hussain, M. Z., Chow, C-K., and Mustafa, M. G. Ozone interactions with lung tissue. Am. J. Med. 60: 929–935, 1976.

756. Schnizlein, C. T., Bice, D. E., Rebar, A. H., Wolff, R. K., and Beethe, R. L. Effect of lung damage by acute exposure to nitrogen dioxide on lung immunity in the rat. Environ. Res. 23: 362–370, 1980.

757. Aronow, W. S. Effect of ambient level of carbon monoxide on cardiopulmonary disease (editorial). Chest 74: 1–2, 1978.

758. Hussain, M. Z., Mustafa, M. G., Chow, C. K., and Cross, C. E. Ozone-induced increase of lung proline hydroxylase activity and hydroxyproline content. Chest 69(Suppl): 273–275, 1976.

759. Evans, M. J., Cabral, L. C., Stephens, R. J., and Freeman, G. Acute kinetic response and renewal of the alveolar epithe-

lium following injury by nitrogen dioxide. Chest 65(Suppl.): 62S–64S, 1974.

760. Boatman, E. S. and Frank, R. Morphologic and ultrastructural changes in the lungs of animals during acute exposure to ozone. Chest 65(Suppl.): 9S–11S, 1974.

761. Stephens, R. J., Evans, M. J., Sloan, M. F., and Freeman, G. A comprehensive ultrastructural study of pulmonary injury and repair in the rat resulting from exposures to less than one ppm ozone. Chest 65(Suppl.): 11S–13S, 1974.

762. Lebowitz, M. D., Bendheim, P., Cristea, G., Markovitz, D., Misiaszek, J., Staniec, M., and Van Wyck, D. The effect of air pollution and weather on lung function in exercising children and adolescents. Am. Rev. Respir. Dis. 109: 262–273, 1974.

763. American Thoracic Society. Official statement on Health Effects of Air Pollution. Am. Rev. Respir. Dis. 108: 719–720, 1973.

764. Thurlbeck, W. M., Ryder, R. C., and Sternby, N. A comparative study of the severity of emphysema in necropsy populations in three different countries. Am. Rev. Respir. Dis. 109: 239–248, 1974.

765. Ferris, B. G. Jr., Mahoney, J. R., Patterson, R. M., and First, M. W. Air quality, Berlin, New Hampshire, March 1966–December 1967. Am. Rev. Respir. Dis. 108: 77–84, 1973.

766. Zapletal, A., Jech, J., Paul, T., and Samanek, M. Pulmonary function studies in children living in an air-polluted area. Am. Rev. Respir. Dis. 107: 400–409, 1973.

767. Scott, K. W. M. An autopsy study of bronchial mucous gland hypertrophy in Glasgow. Am. Rev. Respir. Dis. 107: 239–245, 1973.

768. Freeman, G., Crane, S. C., Furiosi, N. J., Stephens, R. J., Evans, M. J., and Moore, W. D. Covert reduction in ventilatory surface in rats during prolonged exposure to subacute nitrogen dioxide. Am. Rev. Respir. Dis. 106: 563–579, 1972.

769. Yokoyama, E. Effect of ventilation with ozone on pressure-volume relationships of excised dogs' lungs. Am. Rev. Respir. Dis. 105: 594–604, 1972.

770. Cohen, C. A., Hudson, A. R., Clausen, J. L., and Knelson, J. H. Respiratory symptoms, spirometry, and oxidant air pollution in nonsmoking adults. Am. Rev. Respir. Dis. 105: 251–261, 1972.

771. Goldstein, E., Peek, N. F., Parks, N. J., Hines, H. H., Steffey, E. P., and Tarkington, B. Fate and distribution of inhaled nitrogen dioxide in rhesus monkeys. Am. Rev. Respir. Dis. 115: 403–412, 1977.

772. Sato, S., Kawakami, M., Maeda, S., and Takashima, T. Scanning electron microscopy of lungs of vitamin E-deficient rats exposed to a low concentration of ozone. Am. Rev. Respir. Dis. 113: 809–821, 1976.

773. McJilton, C. E., Frank, R., and Charlson, R. J. Influence of relative humidity on functional effects of an inhaled SO$_2$-aerosol mixture. Am. Rev. Respir. Dis. 113: 163–169, 1976.

774. Kerr, H. D., Kulle, T. J., McIlhany, M. L., and Swidersky, P. Effects of ozone on pulmonary function in normal subjects. Am. Rev. Respir. Dis. 111: 763–773, 1975.

775. Delucia, A. J., Mustafa, M. G., Hussain, M. Z., and Cross, C. E. Ozone interaction with rodent lung. J. Clin. Invest. 55: 794–802, 1975.

776. Orehek, J., Massari, J. P., Gayrard, P., Grimaud, C., and Charpin, J. Effect of short-term, low-level nitrogen dioxide exposure on bronchial sensitivity of asthmatic patients. J. Clin. Invest. 57: 301–307, 1976.

777. Boatman, E. S., Sato, S., and Frank, R. Acute effects of ozone on cat lungs. II. Structural. Am. Rev. Respir. Dis. 110: 157–169, 1974.

778. Spicer, S. S., Chakrin, L. W., and Wardell, J. R. Jr. Effect of chronic sulfur dioxide inhalation on the carbohydrate histochemistry and histology of the canine respiratory tract. Am. Rev. Respir. Dis. 110: 13–24, 1974.

779. Wolff, R. K., Dolovich, M., Rossman, C. M., and Newhouse, M. T. Sulfur dioxide and tracheobronchial clearance in man. Arch. Environ. Health 30: 521–527, 1975.

780. Hackney, J. D., Linn, W. S., Mohler, J. G., Pedersen, E. E., Breisacher, P., and Russo, A. Experimental studies on human health effects of air pollutants. II. Four-hour exposure

to ozone alone and in combination with other pollutant gases. Arch. Environ. Health 30: 379–384, 1975.

781. Hackney, J. D., Linn, W. S., Law, D. C., Karuza, S. K., Greenberg, H., Buckley, R. D., and Pedersen, E. E. Experimental studies on human health effects of air pollutants. III. Two-hour exposure to ozone alone and in combination with other pollutant gases. Arch. Environ. Health 30: 385–390, 1975.

782. Hirsch, J. A., Swenson, E. W., and Wanner, A. Tracheal mucous transport in beagles after long-term exposure to 1 ppm sulfur dioxide. Arch. Environ. Health 30: 249–253, 1975.

783. Alarie, Y., Krumm, A. A., Busey, W. M., Ulrich, C. E., and Kantz, R. J. II. Long-term exposure to sulfur dioxide, sulfuric acid mist, fly ash, and their mixtures. Arch. Environ. Health 30: 254–262, 1975.

784. Kagawa, J. and Toyama, T. Photochemical air pollution. Its effects on respiratory function of elementary school children. Arch. Environ. Health 30: 117–122, 1975.

785. Kagawa, J. and Toyama, T. Effects of ozone and brief exercise on specific airway conductance in man. Arch. Environ. Health 30: 36–39, 1975.

786. Penha, P. D. and Werthamer, S. Pulmonary lesions induced by long-term exposure to ozone. Arch. Environ. Health 29: 282–289, 1974.

787. Freeman, G., Juhos, L. T., Furiosi, N. J., Mussenden, R., Stephens, R. J., and Evans, M. J. Pathology of pulmonary disease from exposure to interdependent ambient gases (nitrogen dioxide and ozone). Arch. Environ. Health 29: 203–210, 1974.

788. Andersen, I., Lundqvist, G. R., Jensen, P. L., and Proctor, D. F. Human response to controlled levels of sulfur dioxide. Arch. Environ. Health 28: 31–39, 1974.

789. Goldstein, B. D., Lai, L. Y., and Cuzzi-Spada, R. Potentiation of complement-dependent membrane damage by ozone. Arch. Environ. Health 28: 40–42, 1974.

790. Durham, W. H. Air pollution and student health. Arch. Environ. Health 28: 241–254, 1974.

791. Hammer, D. I., Hasselblad, V., Portnoy, B., and Wehrle, P. F. Los Angeles student nurse study. Arch. Environ. Health 28: 255–260, 1974.

792. Fenters, J. D., Findlay, J. C., Port, C. D., Ehrlich, R., and Coffin, D. L. Chronic exposure to nitrogen dioxide. Arch. Environ. Health 27: 85–89, 1973.

793. Sherwin, R. P. Protein content of lung lavage fluid of guinea pigs exposed to 0.4 ppm nitrogen dioxide. Arch. Environ. Health 27: 90–93, 1973.

794. French, J. G., Lowrimore, G., Nelson, W. C., Finklea, J. F., English, T., and Hertz, M. The effect of sulfur dioxide and suspended sulfates on acute respiratory disease. Arch. Environ. Health 27: 129–133, 1973.

795. Ferris, B. G. Jr., Higgins, I. T. T., Higgins, M. W., and Peters, J. M. Sulfur oxides and suspended particulates. Arch. Environ. Health 27: 179–182, 1973.

796. Kinosita, H. and Murakami, A. Control of ciliary motion. Physiol. Rev. 47: 53–82, 1967.

797. Chow, C. K. and Tappel, A. L. Activities of pentose shunt and glycolytic enzymes in lungs of ozone-exposed rats. Arch. Environ. Health 26: 205–208, 1973.

798. Freeman, G., Stephens, R. J., Coffin, D. L., and Stara, J. F. Changes in dogs' lungs after long-term exposure to ozone. Arch. Environ. Health 26: 209–216, 1973.

799. Alarie, Y., Busey, W. M., Krumm, A. A., and Ulrich, E. Long-term continuous exposure to sulfuric acid mist in cynomolgus monkeys and guinea pigs. Arch. Environ. Health 27: 16–24, 1973.

800. Lewis, T. R., Moorman, W. J., Ludmann, W. F., and Campbell, K. I. Toxicity of long-term exposure to oxides of sulfur. Arch. Environ. Health 26: 16–21, 1973.

801. Gardner, D. E., Lewis, T. R., Alpert, S. M., Hurst, D. J., and Coffin, D. L. The role of tolerance in pulmonary defense mechanisms. Arch. Environ. Health 25: 432–438, 1972.

802. Yokoyama, E. and Frank, R. Respiratory uptake of ozone in dogs. Arch. Environ. Health 25: 132–138, 1972.

803. Stephens, R. J., Freeman, G., and Evans, M. J. Early response of lungs to low levels of nitrogen dioxide. Arch. Environ. Health 24: 160–179, 1972.

804. Evans, M. J., Stephens, R. J., Cabral, L. J., and Freeman, G. Cell renewal in lungs of rats exposed to low levels of NO₂. Arch. Environ. Health 24: 180–188, 1972.

805. Alpert, S. M. and Lewis, T. R. Unilateral pulmonary function study of ozone toxicity in rabbits. Arch. Environ. Health 23: 451–458, 1971.

806. Evans, M. J., Mayr, W., Bils, R. F., and Loosli, C. G. Effects of ozone on cell renewal in pulmonary alveoli of aging mice. Arch. Environ. Health 21: 450–453, 1971.

807. Yuen, T. G. H. and Sherwin, R. P. Hyperplasia of type 2 pneumocytes and nitrogen dioxide (10 ppm) exposure. Arch. Environ. Health 22: 178–188, 1971.

808. Bils, R. F. Ultrastructural alterations of alveolar tissue of mice. III. Ozone. Arch. Environ. Health 20: 468–480, 1970.

809. Henry, M. C., Findlay, J., Spangler, J., and Ehrlich, R. Chronic toxicity of NO₂ in squirrel monkeys. Arch. Environ. Health 20: 566–570, 1970.

810. Biersteker, K. and van Leewen, P. Air pollution and peak flow rates of schoolchildren. Arch. Environ. Health 20: 382–384, 1970.

811. Werthamer, S., Schwarz, L. H., Carr, J. J., and Soskind, L. Ozone-induced pulmonary lesions. Arch. Environ. Health 20: 16–21, 1970.

812. Mustafa, M. G. and Tierney, D. F. Biochemical and metabolic changes in the lung with oxygen, ozone, and nitrogen toxicity. Am. Rev. Respir. Dis. 118: 1061–1090, 1978.

813. Lum, H., Schwartz, L. W., Dungworth, D. L., and Tyler, W. S. A comparative study of cell renewal after exposure to ozone or oxygen. Am. Rev. Respir. Dis. 118: 335–345, 1978.

814. Levy, D., Gent, M., and Newhouse, M. T. Relationship between acute respiratory illness and air pollution levels in an industrial city. Am. Rev. Respir. Dis. 116: 167–173, 1977.

815. Ishikawa, S., Bowden, D. H., Fisher, V., and Wyatt, J. P. The emphysema profile in two midwestern cities in North America. Arch. Environ. Health 18: 660–666, 1969.

816. Koenig, J. Q., Pierson, W. E., and Frank, R. Acute effects of inhaled SO₂ plus NaCl droplet aerosol on pulmonary function in asthmatic adolescents. Environ. Res. 22: 145–153, 1980.

817. Blank, M. L., Dalbey, W., Nettesheim, P., Price, J., Creasia, D., and Snyder, F. Sequential changes in phospholipid composition and synthesis in lungs exposed to nitrogen dioxide. Am. Rev. Respir. Dis. 117: 273–280, 1978.

818. Last, J. A., Jennings, M. D., Schwartz, L. W., and Cross, C. E. Glycoprotein secretion by tracheal explants cultured from rats exposed to ozone. Am. Rev. Respir. Dis. 116: 695–703, 1977.

819. Van Der Lende, R., Huygen, C., Jansen-Koster, E. J., Knijpstra, S., Peset, R., Visser, B. F., Wolfs, E. H. E., and Orie, N. G. M. A temporary decrease in the ventilatory function of an urban population during an acute increase in air pollution. Bull. Physiopathol. Respir. 11: 31–43, 1975.

820. Mastrangelo, G. and Clonfero, E. Influence de la pollution sur la fonction respiratoire. Enquête chez les enfants de l'agglomeration de Venise. Bull. Eur. Physiopathol. Respir. 12: 319–331, 1976.

821. Quanjer, P. H., Van Der Maas, L. J., Van Hartevelt, J. H., and Van Der Lende, R. Maximal expiratory flow-volume curves in a follow-up study. Scand. J. Respir. Dis. 57: 309–310, 1976.

822. Voison, C., Aerts, C., Jakubczak, E., Houdret, J. L., and Tonnel, A. B. Effets du bioxyde d'azote sur les macrophages alvéolaires en survie en phase gazeuse. Bull. Eur. Physiopathol. Respir. 13: 137–144, 1977.

823. Woolcock, A. J., Leeder, S. R., Armstrong, J. G., Peat, J. K., Colman, M., and Cullen, K. J. The single breath nitrogen test in rural and urban smokers and non-smokers. Bull. Eur. Physiopathol. Respir. 14: 127–135, 1978.

824. Becklake, M. R., Soucie, J., Gibbs, G. W., and Ghezzo, H. Respiratory health status of children in three Quebec urban communities: an epidemiologic study. Bull. Eur. Physiopathol. Respir. 14: 205–221, 1978.

825. Azoulay, E., Soler, P., and Blayo, M. C. The absence of lung damage in rats after chronic exposure to 2 ppm nitrogen dioxide. Bull. Eur. Physiopathol. Respir. 14: 311–325, 1978.

826. Ronchetti, R., Criscione, S., Macri, F., Tramutoli, G. M., Martinez, F., Tripodi, S., Barretta, A., and Penacchia, M.

Respiratory function and environmental factors in children: epidemiologic survey of Italian schoolchildren. Bull. Eur. Physiopathol. Respir. 16: 3P–4P, 1980.

827. Wuthe, H., Bergmann, K. C., Muller, E., Merker, G., and Vogel, G. Differences of lung function in children living in a rural area and in a highly polluted area. Bull. Eur. Physiopathol. Respir. 16: 4P–5P, 1980.

828. Melia, R. J. W., Florey, C. D. V., Chinn, S., Goldstein, B. D., Brooks, A. G. F., John, H. H., Clark, D., Craighead, I. B., and Webster, X. The relation between indoor air pollution from nitrogen dioxide and respiratory illness in primary schoolchildren. Bull. Eur. Physiopathol. Respir. 16: 7P–8P, 1980.

829. Van der Lende, R., Kok, T. J., Reig, R. P., Quanjer, P. H., Schouten, J. P., and Orie, N. G. M. Decreases in VC and FEV₁ with time: indicators for effects of smoking and air pollution. Bull. Eur. Physiopathol. Respir. 17: 775–792, 1981.

830. Boucher, R. C. Mechanisms of pollutant-induced airways toxicity. In: Clinics in Chest Medicine, Vol. 2, No. 3. Occupational Lung Diseases II. W. B. Saunders, Philadelphia, 1981.

831. Aubry, F., Gibbs, G. W., and Becklake, M. R. Air pollution and health in three urban communities. Arch. Environ. Health 34: 360–368, 1979.

832. Puchelle, E., Zahm, J. M., and Sadoul, P. Mucociliary frequency of frog palate epithelium. Am. J. Physiol. 242: C31–C35, 1982.

833. Bedi, J. F., Folinsbee, L. J., Horvath, S. M., and Ebenstein, R. S. Human exposure to sulfur dioxide and ozone: absence of a synergistic effect. Arch. Environ. Health 34: 233–239, 1979.

834. King, M. Measurement of mucociliary clearance using animal models. Excerpta Medica (Asia Pacific Congress Series) 33: 2–10, 1984.

835. Hackney, J. D., Linn, W. S., Karuza, S. K., Buckley, R. D., Law, D. C., Bates, D. V., Hazucha, M., Pengelly, L. D., and Silverman, F. Effects of ozone exposures in Canadians and southern Californians. Evidence for adaptation? Arch. Environ. Health 32: 110–116, 1977.

836. Plopper, C. G., Dungworth, D. L., Tyler, W. S., and Chow, C. K. Pulmonary alterations in rats exposed to 0.2 and 0.1 ppm ozone: a correlated morphological and biochemical study. Arch. Environ. Health 34: 390–395, 1979.

837. Srizankar, E. V. and Patterson, L. K. Reactions of ozone with fatty acid monolayers: a model system for disruption of lipid molecular assemblies by ozone. Arch. Environ. Health 34: 346–349, 1979.

838. Kleinerman, J. Effects of nitrogen dioxide on elastin and collagen contents of lung. Arch. Environ. Health 34: 228–232, 1979.

839. Sherwin, R. P. and Layfield, L. J. Protein leakage in the lungs of mice exposed to 0.5 ppm nitrogen dioxide. Arch. Environ. Health 31: 50–52, 1976.

840. Comstock, G. W., Meyer, M. B., Helsing, K. J., and Tockman, M. S. Respiratory effects of household exposures to tobacco smoke and gas cooking. Am. Rev. Respir. Dis. 124: 143–148, 1981.

841. Detels, R., Sayre, J. W., Coulson, R. H., Rokaw, S. N., Massey, F. J. Jr., Tashkin, D. P., and Wu, M-M. The UCLA population studies of chronic obstructive respiratory disease. IV. Respiratory effect of long-term exposure to photochemical oxidants, nitrogen dioxide, and sulfates on current and never smokers. Am. Rev. Respir. Dis. 124: 673–680, 1981.

842. Hasselblad, V., Humble, C. G., Graham, M. G., and Anderson, H. S. Indoor environmental determinants of lung function in children. Am. Rev. Respir. Dis. 123: 479–485, 1981.

843. Ranga, V., Kleinerman, J., Ip, M. P. C., and Collins, A. M. The effect of nitrogen dioxide on tracheal uptake and transport of horseradish peroxidase in the guinea pig. Am. Rev. Respir. Dis. 122: 483–490, 1980.

844. Kenoyer, J. L., Phalen, R. F., and Davis, J. R. Particle clearance from the respiratory tract as a test of toxicity: effect of ozone on short and long term clearance. Exp. Lung Res. 2: 111–120, 1981.

845. Kreisman, H., Mitchell, C. A., Hosein, H. R., and Bouhuys, A. Effect of low concentrations of sulfur dioxide on respiratory funtion in man. Lung 154: 25–34, 1976.

846. Bates, D. V. Air pollution: political initiative, scientific reality, and the process of decision-making. Lung 156: 87–94, 1979.

847. De Nevers, N. Human health effects and air pollution control philosophies. Lung 156: 95–107, 1979.

848. Johnson, D. A. Ozone inactivation of human alpha₁-proteinase inhibitor. Am. Rev. Respir. Dis. 121: 1031–1038, 1980.

849. McCord, J. M. and Fridovich, I. The biology and pathology of oxygen radicals. Ann. Intern. Med. 89: 122–127, 1978.

850. Reed, D., Glaser, S., and Kaldor, J. Ozone toxicity symptoms among flight attendants. Am. J. Indust. Med. 1: 43–54, 1980.

851. Ozone in smog (editorial). Lancet ii: 1077–1078, 1975.

852. Snashall, P. D. and Baldwin, C. Mechanisms of sulphur dioxide induced bronchoconstriction in normal and asthmatic man. Thorax 37: 118–123, 1982.

853. McCarthy, D. S. and Craig, D. B. Why the difference in closing volume? (letter to editor). Lancet ii: 1321, 1972.

854. Lambert, P. M. and Reid, D. D. Smoking, air pollution, and bronchitis in Britain. Lancet i: 853–857, 1970.

855. Avol, E. L., Jones, M. P., Bailey, R. M., Chang, N-M. M., Kleinman, M. T., Linn, W. S., Bell, K. A., and Hackney, J. D. Controlled exposures of human volunteers to sulfate aerosols. Am. Rev. Respir. Dis. 120: 319–327, 1979.

856. Lippmann, M., Lioy, P. J., Leikauf, G., Green, K. B., Baxter, D., Morandi, M., Pasternack, B. S., Fife, D., and Speizer, F. E. Effect of ozone on the pulmonary function of children. In: Lee, S. D., Mustafa, M. G., and Mehlman, M. A. (eds.). Advances in Modern Environmental Toxicology, Vol. 5. Princeton Scientific Publishers, Princeton, 1983.

857. Photochemical Air Pollution: Formation, transport and effects. Ottawa, National Research Council of Canada, Report No. 14096, 1975.

858. Bates, D. V., Bell, G. M., Burnham, C. D., Hazucha, M., Mantha, J., Pengelly, L. D., and Silverman, F. Short-term effects of ozone on the lung. J. Appl. Physiol. 32: 176–181, 1972.

859. Hazucha, M., Silverman, F., Parent, C., Field, S., and Bates, D. V. Pulmonary function in man after short-term exposure to ozone. Arch. Environ. Health 27: 183–188, 1973.

860. Hazucha, M. and Bates, D. V. Combined effect of ozone and sulphur dioxide on human pulmonary function. Nature 257: 50–51, 1975.

861. Ferris, B. G. Jr., Speizer, F. E., and Ware, J. H. Uses of tests of pulmonary function to measure effect of air pollutants. In: Berg, G. G. and Maillie, H. D. (eds.). Measurement of Risks. Plenum Publishing Corp. New York and London, 1981.

862. Hackney, J. D. and Linn, W. S. Experimental evaluation of air pollutants in humans as a basis for estimating risk. In: Berg, G. G. and Maillie, H. D. (eds.). Measurement of Risks. Plenum Publishing Corp., New York and London, 1981.

863. Linn, W. S., Medway, D. A., Anzar, U. T., Valencia, L. M., Spier, C. E., Tsao, F. S-D., Fischer, D. A., and Hackney, J. D. Persistence of adaptation to ozone in volunteers exposed repeatedly for six weeks. Am. Rev. Respir. Dis. 125: 491–495, 1982.

864. Linn, W. S., Bailey, R. M., Shamoo, D. A., Venet, T. G., Wightman, L. H., and Hackney, J. D. Respiratory responses of young adult asthmatics to sulfur dioxide exposure under simulated ambient conditions. Environ. Res. 29: 220–232, 1982.

865. Linn, W. S., Chang, Y. T. C., Julin, D. R., Spier, C. E., Anzar, U. T., Mazur, S. F., Trim, S. C., Avol, E. L., and Hackney, J. D. Short-term human health effects of ambient air in a pollutant source area. Lung 160: 219–227, 1982.

866. Linn, W. S., Avol, E. A., and Hackney, J. D. Effects of ambient oxidant pollutants on humans: a movable environmental chamber study. In: Lee, S. D., Mustafa, M. G., and Mehlman, M. A. (eds.). Advances in Modern Environmental Toxicology, Vol. 5. Princeton Scientific Publishers, Princeton, 1983.

867. Linn, W. S., Fischer, D. A., Medway, D. A., Anzar, U. T., Spier, C. E., Valencia, L. M., Venet, T. G., and Hackney, J. D. Short-term respiratory effects of 0.12 ppm ozone

exposure in volunteers with chronic obstructive pulmonary disease. Am. Rev. Respir. Dis. 125: 658–663, 1982.

868. Kleinman, M. T., Bailey, R. M., Chang, Y-T. C., Clark, K. W., Jones, M. P., Linn, W. S., and Hackney, J. D. Exposures of human volunteers to a controlled atmospheric mixture of ozone, sulfur dioxide and sulfuric acid. Am. Indust. Hyg. Assoc. J. 42: 61–69, 1981.

869. Melia, R. J. W., Florey, C. D. V., and Chinn, S. The relation between respiratory illness in primary schoolchildren and the use of gas for cooking. I. Results from a national survey. Int. J. Epidemiol. 8: 333–338, 1979.

870. Bates, D. V. Anyone for the Beach? (editorial). Am. Rev. Respir. Dis. 125: 621–622, 1982.

871. Bromberg, P. A. and Hazucha, M. A. Is "adaptation" to ozone protective? (editorial). Am. Rev. Respir. Dis. 125: 489–490, 1982.

872. Lipfert, F. W. Sulfur oxides, particulates, and human mortality; synopsis of statistical correlations. J. Air Pollution Control Assn. 30: 366–371, 1980.

873. Bates, D. V. Effects of irritant gases on maximal exercise performance. In: Cerretelli, P. and Whipp, B. (eds.). Exercise Bioenergetics and Gas Exchange. Elsevier/North-Holland Biomedical Press, Amsterdam, 1980.

874. Farrell, B. P., Kerr, H. D., Kulle, T. J., Sauder, L. R., and Young, J. L. Adaptation in human subjects to the effects of inhaled ozone after repeated exposures. Am. Rev. Respir. Dis. 119: 725–730, 1979.

875. Horvath, S. M., Gliner, J. A., and Folinsbee, L. J. Adaptation to ozone: duration of effect. Am. Rev. Respir. Dis. 123: 496–499, 1981.

876. Linn, W. S., Jones, M. P., Bachmayer, E. A., Spier, C. E., Mazur, S. F., Avol, E. L., and Hackney, J. D. Short term respiratory effects of polluted ambient air: a laboratory study of volunteers in a high-oxidant community. Am. Rev.Respir. Dis. 121: 243–252, 1980.

877. Khan, A. U. The role of air pollution and weather changes in childhood asthma. Ann. Allergy 39: 397–400, 1977.

878. Kurata, J. H., Glovsky, M. M., Newcomb, R. L., and Easton, J. G. A multifactorial study of patients with asthma. 2. Air pollution, animal dander, and asthma symptoms. Ann. Allergy 37: 398–409, 1976.

879. Rokaw, S. N., Detels, R., Coulson, A. H., Sayre, J. W., Tashkin, D. P., Allwright, S. S., and Massey, F. J. Jr. The UCLA population studies of chronic obstructive respiratory disease. 3. Comparison of pulmonary function in three communities exposed to photochemical oxidants, multiple primary pollutants, or minimal pollutants. Chest 78: 252–262, 1980.

880. Linn, W. S., Hackney, J. D., Pedersen, E. E., Breisacher, P., Patterson, J. V., Mulry, C. A., and Coyle, J. F. Respiratory function and symptoms in urban office workers in relation to oxidant air pollution exposure. Am. Rev. Respir. Dis. 114: 477–483, 1976.

881. Mahoney, L. E. Windflow and respiratory mortality in Los Angeles. Arch. Environ. Health 22: 344–347, 1971.

882. Mellick, P. W., Dungworth, D. L., Schwartz, L. W., and Tyler, W. S. Short term morphologic effects of high ambient levels of ozone on lungs of rhesus monkeys. Lab. Invest. 36: 82–90, 1977.

883. Keller, M. D., Lanese, R. R., Mitchell, R. I., and Cote, R. W. Respiratory illness in households using gas and electricity for cooking. Environ. Res. 19: 495–503, 1979.

884. Tashkin, D. P., Calvarese, B. M., Simmons, M. S., and Shapiro, B. J. Respiratory status of seventy-four habitual marijuana smokers. Chest 78: 699–706, 1980.

885. Davies, A., Dixon, M., Penman, R., Widdicombe, J. G., and Wise, J. C. M. Effect of repeated exposures to high concentrations of sulphur dioxide on respiratory reflexes in rabbits. Bull. Eur. Physiopathol. Respir. 14: 41–52, 1978.

886. Frager, N. B., Phalen, R. F., and Kenoyer, J. L. Adaptation to ozone in reference to mucociliary clearance. Arch. Environ. Health 34: 51–57, 1979.

887. Lucas, A. M. and Douglas, L. C. Principles underlying ciliary activity in the respiratory tract. Arch. Otolaryngol. 20: 528–541, 1934.

888. Yoneda, K. Mucous blanket of rat bronchus: an ultrastructural study. Am. Rev. Respir. Dis. 114: 837–842, 1976.

889. Reissig, M., Bang, B. G., and Bang, F. B. Ultrastructure of the mucociliary interface in the nasal mucosa of the chicken. Am. Rev. Respir. Dis. 117: 327–341, 1978.

890. Sanderson, M. J. and Sleigh, M. A. Ciliary activity of cultured rabbit tracheal epithelium: beat pattern and metachrony. J. Cell Sci. 47: 331–347, 1981.

891. Van As, A. Pulmonary airway clearance mechanisms: a reappraisal (editorial). Am. Rev. Respir. Dis. 115: 721–726, 1977.

892. Ross, S. M. and Corrsin, S. Results of an analytical model of mucociliary pumping. J. Appl. Physiol. 37: 333–340, 1974.

893. Blake, J. On the movement of mucus in the lung. J. Biomech. 8: 179–190, 1975.

894. Iravani, J. and Melville, G. N. Wirkung von Pharmaka und Milieuanderungen auf die Flimmertatigkeit der Atemwege. Respiration 32: 157–164, 1975.

895. Van As, A. and Avner, B. P. Autonomic control of ciliary frequency (abstract). Am. Rev. Respir. Dis. 125: 159, 1982.

896. Maurer, D. R., Sielczak, M., Oliver, W. Jr., Abraham, W. A., and Wanner, A. Role of ciliary motility in acute allergic mucociliary dysfunction. J. Appl. Physiol. 52: 1018–1023, 1982.

897. Rutland, J., Griffin, W., and Cole, P. Nasal brushing and measurement of ciliary beat frequency. Chest 80(Suppl.): 865–867, 1981.

898. Hee, J. and Guillerm, R. Influence des facteurs de l'environment sur l'activite ciliaire et le transport du mucus. Bull. Eur. Physiopathol. Respir. 9: 377–393, 1973.

899. Dulfano, M. J. Cilia inhibitory factor in sputum (abstract). Am. Rev. Respir. Dis. 121: 334, 1980.

900. Carlson, H. E. and Robbins, J. Effects of hormones and nucleotides on ciliary beating in frog esophagus and guinea pig trachea. Life Sci. 14: 2413–2426, 1974.

901. Sleigh, M. A. Some aspects of the comparative physiology of cilia. Am. Rev. Respir. Dis. 93(Suppl.): 16–31, 1966.

902. Boucher, R. C., Stutts, M. J., and Gatzy, J. T. Regional differences in bioelectric properties and ion flow in excised canine airways. J. Appl. Physiol. 51: 705–714, 1981.

903. Gilboa, A. and Silberberg, A. Characterization of epithelial mucus and its function in clearance by ciliary propulsion. In: Aharonson, E. F., Ben-David, A., and Klingberg, M. A. (eds.). Air Pollution and the Lung. Wiley, New York, 1976.

904. Rutland, J. and Cole, P. J. Nasal mucociliary clearance and ciliary beat frequency in cystic fibrosis compared with sinusitis and bronchiectasis. Thorax 36: 654–658, 1981.

905. Konietzko, N., Nakhosteen, J. A., Mizera, W., Kasparek, R., and Hesse, H. Ciliary beat frequency of biopsy samples taken from normal persons and patients with various lung diseases. Chest 80(Suppl.): 855–857, 1981.

906. Serafini, S. M. and Michaelson, E. D. Length and distribution of cilia in human and canine airways. Bull. Eur. Physiopathol. Respir. 13: 551–559, 1977.

907. Stewart, W. C. Weight-carrying capacity and excitability of excised ciliated epithelium. Am. J. Physiol. 152: 1–5, 1948.

908. Sade, J., Eliezer, N., Silberberg, A., and Nevo, A. C. The role of mucus in transport by cilia. Am. Rev. Respir. Dis. 102: 48–52, 1970.

909. King, M., Kelly, S., and Cosio, M. Alteration of airway reactivity by mucus. Respir. Physiol. 62: 47–59, 1985.

910. King, M., Gilboa, A., Meyer, F. A., and Silberberg, A. On the transport of mucus and its rheologic simulants in ciliated systems. Am. Rev. Respir. Dis. 110: 740–745, 1974.

911. King, M. Is cystic fibrosis mucus abnormal? Pediat. Res. 15: 120–122, 1981.

912. Shih, C. K., Litt, M., Khan, M. A., and Wolf, D. P. Effect of nondialyzable solids concentration and viscoelasticity on ciliary transport of tracheal mucus. Am. Rev. Respir. Dis. 115: 989–995, 1977.

913. Meyer, F. A. and Gelman, R. A. Mucociliary transference rate and mucus viscoelasticity: dependence on dynamic storage and loss modulus. Am. Rev. Respir. Dis. 120: 553–557, 1979.

914. Puchelle, E., Girard, F., and Zahm, J. M. Rhéologie des sécrétions bronchiques et transport muco-ciliaire. Bull. Eur. Physiopathol. Respir. 12: 771–779, 1976.

915. Chen, T. M. and Dulfano, M. J. Mucus viscoelasticity and mucociliary transport rate. J. Lab. Clin. Med. 91: 423–431, 1978.

916. Giordano, A. M., Holsclaw, D., and Litt, M. Mucus rheology and mucociliary clearance: normal physiologic state. Am. Rev. Respir. Dis. 118: 245–250, 1978.

917. King, M. Interrelation between mechanical properties of mucus and mucociliary transport: effect of pharmacologic interventions. Biorheology 16: 57–68, 1979.

918. King, M. Relationship between mucus viscoelasticity and ciliary transport in guaran gel/frog palate model system. Biorheology 17: 249–254, 1980.

919. Zanjanian, M. H. Expectorants and antitussive agents: are they helpful? Ann. Allergy 44: 290–295, 1980.

920. Nadel, J. A. Autonomic control of airway smooth muscle and airway secretions. Am. Rev. Respir. Dis. 115(Suppl.): 117–126, 1977.

921. King, M. and Viires, N. Effect of methacholine chloride on rheology and transport of canine tracheal mucus. J. Appl. Physiol. 47: 26–31, 1979.

922. King, M., Cohen, C., and Viires, N. Influence of vagal tone on rheology and transportability of canine tracheal mucus. Am. Rev. Respir. Dis. 120: 1215–1219, 1979.

923. Basbaum, C. B., Ueki, I., Brezina, L., and Nadel, J. A. Tracheal submucosal gland serous cells stimulated in vitro with adrenergic and cholinergic agonists: a morphometric study. Cell Tissue Res. 220: 481–498, 1981.

924. Puchelle, E., Zahm, J. M., Polu, J. M., and Sadoul, P. Drug effects on viscoelasticity of mucus. Eur. J. Respir. Dis. 110(Suppl.): 195–208, 1980.

925. Charman, J. and Reid, L. Sputum viscosity in chronic bronchitis, bronchiectasis, asthma, and cystic fibrosis. Biorheology 9: 185–199, 1972.

926. Lopez-Vidriero, M. T. and Reid, L. Chemical markers of mucous and serum glycoproteins and their relation to viscosity in mucoid and purulent sputum from various hypersecretory diseases. Am. Rev. Respir. Dis. 117: 465–477, 1978.

927. Dulfano, M. J. and Adler, K. B. Physical properties of sputum. VII. Rheologic properties and mucociliary transport. Am. Rev. Respir. Dis. 112: 341–347, 1975.

928. Newhouse, M., Sanchis, J., and Bienenstock, J. Lung defense mechanisms. N. Engl. J. Med. 295: 990–998, 1045–1052, 1976.

929. Robertson, B. Basic morphology of the pulmonary defence system. In: Belin, L., Jarrholm, B., Larsson, S., and Thiringer, G. (eds.). Chest Diseases and the Working Environment. Eur. J. Respir. Dis. 61(Suppl. 107): 21–40, 1980.

930. Camner, P. Alveolar clearance. In: Belin, L., Jarrholm, B., Larsson, S., and Thiringer, G. (eds.). Chest Diseases and the Working Environment. Eur. J. Respir. Dis. 61(Suppl. 107): 59–72, 1980.

931. Richardson, P. S. and Peatfield, A. C. Reflexes concerned in the defence of the lungs. Bull. Eur. Physiopathol. Respir. 17: 979–1012, 1981.

932. Leikauf, G. D., Ueki, I. F., and Nadel, J. A. Autonomic regulation of viscoelasticity of cat tracheal gland secretion. J. Appl. Physiol. 56: 426–430, 1984.

933. Iravani, J. and Melville, G. N. Mucociliary activity in the respiratory tract as influenced by prostaglandin E$_1$. Respiration 32: 305–315, 1975.

934. Toremalm, N-G. Factors influencing the mucociliary activity in the respiratory tract. In: Belin, L., Jarrholm, B., Larsson, S., and Thiringer, G. (eds.). Chest Diseases and the Working Environment. Eur. J. Respir. Dis. 61(Suppl. 107): 41–49, 1980.

935. Adler, K., Wooten, O., Philipoff, W., Lerner, E., and Dulfano, M. J. Physical properties of sputum. III. Rheologic variability and intrinsic relationships. Am. Rev. Respir. Dis. 106: 100–108, 1972.

936. Puchelle, E., Pham, Q. T., Caraux, G., and Zahm, J. M. Etat rhéologique des sécrétions bronchiques chez le bronchiteux chronique. Bull. Physiopathol. Respir. 9: 143–159, 1973.

937. Pham, Q. T., Peslin, R., Puchelle, E., Salmon, D., Caraux, G., and Benis, A. M. Fonction réspiratoire et état rhéologique des sécrétions récueilllés pendant l'expectoration spontanée et dirigée. Bull. Physiopathol. Respir. 9: 293–311, 1973.

938. Medici, T. C., Chodosh, S., Ishikawa, S., and Enslein, K. Physical properties of sputum and respiratory function in chronic bronchial disease. Bull. Physiopathol. Respir. 9: 315–323, 1973.

939. Lopez-Vidriero, M. Individual and group correlations of sputum viscosity and airways obstruction. Bull. Physiopathol. Respir. 9: 339–346, 1973.

940. Puchelle, E., Aug, F., Zahm, J. M., and Bertrand, A. Comparison of nasal and bronchial mucociliary clearance in young non-smokers. Clin. Sci. 62: 13–16, 1982.

941. Andersen, I., Camner, P., Jensen, P. L., Philipson, K., and Proctor, D. F. A comparison of nasal and tracheobronchial clearance. Arch. Environ. Health 29: 290–293, 1974.

942. Asmundsson, T. and Kilburn, K. H. Mucociliary clearance rates at various levels in dog lungs. Am. Rev. Respir. Dis. 102: 388–397, 1970.

943. Serafini, S. M., Wanner, A., and Michaelson, E. D. Mucociliary transport in central and intermediate size airways: effect of aminophyllin. Bull. Eur. Physiopathol. Respir. 12: 415–422, 1976.

944. Foster, W. M., Langenback, E., and Bergofsky, E. H. Measurement of tracheal and bronchial mucus velocities in man: relation to lung clearance. J. Appl. Physiol. 48: 965–971, 1980.

945. Low, P. M. P., Luk, C. K., Dulfano, M. J., and Finch, P. J. P. Ciliary beat frequency of human respiratory tract by different sampling techniques. Am. Rev. Respir. Dis. 130: 497–498, 1984.

946. Albert, R. E., Berger, J., Sanborn, K., and Lippmann, M. Effects of cigarette smoke components on bronchial clearance in the donkey. Arch. Environ. Health 29: 96–101, 1974.

947. Cruz, R. S., Landa, J., Hirsch, J., and Sackner, M. A. Tracheal mucous velocity in normal man and patients with obstructive lung disease: effects of terbutaline. Am. Rev. Respir. Dis. 109: 458–463, 1974.

948. Bohning, D. E., Albert, R. E., Lippmann, M., and Foster, W. M. Tracheobronchial particle deposition and clearance. Arch. Environ. Health 30: 457–462, 1975.

949. Pavia, D. and Thomson, M. L. Unimpaired mucociliary clearance in the lung of a centenarian smoker (letter to editor). Lancet ii: 101–102, 1970.

950. Sackner, M. A., Hirsch, J. A., Epstein, S., and Rywlin, A. M. Effect of oxygen in graded concentrations upon tracheal mucous velocity. Chest 69: 164–167, 1976.

951. Saketkhoo, K., Januszkiewicz, A., and Sackner, M. A. Effects of drinking hot water, cold water, and chicken soup on nasal mucous velocity and nasal airflow resistance. Chest 74: 408–410, 1978.

952. Pavia, D., Bateman, J. R. M., Sheahan, N. F., Agnew, J. E., Newman, S. P., and Clarke, S. W. Techniques for measuring lung mucociliary clearance. In: Berglund, E., Nilsson, B. S., Mossberg, B., and Bake, B. (eds.). Cough and Expectoration. Eur. J. Respir. Dis. 61(Suppl. 110): 157–168, 1980.

953. Mossberg, B. Human tracheobronchial clearance by mucociliary transport and cough. In: Belin, L., Jarrholm, B., Larsson, S., and Thiringer, G. (eds.). Chest Diseases and the Working Environment. Eur. J. Respir. Dis. 61(Suppl. 107): 51–58, 1980.

954. Puchelle, E., Zahm, J. M., Girard, F., Bertrand, A., Polu, J. M., Aug, F., and Sadoul, P. Mucociliary transport in vivo and in vitro. Eur. J. Respir. Dis. 61: 254–264, 1980.

955. Sanchis, J., Dolovich, M., Rossman, C., Wilson, W., and Newhouse, M. Pulmonary mucociliary clearance in cystic fibrosis. N. Engl. J. Med. 288: 651–654, 1973.

956. Wood, R. E., Wanner, A., Hirsch, J., and Farrell, P. M. Tracheal mucociliary transport in patients with cystic fibrosis and its stimulation by terbutaline. Am. Rev. Respir. Dis. 111: 733–738, 1975.

957. Yeates, D. B., Aspin, N., Bryan, A. C., and Levison, H. Regional clearance of ions from the airways of the lung. Am. Rev. Respir. Dis. 107: 602–608, 1973.

958. Bateman, J. R. M., Pavia, D., and Clarke, S. W. The retention of lung secretions during the night in normal subjects. Clin. Sci. 55: 523–527, 1978.

959. Mezey, R. J., Cohn, M. A., Fernandez, R. J., Januszkiewicz, A. J., and Wanner, A. Mucociliary transport in allergic patients with antigen-induced bronchospasm. Am. Rev. Respir. Dis. 118: 677–684, 1978.

960. King, M. Rheological requirements for optimal clearance of secretions: ciliary transport versus cough. In: Berglund, E., Nilsson, B. S., Mossberg, B., and Bake, B. (eds.). Cough and Expectoration. Eur. J. Respir. Dis. 61(Suppl. 110): 39–42, 1980.

961. Camner, P., Mossberg, B., and Philipson, K. Tracheobronchial clearance and chronic obstructive lung disease. Scand. J. Respir. Dis. 54: 272–281, 1973.

962. Mossberg, B., Philipson, K., Strandberg, K., and Camner, P. Clearance by voluntary coughing and its relationship to subjective assessment and effect of intravenous bromhexine. Eur. J. Respir. Dis. 62: 173–179, 1981.

963. Oldenburg, F. A. Jr., Dolovich, M. B., Montgomery, J. M., and Newhouse, M. T. Effects of postural drainage, exercise, and cough on mucus clearance in chronic bronchitis. Am. Rev. Respir. Dis. 120: 739–745, 1979.

964. Bateman, J. R. M., Newman, S. P., Daunt, K. M., Sheahan, N. F., Pavia, D., and Clarke, S. W. Is cough as effective as chest physiotherapy in the removal of excessive tracheobronchial secretions? Thorax 36: 683–687, 1981.

965. Camner, P., Mossberg, B., Philipson, K., and Strandberg, K. Elimination of test particles from the human tracheobronchial tree by voluntary coughing. Scand. J. Respir. Dis. 60: 56–62, 1979.

966. Berkowitz, H., Reichel, J., and Shim, C. The effect of ethanol on the cough reflex. Clin. Sci. 45: 527–531, 1973.

967. Byrd, R. B. and Burns, J. R. Cough dynamics in the postthoracotomy state. Chest 67: 654–657, 1975.

968. Pryor, J. A., Webber, B. A., Hodson, M. E., and Batten, J. C. Evaluation of the forced expiration technique as an adjunct to postural drainage in treatment of cystic fibrosis. Br. Med. J. 2: 417–418, 1979.

969. Flower, K. A., Eden, R. I., Lomax, L., Mann, N. M., and Burgess, J. New mechanical aid to physiotherapy in cystic fibrosis. Br. Med. J. 2: 630–631, 1979.

970. Cochrane, G. M., Webber, B. A., and Clarke, S. W. Effects of sputum on pulmonary function. Br. Med. J. 2: 1181–1183, 1977.

971. Ozone and Other Photochemical Oxidants. National Academy Press, Washington, D.C., 1977.

972. Frederick, E. R., for the Air Pollution Control Association (ed.). Ozone/Oxidants: Interactions with the Total Environment. Proceedings of a specialty conference October 14–17, 1979, Gallena Plaza, Houston, Texas, 1979.

973. Rubinfeld, A. R. and Pain, M. C. F. Respiratory disability in worker's compensation claimants. Med. J. Austral. 1: 119–121, 1983.

974. O'Brien, R. J. and Drizd, T. A. Basic data on spirometry in adults 25–74 years of age. In: Vital and Health Statistics, series 11. DHSS Publication No. (PHS) 81–1672, 1981.

975. Bates, D. V. Introduction to the discussion. In: Sadoul, P., Milic-Emili, J., Simonsson, B. G., and Clark, T. J. H. (eds.). Small Airways in Health and Disease. Excerpta Medica, Amsterdam, 1979.

976. Green, M. Bronchiolitis. In: Sadoul, P., Milic-Emili, J., Simonsson, B. G., and Clark, T. J. H. (eds.). Small Airways in Health and Disease. Excerpta Medica, Amsterdam, 1979.

977. Bates, D. V. Chronic bronchitis and emphysema: the search for their natural history. In: Macklem, P. T. and Permutt, S. The Lung in Transition between Health and Disease. Marcel Dekker, New York and Basel, 1979.

978. Campbell, E. J. M. Physical signs of diffuse airways obstruction and lung distension. Thorax 24: 1–3, 1969.

979. Godfrey, S., Edwards, R. H. T., Campbell, E. J. M., Armitage, P., and Oppenheimer, E. A. Repeatability of physical signs in airways obstruction. Thorax 24: 4–9, 1969.

980. Godfrey, S., Edwards, R. H. T., Campbell, E. J. M., and Newton-Howes, J. Clinical and physiological association of some physical signs observed in patients with chronic airways obstruction. Thorax 25: 285–287, 1970.

981. Bates, D. V., Anthonisen, N. R., Bass, H., Heckscher, T., and Oriol, A. Recent observations on the measurement of regional V/Q ratios in chronic lung disease. In: Cumming, G. and Hunt, L. B. (eds.). Form and Function in the Human Lung. Williams & Wilkins Co., Baltimore, 1968.

982. Mendella, L. A., Manfreda, J., Warren, C. P. W., and Anthonisen, N. R. Steroid response in chronic obstructive pulmonary disease. Ann. Intern. Med. 96: 17–21, 1982.

983. Mills, F. C., Parsons, W. D., Pare, J. A. P., and Bates, D. V. The physical status of men in the lowest income group in the sixth decade of life. Can. Med. Assn. J. 89: 281–288, 1963.

984. Anthonisen, N. R., Bass, H., Oriol, A., Place, R. E. G., and Bates, D. V. Regional lung function in patients with chronic bronchitis. Clin. Sci. 35: 495–512, 1968.

985. Macklem, P. T. and Becklake, M. R. The relationship between the mechanical and diffusing properties of the lung in health and disease. Am. Rev. Respir. Dis. 87: 47–52, 1963.

986. Ward, H., Bates, D. V., Paul, G. I., Snidal, D., Gordon, C. A., and Woolf, C. A. Twenty-year follow-up of chronic bronchitics in three Canadian cities. (In preparation)

987. Eriksson, S., Moestrup, T., and Hagerstrand, I. Liver, lung, and malignant disease in heterozygous (PiMZ) alpha₁-antitrypsin deficiency. Acta Med. Scand. 198: 243–247, 1975.

988. Thurlbeck, W. M. T. Changes in lung structure. In: Macklem, P. T. and Permutt, S. (eds.). The Lung in the Transition between Health and Disease. Marcel Dekker, New York and Basel, 1979.

989. Mead, J. Problems in interpreting common tests of pulmonary mechanical function. In: Macklem, P. T. and Permutt, S. (eds.). The Lung in the Transition between Health and Disease. Marcel Dekker, New York and Basel, 1979.

990. Young, I. H. and Woolcock, A. J. Arterial blood gas tension changes at the start of exercise in chronic obstructive pulmonary disease. Am. Rev. Respir. Dis. 119: 213–221, 1979.

991. Postma, D. S., Burema, J., Gimeno, F., May, J. F., Smit, J. M., Steenhuis, E. J., Weele, L. T. V. D., and Sluiter, H. J. Prognosis in severe chronic obstructive pulmonary disease. Am. Rev. Respir. Dis. 119: 357–367, 1979.

992. Buist, A. S., Sexton, G. J., Azzam, A-M. H., and Adams, B. E. Pulmonary function in heterozygotes for alpha₁-antitrypsin deficiency: a case-control study. Am. Rev. Respir. Dis. 120: 759–766, 1979.

993. Minh, V-D., Lee, H. M., Dolan, G. F., Light, R. W., Bell, J., and Vasquez, P. Hypoxemia during exercise in patients with chronic obstructive pulmonary disease. Am. Rev. Respir. Dis. 120: 787–794, 1979.

994. Gibson, G. J., Pride, N. B., Davis, J., and Schroter, R. C. Exponential description of the static pressure-volume curve of normal and diseased lungs. Am. Rev. Respir. Dis. 120: 799–811, 1979.

995. Palmer, K. N. V. Chronic obstructive lung disease (letter to editor). Lancet ii: 1294–1295, 1971.

996. Hughes, J. A., Hutchison, D. C. S., Bellamy, D., Dowd, D. E., Ryan, K. C., and Hugh-Jones, P. The influence of cigarette smoking and its withdrawal on the annual change of lung function in pulmonary emphysema. Q. J. Med. 51: 115–124, 1982.

997. Berend, N., Skoog, C., and Thurlbeck, W. M. Exponential analysis of lobar pressure-volume characteristics. Thorax 36: 452–455, 1981.

998. Weitzenblum, E., Hirth, C., Duculone, A., Mirhom, R., Rasaholinjanahary, J., and Erhart, M. Prognostic value of pulmonary artery pressure in chronic obstructive pulmonary disease. Thorax 36: 752–758, 1981.

999. Hughes, J. A., Hutchison, D. C. S., Bellamy, D., Dowd, D. E., Ryan, K. C., and Hugh-Jones, P. Annual decline of lung function in pulmonary emphysema: influence of radiological distribution. Thorax 37: 32–37, 1981.

1000. Rutland, R. J. A., Pang, J. A., and Geddes, D. M. Carbimazole and exercise tolerance in chronic airflow obstruction. Thorax 37: 64–67, 1982.

1001. Fletcher, C. M. and Pride, N. B. What does "chronic bronchitis" mean? British Thoracic Association and the Thoracic Society Proceedings. Thorax 37: 228, 1982.

1002. Pereira, R. P., Hunter, D., and Pride, N. B. Use of lung pressure-volume curves and helium-sulphur hexafluoride washout to detect emphysema in subjects with mild airflow obstruction. Thorax 36: 29–37, 1981.

1003. Cockcroft, A. E., Saunders, M. J., and Berry, G. Randomised controlled trial of rehabilitation in chronic respiratory disability. Thorax 36: 200–203, 1981.

1004. Woodcock, A. A., Gross, E. R., and Geddes, D. M. Oxygen relieves breathlessness in "pink puffers." Lancet i: 907–909, 1981.

1005. Long term domiciliary oxygen therapy in chronic hypoxic cor pulmonale complicating chronic bronchitis and emphysema. Report of MRC Working Party. Sir Charles Stuart-Harris, chairman. Lancet i: 681–685, 1981.

1006. British phlegm, British bronchi (editorial). Lancet i: 403–405, 1977.

1007. Stevens, P. M., Hnilica, V. S., Johnson, P. C., and Bell, R. L. Pathophysiology of hereditary emphysema. Ann. Intern. Med. 74: 672–680, 1971.

1008. Nocturnal Oxygen Therapy Trial Group. Continuous or nocturnal oxygen therapy in hypoxemic chronic obstructive lung disease. A clinical trial. Ann. Intern. Med. 93: 391–398, 1980.

1009. Karpick, R. J., Pratt, P. C., Asmundsson, T., and Kilburn, K. H. Pathological findings in respiratory failure. Ann. Intern. Med. 72: 189–197, 1970.

1010. Duffell, G. M., Marcus, J. H., and Ingram, R. H. Jr. Limitation of expiratory flow in chronic obstructive pulmonary disease. Ann. Intern. Med. 72: 365–374, 1970.

1011. Peach, H. and Pathy, M. S. Follow-up study of disability among elderly patients discharged from hospital with exacerbations of chronic bronchitis. Thorax 36: 585–589, 1981.

1012. Kueppers, F. and Donhardt, A. Obstructive lung disease in heterozygotes for alpha-1 antitrypsin deficiency. Ann. Intern. Med. 80: 209–212, 1974.

1013. Woodcock, A. A., Gross, E. R., and Geddes, D. M. Drug treatment of breathlessness: contrasting effects of diazepam and promethazine in pink puffers. Br. Med. J. 283: 343–346, 1981.

1014. Sinclair, D. J. M. and Ingram, C. G. Controlled trial of supervised exercise training in chronic bronchitis. Br. Med. J. 1: 519–521, 1980.

1015. McGavin, C. R., Gupta, S. P., and McHardy, G. J. R. Twelve-minute walking test for assessing disability in chronic bronchitis. Br. Med. J. 1: 822–823, 1976.

1016. Muller, J. and Radwan, L. The effect of voluntary hyperventilation on arterial blood gases and gas exchange in patients with chronic obstructive lung disease. Scand. J. Respir. Dis. 57: 129–138, 1976.

1017. Schaanning, J. Ventilatory and heart rate adjustments during submaximal and maximal exercise in patients with chronic obstructive lung disease. Scand. J. Respir. Dis. 57: 63–72, 1976.

1018. Varpela, E. and Salorinne, Y. Respiratory disease profile in 22 patients with alpha$_1$-antitrypsin deficiencies. Scand. J. Respir. Dis. 89(Suppl.): 251–260, 1974.

1019. Evans, C. C., Ridyard, J. B., and Ogilvie, C. M. Regional lung function in chronic airways obstruction. In: Regional Lung Function and Closing Volume. Scand. J. Respir. Dis. 85(Suppl.): 75–82, 1974.

1020. Pham, Q. T., Uffholtz, H., and Schrijen, F. Respiratory disturbances in chronic bronchitis. Scand. J. Respir. Dis. 55: 209–217, 1974.

1021. Kiviloog, J., Irnell, L., and Eklund, G. The prevalence of bronchial asthma and chronic bronchitis in smokers and non-smokers in a representative local Swedish population. Scand. J. Respir. Dis. 55: 262–276, 1974.

1022. Kok-Jensen, A., Sorensen, E., and Damsgaard, T. Prognosis in severe chronic obstructive pulmonary disease. Scand. J. Respir. Dis. 55: 120–128, 1974.

1023. Brundin, A. Physical training in severe chronic obstructive lung disease. II. Observations on gas exchange. Scand. J. Respir. Dis. 55: 37–46, 1974.

1024. Brundin, A. Physical training in severe chronic obstructive lung disease. I. Clinical course, physical working capacity and ventilation. Scand. J. Respir. Dis. 55: 25–36, 1974.

1025. Kauffmann, F., Brille, D., and Lellouch, J. Evaluation de la valeur pronostique de la toux, de l'expectoration chronique et de valeurs spirographiques par l'étude de la mortalite chez 1,487 hommes au travail en 1960–1961. Bull. Physiopathol. Respir. 11: 45–64, 1975.

1026. Kok-Jensen, A. Simple electrocardiographic features of importance for prognosis in severe chronic bronchial obstruction. Scand. J. Respir. Dis. 56: 273–284, 1975.

1027. Kiviloog, J., Irnell, L., and Eklund, G. Course and severity of bronchial asthma and chronic bronchitis in a local Swedish population sample. Scand. J. Respir. Dis. 56: 129–137, 1975.

1028. Kiviloog, J., Irnell, L., and Eklund, G. Ventilatory capacity, working capacity, and exercise-induced bronchoconstriction in a population sample of subjects with bronchial asthma or chronic bronchitis. Scand. J. Respir. Dis. 56: 73–83, 1975.

1029. Kokkola, K. and Vuorio, M. Diurnal variation of respiratory function in patients with severe airways obstruction. Scand. J. Respir. Dis. 54: 137–141, 1973.

1030. Sawicki, F. and Twardowska, L. Mortality within a sample of an adult population in Cracow followed-up for 5 years. Bull. Physiopathol. Respir. 10: 681–697, 1974.

1031. Berry, G. Longitudinal observations. Their usefulness and limitations with special reference to the forced expiratory volume. Bull. Physiopathol. Respir. 10: 643–655, 1974.

1032. Sorbini, C-A., Casucci, G., Marchesi, N., and Muiesan, G. La mésure de la DLCO par la methode en steady-state, en estimant la PCO$_2$ par le technique de "rebreathing." In: Sadoul, P. (ed.). Le Transfert de l'Oxyde de Carbone. Soc. Eur. Physiopathol. Respir. Masson et Cie, Paris, 1969.

1033. Colomer, P. R. and Schrijen, F. Hemodynamique pulmonaire à l'exercise et puissance maximale tolerée dans les bronchopneumopathies chroniques. Bull. Physiopathol. Respir. 10: 301–314, 1974.

1034. Gimenez, M., Colomer, P. R., Hennequin, R., and Saunier, C. Hyperlactacidemie et hemodynamique pulmonaire à l'exercise modere chez les insuffisants respiratoires chroniques. Bull. Physiopathol. Respir. 10: 281–300, 1974.

1035. Fletcher, C. M. Causes and development of chronic airways obstruction and its further investigation. Bull. Physiopathol. Respir. 9: 1131–1148, 1973.

1036. Ferris, B. G. Jr. Geographic distribution of chronic bronchitis. Bull. Physiopathol. Respir. 9: 1121–1129, 1973.

1037. Zapol, W. M., Trelstad, R. L., Coffey, J. W., Tsai, I., and Salvador, R. A. Pulmonary fibrosis in severe acute respiratory failure. Am. Rev. Respir. Dis. 119: 547–554, 1979.

1038. Anthonisen, N. R., Heckscher, T., Bass, H., Oriol, A., and Bates, D. V. Studies of regional lung function in chronic bronchitis with emphysema. Bull. Physiopathol. Respir. 9: 1025–1044, 1973.

1039. Hatzfeld, C. Distribution gazeuse dans la bronchite chronique et l'emphysème pulmonaire—compartements bien et mal ventilés. Bull. Physiopathol. Respir. 9: 997–1023, 1973.

1040. Schuren, K. P. and Huttemann, U. Chronic obstructive lung disease: pulmonary circulation and right ventricular function in two different clinical types. Bull. Physiopathol. Respir. 9: 716–724, 1973.

1041. Harris, L. The discriminatory value of single breath carbon monoxide diffusion coefficient (kCO) in chronic airways obstruction. Bull. Physiopathol. Respir. 9: 473–480, 1973.

1042. Teculescu, D. B., Racoveanu, C., and Pacuraru, R. Alveolar nitrogen plateau in "bronchitic" and "emphysematous" obstructive lung disease. Scand. J. Respir. Dis. 52: 199–211, 1971.

1043. Weitzenblum, E., El Gharbi, T., Vandevenne, A., Bleger, A., Hirth, C., and Oudet, P. Pulmonary hemodynamic changes during muscular exercise in 'non-decompensated' chronic bronchitis. Bull. Physiopathol. Respir. 8: 49–71, 1972.

1044. Desmeules, M., Peslin, R., Saraiva, C., Uffholtz, H., and Sadoul, P. Propriétes statiques et dynamiques pulmonaires dans la bronchite chronique et l'emphysème. Bull. Physiopathol. Respir. 7: 395–409, 1971.

1045. Teculescu, D. B., Stanescu, D. C., and Racoveanu, C. Static mechanical properties of the lung in "bronchitic" and "emphysematous" obstructive lung disease. Bull. Physiopathol. Respir. 7: 375–393, 1971.

1046. Bignon, J., Pariente, R., and Brouet, G. Fréquence autopsique des thrombo-embolies pulmonaires au stade terminal des bronchopneumopathies chroniques obstructives. Bull. Physiopathol. Respir. 6: 405–424, 1970.

1047. Roussos, C. Respiratory muscle fatigue in the hypercapnic patient. Bull. Eur. Physiopathol. Respir. 15(Suppl.): 117–123, 1979.

1048. Rossoff, L. J., Csima, A., and Zamel, N. Reproducibility of maximum expiratory flow in severe chronic obstructive pulmonary disease. Bull. Eur. Physiopathol. Respir. 15: 1129–1136, 1979.

1049. Thiriet, M., Douguet, D., Bonnet, J. C., Canonne, C., and Hatzfeld, C. Influence du melange He-O₂ sur la mixique dans les bronchopneumopathies obstructives chroniques. Bull. Eur. Physiopathol. Respir. 15: 1053–1068, 1979.

1050. Rochester, D. F., Arora, N. S., Braun, N. M. T., and Goldberg, S. K. The respiratory muscles in chronic obstructive pulmonary disease (COPD). Bull. Eur. Physiopathol. Respir. 15: 951–975, 1979.

1051. Massin, N., Westphal, J. C., Schrijen, F., Polu, J. M., and Sadoul, P. Valeur pronostique du bilan hemodynamique des bronchiteux chroniques. Bull. Eur. Physiopathol. Respir. 15: 821–837, 1979.

1052. Zielinski, J. Intrathoracic pressure variations and pulmonary artery pressure in patients with chronic obstructive lung disease. Bull. Eur. Physiopathol. Respir. 15: 397–405, 1979.

1053. Ruhle, K. H., Fischer, J., and Matthys, H. Exercise limiting factors in patients with chronic obstructive lung disease. Bull. Eur. Physiopathol. Respir. 15: 357, 1979.

1054. Vu-Dinh, M., Lee, H. M., Vasquez, P., Shepard, J. W., and Bell, J. W. Relation of VO₂max to cardiopulmonary function in patients with chronic obstructive lung disease. Bull. Eur. Physiopathol. Respir. 15: 359–375, 1979.

1055. Lockhart, A. Facteurs limitant l'exercise dans les bronchopneumopathies obstructives chroniques. Bull. Eur. Physiopathol. Respir. 15: 305–317, 1979.

1056. Derenne, J. P., Lochon, B., Neukirch, F., Lochon, C., Despres, M., Bidart, J. M., Legrand, A., Murciano, D., and Pariente, R. Rélation entre acidose metabolique et gaz du sang à l'exercise chez les insuffisants respiratoires chroniques. Effets de l'entrainement. Bull. Eur. Physiopathol. Respir. 15: 243–257, 1979.

1057. Magnusen, H., Hartmann, V., and Holle, J. P. Decrease of PaO₂ during exercise in patients with emphysema and lung fibrosis. Evidence for different intrapulmonary diffusive resistances. Bull. Eur. Physiopathol. Respir. 15: 153–160, 1979.

1058. Smidt, U., Worth, H., and Petro, W. Ventilatory limitation of exercise in patients with chronic bronchitis and/or emphysema. Bull. Eur. Physiopathol. Respir. 15: 95–101, 1979.

1059. Grassino, A., Gross, P., Macklem, P. T., Roussos, C., and Zagelbaum, G. Inspiratory muscle fatigue as a factor limiting exercise. Bull. Eur. Physiopathol. Respir. 15: 105–111, 1979.

1060. Hannhart, B., Peslin, R., Bohadana, A., and Teculescu, D. Limitations ventilatoires de l'exercise chez le malade obstructif. Bull. Physiopathol. Respir. 15: 75–87, 1979.

1061. Sergysels, R., Degre, S., Garcia-Herreros, P., Willeput, R., and De Coster, A. Le profil ventilatoire à l'exercise dans les bronchopathies chroniques obstructives. Bull. Eur. Physiopathol. Respir. 15: 57–70, 1979.

1062. Schaanning, J. Respiratory cycle time duration during exercise in patients with chronic obstructive lung disease. Scand. J. Respir. Dis. 59: 313–318, 1978.

1063. Rasmussen, F. V., Borchsenius, L., Winslow, J. B., and Ostergaard, E. R. Associations between housing conditions, smoking habits and ventilatory lung function in men with clean jobs. Scand. J. Respir. Dis. 59: 264–276, 1978.

1064. Mossberg, B., Philipson, K., and Camner, P. Tracheobronchial clearance in patients with emphysema associated with alpha₁-antitrypsin deficiency. Scand. J. Respir. Dis. 59: 1–7, 1978.

1065. Hale, T., Cumming, G., and Spriggs, J. The effects of physical training in chronic obstructive pulmonary disease. Bull. Eur. Physiopathol. Respir. 14: 593–608, 1978.

1066. Stanescu, D. C., Veriter, C., and Brasseur, L. Airway conductance: the most sensitive index of abnormality in long-term smokers. Bull. Eur. Physiopathol. Respir. 14: 383–399, 1978.

1067. Girard, F., Aug, F., Camara, M., Bohadana, A. B., Bagrel, A., Museur, G., and Abraham, S. Bilan pulmonaire et deficit heterozygote en alpha₁-antitrypsin au sein d'une population active générale. Bull. Eur. Physiopathol. Respir. 14: 11–22, 1978.

1068. Kok-Jensen, A. and Ebbehoj, K. Prognosis of chronic obstructive lung disease in relation to radiology and electrocardiogram. Scand. J. Respir. Dis. 58: 304–310, 1977.

1069. Schrijen, F. and Jezek, V. Haemodynamics and pulmonary wedge angiography findings in chronic bronchopulmonary disease. Scand. J. Respir. Dis. 58: 151–158, 1977.

1070. Kabondo, P. and Orehek, J. Reversibilité de l'obstruction bronchique dans l'asthme et bronchite chronique. Bull. Eur. Physiopathol. Respir. 13: 829–836, 1977.

1071. Shephard, R. J. On the design and effectiveness of training regimes in chronic obstructive lung disease. Bull. Eur. Physiopathol. Respir. 13: 457–469, 1977.

1072. Teculescu, D., Manicatide, M., and Racoveanu, C. Ventilatory impairment and hypoxemia in chronic non-specific lung disease. Bull. Eur. Physiopathol. Respir. 13: 445–455, 1977.

1073. Degre, S., Sergysels, R., De Coster, A., Denolin, H., and Degre-Coustry, C. Effets thérapeutiques de l'entrainement physique chez les patients en insuffisance respiratoire chronique. Bull. Eur. Physiopathol. Respir. 13: 445–455, 1977.

1074. Brown, H. V., Wasserman, K., and Whipp, B. J. Strategies of exercise testing in chronic lung disease. Bull. Eur. Physiopathol. Respir. 13: 409–423, 1977.

1075. Denolin, H. Exercise et pneumopathies chroniques. Bull. Eur. Physiopathol. Respir. 13: 325–328, 1977.

1076. Smidt, U. Emphysema as a possible explanation for the alteration of expiratory PO₂ and PCO₂ curves. Bull. Eur. Physiopathol. Respir. 12: 605–624, 1976.

1077. Parent, J. G., Schrijen, F., and Viana, R. A. Indices radiologiques d'hypertension pulmonaire dans la maladie obstructive chronique. Bull. Eur. Physiopathol. Respir. 12: 637–650, 1976.

1078. Delaunois, L., Lulling, J., and Prignot, J. Diagnostic differentiel des bronchopneumopathies obstructives chroniques. Bull. Eur. Pathophysiol. Respir. 12: 453–466, 1976.

1079. Oxhoj, H., Bake, B., and Wilhelmsen, L. Spirometry and flow-volume curves in 10-year follow up in men born 1913. Scand. J. Respir. Dis. 57: 310–312, 1976.

1080. Larsson, C., Dirksen, H., Sundstrom, G., and Eriksson, S. Lung function studies in asymptomatic individuals with moderately (PiSZ) and severely (PiZ) reduced levels of alpha₁-antitrypsin. Scand. J. Respir. Dis. 57: 267–280, 1976.

1081. Spiro, S. G., Hahn, H. L., Edwards, R. H. T., and Pride, N. B. Cardiorespiratory adaptations at the start of exercise in normal subjects and in patients with chronic obstructive bronchitis. Clin. Sci. 47: 165–172, 1974.

1082. Hughes, J. M. B., Grant, B. J. B., Greene, R. E., Iliff, L. D., and Milic-Emili, J. Inspiratory flow rate and ventilation distribution in normal subjects and in patients with simple chronic bronchitis. Clin. Sci. 43: 583–595, 1972.

1083. Ramsey, J. M. Carbon monoxide, tissue hypoxia, and sensory psychomotor response in hypoxemic subjects. Clin. Sci. 42: 619–625, 1972.

1084. Cayton, R. M. and Howard, P. Peripheral airways resistance, static recoil and the forced expiratory volume. Clin. Sci. 42: 505–514, 1972.

1085. Sutinen, S., Paakko, P., Lohela, P., and Lahti, R. Pattern recognition in radiographs of excised air-inflated lungs. IV. Emphysema alone and with other common lesions. Eur. J. Respir. Dis. 62: 297–314, 1981.

1086. Cutillo, A., Bigler, A. H., Perondi, R., Turiel, M., Watanabe, S., and Renzetti, A. D. Jr. Exercise and distribution of inspired gas in patients with obstructive lung disease. Bull. Eur. Physiopathol. Respir. 17: 891–901, 1981.

1087. Anderson, L. H. and Rasmussen, F. V. Underestimation of closing volume with increase in airflow obstruction. Bull. Eur. Physiopathol. Respir. 17: 823–836, 1981.

1088. Gelb, A. F. and Zamel, N. Lung recoil and density dependence of maximum expiratory flow in emphysema. Bull. Eur. Physiopathol. Respir. 17: 793–798, 1981.

1089. Sergysels, R., Van Meerhaege, A., Scano, G., Denaut, M., Willeput, R., Messin, R., and De Coster, A. Respiratory drive during exercise in chronic obstructive lung disease. Bull. Eur. Physiopathol. Respir. 17: 755–766, 1981.

1090. Ameille, J., Chambille, B., Orvoen-Frija, E., Jacquemin, C., and Rochemaure, J. Entrainement sur tapis roulant chez des insuffisants respiratoires chroniques obstructifs. Bull. Eur. Physiopathol. Respir. 17: 741–753, 1981.

1091. Ravez, P., Kaminsky, P., Chau, N., Schrijen, F., and Sadoul, P. Bilan hémodynamique dans la bronchite chronique peu avancée. Bull. Eur. Physiopathol. Respir. 17: 351–363, 1981.

1092. Huhti, E. and Ikkala, J. A 10-year follow-up study of respiratory symptoms and ventilatory function in a middle-aged rural population. Eur. J. Respir. Dis. 61: 33–45, 1980.

1093. Staub, N. C. and Conhaim, R. L. An anatomical basis for very low ventilation/perfusion units in the lung. In: Piiper, J. and Scheid, P. (eds.). Progress in Respiration Research, Vol. 16. S. Karger, Basel, 1981.

1094. Anderson, S. D., Connolly, N. M., and Godfrey, S. Comparison of bronchoconstriction induced by cycling and running. Thorax 26: 396–401, 1971.

1095. Hutchison, D. C. S. A survey of alpha₁-antitrypsin deficiency by the British Thoracic Association. Bull. Eur. Physiopathol. Respir. 16(Suppl.): 315–319, 1980.

1096. Smidt, U., Worth, H., and Busch, A. Limitation of ergometric work and respiratory muscle fatigue Bull. Eur. Physiopathol. Respir. 16: 211P–212P, 1980.

1097. Kanaev, N. N. and Laskin, G. M. Clinical significance of the ratio between breath-holding and steady-state diffusing capacity in patients with chronic bronchitis and diffuse lung fibrosis. Bull. Eur. Physiopathol. Respir. 16: 521–532, 1980.

1098. Lavender, J. P. and Cunningham, D. A. Clinical value of krypton-81M and technetium-99M perfusion lung scanning. Bull. Eur. Physiopathol. Respir. 16: 309–320, 1980.

1099. Harf, A. and Meignan, M. Le calcul des rapports ventilationperfusion pulmonaires regionaux: une aide au diagnostic des embolies pulmonaires. Bull. Eur. Physiopathol. Respir. 16: 299–308, 1980.

1100. Vandevenne, A., Weitzenblum, E., Moyses, B., Durin, M., and Rasaholinjanahary, J. Modifications de la fonction pulmonaire regionale au cours de la ventilation abdomino-diaphragmatique a frequence basse et grand volume courant. Bull. Eur. Physiopathol. Respir. 16: 171–184, 1980.

1101. Gulsvik, A. Prevalence and manifestations of obstructive lung disease in the city of Oslo. Scand. J. Respir. Dis. 60: 286–296, 1979.

1102. Gulsvik, A. Prevalence of respiratory symptoms in the city of Oslo. Scand. J. Respir. Dis. 60: 275–285, 1979.

1103. Gulsvik, A. and Fagerhol, M. K. Alpha₁-antitrypsin phenotypes and obstructive lung disease in the city of Oslo. Scand. J. Respir. Dis. 60: 267–274, 1979.

1104. Andersen, J. B., Dragsted, L., Kann, T., Johansen, S. H., Nielsen, K. B., Karbo, E., and Bentzen, L. Resistive breathing training in severe chronic obstructive pulmonary disease. Scand. J. Respir. Dis. 60: 151–156, 1979.

1105. Weitzenblum, E., Muzet, A., Erhart, M., Sautegeau, A., and Weber, L. Variations nocturnes des gaz du sang et de la pression arterielle pulmonaire chez les bronchitiques chroniques insuffisants respiratoire. Nouv. Presse Med. 11: 1119–1122, 1982.

1106. Pieler, R. Deutung simultaner pulmonaler ein-und Auswashkurven von Helium, Argon und Schwefelhexafluorid. Atemwegs und Lungenkrankheiten 6: 28–29, 1980.

1107. Semple, P. D. A., Reid, C. B., and Thompson, W. D. Widespread panacinar emphysema with alpha₁-antitrypsin deficiency. Br. J. Dis. Chest 74: 289–295, 1980.

1108. Bradley, B. L., Forman, J. W., and Miller, W. C. Lowdensity gas breathing during exercise in chronic obstructive lung disease. Respiration 40: 311–316, 1980.

1109. Wanner, A., Hirsch, J. A., Greeneltch, D. E., Swenson, E. W., and Fore, T. Tracheal mucous velocity in beagles after chronic exposure to cigarette smoke. Arch. Environ. Health 27: 370–371, 1973.

1110. Rizzatto, G., Ferrara, A., Bertoli, L., Merlini, R., and Mantero, O. Relationship between chronic $PaCO_2$ and total body buffering capacity in patients with chronic obstructive lung disease. Respiration 39: 206–212, 1980.

1111. Dutu, S., Jienescu, Z., and Baicoianu, S. Etude epidemiologique de la bronchite chronique dans une population agée de 60 à 85 ans. Respiration 39: 49–59, 1980.

1112. Sergysels, R., De Coster, A., Degre, S., and Denolin, H. Functional evaluation of a physical rehabilitation program including breathing exercises and bicycle training in chronic obstructive lung disease. Respiration 38: 105–111, 1979.

1113. Magnussen, H., Holle, J. P., Hartmann, V., and Schoenen, J. D. Dco at various breath-holding times: comparison in patients with chronic bronchial asthma and emphysema. Respiration 37: 177–184, 1979.

1114. Bohadana, A. B., Peslin, R., Uffholtz, H., and Girard, F.

Profil clinique et fonctionel pulmonaire d'homozygotes (PiZ) deficitaires en alpha₁ antitrypsine. Respiration 37: 167–176, 1979.

1115. Weitzenblum, E., Hirth, C., Parini, J. P., Rasaholinjanahary, J., and Oudet, P. Clinical, functional and pulmonary hemodynamic course of patients with chronic obstructive pulmonary disease followed-up over 3 years. Respiration 36: 1–9, 1979.

1116. Devos, P., Demedts, M., Vandercruys, A., Cosemans, J., and De Roo, M. Comparison of ¹³³Xe washout curves after bolus inhalation, perfusion, and equilibration. Respiration 35: 115–121, 1978.

1117. Rampulla, C., Rizzato, G., Mantero, O., Benza, G. C., Scacciante, L., and Morpurgo, M. Regional lung perfusion and pulmonary artery pressure in chronic obstructive lung disease. Respiration 33: 372–380, 1976.

1118. Neukirch, F., Du Perron, M. C., Verdier, F., Legrand, M., Breant, J., Fleury, M. F., Marion, C., and Drutel, P. Etude statistique des correlations entre les criteres spirographiques et les pressions partielles d'oxygene et d'anhydride carbonique dans le sang arteriel. Respiration 32: 165–178, 1975.

1119. Rufener-Press, C., Rey, P., and Press, P. Une étude epidemiologique de la bronchite chronique à Génève. Respiration 30: 458–516, 1973.

1120. Neukirch, F., Breant, J., Fleury, M. F., Marion, C., Du Perron, M. C., Verdier, F., Legrand, M., and Drutel, P. Etude statistique des correlations entre les criteres spirographiques et les pressions partielles d'oxygene et d'anhydride carbonique dans le sang arteriel. Respiration 34: 285–294, 1977.

1121. Teculescu, D. B., Racoveanu, C., and Manicatide, M. M. Transfer factor for the lung and the 'emphysema score.' Respiration 30: 311–328, 1973.

1122. Weitzenblum, E., Vandevenne, A., Hirth, C., Parini, J. P., Roeslin, N., and Oudet, P. L'hemodynamique pulmonaire au cours de l'exercise musculaire chez les bronchiteux chroniques. Respiration 30: 64–88, 1973.

1123. Parot, S., Saunier, C., Gautier, H., Milic-Emili, J., and Sadoul, P. Breathing pattern and hypercapnia in patients with chronic obstructive pulmonary disease. Am. Rev. Respir. Dis. 121: 985–991, 1980.

1124. Colebatch, H. J. H. and Greaves, I. A. Exponential analysis of lung elastic behaviour (letter to editor). Am. Rev. Respir. Dis. 121: 898, 1980.

1125. Astin, T. W. Airways obstruction and arterial blood gas tensions in chronic obstructive lung disease. Respiration 29: 74–82, 1972.

1126. Weitzenblum, E., Roeslin, N., and Hirth, C. Mésures de mecanique ventilatoire dans la bronchite chronique et l'emphysème evolués. Etude comparative. Poumon Coeur 34: 27–35, 1978.

1127. Kreukniet, J. Death rate and pulmonary function in patients with chronic non-specific lung disease (CNSLD) after a 10-year follow-up. Respiration 28: 314–330, 1971.

1128. Weitzenblum, E., Rasaholinjanahary, J., Meyer, P. D., Hirth, C., and Oudet, P. Evolution clinique, fonctionelle et hemodynamique de bronchiteux chronique au stade du "coeur pulmonaire chronique." Poumon Coeur 32: 299–305, 1976.

1129. Yernault, J-C., Robience, Y., Denaut, M., De Coster, A., and Englert, M. Distribution régionale de la ventilation et de la perfusion dans les broncho-pneumopathies chroniques debutantes. Poumon Coeur 31: 241–248, 1975.

1130. Bignon, J. and Depierre, A. L'obstruction des petits voies aeriennes: essai de correlations structure-fonction. Poumon Coeur 31: 233–240, 1975.

1131. Milne, J. S. and Williamson, J. Respiratory symptoms and smoking habits in older people with age and sex differences. Respiration 29: 359–370, 1972.

1132. Postma, D. S. and Sluiter, H. J. Predictors of mortality in chronic obstructive pulmonary disease (letter to editor). Am. Rev. Respir. Dis. 121: 1056–1057, 1980.

1133. Sergysels, R., Etien, J-L., Schandevyl, W., and Hennebert, A. Le comportement à l'effort des patients atteints de bronchopneumopathie obstructive au stade d'hypoxie et d'hypercapnie chroniques. Poumon Coeur 31: 35–45, 1975.

1134. Third International Symposium on Asthma and Chronic Bronchitis in Children and Their Prognosis into Adult Life, Davos, 1969. Respiration 27(Suppl.): 1970.

1135. Weitzenblum, E., Roeslin, N., Hirth, C., and Oudet, P. Etude comparative des données cliniques et de la fonction respiratoire entre la bronchite chronique et l'emphyseme "primitif." Respiration 27: 493–510, 1970.

1136. Belman, M. J. and Mittman, C. Ventilatory muscle training improves exercise capacity in chronic obstructive pulmonary disease patients. Am. Rev. Respir. Dis. 121: 273–280, 1980.

1137. Greaves, I. A. and Colebatch, H. J. H. Elastic behaviour and structure of normal and emphysematous lungs postmortem. Am. Rev. Respir. Dis. 121: 127–136, 1980.

1138. Littner, M. R., McGinty, D. J., and Arand, D. L. Determinants of oxygen desaturation in the course of ventilation during sleep in chronic obstructive pulmonary disease. Am. Rev. Respir. Dis. 122: 849–857, 1980.

1139. Fleetham, J. A., Mezon, B., West, P., Bradley, C. A., Anthonisen, N. R., and Kryger, M. H. Chemical control of ventilation and sleep arterial oxygen desaturation in patients with COPD. Am. Rev. Respir. Dis. 122: 583–589, 1980.

1140. Thurlbeck, M. W. Smoking, airflow limitation, and the pulmonary circulation (editorial). Am. Rev. Respir. Dis. 122: 183–186, 1980.

1141. Fleetham, J. A. and Kryger, M. H. Sleep disorders in chronic airflow obstruction. In: Mathay, R. A. (ed.). Chronic Obstructive Lung Diseases. Med. Clin. North Am. 65: 549–561, 1981.

1142. Fanta, C. H. and Ingram, R. H. Jr. Airway responsiveness and chronic airway obstruction. In: Matthay, R. A. (ed.). Chronic Obstructive Lung Diseases. Med. Clin. North Am. 65: 473–487, 1981.

1143. Burrows, B. An overview of obstructive lung diseases. In: Matthay, R. A. (ed.). Chronic Obstructive Lung Diseases. Med. Clin. North Am. 65: 455–471, 1981.

1144. Pardy, R. L., Rivington, R. N., Despas, P. J., and Macklem, P. T. The effects of inspiratory muscle training on exercise performance in chronic airflow limitation. Am. Rev. Respir. Dis. 123: 426–433, 1981.

1145. Pardy, R. L., Rivington, R. N., Despas, P. J., and Macklem, P. T. Inspiratory muscle training compared with physiotherapy in patients with chronic airflow limitation. Am. Rev. Respir. Dis. 123: 421–425, 1981.

1146. Irwin, R. S., Corrao, W. M., and Pratter, M. R. Chronic persistent cough in the adult: the spectrum and frequency of causes and successful outcome of specific therapy. Am. Rev. Respir. Dis. 123: 413–417, 1981.

1147. Belman, M. J. and Kendregan, B. A. Exercise training fails to increase skeletal muscle enzymes in patients with chronic obstructive pulmonary disease. Am. Rev. Respir. Dis. 123: 256–261, 1981.

1148. Petty, T. L., Silvers, G. W., and Stanford, R. E. Functional correlations with mild and moderate emphysema in excised human lungs. Am. Rev. Respir. Dis. 124: 700–704, 1981.

1149. Berend, N. Lobar distribution of bronchiolar inflammation in emphysema. Am. Rev. Respir. Dis. 124: 218–220, 1981.

1150. Grimby, G. and Stiksa, J. Flow-volume curves and breathing patterns during exercise in patients with obstructive lung disease. Scand. J. Clin. Lab. Invest. 25: 303–313, 1970.

1151. Madison, R., Mittman, C., Afifi, A. A., and Zelman, R. Risk factors for obstructive lung disease. Am. Rev. Respir. Dis. 124: 149–153, 1981.

1152. Bignon, J. Bronchite Chronique et Emphyseme: Mechanismes, Clinique, Traitement. Flammarion Medicine-Sciences, Paris, 1982.

1153. Cochrane, G. M., Prior, J. G., and Wolff, C. B. Respiratory arterial pH and PCO_2 oscillations in patients with chronic obstructive airways disease. Clin. Sci. 61: 693–702, 1981.

1154. Garrard, C. S. and Lane, D. J. The pattern of breathing in patients with chronic airflow obstruction. Clin. Sci. 56: 215–221, 1979.

1155. Schrijen, F. and Jezek, V. Hemodynamic variables during repeated exercise in chronic lung disease. Clin. Sci. 55: 485–490, 1978.

1156. Eiser, N. M., Jones, H. A., and Hughes, J. M. B. Effect of 30% oxygen on local matching of perfusion and ventilation in chronic airways obstruction. Clin. Sci. 53: 387–395, 1977.

1157. Ferris, B. G. Epidemiology standardisation project. Am. Rev. Respir. Dis. 118(Suppl.): 120, 1978.

1158. Pinuera, R. F., Woolcock, A. J., Green, W., and Crockett, A. J. Pulmonary function in alpha$_1$-antitrypsin deficiency. Aust. N.Z. J. Med. 2: 159–167, 1972.

1159. Mittman, C. The PiMZ phenotype: is it a significant risk factor for the development of chronic obstructive lung disease? (editorial). Am. Rev. Respir. Dis. 118: 649–652, 1978.

1160. Golden, J. A., Nadel, J. A., and Boushey, H. A. Bronchial hyperirritability in healthy subjects after exposure to ozone. Am. Rev. Respir. Dis. 118: 287–294, 1978.

1161. Bradley, B. L., Garner, A. E., Billu, D., Mestas, J. M., and Forman, J. Oxygen-assisted exercise in chronic obstructive lung disease. Am. Rev. Respir. Dis. 118: 239–243, 1978.

1162. Kosarevic, D., Laban, M., Budimir, M., Vojvodic, N., Roberts, A., Gordon, T., and McGee, D. L. Intermediate alpha$_1$-antitrypsin deficiency and chronic obstructive pulmonary disease in Yugoslavia. Am. Rev. Respir. Dis. 117: 1039–1043, 1978.

1163. Mithoefer, J. C., Ramirez, C., and Cook, W. The effect of mixed venous oxygenation on arterial blood in chronic obstructive pulmonary disease. Am. Rev. Respir. Dis. 117: 259–264, 1978.

1164. Chan-Yeung, M., Ashley, M. J., Corey, P., and Maledy, H. Pi phenotypes and the prevalence of chest symptoms and lung function abnormalities in workers employed in dusty industries. Am. Rev. Respir. Dis. 117: 239–245, 1978.

1165. Leaver, D. G., Tattersfield, A. E., and Pride, N. B. Contributions of loss of lung recoil and of enhanced airways collapsibility to the airflow obstruction of chronic bronchitis and emphysema. J. Clin. Invest. 52: 2117–2128, 1973.

1166. Galdston, M., Melnick, E. L., Goldring, R. M., Levytska, V., Curasi, C. A., and Davis, A. L. Interactions of neutrophil elastase, serum trypsin inhibitory activity, and smoking history as risk factors for chronic obstructive pulmonary disease in patients with MM, MZ, and ZZ phenotypes for alpha$_1$-antitrypsin. Am. Rev. Respir. Dis. 116: 837–846, 1977.

1167. Higgins, M. W., Keller, J. B., and Metzner, H. L. Smoking, socioeconomic status, and chronic respiratory disease. Am. Rev. Respir. Dis. 116: 403–410, 1977.

1168. Niewohner, D. E. and Kleinerman, J. Morphometric study of elastic fibers in normal and emphysematous human lungs. Am. Rev. Respir. Dis. 115: 15–21, 1977.

1169. Lertzman, M. M. and Cherniack, R. M. Rehabilitation of patients with chronic obstructive pulmonary disease. Am. Rev. Respir. Dis. 114: 1145–1165, 1976.

1170. Shigeoka, J. W., Hall, W. J., Hyde, R. W., Schwartz, R. H., Mudholkar, G. S., Speers, D. M., and Lin, C-C. The prevalence of alpha$_1$-antitrypsin heterozygotes (Pi MZ) in patients with obstructive pulmonary disease. Am. Rev. Respir. Dis. 114: 1077–1084, 1976.

1171. Rawlings, W. Jr., Kreiss, P., Levy, D., Cohen, B., Menkes, H., Brashears, S., and Permutt, S. Clinical, epidemiologic, and pulmonary function studies in alpha$_1$-antitrypsin-deficient subjects of Pi Z type. Am. Rev. Respir. Dis. 114: 945–953, 1976.

1172. Anderson, H. R. Respiratory abnormalities and ventilatory capacity in a Papua New Guinea island community. Am. Rev. Respir. Dis. 114: 537–548, 1976.

1173. Tager, I. B., Rosner, B., Tishler, P. V., Speizer, F. E., and Kass, E. H. Household aggregation of pulmonary function and chronic bronchitis. Am. Rev. Respir. Dis. 114: 485–492, 1976.

1174. Butler, C. Lung surface area in various morphologic forms of human emphysema. Am. Rev. Respir. Dis. 114: 347–352, 1976.

1175. Dosman, J., Bode, F., Ghezzo, R. H., Martin, R., and Macklem, P. T. The relationship between symptoms and functional abnormalities in clinically healthy cigarette smokers. Am. Rev. Respir. Dis. 114: 297–304, 1976.

1176. Butler, C. Diaphragmatic changes in emphysema. Am. Rev. Respir. Dis. 114: 155–159, 1976.

1177. Lebowitz, M. D. and Burrows, B. Comparison of questionnaires: the BMRC and NHLI respiratory questionnaires and a new self-completion questionnaire. Am. Rev. Respir. Dis. 113: 627–635, 1976.

1178. Cox, D. W., Hoeppner, V. H., and Levison, H. Protease

inhibitors in patients with chronic obstructive pulmonary disease: the alpha$_1$-antitrypsin heterozygote controversy. Am. Rev. Respir. Dis. 113: 601–606, 1976.

1179. Musk, A. W. and Robertson, P. W. Pulmonary elastic recoil and diffusing capacity in subjects with intermediate concentrations of alpha-1 antitrypsin. Aust. N. Z. J. Med. 6: 284–287, 1976.

1180. Mork, T. Bronchitis in the United Kingdom and the United States of America. J. Chron. Dis. 23: 345–350, 1970.

1181. Haenszel, W. and Hougen, A. Prevalence of respiratory symptoms in Norway. J. Chron. Dis. 25: 519–544, 1972.

1182. Schlesselman, J. J. Planning a longitudinal study: II. Frequency of measurement and study duration. J. Chron. Dis. 26: 561–570, 1973.

1183. Higgins, M. and Keller, J. Familial occurrence of chronic respiratory disease and familial resemblance in ventilatory capacity. J. Chron. Dis. 28: 239–251, 1975.

1184. Burrows, B. and Lebowitz, M. D. Characteristics of chronic bronchitis in a warm, dry region. Am. Rev. Respir. Dis. 112: 365–370, 1975.

1185. Thurlbeck, W. M., Malaka, D., and Murphy, K. Goblet cells in the peripheral airways in chronic bronchitis. Am. Rev. Respir. Dis. 112: 65–69, 1975.

1186. Klayton, R., Fallat, R., and Cohen, A. B. Determinants of chronic obstructive pulmonary disease in patients with intermediate levels of alpha$_1$-antitrypsin. Am. Rev. Respir. Dis. 112: 71–75, 1975.

1187. Barnett, T. B., Gottovi, D., and Johnson, A. M. Protease inhibitors in chronic obstructive pulmonary disease. Am. Rev. Respir. Dis. 111: 587–593, 1975.

1188. Abboud, R. T. and Morton, J. W. Comparison of maximal mid-expiratory flow, flow volume curves, and nitrogen closing volumes in patients with mild airway obstruction. Am. Rev. Respir. Dis. 111: 405–417, 1975.

1189. Ebert, R. V. and Terracio, M. J. The bronchiolar epithelium in cigarette smokers. Am. Rev. Respir. Dis. 111: 4–11, 1975.

1190. Niewohner, D. E., Knoke, J. D., and Kleinerman, J. Peripheral airways as a determinant of ventilatory function in the human lung. J. Clin. Invest. 60: 139–151, 1977.

1191. Wehr, K. L. and Johnson, R. L. Jr. Maximal oxygen consumption in patients with lung disease. J. Clin. Invest. 58: 880–890, 1976.

1192. Hall, W. J., Hyde, R. W., Schwartz, R. H., Mudholkar, G. S., Webb, D. R., Chaubey, Y. P., and Townes, P. L. Pulmonary abnormalities in intermediate alpha-1-antitrypsin deficiency. J. Clin. Invest. 58: 1069–1077, 1976.

1193. Cooper, D. M., Hoeppner, V., Cox, D., Zamel, N., Bryan, A. C., and Levison, H. Lung function in alpha$_1$-antitrypsin heterozygotes (Pi type MZ). Am. Rev. Respir. Dis. 110: 708–715, 1974.

1194. Degre, S., Sergysels, R., Messin, R., Vandermoten, P., Salhadin, P., Denolin, H., and De Coster, A. Hemodynamic responses to physical training in patients with chronic lung disease. Am. Rev. Respir. Dis. 110: 395–402, 1974.

1195. Thurlbeck, W. M., Pun, R., Toth, J., and Frazer, R. G. Bronchial cartilage in chronic obstructive lung disease. Am. Rev. Respir. Dis. 109: 73–80, 1974.

1196. Boushy, S. F., Thompson, H. K. Jr., North, L. B., Beale, A. R., and Snow, T. R. Prognosis in chronic obstructive pulmonary disease. Am. Rev. Respir. Dis. 108: 1373–1383, 1973.

1197. Bates, D. V. The fate of the chronic bronchitic: a report of the ten-year follow-up in the Canadian Department of Veteran's Affairs coordinated study of chronic bronchitis. Am. Rev. Respir. Dis. 108: 1043–1065, 1973.

1198. Boushy, S. F., North, L. B., and Fagan, T. J. The role of parenchymal and airway disease in limiting forced expiratory flows in chronic obstructive pulmonary disease. Am. Rev. Respir. Dis. 108: 870–878, 1973.

1199. Ishikawa, S. and Hayes, J. A. Functional morphometry of the diaphragm in patients with chronic obstructive lung disease. Am. Rev. Respir. Dis. 108: 135–138, 1973.

1200. Lanyi, M. Classification of chronic obstructive pulmonary diseases (letter to editor). Am. Rev. Respir. Dis. 107: 1076, 1973.

1201. Weibel, E. A simplified morphometric method for estimating diffusing capacity in normal and emphysematous human lungs. Am. Rev. Respir. Dis. 107: 579–588, 1973.

1202. Matsuba, K. and Thurlbeck, W. M. Disease of the small airways in chronic bronchitis. Am. Rev. Respir. Dis. 107: 552–558, 1973.

1203. Gelb, A. F., Gold, W. M., Wright, R. R., Bruch, H. R., and Nadel, J. A. Physiologic diagnosis of subclinical emphysema. Am. Rev. Respir. Dis. 107: 50–65, 1973.

1204. Kass, I., O'Brien, L. E., Zamel, N., and Dyksterhuis, J. E. Lack of correlation between clinical background and pulmonary function tests in patients with chronic obstructive pulmonary diseases. Am. Rev. Respir. Dis. 107: 64–69, 1973.

1205. Knudson, R. J., Mead, J., Goldman, M. D., Schwaber, J. R., and Wohl, M. E. The failure of indirect indices of elastic lung recoil. Am. Rev. Respir. Dis. 107: 70–82, 1973.

1206. Kass, I. A way to classify chronic obstructive pulmonary disease (letter to editor). Am. Rev. Respir. Dis. 106: 622–623, 1972.

1207. Ostrow, D. N. and Cherniack, R. M. The mechanical properties of the lungs in intermediate deficiency of alpha$_1$-antitrypsin. Am. Rev. Respir. Dis. 106: 377–383, 1972.

1208. Black, L. F., Hyatt, R. E., and Stubbs, S. E. Mechanism of expiratory airflow limitation in chronic obstructive pulmonary disease associated with alpha$_1$-antitrypsin deficiency. Am. Rev. Respir. Dis. 105: 891–899, 1972.

1209. Jain, B. P., Pande, J. N., and Guleria, J. S. Membrane diffusing capacity and pulmonary capillary blood volume in chronic obstructive lung disease. Am. Rev. Respir. Dis. 105: 900–907, 1972.

1210. Ingram, R. H. Jr., Miller, R. B., and Tate, L. A. Ventilatory response to carbon dioxide and to exercise in relation to the pathophysiologic type of chronic obstructive pulmonary disease. Am. Rev. Respir. Dis. 105: 541–551, 1972.

1211. Marcus, J. H., Ingram, R. H. Jr., and McLean, R. L. The threshold of anaerobic metabolism in chronic obstructive pulmonary disease. Am. Rev. Respir. Dis. 104: 490–498, 1971.

1212. Matsuba, K. and Thurlbeck, W. M. The number and dimensions of small airways in nonemphysematous lungs. Am. Rev. Respir. Dis. 104: 516–524, 1971.

1213. Takizawa, T. and Thurlbeck, W. M. Muscle and mucous gland size in the major bronchi of patients with chronic bronchitis, asthma, and asthmatic bronchitis. Am. Rev. Respir. Dis. 104: 331–336, 1971.

1214. Takizawa, T. and Thurlbeck, W. M. A comparison of four methods of assessing the morphologic changes in chronic bronchitis. Am. Rev. Respir. Dis. 103: 774–783, 1971.

1215. Jones, N. L., Jones, G., and Edwards, R. H. T. Exercise tolerance in chronic airway disease. Am. Rev. Respir. Dis. 103: 477–491, 1971.

1216. Stone, D. J., Keltz, H., and Samortin, T. The effect of beta-adrenergic inhibition on respiratory gas exchange and lung function. Am. Rev. Respir. Dis. 103: 503–508, 1971.

1217. Vyas, M. N., Banister, E. W., Morton, J. W., and Grzybowski, S. Response to exercise in patients with chronic airway obstruction I. Effects of exercise training. Am. Rev. Respir. Dis. 103: 390–400, 1971.

1218. Vyas, M. N., Banister, E. W., Morton, J. W., and Grzbowski, S. Response to exercise in patients with chronic airway obstruction II. Effects of breathing 40 per cent oxygen. Am. Rev. Respir. Dis. 103: 401–412, 1971.

1219. Tammeling, G. J., Sluiter, H. J., Hilvering, C., and Berg, W. C. Transpulmonary pressure at full inspiration and dynamics of the airways in patients with obstructive lung disease. Am. Rev. Respir. Dis. 103: 38–48, 1971.

1220. Falk, G. A., Siskind, G. W., and Smith, J. P. Jr. Chronic obstructive pulmonary disease: a subgroup of patients identified by serum alpha$_1$-antitrypsin and immunoglobulin concentrations. Am. Rev. Respir. Dis. 103: 18–25, 1971.

1221. Tulou, P. P. and Walsh, P. M. Measurement of alveolar carbon dioxide tension at maximal expiration as an estimate of arterial carbon dioxide tension in patients with airway obstruction. Am. Rev. Respir. Dis. 102: 921–926, 1970.

1222. Park, S. S., Janis, M., Shim, C. S., and Williams, M. H. Jr. Relationship of bronchitis and emphysema to altered pulmonary function. Am. Rev. Respir. Dis. 102: 927–936, 1970.

1223. Butler, C. II and Kleinerman, J. Capillary density: alveolar diameter, a morphometric approach to ventilation and perfusion. Am. Rev. Respir. Dis. 102: 886–894, 1970.

1224. Deutscher, S. and Higgins, M. W. The relationship of parental longevity to ventilatory function and prevalence of chronic nonspecific respiratory disease among sons. Am. Rev. Respir. Dis. 102: 180–189, 1970.

1225. Nicholas, J. J., Gilbert, R., Gabe, R., and Auchincloss, J. H. Jr. Evaluation of an exercise program for patients with chronic obstructive pulmonary disease. Am. Rev. Respir. Dis. 102: 1–9, 1970.

1226. Morse, J. O. Alpha₁-antitrypsin deficiency. N. Engl. J. Med. 299: 1045–1048, 1099–1105, 1978.

1227. Knudson, R. J. Familial emphysema discovered by James Jackson, Jr. (letter to editor). N. Engl. J. Med. 300: 374, 1979.

1228. Morse, J. O., Lebowitz, M. D., Knudson, R. J., and Burrows, B. Relation of protease inhibitor phenotypes to obstructive lung diseases in a community. N. Engl. J. Med. 296: 1190–1194, 1977.

1229. Morse, J. O., Lebowitz, M. D., Knudson, R. J., and Burrows, B. A community study of the relation of alpha₁-antitrypsin levels to obstructive lung diseases. N. Engl. J. Med. 292: 278–281, 1975.

1230. Burrows, B., Kettel, L. J., Niden, A. H., Rabinowitz, M., and Diener, C. F. Patterns of cardiovascular dysfunction in chronic obstructive lung disease. N. Engl. J. Med. 286: 912–918, 1972.

1231. Auerbach, O., Hammond, E. C., Garfinkel, L., and Benante, C. Relation of smoking and age to emphysema. N. Engl. J. Med. 286: 853–857, 1972.

1232. Colp, C., Park, S. S., and Williams, M. H. Jr. Emphysema with little airway obstruction. Am. Rev. Respir. Dis. 101: 615–619, 1970.

1233. Anderson, A. E. Jr., Furlaneto, J. A., and Foraker, A. G. Bronchopulmonary derangements in nonsmokers. Am. Rev. Respir. Dis. 101: 518–527, 1970.

1234. Penman, R. W. B., O'Neill, R. P., and Begley, L. Lung elastic recoil and airway resistance as factors limiting forced expiratory flow. Am. Rev. Respir. Dis. 101: 528–535, 1970.

1235. Barter, C. E., Campbell, A. H., and Tandon, M. K. Factors affecting the decline of FEV₁ in chronic bronchitis. Aust. N.Z. J. Med. 4: 339–345, 1974.

1236. Kearley, R., Wynne, J. W., Block, A. J., Boysen, P. G., Lindsey, S., and Martin, C. The effect of low flow oxygen on sleep-disordered breathing and oxygen desaturation. Chest 78: 682–685, 1980.

1237. Olvey, S. K., Reduto, L. A., Stevens, P. M., Deaton, W. J., and Miller, R. R. First pass radionuclide assessment of right and left ventricular ejection fraction in chronic pulmonary disease. Chest 78: 4–9, 1980.

1238. Gertz, I., Hedenstierna, G., and Wester, P. O. Improvement in pulmonary function with diuretic therapy in the hypervolemic and polycythemic patient with chronic obstructive pulmonary disease. Chest 75: 146–151, 1979.

1239. Bubis, M. J., Sigurdson, M., McCarthy, D. S., and Anthonisen, N. R. Differences between slow and fast vital capacities in patients with obstructive disease. Chest 77: 626–631, 1980.

1240. Grant, I., Heaton, R. K., McSweeney, A. J., Adams, K. M., and Timms, R. M. Brain dysfunction in COPD. Chest 77(Suppl.): 308–309, 1980.

1241. Sahn, S. A., Nett, L. M., and Petty, T. L. Ten year follow-up of a comprehensive rehabilitation program for severe COPD. Chest 77(Suppl.): 311–314, 1980.

1242. Horton, F. O. III, Mackenthun, A. V., Anderson, P. S. Jr., Patterson, C. D., and Hammarsten, J. F. Alpha₁-antitrypsin heterozygotes (Pi type MZ). Chest 77(Suppl.): 261–264, 1980.

1243. Pride, N. B., Tattersall, S. F., Pereira, R. P., Hunter, D., and Blundell, G. Lung distensibility and airway function in intermediate alpha₁-antitrypsin deficiency (PiMZ). Chest 77(Suppl.): 253–255, 1980.

1244. Boysen, P. G., Block, A. J., Wynne, J. W., Hunt, L. A., and Flick, M. R. Nocturnal pulmonary hypertension in patients with chronic obstructive pulmonary disease. Chest 76: 536–542, 1979.

1245. Barany, J. S., Saltzman, A. R., and Klocke, R. A. Oxygen-related intrapulmonary shunting in obstructive pulmonary disease. Chest 74: 34–38, 1978.

1246. Foster, L. J., Corrigan, K., and Goldman, A. L. Effectiveness of oxygen therapy in hypoxic polycythemic smokers. Chest 73: 572–576, 1978.

1247. Malik, S. K. Chronic bronchitis in North India (letter to editor). Chest 72: 800, 1977.

1248. Chester, E. H., Belman, M. J., Bahler, R. C., Baum, G. L., Schey, G., and Buch, P. The effect of physical training on cardiopulmonary performance in patients with chronic obstructive pulmonary disease. Chest 72: 695–702, 1977.

1249. Boushy, S. F. and North, L. B. Hemodynamic changes in chronic obstructive pulmonary disease. Chest 72: 565–570, 1977.

1250. Thurlbeck, W. M. Aspects of chronic airflow obstruction. Chest 72: 341–349, 1977.

1251. Murphy, M. L., Boger, J., Adamson, J. S. Jr., and Rubin, S. Evaluation of cardiac size in chronic bronchitis and pulmonary emphysema. Chest 71: 712–717, 1977.

1252. Bracchi, G., Barbaccia, P., Vezzoli, F., Marazzini, L., and Longhini, E. Peripheral pulmonary wedge angiography in chronic obstructive pulmonary disease. Chest 71: 718–724, 1977.

1253. Saltzman, H. P., Ciulla, E. M., and Kuperman, A. S. The spirographic "kink." Chest 69: 51–55, 1976.

1254. Dayton, L. M., McCullough, R. E., Scheinhorn, D. J., and Weil, J. V. Symptomatic and pulmonary response to acute phlebotomy in secondary polycythemia. Chest 68: 785–790, 1975.

1255. Lilker, E. S., Karnick, A., and Lerner, L. Portable oxygen in chronic obstructive lung disease with hypoxaemia and cor pulmonale. Chest 68: 236–241, 1975.

1256. McCarthy, D. S., Robertson, M., and Simon, G. Diagnosis of emphysema. Chest 68: 46–50, 1975.

1257. Pulmonary Terms and Symbols. A report of the ACCP–ATS Joint Committee on Pulmonary Nomenclature. Chest 67: 583–593, 1975.

1258. Nordstrom, L. A., MacDonald, F., and Gobel, F. L. Effect of propranolol on respiratory function and exercise tolerance in patients with chronic obstructive lung disease. Chest 67: 287–292, 1975.

1259. Sherter, C. B., Jabbour, S. M., Kovnat, D. M., and Snider, G. L. Prolonged rate of decay of arterial PO₂ following oxygen breathing in chronic airways obstruction. Chest 67: 259–261, 1975.

1260. Alpert, J. S., Bass, H., Szucs, M. M., Banas, J. S., Dalen, J. E., and Dexter, L. Effects of physical training on hemodynamics and pulmonary function at rest and during exercise in patients with chronic obstructive pulmonary disease. Chest 66: 647–651, 1974.

1261. Mithoefer, J. C., Holford, F. D., and Keighley, J. F. H. The effect of oxygen administration on mixed venous oxygenation in chronic obstructive pulmonary disease. Chest 66: 122–132, 1974.

1262. Houstek, J., Copova, M., Zapletal, A., Tomasova, H., and Samanek, M. Alpha₁-antitrypsin deficiency in a child with chronic lung disease. Chest 64: 773–776, 1973.

1263. Bates, D. V. The prevention of emphysema. Chest 65: 437–441, 1974.

1264. Tandon, M. K. Correlations of electrocardiographic features with airway obstruction in chronic bronchitis. Chest 63: 146–148, 1973.

1265. Depierre, A., Bignon, J., Lebeau, A., and Brouet, G. Quantitative study of parenchyma and small conductive airways in chronic nonspecific lung disease. Chest 62: 699–708, 1972.

1266. Gottlieb, L. S. and Balchum, O. J. Course of chronic obstructive pulmonary disease following first onset of respiratory failure. Chest 63: 5–8, 1973.

1267. Ingram, R. H. Jr., Miller, R. B., and Tate, L. A. Arterial carbon dioxide changes during voluntary hyperventilation in chronic obstructive pulmonary disease. Chest 62: 14–18, 1972.

1268. Krumholz, R. A., Burnham, G. M., and DeLong, J. F. Lung scan utilization in the diagnosis of pulmonary disease. Chest 62: 4–8, 1972.

1269. Quaife, M. A. and Kass, I. Correlation of the ventilation and perfusion aspects of chronic obstructive pulmonary disease: a review of 100 cases. Chest 61: 459–464, 1972.

1270. Pump, K. K. The aged lung. Chest 60: 571–577, 1971.

1271. Mittman, C., Lieberman, J., Marasso, F., and Miranda, A. Smoking and chronic obstructive lung disease in alpha$_1$-antitrypsin deficiency. Chest 60: 214–221, 1971.

1272. Petty, T. L., Brink, G. A., Miller, M. W., and Corsello, P. R. Objective functional improvement in chronic airway obstruction. Chest 57: 216–223, 1970.

1273. Dunnill, M. S. The contribution of morphology to the study of chronic obstructive lung disease. Am. J. Med. 57: 506–519, 1974.

1274. Hsieh, Y-C., Frayser, R., and Ross, J. C. The effect of cold air inhalation on respiratory gas exchange during exercise in patients with chronic obstructive pulmonary disease. Chest 57: 18–21, 1970.

1275. Slutsky, R. A., Ackerman, W., Karliner, J. S., Ashburn, W. L., and Moser, K. M. Right and left ventricular dysfunction in patients with chronic obstructive lung disease. Am. J. Med. 68: 197–205, 1980.

1276. Kanner, R. E., Renzetti, A. D. Jr., Klauber, M. R., Smith, C. B., and Golden, C. A. Variables associated with changes in spirometry in patients with obstructive lung diseases. Am. J. Med. 67: 44–50, 1979.

1277. Wynne, J. W., Block, A. J., Hemenway, J., Hunt, L. A., and Flick, M. R. Disordered breathing and oxygen desaturation during sleep in patients with chronic obstructive lung disease (COLD). Am. J. Med. 66: 573–579, 1979.

1278. Aranow, W. S., Ferlinz, J., and Glauser, F. Effect of carbon monoxide on exercise performance in chronic obstructive pulmonary disease. Am. J. Med. 63: 904–908, 1977.

1279. Briscoe, W. A. and King, T. K. C. Analysis of the disturbance in oxygen transfer in hypoxic lung disease. Am. J. Med. 57: 349–360, 1974.

1280. King, M., Brock, G., and Lundell, C. Clearance of mucus by simulated cough. J. Appl. Physiol. 58: 1776–1782, 1985.

1281. Isawa, T., Teshima, T., Hirano, T., Ebina, A., and Konno, K. Mucociliary clearance mechanism in smoking and nonsmoking normal subjects. J. Nucl. Med. 25: 352–359, 1984.

1282. Emirgil, C., Sobol, B. J., Herbert, W. H., and Trout, K. W. Routine pulmonary function studies as a key to the status of the lesser circulation in chronic obstructive pulmonary disease. Am. J. Med. 50: 191–199, 1971.

1283. Marcus, J. H., McLean, R. L., Duffell, G. M., and Ingram, R. H. Exercise performance in relation to the pathophysiologic type of chronic obstructive pulmonary disease. Am. J. Med. 49: 14–22, 1970.

1284. Mungall, I. P. F. and Hainsworth, R. An objective assessment of the value of exercise training to patients with chronic obstructive airways disease. Q. J. Med. 49: 77–85, 1980.

1285. Howard, P. A long-term follow-up of respiratory symptoms and ventilatory function in a group of working men. Br. J. Ind. Med. 27: 326–333, 1970.

1286. Silvers, G. W., Petty, T. L., and Stanford, R. E. Elastic recoil changes in early emphysema. Thorax 35: 490–495, 1980.

1287. Douglas, A. N. Quantitative study of bronchial mucous gland enlargement. Thorax 35: 198–201, 1980.

1288. Sergysels, R., Willeput, R., Lenders, D., Vachaudez, J-P., Schandevyl, W., and Hennebert, A. Low frequency breathing at rest and during exercise in severe chronic obstructive bronchitis. Thorax 34: 536–539, 1979.

1289. Mungall, I. P. F. and Hainsworth, R. Assessment of respiratory function in patients with chronic obstructive airways disease. Thorax 34: 254–258, 1979.

1290. Johnson, A. N., Cooper, D. F., and Edwards, R. H. T. Exertion of stairclimbing in normal subjects and in patients with chronic obstructive bronchitis. Thorax 32: 711–716, 1977.

1291. Lawther, P. J., Brooks, A. G. F., and Waller, R. E. Respiratory function measurements in a cohort of medical students: a ten-year follow-up. Thorax 33: 773–778, 1978.

1292. Leitch, A. G., Hopkin, J. M., Ellis, D. A., Merchant, S., and McHardy, G. J. R. The effect of aerosol ipratropium bromide and salbutamol on exercise tolerance in chronic bronchitis. Thorax 33: 711–713, 1978.

1293. Tandon, M. K. Adjunct treatment with yoga in chronic severe airways obstruction. Thorax 33: 514–517, 1978.

1294. Thurlbeck, W. Diaphragm and body weight in emphysema. Thorax 33: 483–487, 1978.

1295. Cookson, J. B. and Mataka, G. Prevalence of chronic bronchitis in Rhodesian Africans. Thorax 33: 328–334, 1978.

1296. Musk, A. W., Gandevia, B., and Palmer, F. J. Peripheral pooling of bronchographic contrast material: evidence of its relationship to smoking and emphysema. Thorax 33: 193–200, 1978.

1297. McGavin, C. R., Gupta, S. P., Lloyd, E. L., and McHardy, G. J. R. Physical rehabilitation for the chronic bronchitic: results of a controlled trial of exercises in the home. Thorax 32: 307–311, 1977.

1298. Mittman, C. Alpha$_1$-antitrypsin deficiency and other genetic factors in lung disease. In: Macklem, P. T. and Permutt, S. (eds.). The Lung in Transition between Health and Disease. Marcel Dekker, New York and Basel, 1979.

1299. Cole, R. B., Nevin, N. C., Blundell, G., Merrett, J. D., McDonald, J. R., and Johnston, W. P. Relation of alpha-1-antitrypsin phenotype to the performance of pulmonary function tests and to the prevalence of respiratory illness in a working population. Thorax 31: 149–157, 1976.

1300. Ogilvie, A. G. Bronchography in chronic bronchitis. Thorax 30: 631–635, 1975.

1301. Spiro, S. G., Hahn, H. L., Edwards, R. H. T., and Pride, N. B. An analysis of the physiological strain of submaximal exercise in patients with chronic obstructive bronchitis. Thorax 30: 415–425, 1975.

1302. Joshi, R. C., Madan, R. N., and Brash, A. A. Prevalence of chronic bronchitis in an industrial population in North India. Thorax 30: 61–67, 1975.

1303. Leaver, D. G., Tattersfield, A. E., and Pride, N. B. Bronchial and extrabronchial factors in chronic airflow obstruction. Thorax 29: 394–400, 1974.

1304. Martelli, N. A., Goldman, E., and Roncoroni, A. J. Lower-zone emphysema in young patients without alpha$_1$-antitrypsin deficiency. Thorax 29: 237–244, 1974.

1305. Anderson, A. E. Jr. and Foraker, A. G. Centrilobular emphysema and panlobular emphysema: two different diseases. Thorax 28: 547–550, 1973.

1306. Barter, C. E., Hugh-Jones, P., Laws, J. W., and Crosbie, W. A. Radiology compared with xenon-133 scanning and bronchoscopic lobar sampling as methods for assessing regional lung function in patients with emphysema. Thorax 28: 29–40, 1973.

1307. Caird, F. I. and Akhtar, A. J. Chronic respiratory disease in the elderly. Thorax 27: 764–768, 1972.

1308. Simon, G., Pride, N. B., Jones, N. L., and Raimondi, A. C. Relation between abnormalities in the chest radiograph and changes in pulmonary function in chronic bronchitis and emphysema. Thorax 28: 15–23, 1973.

1309. Cocking, J. B. and Darke, C. S. Blood volume studies in chronic obstructive non-specific lung disease. Thorax 27: 44–51, 1972.

1310. Bignon, J., Andre-Bougaran, J., and Brouet, G. Parenchymal, bronchiolar, and bronchial measurements in centrilobular emphysema. Thorax 25: 556–567, 1970.

1311. Jones, M. C. and Thomas, G. O. Alpha$_1$-antitrypsin deficiency and pulmonary emphysema. Thorax 26: 652–662, 1971.

1312. Sharp, J. T., Paul, O., McKean, H., and Best, W. R. A longitudinal study of bronchitic symptoms and spirometry in a middle-aged, male, industrial population. Am. Rev. Respir. Dis. 108: 1066–1077, 1973.

1313. Scott, K. W. M. A pathological study of the lungs and heart in fatal and nonfatal chronic airways obstruction. Thorax 31: 70–79, 1976.

1314. Hodson, M. E., Simon, G., and Batten, J. C. Radiology of uncomplicated asthma. Thorax 29: 296–303, 1974.

1315. Simonsson, B. G., Skoogh, B-E., and Ekstrom-Jodal, B. Exercise-induced airways constriction. Thorax 27: 169–180, 1972.

1316. Kanner, R. E., Klauber, M. R., Watanabe, S., Renzetti, A. D. Jr., and Bigler, A. Pathologic patterns of chronic obstructive pulmonary disease in patients with normal and deficient levels of alpha$_1$-antitrypsin. Am. J. Med. 54: 706–712, 1973.

1317. Johnston, R. N., McNeill, R. S., Smith, D. H., Legge, J. S., and Fletcher, F. Chronic bronchitis: Measurements and observations over 10 years. Thorax 31: 25–29, 1976.

1318. Howard, P. and Astin, T. W. Precipitous fall in the forced expiratory volume. Thorax 24: 492–495, 1969.

1319. Holma, B. and Kjaer, G. Alcohol, housing, and smoking in relation to respiratory symptoms. Environ. Res. 21: 126–142, 1980.

1320. Geddes, D. M., Corrin, B., Brewerton, D. A., Davies, R. J., and Turner-Warwick, M. Progressive airway obliteration in adults and its association with rheumatoid disease. Q. J. Med. 46: 427–444, 1977.

1321. Fletcher, C. M. and Peto, R. The natural history of chronic airflow obstruction. Br. Med. J. 1: 1645–1648, 1977.

1322. Fallat, R. J., Powell, M. R., Kueppers, F., and Lilker, E. Xe^{133} ventilatory studies in alpha$_1$ antitrypsin deficiency. J. Nucl. Med. 14: 5–13, 1973.

1323. Diener, C. F. and Burrows, B. Further observations on the course and prognosis of chronic obstructive lung disease. Am. Rev. Respir. Dis. 111: 719–724, 1975.

1324. Black, L. F. and Kueppers, F. Alpha$_1$-antitrypsin deficiency in nonsmokers. Am. Rev. Respir. Dis. 117: 421–428, 1978.

1325. Sadoul, P. and Tournier, J. M. Respiratory functional disturbances in alpha$_1$-antitrypsin deficits. Bull. Eur. Physiopathol. Respir. 16(Suppl.): 293–297, 1980.

1326. Boushy, S. F., Abounrad, M. H., North, L. B., and Helgason, A. H. Lung recoil pressure, airway resistance, and forced flows related to morphologic emphysema. Am. Rev. Respir. Dis. 104: 551–561, 1971.

1327. Martelli, N. A., Hutchison, D. C. S., and Barter, C. E. Radiological distribution of pulmonary emphysema. Thorax 29: 81–89, 1974.

1328. Anderson, J. A., Dunnill, M. S., and Ryder, R. C. Dependence of the incidence of emphysema on smoking history, age, and sex. Thorax 27: 547–551, 1972.

1329. Turino, G. M., Keller, S., Chrzanowski, P., Osman, M., Cerreta, J., and Mandl, I. Lung elastin content in normal and emphysematous lungs. Bull. Eur. Physiopathol. Respir. 16(Suppl.): 43–56, 1980.

1330. Steele, R. H. and Heard, B. E. Size of the diaphragm in chronic bronchitis. Thorax 28: 55–60, 1973.

1331. Scott, K. W. M. and Steiner, G. M. Postmortem assessment of chronic airways obstruction by tantalum bronchography. Thorax 30: 405–414, 1975.

1332. Wagner, P. D., Dantzker, D. R., Dueck, R., Clausen, J. L., and West, J. B. Ventilation-perfusion inequality in chronic obstructive pulmonary disease. J. Clin. Invest. 59: 203–216, 1977.

1333. Gimenez, M., Martin, R., and Peslin, R. Incidences mecaniques de la rééducation respiratoire de bronchiteux chroniques. Bull. Physiopathol. Respir. 7: 586–599, 1971.

1334. Campbell, E. J. M. Respiratory failure. Definition, mechanisms and recent developments. Bull. Eur. Physiopathol. Respir. 15(Suppl.): 1–12, 1979.

1335. Cochrane, G. M. and Clark, T. J. H. A survey of asthma mortality in patients between ages 35 and 64 in the Greater London hospitals in 1971. Thorax 30: 300–305, 1975.

1336. King, A. J., Cooke, N. J., Leitch, A. G., and Flenley, D. C. The effects of 30 per cent oxygen on the respiratory response to treadmill exercise in chronic respiratory failure. Clin. Sci. 44: 151–162, 1973.

1337. Bradley, G. W. and Crawford, R. Regulation of breathing during exercise in normal subjects and in chronic lung disease. Clin. Sci. 51: 575–582, 1976.

1338. Grover, R. F. and Reeves, J. T. Oxygen transport in man during hypoxia: high altitude compared with chronic lung disease. Bull. Eur. Physiopathol. Respir. 15: 121–128, 1979.

1339. Patakas, D., Louridas, G., and Kakavelas, E. Reduced baroreceptor sensitivity in patients with chronic obstructive pulmonary disease. Thorax 37: 292–295, 1982.

1340. Petty, T. L., Pierson, D. J., Dick, N. P., Hudson, L. D., and Walker, S. H. Follow-up evaluation of a prevalence study for chronic bronchitis and chronic airway obstruction. Am. Rev. Respir. Dis. 114: 881–890, 1976.

1341. Carson, J. L., Collier, A. M., and Hu, S. C. S. Acquired ciliary defects in nasal epithelium of children with acute viral upper respiratory infections. N. Engl. J. Med. 312: 463–468, 1985.

1342. Bates, D. V., Woolf, C. R., and Paul, G. I. Chronic bronchitis. A report on the first two stages of the co-ordinated study of chronic bronchitis in the Department of Veteran's Affairs, Canada. Med. Serv. J. Can. 18: 211–303, 1962.

1343. Bates, D. V., Gordon, C. A., Paul, G. I., Place, R. E. G., Snidal, D. P., and Woolf, C. R. Chronic bronchitis. Report on the third and fourth stages of the co-ordinated study of chronic bronchitis in the Department of Veteran's Affairs, Canada. Med. Serv. J. Can. 22: 5–59, 1966.

1344. Eriksson, S., Hedenstierna, G., and Soderholm, B. Lung function in homozygous alpha$_1$-antitrypsin deficiency: mechanics and regional function in an asymptomatic male. In: Mittman, C. (ed.). Pulmonary Emphysema and Proteolysis. Academic Press, New York, 1972.

1345. Hudgel, D. W., Langston, L. Jr., Selner, J. C., and McIntosh, K. Viral and bacterial infections in adults with chronic asthma. Am. Rev. Respir. Dis. 120: 393–397, 1979.

1346. Kelsen, S. G., Fleegler, B., and Altose, M. D. The respiratory neuromuscular response to hypoxia, hypercapnia, and obstruction to airflow in asthma. Am. Rev. Respir. Dis. 120: 517–527, 1979.

1347. Paterson, J. W., Woolcock, A. J., and Shenfield, G. M. Bronchodilator drugs. Am. Rev. Respir. Dis. 120: 1149–1188, 1979.

1348. Barnes, P. J., Wilson, N. M., and Brown, M. J. A calcium antagonist, nifedipine, modifies exercise-induced asthma. Thorax 36: 726–730, 1981.

1349. Jenkins, P. F., Benfield, G. F. A., and Smith, A. P. Predicting recovery from acute severe asthma. Thorax 36: 835–841, 1981.

1350. Beaupre, A. and Orehek, J. Factors influencing the bronchodilator effect of a deep inspiration in asthmatic patients with provoked bronchoconstriction. Thorax 37: 124–128, 1982.

1351. Stellman, J. L., Spicer, J. E., and Cayton, R. M. Morbidity from chronic asthma. Thorax 36: 218–221, 1982.

1352. Partridge, M. R., Watson, A. C., and Saunders, K. B. Moment analysis of the flow-time curve after breathing gases of different densities. Thorax 36: 38–44, 1981.

1353. Karetzky, M. S. Asthma mortality associated with pneumothorax and intermittent positive-pressure breathing. Lancet ii: 828–829, 1975.

1354. Reversibility of asthma (editorial). Lancet i: 1327, 1974.

1355. Long-term prognosis in asthma (editorial). Lancet ii: 1015, 1977.

1356. Goodall, R. J. R., Earis, J. E., Cooper, D. N., Bernstein, A., and Temple, J. G. Relationship between asthma and gastro-oesophageal reflux. Thorax 36: 116–121, 1981.

1357. Morris, M. J. and Lane, D. J. Tidal expiratory flow patterns in airflow obstruction. Thorax 36: 135–142, 1981.

1358. Anderson, S. D., Bye, P. T. P., Schoeffel, R. E., Seale, J. P., Taylor, K. M., and Ferris, L. Arterial plasma histamine levels at rest, and during and after exercise in patients with asthma: effects of terbutaline aerosol. Thorax 36: 259–267, 1981.

1359. Neijens, H. J., Wesselius, T., and Kerrebijn, K. F. Exercise-induced bronchoconstriction as an expression of bronchial hyperreactivity: a study of its mechanisms in children. Thorax 36: 517–522, 1981.

1360. Partridge, M. R. and Saunders, K. B. Site of action of ipratropium bromide and clinical and physiological determinants of response in patients with asthma. Thorax 36: 530–533, 1981.

1361. Tweeddale, P. M., Godden, D. J., and Grant, I. W. B. Hyperventilation or exercise to induce asthma? Thorax 36: 596–598, 1981.

1362. Morris, M. J. Asthma—expiratory dyspnoea? Br. Med. J. 283: 838–839, 1981.

1363. Hudgel, D. W. and Weil, J. V. Asthma associated with decreased hypoxic ventilatory drive. A family study. Ann. Intern. Med. 80: 622–625, 1974.

1364. Orehek, J., Gayrard, P., Grimaud, C., and Charpin, J. Effect of maximal respiratory manoeuvres on bronchial sensitivity of asthmatic patients as compared to normal people. Br. Med. J. 1: 123–125, 1975.

1365. Palmer, K. N. V. and Kelman, G. R. Pulmonary function in asthmatic patients in remission. Br. Med. J. 1: 485–486, 1975.

1366. Burr, M. L., Charles, T. J., Roy, K., and Seaton, A. Asthma in the elderly: an epidemiological survey. Br. Med. J. 1: 1041–1044, 1979.

1367. Hetzel, M. R., Clark, T. J. H., and Branthwaite, M. A. Asthma: analysis of sudden deaths and ventilatory arrests in hospital. Br. Med. J. 1: 808–811, 1977.

1368. Kerrebijn, K. F., Fioole, A. C., and van Bentveld, R. D. W. Lung function in asthmatic children after year or more without symptoms or treatment. Br. Med. J. 1: 886–888, 1978.

1369. Bianco, S., Griffin, J. P., Kamburoff, P. L., and Prime, F. J. Prevention of exercise-induced asthma by indoramin. Br. Med. J. 4: 18–20, 1970.

1370. Wagner, P. D. and West, J. B. Changes in ventilation-perfusion relationships and gas exchange. In: Macklem, P. T. and Permutt, S. (eds.). The Lung in Transition between Health and Disease. Marcel Dekker, New York and Basel, 1979.

1371. Kjellen, G., Tibbling, L., and Wranne, B. Bronchial obstruction after oesophageal acid perfusion in asthmatics. Clin. Physiol. 1: 285–292, 1981.

1372. Smith, A. P. Patterns of recovery from acute severe asthma. Br. J. Dis. Chest 75: 132–140, 1981.

1373. Schofield, N. McC., Green, M., and Davies, R. J. Response of the lung airway to exercise testing in asthma and rhinitis. Br. J. Dis. Chest 74: 155–163, 1980.

1374. Kivity, S. and Souhrada, J. F. Hyperpnea: the common stimulus for bronchospasm in asthma during exercise and voluntary isocapnic hyperpnea. Respiration 40: 169–177, 1980.

1375. Todisco, T., Grassi, V., Sorbini, C. A., Dottorini, M., de Benedictis, F. M., Castellucci, G., and Romano, S. Circadian rhythm of respiratory functions in asthmatics. Respiration 40: 128–135, 1980.

1376. Toth, A. and Vastag, E. Site of bronchospasm in exercise-induced asthma. Respiration 39: 251–255, 1980.

1377. Ahonen, A. Analysis of the changes in ECG during status asthmaticus. Respiration 37: 85–90, 1979.

1378. Nanchev, L. A forced expiration end-segment flow rate to improve diagnosis of reversible bronchial obstruction. Respiration 36: 73–77, 1978.

1379. Fish, J. E., Kehoe, T. J., and Cugell, D. W. Effect of deep inspiration on maximum flow rates in asthmatic subjects. Respiration 36: 57–63, 1978.

1380. Beil, M. and de Kock, M. A. Role of alpha-adrenergic receptors in exercise-induced bronchoconstriction. Respiration 35: 78–86, 1978.

1381. Chen, W. Y. and Horton, D. J. Heat and water loss from the airways and exercise-induced asthma. Respiration 34: 305–313, 1977.

1382. Marazzini, L., Galli, G., Vezzoli, F., and Longhini, E. Drive and performance of ventilatory system during rebreathing. Respiration 34: 50–60, 1977.

1383. Fueki, R., Kleisbauer, J-P., Feliciano, J-M., Poirier, R., Cohen, G., and Laval, P. Etude analytique des boucles débit/volume chez les asthmatiques et de leur application lors d'épreuves pharmacodynamiques. Respiration 33: 425–435, 1976.

1384. Roncoroni, A. J., Adrogue, H. J. A., de Obrutsky, C. W., Marchiso, M. L., and Herrera, M. R. Metabolic acidosis in status asthmaticus. Respiration 33: 85–94, 1976.

1385. Melville, G. N. and Iravani, J. Resistance and blood gas tensions in bronchial asthma. Respiration 31: 381–389, 1974.

1386. Peel, E. T. and Gibson, G. J. Effect of long-term inhaled salbutamol therapy on the provocation of asthma by histamine. Am. Rev. Respir. Dis. 121: 973–978, 1980.

1387. Deal, E. C. Jr., McFadden, E. R. Jr., Ingram, R. H. Jr., Breslin, F. J., and Jaeger, J. J. Airway responsiveness to cold air and hyperpnea in normal subjects and in those with hay fever and asthma. Am. Rev. Respir. Dis. 121: 621–628, 1980.

1388. Martin, J., Powell, E., Shore, S., Emrich, J., and Engel, L. A. The role of respiratory muscles in the hyperinflation of bronchial asthma. Am. Rev. Respir. Dis. 121: 441–447, 1980.

1389. Charan, N. B., Hildebrandt, J., and Butler, J. Alveolar gas compression in smokers and asthmatics. Am. Rev. Respir. Dis. 121: 291–295, 1980.

1390. Loke, J., Ganeshananthan, M., Palm, C. R., and Motoyama,

E. K. Site of airway obstruction in asymptomatic asthmatic children. Lung 159: 35–42, 1981.

1391. McFadden, E. R. Jr. An analysis of exercise as a stimulus for the production of airway obstruction. Lung 159: 3–11, 1981.

1392. Fazio, F., Palla, A., Santolicandro, A., Solfanelli, S., Fornai, E., and Giuntini, C. Studies of regional ventilation in asthma using ^{81M}Kr. Lung 156: 185–194, 1979.

1393. Burrows, B., Hasan, F. M., Barbee, R. A., Halonen, M., and Lebowitz, M. D. Epidemiologic observations on eosinophilia and its relation to respiratory disorders. Am. Rev. Respir. Dis. 122: 709–719, 1980.

1394. Weiss, S. T., Tager, I. B., Speizer, F. E., and Rosner, B. Persistent wheeze. Its relation to respiratory illness, cigarette smoking, and level of pulmonary function in a population sample of children. Am. Rev. Respir. Dis. 122: 697–707, 1980.

1395. Martin, A. J., Landau, L. I., and Phelan, P. D. Lung function in young adults who had asthma in childhood. Am. Rev. Respir. Dis. 122: 609–616, 1980.

1396. Oberger, E. and Engstrom, I. Blood gases and acid-base balance in children with bronchial asthma. Lung 155: 111–122, 1978.

1397. Lisboa, C., Jardim, J., Angus, E., and Macklem, P. T. Is extrathoracic airway obstruction important in asthma? Am. Rev. Respir. Dis. 122: 115–121, 1980.

1398. Fairshter, R. D. and Wilson, A. F. Relationship between the site of airflow limitation and localization of the bronchodilator response in asthma. Am. Rev. Respir. Dis. 122: 27–32, 1980.

1399. Holtzmann, M. J., Sheller, J. R., Dimeo, M., Nadel, J. A., and Boushey, H. A. Effect of ganglionic blockade on bronchial reactivity in atopic subjects. Am. Rev. Respir. Dis. 122: 17–25, 1980.

1400. Breslin, F. J., McFadden, E. R. Jr., and Ingram, R. H. Jr. The effects of cromolyn sodium on the airway response to hyperpnea and cold air in asthma. Am. Rev. Respir. Dis. 122: 11–16, 1980.

1401. Orehek, J., Nicoli, M. M., Delpierre, S., and Beaupre, A. Influence of the previous deep inspiration on the spirometric measurement of provoked bronchoconstriction in asthma. Am. Rev. Respir. Dis. 123: 269–272, 1981.

1402. Fanta, C. H., McFadden, E. R. Jr., and Ingram, R. H. Jr. Effects of cromolyn sodium on the response to respiratory heat loss in normal subjects. Am. Rev. Respir. Dis. 123: 161–164, 1981.

1403. Gottfried, S. B., Altose, M. D., Kelsen, S. G., and Cherniack, N. S. Perception of changes in airflow resistance in obstructive pulmonary disorders. Am. Rev. Respir. Dis. 124: 566–570, 1981.

1404. Tabachnik, E., Muller, N. L., Levison, H., and Bryan, A. C. Chest wall mechanics and pattern of breathing during sleep in asthmatic adolescents. Am. Rev. Respir. Dis. 124: 269–273, 1981.

1405. Barnes, P. J. and Brown, M. J. Venous plasma histamine in exercise- and hyperventilation-induced asthma in man. Clin. Sci. 61: 159–162, 1981.

1406. Saunders, K. B. and Rudolf, M. The interpretation of different measurements of airways obstruction in the presence of lung volume changes in bronchial asthma. Clin. Sci. Mol. Med. 54: 313–321, 1978.

1407. Rubinfeld, A. R. and Pain, M. C. F. Bronchial provocation in the study of sensations associated with disordered breathing. Clin. Sci. Mol. Med. 52: 423–428, 1977.

1408. Smith, A. P., Cuthbert, M. F., and Dunlop, L. S. Effects of inhaled prostaglandins E_1, E_2, and $F_{2\alpha}$ on the airway resistance of healthy and asthmatic man. Clin. Sci. Mol. Med. 48: 421–430, 1975.

1409. Ellul-Micallef, R., Borthwick, R. C., and McHardy, G. J. R. The time-course of response to prednisolone in chronic bronchial asthma. Clin. Sci. Mol. Med. 47: 105–117, 1974.

1410. Godfrey, S., Zeidifard, E., Brown, K., and Bell, J. H. The possible site of action of sodium cromoglycate assessed by exercise challenge. Clin. Sci. Mol. Med. 46: 265–272, 1974.

1411. Jaffe, P., Konig, P., Ijaduola, O., Walker, S., and Godfrey, S. Relationship between plasma cortisol and peak expiratory flow rate in exercise-induced asthma and the effect of sodium cromoglycate. Clin. Sci. 45: 533–541, 1973.

1412. Oberger, E. and Engstrom, I. Long-term treatment with

corticosteroids and ACTH in asthmatic children. Eur. J. Respir. Dis. 62: 256–267, 1981.

1413. Inbar, O., Alvarez, D. X., and Lyons, H. A. Exercise-induced asthma—a comparison between two modes of exercise stress. Eur. J. Respir. Dis. 62: 160–167, 1981.

1414. Newman, S. P., Pavia, D., and Clarke, S. W. How should a pressurized beta-adrenergic bronchodilator be inhaled? Eur. J. Respir. Dis. 62: 3–21, 1981.

1415. Kiers, A., Van Der Mark, Th. W., Woldring, M. G., and Peset, R. Changes in functional residual capacity during exercise in patients with exercise-induced asthma. Bull. Eur. Physiopathol. Respir. 17: 869–878, 1981.

1416. Denjean, A., Cerrina, J., and Lockhart, A. Asthma postexercise. Bull. Eur. Physiopathol. Respir. 17: 847–867, 1981.

1417. Matthys, H., Vastag, E., Kohler, D., Daikeler, G., and Fischer, J. Mucociliary clearance in patients with chronic bronchitis and bronchial carcinoma. Respiration 44: 329–337, 1983.

1418. Laitinen, L. A. and Kava, T. Bronchial reactivity following uncomplicated influenza A infection in healthy subjects and in asthmatic patients. In: Proceedings of a Meeting on Bronchial Hyperreactivity Syndrome. Eur. J. Respir. Dis. 106(Suppl.): 61, 51–58, 1980.

1419. Graff-Lonnevig, V., Bevegard, S., and Eriksson, B. O. Ventilation and pulmonary gas exchange at rest and during exercise in boys with bronchial asthma. Eur. J. Respir. Dis. 61: 357–366, 1980.

1420. Bagg, L. R. and Hughes, D. T. D. Diurnal variation in peak expiratory flow in asthmatics. Eur. J. Respir. Dis. 61: 298–302, 1980.

1421. Andersen, L. H. and Haghfelt, T. Regional lung function in asthmatics in remission, before and after fenoterol. Bull. Eur. Physiopathol. Respir. 16: 215–228, 1980.

1422. Chen, W. Y., Weiser, P. C., and Chai, H. Airway cooling. Scand. J. Respir. Dis. 60: 144–150, 1979.

1423. Prefaut, Ch., Lloret, M. C., Tronc, J. F., Michel, F. B., and Chardon, G. Density dependence of the maximal expiratory flow volume curves in normal and asthmatic children. Scand. J. Respir. Dis. 60: 109–118, 1979.

1424. Dahl, R. and Henriksen, J. M. Inhibition of exercise-induced bronchoconstriction by nebulised sodium cromoglycate in patients with bronchial asthma. Scand. J. Respir. Dis. 60: 51–55, 1979.

1425. Graff-Lonnevig, V., Bevegard, S., and Eriksson, B. O. Cardiac output and blood pressure at rest and during exercise in boys with bronchial asthma. Scand. J. Respir. Dis. 60: 36–43, 1979.

1426. Poukkula, A. Prognosis for adult asthmatics. Scand. J. Respir. Dis. 100(Suppl.): 1977.

1427. Poppius, H. and Stenius, B. Changes in arterial oxygen saturation in patients with hyperreactive airways during a histamine inhalation test. Scand. J. Respir. Dis. 58: 1–4, 1977.

1428. Seale, J. P., Anderson, S. D., and Lindsay, D. A. A trial of an alpha-adrenoreceptor blocking drug (indoramin) in exercise-induced bronchoconstriction. Scand. J. Respir. Dis. 57: 261–266, 1976.

1429. Mossberg, B., Strandberg, K., Philipson, K., and Camner, P. Tracheobronchial clearance in bronchial asthma: response to beta-adrenergic stimulation. Scand. J. Respir. Dis. 57: 119–128, 1976.

1430. Anderson, S. D., Pojer, R., Smith, I. D., and Temple, D. Exercise-related changes in plasma levels of 15-keto-13,14-dihydro-prostaglandin $F_{2\alpha}$ and noradrenaline in asthmatic and normal subjects. Scand. J. Respir. Dis. 57: 41–48, 1976.

1431. Lissac, J., Labrousse, J., Tenaillon, A., Bousser, J. P., Labrousse, F., and Jacquot, Ch. Les desordres acido-basiques dans l'état de mal asthmatique. Bull. Physiopathol. Respir. 11: 745–756, 1975.

1432. Bulow, K. B., Lindell, S. E., and Arborelius, M. Jr. Predominantly unilateral asthma studied with Xe^{133} radiospirometry. Scand. J. Respir. Dis. 56: 223–230, 1975.

1433. Simonsson, B. G., Jonson, B., and Strom, B. Bronchodilatory and circulatory effects of inhaling increasing doses of an anticholinergic drug, ipratropium bromide (SCH 1000). Scand. J. Respir. Dis. 56: 138–149, 1975.

1434. Kiviloog, J. Bronchial reactivity to exercise and methacholine in bronchial asthma. Scand. J. Respir. Dis. 54: 359–368, 1973.

1435. Poppius, H. and Salorinne, Y. Comparative trial of salbutamol and an anticholinergic drug, SCH 1000, in prevention of exercise-induced asthma. Scand. J. Respir. Dis. 54: 142–147, 1973.

1436. Said, S. I. The prostaglandins in relation to the lung: regulators of function, mediators of disease, or therapeutic agents? Bull. Physiopathol. Respir. 10: 411–418, 1974.

1437. Stanescu, D. C., Frans, A., and Brasseur, L. Acute increase of total lung capacity in asthma following histamine aerosols. Bull. Physiopathol. Respir. 9: 523–530, 1973.

1438. Hedstrand, U. The optimal frequency of breathing in bronchial asthma. Scand. J. Respir. Dis. 52: 217–221, 1971.

1439. Granerus, G., Simonsson, B. G., Skoogh, B-E., and Wetterqvist, H. Exercise-induced bronchoconstriction and histamine release. Scand. J. Respir. Dis. 52: 131–136, 1971.

1440. Gayrard, P., Orehek, J., and Charpin, J. Effets de différents produits bronchodilatateurs sur la conductance des voies aeriennes dans l'asthme, lors d'un blocage beta-adrenergique provoque. Bull. Physiopathol. Respir. 8: 625–640, 1972.

1441. Macleod, J. P., Taylor, N. W. G., and Macklem, P. T. Phase differences between gas displacements by the thorax and at the airway opening. Bull. Physiopathol. Respir. 7: 433–440, 1971.

1442. Despas, P. J., Leroux, M., and Macklem, P. T. Site of airway obstruction in asthma as determined by measuring maximal expiratory flow breathing air and a helium-oxygen mixture. J. Clin. Invest. 51: 3235–3243, 1972.

1443. Burki, N. K., Mitchell, K., Chaudhary, B. A., and Zechman, F. W. The ability of asthmatics to detect added resistive loads. Am. Rev. Respir. Dis. 117: 71–75, 1978.

1444. Edmunds, A. T., Tooley, M., and Godfrey, S. The refractory period after exercise-induced asthma: its duration and relation to the severity of exercise. Am. Rev. Respir. Dis. 117: 247–254, 1978.

1445. Mellis, C. M., Kattan, M., Keens, T. G., and Levison, H. Comparative study of histamine and exercise challenges in asthmatic children. Am. Rev. Respir. Dis. 117: 911–915, 1978.

1446. Horton, D. J., Suda, W. L., Kinsman, R. A., Souhrada, J., and Spector, S. L. Bronchoconstrictive suggestion in asthma: a role for airways hyperreactivity and emotions. Am. Rev. Respir. Dis. 117: 1029–1038, 1978.

1447. Shturman-Ellstein, R., Zeballos, R. J., Buckley, J. M., and Souhara, J. F. The beneficial effect of nasal breathing on exercise-induced bronchoconstriction. Am. Rev. Respir. Dis. 118: 65–73, 1978.

1448. Wagner, P. D., Dantzker, D. R., Iacovoni, V. E., Tomlin, W. C., and West, J. B. Ventilation-perfusion inequality in asymptomatic asthma. Am. Rev. Respir. Dis. 118: 511–524, 1978.

1449. Rubinfeld, A. R., Wagner, P. D., and West, J. B. Gas exchange during acute experimental canine asthma. Am. Rev. Respir. Dis. 118: 525–536, 1978.

1450. Mildon, A., Leroux, M., Hutcheon, M., and Zamel, N. The site of airways obstruction in exercise-induced asthma. Am. Rev. Respir. Dis. 110: 409–414, 1974.

1451. Strauss, R. H., McFadden, E. R. Jr., Ingram, R. H. Jr., Deal, E. C. Jr., and Jaeger, J. J. Influence of heat and humidity on the airway obstruction induced by exercise in asthma. J. Clin. Invest. 61: 433–440, 1978.

1452. Mathe, A. A. and Hedqvist, P. Effect of prostaglandins $F_{2\alpha}$ and E_2 on airway conductance in healthy subjects and asthmatic patients. Am. Rev. Respir. Dis. 111: 313–320, 1975.

1453. Gayrard, P., Orehek, J., Grimaud, C., and Charpin, J. Bronchoconstrictor effects of a deep inspiration in patients with asthma. Am. Rev. Respir. Dis. 111: 433–439, 1975.

1454. Kreisman, H., Van de Wiel, W., and Mitchell, C. A. Respiratory function during prostaglandin-induced labor. Am. Rev. Respir. Dis. 111: 564–565, 1975.

1455. Landau, L. I., Taussig, L. M., Macklem, P. T., and Beaudry, P. H. Contribution of inhomogeneity of lung units to the maximal expiratory flow-volume curve in children with asthma and cystic fibrosis. Am. Rev. Respir. Dis. 111: 725–731, 1975.

1456. Cropp, G. J. A. The role of the parasympathetic nervous system in the maintenance of chronic airway obstruction in asthmatic children. Am. Rev. Respir. Dis. 112: 599–605, 1975.

1457. Sobol, B. J. and Emirgil, C. Pulmonary function in ambulatory asthmatics. J. Chron. Dis. 29: 233–242, 1976.

1458. Cade, J. F. and Pain, M. C. F. Pulmonary function during clinical remission of asthma—how reversible is asthma? Aust. N. Z. J. Med. 3: 545–551, 1973.

1459. Chan-Yeung, M., Abboud, R., Tsao, M. S., and Maclean, L. Effect of helium on maximal expiratory flow in patients with asthma before and during induced bronchoconstriction. Am. Rev. Respir. Dis. 113: 433–443, 1976.

1460. Siegler, D., Fukuchi, Y., and Engel, L. Influence of bronchomotor tone on ventilation distribution and airway closure in asymptomatic asthma. Am. Rev. Respir. Dis. 114: 123–130, 1976.

1461. Anderson, S. D., Seale, J. P., Rozea, P., Bandler, L., Theobald, G., and Lindsay, D. A. Inhaled and oral salbutamol in exercise-induced asthma. Am. Rev. Respir. Dis. 114: 493–500, 1976.

1462. Allegra, L., Abraham, W. M., Chapman, G. A., and Wanner, A. Duration of mucociliary dysfunction following antigen challenge. J. Appl. Physiol. 55: 726–730, 1983.

1463. Haynes, R. L., Ingram, R. H. Jr., and McFadden, E. R. Jr. An assessment of the pulmonary response to exercise in asthma and an analysis of the factors influencing it. Am. Rev. Respir. Dis. 114: 739–752, 1976.

1464. Zackon, H., Despas, P. J., and Anthonisen, N. R. Occlusion pressure responses in asthma and chronic obstructive pulmonary disease. Am. Rev. Respir. Dis. 114: 917–927, 1976.

1465. Fish, J. E., Rosenthal, R. R., Summer, W. R., Menkes, H., Norman, P. S., and Permutt, S. The effect of atropine on acute antigen-mediated airway constriction in subjects with allergic asthma. Am. Rev. Respir. Dis. 115: 371–379, 1977.

1466. Sackner, M. A., Silva, G., Zucker, C., and Marks, M. B. Long-term effects of metaproterenol in asthmatic children. Am. Rev. Respir. Dis. 115: 945–953, 1977.

1467. Cooper, D. M., Doron, I., Mansell, A. L., Bryan, A. C., and Levison, H. The relative sensitivity of closing volume in children with asthma and cystic fibrosis. Am. Rev. Respir. Dis. 109: 519–524, 1974.

1468. Gimeno, F., Quanjer, Ph. H., Berg, W. C., Sluiter, H. J., and Tammeling, G. J. Drug-resistant postexercise airway obstruction. Am. Rev. Respir. Dis. 108: 960–963, 1973.

1469. Fanburg, B. L. Prostaglandins and the lung. Am. Rev. Respir. Dis. 108: 482–489, 1973.

1470. Tam, C. H., Mansell, A. L., Levison, H., Reilly, B. J., and Aspin, N. Dynamic regional lung function studies in patients with asthma and cystic fibrosis. Am. Rev. Respir. Dis. 108: 283–293, 1973.

1471. Chick, T. W., Nicholson, D. P., and Johnson, R. L. Jr. Effects of isoproterenol on distribution of ventilation and perfusion in asthma. Am. Rev. Respir. Dis. 107: 869–873, 1973.

1472. Allen, T. W., Addington, W., Rosendal, T., and Cugell, D. W. Alveolar carbon dioxide and airway resistance in patients with postexercise bronchospasm. Am. Rev. Respir. Dis. 107: 816–821, 1973.

1473. McCarthy, D. and Milic-Emili, J. Closing volume in asymptomatic asthma. Am. Rev. Respir. Dis. 107: 559–570, 1973.

1474. Hossain, S. Quantitative measurement of bronchial muscle in men with asthma. Am. Rev. Respir. Dis. 107: 99–109, 1973.

1475. Olive, J. T. Jr. and Hyatt, R. E. Maximal expiratory flow and total respiratory resistance during induced bronchoconstriction in asthmatic subjects. Am. Rev. Respir. Dis. 106: 366–376, 1972.

1476. Anderson, S. D., McEvoy, J. D. S., and Bianco, S. Changes in lung volumes and airway resistance after exercise in asthmatic subjects. Am. Rev. Respir. Dis. 106: 30–37, 1972.

1477. Stolley, P. D. Asthma mortality. Am. Rev. Respir. Dis. 105: 883–890, 1972.

1478. Lindsay, D. A. and Read, J. Pulmonary vascular responsiveness in the prognosis of chronic obstructive lung disease. Am. Rev. Respir. Dis. 105: 242–250, 1972.

1479. Chan-Yeung, M. M. W., Vyas, M. N., and Grzbowski, S.

Exercise-induced asthma. Am. Rev. Respir. Dis. 104: 915–923, 1971.

1480. Woolcock, A. J., Rebuck, A. S., Cade, J. F., and Read, J. Lung volume changes in asthma measured concurrently by two methods. Am. Rev. Respir. Dis. 104: 703–709, 1971.

1481. Stanescu, D. Measurement of total lung volume by helium dilution (letter to editor). Am. Rev. Respir. Dis. 104: 134–135, 1971.

1482. Renzetti, A. D. Jr. Measurement of total lung volume by helium dilution (letter to editor). Am. Rev. Respir. Dis. 104: 135, 1971.

1483. Curran, W. S. and Graham, W. G. B. Long term effects of glomectomy. Am. Rev. Respir. Dis. 103: 566–568, 1971.

1484. Levine, G., Housley, E., Macleod, P., and Macklem, P. T. Gas exchange abnormalities in mild bronchitis and asymptomatic asthma. N. Engl. J. Med. 282: 1277–1282, 1970.

1485. Fisher, H. K., Holton, P., Buxton, R. S. J., and Nadel, J. A. Resistance to breathing during exercise-induced asthma attacks. Am. Rev. Respir. Dis. 101: 885–896, 1970.

1486. Ingram, R. H. Jr., Krumpe, P. E., Duffell, G. M., and Maniscalo, B. Ventilation-perfusion changes after aerosolized isoproterenol in asthma. Am. Rev. Respir. Dis. 101: 364–370, 1970.

1487. Weng, T-R., Langer, H. M., Featherby, E. A., and Levison, H. Arterial blood gas tensions and acid-base balance in symptomatic and asymptomatic asthma in childhood. Am. Rev. Respir. Dis. 101: 274–282, 1970.

1488. Cockcroft, D. W. and Berscheid, B. A. Volume adjustment of maximal midexpiratory flow. Chest 78: 595–600, 1980.

1489. Horton, D. J. and Chen, W. Y. Effects of breathing warm humidified air on bronchoconstriction induced by body cooling and by inhalation of methacholine. Chest 75: 24–28, 1979.

1490. Lonky, S. A. and Tisi, G. M. Determining changes in airway caliber in asthma: the role of submaximal flow rates. Chest 77: 741–748, 1980.

1491. Ashutosh, K., Mead, G., Dickey, J. C. Jr., Berman, P., and Kuppinger, M. Density dependence of expiratory flow and bronchodilator response in asthma. Chest 77: 68–75, 1980.

1492. Burki, N. K. Resting ventilatory pattern, mouth occlusion pressure, and the effects of aminophylline in asthma and chronic airways obstruction. Chest 76: 629–635, 1979.

1493. Hudgel, D. W., Capehart, M., and Hirsch, J. E. Ventilation response and drive during hypoxia in adult patients with asthma. Chest 76: 294–299, 1979.

1494. Keens, T. G., Mansell, A., Krastins, I. R. B., Levison, H., Bryan, A. C., Hyland, R. H., and Zamel, N. Evaluation of the single-breath diffusing capacity in asthma and cystic fibrosis. Chest 76: 41–44, 1979.

1495. Permutt, S. What should we measure to evaluate bronchodilator drug response? Chest 73(Suppl.): 944–947, 1978.

1496. Chang, K. C., Morrill, C. G., and Chai, H. Impaired response to hypoxia after bilateral carotid body resection for treatment of bronchial asthma. Chest 73: 667–669, 1978.

1497. Sherter, C. B., Connolly, J. J., and Schilder, D. P. The significance of volume-adjusting the maximal midexpiratory flow in assessing the response to a bronchodilator drug. Chest 73: 568–571, 1978.

1498. Kelsen, S. G., Fleegler, B., Altose, M. D., Gottfried, S., and Cherniack, N. S. Effects of hypercapnia and flow resistive loading on respiratory activity in asthma and chronic obstructive lung disease. Chest 73(Suppl.): 288–290, 1978.

1499. Light, R. W., Conrad, S. A., and George, R. B. The one best test for evaluating the effects of bronchodilator therapy. Chest 72: 512–516, 1977.

1500. Rubinfeld, A. R. and Pain, M. C. F. Conscious perception of bronchospasm as a protective phenomenon in asthma. Chest 72: 154–158, 1977.

1501. Rubin, A-H. E., Mansur, A., Schey, G., Shahor, Y., and Bruderman, I. Reversibility of small airway obstruction after therapy with salbutamol. Chest 71: 470–472, 1977.

1502. Cooper, D. M., Cutz, E., and Levison, H. Occult pulmonary abnormalities in asymptomatic asthmatic children. Chest 71: 361–365, 1977.

1503. Riley, D. J., Fisher, A. B., Hansell, J. R., and Brody, J. S. Regional bronchoconstriction in asthma. Chest 70: 715–718, 1976.

1504. Popa, V. T. and Werner, P. Dose-related dilatation of airways after inhalation of metaproterenol sulfate. Chest 70: 205–211, 1976.

1505. Shaw, J. O. and Moser, K. M. The current status of prostaglandins and the lungs. Chest 68: 75–80, 1975.

1506. Newball, H. H. The unreliability of the maximal midexpiratory flow as an index of acute airway changes. Chest 67: 311–314, 1975.

1507. Thurlbeck, W. M. A pathologist looks at respiratory failure due to obstructive lung disease. Chest 58: 408–414, 1970.

1508. Shim, C. S. and Williams, M. H. Jr. Evaluation of the severity of asthma: patients versus physicians. Am. J. Med. 68: 11–13, 1980.

1509. Tashkin, D. P., Trevor, E., Chopra, S. K., and Taplin, G. V. Sites of airway dilatation in asthma following inhaled versus subcutaneous terbutaline. Am. J. Med. 68: 14–26, 1980.

1510. Wanner, A. The role of mucociliary dysfunction in bronchial asthma. Am. J. Med. 67: 477–485, 1979.

1511. Westerman, D. E., Benatar, S. R., Potgeiter, P. D., and Ferguson, A. D. Identification of the high-risk asthmatic patient. Am. J. Med. 66: 565–572, 1979.

1512. Weitzman, R. H. and Wilson, A. F. Diffusing capacity and over-all ventilation:perfusion in asthma. Am. J. Med. 57: 767–774, 1974.

1513. Peress, L., Sybrecht, G., and Macklem, P. T. The mechanism of increase in total lung capacity during acute asthma. Am. J. Med. 61: 165–169, 1976.

1514. McFadden, E. R., Kiser, R., deGroot, W. J., Holmes, B., Kiker, R., and Viser, G. A controlled study of the effects of single doses of hydrocortisone on the resolution of acute attacks of asthma. Am. J. Med. 60: 52–59, 1976.

1515. Gazioglu, K., Condemi, J. J., Hyde, R. W., and Kaltreider, N. L. Effect of isoproterenol on gas exchange during air and oxygen breathing in patients with asthma. Am. J. Med. 50: 185–190, 1971.

1516. Wilson, A. F., Surprenant, E. L., Beall, G. N., Siegel, S. C., Simmons, D. H., and Bennett, L. R. The significance of regional pulmonary function changes in bronchial asthma. Am. J. Med. 48: 416–423, 1970.

1517. Rubinfeld, A. R. and Pain, M. C. F. Perception of asthma. Lancet i: 882–883, 1976.

1518. Zielinski, J., Chodosowska, E., Radomyski, A., Araszkiewicz, Z., and Kozlowski, S. Plasma catecholamines during exercise-induced bronchoconstriction in bronchial asthma. Thorax 35: 823–827, 1980.

1519. Schnall, R. P. and Landau, L. I. Protective effects of repeated short sprints in exercise-induced asthma. Thorax 35: 828–832, 1980.

1520. Hetzel, M. R. and Clark, T. J. H. Comparison of normal and asthmatic circadian rhythms in peak expiratory flow rate. Thorax 35: 732–738, 1980.

1521. Hartley, J. P. R. and Nogrady, S. G. Effect of an inhaled antihistamine on exercise-induced asthma. Thorax 35: 675–679, 1980.

1522. Fairfax, A. J., McNabb, W. R., Davies, H. J., and Spiro, S. G. Slow-release oral salbutamol and aminophylline in nocturnal asthma: relation of overnight changes in lung function and plasma drug levels. Thorax 35: 526–530, 1980.

1523. Thomson, N. C. and Kerr, J. W. Effect of inhaled H1 and H2 receptor antagonists in normal and asthmatic subjects. Thorax 35: 428–434, 1980.

1524. Bateman, J. R. M., Siegler, D., Wagstaff, D., and Clarke, S. W. Comparison of serial electrocardiographic and vectorcardiographic changes during recovery from status asthmaticus. Thorax 35: 355–358, 1980.

1525. McCarthy, D. S. and Sigurdson, M. Lung elastic recoil and reduced airflow in clinically stable asthma. Thorax 35: 298–302, 1980.

1526. Schoeffel, R. E., Anderson, S. D., Gillam, I., and Lindsay, D. A. Multiple exercise and histamine challenge in asthmatic patients. Thorax 35: 164–170, 1980.

1527. Gayrard, P., Orehek, J., Grimaud, Ch., and Charpin, J. Mechanisms of the bronchoconstrictor effects of deep inspiration in asthmatic patients. Thorax 34: 234–240, 1979.

1528. Hetzel, M. R. and Clark, T. J. H. Does sleep cause nocturnal asthma? Thorax 34: 749–754, 1979.

1529. Hartley, J. P. R. Exercise-induced asthma (editorial). Thorax 34: 571–574, 1979.

1530. Chopra, S. K., Taplin, G. V., Tashkin, D. P., Trevor, E., and Elam, D. Imaging sites of airway obstruction and measuring functional responses to bronchodilator treatment in asthma. Thorax 34: 493–500, 1979.

1531. Bellamy, D. and Collins, J. V. "Acute" asthma in adults. Thorax 34: 36–39, 1979.

1532. Bateman, J. R. M. and Clarke, S. W. Sudden death in asthma. Thorax 34: 40–44, 1979.

1533. Thomson, N. C., Patel, K. R., and Kerr, J. W. Sodium cromoglycate and ipratropium bromide in exercise-induced asthma. Thorax 33: 694–699, 1978.

1534. Holmes, P. W., Campbell, A. H., and Barter, C. E. Acute changes in lung volumes and lung mechanics in asthma and in normal subjects. Thorax 33: 394–400, 1978.

1535. Seaton, A. Asthma—contrasts in care (editorial). Thorax 33: 1–2, 1978.

1536. Soutar, C. A., Carruthers, M., and Pickering, C. A. C. Nocturnal asthma and urinary adrenaline and noradrenaline excretion. Thorax 32: 677–683, 1977.

1537. Hetzel, M. R., Clark, T. J. H., and Houston, K. Physiological patterns in early morning asthma. Thorax 32: 418–423, 1977.

1538. Cockcroft, D. W., Killian, D. N., Mellon, J. J. A., and Hargreave, F. C. Protective effect of drugs on histamine-induced asthma. Thorax 32: 429–437, 1977.

1539. Rubinfeld, A. R. and Pain, M. C. F. How mild is mild asthma? Thorax 32: 177–181, 1977.

1540. Mellis, C. M. and Phelan, P. D. Asthma deaths in children—a continuing problem. Thorax 32: 29–34, 1977.

1541. Godfrey, S. and Konig, P. Inhibition of exercise-induced asthma by different pharmacological pathways. Thorax 31: 137–143, 1976.

1542. Kerr, A. A. Dead space ventilation in normal children and children with obstructive airways disease. Thorax 31: 63–69, 1976.

1543. Morgan, E. J. and Hall, D. R. Abnormalities of lung function in hay fever. Thorax 31: 80–86, 1976.

1544. Gayrard, P., Orehek, J., Grimaud, C., and Charpin, J. Beta-adrenergic function in airways of healthy and asthmatic subjects. Thorax 30: 657–662, 1975.

1545. Burr, M. L., St. Leger, A. S., Bevan, C., and Merrett, T. G. A community survey of asthmatic characteristics. Thorax 30: 663–668, 1975.

1546. Soutar, C. A., Costello, J., Ijaduola, O., and Turner-Warwick, M. Nocturnal and morning asthma. Thorax 30: 436–440, 1975.

1547. Funahashi, A., Melville, G. N., and Hamilton, L. H. Ability of single-breath nitrogen closing volume to detect early airway obstruction. Thorax 30: 220–224, 1975.

1548. Miller, G. J., Davies, B. H., Cole, T. J., and Seaton, A. Comparison of the bronchial response to running and cycling in asthma using an improved definition of the response to work. Thorax 30: 306–311, 1975.

1549. Ellul-Micallef, R. and Fenech, F. F. Intravenous prednisolone in chronic bronchial asthma. Thorax 30: 312–315, 1975.

1550. Bye, P. T. P., Anderson, S. D., Daviskas, E., Marty, J. J., and Sampson, D. Plasma cyclic AMP levels in response to exercise and terbutalin sulphate aerosol in normal and asthmatic subjects. Eur. J. Respir. Dis. 61: 287–297, 1980.

1551. Stone, R. W., Comstock, G. W., Tonascia, J. A., and Chandra, V. Prediction value of respiratory findings. Bull. Eur. Physiopathol. Respir. 14: 189–196, 1978.

1552. Minor, T. E., Dick, E. C., Baker, J. W., Ouellette, J. J., Cohen, M., and Reed, C. E. Rhinovirus and influenza type A infections as precipitants of asthma. Am. Rev. Respir. Dis. 113: 149–153, 1976.

1553. Clarke, C. W. Relationships of bacterial and viral infections to exacerbations of asthma. Thorax 34: 344–347, 1979.

1554. Antic, R. and Macklem, P. T. The influence of clinical factors on site of airway obstruction in asthma. Am. Rev. Respir. Dis. 114: 851–859, 1976.

1555. Juniper, E. F., Frith, P. A., and Hargreave, F. E. Long-term stability of bronchial responsiveness to histamine. Thorax 37: 292–295, 1982.

1556. Beaudry, C. and Laplante, L. Severe allergic pneumonitis from hydrochlorothiazide. Ann. Intern. Med. 78: 251–253, 1973.

1557. Holoye, P. Y., Luna, M. A., MacKay, B., and Bedrossian,

C. W. M. Bleomycin hypersensitivity pneumonitis. Ann. Intern. Med. 88: 47–49, 1978.

1558. Hodges, G. R., Fink, J. N., and Schlueter, D. P. Hypersensitivity pneumonitis caused by a contaminated cool-mist vaporizer. Ann. Intern. Med. 80: 501–504, 1974.

1559. Schlueter, D. P., Fink, J. N., and Hensley, G. T. Wood-pulp worker's disease: a hypersensitivity pneumonitis caused by 'Alternaria.' Ann. Intern. Med. 77: 907–914, 1972.

1560. Harper, L. O., Burrell, R. G., Lapp, N. L., and Morgan, W. K. C. Allergic alveolitis due to pituitary snuff. Ann. Intern. Med. 73: 581–584, 1970.

1561. Katila, M-L., Mantyjarvi, R. A., and Ojanen, T. H. Sensitisation against environmental antigens and respiratory symptoms in swine workers. Br. J. Ind. Med. 38: 334–338, 1981.

1562. Patterson, R., Wang, J. L. F., Fink, J. N., Calvanico, N. J., and Roberts, M. IgA and IgG antibody activities of serum and bronchoalveolar fluid from symptomatic and asymptomatic pigeon breeders. Am. Rev. Respir. Dis. 120: 1113–1118, 1979.

1563. Bernardo, J., Hunninghake, G. W., Gadek, J. E., Ferrans, V. J., and Crystal, R. G. Acute hypersensitivity pneumonitis: serial changes in lung lymphocyte subpopulations after exposure to antigen. Am. Rev. Respir. Dis. 120: 985–994, 1979.

1564. Bureau, M. A., Fecteau, C., Patriquin, H., Rola-Pleszczynski, M., Masse, S., and Begin, R. Farmer's lung in early childhood. Am. Rev. Respir. Dis. 119: 671–675, 1979.

1565. Braun, S. R., doPico, G. A., Tsiatis, A., Horvath, E., Dickie, H., and Rankin, J. Farmer's lung disease: long-term clinical and physiologic outcome. Am. Rev. Respir. Dis. 119: 185–191, 1979.

1566. Sovijarvi, A. R. A., Kuusisto, P., Muittari, A., and Kauppinen-Walin, K. Trapped air in extrinsic allergic alveolitis. Respiration 40: 57–64, 1980.

1567. Petro, W., Muller, E., Wuthe, H., Bergmann, K. C., Unger, U., and Vogel, J. Site and type of impaired lung function in extrinsic allergic alveolitis. Respiration 39: 87–96, 1980.

1568. Petro, W., Muller, E., Bergmann, K-C., Unger, U., and Vogel, J. Impaired CO transfer factors in bird fancier's lung. Lung 155: 269–276, 1978.

1569. Lupi-Herrera, E., Sandoval, J., Bialostozky, D., Seoane, M., Martinez, M. L., Bonetti, P. F., Reyes, P., and Barrios, R. Extrinsic allergic alveolitis caused by pigeon breeding at a high altitude (2,240 meters). Am. Rev. Respir. Dis. 124: 602–607, 1981.

1570. Tukianen, P., Taskinen, E., Korhola, O., and Valle, M. Farmer's lung. Eur. J. Respir. Dis. 61: 3–11, 1980.

1571. Khan, Z. U., Sandhu, R. S., Randhawa, H. S., and Parkash, D. Allergic bronchopulmonary aspergillosis in a cane-sugar mill. Scand. J. Respir. Dis. 58: 129–133, 1977.

1572. Pepys, J. Clinical and therapeutic significance of patterns of allergic reactions of the lungs to extrinsic agents. Am. Rev. Respir. Dis. 116: 569–572, 1977.

1573. Allen, D. H., Williams, G. V., and Woolcock, A. J. Bird breeder's hypersensitivity pneumonitis: progress studies of lung function after cessation of exposure to the provoking antigen. Am. Rev. Respir. Dis. 114: 555–566, 1976.

1574. Warren, C. P. W. and Tse, K. S. Extrinsic allergic alveolitis owing to hypersensitivity to chickens—significance of sputum precipitins. Am. Rev. Resp. Dis. 109: 672–677, 1974.

1575. Riley, D. J. and Saldana, M. Pigeon breeder's lung. Am. Rev. Respir. Dis. 107: 456–460, 1973.

1576. Chan-Yeung, M., Gryzbowski, S., and Schonell, M. Mushroom worker's lung. Am. Rev. Respir. Dis. 105: 819–822, 1972.

1577. Cortez, L. M. and Pankey, G. A. Acute pulmonary hypersensitivity to furazolidone. Am. Rev. Respir. Dis. 105: 823–826, 1972.

1578. Banaszak, E. F., Thiede, W. H., and Fink, J. N. Hypersensitivity pneumonitis due to contamination of an air conditioner. N. Engl. J. Med. 283: 271–276, 1970.

1579. Ho, D., Tashkin, D. P., Bein, M. E., and Sharma, O. Pulmonary infiltrates with eosinophilia associated with tetracycline. Chest 76: 33–36, 1979.

1580. Karr, R. M., Kohler, P. F., and Salvaggio, J. E. Hypersensitivity pneumonitis and extrinsic asthma. Chest 74: 98–102, 1978.

1581. Dodge, R. R., Reed, C. E., and Barbee, R. A. The absence of a relationship between serum precipitins and pulmonary disease in a community. Chest 73: 608–612, 1978.

1582. Warren, W. P. Hypersensitivity pneumonitis due to exposure to budgerigars. Chest 62: 170–174, 1972.

1583. Arnow, P. M., Fink, J. N., Schlueter, D. P., Barboriak, J. J., Mallison, G., Said, S. I., Martin, S., Unger, G. F., Scanlon, G. T., and Kurup, V. P. Early detection of hypersensitivity pneumonitis in office workers. Am. J. Med. 64: 236–242, 1978.

1584. Yocum, M. W., Saltzman, A. R., Strong, D. M., Donaldson, J. C., Ward, G. W., Walsh, F. M., Cobb, O. M., and Elliott, R. C. Extrinsic allergic alveolitis after Aspergillus fumigatus inhalation. Am. J. Med. 61: 939–945, 1976.

1585. Allen, D. H., Basten, A., Williams, G. V., and Woolcock, A. Familial hypersensitivity pneumonitis. Am. J. Med. 59: 505–514, 1975.

1586. Pether, J. V. S. and Greatorex, F. B. Farmer's lung disease in Somerset. Br. J. Ind. Med. 33: 265–268, 1976.

1587. Warren, C. P. W., Tse, K. S., and Cherniack, R. M. Mechanical properties of the lungs in extrinsic allergic alveolitis. Thorax 33: 315–321, 1978.

1588. Ross, P. J., Seaton, A., Foreman, H. M., and Evans, W. H. M. Pulmonary calcification following smallpox handler's lung. Thorax 29: 659–665, 1974.

1589. Warren, C. P. W. Extrinsic allergic alveolitis: a disease commoner in non-smokers. Thorax 32: 567–569, 1977.

1590. Howie, A. D., Boyd, G., and Moran, F. Pulmonary hypersensitivity to ramin (Gonystylus bancanus). Thorax 31: 585–587, 1976.

1591. Smyth, J. T., Adkins, G. E., Lloyd, M., Moore, B., and McWhite, E. Farmer's lung in Devon. Thorax 30: 197–203, 1975.

1592. Van Toorn, D. W. Coffee worker's lung. Thorax 25: 399–405, 1970.

1593. Jackson, E. and Welch, K. M. A. Mushroom worker's lung. Thorax 25: 25–30, 1970.

1594. Warren, C. P. W., Tse, K. S., and Cherniack, R. M. Mechanical properties of the lung in extrinsic allergic alveolitis. Thorax 33: 315–321, 1978.

1595. Madsen, D., Klock, L. E., Wenzel, F. J., Robbins, L., and Schmidt, C. D. The prevalence of farmer's lung in an agricultural population. Am. Rev. Respir. Dis. 113: 171–174, 1976.

1596. Hendrick, D. J., Faux, J. A., and Marshall, R. Budgerigar-fancier's lung: the commonest variety of allergic alveolitis in Britain. Br. Med. J. 2: 81–84, 1978.

1597. Boyd, M. J., Williams, I. P., Turton, C. W. G., Brooks, N., Leech, G., and Millard, F. J. C. Echocardiographic method for the estimation of pulmonary artery pressure in chronic lung disease. Thorax 35: 914–919, 1980.

1598. Morris, M. J., Smith, M. M., and Clarke, B. G. Lung mechanics after cardiac valve replacement. Thorax 35: 453–460, 1980.

1599. Scott, K. W. M. A clinicopathological study of fatal airways obstruction. Thorax 31: 693–701, 1976.

1600. Edwards, C. W. Left ventricular hypertrophy in emphysema. Thorax 29: 75–80, 1974.

1601. Vereerstraeten, J., Schoutens, A., Tombroff, M., and De Koster, J. P. Value of measurement of alveolo-arterial gradient of P_{CO_2} compared to pulmonary scan in diagnosis of thromboembolic pulmonary disease. Thorax 28: 306–312, 1973.

1602. Schmock, C. L., Pomerantz, B., Mitchell, R. S., Pryor, R., and Maisel, J. C. The electrocardiogram in emphysema with and without chronic airways obstruction. Chest 60: 328–334, 1971.

1603. Shuck, J. W., Walder, J. S., Kam, T. H., and Thomas, H. M. Chronic persistent pulmonary embolism. Am. J. Med. 69: 790–794, 1980.

1604. De Troyer, A., Estenne, M., and Yernault, J. C. Disturbance of respiratory muscle function in patients with mitral valve disease. Am. J. Med. 69: 867–873, 1980.

1605. Overland, E. S., Nolan, A. J., and Hopewell, P. C. Alteration of pulmonary function in intravenous drug abusers. Am. J. Med. 68: 231–237, 1980.

1606. Robertson, C. H., Reynolds, R. C., and Wilson, J. E. III.

Pulmonary hypertension and foreign body granulomas in intravenous drug abusers. Am. J. Med. 61: 657–664, 1976.

1607. Schlozman, D. L., Kerby, G. R., and Ruth, W. E. Chronic pulmonary artery thrombosis with features of unilateral hyperlucent lung syndrome. Am. J. Med. 50: 547–551, 1971.

1608. Walcott, G., Burchell, H. B., and Brown, A. L. Primary pulmonary hypertension. Am. J. Med. 49: 70–79, 1970.

1609. Avery, W. G., Samet, P., and Sackner, M. A. The acidosis of pulmonary edema. Am. J. Med. 48: 320–324, 1970.

1610. Arciniegas, E., Hakimi, M., Hertzler, J. H., Farooki, Z. Q., and Green, E. W. Surgical management of congenital vascular rings. J. Thorac. Cardiovasc. Surg. 77: 721–727, 1979.

1611. Thadani, U., Burrow, C., Whitaker, W., and Heath, D. Pulmonary veno-occlusive disease. Q. J. Med. 44: 133–159, 1975.

1612. Oh, K. S., Park, S. C., Galvis, A. G., Young, L. W., Neches, W. H., and Zuberbuhler, J. R. Pulmonary hyperinflation in ventricular septal defect. J. Thorac. Cardiovasc. Surg. 76: 706–709, 1978.

1613. Dye, T. E., Saab, S. B., Almond, C. H., and Watson, L. Sclerosing mediastinitis with occlusion of pulmonary veins. J. Thorac. Cardiovasc. Surg. 74: 137–141, 1977.

1614. Sade, R. M., Williams, R. G., Castaneda, A. R., and Treves, S. Abnormalities of regional lung function associated with ventricular septal defect and pulmonary artery band. J. Thorac. Cardiovasc. Surg. 71: 572–580, 1976.

1615. Sproule, B. J., Brady, J. L., and Gilbert, J. A. L. Studies on the syndrome of fat embolization. Can. Med. Assoc. J. 90: 1243–1247, 1964.

1616. Singh, T., Dinda, P., Chatterjee, S. S., Riding, W. D., and Patel, T. K. Pulmonary function studies before and after closed mitral valvotomy. Am. Rev. Respir. Dis. 101: 62–66, 1970.

1617. Wilson, J. R., Mason, U. G. III, Bahler, R. C., Chester, E. H., Picken, J. J., and Baum, G. L. Vectorcardiographic detection of early hemodynamic abnormalities in chronic obstructive pulmonary disease. Chest 76: 160–165, 1979.

1618. Hales, C. A. and Kazemi, H. Pulmonary function after uncomplicated myocardial infarction. Chest 72: 350–358, 1977.

1619. Neuhaus, A., Bentz, R. R., and Weg, J. G. Pulmonary embolism in respiratory failure. Chest 73: 460–465, 1978.

1620. Shelton, D. M., Keal, E., and Reid, L. The pulmonary circulation in chronic bronchitis and emphysema. Chest 71(Suppl.): 303–306, 1977.

1621. Banyai, A. L. Editorial. Pulmonary fat embolism. Chest 69: 355, 1976.

1622. Wagenvoort, C. A. Pulmonary veno-occlusive disease. Chest 69: 82–86, 1976.

1623. Murphy, M. L. and Hutcheson, F. The electrocardiographic diagnosis of right ventricular hypertrophy in chronic obstructive pulmonary disease. Chest 65: 622–627, 1974.

1624. Auerbach, O., Garfinkel, L., and Hammond, E. C. Relation of smoking and age to findings in lung parenchyma: a microscopic study. Chest 65: 29–35, 1974.

1625. Soin, J. S., Wagner, H. N. Jr., Thomashaw, D., and Brown, T. C. Increased sensitivity of regional measurements in early detection of narcotic lung disease. Chest 67: 325–330, 1975.

1626. Camargo, G. and Colp, C. Pulmonary function studies in ex-heroin users. Chest 67: 331–334, 1975.

1627. Shinnick, J. P. and Cudkowicz, L. A problem in pulmonary hypertension. Chest 65: 69–75, 1974.

1628. Rebuck, A. S. and Vandenberg, R. A. The relationship between pulmonary arterial pressure and physiologic dead space in patients with obstructive lung disease. Am. Rev. Respir. Dis. 107: 423–428, 1973.

1629. Davidson, F. F. and Murray, J. F. Use of pulmonary diffusing capacity measurements to detect unsuspected fat embolism. Am. Rev. Respir. Dis. 106: 715–720, 1972.

1630. Al Bazzaz, F. J. and Kazemi, H. Arterial hypoxemia and distribution of pulmonary perfusion after uncomplicated myocardial infarction. Am. Rev. Respir. Dis. 106: 721–728, 1972.

1631. Ishikawa, S., Fattal, G. A., Popiewicz, J., and Wyatt, J. P. Functional morphometry of myocardial fibers in cor pulmonale. Am. Rev. Respir. Dis. 105: 358–367, 1972.

1632. Wood, T. E., McLeod, P., Anthonisen, N. R., and Macklem,

P. T. Mechanics of breathing in mitral stenosis. Am. Rev. Respir. Dis. 104: 52–60, 1971.

1633. Cullen, J. H., Kaemmerlen, J. T., Daoud, A., and Katz, H. L. A prospective clinical-pathologic study of the lungs and heart in chronic obstructive pulmonary disease. Am. Rev. Respir. Dis. 102: 190–204, 1970.

1634. Celli, B. and Khan, M. A. Mercury embolization of the lung. N. Engl. J. Med. 295: 883–885, 1976.

1635. Hales, C. A. and Kazemi, H. Small-airways function in myocardial infarction. N. Engl. J. Med. 290: 761–765, 1974.

1635a. Edelman, N. H., Lahiri, S., Braudo, L., Cherniack, N. S., and Fishman, A. P. The blunted ventilatory response to hypoxia in cyanotic congenital heart disease. N. Engl. J. Med. 282: 405–411, 1970.

1636. Moser, K. M. Pulmonary embolism. Am. Rev. Respir. Dis. 115: 829–852, 1977.

1637. De Troyer, A., Yernault, J-C., and Englert, M. Mechanics of breathing in patients with atrial septal defect. Am. Rev. Respir. Dis. 115: 413–421, 1977.

1638. Fishman, A. P. Chronic cor pulmonale. Am. Rev. Respir. Dis. 114: 775–794, 1976.

1639. Mitchell, R. S., Stanford, R. E., Silvers, G. W., and Dart, G. The right ventricle in chronic airway obstruction: a clinicopathologic study. Am. Rev. Respir. Dis. 114: 147–154, 1976.

1640. Vaughan, T. R. Jr., DeMarino, E. M., and Staub, N. C. Indicator dilution lung water and capillary blood volume in prolonged heavy exercise in normal men. Am. Rev. Respir. Dis. 113: 757–762, 1976.

1641. McKeen, C. R., Brigham, K. L., Bowers, R. E., and Harris, T. R. Pulmonary vascular effects of fat emulsion infusion in unanaesthetized sheep. J. Clin. Invest. 61: 1291–1297, 1978.

1642. Dawson, A., Rocamora, J. M., and Morgan, J. R. Regional lung function in chronic pulmonary congestion with and without mitral stenosis. Am. Rev. Respir. Dis. 113: 51–59, 1976.

1643. Interiano, B., Hyde, R. W., Hodges, M., and Yu, P. N. Interrelation between alterations in pulmonary mechanics and hemodynamics in acute myocardial infarction. J. Clin. Invest. 52: 1994–2006, 1973.

1644. Sutherland, P. W., Cade, J. F., and Pain, M. C. F. Pulmonary extravascular fluid volume and hypoxaemia in myocardial infarction. Aust. N.Z. J. Med. 2: 141–145, 1971.

1645. Bass, H. Regional pulmonary function in patients with pulmonary embolism. Bull. Physiopathol. Respir. 6: 123–134, 1970.

1646. Schrijen, F. and Jezek, V. Spirographie et échanges gazeuses à long terme après embolie pulmonaire. Bull. Physiopathol. Respir. 6: 195–210, 1970.

1647. Bignon, J., Pariente, R., and Brouet, G. Fréquence autopsique des thrombo-embolies pulmonaires au stade terminal des bronchopneumopathies chroniques obstructives. Bull. Physiopathol. Respir. 6: 405–424, 1970.

1648. Stanek, V., Oppelt, A., Jebavy, P., and Widimsky, J. A contribution to the mechanism of the distribution of pulmonary blood flow in patients with mitral stenosis. Bull. Physiopathol. Respir. 7: 913–924, 1971.

1649. Turino, G. M., Pine, M. B., Shubrooks, S. J. Jr., and Carey, J. P. The volume of extravascular water of the lung in normal man and in disease. Bull. Physiopathol. Respir. 7: 1161–1179, 1971.

1650. Gourgon, R., Motte, G., Gueris, J., Masquet, C., Lemaire, F., Christeler, P., and Lorente, P. Les oedemes pulmonaires precoces de l'infarctus du myocarde. Bull. Physiopathol. Respir. 7: 1257–1277, 1971.

1651. Gazioglu, K. Pulmonary diffusing capacity and capillary blood volume in valvular heart disease. Bull. Physiopathol. Respir. 9: 631–634, 1973.

1652. Schuren, K. P. and Huttemann, U. Chronic obstructive lung disease: pulmonary circulation and right ventricular function in two different clinical types. Bull. Physiopathol. Respir. 9: 716–724, 1973.

1653. Lockhart, A. Hemodynamique pulmonaire dans la bronchite chronique. Bull. Physiopathol. Respir. 9: 1069–1099, 1973.

1654. Demedts, M., Sniderman, A., Utz, G., Palmer, W. H., and Becklake, M. R. Lung volumes including closing volume, and arterial blood gas measurements in acute ischaemic left heart failure. Bull. Physiopathol. Respir. 10: 11–25, 1974.

1655. Stratta, P., Cardellino, G., Garbagni, R., Grassini, G., and Tartara, D. La diffusion du CO dans la sténose mitrale, dans la communication interauriculaire et dans l'hypertension pulmonaire primitive. In: Sadoul, P. (ed.). Le Transfert de l'Oxyde de Carbone. Soc. Eur. Physiopathol. Respir. Masson et Cie, Paris, 1969.

1656. Wattel, F., Lefevre, J., Chopin, C., Lottin, D., Raviart, B., and Lefranc, M. F. Etude isotopique des perturbations hydro-electriques chez l'insuffisant respiratoire chronique decompense. Bull. Physiopathol. Respir. 11: 683–707, 1975.

1657. Denolin, H. and Arhirii, M. (ed.). Nomenclature and definitions in respiratory physiology and clinical aspects of chronic lung disease. Bull. Physiopathol. Respir. 11: 937–959, 1975.

1658. Bjarke, B. Spirometric data, pulmonary ventilation and gas exchange at rest and during exercise in adult patients with tetralogy of Fallot. Scand. J. Respir. Dis. 55: 47–61, 1974.

1659. Parent, J. G., Schrijen, F., and Viana, R. A. Indices radiologiques d'hypertension pulmonaire dans la maladie obstructive chronique. Bull. Eur. Physiopathol. Respir. 12: 637–650, 1976.

1660. Chronic lung diseases leading to cor pulmonale. World Health Organization. Florence, Dec 6–7, 1976. Bull. Physiopathol. Respir. 14: 1P–9P, 1978.

1661. Gabinski, C., Courty, G., Besse, P., and Castaing, R. La fonction ventriculaire gauche au cours des bronchopneumopathies chroniques obstructives. Bull. Eur. Physiopathol. Respir. 15: 755–772, 1979.

1662. Schrijen, F. and Urtiaga, B. Le volume sanguin pulmonaire dans les bronchopneumopathies chroniques. Bull. Eur. Physiopathol. Respir. 16: 637–644, 1980.

1663. Riedel, M., Stanek, V., and Widimsky, J. Spirometry and gas exchange in chronic pulmonary thromboembolism. Bull. Eur. Physiopathol. Respir. 17: 209–221, 1981.

1664. Yernault, J-C. and Vandivivere, J. Infuence des cardiopathies sur la fonction pulmonaire régionale. Bull. Eur. Physiopathol. Respir. 16: 411–420, 1980.

1665. Riedel, M., Widimsky, J., and Stanek, V. Steady-state pulmonary transfer factor in chronic thromboembolic disease. Bull. Eur. Physiopathol. Respir. 16: 469–477, 1980.

1666. Corris, P. A., Nariman, S., and Gibson, G. J. Nifedipine in the prevention of asthma induced by exercise and histamine. Am. Rev. Respir. Dis. 128: 991–992, 1983.

1667. Dantzker, D. R. and Bower, J. S. Gas exchange in obliterative pulmonary vascular disease. In: Piiper, J. and Scheid, P. (eds.). Gas exchange function in normal and diseased lungs. Progress in Respiration Research, Vol. 16. S. Karger, Basel, 1981.

1668. Jezek, V. and Schrijen, F. Left ventricular function in chronic obstructive pulmonary disease with and without cardiac failure. Clin. Sci. 45: 267–279, 1973.

1669. Collins, J. V., Cochrane, G. M., Davis, J., Benatar, S. R., and Clark, T. J. H. Some aspects of pulmonary function after rapid saline infusion in healthy subjects. Clin. Sci. 45: 407–410, 1973.

1670. Tattersfield, A. E., McNicol, M. W., and Sillett, R. W. Relationship between haemodynamic and respiratory function in patients with myocardial infarction and left ventricular failure. Clin. Sci. 42: 751–768, 1972.

1671. Taylor, M. R. H. The ventilatory response to hypoxia during exercise in cyanotic congenital heart disease. Clin. Sci. 45: 99–105, 1973.

1672. Spierer, M. The ventilatory response to carbon dioxide in patients who have recovered from cardiogenic pulmonary oedema. Clin. Sci. 47: 285–288, 1974.

1673. Collins, J. V., Clark, T. J. H., and Brown, D. J. Airway function in healthy subjects and patients with left heart disease. Clin. Sci. 49: 217–228, 1975.

1674. Campbell, R. H. A., Brand, H. L., Cox, J. R., and Howard, P. Body weight and body water in chronic cor pulmonale. Clin. Sci. 49: 323–335, 1975.

1675. Levinson, R., Epstein, M., Sackner, M. A., and Begin, R. Comparison of the effects of water immersion and saline infusion on central hemodynamics in man. Clin. Sci. 52: 343–350, 1977.

1676. Raffestin, B., Valette, H., Hebert, J. L., Duhaze, P., and

Lockhart, A. Pulmonary blood volume in chronic bronchitis. Clin. Sci. 53: 587–593, 1977.

1677. Patrick, J. M., Tutty, J., and Pearson, S. B. Propranolol and the ventilatory response to hypoxia and hypercapnia in normal man. Clin. Sci. 55: 491–497, 1978.

1678. Reed, J. W., Ablett, M., and Cotes, J. E. Ventilatory responses to exercise and to carbon dioxide in mitral stenosis before and after valvulotomy: causes of tachypnoea. Clin. Sci. 54: 9–16, 1978.

1679. Yernault, J-C., Englert, M., and De Troyer, A. Mechanical and diffusing lung properties in patients with rheumatic valve disease. In: Giuntini, C. and Panuccio, P. (eds.). Cardiac Lung. Proceedings of an international congress, Firenze, 1976. Piccin Editore, Padova, Italy, 1979.

1680. Thoma, R., Niehues, B., Behrenbeck, D. W., and Siemon, G. CO diffusing components and closing capacity in valvular heart disease. In: Giuntini, C. and Panuccio, P. (eds.). Cardiac Lung. Proceedings of an international congress, Firenze, 1976. Piccin Editore, Padova, Italy, 1979.

1681. Mariani, M., Barsotti, A., Balbarini, A., Marini, C., Fornai, C., and Giuntini, C. Gas exchange in relation to pulmonary hemodynamics and function in patients with left heart valvular disease. In: Giuntini, C. and Panuccio, P. (eds.). Cardiac Lung. Proceedings of an international congress, Firenze, 1976. Piccin Editore, Padova, Italy, 1979.

1682. Stanek, V., Yebavy, P., Malek, I., Oppelt, A., and Widimsky, J. Regional lung function in patients with valvular heart disease. In: Giuntini, C. and Panuccio, P. (eds.). Cardiac Lung. Proceedings of an international congress, Firenze, 1976. Piccin Editore, Padova, Italy, 1979.

1683. Strieder, D. J. Exercise performance in tetralogy of Fallot. In: Giuntini, C. and Panuccio, P. (eds.). Cardiac Lung. Proceedings of an international congress, Firenze, 1976. Piccin Editore, Padova, Italy, 1979.

1684. De Troyer, A., Yernault, J-C., Polis, O., and Englert, M. Lung mechanics in left to right shunts in relation to haemodynamic data and diffusing capacity. In: Giuntini, C. and Panuccio, P. (eds.). Cardiac Lung. Proceedings of an international congress, Firenze, 1976. Piccin Editore, Padova, Italy, 1979.

1685. Thoma, R., Niehues, B., Behrenbeck, D. W., and Siemon, G. CO diffusing components and closing capacity in congenital heart disease. In: Giuntini, C. and Panuccio, P. (eds.). Cardiac Lung. Proceedings of an international congress, Firenze, 1976. Piccin Editore, Padova, Italy, 1979.

1686. Santolicandro, A., Palla, A., Fornai, E., Barsotti, A., Mariani, M., and Giuntini, C. Regional lung ventilation and perfusion in patients with congenital heart disease with shunt. In: Giuntini, C. and Panuccio, P. (eds.). Cardiac Lung. Proceedings of an international congress, Firenze, 1976. Piccin Editore, Padova, Italy, 1979.

1687. Wilhelmsen, L., Tibblin, G., Grimby, G., Bjure, J., Ekstrom-Jodal, B., and Aurell, M. Relationship between dyspnea and later manifestations of clinical coronary heart disease and death. In: Giuntini, C. and Panuccio, P. (eds.). Cardiac Lung. Proceedings of an international congress, Firenze, 1976. Piccin Editore, Padova, Italy, 1979.

1688. Giuntini, C., Pistolesi, M., Begliomini, E., Pollastri, A., Ballestra, A. M., and Maseri, A. Chest X-ray versus dilution method in the assessment of pulmonary edema in patients with coronary heart disease. In: Giuntini, C. and Panuccio, P. (eds.). Cardiac Lung. Proceedings of an international congress, Firenze, 1976. Piccin Editore, Padova, Italy, 1979.

1689. Hyde, R. W., Gray, B. A., Interiano, M., Hodges, M., and Yu, P. N. Relation between pulmonary vascular hemodynamics and pulmonary function in angina pectoris and myocardial infarction. In: Giuntini, C. and Panuccio, P. (eds.). Cardiac Lung. Proceedings of an international congress, Firenze, 1976. Piccin Editore, Padova, Italy, 1979.

1690. Malek, I., Stanek, V., Pavlovic, J., and Widimsky, J. Hemodynamics and pulmonary function in acute myocardial infarction. In: Giuntini, C. and Panuccio, P. (eds.). Cardiac Lung. Proceedings of an international congress, Firenze, 1976. Piccin Editore, Padova, Italy, 1979.

1691. Ballestra, A. M., Pistolesi, M., Maseri, A., and Giuntini, C. Mechanisms of arterial hypoxemia in acute myocardial infarction. In: Giuntini, C. and Panuccio, P. (eds.). Cardiac Lung.

Proceedings of an international congress, Firenze, 1976. Piccin Editore, Padova, Italy, 1979.

1692. Muir, A. L. The lung in cardiogenic shock. In: Giuntini, C. and Panuccio, P. (eds.). Cardiac Lung. Proceedings of an international congress, Firenze, 1976. Piccin Editore, Padova, Italy, 1979.

1693. Siemon, G., Niehues, B., Behrenbeck, D. W., and Thoma, R. Lung function in coronary heart disease. In: Giuntini, C. and Panuccio, P. (eds.). Cardiac Lung. Proceedings of an international congress, Firenze, 1976. Piccin Editore, Padova, Italy, 1979.

1694. Ressl, J., Jandova, R., and Widimsky, J. Central hemodynamics and pulmonary function in patients 3 to 5 months after acute myocardial infarction. In: Giuntini, C. and Panuccio, P. (eds.). Cardiac Lung. Proceedings of an international congress, Firenze, 1976. Piccin Editore, Padova, Italy, 1979.

1695. Sorbini, C. A., Grassi, V., Todisco, T., Ansidei, V., Boschetti, E., Dottorini, M., and Muiesan, G. Pulmonary function in congestive heart disease due to chronic ischemic heart disease. In: Giuntini, C. and Panuccio, P. (eds.). Cardiac Lung. Proceedings of an international congress, Firenze, 1976. Piccin Editore, Padova, Italy, 1979.

1696. Book, K. and Holmgren, H. Long term changes in pulmonary function following cardiac surgery. In: Giuntini, C. and Panuccio, P. (eds.). Cardiac Lung. Proceedings of an international congress, Firenze, 1976. Piccin Editore, Padova, Italy, 1979.

1697. Kral, B. Changes in regional lung function following valvular heart surgery. In: Giuntini, C. and Panuccio, P. (eds.). Cardiac Lung. Proceedings of an international congress, Firenze, 1976. Piccin Editore, Padova, Italy, 1979.

1698. Dantzker, A. and Bower, J. S. Partial reversibility of chronic pulmonary hypertension caused by pulmonary thromboembolic disease. Am. Rev. Respir. Dis. 124: 129–131, 1981.

1699. Schrijen, F. and Urtiaga, B. Pulmonary blood volume in chronic lung disease. Chest 81: 544–549, 1982.

1700. Matthay, R. A. and Berger, H. J. Cardiovascular performance in chronic obstructive pulmonary disease. Med. Clin. North Am. 65(3): 489–524, 1981.

1701. Jebavy, P., Widimsky, J., and Stanek, V. Distribution of inspired gas and pulmonary diffusing capacity at rest and during graded exercise in patients with mitral stenosis. Respiration 28: 216–235, 1971.

1702. Weitzenblum, E., Hirth, C., Roeslin, N., Vandevenne, A., and Oudet, P. Les modifications hemodynamiques pulmonaires au cours de l'insuffisance respiratoire aigue des bronchopneumopathies chroniques. Respiration 28: 539–554, 1971.

1703. Stanek, V., Widimsky, J., and Jebavy, P. Respiratory function in recurrent pulmonary embolism. Respiration 30: 223–233, 1973.

1704. Schuren, K. P. and Huttemann, U. Effect of respiratory and hemodynamic abnormalities on the electrocardiogram in chronic obstructive lung disease. Respiration 30: 234–245, 1973.

1705. Simon, H., Ferlinz, R., Fricke, G., Esser, H., Stadeler, H. J., Endres, P., and Kikis, D. Pulmonalarterien Mitteldruck und Lungenfunktion beim chronisch obstruktiven Syndrom. Respiration 30: 552–560, 1973.

1706. Pande, J. N., Gupta, S. P., and Guleria, J. S. Clinical significance of the measurement of membrane diffusing capacity and pulmonary capillary blood volume. Respiration 32: 317–324, 1975.

1707. Jebavy, P., Hurych, J., and Widimsky, J. Influence of pulmonary hypertension on pulmonary diffusing capacity in patients with mitral stenosis. Respiration 35: 1–7, 1978.

1708. Roux, J. J., Deveze, J. L., Escojido, H., and Ohresser, P. Fonction ventriculaire gauche de l'insuffisance respiratoire chronique au decours d'une decompensation aigue. Respiration 38: 43–49, 1979.

1709. Bucca, C., Rolla, G., Pecchio, O., Ratti, C., Accotino, G., and Galeasso, B. Systemic arterial hypertension and small airways function. Respiration 39: 188–192, 1980.

1710. Hutsebaut, J., Scano, G., Garcia-Herreros, P., Degre, S., De Coster, A., and Sergysels, R. Hemodynamic characteristics in chronic obstructive lung disease as related to cardiac size. Respiration 41: 25–32, 1981.

1711. Metanov, L., Bachtchevandjieva, R., and Kirkova, T. Influ-

ence d'une hemodynamique pulmonaire perturbée sur l'obstruction bronchique precoce chez les patients souffrant de troubles mitraux. Respiration 42: 25–29, 1981.

1712. Rolla, G., Bucca, C., Sclavo, M., Borello, G., and Bellone, E. Relation between respiratory function and pulmonary hemodynamics before and after intravenous administration of furosemide in acute myocardial infarction. Respiration 42: 161–167, 1981.

1713. Fazio, F. and Wollmer, P. Clinical ventilation-perfusion scintigraphy. Clin. Physiol. 1: 323–327, 1981.

1714. Fulop, M., Horowitz, M., Aberman, A., and Jaffe, E. R. Lactic acidosis in pulmonary edema due to left ventricular failure. Ann. Intern. Med. 79: 180–186, 1973.

1715. Aberman, A. and Fulop, M. The metabolic and respiratory acidosis of acute pulmonary edema. Ann. Intern. Med. 76: 173–184, 1972.

1716. McHugh, T. J., Forrester, J. S., Adler, L., Zion, D., and Swan, H. J. C. Pulmonary vascular congestion in acute myocardial infarction: hemodynamic and radiologic correlations. Ann. Intern. Med. 76: 29–33, 1972.

1717. Murphy, M. L., Adamson, J., and Hutcheson, F. Left ventricular hypertrophy in patients with chronic bronchitis and emphysema. Ann. Intern. Med. 81: 307–313, 1974.

1718. Moser, K. M., Guisan, M., Cuomo, A., and Ashburn, W. L. Differentiation of pulmonary vascular from parenchymal disease by ventilation/perfusion scintiphotography. Ann. Intern. Med. 75: 597–605, 1971.

1719. Pulmonary veno-occlusive disease (editorial). Lancet ii: 566–567, 1979.

1720. Pajewski, M., Reif, R., Manor, H., Starinsky, R., and Katzir, D. Pulmonary veno-occlusive disease in a unilateral hypertransradiant lung. Thorax 36: 397–399, 1981.

1721. Horsfield, K. and Thomas, M. Morphometry of pulmonary arteries from angiograms in chronic obstructive lung disease. Thorax 36: 360–365, 1981.

1722. Schor, R. A., Shames, D. M., Weber, P. M., and Dos Remedios, L. V. Regional ventilation studies with Kr^{81m} and Xe^{133}: a comparative analysis. J. Nucl. Med. 19: 348–353, 1978.

1723. Yernault, J-C. and De Troyer, A. Mechanics of breathing in patients with aortic valve disease. Bull. Eur. Physiopathol. Respir. 16: 491–499, 1980.

1724. Macarthur, C. G. C., Hunter, D., and Gibson, G. J. Ventilatory function in the Eisenmenger syndrome. Thorax 34: 348–353, 1979.

1725. Anthonisen, N. R. and Smith, H. J. Respiratory acidosis as a consequence of pulmonary edema. Ann. Intern. Med. 62: 991–999, 1965.

1726. Sanderson, J. E., Spiro, S. G., Hendry, A. T., and Turner-Warwick, M. A case of pulmonary veno-occlusive disease responding to treatment with azathioprine. Thorax 32: 140–148, 1977.

1727. Yernault, J-C. and De Troyer, A. Mechanics of breathing in patients with primary pulmonary hypertension (letter to editor). Am. Rev. Respir. Dis. 119: 320–321, 1979.

1728. Trell, E. Pulmonary hypertension in disorders of the left heart. Scand. J. Clin. Lab. Invest. 31: 409–418, 1973.

1729. Andersen, N. B. and Ghia, J. Pulmonary function, cardiac status, and postoperative course in relation to cardiopulmonary bypass. J. Thorac. Cardiovasc. Surg. 59: 474–483, 1970.

1730. Rabelo, R. C., Oliviera, S. A., Tanaka, H., Weigl, D. R., Verginelli, G., and Zerbini, E. J. The influence of the nature of the prime on postperfusion pulmonary changes. J. Thorac. Cardiovasc. Surg. 66: 782–793, 1973.

1731. Rea, H. H., Harris, E. A., Seelye, E. R., Whitlock, R. M. L., and Withy, S. J. The effects of cardiopulmonary bypass upon pulmonary gas exchange. J. Thorac. Cardiovasc. Surg. 75: 104–120, 1978.

1732. Asada, S. and Yamaguchi, M. Fine structural change in the lung following cardiopulmonary bypass. Chest 59: 478–483, 1971.

1733. Braun, S. R., Birnbaum, M. L., and Chopra, P. S. Pre- and postoperative pulmonary function abnormalities in coronary artery revascularization surgery. Chest 73: 316–320, 1978.

1734. Cain, H. D., Stevens, P. M., and Adaniya, R. Preoperative pulmonary function and complications after cardiovascular surgery. Chest 76: 130–135, 1979.

1735. Foliguet, B. and Helmer, J. Le poumon de CEC. Complication de la chirurgie cardiaque. Bull. Physiopathol. Respir. 11: 353–392, 1975.

1736. Buhlmann, A. A. and Frick, P. Acute respiratory distress, consequent to cardiac surgery with relation to the preoperative hemodynamics and pulmonary function pattern (288 adults). In: Giuntini, C. and Panuccio, P. (eds.). Cardiac Lung. Proceedings of an international congress, Firenze, 1976. Piccin Editore, Padova, Italy, 1979.

1737. Henriksen, J. M. and Dahl, R. Effects of inhaled budenoside alone and in combination with low-dose terbutaline in children with exercise-induced asthma. Am. Rev. Respir. Dis. 128: 993–997, 1983.

1738. Prior, A. L., Efthimiou, J. J., and Yates, A. K. Local excision of pulmonary arteriovenous fistulae including the feeding artery and draining vein. Thorax 34: 662–664, 1979.

1739. Loebl, E. C., Platt, M. R., Mills, L. J., and Estrera, A. S. Pulmonary resection for a traumatic pulmonary arteriovenous fistula. J. Thorac. Cardiovasc. Surg. 77: 674–676, 1979.

1740. Honey, M. Anomalous pulmonary venous drainage of right lung to inferior vena cava ("scimitar syndrome"): clinical spectrum in older patients and role of surgery. Q. J. Med. 46: 463–483, 1977.

1741. Harrow, E. M., Beach, P. M., Wise, J. R. Jr., Lynch, C., Graham, W. G. B., and Wight, G. Pulmonary arteriovenous fistula. Chest 73: 92–94, 1978.

1742. Kawai, C., Ishikawa, K., Kato, M., Ishii, Y., and Nakao, K. "Pulmonary pulseless disease": pulmonary involvement in so-called Takayasu's disease. Chest 73: 651–657, 1978.

1743. Kleiner, J. P. and Kmiecik, J. Hypoxemia with a nonresolving pulmonary infiltrate. Chest 78: 327–329, 1980.

1744. Huseby, J. S., Culver, B. H., and Butler, J. Pulmonary arteriovenous fistulas: increase in shunt at high lung volumes. Am. Rev. Respir. Dis. 115: 229–232, 1977.

1745. Paramelle, B., Hohn, B., Parent, B., Coulomb, M., Mikler, F., and Paramelle, F. La fonction respiratoire au cours des obstructions chroniques des gros troncs arterielles pulmonaires. Poumon Coeur 32: 205–212, 1976.

1746. Laros, C. D. Shunts in and over the lungs. Respiration 29: 24–39, 1972.

1747. Genovesi, M. G., Tierney, D. F., Taplin, G. V., and Eisenberg, H. An intravenous radionuclide method to evaluate hypoxemia caused by abnormal alveolar vessels. Am. Rev. Respir. Dis. 114: 59–65, 1976.

1748. Bruya, T. E., Keppel, J. F., D'Silva, R., and Barker, A. F. Longitudinal evaluation of a patient with arteriovenous fistulas. Chest 76: 603–605, 1979.

1749. Shannon, D. C. and Kazemi, H. Distribution of lung function in patients with anomalies of the pulmonary circulation. J. Thorac. Cardiovasc. Surg. 64: 26–30, 1972.

1750. Rice, D. L., Bedrossian, C., Blair, H. T., and Miller, W. C. Closing volumes with variations in pulmonary capillary wedge pressure. Am. Rev. Respir. Dis. 123: 513–516, 1981.

1751. Holl, J. E., Kolbeck, R. C., and Speir, W. A. Jr. Pulmonary vascular responsiveness to histamine: exquisite sensitivity of small intrapulmonary arteries. Am. Rev. Respir. Dis. 122: 909–913, 1980.

1752. Sudhakaran, K., Viswanathan, R., and Subramanian, T. A. V. Plasma histamine levels under hypoxic stress. Respiration 37: 91–96, 1979.

1753. Viswanathan, R., Lodi, S. T. K., Subramanian, S., and Radha, T. G. Pulmonary vascular response to ventilation hypercapnia in man. Respiration 33: 165–178, 1976.

1754. Muir, A. L. Radionuclide determined pulmonary blood volume in ischemic heart disease. Thorax 36: 922–927, 1981.

1755. Collins, R. L., Turner, R. A., Johnson, A. M., Whitley, N. O., and McLean, R. L. Obstructive pulmonary disease in rheumatoid arthritis. Arthritis Rheum. 19: 623–628, 1976.

1756. Kan, W. O., Ledsome, J. R., and Bolter, C. P. Pulmonary arterial distension and activity in phrenic nerve of anesthetized dogs. J. Appl. Physiol. 46: 625–631, 1979.

1757. Pride, N. B. Tests of small airway function in the natural history of chronic airflow obstruction in smokers. In: Sadoul, P., Milic-Emili, J., Simonsson, B. G., and Clark, T. J. H. (eds.). Small Airways in Health and Disease. Proceedings of a Symposium, Copenhagen, March 1979. Excerpta Medica, Amsterdam, 1979.

1758. Bouhuys, A., Beck, G. J., and Schoenberg, J. B. Lung function: normal values and risk factors. In: Sadoul, P., Milic-Emili, J., Simonsson, B. G., and Clark, T. J. H. (eds.). Small Airways in Health and Disease. Proceedings of a Symposium, Copenhagen, March 1979. Excerpta Medica, Amsterdam, 1979.

1759. Laitinen, O., Nissila, M., Salorinne, Y., and Aalto, P. Pulmonary involvement in patients with rheumatoid arthritis. Scand. J. Respir. Dis. 56: 297–304, 1975.

1760. Veevaete, F., Van Der Straeten, M., De Vos, M., and Roels, H. Allergic granulomatous angiitis. Scand. J. Respir. Dis. 59: 287–296, 1978.

1761. Arnalich, F., De Andres, S. R., Gil, A., Puig, J. G., Barbado, J., and Vazquez, J. J. Pulmonary function in systemic lupus erythematosus patients without respiratory symptoms. Bull. Eur. Physiopathol. Respir. 15: 649–657, 1979.

1762. Greening, A. P. and Hughes, J. M. B. Serial estimations of carbon monoxide diffusing capacity in intrapulmonary haemorrhage. Clin. Sci. 60: 507–512, 1981.

1763. Herzog, C. A., Miller, R. R., and Hoidal, J. R. Bronchiolitis and rheumatoid arthritis. Am. Rev. Respir. Dis. 124: 636–639, 1981.

1764. Florin-Christensen, A., Doniach, D., and Newcomb, P. B. Alpha-chain disease with pulmonary manifestations. Br. Med. J. 2: 413–415, 1974.

1765. Schernthaner, G., Kummer, F., Scherak, O., and Kolarz, G. Respiratory function in rheumatoid arthritis (letter to editor). Br. Med. J. 4: 43, 1975.

1766. Armstrong, J. G. and Steele, R. H. Localised pulmonary arteritis in rheumatoid disease. Thorax 37: 313–314, 1982.

1767. Segal, I., Fink, G., Machtey, I., Gura, V., and Spitzer, S. A. Pulmonary function abnormalities in Sjogren's syndrome and the sicca complex. Thorax 36: 286–289, 1981.

1768. Eisenberg, H., Dubois, E. L., Sherwin, R. P., and Balchum, O. J. Diffuse interstitial lung disease in systemic lupus erythematosus. Ann. Intern. Med. 79: 37–45, 1973.

1769. Perrault, J. L., Janis, M., and Wolinsky, H. Resolution of chronic eosinophilic pneumonia with corticosteroid therapy. Ann. Intern. Med. 74: 951–954, 1971.

1770. Edwards, C. W. Vasculitis and granulomatosis of the respiratory tract (editorial). Thorax 37: 81–87, 1982.

1771. Fairfax, A. J., Haslam, P. L., Pavia, D., Sheahan, N. F., Bateman, J. R. M., Agnew, J. E., Clarke, S. W., and Turner-Warwick, M. Pulmonary disorders associated with Sjogren's syndrome. Q. J. Med. 50: 279–295, 1981.

1772. Newball, H. H. and Brahim, S. A. Chronic obstructive airway disease in patients with Sjogren's syndrome. Am. Rev. Respir. Dis. 115: 295–304, 1977.

1773. Helman, C. A., Keeton, G. R., and Benatar, S. R. Lymphoid interstitial pneumonia with associated chronic active hepatitis and renal tubular acidosis. Am. Rev. Respir. Dis. 115: 161–164, 1977.

1774. Katzenstein, A-L., Liebow, A. A., and Friedman, P. J. Bronchocentric granulomatosis, mucoid impaction, and hypersensitivity reactions to fungi. Am. Rev. Respir. Dis. 111: 497–537, 1975.

1775. Allue, X., Wise, M. B., and Beaudry, P. H. Pulmonary function studies in idiopathic pulmonary hemosiderosis in children. Am. Rev. Respir. Dis. 107: 410–415, 1973.

1776. Roberts, L. N., Montessori, G., and Patterson, J. G. Idiopathic pulmonary hemosiderosis. Am. Rev. Respir. Dis. 106: 904–908, 1972.

1777. Gross, M., Esterly, J. R., and Earle, R. H. Pulmonary alterations in systemic lupus erythematosus. Am. Rev. Respir. Dis. 105: 572–577, 1972.

1778. Elliott, M. L. and Kuhn, C. Idiopathic pulmonary hemosiderosis. Am. Rev. Respir. Dis. 102: 895–904, 1970.

1779. Cohen, J. M., Miller, A., and Spiera, H. Interstitial pneumonitis complicating rheumatoid arthritis. Chest 72: 521–524, 1977.

1780. Strimlan, C. V., Rosenow, E. C. III, Divertie, M. B., and Harrison, E. G. Jr. Pulmonary manifestations of Sjogren's syndrome. Chest 70: 354–361, 1976.

1781. Murphy, D. M. F., Fairman, R. P., Lapp, N. L., and Morgan, W. K. C. Severe airway disease due to inhalation of fumes from cleansing agents. Chest 69: 372–376, 1976.

1782. Rogers, R. M., Christiansen, J. R., Coalson, J. J., and

Patterson, C. D. Eosinophilic pneumonia. Chest 68: 665–671, 1975.

1783. Matthay, R. A. and Petty, T. L. Treatment of acute lupus pneumonitis with azothioprine. Chest 66: 219–220, 1974.

1784. Frank, S. T., Weg, J. G., Harkleroad, L. E., and Fitch, R. F. Pulmonary dysfunction in rheumatoid disease. Chest 63: 27–34, 1973.

1785. Rosenberg, D. M., Weinberger, S. E., Fulmer, J. D., Flye, M. W., Fauci, A. S., and Crystal, R. G. Functional correlates of lung involvement in Wegener's granulomatosis. Am. J. Med. 69: 387–394, 1980.

1786. Gibson, G. J., Edmonds, J. P., and Hughes, G. R. V. Diaphragm function and lung involvement in systemic lupus erythematosus. Am. J. Med. 63: 926–932, 1977.

1787. Donald, K. J., Edwards, R. L., and McEvoy, J. D. S. Alveolar capillary basement membrane lesions in Goodpasture's syndrome and idiopathic pulmonary hemosiderosis. Am. J. Med. 59: 642–649, 1975.

1788. Bedrossian, C. W. M., Greenberg, S. D., and Williams, L. J. Ultrastructure of the lung in Loeffler's pneumonia. Am. J. Med. 58: 438–443, 1975.

1789. Proskey, A. J., Weatherbee, L., Easterling, R. E., Greene, J. A., and Weller, J. M. Goodpasture's syndrome. Am. J. Med. 48: 162–173, 1970.

1790. Lee, P., Urowitz, M. B., Bookman, A. A. M., Koehler, B. E., Smythe, H. A., Gordon, D. A., and Ogryzlo, M. A. Systemic lupus erythematosus. Q. J. Med. 46: 1–32, 1977.

1791. Hills, E. A. and Geary, M. Membrane diffusing capacity and pulmonary capillary volume in rheumatoid disease. Thorax 35: 851–855, 1980.

1792. Fox, B. and Seed, W. A. Chronic eosinophilic pneumonia. Thorax 35: 570–580, 1980.

1793. Hills, E. A., Davies, S., and Geary, M. Frequency dependence of dynamic compliance in patients with rheumatoid arthritis. Thorax 34: 755–761, 1979.

1794. Lipscomb, D. J., Patel, K., and Hughes, J. M. B. Interpretation of increases in the transfer coefficient for carbon monoxide (TLco/VA or Kco). Thorax 33: 728–733, 1978.

1795. Nesarajah, M. S. Pulmonary function in tropical eosinophilia before and after treatment with diethylcarbamazine. Thorax 30: 574–577, 1975.

1796. Poh, S. C. The course of lung function in treated tropical pulmonary eosinophilia. Thorax 29: 710–712, 1974.

1797. Macfarlane, A. and Davies, D. Diffuse lymphoid interstitial pneumonia. Thorax 28: 768–776, 1973.

1798. Laitinen, O., Nissila, M., Salorinne, Y., and Aalto, P. Pulmonary involvement in patients with rheumatoid arthritis. Scand. J. Respir. Dis. 56: 297–304, 1975.

1799. Rodriguez-Roisin, R., Pares, A., Bruguera, M., Coll, J., Picado, C., Agusti-Ovidal, A., Burgos, F., and Rodes, J. Pulmonary involvement in primary biliary cirrhosis. Thorax 36: 208–212, 1981.

1800. Ahonen, A. V., Stenius-Aarniala, B. S. M., Viljanen, B. C., Halttunen, P. E. A., Oksa, P., and Mattson, K. V. Obstructive lung disease in Behçet's syndrome. Scand. J. Respir. Dis. 59:44–50, 1978.

1801. Scherak, O., Schernthaner, G., Hofner, W., Kolarz, G., and Kummer, F. Lungen Veranderungen bei der progredient chronischen Polyarthritis. Respiration 34: 162–170, 1977.

1802. Bake, B. Small airways—related to tobacco smoking. In: Sadoul, P., Milic-Emili, J., Simonsson, B. G., and Clark, T. J. H. (eds.). Small Airways in Health and Disease. Proceedings of a Symposium, Copenhagen, March 1979. Excerpta Medica, Amsterdam, 1979.

1803. Turner-Warwick, M., Burrows, B., and Johnson, A. Cryptogenic fibrosing alveolitis: response to corticosteroid treatment and its effect on survival. Thorax 35: 593–599, 1980.

1804. Turner-Warwick, M., Burrows, B., and Johnson, A. Cryptogenic fibrosing alveolitis: clinical features and their influence on survival. Thorax 35: 171–180, 1980.

1805. Kaufmann, J. M., Cuvelier, C. A., and Van Der Straeten, M. Mycoplasma pneumonia with fulminant evolution into diffuse interstitial fibrosis. Thorax 35: 140–144, 1980.

1806. De Troyer, A. and Yernault, J-C. Inspiratory muscle force in normal subjects and patients with interstitial lung disease. Thorax 35: 92–100, 1980.

1807. Pratt, D. S., Schwartz, M. I., May, J. J., and Dreisen, R. B. Rapidly fatal pulmonary fibrosis: the accelerated variant of interstitial pneumonitis. Thorax 34: 587–593, 1979.

1808. Bagg, L. R. and Hughes, D. T. D. Serial pulmonary function tests in progressive systemic sclerosis. Thorax 34: 224–228, 1979.

1809. Levin, P. J., Klaff, L. J., Rose, A. G., and Ferguson, A. D. Pulmonary effects of contact exposure to paraquat: a clinical and experimental study. Thorax 34: 150–160, 1979.

1810. Chopra, S. K., Taplin, G. V., Tashkin, D. P., and Elam, D. Lung clearance of soluble radioaerosols of different molecular weights in systemic sclerosis. Thorax 34: 63–67, 1979.

1811. Mark, G. J., Lehimgar-Zadeh, A., and Ragsdale, B. D. Cyclophosphamide pneumonitis. Thorax 33: 89–93, 1978.

1812. Davies, D., Crowther, J. S., and MacFarlane, A. Idiopathic progressive pulmonary fibrosis. Thorax 30: 316–325, 1975.

1813. Smith, P. and Heath, D. Paraquat lung: a reappraisal. Thorax 29: 643–653, 1974.

1814. Jones, G. R. and Malone, D. N. S. Sulphasalazine-induced lung disease. Thorax 27: 713–717, 1972.

1815. Stack, B. H. R., Choo-Kang, Y. F. J., and Heard, B. E. The prognosis of cryptogenic fibrosing alveolitis. Thorax 27: 535–542, 1972.

1816. Gardiner, A. J. S. Pulmonary oedema in paraquat poisoning. Thorax 27: 132–136, 1972.

1817. Thompson, P. L. and Mackay, I. R. Fibrosing alveolitis and polymyositis. Thorax 25: 504–507, 1970.

1818. Russell, D. C., Maloney, A., and Muir, A. L. Progressive generalised scleroderma: Respiratory failure from primary chest wall involvement. Thorax 36: 219–220, 1981.

1819. Rudders, R. A. and Hensley, G. T. Bleomycin pulmonary toxicity. Chest 63: 626–628, 1973.

1820. Dohner, V. A., Ward, H. P., and Standord, E. Alveolitis during procarbazine, vincristine and cyclophosphamide therapy. Chest 62: 636–639, 1972.

1821. Capron, J. P., Marti, R., Rey, J. L., Dupas, J. L., Capron, D., Delamarre, J., and Potet, F. Fibrosing alveolitis and hepatitis B surface antigen-associated chronic active hepatitis in a patient with immunoglobulin A deficiency. Am. J. Med. 66: 874–878, 1979.

1822. Garay, S. M., Gardella, J. E., Fazzini, E. P., and Goldring, R. M. Hermansky-Pudlak syndrome. Am. J. Med. 66: 737–747, 1979.

1823. Bjerke, R. D., Tashkin, D. P., Clements, P. J., Chopra, S. K., Gong, H., and Bein, M. Small airways in progressive systemic sclerosis (PSS). Am. J. Med. 66: 201–209, 1979.

1824. Winterbauer, R. H., Hammar, S. P., Hallman, K. O., Hays, J. E., Pardee, N. E., Morgan, E. H., Allen, J. D., Moores, K. D., Bush, W., and Walker, J. H. Diffuse interstitial pneumonitis. Am. J. Med. 65: 661–672, 1978.

1825. Young, R. H. and Mark, G. J. Pulmonary vascular changes in scleroderma. Am. J. Med. 64: 998–1004, 1978.

1826. Sostman, H. D., Matthay, R. A., and Putnam, C. E. Cytotoxic drug-induced lung disease. Am. J. Med. 62: 608–615, 1977.

1827. Duncan, P. E., Griffin, J. P., Garcia, A., and Kaplan, S. B. Fibrosing alveolitis in polymyositis. Am. J. Med. 57: 621–626, 1974.

1828. Bone, R. C., Wolfe, J., Sobonya, R. E., Kerby, G. R., Stechschulte, D., Ruth, W. E., and Welch, M. Desquamative interstitial pneumonia following long-term nitrofurantoin therapy. Am. J. Med. 60: 697–701, 1976.

1829. Fairshter, R. D. and Wilson, A. F. Paraquat poisoning. Am. J. Med. 59: 751–754, 1975.

1830. Renzetti, A. D., Kobayashi, T., Bigler, A., and Mitchell, M. N. Regional ventilation and perfusion in silicosis and in the alveolar-capillary block syndrome. Am. J. Med. 49: 5–13, 1970.

1831. Davies, B. H. and Tuddenham, E. G. D. Familial pulmonary fibrosis associated with oculocutaneous albinism and platelet function defect: a new syndrome. Q. J. Med. 45: 219–232, 1976.

1832. Brown, C. H. and Turner-Warwick, M. The treatment of cryptogenic fibrosing alveolitis with immunosuppressant drugs. Q. J. Med. 40: 289–302, 1971.

1833. Keogh, B. A. and Crystal, R. G. Pulmonary function testing in interstitial pulmonary disease. Chest 78: 856–865, 1980.

1834. Javaheri, S., Lederer, D. H., Pella, J. A., Mark, G. J., and

Levine, B. W. Idiopathic pulmonary fibrosis in monozygotic twins. Chest 78: 591–594, 1980.

1835. Goucher, G., Rowland, V., and Hawkins, J. Melphalan-induced pulmonary interstitial fibrosis. Chest 77: 805–806, 1980.

1836. McCarthy, D. S., Ostrow, D. N., and Hershfield, E. S. Chronic obstructive pulmonary disease following idiopathic pulmonary fibrosis. Chest 77: 473–477, 1980.

1837. Whipp, B. J. Tenets of the exercise hyperpnea and their degree of corroboration. Chest 73(Suppl.): 274–276, 1978.

1838. Crittenden, D., Tranum, B. L., and Haut, A. Pulmonary fibrosis after prolonged therapy with 1,3-bis(2-chloroethyl)-1-nitrosourea. Chest 72: 372–373, 1977.

1839. Carrington, C. B. Conference summary. Chest 69(Suppl.): 322–328, 1976.

1840. Thurlbeck, W. M. and Thurlbeck, S. M. Pulmonary effects of paraquat poisoning. Chest 69(Suppl.): 276–280, 1976.

1841. Bone, R. C., Wolfe, J., Sobonya, R. E., Kerby, G. R., Stechschulte, D., Ruth, W. E., and Welch, M. Desquamative interstitial pneumonia following chronic nitrofurantoin therapy. Chest 69(Suppl.): 296–297, 1976.

1842. Green, G. M., Graham, W. G. B., Hanson, J. S., Gump, D. W., Phillips, C. A., Brody, A. R., Sylvester, D. W., Landis, J. N., Davis, G. S., and Craighead, J. E. Correlated studies of interstitial pulmonary disease. Chest 69(Suppl.): 263, 1976.

1843. Fulmer, J. D., Roberts, W. C., and Crystal, R. G. Diffuse fibrotic lung disease: a correlative study. Chest 69(Suppl.): 263–265, 1976.

1844. Chester, E. H., Fleming, G. M., and Montenegro, H. Effect of steroid therapy on gas exchange abnormalities in patients with diffuse interstitial lung disease. Chest 69(Suppl.): 269–271, 1976.

1845. Weese, W. C., Levine, B. W., and Kazemi, H. Interstitial lung disease resistant to corticosteroid therapy. Chest 67: 57–60, 1975.

1846. Hazlett, D. R., Ward, G. W. Jr., and Madison, D. S. Pulmonary function loss in diphenylhydantoin therapy. Chest 66: 660–664, 1974.

1847. Hudson, A. R., Halprin, G. M., Miller, J. A., and Kilburn, K. H. Pulmonary interstitial fibrosis following alveolar proteinosis. Chest 65: 700–702, 1974.

1848. Frazier, A. R. and Miller, R. D. Interstitial pneumonitis in association with polymyositis and dermatomyositis. Chest 65: 403–407, 1974.

1849. Cassan, S. M., Divertie, M. B., and Brown, A. L. Jr. Fine structural morphometry on biopsy specimens of human lung. Chest 65: 275–278, 1974.

1850. Patchefsky, A. S., Atkinson, W. G., Hoch, W. S., Gordon, G., and Lipshitz, H. I. Interstitial pulmonary fibrosis and von Recklinghausen's disease. An ultrastructural and immunofluorescent study. Chest 64: 459–464, 1973.

1851. Rhodes, M. L. Desquamative interstitial pneumonia. Am. Rev. Respir. Dis. 108: 950–954, 1973.

1852. Ayotte, B., Friesen, W. O., Rosenhamer, G., and McIlroy, M. B. A new method of measuring pulmonary diffusing capacity for oxygen in patients with diffuse lung disease. Am. Rev. Respir. Dis. 108: 587–592, 1973.

1853. Israel, K. S., Brashear, R. E., Sharma, H. M., Yum, M. N., and Glover, J. L. Pulmonary fibrosis and nitrofurantoin. Am. Rev. Respir. Dis. 108: 353–356, 1973.

1854. Ostrow, D. and Cherniack, R. M. Resistance to airflow in patients with diffuse interstitial lung disease. Am. Rev. Respir. Dis. 108: 205–210, 1973.

1855. Pascual, R. S., Mosher, M. B., Sikand, R. S., De Conti, R. C., and Bouhuys, A. Effects of bleomycin on pulmonary function in man. Am. Rev. Respir. Dis. 108: 211–217, 1973.

1856. Topilow, A. A., Rothenberg, S. P., and Cottrell, T. S. Interstitial pneumonia after prolonged treatment with cyclophosphamide. Am. Rev. Respir. Dis. 108: 114–117, 1973.

1857. Fisher, H. K., Clements, J. A., and Wright, R. R. Enhancement of oxygen toxicity by the herbicide paraquat. Am. Rev. Respir. Dis. 107: 246–252, 1973.

1858. McCarthy, D. and Cherniack, R. M. Regional ventilation-perfusion and hypoxia in cryptogenic fibrosing alveolitis. Am. Rev. Respir. Dis. 107: 200–208, 1973.

1859. Perez-Guerra, F., Harkleroad, L. E., Walsh, R. E., and

Costanzi, J. J. Acute bleomycin lung. Am. Rev. Respir. Dis. 106: 909–913, 1972.

1860. Kuplic, J. B., Higley, C. S., and Niewohner, D. E. Pulmonary ossification associated with long-term busulfan therapy in chronic myeloid leukemia. Am. Rev. Respir. Dis. 106: 759–762, 1972.

1861. Olsen, G. N. and Swenson, E. W. Polymyositis and interstitial lung disease. Am. Rev. Respir. Dis. 105: 611–617, 1972.

1862. Cohen, R. and Overfield, E. M. The diffusion component of arterial hypoxemia. Am. Rev. Respir. Dis. 105: 532–540, 1972.

1863. Barrocas, M., Nuchprayoon, C. V., Claudio, M., King, F. W., Danon, J., and Sharp, J. T. Gas exchange abnormalities in diffuse lung disease. Am. Rev. Respir. Dis. 104: 72–87, 1971.

1864. Schwarz, M. I., Whitcomb, M. E., and French, J. B. Significance of an isolated reduction in residual volume. Am. Rev. Respir. Dis. 103: 430–432, 1971.

1865. Carrington, C. B., Gaensler, E. A., Coutu, R. E., Fitzgerald, M. X., and Gupta, R. G. Natural history and treated course of usual and desquamative interstitial pneumonia. N. Engl. J. Med. 298: 801–809, 1978.

1866. Epler, G. R., McLoud, T. C., Gaensler, E. A., Mikus, J. P., and Carrington, C. B. Normal chest roentgenograms in chronic diffuse infiltrative lung disease. N. Engl. J. Med. 298: 934–939, 1978.

1867. Winterbauer, R. H., Wilske, K. R., and Wheelis, R. F. Diffuse pulmonary injury associated with gold treatment. N. Engl. J. Med. 294: 919–921, 1976.

1868. Miller, A., Langer, A. M., Teirstein, A. S., and Selikoff, I. J. "Nonspecific" interstitial pulmonary fibrosis. N. Engl. J. Med. 292: 91–93, 1975.

1869. Case records of the Massachusetts General Hospital. Case 22-1974. N. Engl. J. Med. 290: 1309–1314, 1974.

1870. Wehr, K. L. and Johnson, R. L. Jr. Maximal oxygen consumption in patients with lung disease. J. Clin. Invest. 58: 880–890, 1976.

1871. Fulmer, J. D., Roberts, W. C., Von Gal, E. R., and Crystal, R. G. Small airways in idiopathic pulmonary fibrosis. J. Clin. Invest. 60: 595–610, 1977.

1872. Fulmer, J. D., Roberts, W. C., Von Gal, E. R., and Crystal, R. G. Morphologic-physiologic correlates of the severity of fibrosis and degree of cellularity in idiopathic pulmonary fibrosis. J. Clin. Invest. 63: 665–676, 1979.

1873. Gibson, G. J. and Pride, N. B. Pulmonary mechanics in fibrosing alveolitis. Am. Rev. Respir. Dis. 116: 637–647, 1977.

1874. Line, B. R., Fulmer, J. D., Reynolds, H. Y., Roberts, W. C., Jones, A. E., Harris, E. K., and Crystal, R. G. Gallium-67 citrate scanning in the staging of idioipathic pulmonary fibrosis: correlation with physiologic and morphologic features and bronchoalveolar lavage. Am. Rev. Respir. Dis. 118: 355–365, 1978.

1875. Vale, J. R. Effect of exercise and O_2 breathing on gas exchange in chronic bronchitis and in diffuse, restrictive pulmonary disease. Scand. J. Respir. Dis. 51: 316–332, 1970.

1876. Vale, J. R. Respiratory function in sarcoidosis and other interstitial lung diseases with similar radiological appearances. Scand. J. Respir. Dis. 52: 3–12, 1971.

1877. Ruikka, I., Vaissalo, T., and Saarimaa, H. Progressive pulmonary fibrosis during nitrofurantoin therapy. Scand. J. Respir. Dis. 52: 162–166, 1971.

1878. Gimenez, M., Uffholtz, H., and Schrijen, F. Reponses ventilatoires et cardio-respiratoires des restrictifs à l'exercice musculaire. Bull. Eur. Physiopathol. Respir. 13: 355–367, 1977.

1879. Sovijarvi, A. R. A., Lemola, M., Stenius, B., and Idanpaan-Heikkila, J. Nitrofurantoin-induced acute, subacute and chronic pulmonary reactions. A report of 66 cases. Scand. J. Respir. Dis. 58: 41–50, 1977.

1880. Jones, N. L. and Rebuck, A. S. Tidal volume during exercise in patients with diffuse fibrosing alveolitis. Bull. Eur. Physiopathol. Respir. 15: 321–327, 1979.

1881. Weitzenblum, E., Hirth, C., Rasaholinjanahary, J., Mirhom, R., and Roegel, E. Interet de l'epreuve d'exercice musculaire dans les pneumopathies interstitielles diffuses. Bull. Eur. Physiopathol. Respir. 15: 329–339, 1979.

1882. Briscoe, W. A. Does impaired diffusion for oxygen exist in diseased lungs? Bull. Eur. Physiopathol. Respir. 15: 805–811, 1979.

1883. Thomas, H. M. III, Austin, J. H. M., Yount, B. G. Jr., and Enson, Y. Redistribution of pulmonary blood flow in interstitial lung diseases: the chest radiograph as a physiologic tool. Bull. Eur. Physiopathol. Respir. 15: 1079–1089, 1979.

1884. Terho, E. O., Torkko, M., and Valta, R. Pulmonary damage associated with gold therapy. Scand. J. Respir. Dis. 60: 345–349, 1979.

1885. Gaultier, G., Chaussain, M., Boule, M., Buvry, A., Allaire, Y., Perret, L., and Girard, F. Lung function in interstitial lung diseases in children. Bull. Eur. Physiopathol. Respir. 16: 57–66, 1980.

1886. Jekek, V., Fucik, J., Michaljanic, A., and Jezkova, L. The prognostic significance of functional tests in kryptogenic fibrosing alveolitis. Bull. Eur. Physiopathol. Respir. 16: 711–720, 1980.

1887. Wagner, P. D. Distribution of diffusing capacity (letter to editor). Bull. Eur. Physiopathol. Respir. 16: 151P, 1980.

1888. Briscoe, W. A. Author's response. Bull. Eur. Physiopathol. Respir. 16: 152P, 1980.

1889. Wagner, P. D. Multiple inert gas techniques: results in normal subjects and patients. In: Piiper, J. and Scheid, P. (eds.). Gas Exchange Function in Normal and Diseased Lungs. Progress in Respiration Research, Vol. 16. S. Karger, Basel, 1981.

1890. Renzi, G., Milic-Emili, J., and Grassino, A. E. The pattern of breathing in diffuse lung fibrosis. Bull. Eur. Physiopathol. Respir. 18: 461–472, 1982.

1891. Murphy, D. M. F., Hall, D. R., Petersen, M. R., and Lapp, N. L. The effect of diffuse pulmonary fibrosis on lung mechanics. Bull. Eur. Physiopathol. Respir. 17: 27–41, 1981.

1892. Holmberg, L. and Boman, G. Pulmonary reactions to nitrofurantoin. Eur. J. Respir. Dis. 62: 180–189, 1981.

1893. Stockley, R. A. and Lee, K. D. Estimation of the resting reflex hypoxic drive to respiration in patients with diffuse pulmonary infiltration. Clin. Sci. 50: 109–114, 1976.

1894. Savoy, J., Dhingra, S., and Anthonisen, N. R. Role of vagal airway reflexes in control of ventilation in pulmonary fibrosis. Clin. Sci. 61: 781–784, 1981.

1895. Rudd, R. M., Haslam, P. L., and Turner-Warwick, M. Cryptogenic fibrosing alveolitis. Am. Rev. Respir. Dis. 124: 1–8, 1981.

1896. Wagner, P. D. Ventilation-perfusion inequality and gas exchange during exercise in lung disease. In: Dempsey, J. A. and Reed, C. E. (eds.). Muscular Exercise and the Lung. Univ. of Wisconsin Press, Madison, 1977.

1897. Mohsenifar, Z., Tashkin, D. P., Levy, S. E., Bjerke, R. D., Clements, P. J., and Furst, D. Lack of sensitivity of measurements of VD/VT at rest and during exercise in detection of hemodynamically significant pulmonary vascular abnormalities in collagen vascular disease. Am. Rev. Respir. Dis. 123: 508–512, 1981.

1898. McCormick, J., Cole, S., Lahirir, B., Knauft, F., Cohen, S., and Yoshida, T. Pneumonitis caused by gold salt therapy: evidence for the role of cell-mediated immunity in its pathogenesis. Am. Rev. Respir. Dis. 122: 145–152, 1980.

1899. Weitzenblum, E., El Gharbi, T., Hirth, C., Parini, J. P., and Oudet, P. Les troubles des echanges gazeux dans les fibroses pulmonaires interstitielles diffuses: importance de l'effet shunt. Poumon Coeur 29: 569–579, 1973.

1900. Prefaut, Ch., Devaux, D., and Chardon, G. Le diagnostic fonctionnel des fibroses pulmonaires interstitielles diffuses. Poumon Coeur 29: 553–565, 1973.

1901. Bollinelli, R., Rouch, Y., Fabre, J., Carles, P., and Alves, M. Les echanges pulmonaires dans les fibroses interstitielles diffuses d'evolution lente. Correlations radio-fonctionelles et anatomo-fonctionelles. Poumon Coeur 29: 581–595, 1973.

1902. Galy, P., Brune, J., Wiesendanger, T., Rousset, H., and Serin, D. Fibroses pulmonaires interstitielles diffuses d'evolution lente. Fibroses cryptogeniques. Poumon Coeur 29: 649–654, 1973.

1903. Rinderknecht, J., Shapiro, L., Krauthammer, M., Taplin, G., Wasserman, K., Uszler, J. M., and Effros, R. M. Accelerated clearance of small solutes from the lungs in interstitial lung disease. Am. Rev. Respir. Dis. 121: 105–117, 1980.

1904. Hutas, I., Urai, L., Boszormenyi-Nagy, G., and Grosz, A. Atemfunktionsprufungen bei Sklerodermie (progressiven Systemsklerose). Respiration 30: 141–152, 1973.

1905. Roncoroni, A. J., Casas, J. C. F., Puy, R. J. M., Goldman, E., and Olmedo, G. Idiopathic interstitial pulmonary fibrosis with hypercapnia. Respiration 32: 405–414, 1975.

1906. Renzi, G. D. and Lopez-Majano, V. Early diagnosis of interstitial fibrosis. Respiration 33: 294–302, 1976.

1907. Todisco, T., Matthys, H., and Cegla, U. H. Clinical determination of airway closure, comparison of three methods in patients with lung fibrosis. Respiration 34: 197–204, 1977.

1908. Israel, R. H., Gross, R. A., and Bomba, P. A. Adult respiratory distress syndrome associated with acute nitrofurantoin toxicity. Respiration 39: 318–322, 1980.

1909. Spiro, S. G., Dowdeswell, I. R. G., and Clark, T. J. H. An analysis of submaximal exercise responses in patients with sarcoidosis and fibrosing alveolitis. Br. J. Dis. Chest 75: 169–180, 1981.

1910. Costabel, U. and Matthys, H. Different therapies and factors influencing response to therapy in idiopathic diffuse fibrosing alveolitis. Respiration 42: 141–149, 1981.

1911. Tan, C. S. H. and Tashkin, D. P. Supernormal maximal midexpiratory flow rates in diffuse interstitial lung disease. Respiration 42: 200–208, 1981.

1912. James, D. W., Whimster, W. F., and Hamilton, E. B. D. Gold lung. Br. Med. J. 1: 1523–1524, 1978.

1913. Cummiskey, J., Keelan, P., and Weir, D. G. Coeliac disease and diffuse pulmonary disease (letter to editor). Br. Med. J. 1: 1401, 1976.

1914. Millar, J. W. Infectious mononucleosis and fibrosing alveolitis. Br. Med. J. 1: 612, 1977.

1915. Thurston, J. G. B., Marks, P., and Trapnell, D. Lung changes associated with phenylbutazone treatment. Br. Med. J. 2: 1422–1423, 1976.

1916. Geddes, D. M. and Brostoff, J. Pulmonary fibrosis associated with hypersensitivity to gold salts. Br. Med. J. 1: 1444, 1976.

1917. Erwteman, T. M., Braat, M. C. P., and van Aken, W. G. Interstitial pulmonary fibrosis: a new side effect of practolol. Br. Med. J. 2: 297–298, 1977.

1918. Musk, A. W. and Pollard, J. A. Pindolol and pulmonary fibrosis. Br. Med. J. 2: 581–582, 1979.

1919. Ross, G. Letter from Spain: a deadly oil. Br. Med. J. 283: 424–425, 1981.

1920. Butler, P., Chahal, P., Hudson, N. M., and Hubner, P. J. B. Pulmonary hypertension after lung irradiation in infancy. Br. Med. J. 283: 1365, 1981.

1921. Braude, A. C., Downar, E., Chamberlain, D. W., and Rebuck, A. S. Tocainide-associated interstitial pneumonitis. Thorax 37: 309–310, 1982.

1922. Beaumont, F., Jansen, H. M., Elema, J. D., Tenkate, L. P., and Sluiter, H. J. Simultaneous occurrence of pulmonary interstitial fibrosis and alveolar cell carcinoma in one family. Thorax 36: 252–258, 1981.

1923. Orwoll, E. S., Kiessling, P. J., and Patterson, J. R. Interstitial pneumonia from mitomycin. Ann. Intern. Med. 89: 352–355, 1978.

1924. Gross, N. J. Pulmonary effects of radiation therapy. Ann. Intern. Med. 86: 81–92, 1977.

1925. Crystal, R. G. (moderator). Idiopathic pulmonary fibrosis. NIH Conference. Ann. Intern. Med. 85: 769–788, 1976.

1926. Benoist, M. R., Lemerle, J., Jean, R., Rufin, P., Scheinmann, P., and Paupe, J. Effects on pulmonary function of whole lung irradiation for Wilm's tumour in children. Thorax 37: 175–180, 1982.

1927. Pande, J. N. Interrelationship between lung volume, expiratory flow, and lung transfer factor in fibrosing alveolitis. Thorax 36: 858–862, 1981.

1928. Bass, B. H. Hydralazine lung. Thorax 36: 695–696, 1981.

1929. Keogh, B. A. and Crystal, R. G. Alveolitis: the key to the interstitial lung disorders (editorial). Thorax 37: 1–10, 1982.

1930. Wagner, P. D., Dantzker, D. R., Dueck, R., de Polo, J. L., Wasserman, K., and West, J. B. Distribution of ventilation-perfusion ratios in patients with interstitial lung disease. Chest 69(Suppl.): 256–257, 1976.

1931. Auchincloss, J. H. Jr., Ashutosh, K., Rana, S., Peppi, D., Johnson, L. W., and Gilbert, R. Effect of cardiac, pulmonary, and vascular disease on one minute oxygen uptake. Chest 70: 486–493, 1976.

1932. Salerni, R., Rodnan, G. P., Leon, D. F., and Shaver, J. A. Pulmonary hypertension in the CREST syndrome variant of progressive systemic sclerosis (scleroderma). Ann. Intern. Med. 86: 394–399, 1977.

1933. Cullinan, S. A. and Bower, G. C. Acute pulmonary hypersensitivity to carbamazepine. Chest 68: 580–581, 1975.

1934. Popper, K. Unended Quest. Fontana Publications, William Collins Sons & Co., Glasgow, 1976.

1935. Carrington, C. B., Gaensler, E. A., Mikus, J. P., Schachter, A. W., Burke, G. W., and Goff, A. M. Structure and function in sarcoidosis. Ann. N.Y. Acad. Sci. 278: 265–283, 1976.

1936. Saumon, G., Georges, R., Loiseau, A., and Turiaf, J. Membrane diffusing capacity and pulmonary capillary blood volume in pulmonary sarcoidosis. Ann. N.Y. Acad. Sci. 278: 284–291, 1976.

1937. Miller, A., Chuang, M., Teirstein, A. S., and Siltzbach, L. E. Pulmonary function in stage I and II pulmonary sarcoidosis. Ann. N.Y. Acad. Sci. 278: 292–300, 1976.

1938. Colp, C., Park, S. S., and Williams, M. H. Jr. Pulmonary function follow-up of 120 patients with sarcoidosis. Ann. N.Y. Acad. Sci. 278: 301–307, 1976.

1939. Line, B. R., Hunninghake, G. W., Keogh, B. A., Jones, A. E., Johnston, G. S., and Crystal, R. G. Gallium-67 scanning to stage the alveolitis of sarcoidosis; correlation with clinical studies, pulmonary function studies, and bronchoalveolar lavage. Am. Rev. Respir. Dis. 123: 440–446, 1981.

1940. Radwan, L., Grebska, E., and Koziorowski, A. Small airways function in pulmonary sarcoidosis. Scand. J. Respir. Dis. 59: 37–43, 1978.

1941. Marshall, R. and Karlish, A. J. Lung function in sarcoidosis. Thorax 26: 402–405, 1971.

1942. Battesti, J. P., Georges, R., Basset, F., and Saumon, G. Chronic cor pulmonale in pulmonary sarcoidosis. Thorax 33: 76–84, 1978.

1943. Levinson, R. S., Metzger, L. F., Stanley, N. N., Kelsen, S. G., Altose, M. D., Cherniack, N. S., and Brody, J. S. Airway function in sarcoidosis. Am. J. Med. 62: 51–59, 1977.

1944. Emirgil, C., Sobol, B. J., Herbert, W. H., and Trout, K. The lesser circulation in pulmonary fibrosis secondary to sarcoidosis and its relation to respiratory function. Chest 60: 371–378, 1971.

1945. Westcott, J. L. and Noehren, T. H. Bronchial stenosis in chronic sarcoidosis. Chest 63: 893–897, 1973.

1946. Damuth, T. E., Bower, J. S., Cho, K., and Dantzker, D. R. Major pulmonary artery stenosis causing pulmonary hypertension in sarcoidosis. Chest 78: 888–893, 1980.

1947. Winterbauer, R. H. and Hutchinson, J. F. Use of pulmonary function tests in the management of sarcoidosis. Chest 78: 640–647, 1980.

1948. Olsson, T., Bjornstad-Pettersen, H., and Stjernberg, N. L. Bronchostenosis due to sarcoidosis. Chest 75: 663–666, 1979.

1949. Rosen, Y., Athanassiades, T. J., Moon, S., and Lyons, H. A. Nongranulomatous interstitial pneumonitis in sarcoidosis. Chest 74: 122–125, 1978.

1950. Colp, C. R. Treatment of sarcoidosis (letter to editor). Chest 72: 547–548, 1977.

1951. DeRemee, R. A. Treatment of sarcoidosis (letter to editor). Chest 72: 548, 1977.

1952. Onal, E., Lopata, M., and Lourenco, R. V. Nodular pulmonary sarcoidosis. Chest 72: 296–300, 1977.

1953. Divertie, M. B., Cassan, S. M., and Brown, A. L. Ultrastructural morphometry of the blood-air barrier in pulmonary sarcoidosis. Chest 69: 154–157, 1976.

1954. Arnett, J. C. Jr. and Hatch, H. B. Jr. Pulmonary sarcoidosis presenting as bronchial carcinoma. Chest 67: 729–731, 1975.

1955. Sahn, S. A., Schwarz, M. I., and Lakshminarayan, S. Sarcoidosis: the significance of an acinar pattern on chest roentgenogram. Chest 65: 684–687, 1974.

1956. Carasso, B. Sarcoidosis of the larynx causing airway obstruction. Chest 65: 693–695, 1974.

1957. Young, R. C., Headings, V. E., Bose, S., Harden, K. A., Crockett, E. D., and Hackney, R. L. Jr. Alpha$_1$ antitrypsin levels in sarcoidosis: relationship to disease activity. Chest 64: 39–45, 1973.

1958. Miller, A., Teirstein, A. S., Jackler, I., Chuang, M., and

Siltzbach, L. E. Airway function in chronic pulmonary sarcoidosis with fibrosis. Am. Rev. Respir. Dis. 109: 179–189, 1974.

1959. Nelson, D. G. and Loudon, R. G. Sarcoidosis with pleural involvement. Am. Rev. Respir. Dis. 108: 647–651, 1973.

1960. Gracey, D. R., Divertie, M. B., and Brown, A. L. Jr. Alveolar capillary membrane in sarcoidosis: an electron microscopic study. Am. Rev. Respir. Dis. 106: 617–621, 1972.

1961. Di Benedetto, R. and Lefrak, S. Systematic sarcoidosis with severe involvement of the upper respiratory tract. Am. Rev. Respir. Dis. 102: 801–807, 1970.

1962. DeRemee, R. A. and Anderson, H. A. Sarcoidosis (letter to editor). Am. Rev. Respir. Dis. 112: 151, 1975.

1963. Mitchell, D. N. and Scadding, J. G. Sarcoidosis (letter to editor). Am. Rev. Respir. Dis. 112: 151–152, 1975.

1964. Mitchell, D. N. and Scadding, J. G. Sarcoidosis. Am. Rev. Respir. Dis. 110: 774–802, 1974.

1965. Benatar, S. R. and Clark, T. J. H. Pulmonary function in a case of endobronchial sarcoidosis. Am. Rev. Respir. Dis. 110: 490–496, 1974.

1966. Georges, R. and Basset, G. Différence de pression alveoloarterielle d'oxygene (A-a)DO$_2$ dans les fibroses et infiltrations interstitielles diffuses du poumon. Bull. Physiopathol. Respir. 6: 525–530, 1970.

1967. Thygesen, K. and Viskum, K. Manifestations and course of the disease in intrathoracic sarcoidosis. Scand. J. Respir. Dis. 53: 174–180, 1972.

1968. Viskum, K. and Thygesen, K. Vital prognosis in intrathoracic sarcoidosis. Scand. J. Respir. Dis. 53: 181–186, 1972.

1969. Renzi, G., Anthonisen, N. R., Grassino, A., Knight, L., and Martin, R. R. Regional lung function in sarcoidosis. Scand. J. Respir. Dis. 85(Suppl.): 64–74, 1974.

1970. Kaneko, K. and Sharma, O. P. Airway obstruction in pulmonary sarcoidosis. Bull. Eur. Physiopathol. Respir. 13: 231–240, 1977.

1971. Weitzenblum, E., Moyses, B., Hirth, C., Meunier-Carus, J., Methlin, G., and Oudet, P. Regional pulmonary function in sarcoidosis. Scand. J. Respir. Dis. 58: 17–26, 1977.

1972. Selroos, O. and Klockars, M. Serum lysozyme in sarcoidosis. Scand. J. Respir. Dis. 58: 110–116, 1977.

1973. De Troyer, A., Yernault, J-C., Dierckx, P., Englert, M., and De Coster, A. Lung and airway mechanics in early pulmonary sarcoidosis. Bull. Eur. Physiopathol. Respir. 14: 299–310, 1978.

1974. Gronhagen-Riska, C., Kurppa, K., Fyhrquist, F., and Selroos, O. Angiotensin-converting enzyme and lysozyme in silicosis and asbestosis. Scand. J. Respir. Dis. 59: 228–231, 1978.

1975. Gronhagen-Riska, C. Angiotensin-converting enzyme. Scand. J. Respir. Dis. 60: 83–93, 1979.

1976. Gronhagen-Riska, C., Selroos, O., Wagar, G., and Fyhrquist, F. Angiotensin-converting enzyme. Scand. J. Respir. Dis. 60: 94–101, 1979.

1977. Selroos, O. and Sellergren, T-L. Corticosteroid therapy of pulmonary sarcoidosis. Scand. J. Respir. Dis. 60: 215–221, 1979.

1978. Selroos, O. and Gronhagen-Riska, C. Angiotensin-converting enzyme. Scand. J. Respir. Dis. 60: 328–336, 1979.

1979. Bower, J. S., Belen, J. E., Weg, J. G., and Dantzker, D. R. Manifestations and treatment of laryngeal sarcoidosis. Am. Rev. Respir. Dis. 122: 325–332, 1980.

1980. Huang, C. T., Heurich, A. E., Rosen, Y., Moon, S., and Lyons, H. A. Pulmonary sarcoidosis. Respiration 37: 337–345, 1979.

1981. Miller, A. The vanishing lung syndrome associated with pulmonary sarcoidosis. Br. J. Dis. Chest. 75: 209–214, 1981.

1982. Renzi, G. D., Renzi, P. M., Lopez-Majano, V., and Dutton, R. E. Airway function in sarcoidosis: effect of short-term steroid therapy. Respiration 42: 98–104, 1981.

1983. Iles, P. B. Multiple bronchial stenoses: treatment by mechanical dilatation. Thorax 36: 784–786, 1981.

1984. Hadfield, J. W., Page, R. L., Flower, C. D. R., and Stark, J. E. Localised airway narrowing in sarcoidosis. Thorax 37: 443–447, 1982.

1985. Schoenberger, C. I., Line, B. R., Keogh, B. A., Hunninghake, G. W., and Crystal, R. G. Lung inflammation in sarcoidosis: comparison of serum angiotensin-converting enzyme levels with bronchoalveolar lavage and gallium-67 scanning assessment of the T lymphocyte alveolitis. Thorax 37: 19–25, 1982.

1986. Lieberman, J., Nosal, A., Schlessner, L. A., and Sastre-Foken, A. Serum angiotensin-converting enzyme for diagnosis and therapeutic evaluation of sarcoidosis. Am. Rev. Resp. Dis. 120: 329–335, 1979.

1987. Hunninghake, G. W., Fulmer, J. D., Young, R. C. Jr., Gadek, J. E., and Crystal, R. G. Localisation of the immune response in sarcoidosis. Am. Rev. Respir. Dis. 120: 49–57, 1979.

1988. Keens, T. G., Krastins, I. R. B., Wannamaker, E. M., Levison, H., Crozier, D. N., and Bryan, A. C. Ventilatory muscle endurance training in normal subjects and patients with cystic fibrosis. Am. Rev. Respir. Dis. 116: 853–860, 1977.

1989. Corey, M., Levison, H., and Crozier, D. Five- to seven-year course of pulmonary function in cystic fibrosis. Am. Rev. Respir. Dis. 114: 1085–1092, 1976.

1990. Neuberger, N., Levison, H., and Kruger, K. Transit time analysis of the forced expiratory vital capacity in cystic fibrosis. Am. Rev. Respir. Dis. 114: 753–759, 1976.

1991. Wayne, K. S. and Taussig, L. M. Probable familial congenital bronchiectasis due to cartilage deficiency (Williams-Campbell syndrome). Am. Rev. Respir. Dis. 114: 15–22, 1976.

1992. Corbet, A., Ross, J., Popkin, J., and Beaudry, P. Relationship of arterial-alveolar nitrogen tension to alveolar-arterial oxygen tension, lung volume, flow measurements, and diffusing capacity in cystic fibrosis. Am. Rev. Respir. Dis. 112: 513–519, 1975.

1993. Mansell, A., Dubrawsky, C., Levison, H., Bryan, A. C., and Crozier, D. N. Lung elastic recoil in cystic fibrosis. Am. Rev. Respir. Dis. 109: 190–197, 1974.

1994. Landau, L. I. and Phelan, P. D. The spectrum of cystic fibrosis. Am. Rev. Respir. Dis. 108: 593–602, 1973.

1995. Poe, R. H., Wellman, H. N., Berke, R. A., Vassallo, C. L., and Domm, B. M. Perfusion-ventilation scintiphotography in bullous disease of the lung. Am. Rev. Respir. Dis. 107: 946–954, 1973.

1996. Chang, N., Levison, H., Cunningham, K., Crozier, D. N., and Grosett, O. An evaluation of nightly mist tent therapy for patients with cystic fibrosis. Am. Rev. Respir. Dis. 107: 672–675, 1973.

1997. Pride, N. B., Barter, C. E., and Hugh-Jones, P. The ventilation of bullae and the effect of their removal on thoracic gas volumes and tests of over-all pulmonary function. Am. Rev. Respir. Dis. 107: 83–98, 1973.

1998. Wood, L. D. H., Prichard, S., Weng, T. R., Kruger, K., Bryan, A. C., and Levison, H. Relationship between anatomic dead space and body size in health, asthma, and cystic fibrosis. Am. Rev. Respir. Dis. 104: 215–222, 1971.

1999. Sanchis, J., Dolovich, M., Rossman, C., Wilson, W., and Newhouse, M. Pulmonary mucociliary clearance in cystic fibrosis. N. Engl. J. Med. 288: 651–654, 1973.

2000. Tenholder, M. F., Jones, P. A., Matthews, J. I., and Hooper, R. G. Bullous emphysema. Chest 77: 802–806, 1980.

2001. Fink, R. J., Doershuk, C. F., Tucker, A. S., Stern, R. C., Boat, T. F., and Matthews, L. W. Pulmonary function and morbidity in 40 adult patients with cystic fibrosis. Chest 74: 643–647, 1978.

2002. Harris, J. Severe bullous emphysema. Chest 70: 658–660, 1976.

2003. Longstreth, G. F., Weitzman, S. A., Browning, R. J., and Lieberman, J. Bronchiectasis and homozygous alpha₁-antitrypsin deficiency. Chest 67: 233–235, 1975.

2004. Gross, D., Zidulka, A., O'Brien, C., Wight, D., Fraser, R., Rosenthal, L., and King, M. Peripheral mucociliary clearance with high-frequency chest wall compression. J. Appl. Physiol. 58: 1157–1163, 1985.

2005. Tomashefski, J. F., Christoforidis, A. J., and Abdullah, A. K. Cystic fibrosis in young adults. Chest 57: 28–36, 1970.

2006. DiSant'agnese, P. A. and Davis, P. B. Cystic fibrosis in adults. Am. J. Med. 66: 121–132, 1979.

2007. Mitchell-Heggs, P., Mearns, M., and Batten, J. C. Cystic fibrosis in adolescents and adults. Q. J. Med. 45: 479–504, 1976.

2008. Pride, N. B., Hugh-Jones, P., O'Brien, E. N., and Smith, L. A. Changes in lung function following the surgical treatment of bullous emphysema. Q. J. Med. 39: 49–69, 1970.

2009. Braun, S. R., doPico, G. A., Birnbaum, M. L., and Pellett, J. R. Bullae and severe generalised disease. J. Thorac. Cardiovasc. Surg. 65: 926–929, 1973.

2010. Fitzgerald, M. X., Keelan, P. J., Cugell, D. W., and Gaensler, E. A. Long-term results of surgery for bullous emphysema. J. Thorac. Cardiovasc. Surg. 68: 566–587, 1974.

2011. Gunstensen, J. and McCormack, R. J. M. The surgical management of bullous emphysema. J. Thorac. Cardiovasc. Surg. 65: 920–925, 1973.

2012. Pande, J. N., Jain, B. P., Gupta, R. G., and Guleria, J. S. Pulmonary ventilation and gas exchange in bronchiectasis. Thorax 26: 727–733, 1971.

2013. Mearns, M. and Simon, G. Patterns of lung and heart growth as determined from serial radiographs of 76 children with cystic fibrosis. Thorax 28: 537–546, 1973.

2014. Landau, L. I., Phelan, P. D., and Williams, H. E. Ventilatory mechanics in patients with bronchiectasis starting in childhood. Thorax 29: 304–312, 1974.

2015. Sanderson, J. M., Kennedy, M. C. S., Johnson, M. F., and Manley, D. C. E. Bronchiectasis: results of surgical and conservative management. Thorax 29: 407–416, 1974.

2016. Ryland, D. and Reid, L. The pulmonary circulation in cystic fibrosis. Thorax 30: 285–292, 1975.

2017. Disability and pneumoconiosis (editorial). Br. Med. J. ii: 478, 1970.

2018. Gibson, G. J. Familial pneumothoraces and bullae. Thorax 32: 88–90, 1977.

2019. Macarthur, A. M. and Fountain, S. W. Intracavity suction and drainage in the treatment of emphysematous bullae. Thorax 32: 668–672, 1977.

2020. Nogrady, S. G., Evans, W. V., and Davies, B. H. Reversibility of airways obstruction in bronchiectasis. Thorax 33: 635–637, 1978.

2021. Ripe, E. Bronchiectasis. I. A follow-up study after surgical treatment. Scand. J. Respir. Dis. 52: 96–112, 1971.

2022. Ripe, E., Selander, H., and Wolodarski, J. Bronchiectasis. II. A model for prognosticating the results of surgery. Scand. J. Respir. Dis. 52: 113–120, 1971.

2023. Sackner, M. A. and Landa, J. Bullous disease of the lung: with relatively unimpaired ventilation and minimal or absent hyperinflation. Bull. Physiopathol. Respir. 9: 945–960, 1973.

2024. Galy, P., Brune, J., Dorsit, G., Wiesendanger, T., and Brune, A. Interpretation de l'abaissement de DL_{co}/VA dans les emphysemes radiologiquement bulleux. In: Sadoul, P. (ed.). Le Transfert de l'Oxyde de Carbone. Soc. Eur. Physiopathol. Respir. Masson et Cie, Paris, 1969.

2025. Denolin, H. and Arhirii, M. Nomenclature and definitions in respiratory physiology and clinical aspects of chronic lung disease. Bull. Physiopathol. Respir. 11: 937–959, 1975.

2026. Mossberg, B., Afzelius, B. A., Eliason, R., and Camner, P. On the pathogenesis of obstructive lung disease. A study of the immotile-cilia syndrome. Scand. J. Respir. Dis. 59: 55–65, 1978.

2027. Kollberg, H., Mossberg, B., Afzelius, B. A., Philipson, K., and Camner, P. Cystic fibrosis compared with the immotile-cilia syndrome. Scand. J. Respir. Dis. 59: 297–306, 1978.

2028. Zapletal, A., Houstek, J., Samanek, M., Vavrova, V., and Srajer, J. Lung function abnormalities in cystic fibrosis and changes during growth. Bull. Eur. Physiopathol. Respir. 15: 575–592, 1979.

2029. Boye, N. P., Skarpaas, I. J. K., and Fausa, O. Cystic fibrosis in adult patients. Eur. J. Respir. Dis. 61: 227–232, 1980.

2030. Coates, A. L., Desmond, K. J., Milic-Emili, J., and Beaudry, P. H. Ventilation, respiratory center output, and contribution of the rib cage and abdominal components to ventilation during CO_2 rebreathing in children with cystic fibrosis. Am. Rev. Respir. Dis. 124: 526–530, 1981.

2031. Corkey, C. W. B., Levison, H., and Turner, J. A. P. The immotile cilia syndrome. Am. Rev. Respir. Dis. 124: 544–548, 1981.

2032. Muller, N. L., Francis, P. W., Gurwitz, D., Levison, H., and Bryan, A. C. Mechanism of hemoglobin desaturation during rapid-eye-movement sleep in normal subjects and in patients with cystic fibrosis. Am. Rev. Respir. Dis. 121: 463–469, 1980.

2033. Roeslin, N., Weitzenblum, E., and Meunier-Carus, J. Evolution post operatoire de la fonction respiratoire dans une serie d'emphyseme bulleux. Poumon Coeur 30: 349–355, 1974.

2034. Rossman, C. M., Forrest, J. B., Ruffin, R. E., and Newhouse, M. T. Immotile cilia syndrome in persons with and without Kartagener's syndrome. Am. Rev. Respir. Dis. 121: 1011–1016, 1980.

2035. Fitzgerald, M. X., Keelan, P. J., and Gaensler, E. A. Surgery for bullous emphysema. Respiration 30: 187–200, 1973.

2036. Haluszka, J. and Scislicki, A. Bronchial lability in children suffering from some diseases of the bronchi. Respiration 32: 217–226, 1975.

2037. Weller, P. H., Bush, E., Preece, M. A., and Matthew, D. J. Short-term effects of chest physiotherapy on pulmonary function in children with cystic fibrosis. Respiration 40: 53–56, 1980.

2038. Svenonius, E., Arborelius, M. Jr., Kautto, R., Kornfalt, R., and Lindberg, T. Lung function in cystic fibrosis. Respiration 40: 226–232, 1980.

2039. Flower, K. A., Eden, R. I., Lomax, L., Mann, N. M., and Burgess, J. New mechanical aid to physiotherapy in cystic fibrosis. Br. Med. J. 2: 630–631, 1979.

2040. Pryor, J. A., Webber, B. A., Hodson, M. E., and Batten, J. C. Evaluation of the forced expiration technique as an adjunct to postural drainage in treatment of cystic fibrosis. Br. Med. J. 2: 417–418, 1979.

2041. Bateman, E. D., Westerman, D. E., Hewitson, R. P., and Ferguson, A. D. Pneumonectomy for massive ventilated lung cysts. Thorax 36: 554–556, 1981.

2042. Shneerson, J. M. Lung, bullae, bronchiectasis, and Hashimoto's disease associated with ulcerative colitis treated by colectomy. Thorax 36: 313–314, 1981.

2043. Potgieter, P. D., Benatar, S. R., Hewitson, R. P., and Ferguson, A. D. Surgical treatment of bullous lung disease. Thorax 36: 885–890, 1981.

2044. Nelson, L. A., Callerame, M. L., and Schwartz, R. H. Aspergillosis and atopy in cystic fibrosis. Am. Rev. Respir. Dis. 120: 863–873, 1979.

2045. Ellis, D. A., Thornley, P. E., Wightman, A. J., Walker, M., Chalmers, J., and Crofton, J. W. Present outlook in bronchiectasis: clinical and social study and review of factors influencing prognosis. Thorax 36: 659–664, 1981.

2046. Feldman, J., Traver, G. A., and Taussig, L. M. Maximal expiratory flows after postural drainage. Am. Rev. Resp. Dis. 119: 239–245, 1979.

2047. Cochrane, G. M., Webber, B. A., and Clarke, S. W. Effects of sputum on pulmonary function. Br. Med. J. 2: 1181–1183, 1977.

2048. Pivoteau, C. and Dechoux, J. Le retentissement fonctionnel des pneumoconiose à opacites fines des mineurs de charbon sans troubles ventilatoires. Respiration 29: 161–172, 1972.

2049. Hildick-Smith, M. Natural history of coal-worker's pneumoconiosis in men over 65. J. R. Coll. Physicians Lond. 17: 111–114, 1983.

2050. Lyons, J. P., Ryder, R., Campbell, H., and Gough, J. Pulmonary disability in coalworker's pneumoconiosis. Br. Med. J. 1: 713–716, 1972.

2051. Hurley, J. F., Burns, J., Copland, L., Dodgson, J., and Jacobsen, M. Coalworkers' simple pneumoconiosis and exposure to dust at 10 British coalmines. Br. J. Ind. Med. 39: 120–127, 1982.

2052. Musk, A. W., Cotes, J. E., Bevan, C., and Campbell, M. J. Relationship between type of simple coalworker's pneumoconiosis and lung function. A nine-year follow-up study of subjects with small rounded opacities. Br. J. Ind. Med. 38: 313–320, 1981.

2053. Shennan, D. H., Washington, J. S., Thomas, D. J., Dick, J. A., Kaplan, Y. S., and Bennett, J. G. Factors predisposing to the development of progressive massive fibrosis in coal miners. Br. J. Ind. Med. 38: 321–326, 1981.

2054. Copland, L., Burns, J., and Jacobsen, M. Classification of chest radiographs for epidemiological purposes by people not experienced in the radiology of pneumoconiosis. Br. J. Ind. Med. 38: 254–261, 1981.

2055. Jain, B. L. and Patrick, J. M. Ventilatory function in Nigerian coal miners. Br. J. Ind. Med. 38: 275–280, 1981.

2056. Hankinson, J. L., Palmes, E. D., and Lapp, N. L. Pulmonary air space in coal miners. Am. Rev. Respir. Dis. 119: 391–397, 1979.

2057. Lapp, N. L. and Seaton, A. Lung mechanics in coal worker's pneumoconiosis. In: Coal Worker's Pneumoconiosis. Ann. N.Y. Acad. Sci. 200: 433–454, 1972.

2058. Rasmussen, D. L. Patterns of physiological impairment in coal worker's pneumoconiosis. In: Coal Worker's Pneumoconiosis. Ann. N.Y. Acad. Sci. 200: 455–462, 1972.

2059. Morgan, W. K. C., Seaton, A., Burgess, D. B., Lapp, N. L., and Reger, R. Lung volumes in working coal miners. In: Coal Worker's Pneumoconiosis. Ann. N.Y. Acad. Sci. 200: 478–493, 1972.

2060. Higgins, I. T. T. Chronic respiratory disease in mining communities. In: Coal Worker's Pneumoconiosis. Ann. N.Y. Acad. Sci. 200: 197–210, 1972.

2061. Ulmer, W. T. and Reichel, G. Functional impairment in coal worker's pneumoconiosis. In: Coal Worker's Pneumoconiosis. Ann. N.Y. Acad. Sci. 200: 405–412, 1972.

2062. Kremer, R. Pulmonary hemodynamics in coal worker's pneumoconiosis. In: Coal Worker's Pneumoconiosis. Ann. N.Y. Acad. Sci. 200: 413–432, 1972.

2063. Beil, M., Knorpp, K., and Ulmer, W. T. Verschlussvolumen und Resistance-Lungenvolumen-Beziehung bei kleinknotiger Anthrakosilikose. Lung 154: 75–87, 1976.

2064. Selikoff, I. J., Key, M. M., and Lee, D. H. K. (eds.). Coal Worker's Pneumoconiosis. Ann. N.Y. Acad. Sci. 200: 1–861, 1972.

2065. Morgan, W. K. C., Reger, R., Burgess, D. B., and Shoub, E. A comparison of the prevalence of coal worker's pneumoconiosis and respiratory impairment in Pennsylvania bituminous and anthracite miners. In: Coal Worker's Pneumoconiosis. Ann. N.Y. Acad. Sci. 200: 252–259, 1972.

2066. Brooks, S. M. An approach to patients suspected of having an occupational pulmonary disease. Clin. Chest Med. 2(2): 171–178, 1981.

2067. Love, R. G. and Miller, B. G. Longitudinal study of lung function in coal-miners. Thorax 37: 193–197, 1982.

2068. Fairman, R. P., O'Brien, R. J., Swecker, S., Amandus, H. E., and Shoub, E. P. Respiratory status of surface coal miners in the United States. Arch. Environ. Health 32: 211–215, 1977.

2069. Musk, A. W., Bevan, C., Campbell, M. J., and Cotes, J. E. Factors contributing to the clinical grade of breathlessness in coalworkers with pneumoconiosis. Bull. Eur. Physiopathol. Respir. 15: 343–353, 1979.

2070. Smidt, U., Worth, H., and Busch, A. Limitation of ergometric work and respiratory muscle fatigue. Bull. Eur. Physiopathol. Respir. 16: 211P–212P, 1980.

2071. Lyons, J. P., Ryder, R., Seal, R. M. E., and Wagner, J. C. Emphysema in smoking and non-smoking coalworkers with pneumoconiosis. Bull. Eur. Physiopathol. Respir. 17: 75–85, 1981.

2072. Robience, Y., Yernault, J. C., Libert, P., Denaut, M., Halloy, J. L., and Richez, M. La fonction pulmonaire regionale chez les houilleurs. Bull. Eur. Physiopathol. Respir. 14: 23–30, 1978.

2073. Murphy, D. M. F., Hall, D. R., Petersen, M. R., and Lapp, N. L. The effects of coal worker's pneumoconiosis on lung mechanics. Bull. Eur. Physiopathol. Respir. 14: 61–74, 1978.

2074. Smidt, U., Worth, H., and Petro, W. Ventilatory limitation of exercise in patients with chronic bronchitis and/or emphysema. Bull. Eur. Physiopathol. Respir. 15: 95–101, 1979.

2075. Frans, A., Veriter, C., and Brasseur, L. Pulmonary diffusing capacity for carbon monoxide in simple coalworkers pneumoconiosis. Bull. Physiopathol. Respir. 11: 479–502, 1975.

2076. Frans, A., Veriter, C., Gerin-Portier, N., and Brasseur, L. Blood gases in simple coalworkers pneumoconiosis. Bull. Physiopathol. Respir. 11: 503–526, 1975.

2077. Lapp, N. L. and Morgan, W. K. C. Cardio-respiratory function in United States coal workers. Bull. Physiopathol. Respir. 11: 527–559, 1975.

2078. Muir, D. C. F. Pulmonary function in miners working in British collieries: epidemiological investigation by the National Coal Board. Bull. Physiopathol. Respir. 11: 404–414, 1975.

2079. Ulmer, W. T. Chronic obstructive airway disease in pneumoconiosis in comparison to chronic obstructive airway disease in non dust-exposed workers. Bull. Physiopathol. Respir. 11: 415–447, 1975.

2080. Lamb, D. Physiological/pathological correlations in coal worker's pneumoconiosis. Bull. Physiopathol. Respir. 11: 471–478, 1975.

2081. Worth, G., Muysers, K., Smidt, U., and Gasthaus, L. The epidemiology of bronchopulmonary symptoms in coal miners, foundry workers, chemical workers, and bakers. Bull. Physiopathol. Respir. 6: 617–636, 1970.

2082. Marek, L. and Kujawska, A. L'influence des lesions pneumoconiotiques precoces sur la fonction respiratoire. Bull. Physiopathol. Respir. 9: 1173–1187, 1973.

2083. Unge, G. and Mellner, C. Caplan's syndrome—a clinical study of 13 cases. Scand. J. Respir. Dis. 56: 287–291, 1975.

2084. Morgan, W. K. C., Handelsman, L., Kibelstis, J., Lapp, N. L., and Reger, R. Ventilatory capacity and lung volumes of US coal miners. Arch. Environ. Health 28: 182–189, 1974.

2085. Morgan, W. K. C., Burgess, D. B., Jacobson, G., O'Brien, R. J., Pendergrass, E. P., Reger, R. B., and Shoub, E. P. The prevalence of coal worker's pneumoconiosis in US coal miners. Arch. Environ. Health 27: 221–226, 1973.

2086. Seaton, A., Lapp, N. L., and Morgan, W. K. C. Lung mechanics and frequency dependence of compliance in coal miners. J. Clin. Invest. 51: 1203–1211, 1972.

2087. Hankinson, J. L., Reger, R. B., and Morgan, W. K. C. Maximal expiratory flows in coal miners. Am. Rev. Respir. Dis. 116: 175–180, 1977.

2088. Love, R. G. and Muir, D. C. F. Aerosol deposition and airway obstruction. Am. Rev. Respir. Dis. 114: 881–890, 1976.

2089. Lapp, N. L., Block, J., Boehlecke, B., Lippmann, M., Morgan, W. K. C., and Reger, R. B. Closing volume in coal miners. Am. Rev. Respir. Dis. 113: 155–161, 1976.

2090. Reger, R. B., Amandus, H. E., and Morgan, W. K. C. On the diagnosis of coalworker's pneumoconiosis. Am. Rev. Respir. Dis. 108: 1186–1191, 1973.

2091. Kibelstis, J. A., Morgan, E. J., Reger, R., Lapp, N. L., Seaton, A., and Morgan, W. K. C. Prevalence of bronchitis and airway obstruction in American bituminous coal miners. Am. Rev. Respir. Dis. 108: 886–893, 1973.

2092. Lapp, N. L., Seaton, A., Kaplan, K. C., Hunsaker, M. R., and Morgan, W. K. C. Pulmonary hemodynamics in symptomatic coal miners. Am. Rev. Respir. Dis. 104: 418–426, 1971.

2093. Seaton, A., Lapp, N. L., and Chang, C. H. J. Lung perfusion scanning in coal workers pneumoconiosis. Am. Rev. Respir. Dis. 103: 338–349, 1971.

2094. Reger, R. B. and Morgan, W. K. C. On the factors influencing consistency in the radiologic diagnosis of pneumoconiosis. Am. Rev. Respir. Dis. 102: 905–915, 1970.

2095. Ashford, J. R., Morgan, D. C., Rae, S., and Sowden, R. R. Respiratory symptoms in British coal miners. Am. Rev. Respir. Dis. 102: 370–381, 1970.

2096. Liddell, F. D. K. Radiological assessment of small pneumoconiotic opacities. Br. J. Ind. Med. 34: 85–94, 1977.

2097. Amandus, H. E., Lapp, N. L., Jacobson, G., and Reger, R. B. Significance of irregular small opacities in radiographs of coalminers in the USA. Br. J. Ind. Med. 33: 13–17, 1976.

2098. Waters, W. E., Cochrane, A. L., and Moore, F. Mortality in punctiform type of coalworker's pneumoconiosis. Br. J. Ind. Med. 31: 196–200, 1974.

2099. Cotes, J. E. and Field, G. B. Lung gas exchange in simple pneumoconiosis of coal workers. Br. J. Ind. Med. 29: 268–273, 1972.

2100. Lowe, C. R. and Khosla, T. Chronic bronchitis in ex-coal miners working in the steel industry. Br. J. Ind. Med. 29: 45–49, 1972.

2101. Elmes, P. C. International classification of radiographs of pneumoconioses. Br. J. Ind. Med. 28: 90–93, 1971.

2102. Williams, T. J., Raval, B., and Ahmad, D. Progressive massive fibrosis developing after brief coal dust exposure: evaluation with CT scanning and radionuclide angiocardiocardiography. J. Occup. Med. 22: 21–24, 1980.

2103. Morgan, W. K. C., Lapp, L., and Seaton, A. Respiratory impairment in simple coal worker's pneumoconiosis. J. Occup. Med. 14: 839–844, 1972.

2104. Hyatt, R. E. Pulmonary function in coal miners' pneumoconiosis. J. Occup. Med. 13: 123–130, 1971.

2105. Constantinidis, K., Musk, A. W., Jenkins, J. P. R., and Berry, G. Pulmonary function in coal workers with Caplan's syndrome and non-rheumatoid complicated pneumoconiosis. Thorax 33: 764–768, 1978.

2106. Lyons, J. P. and Campbell, H. Evolution of disability in coalworker's pneumoconiosis. Thorax 31: 527–533, 1976.

2107. McKenzie, H. I., Outhred, K. G., and Glick, M. Postmortem evaluation of the use of diaphragmatic excursus in assessment of pulmonary emphysema in coal miners. Thorax 27: 359–364, 1972.

2108. Morgan, W. K. C., Burgess, D. B., Lapp, N. L., and Seaton, A. Hyperinflation of the lungs in coal miners. Thorax 26: 585–590, 1971.

2109. Seaton, A., Lapp, N. L., and Morgan, W. K. Relationship of pulmonary impairment in simple coalworkers pneumoconiosis to type of radiographic opacity. Br. J. Ind. Med. 29: 50–55, 1972.

2110. Ryder, R., Lyons, J. P., Campbell, H., and Gough, J. Emphysema in coal worker's pneumoconiosis. Br. Med. J. ii: 481–487, 1970.

2111. Rogan, J. M., Attfield, M. D., Jacobsen, M., Rae, S., Walker, D. D., and Walton, W. H. Role of dust in the working environment in the development of chronic bronchitis in British coal miners. Br. J. Ind. Med. 30: 217–226, 1973.

2112. Rom, W. N., Kanner, R. E., Renzetti, A. D. Jr., Shigeoka, J. W., Barkman, H. W., Nichols, M., Turner, W. A., Coleman, M., and Wright, W. E. Respiratory disease in Utah coal miners. Am. Rev. Respir. Dis. 123: 372–377, 1981.

2113. Muir, D. C. F., Burns, J., Jacobsen, M., and Walton, W. H. Pneumoconiosis and chronic bronchitis. Br. Med. J. ii: 424–427, 1977.

2114. Lyons, J. P., Ryder, R. C., Campbell, H., Clarke, W. G., and Gough, J. Significance of irregular opacities in the radiology of coalworker's pneumoconiosis. Br. J. Ind. Med. 31: 36–44, 1974.

2115. Lainhart, W. S., Doyle, H. N., Enterline, P. E., Henschel, A., and Kendrick, M. A. Pneumoconiosis in Appalachian bituminous coal miners. PHS Publication Number 2000. US Dept. of HEW, Public Health Service. Bureau of Occupational Safety & Health, Cincinnati, 1969.

2116. Jacobsen, M. New data on the relationship between simple pneumoconiosis and exposure to coal mine dust. Chest 78(Suppl.): 408–410, 1980.

2117. Bates, D. V., Pham, Q. T., Chau, N., Pivoteau, C., Dechoux, J., and Sadoul, P. A longitudinal study of pulmonary function in coal miners in Lorraine, France. Am. J. Ind. Med. 8: 21–32, 1985.

2118. Sadoul, P. Fonctions respiratoires et pneumoconioses. Bull. Physiopathol. Respir. 11: 403–414, 1975.

2119. Fox, A. J., Tombleson, J. B. L., Watt, A., and Wilkie, A. G. A survey of respiratory disease in cotton operatives. Part 2. Symptoms, dust estimations, and the effect of smoking habit. Br. J. Ind. Med. 30: 48–53, 1973.

2120. Henderson, Y. and Haggard, H. W. Noxious Gases. 2nd ed. Reinhold Publishing Corp., New York, 1943.

2121. Hodge, H. C. and Smith, F. A. Occupational fluoride exposure. J. Occup. Med. 19: 12–39, 1977.

2122. Akbarkhanzadeh, F. Long-term effects of welding fumes upon respiratory symptoms and pulmonary function. J. Occup. Med. 22: 337–341, 1980.

2123. Axelson, O., Dahlgren, E., Jansson, C-D., and Rehnlund, S. O. Arsenic exposure and mortality: a case-referent study from a Swedish copper smelter. Br. J. Ind. Med. 35: 8–15, 1978.

2124. Beach, F. X. M., Sherwood Jones, E., and Scarrow, G. D. Respiratory effects of chlorine gas. Br. J. Ind. Med. 26: 231–236, 1969.

2125. Berry, G., McKerrow, C. B., Molyneux, M. K. B., Rossiter, C. E., and Tombleson, J. B. L. A study of the acute and chronic changes in ventilatory capacity of workers in Lancashire cotton mills. Br. J. Ind. Med. 30: 25–36, 1973.

2126. Brubaker, R. E. Pulmonary problems associated with the use of polytetrafluoroethylene (PTFE). J. Occup. Med. 19: 693–695, 1977.

2127. Bruce, T., Nystrom, A., Ahlmark, A., and Linderholm, H.

Panel discussion on occupational diseases of the respiratory system. Proceedings of the 23rd Scandinavian Congress for Pulmonary Disease. Scand. J. Resp. Dis. 63(Suppl.): 73–94, 1968.

2128. Chan-Yeung, M., Ashley, M. J., Corey, P., Willson, G., Dorken, E., and Grzybowski, S. A respiratory survey of cedar mill workers. J. Occup. Med. 20: 323–327, 1978.

2129. Chester, E. H., Gillespie, D. G., and Krause, F. D. The prevalence of chronic obstructive lung disease in chlorine gas workers. Am. Rev. Respir. Dis. 99: 365–373, 1969.

2130. Coates, E. O. and Watson, J. H. L. Diffuse interstitial lung disease in tungsten carbide workers. Ann. Intern. Med. 75: 709–716, 1971.

2131. Coates, E. O. and Watson, J. H. L. Pathology of the lung in tungsten carbide workers, using light and electron microscopy. J. Occup. Med. 15: 280–295, 1973.

2132. Discher, D. P. and Breitenstein, B. D. Prevalence of chronic pulmonary disease in aluminum potroom workers. J. Occup. Med. 18: 379–386, 1976.

2133. Ferguson, W. S., Koch, W. C., Webster, L. B., and Gould, J. R. Human physiological response and adaptation to ammonia. J. Occup. Med. 19: 319–326, 1977.

2134. Ellis, E. Workman's compensation and occupational safety: a review and evaluation of current knowledge. J. Occup. Med. 18: 418–425, 1976.

2135. Sadler, R. L. Attributability of death to pneumoconiosis in beneficiaries. Thorax 29: 710–712, 1974.

2136. Fox, A. J., Tombleson, J. B. L., Watt, A., and Wilkie, A. G. A survey of respiratory disease in cotton operatives. Part 1. Symptoms and ventilation test results. Br. J. Ind. Med. 30: 42–47, 1973.

2137. Dinman, B. Occupational health and the reality of risk—an eternal dilemma of tragic choices. J. Occup. Med. 22: 153–157, 1980.

2138. Tauber, J. Instant benzol death. J. Occup. Med. 12: 91–92, 1970.

2139. Behnke, A. R. Medical aspects of pressurized tunnel operations. J. Occup. Med. 12: 101–112, 1970.

2140. Ely, T. S., Pedley, S. F., Hearne, F. T., and Stille, W. T. A study of mortality, symptoms, and respiratory function in humans occupationally exposed to oil mist. J. Occup. Med. 12: 253–261, 1970.

2141. Jorgensen, H. and Svensson, A. Studies on pulmonary function and respiratory tract symptoms of workers in an iron ore mine where diesel trucks are used underground. J. Occup. Med. 12: 348–354, 1970.

2142. McMurrain, K. D. Dermatologic and pulmonary responses in the manufacturing of detergent enzyme products. J. Occup. Med. 12: 416–420, 1970.

2143. Nasr, A. N. M., Ditchek, T., and Scholtens, P. A. The prevalence of radiographic abnormalities in the chests of fiber glass workers. J. Occup. Med. 13: 371–376, 1971.

2144. White, E. S. A case of near fatal ammonia gas poisoning. J. Occup. Med. 13: 549–550, 1971.

2145. Linaweaver, P. G. Jr. Prevention of accidents resulting from exposure to high concentrations of foaming chemicals. J. Occup. Med. 14: 24–30, 1972.

2146. Redmond, C. K., Ciocco, A., Lloyd, J. W., and Rush, H. W. Long-term mortality study of steelworkers. J. Occup. Med. 14: 621–629, 1972.

2147. Brinkman, G. L. and Block, D. L. Chronic bronchitis in a working population. J. Occup. Med. 14: 825–827, 1972.

2148. Bates, D. V. The respiratory bronchiole as a target organ for the effects of dusts and gases. J. Occup. Med. 15: 177–180, 1973.

2149. Merchant, J. A., Lumsden, J. C., Kilburn, K. H., O'Fallon, W. M., Ujda, J. R., Germino, V. H. Jr., and Hamilton, J. D. Dose response studies in cotton textile workers. J. Occup. Med. 15: 222–230, 1973.

2150. Weill, H., Waggenspack, C., Bailey, W., Ziskind, M., and Rossiter, C. Radiographic and physiologic patterns among workers engaged in manufacture of asbestos cement products. J. Occup. Med. 15: 248–252, 1973.

2151. Saslow, A. R. and Clark, P. S. Carbon monoxide poisoning. J. Occup. Med. 15: 490–492, 1973.

2152. Tebbens, B. D. Personal dosimetry versus environmental monitoring. J. Occup. Med. 15: 639–641, 1973.

2153. Wegman, D. H., Pagnotto, L. D., Fine, L. J., and Peters, J. M. A dose-response relationship in TDI workers. J. Occup. Med. 16: 258–260, 1974.

2154. Kuntz, W. D. and McCord, C. P. Polymer-fume fever. J. Occup. Med. 16: 480–482, 1974.

2155. Levy, S. A. and Margolis, S. Siderosilicosis and atypical epithelial hyperplasia. J. Occup. Med. 16: 796–799, 1974.

2156. Amandus, H. E., Lapp, N. L., Morgan, W. K. C., and Reger, R. B. Pulmonary zonal involvement in coal workers' pneumoconiosis. J. Occup. Med. 16: 245–247, 1974.

2157. Holt, P. G. and Nulsen, A. Ozone hazard in UV isolation units. J. Occup. Med. 17: 186–188, 1975.

2158. Cooper, W. C. Radiographic survey of perlite workers. J. Occup. Med. 17: 304–307, 1975.

2159. Zuskin, E. and Bouhuys, A. Byssinosis: airway responses in textile dust exposure. J. Occup. Med. 17: 357–359, 1975.

2160. Montgomery, C. H. and Snyder, H. B. Pulmonary evaluation of sandblasters. J. Occup. Med. 17: 523–527, 1975.

2161. Barnes, R. and Simpson, G. R. Variations of pulmonary function amongst workers in cotton mills. J. Occup. Med. 18: 551–555, 1976.

2162. Cooper, W. C. Pulmonary function in perlite workers. J. Occup. Med. 18: 723–729, 1976.

2163. Pham, Q. T. and Mire, B. Respiratory manifestations and skin reactivity in the detergent industry. J. Occup. Med. 20: 33–38, 1978.

2164. The health manpower situation in occupational medicine. A statement by the New York Academy of Medicine. J. Occup. Med. 20: 57–58, 1978.

2165. Archer, V. E. and Gillam, J. D. Chronic sulfur dioxide exposure in a smelter. II. Indices of chest disease. J. Occup. Med. 20: 88–95, 1978.

2166. Schlueter, D. P., Banaszak, E. F., Fink, J. N., and Barboriak, J. Occupational asthma due to tetrachlorophthalic anhydride. J. Occup. Med. 20: 183–188, 1978.

2167. Ashley, M. J., Corey, P., Chan-Yeung, M., MacLean, L., Maledy, H., and Grzybowski, S. A respiratory survey of cedar mill workers. II. Influence of work-related and host factors on the prevalence of symptoms and pulmonary function abnormalities. J. Occup. Med. 20: 328–332, 1978.

2168. Kelada, F. and Euinton, L. E. Health effects of long-term exposure to sodium sulfate dust. J. Occup. Med. 20: 812–814, 1978.

2169. Morgan, W. K. C. Magnetite pneumoconiosis. J. Occup. Med. 20: 762–763, 1978.

2170. Halen, R. J. The comparability of chest X-ray interpretations and pulmonary function test results by different observers. J. Occup. Med. 20: 670–674, 1978.

2171. Levy, S. A., Storey, J., and Phashko, B. E. Meat worker's asthma. J. Occup. Med. 20: 116–117, 1978.

2172. Gerrard, J. W., Mink, J., Cheung, S-S. C., Tan, L. K-T., and Dosman, J. A. Nonsmoking grain handlers in Saskatchewan: airways reactivity and allergic status. J. Occup. Med. 21: 342–346, 1979.

2173. Gibbs, G. W. and Horowitz, I. Lung cancer mortality in aluminum reduction plant workers. J. Occup. Med. 21: 347–353, 1979.

2174. Milham, S. Mortality in aluminum reduction plant workers. J. Occup. Med. 21: 475–480, 1979.

2175. Braun, S. R. and Tsiatis, A. Pulmonary abnormalities in art glassblowers. J. Occup. Med. 21: 487–489, 1979.

2176. Tola, S., Koskela, R-S., Hernberg, S., and Jarvinen, E. Lung cancer mortality among iron foundry workers. J. Occup. Med. 21: 753–760, 1979.

2177. Lynch, J., Hanis, N. M., Bird, M. G., Murray, K. J., and Walsh, J. P. An association of upper respiratory cancer with exposure to diethyl sulfate. J. Occup. Med. 21: 333–341, 1979.

2178. Felton, J. S., Sargent, E. N., and Gordonson, J. S. Radiographic changes following asbestos exposure: experience with 7,500 workers. J. Occup. Med. 22: 15–20, 1980.

2179. Ringel, E. R., Loring, S. H., McFadden, E. R. Jr., and Ingram, R. H. Jr. Chest wall configurational changes before and during acute obstructive episodes in asthma. Am. Rev. Respir. Dis. 128: 607–610, 1983.

2180. Schenker, M. B. Diesel exhaust—an occupational carcinogen? J. Occup. Med. 22: 41–46, 1980.

2181. Smith, A. B., Brooks, S. M., Blanchard, J., Bernstein, I. L., and Gallagher, J. Absence of airway hyperreactivity to methacholine in a worker sensitized to toluene diisocyanate (TDI). J. Occup. Med. 22: 327–331, 1980.

2182. Williams, M. K. Sickness absence and ventilatory capacity of workers exposed to sulphuric acid mist. Br. J. Ind. Med. 27: 61–66, 1970.

2183. Grundorfer, W. and Raber, A. Progressive silicosis in granite workers. Br. J. Ind. Med. 27: 110–120, 1970.

2184. Molyneux, M. K. B. and Tombleson, J. B. L. An epidemiological study of respiratory symptoms in Lancashire mills, 1963–66. Br. J. Ind. Med. 27: 225–234, 1970.

2185. Gandevia, B. and Milne, J. Occupational asthma and rhinitis due to Western red cedar (*Thuja plicata*), with special reference to bronchial reactivity. Br. J. Ind. Med. 27: 235–244, 1970.

2186. Milne, J., Christophers, A., and De Silva, P. Acute mercurial pneumonitis. Br. J. Ind. Med. 27: 334–338, 1970.

2187. Emara, A. M., El-Ghawabi, S. H., Madkour, O. I., and El-Samra, G. H. Chronic manganese poisoning in the dry battery industry. Br. J. Ind. Med. 28: 78–82, 1971.

2188. Morgan, W. K. C. Disability or disinclination? Chest 75: 712–715, 1979.

2189. Miller, G. J., Hearn, C. E. D., and Edwards, R. H. T. Pulmonary function at rest and during exercise following bagassosis. Br. J. Ind. Med. 28: 152–158, 1971.

2190. Zuskin, E. and Valic, F. Peak flow rate in relation to forced expiratory volume in hemp workers. Br. J. Ind. Med. 28: 159–163, 1971.

2191. Elmes, P. C. and Simpson, M. J. C. Insulation workers in Belfast. 3. Mortality 1940–66. Br. J. Ind. Med. 28: 226–236, 1971.

2192. El Ghawabi, S. H., Mansour, M. B., Youssef, F. L., El Ghawabi, M. H., and El Latif, M. M. A. Decompression sickness in caisson workers. Br. J. Ind. Med. 28: 323–329, 1971.

2193. Walker, D. D., Archibald, R. M., and Attfield, M. D. Bronchitis in men employed in the coke industry. Br. J. Ind. Med. 28: 358–363, 1971.

2194. Valic, F. and Zuskin, E. A comparative study of respiratory function in female non-smoking cotton and jute workers. Br. J. Ind. Med. 28: 364–368, 1971.

2195. Bates, D. V. Disability and compensation. Chest 78(Suppl.): 361–362, 1980.

2196. Lister, W. B. and Wimborne, D. Carbon pneumoconiosis in a synthetic graphite worker. Br. J. Ind. Med. 29: 108–110, 1972.

2197. Fletcher, D. E. A mortality study of shipyard workers with pleural plaques. Br. J. Ind. Med. 29: 142–145, 1972.

2198. Jones, J. G. and Warner, C. G. Chronic exposure to iron oxide, chromium oxide, and nickel oxide fumes of metal dressers in a steelworks. Br. J. Ind. Med. 29: 169–177, 1972.

2199. Ranasinha, K. W. and Uragoda, C. G. Graphite pneumoconiosis. Br. J. Ind. Med. 29: 178–183, 1972.

2200. El-Sadik, Y. M., Moselhi, M., El-Hinady, A. R., and Mostafa, M. N. Study of lung function changes among different grades of byssinosis. Br. J. Ind. Med. 29: 184–187, 1972.

2201. Elwood, R. K., Kennedy, S., Belzberg, A., Hogg, J. C., and Pare, P. D. Respiratory mucosal permeability in asthma. Am. Rev. Respir. Dis. 128: 523–527, 1983.

2202. Valic, F. and Zuskin, E. Effects of different vegetable dust exposures. Br. J. Ind. Med. 29: 293–297, 1972.

2203. McCallum, R. I. Respiratory disease in foundrymen. Br. J. Ind. Med. 29: 341–344, 1972.

2204. Vaskov, L. S. Use of radioisotopes in the study of textile workers with byssinosis and chronic lung damage. Br. J. Ind. Med. 30: 37–41, 1973.

2205. Walton, M. Industrial ammonia gassing. Br. J. Ind. Med. 30: 78–86, 1973.

2206. Lee, W. R. Emergence of occupational medicine in Victorian times. Br. J. Ind. Med. 30: 118–124, 1973.

2207. Nicholls, P. J., Evans, E., Valic, F., and Zuskin, E. Histamine-releasing activity and bronchoconstricting effects of sisal. Br. J. Ind. Med. 30: 142–145, 1973.

2208. Enterline, P., De Coufle, P., and Henderson, V. Respiratory cancer in relation to occupational exposures among retired asbestos workers. Br. J. Ind. Med. 30: 162–166, 1973.

2209. Hill, J. W., Whitehead, W. S., Cameron, J. D., and Hedgecock, G. A. Glass fibers: absence of pulmonary hazard in production workers. Br. J. Ind. Med. 30: 174–179, 1973.

2210. Report of the Advisory Committee on Asbestos Cancers to the Director of the International Agency for Research on Cancer. Br. J. Ind. Med. 30: 180–186, 1973.

2211. Morgan, D. C., Smyth, J. T., Lister, R. W., and Pethybridge, R. J. Chest symptoms and farmer's lung: A community survey. Br. J. Ind. Med. 30: 259–265, 1973.

2212. Zuskin, E. and Valic, F. Respiratory response in simultaneous exposure to flax and hemp dust. Br. J. Ind. Med. 30: 375–380, 1973.

2213. Valic, F. and Zuskin, E. Pharmacological prevention of acute ventilatory capacity reduction in flax dust exposure. Br. J. Ind. Med. 30: 381–384, 1973.

2214. Riddle, H. F. V. Prevalence of respiratory symptoms and sensitization by mould antigens among a group of maltworkers. Br. J. Ind. Med. 31: 31–35, 1974.

2215. Ranga, V., Powers, M. A., Padilla, M., Strope, G. L., Fowler, L., and Kleinerman, J. Effect of allergic bronchoconstriction on airways epithelial permeability to large polar solutes in the guinea pig. Am. Rev. Respir. Dis. 128: 1065–1070, 1983.

2216. Ahmed, T. and Oliver, W. Jr. Does slow-reacting substance of anaphylaxis mediate hypoxic pulmonary vasoconstriction? Am. Rev. Respir. Dis. 127: 566–571, 1983.

2217. Bar-Yishay, E., Ben-Dov, I., and Godfrey, S. Refractory period after hyperventilation-induced asthma. Am. Rev. Respir. Dis. 127: 572–574, 1983.

2218. Uragoda, C. G. A clinical and radiographic study of coir workers. Br. J. Ind. Med. 32: 66–71, 1975.

2219. Adams, W. G. F. Long-term effects on the health of men engaged in the manufacture of tolylene di-isocyanate. Br. J. Ind. Med. 32: 72–78, 1975.

2220. Fairman, R. P., Hankinson, J., Imbus, H., Lapp, N. L., and Morgan, W. K. C. Pilot study of closing volume in byssinosis. Br. J. Ind. Med. 32: 235–238, 1975.

2221. Milne, J. and Brand, S. Occupational asthma after inhalation of dust of the proteolytic enzyme, papain. Br. J. Ind. Med. 32: 302–307, 1975.

2222. Axford, A. T., McKerrow, C. B., Jones, A. P., and Lequesne, P. M. Accidental exposure to isocyanate fumes in a group of firemen. Br. J. Ind. Med. 33: 65–71, 1976.

2223. Doll, R., Mathews, J. D., and Morgan, L. G. Cancers of the lung and nasal sinuses in nickel workers: a reassessment of the period of risk. Br. J. Ind. Med. 34: 102–105, 1977.

2224. Hendrick, D. J. and Lane, D. J. Occupational formalin asthma. Br. J. Ind. Med. 34: 11–18, 1977.

2225. Crosbie, W. A., Clarke, M. B., Cox, R. A. F., McIver, N. K. I., Anderson, I. K., Evans, H. A., Liddle, G. C., Cowan, J. L., Brookings, C. H., and Watson, D. G. Physical characteristics and ventilatory function of 404 commercial divers working in the North Sea. Br. J. Ind. Med. 34: 19–25, 1977.

2226. Musk, A. W. and Gandevia, B. Loss of pulmonary elastic recoil in workers formerly exposed to proteolytic enzyme (alcalase) in the detergent industry. Br. J. Ind. Med. 33: 158–165, 1976.

2227. Uragoda, C. G. An investigation into the health of kapok workers. Br. J. Ind. Med. 34: 181–185, 1977.

2228. Wegman, D. H., Peters, J. M., Pagnotto, L., and Fine, L. J. Chronic pulmonary function loss from exposure to toluene diisocyanate. Br. J. Ind. Med. 34: 196–200, 1977.

2229. Lee, W. R. Some ethical problems of hazardous substances in the working environment. Br. J. Ind. Med. 34: 274–280, 1977.

2230. El Ghawabi, S. H. Respiratory function and symptoms in workers exposed simultaneously to jute and hemp. Br. J. Ind. Med. 35: 16–20, 1978.

2231. Kreyberg, L. Lung cancer in workers in a nickel refinery. Br. J. Ind. Med. 35: 109–116, 1978.

2232. Mustafa, K. Y., Lakha, A. S., Milla, M. H., and Dahoma, U. Byssinosis, respiratory symptoms and spirometric lung function tests in Tanzanian sisal workers. Br. J. Ind. Med. 35: 123–128, 1978.

2233. Seaton, A. and Bishop, C. M. Acute mercury pneumonitis. Br. J. Ind. Med. 35: 258–265, 1978.

2234. Morgan, W. K. C. Industrial bronchitis. Br. J. Ind. Med. 35: 285–291, 1978.

2235. Tukiainen, P., Taskinen, E., Korhola, O., and Valle, M. TruCut needle biopsy in asbestosis and silicosis: correlation of histological changes with radiographic changes and pulmonary function in 41 patients. Br. J. Ind. Med. 35: 292–304, 1978.

2236. Musk, A. W., Smith, T. J., Peters, J. M., and McLaughlin, E. Pulmonary function in firefighters: acute changes in ventilatory capacity and their correlates. Br. J. Ind. Med. 36: 29–34, 1979.

2237. Zuskin, E., Valic, F., and Skuric, Z. Respiratory function in coffee workers. Br. J. Ind. Med. 36: 117–122, 1979.

2238. Ferris, B. G. Jr., Puleo, S., and Chen, H. Y. Mortality and morbidity in a pulp and a paper mill in the United States: a ten-year follow-up. Br. J. Ind. Med. 36: 127–134, 1979.

2239. Saric, M., Zuskin, E., and Gomzi, M. Bronchoconstriction in potroom workers. Br. J. Ind. Med. 36: 211–215, 1979.

2240. Baker, M. D., Irwig, L. M., Johnston, J. R., Turner, D. M., and Bezuidenhout, B. N. Lung function in sisal ropemakers. Br. J. Ind. Med. 36: 216–219, 1979.

2241. Zuskin, E., Valic, F., Butkovic, D., and Bouhuys, A. Lung function in textile workers. Br. J. Indust. Med. 32: 283–288, 1975.

2242. Attfield, M. D. and Ross, D. S. Radiological abnormalities in electric-arc welders. Br. J. Ind. Med. 35: 117–122, 1978.

2243. Miller, A., Teirstein, A. S., Bader, M. E., Bader, R. A., and Selikoff, I. J. Talc pneumoconiosis. Am. J. Med. 50: 395–402, 1971.

2244. Murphy, R. L. H., Gaensler, E. A., Ferris, B. G., Fitzgerald, M., Solliday, N., and Morrisey, W. Diagnosis of "asbestosis." Am. J. Med. 65: 488–498, 1978.

2245. Guenter, C. A., Hanley, D. A., Sproule, B. J., and Coalson, J. J. Rapid onset of emphysema associated with diffuse parenchymal disease. Am. J. Med. 67: 335–338, 1979.

2246. Moskowitz, R. L. Talc pneumoconiosis: a treated case. Chest 58: 37–41, 1970.

2247. Kass, I., Zamel, N., Dobry, C. A., and Holzer, M. Bronchiectasis following ammonia burns of the respiratory tract. Chest 62: 282–285, 1972.

2248. Scott, E. G. and Hunt, W. B. Jr. Silo filler's disease. Chest 63: 701–706, 1973.

2249. Amandus, H. E., Reger, R. B., Pendergrass, E. P., Dennis, J. M., and Morgan, W. K. C. The pneumoconioses: methods of measuring progression. Chest 63: 736–743, 1973.

2250. Horvath, E. P., doPico, G. A., Barbee, R. A., and Dickie, H. A. Nitrogen dioxide—induced pulmonary disease. J. Occup. Med. 20: 103–110, 1978.

2251. Hunt, V. The emergence of the worker's right to know health risks. In: Ng, L. K. Y. and Davis, D. L. (eds.). Strategies for Public Health—Promoting Health and Preventing Disease. Van Nostrand Reinhold, New York, 1981.

2252. Kaltreider, N. L., Elder, M. J., Cralley, L. V., and Colwell, M. O. Health survey of aluminum workers with special reference to fluoride exposure. J. Occup. Med. 14: 531–541, 1972.

2253. Lebowitz, M. D. Occupational exposures in relation to symptomatology and lung function in a community population. Environ. Res. 14: 59–67, 1977.

2254. Hasan, F. M. and Kazemi, H. Chronic beryllium disease: a continuing epidemiologic hazard. Chest 65: 289–293, 1974.

2255. Schmidt-Nowara, W. W., Murphy, R. L. H., and Atkinson, J. D. Lung function after acute toluene di-isocyanate inhalation. Chest 63: 1039–1040, 1973.

2256. Schachter, E. N., Smith, G. J. W., Cohen, G. S., Lee, S. H., Lasser, A., and Gee, J. B. L. Pulmonary granulomas in a patient with pulmonary veno-occlusive disease. Chest 67: 487–489, 1975.

2257. Committee report. The pulmonary response to fiberglass dust. Chest 69: 216–219, 1976.

2258. Lilis, R., Anderson, H., Miller, A., and Selikoff, I. J. Pulmonary changes among vinyl chloride polymerization workers. Chest 69(Suppl.): 299–303, 1976.

2259. Becklake, M. R., Fournier-Massey, G., and Black, R. Lung function profiles in the chrysotile asbestos mines and mills of Quebec. Chest 69(Suppl.): 303, 1976.

2260. Taplin, G. V., Chopra, S., Yanda, R. L., and Elam, D.

Radionuclide lung-imaging procedures in the assessment of injury due to ammonia inhalation. Chest 69: 582–586, 1976.

2261. Jain, S. M., Sapaha, G. C., Khare, K. C., and Dubey, V. S. Silicosis in slate pencil workers. Chest 71: 423–426, 1977.

2262. Genovesi, M. G., Tashkin, D. P., Chopra, S., Morgan, M., and McElroy, C. Transient hypoxemia in firemen following inhalation of smoke. Chest 71: 441–444, 1977.

2263. Tashkin, D. P., Genovesi, M. G., Chopra, S., Coulson, A., and Simmons, M. Respiratory status of Los Angeles firemen. Chest 71: 445–449, 1977.

2264. Chester, E. H., Kaimal, P. J., Payne, C. B. Jr., and Kohn, P. M. Pulmonary injury following exposure to chlorine gas. Chest 72: 247–250, 1977.

2265. Kawakami, M., Sato, S., and Takishima, T. Silicosis in workers dealing with Tonoko. Chest 72: 635–639, 1977.

2266. Dopico, G. A. Asthma due to dust from redwood (*Sequoia sempervirens*). Chest 73: 424–425, 1978.

2267. Rosenthal, T., Baum, G. L., Frand, U., and Molho, M. Poisoning caused by inhalation of hydrogen chloride, phosphorus oxychloride, phosphorus pentachloride, oxalyl chloride, and oxalic acid. Chest 73: 623–626, 1978.

2268. Kirkpatrick, M. B. and Bass, J. B. Severe obstructive lung disease after smoke inhalation. Chest 76: 108–110, 1979.

2269. Mink, J. T., Gerrard, J. W., Cockcroft, D. W., Cotton, D. J., and Dosman, J. A. Increased bronchial reactivity to inhaled histamine in nonsmoking grain workers with normal lung function. Chest 77: 28–31, 1980.

2270. Genovesi, M. G. Effects of smoke inhalation (editorial). Chest 77: 335–336, 1980.

2271. Loke, J., Farmer, W., Matthay, R. A., Putnam, C. E., and Smith, G. J. W. Acute and chronic effects of fire fighting on pulmonary function. Chest 77: 369–373, 1980.

2272. Montague, T. J. and Macneil, A. R. Mass ammonia inhalation. Chest 77: 496–498, 1980.

2273. Schecter, A., Shanske, W., Stenzler, A., Quintilian, H., and Steinberg, H. Acute hydrogen selenide inhalation. Chest 77: 554–555, 1980.

2274. Chester, E. H., Martinez-Catinchi, F. L., Schwartz, H. J., Horowitz, J., Fleming, G. M., Gerblich, A. A., McDonald, E. W., and Brethauer, R. Patterns of airway reactivity to asthma produced by exposure to toluene di-isocyanate. Chest 75(Suppl.): 229–231, 1979.

2275. Fleming, G. M., Chester, E. H., and Montenegro, H. D. Dysfunction of small airways following pulmonary injury due to nitrogen dioxide. Chest 75: 720–721, 1979.

2276. Thiel, H. and Ulmer, W. T. Bakers' asthma: development and possibility for treatment. Chest 78(Suppl.): 400–405, 1980.

2277. Phillips, T. J. G. Compensation for occupational lung disease in the United Kingdom. Chest 78(Suppl.): 363–364, 1980.

2278. Eyssen, G. M. Development of radiographic abnormality in chrysotile miners and millers. Chest 78(Suppl.): 411–414, 1980.

2279. Cordasco, E. M., Demeter, S. L., Kerkay, J., Van Ordstrand, H. S., Lucas, E. V., Chen, T., and Golish, J. A. Pulmonary manifestations of vinyl and polyvinyl chloride (interstitial lung disease). Newer aspects. Chest 78: 828–834, 1980.

2280. Bhattacharjee, J. W., Saxena, R. P., and Zaidi, S. H. Experimental studies on the toxicity of bagasse. Environ. Res. 23: 68–76, 1980.

2281. Adkins, B. Jr., Luginbuhl, G. H., Miller, F. J., and Gardiner, D. E. Increased pulmonary susceptibility to streptococcal infection following inhalation of manganese oxide. Environ. Res. 23: 110–120, 1980.

2282. Oleru, U. G. Pulmonary function of control and industrially exposed Nigerians in asbestos, textile, and toluene diisocyanate-foam factories. Environ. Res. 23: 137–148, 1980.

2283. Segarra, F., Monte, M. B., Ibanez, P. L., and Nicolas, J. P. Asbestosis in a Barcelona fibrocement factory. Environ. Res. 23: 292–300, 1980.

2284. Pain, M. C. F. and Symons, H. S. Bronchial reactivity in occupational asthma. Med. J. Aust. 1: 522–524, 1972.

2285. Schrag, P. E. and Gullett, A. D. Byssinosis in cotton textile mills. Am. Rev. Respir. Dis. 101: 497–503, 1970.

2286. Newhouse, M., Sanchis, J., and Bienenstock, J. Lung defense mechanisms. N. Engl. J. Med. 295: 990–998, 1045–1052, 1976.

2287. Nishimoto, Y., Burrows, B., Miyanishi, M., Katsuta, S., Shigenobu, T., and Kettel, L. J. Chronic obstructive lung disease in Japanese poison gas workers. Am. Rev. Respir. Dis. 102: 173–179, 1970.

2288. Phibbs, B. P., Sundin, R. E., and Mitchell, R. S. Silicosis in Wyoming bentonite workers. Am. Rev. Respir. Dis. 103: 1–17, 1971.

2289. Jodoin, G., Gibbs, G. W., Macklem, P. T., McDonald, J. C., and Becklake, M. R. Early effects of asbestos exposure on lung function. Am. Rev. Respir. Dis. 104: 525–535, 1971.

2290. Dijkman, J. H., Borghans, J. G. A., Savelberg, P. J., and Arkenbout, P. M. Allergic bronchial reactions to inhalation of enzymes of Bacillus subtilis. Am. Rev. Respir. Dis. 107: 387–394, 1973.

2291. Merino, V. L., Lombart, R. L., Marco, R. F., Carnicero, A. B., Guillen, F. G., and Bouhuys, A. Arterial blood gas tensions and lung function during acute responses to hemp dust. Am. Rev. Respir. Dis. 107: 809–815, 1973.

2292. Sidor, R. and Peters, J. M. Differences in ventilatory capacity of Irish and Italian fire fighters. Am. Rev. Respir. Dis. 108: 669–671, 1973.

2293. Chan-Yeung, M., Barton, G. M., MacLean, L., and Grzybowski, S. Occupational asthma and rhinitis due to Western red cedar (Thuja plicata). Am. Rev. Respir. Dis. 108: 1094–1102, 1973.

2294. Pimentel, J. C. A granulomatous lung disease produced by bakelite. Am. Rev. Respir. Dis. 108: 1303–1310, 1973.

2295. Sidor, R. and Peters, J. M. Fire fighting and pulmonary function. Am. Rev. Respir. Dis. 109: 249–254, 1974.

2296. Sidor, R. and Peters, J. M. Prevalence rates of chronic nonspecific respiratory disease in fire fighters. Am. Rev. Respir. Dis. 109: 255–261, 1974.

2297. Villar, T. G. Vineyard sprayer's lung. Am. Rev. Respir. Dis. 110: 545–555, 1974.

2298. Musk, A. W., Gandevia, B., and Williams, B. Respiratory function and the chest radiograph: an epidemiological study of the significance of minor radiographic abnormalities. Aust. N.Z. J. Med. 8: 7–13, 1978.

2299. Morgan, W. K. C. and Lapp, N. L. Respiratory disease in coal miners. Am. Rev. Respir. Dis. 113: 531–559, 1976.

2300. Ziskind, M., Jones, R. N., and Weill, H. Silicosis. Am. Rev. Respir. Dis. 113: 643–665, 1976.

2301. Smith, T. J., Petty, T. L., Reading, J. C., and Lakshminarayan, S. Pulmonary effects of chronic exposure to airborne cadmium. Am. Rev. Respir. Dis. 114: 161–169, 1976.

2302. Chan-Yeung, M. and Abboud, R. Occupational asthma due to California redwood (Sequoia sempervirens) dust. Am. Rev. Respir. Dis. 114: 1027–1031, 1976.

2303. Proctor, D. F. The upper airways. 1. Nasal physiology and defense of the lungs. Am. Rev. Respir. Dis. 115: 97–129, 1977.

2304. Suratt, P. M., Winn, W. C., Brody, A. R., Bolton, W. K., and Giles, R. D. Acute silicosis in tombstone sandblasters. Am. Rev. Respir. Dis. 115: 521–529, 1977.

2305. Lauweryns, J. M. and Baert, J. H. Alveolar clearance and the role of the pulmonary lymphatics. Am. Rev. Respir. Dis. 115: 625–683, 1977.

2306. Musk, A. W., Peters, J. M., Wegman, D. H., and Fine, L. J. Pulmonary function in granite dust exposure: a four-year follow-up. Am. Rev. Respir. Dis. 115: 769–776, 1977.

2307. Dopico, G. A., Reddan, W., Flaherty, D., Tsiatis, A., Peters, M. E., Rao, P., and Rankin, J. Respiratory abnormalities among grain handlers. Am. Rev. Respir. Dis. 115: 915–927, 1977.

2308. Ledsome, J. R. The reflex role of pulmonary arterial baroreceptors. Am. Rev. Respir. Dis. 115(Suppl.): 245–250, 1977.

2309. Friedman, M., Dougherty, R., Nelson, S. R., White, R. P., Sackner, M. A., and Wanner, A. Acute effects of an aerosol hair spray on tracheal mucociliary transport. Am. Rev. Respir. Dis. 116: 281–286, 1977.

2310. Butcher, B. T., Jones, R. N., O'Neill, C. E., Glindmeyer, H. W., Diem, J. E., Dharmarajan, V., Weill, H., and Salvaggio, J. E. Longitudinal study of workers employed in the manufacture of toluene-diisocyanate. Am. Rev. Respir. Dis. 116: 411–421, 1977.

2311. Reichel, G. Disability determination and compensation for pneumoconiosis in West Germany. Chest 78(Suppl.): 365–366, 1980.

2312. Irwig, L. M. and Rocks, P. Lung function and respiratory symptoms in silicotic and nonsilicotic gold miners. Am. Rev. Respir. Dis. 117: 429–435, 1978.

2313. Bush, R. K., Yunginger, J. W., and Reed, C. E. Asthma due to African zebrawood (Microberlinia) dust. Am. Rev. Respir. Dis. 117: 601–603, 1978.

2314. Sprince, N. L., Kanarek, D. J., Weber, A. L., Chamberlin, R. I., and Kazemi, H. Reversible respiratory disease in beryllium workers. Am. Rev. Respir. Dis. 117: 1011–1017, 1978.

2315. Fink, J. N. and Schlueter, D. P. Bathtub refinisher's lung: an unusual response to toluene diisocyanate. Am. Rev. Respir. Dis. 118: 955–959, 1978.

2316. Enterline, P. E. Asbestos and cancer: the international lag (editorial). Am. Rev. Respir. Dis. 118: 975–978, 1978.

2317. Peters, J. M., Murphy, R. L. H., Pagnotto, L. D., and Whittenberger, J. L. Respiratory impairment in workers exposed to "safe" levels of toluene diisocyanate (TDI). Arch. Environ. Health 20: 364–367, 1970.

2318. Ferris, B. G. Jr., Ranadive, M. V., Peters, J. M., Murphy, R. L. H., Burgess, W. A., and Pendergrass, H. P. Prevalence of chronic respiratory disease. Asbestosis in ship repair workers. Arch. Environ. Health 23: 220–225, 1971.

2319. Kaufman, J. and Burkons, D. Clinical, roentgenologic, and physiologic effects of acute chlorine exposure. Arch. Environ. Health 23: 29–34, 1971.

2320. Tucker, A., Faulkner, M. E., and Horvath, S. M. Electrocardiography and lung function in brass instrument players. Arch. Environ. Health 23: 327–334, 1971.

2321. Becklake, M. R., Fournier-Massey, G., Rossiter, C. E., and McDonald, J. C. Lung function in chrysotile asbestos mine and mill workers of Quebec. Arch. Environ. Health 24: 401–409, 1972.

2322. Selikoff, I. J., Nicholson, W. J., and Langer, A. M. Asbestos air pollution. Arch. Environ. Health 25: 1–13, 1972.

2323. Murphy, R. L. H. Jr., Gaensler, E. A., Redding, R. A., Belleau, R., Keelan, P. J., Smith, A. A., Goff, A. M., and Ferris, B. G. Jr. Low exposure to asbestos. Gas exchange in ship pipe coverers and controls. Arch. Environ. Health 25: 253–264, 1972.

2324. Kalacic, I. Chronic nonspecific lung disease in cement workers. Arch. Environ. Health 26: 78–83, 1973.

2325. Kalacic, I. Ventilatory lung function in cement workers. Arch. Environ. Health 26: 84–85, 1973.

2326. Ayres, S. M., Evans, R., Licht, D., Griesbach, J., Reimold, F., Ferrand, E. F., and Criscitiello, A. Health effects of exposure to high concentrations of automotive emissions. Arch. Environ. Health 27: 168–178, 1973.

2327. Brain, J. D. and Valberg, P. A. Models for lung retention based on ICRP Task Group Report. Arch. Environ. Health 28: 1–11, 1974.

2328. Theriault, G. P., Peters, J. M., and Fine, L. J. Pulmonary function in granite shed workers of Vermont. Arch. Environ. Health 28: 18–22, 1974.

2329. Theriault, G. P., Peters, J. M., and Johnson, W. M. Pulmonary function and roentgenographic changes in granite dust exposure. Arch. Environ. Health 28: 23–27, 1974.

2330. Richman, S. I. Meanings of impairment and disability. Chest 78(Suppl.): 367–371, 1980.

2331. Weill, H. Basis for clinical decision-making. Chest 78(Suppl.): 382–383, 1980.

2332. Morgan, W. K. C. Committee Report Workmen's Compensation. Chest 64: 347–349, 1973.

2333. Morgan, W. K. C. Compensation for industrial injury and disease (editorial). Am. Rev. Respir. Dis. 114: 1047–1050, 1976.

2334. Cotes, J. E. Respiratory and cardiac function tests in relation to occupational lung disease. Bull. Physiopathol. Respir. 11: 561–568, 1975.

2335. Cotes, J. E. Assessment of disablement due to impaired respiratory function. Bull. Physiopathol. Respir. 11: 210P–217P, 1975.

2336. Sadoul, P. and Teculescu, D. B. Evaluation du deficit fonctionnel respiratoire. Bull. Eur. Physiopathol. Respir. 14: 475–483, 1978.

2337. Widdicombe, J. G. Dyspnoea. Bull. Eur. Physiopathol. Respir. 15: 437–440, 1979.

2338. Fishman, A. P. Dyspnea. In: Giuntini, C. and Panuccio, P. (eds.). Cardiac Lung. Piccin Editore, Padova, Italy, 1979.

2339. Stark, R. D., Gambles, S. A., and Lewis, J. A. Methods to assess breathlessness in healthy subjects: a critical evaluation and application to analyse the acute effects of diazepam and promethazine on breathlessness induced by exercise or by exposure to raised levels of carbon dioxide. Clin. Sci. 61: 429–439, 1981.

2340. Siegesmund, K. A., Funahashi, A., and Pintar, K. Identification of metals in lung from a patient with interstitial pneumonia. Arch. Environ. Health 28: 345–349, 1974.

2341. Samimi, B., Weill, H., and Ziskind, M. Respirable silica dust exposure of sandblasters and associated workers in steel fabrication yards. Arch. Environ. Health 29: 61–66, 1974.

2342. Kalacic, I. Early detection of expiratory airflow obstruction in cement workers. Arch. Environ. Health 29: 147–149, 1974.

2343. Becklake, M. R., Fournier-Massey, G., McDonald, J. C., Siemiatycki, J., and Rossiter, C. E. Lung function in relation to chest radiographic changes in Quebec asbestos workers. 1. Methods, results and conclusions. Bull. Physiopathol. Respir. 6: 687–699, 1970.

2344. Teculescu, D. B. and Stanescu, D. C. Carbon monoxide transfer factor for the lung in silicosis. Scand. J. Respir. Dis. 51: 150–159, 1970.

2345. Mattson, S-B. and Ringqvist, T. Pleural plaques and exposure to asbestos. Scand. J. Respir. Dis. 75(Suppl.): 1–41, 1970.

2346. Skoogh, B-E., Nadel, J. A., Fabbri, L. M., Sheppard, D., and Holtzmann, M. J. Antihistaminic versus anticholinergic effects of atropine on canine trachealis muscle. Am. Rev. Respir. Dis. 128: 603–606, 1983.

2347. Teculescu, D., Muica, N., and Preda, N. Impairment of pulmonary mixing in simple and complicated silicosis. Bull. Physiopathol. Respir. 11: 447–469, 1975.

2348. Jones, R. N., Weill, H., and Ziskind, M. Pulmonary function in sandblaster's silicosis. Bull. Physiopathol. Respir. 11: 589–595, 1975.

2349. Marek, K. and Kujawska, A. Evolution of functional respiratory disorders in different types of pneumoconiosis. Bull. Physiopathol. Respir. 11: 597–610, 1975.

2350. Rasmussen, F. V., Borchsenius, L., Holstein, B., and Solvsteen, P. Lung function and long-term exposure to cement dust. Scand. J. Respir. Dis. 58: 252–264, 1977.

2351. Samet, J. M., Speizer, F. E., and Gaensler, E. A. Questionnaire reliability and validity in asbestos exposed workers. Bull. Eur. Physiopathol. Respir. 14: 177–188, 1978.

2352. Rossiter, C. E. and Berry, G. The interaction of asbestos exposure and smoking on respiratory health. Bull. Eur. Physiopathol. Respir. 14: 197–204, 1978.

2353. Hillerdal, G. Pleural plaques in a health survey material. Scand. J. Respir. Dis. 59: 257–263, 1978.

2354. Field, G. B. and Owen, P. Respiratory function in an Australian cotton mill. Bull. Eur. Physiopathol. Respir. 15: 455–468, 1979.

2355. Pham, Q. T., Mastrangelo, G., Chau, N., and Haluszka, J. Five year longitudinal comparison of respiratory symptoms and function in steelworkers and unexposed workers. Bull. Eur. Physiopathol. Respir. 15: 469–480, 1979.

2356. Bohadana, A. B., Peslin, R., Poncelet, B., and Hannhart, B. Lung mechanical properties in silicosis and silicoanthracosis. Bull. Eur. Physiopathol. Respir. 16: 521–532, 1980.

2357. Jandova, R. and Widimsky, J. Long-term prognosis of pulmonary hypertension in silicosis. Bull. Eur. Physiopathol. Respir. 16: 128P–131P, 1980.

2358. Hillerdal, G. and Lindgren, A. Pleural plaques: correlation of autopsy findings to radiographic findings and occupational history. Eur. J. Respir. Dis. 61: 315–319, 1980.

2359. Minette, A. (ed.). Bronchial hyperreactivity syndrome: Proceedings of a meeting. Eur. J. Respir. Dis. 61(Suppl. 106): 1980.

2360. Hillerdal, G., Hillerdal, O., and Nou, E. Radiologically visible pleural plaques in a one-year material from a health survey in 1976. A cross sectional study. In: Belin, L., Jarrholm, B., Larsson, S., and Thiringer, G. (eds.). Chest Diseases and the Working Environment. Eur. J. Respir. Dis. 61(Suppl. 106): 89–98, 1980.

2361. Hillerdal, G. Pleural plaques and risk for cancer in the county of Uppsala. In: Belin, L., Jarrholm, B., Larsson, S., and Thiringer, G. (eds.). Chest Diseases and the Working Environment. Eur. J. Respir. Dis. 61(Suppl. 106): 111–118, 1980.

2362. Simonsson, B. G. Bronchial reactivity in occupational asthma and bronchitis. In: Belin, L., Jarrholm, B., Larsson, S., and Thiringer, G. (eds.). Chest Diseases and the Working Environment. Eur. J. Respir. Dis. 61(Suppl. 106): 177–182, 1980.

2363. Richardson, P. S. and Peatfield, A. C. Reflexes concerned in the defence of the lungs. Bull. Eur. Physiopathol. Respir. 17: 979–1012, 1981.

2364. Fridriksson, H. V., Hedenstrom, H., Hillerdal, G., and Malmberg, P. Increased lung stiffness in persons with pleural plaques. Eur. J. Respir. Dis. 62: 412–424, 1981.

2365. Bitterman, P. B., Rennard, S. I., and Crystal, R. G. Environmental lung disease and the interstitium. Clin. Chest Med. 2: 392–412, 1981.

2366. Fine, L. J. and Peters, J. M. Respiratory morbidity in rubber workers. I. Prevalence of respiratory symptoms and disease in curing workers. Arch. Environ. Health 31: 5–9, 1976.

2367. Fine, L. J. and Peters, J. M. Respiratory morbidity in rubber workers. II. Pulmonary function in curing workers. Arch. Environ. Health 31: 10–14, 1976.

2368. Fine, L. J. and Peters, J. M. Studies of respiratory morbidity in rubber workers. III. Respiratory morbidity in pressing workers. Arch. Environ. Health 31: 136–140, 1976.

2369. Fine, L. J., Peters, J. M., Burgess, W. A., and Di Berardinis, L. J. Studies of respiratory morbidity in rubber workers. IV. Respiratory morbidity in talc workers. Arch. Environ. Health 31: 195–200, 1976.

2370. Vitums, V. C., Edwards, M. J., Niles, N. R., Borman, J. O., and Lowry, R. D. Pulmonary fibrosis from amorphous silica dust, a product of silica vapour. Arch. Environ. Health 32: 62–68, 1977.

2371. Oxhoj, H., Bake, B., Wedel, H., and Wilhelmsen, L. Effects of electric arc welding on ventilatory lung function. Arch. Environ. Health 34: 211–217, 1979.

2372. Pratt, P. C., Vollmer, R. T., and Miller, J. A. Epidemiology of pulmonary lesions in nontextile and cotton textile workers: a retrospective autopsy analysis. Arch. Environ. Health 35: 133–138, 1980.

2373. Kamat, S. R., Kamat, G. R., Salpekar, V. Y., and Lobo, E. Distinguishing byssinosis from chronic obstructive pulmonary disease. Results of a prospective five-year study of cotton mill workers in India. Am. Rev. Respir. Dis. 124: 31–40, 1981.

2374. Banks, D. E., Morring, K. L., Boehlecke, B. A., Althouse, R. B., and Merchant, J. A. Silicosis in silica flour workers. Am. Rev. Respir. Dis. 124: 445–450, 1981.

2375. Refsum, H. E. Pulmonary gas exchange during and after exercise of short duration in silicosis. Scand. J. Clin. Lab. Invest. 29(Suppl. 121): 1972.

2376. Graham, W. G., O'Grady, R. V., and Dubuc, B. Pulmonary function loss in Vermont granite workers. Am. Rev. Respir. Dis. 123: 25–28, 1981.

2377. Schachter, E. N., Brown, S., Zuskin, E., Buck, M., Kolack, B., and Bouhuys, A. Airway reactivity in cotton bract-induced bronchospasm. Am. Rev. Respir. Dis. 123: 273–276, 1981.

2378. Pham, Q-T., Mur, J-M., Beigbeider, R., Deniau, R., and Leonet, O. Incidence à long terme de basses teneurs de nuisances gazeuses sur l'appareil respiratoire. Resultats d'une enquete epidemiologique chez les ouvriers des mines de fer du Bassin de Lorraine. Rev. Epidemiol. Sant Publique 25: 255–273, 1977.

2379. Sadoul, P., Horsky, P., Beigbeider, R., Poncelet, B., and Pham, Q-T. La siderose des mineurs de fer lorrains. Arch. Mal. Prof. 40: 15–23, 1979.

2380. Poukkula, A., Huhti, E., and Makarainen, M. Chronic respiratory disease among workers in a pulp mill. A ten year follow-up study. Chest 81: 285–289, 1982.

2381. Higgins, I. T. T., Oh, M. S., and Whittaker, D. E. Chronic respiratory disease in coal miners. Contract HSM 099-71-22. DHHS (NIOSH) Publication No. 81-109. NIOSH Technical Report, April, 1981.

2382. Chan-Yeung, M., Wong, R., Maclean, L., Tan, F., Dorken, E., Schulzer, M., Dennis, R., and Grzybowski, S. Respiratory survey of workers in a pulp and paper mill in Powell

River, British Columbia. Am. Rev. Respir. Dis. 122: 249–257, 1980.

2383. Zuskin, E., Valic, F., and Bouhuys, A. Byssinosis and airway responses due to exposure to textile dust. Lung 154: 17–24, 1976.

2384. Bouhuys, A., Schoenberg, J. B., Beck, G. J., and Schilling, R. S. F. Epidemiology of chronic lung disease in a cotton mill community. Lung 154: 167–186, 1977.

2385. Mitchell, C. A., Charney, M., and Schoenberg, J. B. Early lung disease in asbestos-product workers. Lung 154: 261–272, 1978.

2386. Broder, I., Mintz, S., Hutcheon, M. A., Corey, P. N., and Kuzyk, J. Effect of layoff and rehire on respiratory variables of grain elevator workers. Am. Rev. Respir. Dis. 122: 601–608, 1980.

2387. Teculescu, D. B. and Stanescu, D. C. Pulmonary function in workers with chronic exposure to cadmium oxide fumes. Int. Arch. Arbeitsmed. 26: 335–345, 1970.

2388. Sessa, T., Pecora, L., Vecchione, G., and Mole, R. La fonction cardiorespiratoire dans les suites des bronchopneumopathies par gaz irritants. Poumon Coeur 26: 1097–1107, 1970.

2389. Brun, J., Cassan, G., Kofman, J., and Gilly, J. La siderosclerose des soudeurs à l'arc à forme de fibrose interstitielle diffuse et à forme conglomerative pseudo-tumorale. Poumon Coeur 28: 45–48, 1972.

2390. Sessa, T., Vecchione, C., Mole, R., and Javicoli, N. Hypoxemie et equilibre acide base chez les asbestosiques. Poumon Coeur 30: 135–139, 1974.

2391. Stanescu, D. C., Teculescu, D. B., and Pacuraru, R. Increased N_2 alveolar slope in silicosis. Respiration 27: 228–235, 1970.

2392. Scotti, P. and Aresini, G. Les ductances pulmonaires pour l'evaluation de la capacité de diffusion pulmonaire dans la silicose. Poumon Coeur 31: 309–312, 1975.

2393. Carles, P., Fabre, J., Pujol, M., Duprez, A., and Bollinelli, R. Pneumoconioses complexes chez les prothesistes dentaires. Poumon Coeur 34: 189–192, 1978.

2394. Leophonte, P., Fabre, J., Fortune, J. P., Pincemin, J., and Delaude, A. Les silicatoses pulmonaires. Poumon Coeur 34: 193–201, 1978.

2395. Goff, A. M. and Gaensler, E. A. Asbestosis following brief exposure in cigarette filter manufacture. Respiration 29: 83–93, 1972.

2396. Zedda, S., Aresini, G., Ghezzi, I., and Sartorelli, E. Lung function in relation to radiographic changes in asbestos workers. Respiration 30: 132–140, 1973.

2397. Morrisey, W. L., Gould, I. A., Carrington, C. B., and Gaensler, E. A. Silo-filler's disease. Respiration 32: 81–92, 1975.

2398. Zedda, S., Cirla, A., Aresini, G., and Sala, C. Occupational type test for the etiological diagnosis of asthma due to toluenedi-isocyanate. Respiration 33: 14–21, 1976.

2399. Selikoff, I. J. and Lee, D. H. K. Asbestos and Disease. Academic Press, New York, 1968.

2400. Baur, X., Fruhmann, G., and Von Liebe, V. Persulfat-Asthma und Persulfat-Dermatitis bei zwei Industriearbeitern. Respiration 38: 144–150, 1979.

2401. Woodford, D. M., Coutu, R. E., and Gaensler, E. A. Obstructive lung disease from acute sulfur dioxide exposure. Respiration 38: 238–249, 1979.

2402. Baur, X., Rommelt, H., and Fruhmann, G. On the pathogenesis of isocyanate-induced asthma. Respiration 38: 289–298, 1979.

2403. Rodriguez-Roisin, R., Merchant, J. E. M., Cochrane, G. M., Hickey, B. P. H., Turner-Warwick, M., and Clark, T. J. H. Maximal expiratory flow volume curves in workers exposed to asbestos. Respiration 39: 158–165, 1980.

2404. Epler, G. R., Fitzgerald, M. X., Gaensler, E. A., and Carrington, C. B. Asbestos-related disease from household exposure. Respiration 39: 229–240, 1980.

2405. Smidt, U. and Schnellbacher, F. Autoptisch verifizierte Rechtsherzhypertrophie und die Symptome ihrer Entwicklung bei Silikosekranken. Prax. Klin. Pneumol. 32: 407–416, 1978.

2406. Smidt, U., Worth, G., and Bielert, D. Lung function and clinical findings in cross sectional and longitudinal studies in coal workers from the Ruhr area. Int. Arch. Occup. Environ. Health 40: 45–70, 1977.

2407. Shirai, F., Kudoh, S., Shibuya, A., Sada, K., and Mikami, R. Crackles in asbestos workers: auscultation and lung sound analysis. Br. J. Dis. Chest 75: 386–396, 1981.

2408. Krumpe, P. E., Finley, T. N., and Martinez, N. The search for expiratory obstruction in meat wrappers studied on the job. Am. Rev. Respir. Dis. 119: 611–618, 1979.

2409. Churg, A. and Warnock, M. L. Analysis of the cores of asbestos bodies from members of the general population: patients with probable low-degree exposure to asbestos. Am. Rev. Respir. Dis. 120: 781–786, 1979.

2410. Seaton, A., Lamb, D., Brown, W. R., Sclare, G., and Middleton, W. G. Pneumoconiosis of shale miners. Thorax 36: 412–418, 1981.

2411. Hillerdal, G. Non-malignant asbestos pleural disease. Thorax 36: 669–675, 1981.

2412. Burge, P. S. Occupational asthma in electronics workers caused by colophony fumes: follow-up of affected workers. Thorax 37: 348–353, 1982.

2413. Burge, P. S., Edge, G., Hawkins, R., White, V., and Taylor, A. J. N. Occupational asthma in a factory making flux-cored solder containing colophony. Thorax 36: 828–834, 1981.

2414. Robinson, B. W. S. and Musk, A. W. Benign asbestos pleural effusion: diagnosis and course. Thorax 36: 896–930, 1981.

2415. Slovak, A. J. M. Occupational asthma caused by a plastics blowing agent, azodicarbonamide. Thorax 36: 906–909, 1981.

2416. Graham, V., Coe, M. J. S., and Davies, R. J. Occupational asthma after exposure to a diazonium salt. Thorax 36: 950–951, 1981.

2417. Zuskin, E., Valic, F., and Kanceljak, B. Immunological and respiratory changes in coffee workers. Thorax 36: 9–13, 1981.

2418. Al Zuhair, Y. S., Whitaker, C. J., and Cinkotai, F. F. Ventilatory function in workers exposed to tea and wood dust. Br. J. Ind. Med. 38: 339–345, 1981.

2419. McMillan, G. H. G., Rossiter, C. E., and Deacon, R. Comparison of independent randomised reading of radiographs with direct progression scoring for assessing change in asbestos-related pulmonary and pleural lesions. Br. J. Ind. Med. 39: 60–61, 1982.

2420. Morgan, A. and Holmes, A. Concentrations and characteristics of amphibole fibres in the lungs of workers exposed to crocidolite in the British gas-mask factories, and elsewhere, during the second world war. Br. J. Ind. Med. 39: 62–69, 1982.

2421. Baelum, J., Andersen, I., and Molhave, L. Acute and sub-acute symptoms among workers in the printing industry. Br. J. Ind. Med. 39: 70–75, 1982.

2422. Fawer, R. F., Gardner, A. W., and Oakes, D. Absences attributed to respiratory diseases in welders. Br. J. Ind. Med. 39: 149–152, 1982.

2423. Glyseth, B., Baunan, R. H., and Overaae, L. Analysis of fibres in human lung tissue. Br. J. Ind. Med. 39: 191–195, 1982.

2424. Kauffman, F., Drouet, D., Lellouch, J., and Brille, D. Occupational exposure and 12-year spirometric changes among Paris area workers. Br. J. Ind. Med. 39: 221–232, 1982.

2425. Wegman, D. H., Peters, J. M., Boundy, M. G., and Smith, T. J. Evaluation of respiratory effects in miners and millers exposed to talc free of asbestos and silica. Br. J. Ind. Med. 39: 233–238, 1982.

2426. Froneberg, B., Johnson, P. L., and Landrigan, P. J. Respiratory illness caused by overheating of polyvinyl chloride. Br. J. Ind. Med. 39: 239–243, 1982.

2427. Thomas, H. F., Benjamin, I. T., Elwood, P. C., and Sweetnam, P. M. Further follow-up study of workers from an asbestos cement factory. Br. J. Ind. Med. 39: 273–276, 1982.

2428. Occupation and bronchitis (editorial). Lancet i: 235–236, 1980.

2429. Firemen's lungs (editorial). Lancet i: 439, 1975.

2430. The miners: a special case? (editorial). Lancet i: 81–82, 1974.

2431. Burge, P. S., Newman-Taylor, A. J., Harries, M. G., and O'Brien, I. Toluene diisocyanate (letter to editor). Lancet ii: 96–97, 1978.

2432. Peters, J. M. and Wegman, D. H. Toluene diisocyanate (letter to editor). Lancet ii: 472, 1978.

2433. Ahmad, D., Patterson, R., Morgan, W. K. C., Williams, T., and Zeiss, C. R. Pulmonary haemorrhage and haemolytic anaemia due to trimellitic anhydride. Lancet ii: 328–330, 1979.

2434. Seaton, A., Dodgson, J., Dick, J. A., and Jacobsen, M. Quartz and pneumoconiosis in coal miners. Lancet ii: 1272–1275, 1981.

2435. Ethics in occupational medicine (editorial). Lancet ii: 134, 1980.

2436. Bouhuys, A. and Zuskin, E. Chronic respiratory disease in hemp workers. Ann. Intern. Med. 84: 398–405, 1976.

2437. Wegman, D. H. and Peters, J. M. Polymer fume fever and cigarette smoking. Ann. Intern. Med. 81: 55–57, 1974.

2438. Merchant, J. A., Kilburn, K. H., O'Fallon, W. M., Hamilton, J. D., and Lumsden, J. C. Byssinosis and chronic bronchitis among cotton textile workers. Ann. Intern. Med. 76: 423–433, 1972.

2439. McConnell, L. H., Fink, J. N., Schlueter, D. P., and Schmidt, M. G. Jr. Asthma caused by nickel sensitivity. Ann. Intern. Med. 78: 888–890, 1973.

2440. Liddell, D. Asbestos and public health (editorial). Thorax 36: 241–244, 1981.

2441. Bourne, M. S., Flindt, M. L. H., and Walker, J. M. Asthma due to industrial use of chloramine. Br. Med. J. 2: 10–12, 1979.

2442. Jeffreys, D. B. and Vale, J. A. Malignant mesothelioma and gas-mask assemblers. Br. Med. J. 2: 607, 1978.

2443. Hendrick, D. J. and Lane, D. J. Formalin asthma in hospital staff. Br. Med. J. 1: 607–608, 1975.

2444. Byssinosis: Clinical and Research Issues. National Academy Press, Washington, D.C. 1982.

2445. Jones, N. L. and Campbell, E. J. M. Clinical Exercise Testing. 2nd ed. W. B. Saunders, Philadelphia, 1982.

2446. Ostiguy, G. L. (ed.). Summary of Task Force Report on Occupational Respiratory Disease (pneumoconiosis). Can. Med. Assoc. J. 121: 414–421, 1979.

2447. Zielhuis, R. L. (ed.). Public Health Risks of Exposure to Asbestos. Pergamon Press for the Commission of the European Communities, Oxford, 1977.

2448. Ramazzini, B. On the CCCL Anniversary of His Birth. Pericle Di Pietro, Modena, Italy, 1983.

2449. Hillerdal, G. and Hemmingsson, A. Pulmonary pseudotumours and asbestos. Acta Radiol. Diagn. 21: 615–620, 1980.

2450. Asbestos: Health Risks and Their Prevention. International Labour Office, Geneva, 1974.

2451. Ramazzini, B. De Morbis Artificum: Diseases of Workers. History of Medicine Series. Library of the New York Academy of Medicine. No. 23. Hafner, New York, 1964.

2452. Morgan, W. K. C. and Seaton, A. (eds.). Occupational Lung Diseases. W. B. Saunders, Philadelphia, 1975.

2453. Miller, A., Teirstein, A. S., and Selikoff, I. J. Ventilatory failure due to asbestos pleurisy. Am. J. Med. 75: 911–919, 1983.

2454. Churg, A. and Wright, J. L. Small-airway lesions in patients exposed to nonasbestos mineral dusts. Hum. Pathol. 14: 688–693, 1983.

2455. Karol, M. H. Survey of industrial workers for antibodies to toluene diisocyanate. J. Occup. Med. 23: 741–747, 1981.

2456. Chan-Yeung, M., Lam, S., and Koener, S. Clinical features and natural history of occupational asthma due to Western red cedar (*Thuja plicata*). Am. J. Med. 72: 411–415, 1982.

2457. Cotton, D. J., Graham, B. L., Li, K. Y. R., Froh, F., Barnett, G. D., and Dosman, J. A. Effects of grain dust exposure and smoking on respiratory symptoms and lung function. J. Occup. Med. 25: 131–141, 1983.

2458. Pooley, F. D. Tissue mineral identification. In: Weill, H. and Turner-Warwick, M. (eds.). Occupational Lung Diseases. Marcel Dekker, New York and Basel, 1981.

2459. Gardner, R. M., Hankinson, J. L., and Glindmeyer, H. W. III. Standardisation of spirometry with special emphasis in field testing. In: Weill, H. and Turner-Warwick, M. (eds.). Occupational Lung Diseases. Marcel Dekker, New York and Basel, 1981.

2460. Cotes, J. E. Exercise testing. In: Weill, H. and Turner-Warwick, M. (eds.). Occupational Lung Diseases. Marcel Dekker, New York and Basel, 1981.

2461. McDonald, J. C. Epidemiology. In: Weill, H. and Turner-Warwick, M. (eds.). Occupational Lung Diseases. Marcel Dekker, New York and Basel, 1981.

2462. Field, G. B. Worker surveys. In: Weill, H. and Turner-Warwick, M. (eds.). Occupational Lung Diseases. Marcel Dekker, New York and Basel, 1981.

2463. Berry, G. Statistical analyses. In: Weill, H. and Turner-Warwick, M. (eds.). Occupational Lung Diseases. Marcel Dekker, New York and Basel, 1981.

2464. Block, G., Tse, K. S., Kijek, K., Chan, H., and Chan-Yeung, M. Baker's asthma. Clin. Allergy 13: 359–370, 1983.

2465. Zammit-Tabona, M., Sherkin, M., Kijek, K., Chan, H., and Chan-Yeung, M. Asthma caused by diphenylmethane diisocyanate in foundry workers. Am. Rev. Respir. Dis. 128: 226–230, 1983.

2466. Chan-Yeung, M., Wong, R., Maclean, L., Tan, F., Schulzer, M., Enarson, D., Martin, A., Dennis, R., and Grzybowski, S. Epidemiologic health study of workers in an aluminum smelter in British Columbia. Am. Rev. Respir. Dis. 127: 465–469, 1983.

2467. Chan-Yeung, M., Wong, R., Tan, F., Enarson, D., Schulzer, M., Subbarao, K., Knickerboccker, J., and Grzybowski, S. Epidemiologic health study of workers in an aluminum smelter in Kitimat, BC. Arch. Environ. Health 38: 34–40, 1983.

2468. Redmond, C. K. Cancer mortality among coke oven workers. Environ. Health Perspect. 52: 67–73, 1983.

2469. Wain, J. Samuel Johnson. Viking Press, New York, 1974.

2470. Dosman, J. A. and Cotton, D. J. (eds.). Occupational Pulmonary Disease: Focus on Grain Dust and Health. Academic Press, New York, 1980.

2471. Lednak, W. M., Tyroler, H. A., McMichael, A. J., and Shy, C. M. The occupational determinants of chronic disabling pulmonary disease in rubber workers. J. Occup. Med. 19: 263–268, 1977.

2472. Lee, L-Y., Djokic, T. D., Dumont, C., Graf, P. D., and Nadel, J. A. Mechanism of ozone-induced tachypneic response to hypoxia and hypercapnia in conscious dogs. J. Appl. Physiol. 48: 163–168, 1980.

2473. Mann, B. Pulmonary asbestosis with special reference to an epidemic at Hebden Bridge. J. R. Coll. Physicians Lond. 12: 297–307, 1978.

2474. Findlay, S. R., Stotsky, E., Leiterman, K., Hemady, Z., and Ohman, J. L. Jr. Allergens detected in association with airborne particles capable of penetrating into the peripheral lung. Am. Rev. Respir. Dis. 128: 1008–1012, 1983.

2475. Lee, D. H. K. and Selikoff, I. J. Historical background to the asbestos problem. Environ. Res. 18: 300–314, 1979.

2476. Roemmich, W., Blumenfeld, H. L., and Moritz, H. Evaluating remaining capacity to work in miner applicants with simple pneumoconiosis under 65 yr. of age under Title IV of Public Law 91–173. In: Coal Worker's Pneumoconiosis. Ann. N.Y. Acad. Sci. 200: 608–616, 1972.

2477. Epler, G. R., Saber, F. A., and Gaensler, E. A. Determination of severe impairment (disability) in interstitial lung disease. Am. Rev. Respir. Dis. 121: 647–659, 1980.

2478. Skalpe, I. O. Long-term effects of sulphur dioxide exposure in pulp mills. Br. J. Ind. Med. 21: 69–73, 1964.

2479. Smith, T. J., Peters, J. M., Reading, J. C., and Castle, C. H. Pulmonary impairment from chronic exposure to sulfur dioxide in a smelter. Am. Rev. Respir. Dis. 116: 31–39, 1977.

2480. Smith, T. J., Wagner, W. L., and Moore, D. E. Chronic sulfur dioxide exposure in a smelter. 1. Exposure to SO_2 and dust: 1940–1974. J. Occup. Med. 20: 83–87, 1978.

2481. Archer, V. E. and Gillam, J. D. Chronic sulfur dioxide exposure in a smelter. 2. Indices of chest disease. J. Occup. Med. 20: 88–95, 1978.

2482. Weill, H., George, R., Schwarz, M., and Ziskind, M. Late evaluation of pulmonary function after acute exposure to chlorine gas. Am. Rev. Respir. Dis. 99: 374–379, 1969.

2483. Weiss, W. The forced end-expiratory flow rate in chloromethyl ether workers. J. Occup. Med. 19: 611–614, 1977.

2484. Wessel-Aas, T., Vale, J. R., and Schaaning, J. Occupational disease caused by gas inhalation. Scand. J. Respir. Dis. 63(Suppl.): 95–99, 1968.

2485. Henderson, A. F., Heaton, R. W., Dunlop, L. S., and Costello, J. F. Effects of nifedipine on antigen-induced bronchoconstriction. Am. Rev. Respir. Dis. 127: 549–553, 1983.

2486. Salm, R. and Hughes, E. W. A case of chronic paraffin pneumonitis. Thorax 25: 762–768, 1970.

2487. Morgan, W. K. C., Burgess, D. B., Lapp, N. L., and Seaton, A. Hyperinflation of the lungs in coal miners. Thorax 26: 585–590, 1971.

2488. Valic, F. and Zuskin, E. Byssinosis: a follow-up study of workers exposed to fine grade cotton dust. Thorax 27: 459–462, 1972.

2489. Jones, G. R., Proudfoot, A. T., and Hall, J. I. Pulmonary effects of acute exposure to nitrous fumes. Thorax 28: 61–65, 1973.

2490. Pimentel, J. C. and Avila, R. Respiratory disease in cork workers ("suberosis"). Thorax 28: 409–423, 1973.

2491. Tanser, A. R., Bourke, M. P., and Blandford, A. G. Isocyanate asthma: respiratory symptoms caused by diphenyl-methane di-isocyanate. Thorax 28: 596–600, 1973.

2492. Pimentel, J. C., Avila, R., and Lourenco, A. G. Respiratory disease caused by synthetic fibres: a new occupational disease. Thorax 30: 204–219, 1975.

2493. Warrell, D. A., Harrison, B. D. W., Fawcett, I. W., Mohammed, Y., Mohammed, W. S., Pope, H. M., and Watkins, B. J. Silicosis among grindstone cutters in the north of Nigeria. Thorax 30: 389–398, 1975.

2494. Edwards, C., Macartney, J., Rooke, G., and Ward, F. The pathology of the lung in byssinotics. Thorax 30: 612–623, 1975.

2495. Doig, A. T. Baritosis: a benign pneumoconiosis. Thorax 31: 30–39, 1976.

2496. Klink, K., Herold, B., Burkmann, I., and Julich, H. Atemmechanik und Belastungsdyspnoe bei Silikose. Respiration 32: 135–145, 1975.

2497. Xipell, J. M., Ham, K. N., Price, C. G., and Thomas, D. P. Acute silicolipoproteinosis. Thorax 32: 104–111, 1977.

2498. Jones, R. N., Carr, J., Glindmeyer, H., Diem, J., and Weill, H. Respiratory health and dust levels in cottonseed mills. Thorax 32: 281–286, 1977.

2499. Arnaud, A., Pommier De Santi, P., Garbe, L., Payan, H., and Charpin, J. Polyvinyl chloride pneumoconiosis. Thorax 33: 19–25, 1978.

2500. Burge, P. S., Perks, W., O'Brien, I. M., Hawkins, R., and Green, M. Occupational asthma in an electronics factory. Thorax 34: 13–18, 1979.

2501. Perks, W. H., Burge, P. S., Rehahn, M., and Green, M. Work-related respiratory disease in employees leaving an electronics factory. Thorax 34: 19–22, 1979.

2502. Burge, P. S., Perks, W. H., O'Brien, I. M., Burge, A., Hawkins, R., Brown, D., and Green, M. Occupational asthma in an electronics factory: a case control study to evaluate aetiological factors. Thorax 34: 300–307, 1979.

2503. Burge, P. S., O'Brien, I. M., and Harries, M. G. Peak flow rate records in the diagnosis of occupational asthma due to colophony. Thorax 34: 308–316, 1979.

2504. Burge, P. S., O'Brien, I. M., and Harries, M. G. Peak flow rate records in the diagnosis of occupational asthma due to isocyanates. Thorax 34: 317–323, 1979.

2505. Harries, M. G., Burge, P. S., Samson, M., Taylor, A. J. N., and Pepys, J. Isocyanate asthma: respiratory symptoms due to 1,5-naphthylene di-isocyanate. Thorax 34: 762–766, 1979.

2506. Newman Taylor, A. J. Occupational asthma (editorial). Thorax 35: 241–245, 1980.

2507. Sjogren, I., Hillerdal, G., Andersson, A., and Zetterstrom, O. Hard metal lung disease: importance of cobalt in coolants. Thorax 35: 653–659, 1980.

2508. Unger, K. M., Snow, R. M., Mestas, J. M., and Miller, W. C. Smoke inhalation in firemen. Thorax 35: 838–842, 1980.

2509. Darke, C. S., Knowelden, J., Lacey, J., and Ward, A. M. Respiratory disease of workers harvesting grain. Thorax 31: 190–196, 1976.

2510. Herbert, F. A. and Orford, R. Pulmonary hemorrhage and edema due to inhalation of resins containing tri-mellitic anhydride. Chest 76: 546–551, 1979.

2511. Guyatt, A. R., Douglas, J. S., Zuskin, E., and Bouhuys, A. Lung static recoil and airway obstruction in hemp workers with byssinosis. Am. Rev. Respir. Dis. 108: 1111–1115, 1973.

2512. Bailey, W. C., Brown, M., Buechner, H. A., Weill, H., Ichinose, H., and Ziskind, M. Silico-mycobacterial disease in sandblasters. Am. Rev. Respir. Dis. 110: 115–125, 1974.

2513. Becklake, M. R. Asbestos-related diseases of the lung and other organs: their epidemiology and implications for clinical practice. Am. Rev. Respir. Dis. 114: 187–227, 1976.

2514. Kanarek, D. J., Wainer, R. A., Chamberlin, R. I., Weber, A. L., and Kazemi, H. Respiratory illness in a population exposed to beryllium. Am. Rev. Respir. Dis. 108: 1295–1302, 1973.

2515. Smidt, U. and Worth, G. Principles for the assessment of working disability due to disorders of the lung. Pneumologie 1976(Suppl.): 75–96, 1976.

2516. Smidt, U. Respiratory muscle fatigue as limitation for exercise. Progr. Respir. Res. 11: 215–223, 1979.

2517. Hendrick, D. J. and Fabri, L. Compensating occupational asthma (editorial). Thorax 36: 881–884, 1981.

2518. Smoking, coal, asbestos and the lungs (editorial). Br. Med. J. 283: 457–458, 1981.

2519. Britton, M. G., Hughes, D. T. D., and Phillips, T. J. G. A guide to compensation for asbestos-related diseases. Br. Med. J. 282: 2107–2111, 1981.

2520. Rubinfeld, A. R. and Pain, M. C. F. Respiratory disability in worker's compensation claimants. Med. J. Aust. 1: 119–121, 1983.

2521. McGavin, C. R., Artvinli, M., Naoe, H., and McHardy, G. J. R. Dyspnoea, disability, and distance walked: comparison of estimates of exercise performance in respiratory disease. Br. Med. J. ii: 241–243, 1978.

2522. Kumar, M., Gimenez, M., and Sadoul, P. Exercise studies in cases of silicosis. In preparation, personal communication.

2523. Brugman, T. M., Darnell, M. L., and Hirshman, C. A. Nifedipine aerosol attenuates airway constriction in dogs with hyperreactive airways. Am. Rev. Respir. Dis. 127: 14–17, 1983.

2524. Ogilvie, C. M. Dyspnoea (editorial). Br. Med. J. 287: 160–161, 1983.

2525. Zuskin, E., Valic, F., and Bouhuys, A. Effect of wool dust on respiratory function. Am. Rev. Respir. Dis. 114: 705–709, 1976.

2526. Valic, F., Beritic, D., and Butkovic, D. Respiratory response to tobacco dust exposure. Am. Rev. Respir. Dis. 113: 751–755, 1976.

2527. Davies, R. J., Green, M., and Schofield, N. M. Recurrent nocturnal asthma after exposure to grain dust. Am. Rev. Respir. Dis. 114: 1011–1019, 1976.

2528. Wehr, K. L., Johanson, W. G. Jr., Chapman, J. S., and Pierce, A. K. Pneumoconiosis among activated-carbon workers. Arch. Environ. Health 30: 578–582, 1975.

2529. Ohsaki, Y., Abe, S., Kimura, K., Tsuneta, Y., Mikami, H., and Murao, M. Lung cancer in Japanese chromate workers. Thorax 33: 372–374, 1978.

2530. Churg, A. and Warnock, M. L. Asbestos fibres in the general population. Am. Rev. Respir. Dis. 122: 669–678, 1980.

2531. Lam, S. and Chan-Yeung, M. Ethylenediamine-induced asthma. Am. Rev. Respir. Dis. 121: 151–155, 1980.

2532. Woitowitz, H-J. and Woitowitz, R. H. Clinical experiences with a new beta-sympathicomimetic substance in the provoked attack in occupational asthma. Respiration 29: 549–555, 1972.

2533. Corn, J. K. Byssinosis—an historical perspective. Am. J. Ind. Med. 2: 331–352, 1981.

2534. Goldstein, I. F. and Currie, B. Seasonal patterns of asthma: a clue to etiology. Environ. Res. 33: 201–215, 1984.

2535. Morrow, P. E. Lymphatic drainage of the lung in dust clearance. In: Coal Worker's Pneumoconiosis. Ann. N.Y. Acad. Sci. 200: 46–65, 1972.

2536. Dopico, G. A., Rankin, J., Chosy, L. W., Reddan, W. G., Barbee, R. A., Gee, B., and Dickie, H. A. Respiratory tract disease from thermosetting resins. Study of an outbreak in rubber tire workers. Ann. Intern. Med. 83: 177–184, 1975.

2537. Brown, H. V. and Wasserman, K. Exercise performance in chronic obstructive lung disease. Med. Clin. North Am. 65: 525–548, 1981.

2538. Ison, T. G. Human disability and personal income. In: Studies in Canadian Tort Law. Butterworth & Co., London, 1978.

2539. Smidt, U. and Worth, G. Methods and results of a joint epidemiologic study of CNSLD in 13,000 workers with and without occupational dust exposure. Rev. Inst. Hyg. Mines 29: 1–8, 1974.

2540. Smidt, U. Problems and results in the simultaneous assessment of the role of smoking and occupational dust exposure for chronic bronchitis and pulmonary emphysema. Bronchopneumologie 28: 177–185, 1978.

2541. Saracci, R. Personal-environmental interactions in occupational epidemiology. In: McDonald, J. C. (ed.). Recent Advances in Occupational Health. Churchill Livingstone, London, 1981.

2542. Chovil, A., Sutherland, R. B., and Ojanen, T. H. Respiratory cancer in a cohort of nickel sinter plant workers. Br. J. Ind. Med. 38: 334–338, 1981.

2543. Tabona, M., Chan-Yeung, M., Enarson, D., Maclean, L., Dorken, E., and Schulzer, M. Host factors affecting longitudinal decline in lung spirometry among grain elevator workers. Chest 85: 782–786, 1984.

2544. Block, G. T. and Chan-Yeung, M. Asthma induced by nickel. J.A.M.A. 247: 1600–1602, 1982.

2545. Rotman, H. H., Fliegelman, M. J., Moore, J., Smith, R. G., Angler, D. M., Kowalski, C. J., and Weg, J. G. Effects of low concentrations of chlorine on pulmonary function in man. Presentation to British Thoracic Society, London, Jan. 1981.

2546. Enterline, P. Estimating health risks in studies of the health effects of asbestos. Am. Rev. Respir. Dis. 113: 175–180, 1976.

2547. Berend, N., Woolcock, A. J., and Marlin, G. E. Effects of lobectomy on lung function. Thorax 35: 145–150, 1980.

2548. Nou, E. Quality of survival in bronchial carcinoma. Scand. J. Respir. Dis. 104(Suppl.): 1–226, 1979.

2549. Legge, J. S. and Palmer, K. N. V. Pulmonary function in bronchial carcinoma. Thorax 28: 588–591, 1973.

2550. Hall, D. R. Regional lung function after pneumonectomy. Thorax 29: 425–431, 1974.

2551. Legge, J. S. and Palmer, K. N. V. Effect of lung resection for bronchial carcinoma on pulmonary function in patients with and without chronic obstructive bronchitis. Thorax 30: 563–565, 1975.

2552. Nou, E. and Aberg, T. Quality of survival in patients with surgically treated bronchial carcinoma. Thorax 35: 255–263, 1980.

2553. Bainbridge, E. T. and Matthews, H. R. Hypoxaemia after left thoracotomy for benign oesophageal disease. Thorax 35: 264–268, 1980.

2554. Ogilvie, C. M. Physician among surgeons: thoughts on preoperative assessment (editorial). Thorax 35: 881–883, 1980.

2555. Feofilov, G. L., Siderenko, A. G., and Glock, R. I. Upward displacement of the diaphragm after lung resection. J. Thorac. Cardiovasc. Surg. 69: 315–320, 1975.

2556. Wernly, J. A., DeMeester, T. R., Kirchner, P. T., Myerowitz, P. D., Oxford, D. E., and Golomb, H. M. Clinical value of quantitative ventilation-perfusion lung scans in the surgical management of bronchogenic carcinoma. J. Thorac. Cardiovasc. Surg. 80: 535–543, 1980.

2557. Chiroazzi, N., Weiss, H., Margouleff, D., Farber, S., and Gulotta, S. J. Long-term pulmonary blood flow alterations following relief of partial bronchial obstruction. Am. J. Med. 56: 559–564, 1974.

2558. Hazlett, D. R. and Watson, R. L. Lateral position test: a simple, inexpensive, yet accurate method of studying the separate functions of the lungs. Chest 59: 276–279, 1971.

2559. Boushy, S. F., Billig, D. M., North, L. B., and Helgason, A. H. Clinical course related to preoperative and postoperative pulmonary function in patients with bronchogenic carcinoma. Chest 59: 383–391, 1971.

2560. Ludington, L. G., Verska, J. J., Howard, T., Kypridakis, G., and Brewer, L. A. III. Bronchiolar carcinoma (alveolar cell), another great imitator: a review of 41 cases. Chest 61: 622–628, 1972.

2561. Yang, S-P. and Lin, C-C. Lymphangitic carcinomatosis of the lungs. Chest 62: 179–187, 1972.

2562. Reichel, J. Assessment of operative risk of pneumonectomy. Chest 62: 570–576, 1972.

2563. Kristerson, S., Lindell, S-E., and Svanberg, L. Prediction of pulmonary function loss due to pneumonectomy using ^{133}Xe-radiospirometry. Chest 62: 694–698, 1972.

2564. Ali, M. K., Mountain, C., Miller, J. M., Johnston, D. A., and Schullenberger, C. C. Regional pulmonary function

2565. before and after pneumonectomy using ^{133}xenon. Chest 68: 288–296, 1975.

2565. Lefrak, S. S. Preoperative evaluation for pulmonary resection (editorial). Chest 72: 419–420, 1977.

2566. Boysen, P. G., Block, A. J., Olsen, G. N., Moulder, P. V., Harris, J. O., and Rawitscher, R. E. Prospective evaluation for pneumonectomy using the ^{99m}technetium quantitative perfusion scan. Chest 72: 422–425, 1977.

2567. Walkup, R. H., Vossel, L. F., Griffin, J. P., and Proctor, R. J. Prediction of postoperative pulmonary function with the lateral position test. Chest 77: 24–27, 1980.

2568. Olsen, G. N., Block, A. J., and Tobias, J. A. Prediction of postpneumonectomy pulmonary function using quantitative macroaggregate lung scanning. Chest 66: 13–16, 1974.

2569. Ali, M. K., Mountain, C. F., Ewer, M. S., Johnston, D., and Haynie, T. P. Predicting loss of pulmonary function after pulmonary resection for bronchogenic carcinoma. Chest 77: 337–342, 1980.

2570. Benfield, J. R. A 1980 perspective of lung transplantation (editorial). Chest 78: 548–549, 1980.

2571. Nelems, J. M. B., Rebuck, A. S., Cooper, J. D., Goldberg, M., Halloran, P. F., and Vellend, H. Human lung transplantation. Chest 78: 569–573, 1980.

2572. Stevens, P. M., Johnson, P. C., Bell, R. L., Beall, A. C. Jr., and Jenkins, D. E. Regional ventilation and perfusion after lung transplantation in patients with emphysema. N. Engl. J. Med. 282: 245–249, 1970.

2573. Bates, D. V. The other lung (editorial). N. Engl. J. Med. 282: 277–288, 1970.

2574. Vermeire, P., Tasson, J., Lamont, H., Barbier, F., Versieck, J., and Derom, F. Respiratory function after lung homotransplantation with a ten-month survival in man. Am. Rev. Respir. Dis. 106: 515–527, 1972.

2575. Simons, J., Friedman, J., Theodore, J., Buch, W. S., Lertzman, M., Mark, J. B. D., and Robin, E. D. Pneumonectomy for unilateral lung disease associated with respiratory failure. Am. Rev. Respir. Dis. 108: 652–655, 1973.

2576. Fishman, H. C., Danon, J., Koopot, N., Langston, H. T., and Sharp, J. T. Massive intrapulmonary venoarterial shunting in alveolar cell carcinoma. Am. Rev. Respir. Dis. 109: 124–128, 1974.

2577. Hepper, N. G., Payne, W. S., Sheps, S. G., and Hyatt, R. E. Unilateral hypoperfusion of the lung and carcinoid syndrome due to bronchial carcinoid tumor. Am. Rev. Respir. Dis. 115: 351–357, 1977.

2578. Carrington, C. B., Cugell, D. W., Gaensler, E. A., Marks, A., Redding, R. A., Schaaf, J. T., and Tomasian, A. Lymphangioleiomyomatosis. Am. Rev. Respir. Dis. 116: 977–995, 1977.

2579. Bitker, B. R., Aidan, D. S., and Ladurie, M. le R. Signification de la repartition de la consommation d'oxygene et de la ventilation avant chirurgie thoracique. Bull. Physiopathol. Respir. 6: 687–699, 1970.

2580. Hauge, B. N. Diaphragmatic movement and spirometric volume in patients with one functioning lung. Scand. J. Respir. Dis. 52: 84–99, 1971.

2581. Kristersson, S., Arborelius, M. Jr., Jungqvist, G., Lilja, B., and Svanberg, L. Prediction of ventilatory capacity after lobectomy. Scand. J. Respir. Dis. 54: 315–325, 1973.

2582. Kristersson, S. Preoperative evaluation of differential lung function (^{133}Xe-radiospirometry) in bronchial cancer. In: Regional Lung Function and Closing Volume. Scand. J. Respir. Dis. 85(Suppl.): 110–117, 1974.

2583. Kristerrson, S., Arborelius, M. Jr., Lilja, B., Ohlsson, N. M., and Granqvist, U. Regional lung function in bronchial cancer. In: Regional Lung Function and Closing Volume. Scand. J. Respir. Dis. 85(Suppl.): 134–142, 1974.

2584. Rostad, H. and Vale, J. R. Lung cancer. Scand. J. Respir. Dis. 60: 191–196, 1979.

2585. Bake, B., Larsson, S., and Lofgren, L. Unilateral airway obstruction and distribution of pulmonary flow. Eur. J. Respir. Dis. 61: 46–49, 1980.

2586. Bake, B., Sixt, R., Sorensen, S., and Oxhoj, H. Regional lung function in small cell carcinoma of the lung. Eur. J. Respir. Dis. 61: 50–55, 1980.

2587. Lindell, L., Lindell, S-E., and Svanberg, L. Regional lung function in roentgenologically occult lung cancer. Scand. J. Respir. Dis. 53: 109–113, 1972.

2588. Lindell, S-E. ^{133}Xe-radiospirometry: prediction of lung function after pulmonary resection (editorial). Scand. J. Clin. Lab. Invest. 34: 289–292, 1974.

2589. Bradley, S. L., Dines, D. E., Soule, E. H., and Muhm, J. R. Pulmonary lymphangiomyomatosis. Lung 158: 69–80, 1980.

2590. Jezek, V., Ourednik, A., Lichtenberg, J., and Mostecky, H. Cardiopulmonary function in lung resection performed for bronchogenic cancer in patients above 65 years of age. Respiration 27: 42–50, 1970.

2591. Lopez-Majano, V. and Hooker, D. H. Pulmonary function and lung resection. Respiration 28: 555–568, 1971.

2592. Lockwood, P. Respiratory function and cardiopulmonary complications following thoracotomy for carcinoma of the lung. Respiration 29: 468–479, 1972.

2593. Lockwood, P. The principle of predicting the risk of post-thoracotomy function-related complications in bronchial carcinoma. Respiration 30: 329–344, 1973.

2594. Lockwood, P. Lung function test results and the risk of post-thoracotomy complications. Respiration 30: 529–542, 1973.

2595. Sergysels, R., Denaut, M., De Coster, A., Englert, M., and Yernault, J-C. Pulmonary function in metastatic carcinoma of the lung. Respiration 32: 355–362, 1975.

2596. Mlczoch, J., Zutter, W., Keller, R., and Herzog, H. Influence of lung resection on pulmonary circulation and lung function at rest and on exercise. Respiration 32: 424–435, 1975.

2597. Nicoli, M. M., Jammes, Y., Fornaris, E., Giacchero, G., and Coutant, P. Valeur de l'estimation par le ^{133}Xe des volumes pulmonaires après exercice. Respiration 37: 208–214, 1979.

2598. Laros, K. D. The postpneumonectomy mother. Respiration 39: 185–187, 1980.

2599. Lockwood, P. An improved risk prediction method in bronchial carcinoma surgery. Respiration 39: 166–171, 1980.

2600. Magnussen, H., Holle, J. P., Stiens, R., Mattern, H., Koischwitz, D., and Hartmann, V. Lung function studies in a patient with diffuse pulmonary fibroleiomyomas. Respiration 40: 241–249, 1980.

2601. Lockwood, P. and Westaby, S. Assessment of generalised airway obstruction in patients with carcinoma of the bronchus. Respiration 42: 252–257, 1981.

2602. Tisi, G. M. Preoperative evaluation of pulmonary function. Am. Rev. Respir. Dis. 119: 293–310, 1979.

2603. Veith, F. J., et al. Single lung transplantation in emphysema. Lancet ii: 1138–1139, 1972.

2604. Colman, N. C., Schraufnagel, D. E., Rivington, R. N., and Pardy, R. L. Exercise testing in evaluation of patients for lung resection. Am. Rev. Respir. Dis. 125: 604–606, 1982.

2605. Higenbottam, T., Cochrane, G. M., Clark, T. J. H., Turner, D., Millis, R., and Seymour, W. Bronchial disease in ulcerative colitis. Thorax 35: 581–585, 1980.

2606. Benusiglio, L. N., Stalder, H., and Junod, A. F. Time course of lung function changes in atypical pneumonia. Thorax 35: 586–592, 1980.

2607. Ben-Dov, I., Bar-Yishay, E., and Godfrey, S. Heterogeneity in the response of asthmatic patients to pre-exercise treatment with cromolyn sodium. Am. Rev. Respir. Dis. 127: 113–116, 1983.

2608. Gee, J. B. L. and Fick, R. B. Jr. Bronchoalveolar lavage (editorial). Thorax 35: 1–8, 1980.

2609. Justrabo, E., Genin, R., and Rifle, G. Pulmonary metastatic calcification with respiratory insufficiency in patients on maintenance haemodialysis. Thorax 34: 384–388, 1979.

2610. Sutton, P. P., Parker, R. A., Webber, B. A., Newman, S. P., Garland, N., Lopez-Vidriero, M. T., Pavia, D., and Clarke, S. W. Assessment of the forced expiration technique, postural drainage and directed coughing in chest physiotherapy. Eur. J. Respir. Dis. 64: 62–68, 1983.

2611. Horn, M. E. C., Brain, E. A., Gregg, I., Inglis, J. M., Yealland, S. J., and Taylor, P. Respiratory viral infection and wheezy bronchitis in childhood. Thorax 34: 23–28, 1979.

2612. Freedman, S. Lung volumes and distensibility, and maximum respiratory pressures in thyroid disease before and after treatment. Thorax 33: 785–790, 1978.

2613. Dukes, R. J., Rosenow, E. C. III, and Hermans, P. E.

Pulmonary manifestations of hypogammaglobulinaemia. Thorax 33: 603–607, 1978.

2614. Cormier, Y., Kashima, H., Summer, W., and Menkes, H. Airflow in unilateral vocal cord paralysis before and after Teflon injection. Thorax 33: 57–61, 1978.

2615. O'Byrne, P. M., Thomson, N. C., Morris, M., Roberts, R. S., Daniel, E. E., and Hargreave, F. E. The protective effect of inhaled chlorpheniramine and atropine on bronchoconstriction stimulated by airway cooling. Am. Rev. Respir. Dis. 128: 611–617, 1983.

2616. Stanley, N. N., Williams, A. J., Dewar, C. A., Blendis, L. M., and Reid, L. Hypoxia and hydrothoraces in a case of liver cirrhosis: correlation of physiological, radiographic, scintigraphic, and pathological findings. Thorax 32: 457–471, 1977.

2617. Evans, C. C., Hipkin, L. J., and Murray, G. M. Pulmonary function in acromegaly. Thorax 32: 322–327, 1977.

2618. Malo, J. L., Hawkins, R., and Pepys, J. Studies in chronic allergic bronchopulmonary aspergillosis. 1. Clinical and physiological findings. Thorax 32: 245–261, 1977.

2619. Malo, J. L., Pepys, J., and Simon, G. Studies in chronic allergic bronchopulmonary aspergillosis. 2. Radiological findings. Thorax 32: 262–268, 1977.

2620. Malo, J. L., Inouye, T., Hawkins, R., Simon, G., Turner-Warwick, M., and Pepys, J. Studies in chronic allergic bronchopulmonary aspergillosis. 4. Comparison with a group of asthmatics. Thorax 32: 275–280, 1977.

2621. Holt, S., Ryan, W. F., and Epstein, E. J. Severe mycoplasma pneumonia. Thorax 32: 112–115, 1977.

2622. Scadding, J. W. Fibrosing alveolitis with autoimmune haemolytic anaemia. Thorax 32: 134–139, 1977.

2623. Turner, J. A. McM. and Stanley, N. N. Fragile lung in the Marfan syndrome. Thorax 31: 771–775, 1976.

2624. Funahashi, A., Kutty, A. V. P., and Prater, S. L. Hypoxaemia and cirrhosis of the liver. Thorax 31: 303–308, 1976.

2625. Poh, S. C., Tjia, T. S., and Seah, H. C. Primary diffuse alveolar septal amyloidosis. Thorax 30: 186–191, 1975.

2626. Costello, J. F., Moriarty, D. C., Branthwaite, M. A., Turner-Warwick, M., and Corrin, B. Diagnosis and management of alveolar proteinosis: the role of electron microscopy. Thorax 30: 121–132, 1975.

2627. Lee, H. Y., Stretton, T. B., and Barnes, A. M. The lungs in renal failure. Thorax 30: 46–53, 1975.

2628. Roncoroni, A. J., Puy, R. J. M., Goldman, E., Fonseca, R., and Olmedo, G. Fibrosarcoma of the trachea with severe tracheal obstruction. Thorax 28: 777–781, 1973.

2629. Crosbie, W. A., Lewis, M. L., Ramsay, I. D., and Doyle, D. Pulmonary amyloidosis with impaired gas transfer. Thorax 27: 625–630, 1972.

2630. Stanley, N. N. and Woodgate, D. J. Mottled chest radiograph and gas transfer defect in chronic liver disease. Thorax 27: 315–323, 1972.

2631. Sears, M. R., Chang, A. R., and Taylor, A. J. Pulmonary alveolar microlithiasis. Thorax 26: 704–711, 1971.

2632. Miller, G. J. and Serjeant, G. R. An assessment of lung volumes and gas transfer in sickle-cell anaemia. Thorax 26: 309–315, 1971.

2633. Zundel, W. E. and Prior, A. P. An amyloid lung. Thorax 26: 357–363, 1971.

2634. Utell, M. J., Aquilina, A. T., Hall, W. J., Speers, D. M., Douglas, R. G., Gibb, F. R., Morrow, P. E., and Hyde, R. W. Development of airway reactivity to nitrates in subjects with influenza. Am. Rev. Respir. Dis. 121: 233–241, 1980.

2635. Miller, F. J., Illing, J. W., and Gardner, D. E. Effect of urban ozone levels on laboratory-induced respiratory infections. Toxicol. Lett. 2: 163–169, 1978.

2636. Kattan, M. M., Keens, T. G., Lapierre, J-G., Levison, H., Bryan, A. C., and Reilly, B. J. Pulmonary function abnormalities in symptom-free children after bronchiolitis. Pediatrics 59: 683–688, 1977.

2637. Collett, P. W., Brancatisano, T., and Engel, L. A. Changes in the glottic aperture during bronchial asthma. Am. Rev. Respir. Dis. 128: 719–723, 1983.

2638. Rubin, A. E. and Bruderman, I. Overdistension of lung due to peripheral airways obstruction. Chest 63: 948–951, 1973.

2639. Sackner, M. A. Physiologic features of upper airway obstruction. Chest 62: 414–417, 1972.

2640. O'Brien, T. G. and Sweeney, D. F. Interstitial viral pneumonitis complicated by severe respiratory failure. Chest 63: 314–322, 1973.

2641. Lamy, M. E., Pouthier-Simon, F., and Debacker-Willame, E. Respiratory viral infections in hospital patients with chronic bronchitis. Chest 63: 336–341, 1973.

2642. Lynne-Davies, P., Ganguli, P. C., and Sterns, L. P. Pulmonary function following traumatic rupture of the bronchus. Chest 61: 400–402, 1972.

2643. Stanescu, D. C., Teculescu, D. B., and Racoveanu, C. Lung function in acute pulmonary histoplasmosis. Chest 60: 105–107, 1971.

2644. Mezon, B. J., West, P., Maclean, J. P., and Kryger, M. H. Sleep apnoea in acromegaly. Am. J. Med. 69: 615–618, 1980.

2645. Webster, J. R., Battifora, H., Furey, C., Harrison, R. A., and Shapiro, B. Pulmonary alveolar proteinosis in two siblings with decreased immunoglobulin A. Am. J. Med. 69: 786–789, 1980.

2646. Rosenberg, D. M., Ferrans, V. J., Fulmer, J. D., Line, B. R., Barranger, J. A., Brady, R. O., and Crystal, R. G. Chronic airflow obstruction in Fabry's disease. Am. J. Med. 68: 898–905, 1980.

2647. Nicholls, D., DoPico, G. A., Braun, S., Imbeau, S., Peters, M. E., and Rankin, J. Acute and chronic pulmonary function changes in allergic bronchopulmonary aspergillosis. Am. J. Med. 67: 631–637, 1979.

2648. Kanada, D. J. and Sharma, O. P. Long-term survival with diffuse interstitial pulmonary amyloidosis. Am. J. Med. 67: 879–882, 1979.

2649. Deal, E. C. Jr., Kelsen, S. G., Eberlin, L. B., Salamone, J. A., and Cherniack, N. S. Respiratory effects of bronchoconstriction in anesthetized dogs. Am. Rev. Respir. Dis. 127: 310–315, 1983.

2650. Bombardieri, S., Paoletti, P., Ferri, C., Di Munno, O., Fornai, E., and Giuntini, C. Lung involvement in essential mixed cryoglobulinemia. Am. J. Med. 66: 748–756, 1979.

2651. Rodenstein, D. O., Francis, C., and Stanescu, D. C. Emotional laryngeal wheezing: a new syndrome. Am. Rev. Respir. Dis. 127: 354–356, 1983.

2652. Jay, S. J. Pulmonary alveolar proteinosis. Am. J. Med. 66: 348–354, 1979.

2653. Winberg, C. D., Rose, M. E., and Rappaport, H. Whipple's disease of the lung. Am. J. Med. 65: 873–880, 1978.

2654. Bone, R. C., Henry, J. E., Petterson, J., and Amare, M. Respiratory dysfunction in thrombotic thrombocytopenic purpura. Am. J. Med. 65: 262–270, 1978.

2655. Arnett, E. N., Bacos, J. M., Macher, A. M., Marsh, H. B., Savage, D. D., Fulmer, J. D., and Roberts, W. C. Fibrosing mediastinitis causing pulmonary arterial hypertension without pulmonary venous hypertension. Am. J. Med. 63: 634–643, 1977.

2656. Weisenburger, D., Armitage, J., and Dick, F. Immunoblastic lymphadenopathy with pulmonary infiltrates, hypocomplementemia and vasculitis. Am. J. Med. 63: 849–854, 1977.

2657. Schneider, E. L., Epstein, C. J., Kaback, M. J., and Brandes, D. Severe pulmonary involvement in adult Gaucher's disease. Am. J. Med. 63: 475–480, 1977.

2658. Heinemann, H. O. Alcohol and the lung. Am. J. Med. 63: 81–85, 1977.

2659. Pennington, J. E. and Feldman, N. T. Pulmonary infiltrates and fever in patients with hematologic malignancy. Am. J. Med. 62: 581–587, 1977.

2660. Kryger, M., Bode, F., Antic, R., and Anthonisen, N. Diagnosis of obstruction of the upper and central airways. Am. J. Med. 61: 85–93, 1976.

2661. Ferstenfeld, J. E., Schlueter, D. P., Rytel, M. W., and Molloy, R. P. Recognition and treatment of adult respiratory distress syndrome secondary to viral interstitial pneumonia. Am. J. Med. 58: 709–718, 1975.

2662. Emirgil, C., Sobol, B. J., Heymann, B., Shibutani, K., Reed, A., Varble, A., and Waldie, J. Pulmonary function in alcoholics. Am. J. Med. 57: 69–77, 1974.

2663. Zidulka, A., Despas, P. J., Milic-Emili, J., and Anthonisen, N. R. Pulmonary function with acute loss of excess lung water by hemodialysis in patients with chronic uremia. Am. J. Med. 55: 134–141, 1973.

2664. Rabiner, S. F., Aprill, S. N., and Radner, D. B. Waldenstrom's macroglobulinemia. Am. J. Med. 53: 685–689, 1972.

2665. Oliva, P. B. Severe alveolar hypoventilation in a patient with metabolic alkalosis. Am. J. Med. 52: 817–821, 1972.

2666. Picken, J. J., Niewohner, D. E., and Chester, E. H. Prolonged effects of viral infections of the upper respiratory tract upon small airways. Am. J. Med. 52: 738–746, 1972.

2667. Tuller, M. A. and Mehdi, F. Compensatory hypoventilation and hypercapnia in primary metabolic alkalosis. Am. J. Med. 50: 281–290, 1971.

2668. Lemle, A., Vieira, L. O. B. D., Milward, G. A. F., and Miranda, J. L. Lung function studies in pulmonary South American blastomycosis. Am. J. Med. 48: 434–442, 1970.

2669. Gonzalez-Cueto, D. M., Rigoli, M., Gioseffi, L. M., Lancelle, B., and Martinez, A. Diffuse pulmonary amyloidosis. Am. J. Med. 48: 668–670, 1970.

2670. Murphy, D., Pack, A., and Imrie, C. W. The mechanism of arterial hypoxia occurring in acute pancreatitis. Q. J. Med. 49: 151–163, 1980.

2671. De Troyer, A., Desir, D., and Copinschi, G. Regression of lung size in adults with growth hormone deficiency. Q. J. Med. 49: 329–340, 1980.

2672. Harrison, B. D. W., Millhouse, K. A., Harrington, M., and Nabarro, J. D. N. Lung function in acromegaly. Q. J. Med. 47: 517–532, 1978.

2673. Harrison, B. D. W. Upper airway obstruction—a report on sixteen patients. Q. J. Med. 45: 625–645, 1976.

2674. Dwyer, J. M., Hickie, J. B., and Garvan, J. Pulmonary tuberous sclerosis. Q. J. Med. 40: 115–125, 1971.

2675. Young, R. H., Sandstrom, R. E., and Mark, G. J. Tracheopathia osteoplastica. J. Thorac. Cardiovasc. Surg. 79: 537–541, 1980.

2676. Nagakura, T., Lee, T. H., Assoufi, B. K., Newman-Taylor, A. J., Denison, D. M., and Kay, A. B. Neutrophil chemotactic factor in exercise- and hyperventilation-induced asthma. Am. Rev. Respir. Dis. 128: 294–296, 1983.

2677. Moran, J. F., Jones, R. H., and Wolfe, W. G. Regional pulmonary function during experimental unilateral pneumothorax in the awake state. J. Thorac. Cardiovasc. Surg. 74: 396–402, 1977.

2678. Finucane, K. E., Colebatch, H. J. H., Robertson, M. R., and Gandevia, B. H. The mechanism of respiratory failure in a patient with viral (varicella) pneumonia. Am. Rev. Respir. Dis. 101: 949–958, 1970.

2679. Dutt, A. K. Diaphragmatic paralysis caused by herpes zoster. Am. Rev. Respir. Dis. 101: 755–758, 1970.

2680. Smith, L. J., Ankin, M. G., Katzenstein, A-L., and Shapiro, B. A. Management of pulmonary alveolar proteinosis. Chest 78: 765–770, 1980.

2681. Tenholder, M. F. and Hooper, R. G. Pulmonary infiltrates in leukemia. Chest 78: 468–473, 1980.

2682. Kariman, K., Shelburne, J. D., Gough, W., Zacheck, M. J., and Blackmon, J. A. Pathologic findings and long-term sequelae in Legionnaires' disease. Chest 75: 736–739, 1979.

2683. Cormier, Y., Kashima, H., Summer, W., and Menkes, H. Upper airways obstruction with bilateral vocal cord paralysis. Chest 75: 423–427, 1979.

2684. Prakash, U. B. S., Divertie, M. B., and Banks, P. M. Aggressive therapy in acute respiratory failure from leukemic pulmonary infiltrates. Chest 75: 345–350, 1979.

2685. Sopko, J. A. and Bedell, G. N. A severe, stable obstructive defect in the airways in primary pulmonary histiocytosis X. Chest 75: 205–207, 1979.

2686. Peavy, H. H., Summer, W. R., and Gurtner, G. The effects of acute ethanol ingestion on pulmonary diffusing capacity. Chest 77: 488–492, 1980.

2687. Grant, J. L., Naylor, R. W., and Crandell, W. B. Bronchial adenoma resection with relief of hypoxic pulmonary vasoconstriction. Chest 77: 446–449, 1980.

2688. Vraney, G. A. and Pokorny, C. Pulmonary function in patients with gastroesophageal reflux. Chest 76: 678–680, 1979.

2689. Hall, W. J. and Hall, C. B. Alterations in pulmonary function following respiratory viral infection. Chest 76: 458–465, 1979.

2690. Matthews, J. I. and Hooper, R. G. Idiopathic bronchial stenosis in a young woman. Chest 74: 690–691, 1978.

2691. Davis, H. H., Schwartz, D. J., Lefrak, S. S., Susman, N., and Schainker, B. A. Alveolar-capillary oxygen disequilibrium in hepatic cirrhosis. Chest 73: 507–511, 1978.

2692. De Troyer, A., Naeije, R., Yernault, J-C., and Englert, M. Impairment of pulmonary function in acute pancreatitis. Chest 73: 360–363, 1978.

2693. Murray, H. W., Tuazon, C. U., Kirmani, N., and Sheagren, J. N. The adult respiratory distress syndrome associated with miliary tuberculosis. Chest 73: 37–43, 1978.

2694. Emirgil, C. and Sobol, B. J. Pulmonary function in former alcoholics. Chest 72: 45–51, 1977.

2695. Lewinsohn, G., Bruderman, I., and Bohadana, A. Primary diffuse pulmonary amyloidosis with monoclonal gammopathy. Chest 69: 682–685, 1976.

2696. Rotman, H. H., Liss, H. P., and Weg, J. G. Diagnosis of upper airway obstruction by pulmonary function testing. Chest 68: 796–799, 1975.

2697. Myers, B. D., Rubin, A-H. E., Schey, G., Bruderman, I., Pokroy, N. R., and Levi, J. Functional characteristics of the lung in chronic uraemia treated by renal dialysis therapy. Chest 68: 191–194, 1975.

2698. Bischel, M. D., Scoles, B. G., and Mohler, J. G. Evidence for pulmonary microembolization during hemodialysis. Chest 67: 335–337, 1975.

2699. Homan, W., Harman, E., Braun, N. M. T., Felton, C. P., King, T. K. C., and Smith, J. P. Miliary tuberculosis presenting as acute respiratory failure: treatment by membrane oxygenator and ventricle pump. Chest 67: 366–369, 1975.

2700. Winterbauer, R. H., Riggins, R. C. K., Griesman, F. A., and Bauermeister, D. E. Pleuropulmonary manifestations of Waldenstrom's macroglobulinemia. Chest 66: 368–375, 1974.

2701. Wynne, J. W. and Olsen, G. N. Acute histoplasmosis presenting as the adult respiratory distress syndrome. Chest 66: 158–161, 1974.

2702. Latimer, K. M., O'Byrne, P. M., Morris, M. M., Roberts, R., and Hargreave, F. E. Bronchoconstriction stimulated by airway cooling. Am. Rev. Respir. Dis. 128: 440–443, 1983.

2703. Boushy, S. F. and North, L. B. Pulmonary function in infiltrative lung disease. Chest 64: 448–453, 1973.

2704. Toppell, K. L., Atkinson, R., and Whitcomb, M. E. Lung growth in acromegaly. Am. Rev. Respir. Dis. 108: 1254–1258, 1973.

2705. Yernault, J. C., Englert, M., Sergysels, R., and De Coster, A. Upper airway stenosis: a physiologic study. Am. Rev. Respir. Dis. 108: 996–1000, 1973.

2706. Banner, A. S. Pulmonary function in chronic alcoholism. Am. Rev. Respir. Dis. 108: 851–857, 1973.

2707. Cate, T. R., Roberts, J. S., Russ, M. A., and Pierce, J. A. Effects of common colds on pulmonary function. Am. Rev. Respir. Dis. 108: 858–865, 1973.

2708. Horner, G. J. and Gray, F. D. Jr. Effect of uncomplicated, presumptive influenza on the diffusing capacity of the lung. Am. Rev. Respir. Dis. 108: 866–869, 1973.

2709. Miller, R. D. and Hyatt, R. E. Evaluation of obstructing lesions of the trachea and larynx by flow-volume loops. Am. Rev. Respir. Dis. 108: 475–481, 1973.

2710. Riker, J. B. and Wolinsky, H. Trypsin aerosol treatment of pulmonary alveolar proteinosis. Am. Rev. Respir. Dis. 108: 108–113, 1973.

2711. Zack, M. B. and Kazemi, H. Carbon dioxide retention in mycoplasma pneumonia. Am. Rev. Respir. Dis. 107: 1052–1054, 1973.

2712. Hirsch, M. S. and Hong, C-K. Familial pulmonary histiocytosis-X. Am. Rev. Respir. Dis. 107: 831–835, 1973.

2713. Shear, L. and Brandman, I. S. Hypoxia and hypercapnia caused by respiratory compensation for metabolic acidosis. Am. Rev. Respir. Dis. 107: 836–841, 1973.

2714. Domm, B. M. and Vassallo, C. L. Myxedema coma with respiratory failure. Am. Rev. Respir. Dis. 107: 842–845, 1973.

2715. Roncoroni, A. J., Puy, R. J. M., Goldman, E., Paz, R. R. A., and Fonseca, R. Severe tracheal stenosis by cartilaginous ring dislocation. Am. Rev. Respir. Dis. 107: 274–279, 1973.

2716. Jones, J. S. R., Renzetti, A. D. Jr., and Mitchell, M. M. The maximal breathing capacity in extrathoracic airway obstruction. Am. Rev. Respir. Dis. 106: 925–927, 1972.

2717. Konietzko, N., Schlehe, H., Ruhle, K. H., Overrath, G., Bitter, F., Adam, W. E., and Matthys, H. Regional lung function in different body positions in patients with pulmonary tuberculosis. Am. Rev. Respir. Dis. 106: 548–555, 1972.

2718. Shim, C., Corro, P., Park, S. S., and Williams, M. H. Jr. Pulmonary function studies in patients with upper airway obstruction. Am. Rev. Respir. Dis. 106: 233–238, 1972.

2719. Tong, M. J., Ballantine, T. V. N., and Youel, D. B. Pulmonary function studies in *Plasmodium falciparum* malaria. Am. Rev. Respir. Dis. 106: 23–29, 1972.

2720. Kino, T., Kohara, Y., and Tsun, S. Pulmonary alveolar microlithiasis. Am. Rev. Respir. Dis. 105: 105–110, 1972.

2721. Brashear, R. E., Martin, R. R., and Glover, J. L. Trichinosis and respiratory failure. Am. Rev. Respir. Dis. 104: 245–248, 1971.

2722. Oppenheimer, E. H. and Esterly, J. R. Pulmonary changes in sickle cell disease. Am. Rev. Respir. Dis. 103: 858–859, 1971.

2723. Ramirez-R, J. Alveolar proteinosis: importance of pulmonary lavage. Am. Rev. Respir. Dis. 103: 666–678, 1971.

2724. Zwillich, C. W., Pierson, D. J., Hofeldt, F. D., Lufkin, E. G., and Weil, J. V. Ventilatory control in myxedema and hypothyroidism. N. Engl. J. Med. 292: 662–665, 1975.

2725. Case records of the Massachusetts General Hospital. Case 6-1974. N. Engl. J. Med. 290: 390–396, 1974.

2726. Aberman, A. and Hew, E. Lactic acidosis presenting as acute respiratory failure. Am. Rev. Respir. Dis. 118: 961–963, 1978.

2727. Rubinow, A., Celli, B. R., Cohen, A. S., Rigden, B. G., and Brody, J. S. Localized amyloidosis of the lower respiratory tract. Am. Rev. Respir. Dis. 118: 603–611, 1978.

2728. Little, J. W., Hall, W. J., Douglas, R. G. Jr., Mudholkar, G. S., Speers, D. M., and Patel, K. Airway hyperreactivity and peripheral airway dysfunction in influenza A infection. Am. Rev. Respir. Dis. 118: 295–303, 1978.

2729. Geppert, E. F. and Boushey, H. A. An investigation of the mechanism of ethanol-induced bronchoconstriction. Am. Rev. Respir. Dis. 118: 135–139, 1978.

2730. Martin, R. J., Rogers, R. M., and Myers, N. M. Pulmonary alveolar proteinosis. Am. Rev. Respir. Dis. 117: 1059–1062, 1978.

2731. Lavelle, T. F. Jr., Rotman, H. H., and Weg, J. G. Isoflow-volume curves in the diagnosis of upper airway obstruction. Am. Rev. Respir. Dis. 117: 845–852, 1978.

2732. Schuyler, M. and Niewohner, D. E. Elasticity in juvenile-onset diabetes (letter to editor). Am. Rev. Respir. Dis. 117: 811, 1978.

2733. Scharf, S. M., Feldman, N. T., Goldman, M. D., Haut, H. Z., Bruce, E., and Ingram, R. H. Jr. Vocal cord closure. Am. Rev. Respir. Dis. 117: 391–397, 1978.

2734. Stokes, D., Sigler, A., Khouri, N. F., and Talamo, R. C. Unilateral hyperlucent lung (Swyer-James syndrome) after severe *Mycoplasma pneumoniae* infection. Am. Rev. Respir. Dis. 117: 145–152, 1978.

2735. Collier, A. M., Pimmel, R. L., Hasselblad, V., Clyde, W. A. Jr., Knelson, J. H., and Brooks, J. G. Spirometric changes in normal children with upper respiratory infections. Am. Rev. Respir. Dis. 117: 47–53, 1978.

2736. Daoud, F. S., Reeves, J. T., and Schaefer, J. W. Failure of hypoxic pulmonary vasoconstriction in patients with liver cirrhosis. J. Clin. Invest. 51: 1076–1080, 1972.

2737. Laraya-Cuasay, L. R., DeForest, A., Huff, D., Lischner, H., and Huang, N. N. Chronic pulmonary complications of early influenza virus infection in children. Am. Rev. Respir. Dis. 116: 617–625, 1977.

2738. Schernthaner, G., Haber, P., Kummer, F., and Ludwig, H. Lung elasticity in juvenile-onset diabetes mellitus. Am. Rev. Respir. Dis. 116: 544–546, 1977.

2739. Anthonisen, N. R. and Martin, R. R. Regional lung function in pleural effusion. Am. Rev. Respir. Dis. 116: 201–207, 1977.

2740. Anthonisen, N. R. Regional lung function in spontaneous pneumothorax. Am. Rev. Respir. Dis. 115: 873–876, 1977.

2741. Burrows, B., Knudson, R. J., and Lebowitz, M. D. The relationship of childhood respiratory illness to adult obstructive airway disease. Am. Rev. Respir. Dis. 115: 751–760, 1977.

2742. Proctor, D. F. The upper airways. II. The larynx and trachea. Am. Rev. Respir. Dis. 115: 315–342, 1977.

2743. Bergeron, D., Cormier, Y., and Desmeules, M. Tracheo-bronchopathia osteochondroplastica. Am. Rev. Respir. Dis. 114: 803–806, 1976.

2744. Blair, H. T., Greenberg, S. B., Stevens, P. M., Bilunds, P. A., and Couch, R. B. Effects of rhinovirus infection on pulmonary function of healthy human volunteers. Am. Rev. Respir. Dis. 114: 95–102, 1976.

2745. Brown, R. and Wellman, J. J. Abnormal lung elasticity in juvenile diabetes mellitus (letter to editor). Am. Rev. Respir. Dis. 113: 894, 1976.

2746. Gump, D. W., Phillips, C. A., Forsyth, B. R., McIntosh, K., Lamborn, K. R., and Stouch, W. H. Role of infection in chronic bronchitis. Am. Rev. Respir. Dis. 113: 465–474, 1976.

2747. Ahn, C. H., Nash, D. R., and Hurst, G. A. Ventilatory defects in atypical mycobacteriosis. Am. Rev. Respir. Dis. 113: 273–279, 1976.

2748. Empey, D. W., Laitman, L. A., Jacobs, L., Gold, W. M., and Nadel, J. A. Mechanisms of bronchial hyperreactivity in normal subjects after upper respiratory tract infection. Am. Rev. Respir. Dis. 113: 131–139, 1976.

2749. Hall, W. J., Douglas, R. G. Jr., Hyde, R. W., Roth, F. K., Cross, A. S., and Speers, D. M. Pulmonary mechanics after uncomplicated influenza infection. Am. Rev. Respir. Dis. 113: 141–147, 1976.

2750. Martin, J. G., Shore, S. A., and Engel, L. A. Mechanical load and inspiratory muscle action during induced asthma. Am. Rev. Respir. Dis. 128: 455–460, 1983.

2751. Schuyler, M. R., Niewohner, D. E., Inkley, S. R., and Kohn, R. Abnormal lung elasticity in juvenile diabetes mellitus. Am. Rev. Respir. Dis. 113: 37–41, 1976.

2752. Al-Bazzaz, F., Grillo, H., and Kazemi, H. Response to exercise in upper airway obstruction. Am. Rev. Respir. Dis. 111: 631–640, 1975.

2753. Rosenzweig, D. Y., Dwyer, D. J., Ferstenfeld, J. E., and Rytel, M. W. Changes in small airway function after live attenuated influenza vaccination. Am. Rev. Respir. Dis. 111: 399–403, 1975.

2754. Hebbel, R. P., Kronenberg, R. S., and Eaton, J. W. Hypoxic ventilatory response in subjects with normal and high oxygen affinity hemoglobins. J. Clin. Invest. 60: 1211–1215, 1977.

2755. Hilty-Tammivaara, R. Respiratory function after spontaneous pneumothorax in relation to treatment. Scand. J. Respir. Dis. 51: 105–117, 1970.

2756. Korhonen, O. Overall and regional lung function during bronchopneumonia. Scand. J. Respir. Dis. 53: 280–288, 1972.

2757. Berglund, S. and Arborelius, M. Jr. Lung function and haemodynamics in patients with familial lung changes and haemoglobin Malmo. Scand. J. Respir. Dis. 53: 321–330, 1972.

2758. Reggiani, A., Crepaldi, G., Enzi, G., and Avogardo, P. Comportement du transfert du CO dans les hyperlipemies essentielles. In: Sadonl, P. (ed.). Le Transfert de l'Oxyde de Carbone. Soc. Eur. Physiopathol. Respir. Masson et Cie, Paris, 1969.

2759. Skoogh, B-E. Lung mechanics in pulmonary tuberculosis. II. Airways conductance at different lung volumes. Scand. J. Respir. Dis. 54: 369–378, 1973.

2760. Skoogh, B-E. Lung mechanics in pulmonary tuberculosis. III. Bronchial reactivity. Scand. J. Respir. Dis. 54: 379–387, 1973.

2761. Roncoroni, A. J., Goldman, E., and Puy, R. J. M. Respiratory mechanics in upper airway obstruction. Bull. Physiopathol. Respir. 11: 803–822, 1975.

2762. Bobrowitz, I. D., Rodescu, D., Marcus, H., and Abeles, H. The destroyed tuberculous lung. Scand. J. Respir. Dis. 55: 82–88, 1974.

2763. Schaanning, J. and Sparr, S. Bloodletting and exchange transfusion with dextran 40 in polycythemia secondary to chronic obstructive lung disease. Scand. J. Respir. Dis. 55: 237–244, 1974.

2764. Anthonisen, N. R., Engel, L., Grassino, A., Zidulka, A., Bode, F., Dosman, J., Martin, R. R., and Macklem, P. T. The clinical significance of measurements of closing volume. In: Regional Lung Function and Closing Volume. Scand. J. Respir. Dis. 85(Suppl.): 245–250, 1974.

2765. Danon, G. La fonction respiratoire de sujets drépanocytaires. Bull. Eur. Physiopathol. Respir. 12: 333–348, 1976.

2766. Enzi, G., Bevilacqua, M., and Crepaldi, G. Disturbances in pulmonary gaseous exchange in primary hyperlipoproteinemias. Bull. Eur. Physiopathol. Respir. 12: 433–442, 1976.

2767. Jakab, G. J. Pulmonary defense mechanisms and the interaction between viruses and bacteria in acute respiratory infections. Bull. Eur. Physiopathol. Respir. 13: 119–135, 1977.

2768. Huber, G. L., Pochay, V. E., Mahajan, V. K., McCarthy, C. R., Hinds, W. C., Davies, P., Drath, D. B., and Sornberger, G. C. The effect of chronic exposure to tobacco smoke on the antibacterial defenses of the lung. Bull. Eur. Physiopathol. Respir. 13: 145–156, 1977.

2769. De Troyer, A., Yernault, J-C., Rodenstein, D., Englert, M., and De Coster, A. Pulmonary function in patients with spontaneous pneumothorax. Bull. Eur. Physiopathol. Respir. 14: 31–39, 1978.

2770. Prefaut, Ch., Monteil, A. L., Ramonatxo, M., Slingeneyer, A., Chardon, G., and Mirouze, J. Closing volume and pulmonary gas exchange during peritoneal dialysis. Bull. Eur. Physiopathol. Respir. 14: 755–764, 1978.

2771. Tukainen, P., Poppius, H., and Taskinen, E. Slowly progressive bronchiolitis obliterans. Eur. J. Respir. Dis. 61: 77–83, 1980.

2772. Laitinen, L. A. and Kava, T. Bronchial reactivity following uncomplicated influenza A infection in healthy subjects and in asthmatic patients. In: Proceedings of a meeting on bronchial hyperreactivity syndrome. Eur. J. Respir. Dis. 61(Suppl. 106): 51–58, 1980.

2773. Verdon, F., Van Melle, G., and Perret, C. Respiratory response to acute metabolic acidosis. Bull. Eur. Physiopathol. Respir. 17: 223–235, 1981.

2774. Trenchard, D., Gardner, D., and Guz, A. Role of pulmonary vagal afferent nerve fibres in the development of rapid shallow breathing in lung inflammation. Clin. Sci. 42: 251–263, 1972.

2775. Ramsey, J. M. Carbon monoxide, tissue hypoxia, and sensory psychomotor response in hypoxemic subjects. Clin. Sci. 42: 619–625, 1972.

2776. Miller, G. J., Serjeant, G. R., Sivapragasam, S., and Petch, M. C. Cardio-pulmonary responses and gas exchange during exercise in adults with homozygous sickle-cell disease (sickle-cell anaemia). Clin. Sci. 44: 113–128, 1973.

2777. Harrison, B. D. W. Polycythemia in a selected group of patients with chronic airways obstruction. Clin. Sci. 44: 563–570, 1973.

2778. Van Ypersale De Strihou, C. and Frans, A. The respiratory response to chronic metabolic alkalosis and acidosis in disease. Clin. Sci. 45: 439–448, 1973.

2779. Sahn, S. A., Lakshminarayan, S., Pierson, D. J., and Weil, J. V. Effect of ethanol on the ventilatory responses to oxygen and carbon dioxide in man. Clin. Sci. 49: 33–38, 1975.

2780. Stanescu, D. C., Veriter, C., De Plaen, J. F., Frans, A., Van Ypersele De Strihou, C., and Brasseur, L. Lung function in chronic uraemia before and after removal of excess of fluid by haemodialysis. Clin. Sci. 47: 143–151, 1974.

2781. Stanley, N. N., Salisbury, B. G., McHenry, L. C. Jr., and Cherniack, N. S. Effect of liver failure on the response to ventilation and cerebral circulation to carbon dioxide in man and in the goat. Clin. Sci. 49: 157–169, 1975.

2782. Stanley, N. N., Kelsen, S. G., and Cherniack, N. S. Effect of liver failure on the ventilatory response to hypoxia in man and the goat. Clin. Sci. 50: 25–35, 1976.

2783. Metz, G., Gassull, M. A., Leeds, A. R., Blendis, L. M., and Jenkins, D. J. A. A simple method of measuring breath hydrogen in carbohydrate malabsorption by end-expiratory sampling. Clin. Sci. 50: 237–240, 1976.

2784. Stockley, R. A. and Bishop, J. M. Effect of thyrotoxicosis on the reflex hypoxic respiratory drive. Clin. Sci. 53: 93–100, 1977.

2785. Payne, J., Higenbottam, T., and Guindi, G. Respiratory activity of the vocal cords in normal subjects and patients with airflow obstruction: an electromyographic study. Clin. Sci. 61: 163–167, 1981.

2786. Sanyal, S. K., Mariencheck, W. C., Hughes, W. T., Parvey, L. S., Tsiatis, A. A., and Mackert, P. Course of pulmonary dysfunction in children surviving *Pneumocystis carinii* pneumonitis. Am. Rev. Respir. Dis. 124: 161–166, 1981.

2787. Skatrud, J., Iber, C., Ewart, R., Thomas, G., Rasmussen, H., and Schultze, B. Disordered breathing during sleep in hypothyroidism. Am. Rev. Respir. Dis. 124: 325–329, 1981.

2788. Juhl, B. Pulmonary function investigations on 1011 school children using Wright's peak flow meter. Scand. J. Clin. Lab. Invest. 25: 355–361, 1970.

2789. Lebowitz, M. D. Respiratory symptoms and disease related to alcohol consumption. Am. Rev. Respir. Dis. 123: 16–19, 1981.

2790. Kardel, T. and Rasmussen, S. N. Blood gases and acid-base disturbances of arterial blood in chronic liver disease. Scand. J. Clin. Lab. Invest. 31: 307–309, 1973.

2791. Lee, B. C., Malik, A. B., Barie, P. S., and Minnear, F. L. Effect of acute pancreatitis on pulmonary transvascular fluid and protein exchange. Am. Rev. Respir. Dis. 123: 618–621, 1981.

2792. Aquilina, A. T., Hall, W. J., Douglas, R. G. Jr., and Utell, M. J. Airway reactivity in subjects with viral upper respiratory tract infections: the effects of exercise and cold air. Am. Rev. Respir. Dis. 122: 3–10, 1980.

2793. Gurwitz, D., Corey, M., and Levison, H. Pulmonary function and bronchial reactivity in children after croup. Am. Rev. Respir. Dis. 122: 95–99, 1980.

2794. Burrows, B. and Taussig, L. M. "As the twig is bent, the tree inclines" (perhaps) (editorial). Am. Rev. Respir. Dis. 122: 813–816, 1980.

2795. Michel, F. B., Rousset, G., Grolleau-Raoux, R., Michel, H., Baldet, P., and Vidal, J. Courts-circuits arterio-veineux pulmonaires et cirrhose hepatique. Poumon Coeur 29: 57–65, 1973.

2796. Cormier, Y. F., Camus, P., and Desmeules, M. J. Non-organic acute upper airway obstruction. Am. Rev. Respir. Dis. 121: 147–150, 1980.

2797. Cohen, B. H., Celentano, D. D., Chase, G. A., Diamond, E. L., Ghraves, C. G., Levy, D. A., Menkes, H. A., Meyer, M. B., Permutt, S., and Tockman, M. S. Alcohol consumption and airway obstruction. Am. Rev. Respir. Dis. 121: 205–215, 1980.

2798. Luboshitzky, R. and Barzilai, D. Hypoxemia and pulmonary function in acromegaly. Am. Rev. Respir. Dis. 121: 471–475, 1980.

2799. Gacovin, J. C., Baviera, E., Murat, J. A. G., and Genevrier, R. Amylose pulmonaire diffuse au cours d'une macroglobulinemie de Waldenstrom. Poumon Coeur 30: 403–407, 1974.

2800. Lopez-Majano, V. and Joshi, R. Ch. Indications for decortication. Respiration 27: 565–581, 1970.

2801. Gamsu, G., Borson, D. B., Webb, W. R., and Cunningham, J. H. Structure and function in tracheal stenosis. Am. Rev. Respir. Dis. 121: 519–531, 1980.

2802. Cooper, D. M., Mansell, A. L., Weiner, M. A., Berdon, W. E., Chetty-Baktaviziam, A., Reid, L., and Mellins, R. B. Low lung capacity and hypoxemia in children with thalassemia major. Am. Rev. Respir. Dis. 121: 639–646, 1980.

2803. Petitjean, R., Bierry, J-P., and Burghard, G. Microlithiase alveolaire. Poumon Coeur 31: 145–148, 1975.

2804. Moneger, P. and Oury, M. Evaluation du retentissement fonctionnel des sequelles de la tuberculose pulmonaire. Poumon Coeur 32: 227–232, 1976.

2805. Pasquis, P., Denis, P., Nouvet, G., and Lefrancois, R. Perturbations de la fonction respiratoire après pneumothorax idiopathique. Poumon Coeur 34: 331–333, 1978.

2806. Kaplan, A. I. and Laguarda, R. Cirrhosis of the liver—an unusual cause of severe hypoxemia. Respiration 29: 180–190, 1972.

2807. Lopez-Majano, V. and Dutton, R. E. Factors influencing the diffusing capacity of each lung. Respiration 29: 427–436, 1972.

2808. Zach, M. S., Schnall, R. P., and Landau, L. I. Upper and lower airway hyperreactivity in recurrent croup. Am. Rev. Respir. Dis. 121: 979–983, 1980.

2809. Lopez-Majano, V. Ventilation and transfer of gases in pulmonary tuberculosis. Respiration 30: 48–63, 1973.

2810. Kurgan, J. and Smigla, K. Pulmonary alveolar proteinosis. Respiration 31: 278–286, 1974.

2811. Schomerus, H., Buchta, I., and Arndt, H. Pulmonary function studies and oxygen transfer in patients with liver cirrhosis

and different degrees of portasystemic encephalopathy. Respiration 32: 1–20, 1975.

2812. Arndt, A., Buchta, I., and Schomerus, H. Analysis of factors determining the resistance to diffusion in patients with liver cirrhosis. Respiration 32: 21–31, 1975.

2813. Senyk, J., Arborelius, M. Jr., Lilja, B., and Ohlsson, N-M. Respiratory function in esophageal hiatus hernia. Respiration 32: 93–102, 1975.

2814. Senyk, J., Arborelius, M. Jr., and Lilja, B. Respiratory function in esophageal hiatus hernia. Respiration 32: 103–111, 1975.

2815. Vijaylaxmi, N., Pande, J. N., Gupta, S. P., and Guleria, J. S. Peripheral chemoreceptor insensitivity in chronic severe anemia. Respiration 35: 37–39, 1978.

2816. Boule, M., Gaultier, C., Tournier, G., Allaire, Y., and Girard, F. Lung function in children with recurrent bronchitis. Respiration 38: 127–134, 1979.

2817. Sybrecht, G. W., Koch, G., Tepe, J., and Fabel, H. Lungenfunktion, Gasaustausch und Atem-Regulation bei Patienten mit portokavaler Enzephalopathie. Respiration 39: 307–317, 1980.

2818. Forman, J. W., Ayers, L. N., and Miller, W. C. Pulmonary diffusing capacity in chronic renal disease. Br. J. Dis. Chest. 75: 81–87, 1981.

2819. Simpson, H., Matthew, D. J., Inglis, J. M., and George, E. L. Virological findings and blood gas tensions in acute lower respiratory tract infections in children. Br. Med. J. 2: 629–632, 1974.

2820. Perks, W. H., Horrocks, P. M., Cooper, R. A., Bradbury, S., Allen, A., Baldock, N., Prowse, K., and van't Hoff, W. Sleep apnoea in acromegaly. Br. Med. J. 2: 894–897, 1980.

2821. Pullan, C. R. and Hey, E. N. Wheezing, asthma, and pulmonary dysfunction 10 years after infection with respiratory syncytial virus in infancy. Br. Med. J. 284: 1665–1669, 1982.

2822. Mok, J. Y. Q. and Simpson, H. Outcome of lower respiratory tract infection in infants: preliminary report of seven-year follow-up study. Br. Med. J. 285: 333–337, 1982.

2823. Sims, D. G., Gardner, P. S., Weightman, D., Turner, M. W., and Soothill, J. F. Atopy does not predispose to RSV bronchiolitis or postbronchiolitic wheezing. Br. Med. J. 282: 2086–2088, 1981.

2824. Payne, J., Higenbottam, T., and Guindi, G. Respiratory activity of the vocal cords in normal subjects and patients with airflow obstruction: an electromyographic study. Clin. Sci. 61: 163–167, 1981.

2825. Fridy, W. W., Ingram, R. H. Jr., Hierholzer, J. C., and Coleman, M. T. Airways function during mild viral respiratory illnesses. Ann. Intern. Med. 80: 150–155, 1974.

2826. Cohen, A. A., Stevens, P. M., Greenberg, S. D., and Lemole, G. M. Massive unilateral pulmonary fibrosis. Ann. Intern. Med. 72: 537–542, 1970.

2827. Davidson, F. F. and Glazier, J. B. Unilateral pleuritis and regional lung function. Ann. Intern. Med. 77: 37–42, 1972.

2828. Interiano, B., Stuard, I. D., and Hyde, R. W. Acute respiratory distress syndrome in pancreatitis. Ann. Intern. Med. 77: 923–926, 1972.

2829. Lifschitz, M. D., Brasch, R., Cuomo, A. J., and Menn, S. J. Marked hypercapnia secondary to severe metabolic alkalosis. Ann. Intern. Med. 77: 405–409, 1972.

2830. Conger, J. D., Hammond, W. S., Alfrey, A. C., Contiguglia, S. R., Stanford, R. E., and Huffer, W. E. Pulmonary calcification in chronic dialysis patients. Ann. Intern. Med. 83: 330–336, 1975.

2831. Sagone, A. L. Jr. and Balcerzak, S. P. Smoking as a cause of erythrocytosis. Ann. Intern. Med. 82: 512–515, 1975.

2832. Huseby, J. S. and Hudson, L. D. Miliary tuberculosis and adult respiratory distress syndrome. Ann. Intern. Med. 85: 609–611, 1976.

2833. Iseman, M. D., Schwarz, M. I., and Stanford, R. E. Interstitial pneumonia in angio-immunoblastic lymphadenopathy with dysproteinemia. Ann. Intern. Med. 85: 752–755, 1976.

2834. Yarnell, J. W. G. and St. Leger, A. S. Respiratory infections and their influence on lung function in children: a multiple regression analysis. Thorax 36: 847–851, 1981.

2835. Stradling, J. R. and Lane, D. J. Development of secondary polycythaemia in chronic airways obstruction (editorial). Thorax 36: 321–325, 1981.

2836. Pierce, N. F., Fedson, D. S., Brigham, K. L., Mitra, R. C., Sack, R. B., and Mondal, A. The ventilatory response to acute base deficit in humans. Ann. Intern. Med. 72: 633–640, 1970.

2837. Fanta, C. H. and Drazen, J. M. Calcium blockers and bronchoconstriction (editorial). Am. Rev. Respir. Dis. 127: 673–674, 1983.

2838. Yarnell, J. W. G. and St. Leger, A. S. Respiratory morbidity and lung function in schoolchildren aged 7 to 11 years in South Wales and the west of England. Thorax 36: 842–846, 1981.

2839. Turton, C. W., Williams, G., and Green, M. Cryptogenic obliterative bronchiolitis in adults. Thorax 36: 805–810, 1981.

2840. Smith, M. J. L., Benson, M. K., and Strickland, I. D. Coeliac disease and diffuse interstitial lung disease. Lancet i: 473–475, 1971.

2841. Ramphal, R., Fischlschweiger, W., Shands, J. W. Jr., and Small, P. A. Jr. Murine influenzal tracheitis: a model for the study of influenza and tracheal epithelial repair. Am. Rev. Respir. Dis. 120: 1313–1324, 1979.

2842. Lacronique, J., Roth, C., Battesti, J-P., Basset, F., and Chretien, J. Chest radiological features of pulmonary histiocytosis X: a report based on 50 adult cases. Thorax 37: 104–109, 1982.

2843. O'Connor, S. A., Jones, D. P., Collins, J. V., Heath, R. B., Campbell, M. J., and Leighton, M. H. Changes in pulmonary function after naturally acquired respiratory infection in normal persons. Am. Rev. Respir. Dis. 120: 1087–1093, 1979.

2844. Vracko, R., Thorning, D., and Huang, T. W. Basal lamina of alveolar epithelium and capillaries: quantitative changes with aging and in diabetes mellitus. Am. Rev. Respir. Dis. 120: 973–983, 1979.

2845. Sarosi, G. A. and Davies, S. F. Blastomycosis. Am. Rev. Respir. Dis. 120: 911–938, 1979.

2846. Lebrec, D., Capron, J-P., Dhumeaux, D., and Benhamou, J-P. Pulmonary hypertension complicating portal hypertension. Am. Rev. Respir. Dis. 120: 849–856, 1979.

2847. Wall, M. A., Platt, O. S., and Strieder, D. J. Lung function in children with sickle cell anemia. Am. Rev. Respir. Dis. 120: 210–214, 1979.

2848. Menkes, H. A., Sera, K., Rogers, R. M., Hyde, R. W., Forster, R. E. III, and Dubois, A. B. Pulsatile uptake of CO in the human lung. J. Clin. Invest. 49: 335–345, 1970.

2849. Ruff, F., Hughes, J. M. B., Stanley, N., McCarthy, D., Greene, R., Aronoff, A., Clayton, L., and Milic-Emili, J. Regional lung function in patients with hepatic cirrhosis. J. Clin. Invest. 50: 2403–2413, 1971.

2850. Ayers, L. N., Tierney, D. F., and Imagawa, D. Shortened survival of mice with influenza when given oxygen at one atmosphere. Am. Rev. Respir. Dis. 107: 955–961, 1973.

2851. Johanson, W. G. Jr., Pierce, A. K., and Sanford, J. P. Pulmonary function in uncomplicated influenza. Am. Rev. Respir. Dis. 100: 141–146, 1969.

2852. Lefrak, E. A., Stevens, P. M., Piutha, J., Balsinger, E., Noon, G. P., and Mayor, H. D. Extracorporeal membrane oxygenation for fulminant influenza pneumonia. Chest 66: 385–388, 1974.

2853. Landing, B. H. Congenital malformations and genetic disorders of the respiratory tract. Am. Rev. Respir. Dis. 120: 151–185, 1979.

2854. Gomez-Engler, H. E., Barker, A. F., Klein, R., Dietl, C. A., Macmanus, Q., Torstveit, J., Knight, R., Lawrence, H., and Starr, A., Post-traumatic bronchial stenosis and acute respiratory insufficiency. J. Thorac. Cardiovasc. Surg. 79: 864–867, 1980.

2855. Macklem, P. T., Thurlbeck, W. M., and Fraser, R. G. Chronic obstructive disease of small airways. Ann. Intern. Med. 74: 167–177, 1971.

2856. Rogers, R. M., Levin, D. C., Gray, B. A., and Moseley, L. W. Jr. Physiologic effects of bronchopulmonary lavage in alveolar proteinosis. Am. Rev. Respir. Dis. 118: 255–264, 1978.

2857. Basset, F., Corrin, B., Spencer, H., Lacronique, J., Roth, C., Soler, P., Battesti, J-P., Georges, R., and Chretien, J. Pulmonary histiocytosis X. Am. Rev. Respir. Dis. 118: 811–820, 1978.

2858. Wongchaowart, B., Kennealy, J. A., Crissman, J., and Hawkins, H. Respiratory failure in malignant histiocytosis. Am. Rev. Respir. Dis. 124: 640–642, 1981.

2859. Lebowitz, M. D., Knudson, R. J., and Burrows, B. Tucson epidemiologic study of obstructive lung disease. Am. J. Epidemiol. 102: 137–152, 1975.

2860. Payne, M. and Kjelsberg, M. Respiratory symptoms, lung function and smoking habits in an adult population. Am. J. Public Health 54: 261–277, 1964.

2861. Van der Lende, R. Epidemiology of Chronic Nonspecific Lung Disease (Chronic Bronchitis). Springfield, Charles C Thomas, 1969.

2862. Van der Lende, R., Visser, B. F., Wever-Hess, J., Tammeling, G. J., De Vries, K., and Orie, N. G. M. Epidemiological investigations in the Netherlands into the influence of smoking and atmospheric pollution on respiratory symptoms and lung function disturbance. Pneumologie 149: 119–126, 1973.

2863. Van der Lende, R., Rijcken, B., and Schouten, J. P. Longitudinal versus cross-sectional studies in measuring effects of smoking, air pollution and hyperactivity on VC and FEV_1. Bull. Eur. Physiopathol. Respir. 19: 84, 1983.

2864. Leech, J. A., Ghezzo, H., Stevens, D., and Becklake, M. R. Respiratory pressures and function in young adults. Am. Rev. Respir. Dis. 128: 17–23, 1983.

2865. Epidemiology of Respiratory Disease: Task Force Report. National Institutes of Health Publication 81-2019. US Department of Health and Human Services, Washington, D.C., 1980.

2866. Rom, W. N. (ed.). Environmental and Occupational Medicine. Little, Brown, Boston, 1983.

2867. Last, J. M. (ed.). A Dictionary of Epidemiology. Handbook sponsored by the IEA. Oxford University Press, New York, 1983.

2868. Abramson, J. H. Survey Methods in Community Medicine. Churchill-Livingstone, Edinburgh, 1974.

2869. Monson, R. R. Occupational Epidemiology. CRC Press, Boca Raton, FL, 1980.

2870. McMahon, B. Epidemiology, Principles and Methods. Thomas F. Pugh, Boston, 1970.

2871. Liddell, F. D. K. and McDonald, J. C. Survey design and analysis. In: McDonald, J. C. (ed.). Recent Advances in Occupational Health. Churchill-Livingstone, Edinburgh, 1981.

2872. Sturgess, J. M. The mucus lining of major bronchi in the rabbit lung. Am. Rev. Respir. Dis. 115: 819–827, 1977.

2873. Becklake, M. R. Epidemiologic studies in human populations. In: Witschi, H. P. and Brain, J. D. (eds.). Toxicology of Inhaled Materials, Vol. 1, Sec. C. Springer-Verlag, Berlin, 1984.

2874. Sutton, P. P., Pavia, D., Bateman, J. R. M., and Clarke, S. W. Chest physiotherapy: a review. Eur. J. Respir. Dis. 63: 188–201, 1982.

2875. McDonald, J. C. Conference summary. International Conference on Byssinosis. Chest 79(Suppl.): 134S–136S, 1981.

2876. Clausen, J. L. (ed.). Pulmonary Function Testing Guidelines and Controversies. Academic Press, New York, 1982.

2877. Eisen, E., Wegman, D. H., and Louis, T. A. Effect of selection in a prospective study of forced expiratory volume in Vermont granite workers. Am. Rev. Respir. Dis. 128: 587–591, 1983.

2878. Becklake, M. R. and Permutt, S. Evaluation of tests of lung function for "screening" for early detection of chronic obstructive lung disease. In: Macklem, P. and Permutt, S. (eds.). The Lung in Transition between Health and Disease. Marcel Dekker, New York and Basel, 1979.

2879. Becklake, M. R. Concepts of normality applied to the measurement of lung function. Am. J. Med. 80: 1158–1164, 1986.

2880. Becklake, M. R., Leclerc, M., Strobach, H., and Swift, J. The N2 closing volume test in population studies: sources of variation and reproducibility. Am. Rev. Respir. Dis. 111: 141–147, 1975.

2881. Gardner, R. M. ATS statement—snowbird workshop on standardization of spirometry. Am. Rev. Respir. Dis. 119: 831–838, 1979.

2882. American Thoracic Society. Respiratory care position paper. ATS News 4: 6, 1976.

2883. Glindmeyer, H. W., Diem, J. E., Jones, R. M., and Weill, H. Noncomparability of longitudinally and cross-sectionally determined annual change in spirometry. Am. Rev. Respir. Dis. 125: 544–548, 1982.

2884. Quanjer, Ph. H. (ed.). Standardised lung function testing. Bull. Eur. Physiopathol. Respir. 19(Suppl. 5): 1–95, 1983.

2885. Fournier-Massey, G. and Becklake, M. R. Epreuves de fonction respiratoire. Bull. Physiopathol. Respir. 6: 661–670, 1970.

2886. Stebbings, J. H. Chronic respiratory disease among non-smokers in Hagerstown, Maryland. Environ. Res. 4: 163–192, 1971.

2887. Hughes, A. L. E., Hughes, C. A., and Hughes, D. T. D. Comparison of four spirometers. Thorax 38: 228, 1983.

2888. Weiss, S. T., Tager, I. B., Schenker, M., and Speizer, F. E. The health effects of involuntary smoking. Am. Rev. Respir. Dis. 128: 933–942, 1983.

2889. Ciliary transport vs cough: rheological requirements for optimal clearance of secretions. Eur. J. Respir. Dis. 61(Suppl. 10): 39–42, 1980.

2890. Burrows, B., Cline, M. G., Knudson, R. J., Taussig, L. M., and Lebowitz, M. D. A descriptive analysis of the growth and decline of the FVC and FEV_1. Chest 83: 717–724, 1983.

2891. Ghezzo, R. H. Normalisation of lung function tests for epidemiologic studies. Ph.D. Thesis. McGill University, Montreal, 1982.

2892. Cotes, J. E. Lung Function: Assessment and Applications in Medicine. 4th ed. Blackwell Scientific Publications, Oxford, 1979.

2893. Cole, T. J. Linear and proportional regression models in the prediction of ventilatory function. J. Stat. Soc. Assoc. 132: 297–337, 1975.

2894. Glindmeyer, H. W. Predictable confusion. J. Occup. Med. 23: 845–849, 1981.

2895. Morris, J. F., Koski, A., and Johnson, L. C. Spirometric standards for healthy non-smoking adults. Am. Rev. Respir. Dis. 103: 57–67, 1971.

2896. Miller, A. and Thornton, J. C. The interpretation of spirometric measurements in epidemiologic surveys. Environ. Res. 23: 444–448, 1980.

2897. Conellan, S. J., Carson, R., Holland, T., et al. Role of bronchial hyperreactivity and atopy in enhancing decline of lung function in male smokers. Eur. J. Respir. Dis. 62(Suppl. 113): 130–131, 1981.

2898. Woolcock, A. J., Dowse, G. K., Temple, K., Stanley, H., Alpers, M. P., and Turner, K. J. The prevalence of asthma in the South-Fore people of Papua, New Guinea: a method for field studies of bronchial reactivity. Eur. J. Respir. Dis. 64: 571–581, 1983.

2899. Burrows, B., Lebowitz, M. D., and Knudson, R. J. Epidemiologic evidence that childhood problems predispose to airways disease in the adult (an association between adult and pediatric respiratory disorders). Pediatr. Res. 11: 218–220, 1977.

2900. Napier, J. A. Field methods and response rates in the Tecumseh community health study. Am. J. Public Health 52: 208–216, 1962.

2901. Higgins, M. W., Keller, J. B., Becker, M., Howatt, W., Landis, J. R., Rotman, H., Weg, J. G., and Higgins, I. An index of risk for obstructive airway disease. Am. Rev. Respir. Dis. 125: 144–151, 1982.

2902. Cohen, B. H., et al. A genetic-epidemiologic study of chronic obstructive pulmonary disease. 1. Study design and preliminary observations. Johns Hopkins Med. J. 137: 95–104, 1975.

2903. Speizer, F. E. and Tager, I. B. Epidemiology of mucus hypersecretion and obstructive airways disease. Epidemiol. Rev. 1: 124–141, 1979.

2904. Buist, A. S. Evaluation of lung function: concepts of normality. In: Simmons, D. H. (ed.). Pulmonology, Vol. 4. John Wiley & Sons New York, 1982.

2905. Rea, H. H., Becklake, M. R., and Ghezzo, H. Lung function changes as a reflection of tissue aging in young adults. Bull. Eur. Physiopathol. Respir. 18: 15–19, 1982.

2906. Beck, G. J., Doyle, C. A., and Schachter, E. N. A longitu-dinal study of respiratory health in a rural community. Am. Rev. Respir. Dis. 125: 375–381, 1982.

2907. Diem, J. E., Jones, R. N., Hendrick, D. J., Glindmeyer, H. W., Dharmarajan, V., Butcher, B. T., Salvaggio, J. E., and Weill, H. Five-year longitudinal study of workers employed in a new toluene diisocyanate manufacturing plant. Am. Rev. Respir. Dis. 126: 420–428, 1982.

2908. Oldham, P. D. A note on the analysis of repeated measurements of the same subjects. J. Chron. Dis. 15: 969–977, 1962.

2909. Case records of the Massachusetts General Hospital. Case 22-1977. N. Engl. J. Med. 296: 1279–1287, 1977.

2910. Shy, C. M. Epidemiologic evidence and the United States air quality standards. Am. J. Epidemiol. 110: 661–676, 1979.

2911. Gibbs, G. W. and Lachance, M. Dust exposure in the chrysotile asbestos mines and mills of Quebec. Arch. Environ. Health 24: 189–197, 1972.

2912. McDonald, J. C., Becklake, M. R., Gibbs, G. W., McDonald, A. D., and Rossiter, C. E. The health of chrysotile mine and mill workers in Quebec. Arch Environ. Health 28: 69–71, 1974.

2913. McDonald, J. C., Liddell, F. D. K., Gibbs, G. W., Eyssen, G., and McDonald, A. D. Dust exposure and mortality in chrysotile mining 1919–1975. Br. J. Ind. Med. 37: 11–24, 1980.

2914. Becklake, M. R. Clinical measurements in Quebec chrysotile miners: use for future protection of workers. Ann. N.Y. Acad. Sci. 330: 23–30, 1979.

2915. Becklake, M. R., Thomas, D. T., Liddell, F. D. K., and McDonald, J. C. Follow-up respiratory measurements in Quebec chrysotile asbestos miners and millers. Scand. J. Work Environ. Health 8(Suppl. 1): 105–110, 1982.

2916. Copes, R., Thomas, D., and Becklake, M. R. Temporal patterns of exposure and non-malignant pulmonary abnormality in Quebec chrysotile workers. Arch. Environ. Health 40: 80–87, 1985.

2917. Hernberg, S. The Finnish foundry project: background and general methodology. Scand. J. Work Environ. Health 2(Suppl.): 8–12, 1976.

2918. Karava, R., Hernberg, S., Koskela, R. S., and Luoma, K. Prevalence of pneumoconiosis and chronic bronchitis in foundry workers. Scand. J. Work Environ. Health 2(Suppl.): 64–72, 1976.

2919. Koskela, R. S., Luoma, K., and Hernberg, S. Turnover and health selection among foundry workers. Scand. J. Work Environ. Health 2(Suppl.): 90–105, 1976.

2920. Beck, G. J., Schachter, E. N., Maunder, L. R., and Schilling, R. S. F. A prospective study of chronic lung disease in cotton textile workers. Ann. Intern. Med. 97: 645–651, 1982.

2921. Pare, P. D., Lawson, L. M., and Brooks, L. A. Patterns of response to inhaled bronchodilators in asthmatics. Am. Rev. Respir. Dis. 127: 680–685, 1983.

2922. Vedal, S. and Crapo, R. O. False positive rates of multiple pulmonary function tests in healthy subjects. Bull. Eur. Physiopathol. Respir. 19: 263–266, 1983.

2923. Statement on spirometry. ACCP scientific section recommendations. Chest 83: 547–550, 1983.

2924. Peto, R., Speizer, F. E., Cochrane, A. L., Moore, F., Fletcher, C. M., Tinker, C. M., Higgins, I. T. T., Gray, R. G., Richards, S. M., Gilliland, J., and Norman-Smith, B. The relevance in adults of air-flow obstruction, but not of mucus hypersecretion, to mortality from chronic lung disease. Am. Rev. Respir. Dis. 128: 491–500, 1983.

2925. Van der Lende, R., Kok, T., Peset, R., Quanjer, Ph. H., Schouten, J. P., and Orie, N. G. M. Longterm exposure to air pollution and decline in VC and FEV_1. Chest 80(Suppl.): 26S–27S, 1981.

2926. Ploysongsang, Y., Pare, J. A. P., and Macklem, P. T. Correlation of regional breath sounds with regional ventilation in emphysema. Am. Rev. Respir. Dis. 126: 526–529, 1982.

2927. Loudon, R. G. The lung speaks out (editorial). Am. Rev. Respir. Dis. 126: 411–412, 1982.

2928. Ploysongsang, Y. and Schonfeld, S. A. Mechanism of production of crackles after atelectasis during low-volume breathing. Am. Rev. Respir. Dis. 126: 413–415, 1982.

2929. Workum, P., Holford, S. K., Delbono, E. A., and Murphy, R. L. H. The prevalence and character of crackles (rales) in young women without significant lung disease. Am. Rev. Respir. Dis. 126: 921–923, 1982.

2930. Kraman, S. S. and Austrheim, O. Comparison of lung sound and transmitted sound amplitude in normal men. Am. Rev. Respir. Dis. 128: 451–454, 1983.

2931. Kraman, S. S. Does the vesicular lung sound come only from the lungs? Am. Rev. Respir. Dis. 128: 622–626, 1983.

2932. Campbell, E. J. M. Physical signs of diffuse airways obstruction and lung distension. Thorax 24: 1–3, 1969.

2933. Godfrey, S., Edwards, R. H. T., Campbell, E. J. M., Armitage, P., and Oppenheimer, E. A. Repeatability of physical signs in airways obstruction. Thorax 24: 4–9, 1969.

2934. Godfrey, S., Edwards, R. H. T., Campbell, E. J. M., and Newton-Howes, J. Clinical and physiological association of some physical signs observed in patients with chronic airways obstruction. Thorax 25: 285–287, 1970.

2935. Stubbing, D. G., Mathur, P. N., Roberts, R. S., and Campbell, E. J. M. Some physical signs in patients with chronic airflow obstruction. Am. Rev. Respir. Dis. 125: 549–552, 1982.

2936. Kraman, S. S. Lung sounds: relative sites of origin and comparative amplitudes in normal subjects. Lung 161: 57–64, 1983.

2937. Thacker, R. E. and Kraman, S. S. The prevalence of auscultatory crackles in subjects without lung disease. Chest 81: 672–674, 1982.

2938. Dosani, R. and Kraman, S. S. Lung sound intensity variability in normal men. Chest 83: 615–620, 1983.

2939. Sakula, A. In search of Laennec. J. R. Coll. Physicians Lond. 15: 55–57, 1981.

2940. Hiller, F. C., McCusker, K. T., Mazumder, M. K., Wilson, J. D., and Bone, R. C. Deposition of sidestream cigarette smoke in the human respiratory tract. Am. Rev. Respir. Dis. 125: 406–408, 1982.

2941. Brody, A. R. and Roe, M. W. Deposition pattern of inorganic particles at the alveolar level in the lungs of rats and mice. Am. Rev. Respir. Dis. 128: 724–729, 1983.

2942. Agnew, J. E., Bateman, J. R. M., Pavia, D., and Clarke, S. W. Radionuclide demonstration of ventilatory abnormalities in mild asthma. Clin. Sci. 66: 525–531, 1983.

2943. Tobin, M. J., Jenouri, G., Danta, I., Kim, C., Watson, H., and Sackner, M. A. Response to bronchodilator drug administration by a new reservoir aerosol delivery system and a review of other auxiliary delivery systems. Am. Rev. Respir. Dis. 126: 670–675, 1982.

2944. Gerrity, T. R., Garrard, C. S., and Yeates, D. B. A mathematical model of particle retention in the air-spaces of human lungs. Br. J. Ind. Med. 40: 121–130, 1983.

2945. Agnew, J. E., Bateman, J. R. M., Sheahan, N. F., Lennard-Jones, A. M., Pavia, D., and Clarke, S. W. Effect of oral corticosteroids on mucus clearance by cough and mucociliary transport in stable asthma. Bull. Eur. Physiopathol. Respir. 19: 37–41, 1983.

2946. Lippmann, M., Leikauf, G., Spektor, D., Schlesinger, R. B., and Albert, R. E. The effects of irritant aerosols on mucus clearance from large and small conductive airways. Chest 80(Suppl. 6): 873–876, 1981.

2947. Sutton, P. P., Pavia, D., Bateman, J. R. M., and Clarke, S. W. The effect of oral aminophylline on lung mucociliary clearance in man. Chest 80(Suppl. 6): 889–891, 1981.

2948. Camner, P. Studies on the removal of inhaled particles from the lungs by voluntary coughing. Chest 80(Suppl. 6): 824–825, 1981.

2949. Lopez-Vidriero, M. T. Airway mucus. Chest 80(Suppl. 6): 799–804, 1981.

2950. Marriott, C. The viscoelastic nature of mucus secretion. Chest 80(Suppl. 6): 804–808, 1981.

2951. Dulfano, M. J., Luk, C. K., Beckage, M., and Wooten, O. Ciliary inhibitory effects of asthma patients' sputum. Clin. Sci. 63: 393–396, 1982.

2952. Weiss, T., Dorow, P., and Felix, R. Regional mucociliary removal of inhaled particles in smokers with small airway disease. Respiration 44: 338–345, 1983.

2953. Rensch, H., Von Seefeld, H., Gebhardt, K. F., Renzow, D., and Sell, P-J. Stop and go particle transport in the peripheral airways. Respiration 44: 346–350, 1983.

2954. Agnew, J. E., Little, F., Pavia, D., and Clarke, S. W. Mucus clearance from the airways in chronic bronchitis—smokers and ex-smokers. Bull. Eur. Physiopathol. Respir. 18: 473–484, 1982.

2955. Rossman, C. M., Waldes, R., Sampson, D., and Newhouse, M. T. Effect of chest physiotherapy on the removal of mucus in patients with cystic fibrosis. Am. Rev. Respir. Dis. 126: 131–135, 1982.

2956. Dulfano, M. J. and Luk, C. K. Sputum and ciliary inhibition in asthma. Thorax 37: 646–651, 1982.

2957. Wiggins, J., Elliott, J. A., Stevenson, R. D., and Stockley, R. A. Effect of corticosteroids on sputum sol-phase protease inhibitors in chronic obstructive pulmonary disease. Thorax 37: 652–656, 1982.

2958. Cary, J. M., Krugmeier, R., Newman, B., Ross, B., and Butler, J. Coughs cause systemic blood flow. Thorax 39: 192–195, 1984.

2959. King, M., Phillips, D. M., Gross, D., Vartian, V., Chang, H. K., and Zidulka, A. Enhanced tracheal mucus clearance with high frequency chest wall compression. Am. Rev. Respir. Dis. 128: 511–515, 1983.

2960. Wiggins, J. and Stockley, R. A. Variability in sputum sol phase proteins in chronic obstructive bronchitis. Am. Rev. Respir. Dis. 128: 60–64, 1983.

2961. Desplechain, C., Foliguet, B., Barrat, E., Grignon, G., and Touati, F. Les pores de Kohn des alveoles pulmonaires. Bull. Eur. Physiopathol. Respir. 19: 59–68, 1983.

2962. Moss, I. R., Wald, A., and Ransohoff, J. Respiratory functions and chemical regulation of ventilation in head injury. Am. Rev. Respir. Dis. 109: 2205–215, 1974.

2963. Beeckman, P., Demedts, M., Clarysse, I., and Vanclooster, R. Radiographic evaluation of the influence of age and smoking on thoracic and regional pulmonary dimensions. Lung 161: 39–46, 1983.

2964. Crapo, R. O., Morris, A. H., Clayton, P. D., and Nixon, C. R. Lung volumes in healthy nonsmoking adults. Bull. Eur. Physiopathol. Respir. 18: 419–425, 1982.

2965. Schumaker, P. T., Rhodes, G. R., Newell, J. C., Dutton, R. E., Shah, D. M., Scovill, W. A., and Powers, S. R. Ventilation-perfusion imbalance after head trauma. Am. Rev. Respir. Dis. 119: 33–43, 1979.

2966. Tack, M., Altose, M. D., and Cherniack, N. S. Effect of aging on the perception of resistive ventilatory loads. Am. Rev. Respir. Dis. 126: 463–467, 1982.

2967. Konno, K., Arai, H., Motomiya, M., Nagai, H., Ito, M., Sato, H., and Satoh, K. A biochemical study on glycosaminoglycans (mucopolysaccharides) in emphysematous and in aged lungs. Am. Rev. Respir. Dis. 126: 797–801, 1982.

2968. Beck, G. J., Doyle, C. A., and Schachter, E. N. A longitudinal study of respiratory health in a rural community. Am. Rev. Respir. Dis. 125: 375–381, 1982.

2969. Knudson, R. J., Lebowitz, M. D., Holberg, C. J., and Burrows, B. Changes in the normal maximal expiratory flow-volume curve with growth and aging. Am. Rev. Respir. Dis. 127: 725–734, 1983.

2970. Patrick, J. M., Bassey, E. J., and Fentem, P. H. The rising ventilatory cost of bicycle exercise in the seventh decade: a longitudinal study of nine healthy men. Clin. Sci. 65: 521–526, 1983.

2971. Bouhuys, A., Beck, G. J., and Schoenberg, J. B. Priorities in prevention of chronic lung disease. Lung 156: 129–148, 1979.

2972. Emirgil, C., Sobol, B. J., Campodonico, S., Herbert, W. H., and Mechkati, R. Pulmonary circulation in the aged. J. Appl. Physiol. 23: 631–640, 1967.

2973. Wagner, P. D., Laravuso, R. B., Uhl, R., and West, J. B. Continuous distributions of ventilation-perfusion ratios in normal subjects breathing air and 100 per cent O_2. J. Clin. Invest. 54: 54–68, 1974.

2974. Harris, E. A., Kenyon, A. M., Nisbet, H. D., Seelye, E. R., and Whitlock, R. M. L. The normal alveolar-arterial oxygen-tension gradient in man. Clin. Sci. Mol. Med. 46: 89–104, 1974.

2975. Hertle, F. H., Georg, E., and Lange, H-J. Die arteriellen Blutgaspartialdrucke und ihr Beziehungen zu alter und anthropometrischen Grossen. Respiration 28: 1–30, 1971.

2976. Druz, W. and Sharp, J. T. Electrical and mechanical activity of the diaphragm accompanying body position in severe chronic obstructive pulmonary disease. Am. Rev. Respir. Dis. 125: 275–280, 1982.

2977. O'Neill, S. and McCarthy, D. S. Postural relief of dyspnoea in severe chronic airflow limitation: relationship to respiratory muscle length. Thorax 38: 595–600, 1983.

2978. Sonnenblick, M., Melzer, E., and Rosin, A. J. Body positional effect on gas exchange in unilateral pleural effusion. Chest 83: 784–786, 1983.

2979. Mahler, D. A., Snyder, P. E., Virgulto, J. A., and Loke, J. Positional dyspnea and oxygen desaturation related to carcinoma of the lung. Chest 83: 826–827, 1983.

2980. Ploysongsang, Y. The lung sounds phase angle test for detection of small airway disease. Respir. Physiol. 53: 203–214, 1983.

2981. Zidulka, A., Braidy, T. F., Rizzi, M. C., and Shiner, R. J. Position may stop pneumothorax progression in dogs. Am. Rev. Respir. Dis. 126: 51–53, 1982.

2982. Marti, Ch. and Ulmer, W. T. Absence of effect of the body position on arterial blood gases. Respiration 43: 41–44, 1982.

2983. Silverstein, D., Michlin, B., Sobel, H. J., and Lavietes, M. H. Right ventricular failure in a patient with diabetic neuropathy (myopathy) and central alveolar hypoventilation. Respiration 44: 460–465, 1983.

2984. Brashear, R. E. Hyperventilation syndrome. Lung 161: 257–273, 1983.

2985. Remolina, C., Khan, A. U., Santiago, T. V., and Edelman, N. H. Positional hypoxemia in unilateral lung disease. N. Engl. J. Med. 304: 523–525, 1981.

2986. Froese, A. B. and Bryan, A. C. Effects of anesthesia and paralysis on diaphragmatic mechanics in man. Anesthesiology 41: 242–255, 1974.

2987. Knudson, R. J. and Kaltenborn, W. T. Evaluation of lung elastic recoil by exponential curve analysis. Respir. Physiol. 46: 29–42, 1981.

2988. Edwards, M. J., Metcalfe, J., Dunham, M. J., and Paul, M. S. Accelerated respiratory response to moderate exercise in late pregnancy. Respir. Physiol. 45: 229–241, 1981.

2989. Prefaut, Ch. and Engel, L. A. Vertical distribution of perfusion and inspired gas in supine man. Respir. Physiol. 43: 209–219, 1981.

2990. Engel, L. A. and Prefaut, C. Cranio-caudal distribution of inspired gas and perfusion in supine man. Respir. Physiol. 45: 43–53, 1981.

2991. Ray, C. S., Sue, D. Y., Bray, G., Hansen, J. E., and Wasserman, K. Effects of obesity on respiratory function. Am. Rev. Respir. Dis. 128: 501–506, 1983.

2992. Lukomsky, G. I., Ovchinnikov, A. A., and Bilal, A. Complications of bronchoscopy. Chest 79: 316–321, 1981.

2993. Burns, D. M., Shure, D., Francoz, R., Kalafer, M., Harrell, J., Witztum, K., and Moser, K. M. The physiologic consequences of saline lobar lavage in healthy human adults. Am. Rev. Respir. Dis. 127: 695–701, 1983.

2994. Freedman, A. R., Mangura, B. T., and Lavietes, M. H. Minute ventilation in asthma. Am. Rev. Respir. Dis. 128: 800–805, 1983.

2995. Faurschou, P., Madsen, F., and Viskum, K. Thoracoscopy: influence of the procedure on some respiratory and cardiac values. Thorax 38: 341–343, 1983.

2996. Perpina, M., Benlloch, E., Marco, V., Abad, F., and Nauffal, D. Effect of thoracentesis on pulmonary gas exchange. Thorax 38: 747–750, 1983.

2997. Bouhuys, A., Beck, G. J., and Schoenberg, J. B. Lung function: normal values and risk factors. In: Sadoul, P., Milic-Emili, J., Simonsson, B. G., and Clark, T. J. H. (eds.). Small Airways in Health and Disease. Symposium, Copenhagen, March, 1979. Excerpta Medica, Amsterdam, 1979.

2998. Yernault, J-C., Englert, M., Sergysels, R., and De Coster, A. Pulmonary mechanics and diffusion after 'shock lung'. Thorax 30: 252–257, 1975.

2999. Screening for adult respiratory disease. Official ATS statement. Am. Rev. Respir. Dis. 128: 768–773, 1983.

3000. Miller, A., Thornton, J. C., Warshaw, R., Anderson, H., Teirstein, A. S., and Selikoff, I. J. Single breath diffusing capacity in a representative sample of the population of Michigan, a large industrial state. Am. Rev. Respir. Dis. 127: 270–277, 1983.

3001. Carel, R. S., Greenstein, A., Ellender, E., Melamed, Y.,

and Kerem, D. Factors affecting ventilatory lung function in young navy selectees. Am. Rev. Respir. Dis. 128: 249–252, 1983.

3002. Campbell, S. C. Estimation of total lung capacity by planimetry of chest radiographs in children 5 to 10 years of age. Am. Rev. Respir. Dis. 127: 106–107, 1983.

3003. Ekwo, E. E., Weinberger, M. M., Dusdieker, L. B., Huntley, W. H., Rodgers, P., and Maxwell, G. A. Airways responses to inhaled isoproterenol in normal children. Am. Rev. Respir. Dis. 127: 108–109, 1983.

3004. Kanner, R. E., Schenker, M. B., Munoz, A., and Speizer, F. E. Spirometry in children: methodology for obtaining optimal results for clinical and epidemiologic studies. Am. Rev. Respir. Dis. 127: 720–724, 1983.

3005. Fedullo, P. F., Moser, K. M., Hartman, M. T., and Ashburn, W. L. Patterns of pulmonary perfusion scans in normal subjects. Am. Rev. Respir. Dis. 127: 776–779, 1983.

3006. Yernault, J-C., Noseda, A., Van Muylem, A., and Estenne, M. Variability of lung elasticity measurements in normal humans. Am. Rev. Respir. Dis. 128: 816–819, 1983.

3007. Pincock, A. C. and Miller, M. R. The effect of temperature on recording spirograms. Am. Rev. Respir. Dis. 128: 894–898, 1983.

3008. O'Brien, R. J. and Drizd, T. A. Roentgenographic determination of total lung capacity: normal values from a national population survey. Am. Rev. Respir. Dis. 128: 949–952, 1983.

3009. Cormier, Y. and Belanger, J. The role of gas exchange in phase IV of the single-breath nitrogen test. Am. Rev. Respir. Dis. 125: 396–399, 1982.

3010. Hubert, H. B., Fabsitz, R. R., Feinleib, M., and Gwinn, C. Genetic and environmental influences on pulmonary function in adult twins. Am. Rev. Respir. Dis. 125: 409–415, 1982.

3011. Townsend, M. C., Du Chene, A. G., and Fallat, R. J. The effects of underrecorded forced expirations on spirometric lung function indexes. Am. Rev. Respir. Dis. 126: 734–737, 1982.

3012. Motoyama, E. K., Hen, J., Tamas, L., and Dolan, T. F. Jr. Spirometry with positive airway pressure. Am. Rev. Respir. Dis. 126: 766–770, 1982.

3013. Baydur, A., Behrakis, P. K., Zin, W. A., Jaeger, M., and Milic-Emili, J. A simple method for assessing the validity of the esophageal balloon technique. Am. Respir. Dis. 126: 788–791, 1982.

3014. Rodenstein, D. O. and Stanescu, D. C. Reassessment of lung volume measurement by helium dilution and by body plethysmography in chronic air-flow obstruction. Am. Rev. Respir. Dis. 126: 1040–1044, 1982.

3015. Shore, S., Milic-Emili, J., and Martin, J. G. Reassessment of body plethysmographic technique for the measurement of thoracic gas volume in asthmatics. Am. Rev. Respir. Dis. 126: 515–520, 1982.

3016. Kauffmann, F. and Drouet, D. Spirometric reference values—what for? (letter to editor). Am. Rev. Respir. Dis. 126: 595, 1982.

3017. Pare, P. D., Harvey, K., Mildenberger, M., and Brooks, L. A. Effects of balloon volume and position on the pressure volume curve of the lung. Clin. Invest. Med. 6: 143–146, 1983.

3018. Russell, N. J., Bagg, L. R., Dobrzynski, J., and Hughes, D. T. D. Clinical assessment of a rebreathing method for measuring pulmonary gas transfer. Thorax 38: 212–215, 1983.

3019. Zimmerman, P. V., Connellan, S. J., Middleton, H. C., Tabona, M. V., Goldman, M. D., and Pride, N. Postural changes in rib cage and abdominal volume-motion coefficients and their effect on the calibration of a respiratory inductance plethysmograph. Am. Rev. Respir. Dis. 127: 209–214, 1983.

3020. Sliman, N. A., Dajani, B. M., and Shubair, K. S. Pulmonary function in normal Jordanian children. Thorax 37: 854–857, 1982.

3021. Armstrong, J. D., Gluck, E. H., Crapo, R. O., Jones, H. A., and Hughes, J. M. B. Lung tissue volume estimated by simultaneous radiographic and helium dilution methods. Thorax 37: 676–679, 1982.

3022. Perks, W. H., Sopwith, T., Brown, D., Jones, C. H., and Green, M. Effects of temperature on Vitalograph spirometer readings. Thorax 38: 592–594, 1983.

3023. Braun, N. M. T., Arora, N. S., and Rochester, D. F. Respiratory muscle and pulmonary function in polymyositis and other proximal myopathies. Thorax 38: 616–623, 1983.

3024. Macnee, W., Power, J., Innes, A., Douglas, N. J., and Sudlow, M. F. The dependence of maximal flow in man on the airway gas physical properties. Clin. Sci. 65: 273–279, 1983.

3025. Pare, P. D., Wiggs, B. J. R., and Coppin, C. A. Errors in the measurement of total lung capacity in chronic obstructive lung disease. Thorax 38: 468–471, 1983.

3026. Forster, R. E. II and Ogilvie, C. M. The single breath carbon monoxide transfer test 25 years on: a reappraisal (editorial). Thorax 38: 1–9, 1983.

3027. Hutchison, A. A., Sum, A. C., Demis, T. A., Erben, A., and Landau, L. I. Moment analysis of multiple breath nitrogen washout in children. Am. Rev. Respir. Dis. 125: 28–32, 1982.

3028. Shaw, R. A., Schonfield, S. A., and Whitcomb, M. E. Progressive and transient hypoxic ventilatory drive tests in healthy subjects. Am. Rev. Respir. Dis. 126: 37–40, 1982.

3029. Higenbottam, T. and Payne, J. Glottis narrowing in lung disease. Am. Rev. Respir. Dis. 125: 746–750, 1982.

3030. Hankinson, J. L. and Gardner, R. M. Standard waveforms for spirometer testing. Am. Rev. Respir. Dis. 126: 362–364, 1982.

3031. Dab, I. Spirometry at adolescence. Bull. Eur. Physiopathol. Respir. 18: 21–29, 1982.

3032. Zapletal, A., Samanek, M., and Paul, T. Upstream and total airway conductance in children and adolescents. Bull. Eur. Physiopathol. Respir. 18: 31–37, 1982.

3033. De Swiniarski, R., Mataame, M., and Tanche, M. Plethysmography study and pulmonary function in well-trained adolescents. Bull. Eur. Physiopathol. Respir. 18: 39–49, 1982.

3034. Palka, M. J. Spirometric predicted values for teenage boys: relation to body composition and exercise performance. Bull. Eur. Physiopathol. Respir. 18: 59–64, 1982.

3035. Hida, W., Sasaki, H., and Takishima, T. Standard values of the maximal expiratory flow-volume curve normalized by total lung capacity. Bull. Eur. Physiopathol. Respir. 18: 117–129, 1982.

3036. Worth, H. and Smidt, U. Phase II of expiratory curves of respiratory and inert gases in normals and in patients with emphysema. Bull. Eur. Physiopathol. Respir. 18: 247–253, 1982.

3037. Zwart, A., Jansen, J. R. C., and Luijendijk, S. C. M. Bohr dead space during helium washout. Bull. Eur. Physiopathol. Respir. 18: 261–272, 1982.

3038. Paiva, M., Van Muylem, A., and Engel, L. A. Slope of phase III in multibreath nitrogen washout and washin. Bull. Eur. Physiopathol. Respir. 18: 273–280, 1982.

3039. Brundler, J. P. and Lewis, C. M. Estimation of lung volume from nitrogen washout curves. Bull. Eur. Physiopathol. Respir. 18: 281–289, 1982.

3040. Ben Jebria, A., Thiriet, M., Bonnet, J. C., Bres, M., Visser, B. F., and Hatzfeld, C. Extraction of tissue compartment from multibreath N2 washout curves in healthy subjects. Bull. Eur. Physiopathol. Respir. 18: 291–302, 1982.

3041. Mertens, P., Paiva, M., Van Muylem, A., and Yernault, J. C. Comparison of nitrogen washin and washout using moment ratio analysis. Bull. Eur. Physiopathol. Respir. 18: 303–307, 1982.

3042. Hughes, J. M. B., Jones, H. A., and Davies, E. E. Applications of multi-breath washin measurements in closed circuit using a mass spectrometer. Bull. Eur. Physiopathol. Respir. 18: 309–317, 1982.

3043. Jones, H. A., Davies, E. E., and Hughes, J. M. B. Influence of flow rate and frequency on the distribution of insoluble gases in the lung during rebreathing. Bull. Eur. Physiopathol. Respir. 18: 319–323, 1982.

3044. Chang, H. K. and Shykoff, B. E. A model simulation of ventilation distributions. Bull. Eur. Physiopathol. Respir. 18: 329–338, 1982.

3045. Denison, D. M. and Waller, J. F. Interpreting the results of regional single-breath studies from the patient's point of view. Bull. Eur. Physiopathol. Respir. 18: 339–351, 1982.

3046. Wagner, P. D. Information content of inert gas elimination techniques. Bull. Eur. Physiopathol. Respir. 18: 361–372, 1982.

3047. Chaussian, M., Denjean, A., Lebeau, C., De Lattre, J., and Badoual, J. Lung transfer factor for CO at rest in normal children by a steady-state method. Bull. Eur. Physiopathol. Respir. 18: 403–410, 1982.

3048. Tweeddale, P. M., Merchant, S., Leslie, M. J., and McHardy, G. J. R. Quality control in pulmonary function testing. A help or a hindrance? Bull. Eur. Physiopathol. Respir. 18: 485–490, 1982.

3049. Brown, C. and Borth, F. M. A comparative study of two methods of calibrating spirometers for use in field surveys. Bull. Eur. Physiopathol. Respir. 18: 673–677, 1982.

3050. Sulotto, F., Romano, C., and Guazzotti, T. A computerized interpretation of standard pulmonary function tests. Bull. Eur. Physiopathol. Respir. 18: 583–599, 1982.

3051. Zeck, R. T., Solliday, N. H., Celic, L., and Cugell, D. W. Variability of the volume of isoflow. Chest 79: 269–272, 1981.

3052. Lebowitz, M. D., Knudson, R. J., Robertson, G., and Burrows, B. Significance of intraindividual changes in maximum expiratory flow volume and peak expiratory flow measurements. Chest 81: 566–570, 1982.

3053. Landser, F. J., Clement, J., and Van De Woestijne, K. P. Normal values of total respiratory resistance and reactance determined by forced oscillations. Chest 81: 586–591, 1982.

3054. Eichenhorn, M. S., Beauchamp, R. K., Harper, P. A., and Ward, J. C. An assessment of three portable peak flow meters. Chest 82: 306–309, 1982.

3055. Felton, C., Rose, G. L., Cassidy, S. S., and Johnson, R. L. Jr. Comparison of lung diffusing capacity during rebreathing and during slow exhalation. Respir. Physiol. 43: 13–22, 1981.

3056. Ratner, E. R. and Wagner, P. D. Resolution of the multiple inert gas method for estimating VA/Q maldistribution. Respir. Physiol. 49: 293–313, 1982.

3057. Martin, B. J. and Thomas, C. M. Variation among normal persons in short-term ventilatory capacity. Respiration 43: 23–28, 1982.

3058. Schulzer, M., Chan-Yeung, M., and Tan, F. On the possible significance of the quadratic effect of age on lung-function measurements. Can. J. Stat. 10: 293–303, 1982.

3059. Knudson, R. J., Schroter, R. C., Knudson, D. E., and Sugihara, S. Influence of airway geometry on expiratory flow limitation and density dependence. Respir. Physiol. 52: 113–123, 1983.

3060. Knudson, R. J. and Schroter, R. C. A consideration of density dependence of maximum expiratory flow. Respir. Physiol. 52: 125–136, 1983.

3061. Rodenstein, D. O., Goncette, L., and Stanescu, D. C. Extrathoracic airways changes during plethysmographic measurements of lung volume. Respir. Physiol. 52: 217–227, 1983.

3062. Shigeoka, J. W., Gardner, R. M., and Barkman, H. W. A portable volume/flow calibrating syringe. Chest 82: 598–601, 1982.

3063. Berend, N., Nelson, N. A., Rutland, J., Marlin, G. E., and Woolcock, A. J. The maximum expiratory flow-volume curve with air and a low-density gas mixture. Chest 80: 23–30, 1981.

3064. Clement, J., Landser, F. J., and Van De Woestijne, K. P. Total resistance and reactance in patients with respiratory complaints with and without airways obstruction. Chest 83: 215–220, 1983.

3065. Tobin, M. J., Jenouri, G., Lind, B., Watson, H., Schneider, A., and Sackner, M. A. Validation of respiratory inductive plethysmography in patients with pulmonary disease. Chest 83: 615–620, 1983.

3066. Cormier, Y. and Belanger, J. Quantification of the effect of gas exchange on the slope of Phase III. Bull. Eur. Physiopathol. Respir. 19: 13–16, 1983.

3067. Stam, H., Versprille, A., and Bogaard, J. M. The components of the carbon monoxide diffusing capacity in man dependent on alveolar volume. Bull. Eur. Physiopathol. Respir. 19: 17–22, 1983.

3068. Schrader, P. C., Quanjer, Ph. H., Van Zomeren, B. C., De Groodt, E. G., Wever, A. M. J., and Wise, M. E. Selection of variables from maximum expiratory flow-volume curves. Bull. Eur. Physiopathol. Respir. 19: 43–49, 1983.

3069. Begin, P. and Peslin, R. Mesure plethysmographiques du volume gazeux intrathoracique. Un retour aux hypotheses

3070. Permutt, S. and Menkes, H. A. Spirometry. In: Macklem, P. T. and Permutt, S. (eds.). The Lung in the Transition between Health and Disease. Marcel Dekker, New York and Basel, 1979.

3071. DeGroodt, E. G., Quanjer, P. H., and Wise, M. E. Influence of external resistance and minor flow variations on single breath nitrogen test and residual volume. Bull. Eur. Physiopathol. Respir. 19: 267–272, 1983.

3072. Boutros-Toni, F., Pigearias, B., Konate, P., and Lonsdorfer, J. Valeurs de reference spirometriques des femmes melanodermes. Bull. Eur. Physiopathol. Respir. 19: 331–338, 1983.

3073. Harris, E. A. and Whitlock, R. M. L. Fractional carbon monoxide uptake and "diffusing capacity" in models of pulmonary maldistribution. Bull. Eur. Physiopathol. Respir. 19: 427–432, 1983.

3074. Harris, E. A. and Whitlock, R. M. L. Prediction equations for fractional CO uptake derived from 50 healthy subjects. Bull. Eur. Physiopathol. Respir. 19: 433–438, 1983.

3075. Pedersen, O. F., Naeraa, N., Lyager, S., Hilberg, C., and Larsen, L. A device for evaluation of flow recording equipment. Bull. Eur. Physiopathol. Respir. 19: 515–520, 1983.

3076. Engel, L. A. Intraregional ventilation distribution. Bull. Eur. Physiopathol. Respir. 18: 181–188, 1982.

3077. Paiva, M. Model analysis of inert gas mixing in the lung. Bull. Eur. Physiopathol. Respir. 18: 189–210, 1982.

3078. Allen, T. W., Addington, W., Rosendal, T., and Cugell, D. W. Alveolar carbon dioxide and airway resistance in patients with postexercise bronchospasm. Am. Rev. Respir. Dis. 107: 816–821, 1973.

3079. Pimmel, R. L., Fullton, J. M., Ginsberg, J. F., Hazucha, M. J., Haak, E. D., McDonnell, W. F., and Bromberg, P. A. Correlation of airway resistance with forced random noise parameters. J. Appl. Physiol. 51: 33–39, 1981.

3080. Nagels, J., Landser, F. J., Van Der Linden, L., Clement, J., and Van De Woestijne, K. P. Mechanical properties of lungs and chest wall during spontaneous breathing. J. Appl. Physiol. 49: 408–416, 1980.

3081. Tsai, M. J., Pimmel, R. L., Stiff, E. J., Bromberg, P. A., and Hamlin, R. L. Respiratory parameter estimation using forced oscillation impedance data. J. Appl. Physiol. 43: 322–330, 1977.

3082. Pimmel, R. L., Tsai, M. J., Winter, D. C., and Bromberg, P. A. Estimating central and peripheral respiratory resistance. J. Appl. Physiol. 45: 375–380, 1978.

3083. Malo, J-L., Pineau, L., Cartier, A., and Martin, R. R. Reference values of the provocative concentrations of methacholine that cause 6 per cent and 20 per cent changes in forced expiratory volume in one second in a normal population. Am. Rev. Respir. Dis. 128: 8–11, 1983.

3084. Parham, W. M., Shepard, R. H., Norman, P. S., and Fish, J. E. Analysis of time course and magnitude of lung inflation effects on airway tone: relation to airway reactivity. Am. Rev. Respir. Dis. 128: 240–245, 1983.

3085. Vincenc, K. S., Black, J. L., Armour, C. L., Donnelly, P. D., and Woolcock, A. J. Comparison of in vivo and in vitro responses to histamine in human airways. Am. Rev. Respir. Dis. 128: 875–879, 1983.

3086. Pratter, M. R., Woodman, T. F., Irwin, R. S., and Johnson, B. Stability of stored methacholine chloride solutions. Am. Rev. Respir. Dis. 126: 717–719, 1982.

3087. Chung, K. F., Morgan, B., Keyes, S. J., and Snashall, P. D. Histamine dose-response relationships in normal and asthmatic subjects. Am. Rev. Respir. Dis. 126: 849–854, 1982.

3088. Hutchison, A. A., Brigham, K. L., and Snapper, J. R. Effect of histamine on lung mechanics in sheep. Am. Rev. Respir. Dis. 126: 1025–1029, 1982.

3089. Cockcroft, D. W., Berscheid, B. A., and Murdock, K. Y. Measurement of responsiveness to inhaled histamine using FEV_1: comparison of PC20 and threshold. Thorax 38: 523–526, 1983.

3090. Walters, E. H. Prostaglandins and the control of airways responses to histamine in normal and asthmatic subjects. Thorax 38: 188–194, 1983.

3091. Yan, K., Salome, C., and Woolcock, A. J. Rapid method for

measurement of bronchial responsiveness. Thorax 38: 760–765, 1983.

3092. Ben-Dov, I., Amirav, I., Shochina, M., Amitai, I., Bar-Yishay, E., and Godfrey, S. Effect of negative ionisation of inspired air on the response of asthmatic children to exercise and inhaled histamine. Thorax 38: 584–588, 1983.

3093. Cockcroft, D. W. and Berscheid, B. A. Slope of the dose-response curve: usefulness in assessing bronchial responses to inhaled histamine. Thorax 38: 55–61, 1983.

3094. Hariparsad, D., Wilson, N., Dixon, C., and Silverman, M. Reproducibility of histamine challenge tests in asthmatic children. Thorax 38: 258–260, 1983.

3095. Chatham, M., Bleecker, E. R., Smith, P. L., Rosenthal, R. R., Mason, P., and Norman, P. S. A comparison of histamine, methacholine, and exercise airway reactivity in normal and asthmatic subjects. Am. Rev. Respir. Dis. 126: 235–240, 1982.

3096. Eiser, N. M. and Guz, A. Effect of atropine on experimentally-induced airway obstruction in man. Bull. Eur. Physiopathol. Respir. 18: 449–460, 1982.

3097. Michoud, M. C., Ghezzo, H., and Amyot, R. A comparison of pulmonary function tests used for bronchial challenges. Bull. Eur. Physiopathol. Respir. 18: 609–621, 1982.

3098. Massey, D. G., Miyauchi, D., and Fournier-Massey, G. Nebulizer function. Bull. Eur. Physiopathol. Respir. 18: 665–671, 1982.

3099. Bellia, V., Rizzo, A., Amoroso, S., Mirabella, A., and Bonsignore, G. Analysis of dose-response curves in the detection of bronchial hyperreactivity. Respiration 44: 10–18, 1983.

3100. Numeroso, R., Della Torre, F., Radaelli, C., Scarpazza, G., and Ortolani, C. Effect of long-term treatment with sodium cromoglycate on non-specific bronchial hyperreactivity in non-atopic patients with chronic bronchitis. Respiration 44: 109–117, 1983.

3101. Schachter, E. N., Rimar, S., Littner, M., Beck, G. J., and Bouhuys, A. Airway reactivity and exercise in healthy subjects. Chest 81: 461–465, 1982.

3102. Chatham, M., Bleecker, E. R., Norman, P., Smith, P. L., and Mason, P. A screening test for airways reactivity. Chest 82: 15–18, 1982.

3103. Schachter, E. N., Brown, S., Lach, E., and Gerstenhaber, B. Histamine blocking agents in healthy and asthmatic subjects. Chest 82: 143–147, 1982.

3104. Cockcroft, D. W. and Berscheid, B. A. Standardisation of inhalation provocation tests. Chest 82: 572–575, 1982.

3105. Takashima, T., Hida, W., Sasaki, H., Suzuki, S., and Sasaki, T. Direct-writing recorder of the dose-response curves of the airway to methacholine. Chest 80: 600–606, 1981.

3106. Cockcroft, D. W., Berscheid, B. A., and Murdock, K. Y. Unimodal distribution of bronchial responsiveness to inhaled histamine in a random human population. Chest 83: 751–754, 1983.

3107. Eiser, N. M., Kerrebijn, K. F., and Quanjer, P. H. (eds.). SEPCR working group "bronchial hyperreactivity." Guidelines for standardisation of bronchial challenges with (nonspecific) bronchoconstricting agents. Bull. Eur. Physiopathol. Respir. 19: 495–514, 1983.

3108. Cormier, Y., Belanger, J., and Cote, A. Contribution of residual volume to the increased alveolar plateau with bronchoconstriction. Respiration 43: 174–178, 1982.

3109. Tashkin, D. P., Clark, V. A., Coulson, A. H., Bourque, L. B., Simmons, M., Reems, C., Detels, R., and Rokaw, S. Comparison of lung function in young nonsmokers and smokers before and after initiation of the smoking habit. Am. Rev. Respir. Dis. 128: 12–16, 1983.

3110. Schenker, M. B., Samet, J. M., and Speizer, F. E. Risk factors for childhood respiratory disease. Am. Rev. Respir. Dis. 128: 1038–1043, 1983.

3111. Crandall, E. D. (ed.). Fluid balance across alveolar epithelium. Am. Rev. Respir. Dis. 127: S1–S65, 1983.

3112. Davies, S. F., Offord, K. P., Brown, M. G., Campe, H., and Niewohner, D. Urine desmosine is unrelated to cigarette smoking or to spirometric function. Am. Rev. Respir. Dis. 128: 473–475, 1983.

3113. Abboud, R. T., Johnson, A. J., Richter, A. M., and Elwood, R. K. Comparison of in vitro neutrophil elastase release in nonsmokers and smokers. Am. Rev. Respir. Dis. 128: 507–510, 1983.

3114. Sparrow, D., Stefos, T., Bosse, R., and Weiss, S. T. The relationship of tar content to decline in pulmonary function in cigarette smokers. Am. Rev. Respir. Dis. 127: 56–58, 1983.

3115. Hunninghake, G. W. and Crystal, R. G. Cigarette smoking and lung destruction. Am. Rev. Respir. Dis. 128: 833–838, 1983.

3116. Yernault, J-C., Englert, M., Sergysels, R., Degaute, J. P., and De Coster, A. Follow-up of pulmonary function after 'shock lung.' Bull. Eur. Physiopathol. Respir. 13: 241–248, 1977.

3117. McGowan, S. E., Stone, P. J., Calore, J. D., Snider, G. L., and Franzblau, C. The fate of neutrophil elastase incorporated by human alveolar macrophages. Am. Rev. Respir. Dis. 127: 449–455, 1983.

3118. Wright, J. L., Lawson, L. M., Pare, P. D., Wiggs, B. J., Kennedy, S., and Hogg, J. C. Morphology of peripheral airways in current smokers and ex-smokers. Am. Rev. Respir. Dis. 127: 474–477, 1983.

3119. Hoidal, J. R. and Niewohner, D. E. Cigarette smoke inhalation potentiates elastase-induced emphysema in hamsters. Am. Rev. Respir. Dis. 127: 478–481, 1983.

3120. Wallace, J. M., Moser, K. M., Hartman, M. T., and Ashburn, W. L. Patterns of pulmonary perfusion scans in normal subjects. II. The prevalence of abnormal scans in young smokers. Am. Rev. Respir. Dis. 125: 443–447, 1982.

3121. Janoff, A. and Dearing, R. Alpha$_1$-proteinase inhibitor is more sensitive to inactivation by cigarette smoke than is leukocyte elastase. Am. Rev. Respir. Dis. 126: 691–694, 1982.

3122. Kabiraj, M. U., Siminsson, B. G., Groth, S., Bjorklund, A., Bulow, K., and Lindell, S-E. Bronchial reactivity, smoking, and alpha$_1$-antitrypsin. Am. Rev. Respir. Dis. 126: 864–869, 1982.

3123. Ludwig, P. W. and Hoidal, J. R. Alterations in leukocyte oxidative metabolism in cigarette smokers. Am. Rev. Respir. Dis. 126: 977–980, 1982.

3124. Kawakami, Y., Yamamoto, H., Yoshikawa, T., and Shida, A. Respiratory chemosensitivity in smokers. Am. Rev. Respir. Dis. 126: 986–990, 1982.

3125. Hoidal, J. R. and Niewohner, D. E. Lung phagocyte recruitment and metabolic alterations induced by cigarette smoke in humans and in hamsters. Am. Rev. Respir. Dis. 126: 548–552, 1982.

3126. Simani, A. S., Inoue, S., and Hogg, J. C. Penetration of the respiratory epithelium of guinea pigs following exposure to cigarette smoke. Lab. Invest. 31: 75–81, 1984.

3127. Saloojee, Y., Vesey, C. J., Cole, P. V., and Russell, M. Carboxyhaemoglobin and plasma thiocyanate: complementary indicators of smoking behaviour? Thorax 37: 521–525, 1982.

3128. O'Neill, S. and Prichard, J. S. Elastolytic activity of alveolar macrophages in chronic bronchitis: comparison of current and former smokers. Thorax 38: 356–359, 1983.

3129. Jones, J. G., Minty, B. D., Royston, D., and Royston, J. P. Carboxyhaemoglobin and pulmonary epithelial permeability in man. Thorax 38: 129–133, 1983.

3130. Tirlapur, V. G., Gicheru, K., Charalambous, B. M., Evans, P. J., and Mir, M. A. Packed cell volume, haemoglobin, and oxygen saturation changes in healthy smokers and non-smokers. Thorax 38: 785–787, 1983.

3131. Walter, A. and Walter, S. Mast cell density in isolated monkey lungs on exposure to cigarette smoke. Thorax 37: 699–702, 1982.

3132. Enstrom, J. E. Trends in mortality among California physicians after giving up smoking: 1950–79. Br. Med. J. 286: 1101–1105, 1983.

3133. Walter, S. and Walter, A. Basophil degranulation induced by cigarette smoking in man. Thorax 37: 756–759, 1982.

3134. Adams, L., Lee, C., Rawbone, R., and Guz, A. Patterns of smoking: measurement and variability in asymptomatic smokers. Clin. Sci. 65: 383–392, 1983.

3135. Jarvis, M. J., Russell, M. A. H., and Feyerabend, C. Absorption of nicotine and carbon monoxide from passive smoking under natural conditions of exposure. Thorax 38: 829–833, 1983.

3136. Hankins, D., Drage, C., Zamel, N., and Kronenberg, R. Pulmonary function in identical twins raised apart. Am. Rev. Respir. Dis. 125: 119–121, 1982.

3137. Nemery, B., Moavero, N. E., Brasseur, L., and Stanescu, D. C. Changes in lung function after smoking cessation: an assessment from a cross-sectional survey. Am. Rev. Respir. Dis. 125: 122–124, 1982.

3138. Knowles, M. R., Buntin, W. H., Bromberg, P. A., Gatzy, J. T., and Boucher, R. C. Measurements of transepithelial electric potential differences in the trachea and bronchi of human subjects in vivo. Am. Rev. Respir. Dis. 126: 108–112, 1982.

3139. Schenker, M. B., Samet, J. M., and Speizer, F. E. Effect of cigarette tar content and smoking habits on respiratory symptoms in women. Am. Rev. Respir. Dis. 125: 684–690, 1982.

3140. Tobin, M. J. and Sackner, M. A. Monitoring smoking patterns of low and high tar cigarettes with inductive plethysmography. Am. Rev. Respir. Dis. 126: 258–264, 1982.

3141. Baile, E. M., Wright, J. L., Pare, P. D., and Hogg, J. C. The effect of acute small airway inflammation on pulmonary function in dogs. Am. Rev. Respir. Dis. 126: 298–301, 1982.

3142. Teculescu, D. B., Bohadana, A. B., Peslin, R., and Cereceda, J. V. 1-second forced expiratory volume and density dependence in early airflow limitation. Respiration 44: 433–438, 1983.

3143. Tobin, M. J., Schneider, A. W., and Sackner, M. A. Breathing pattern during and after smoking cigarettes. Clin. Sci. 63: 473–483, 1982.

3144. Dosman, J. A., Cotton, D. J., Graham, B. L., Hall, D. L., Li, R., Froh, F., and Barnett, G. D. Sensitivity and specificity of early diagnostic tests of lung function in smokers. Chest 79: 6–11, 1981.

3145. York, E. L. and Jones, R. L. Effects of smoking on regional residual volume in young adults. Chest 79: 12–15, 1981.

3146. Berend, N., Wright, J. L., Thurlbeck, W. M., Marlin, G. E., and Woolcock, A. J. Small airways disease: reproducibility of measurements and correlation with lung function. Chest 79: 263–268, 1981.

3147. Landser, F. J., Clement, J., and Van De Woestijne, K. P. Normal values of total respiratory resistance and reactance determined by forced oscillations. Chest 81: 586–591, 1982.

3148. Sackner, M. A., Rao, A. S. V., Birch, S., Atkins, N., Gibbs, L., and Davis, B. Assessment of density dependent flow-volume parameters in nonsmokers and smokers. Chest 82: 137–142, 1982.

3149. Sackner, M. A., Rao, A. S. V., Birch, S., Atkins, N., Gibbs, L., and Davis, B. Assessment of time-volume and flow-volume components of forced vital capacity. Chest 82: 272–278, 1982.

3150. Tobin, M. J., Jenouri, G., and Sackner, M. A. Effect of naloxone on change of breathing pattern with smoking. Chest 82: 530–537, 1982.

3151. Tobin, M. J., Jenouri, G., and Sackner, M. A. Subjective and objective measurement of cigarette smoke inhalation. Chest 82: 696–700, 1982.

3152. Britt, E. J., Shelhamer, J., Menkes, H., Cohen, B., Meyer, M., and Permutt, S. Sex differences in the decline of pulmonary function with age. Chest 80(Suppl.): 79S–80S, 1981.

3153. Dahms, T. E., Bolin, J. F., and Slavin, R. G. Passive smoking: effects on bronchial asthma. Chest 80: 530–534, 1981.

3154. Hogg, J. C. The effect of smoking on airway permeability (editorial). Chest 83: 1–2, 1983.

3155. Chernick, V. The brain's own morphine and cigarette smoking: the junkie in disguise? (editorial). Chest 83: 2–4, 1983.

3156. Mason, G. R., Uszler, J. M., Effros, R. M., and Reid, E. Rapidly reversible alterations of pulmonary epithelial permeability induced by smoking. Chest 83: 6–11, 1983.

3157. Da Silva, A. M. T. and Hamosh, P. Effect of smoking a cigarette on the density dependence of maximal expiratory flow. Respiration 43: 258–262, 1982.

3158. Cohen, D., Arai, S. F., and Brain, J. D. Smoking impairs long-term clearance from the lung. Science 204: 514–517, 1979.

3159. Auerbach, O., Hammond, E. C., and Garfinkel, L. Changes in bronchial epithelium in relation to cigarette smoking,

1955–1960 vs. 1970–1977. N. Engl. J. Med. 300: 381–386, 1979.

3160. Wright, J. L., Lawson, L. M., Pare, P. D., Kennedy, S., Wiggs, B., and Hogg, J. C. The detection of small airways disease. Am. Rev. Respir. Dis. 129: 989–994, 1984.

3161. Dirksen, H., Janzon, L., and Lindell, S-E. Influence of smoking and cessation of smoking on lung function. In: Regional Lung Function and Closing Volume. Scand. J. Resp. Dis. 85(Suppl.): 266–274, 1974.

3162. Poh, S. C. The effects of opium smoking in cigarette smokers. Am. Rev. Respir. Dis. 106: 239–245, 1972.

3163. Sheppard, D., Epstein, J., Bethel, R. A., Nadel, J. A., and Boushey, H. A. Tolerance to sulfur dioxide-induced bronchoconstriction in subjects with asthma. Environ. Res. 30: 412–419, 1983.

3164. Raub, J. A., Miller, F. J., Graham, J. A., Gardner, D. E., and O'Neill, J. J. Pulmonary function in normal and elastase-treated hamsters exposed to a complex mixture of olefin-ozone-sulfur dioxide reaction products. Environ. Res. 31: 302–310, 1983.

3165. Goldstein, I. F. and Cuzick, J. Daily patterns of asthma in New York City and New Orleans: an epidemiologic investigation. Environ. Res. 30: 211–223, 1983.

3166. Gliner, J. A., Horvath, S. M., and Folinsbee, L. J. Preexposure to low ozone concentrations does not diminish the pulmonary function response on exposure to higher ozone concentrations. Am. Rev. Respir. Dis. 127: 51–55, 1983.

3167. Holtzman, M. J., Fabbri, L. M., O'Byrne, P. M., Gold, B. D., Aizawa, H., Walters, E. H., Alpert, S. E., and Nadel, J. A. Importance of airway inflammation for hyperresponsiveness induced by ozone. Am. Rev. Respir. Dis. 127: 686–690, 1983.

3168. Buist, A. S., Johnson, L. R., Vollmer, W. M., Sexton, G. J., and Kanarek, P. H. Acute effects of volcanic ash from Mount Saint Helens on lung function in children. Am. Rev. Respir. Dis. 127: 714–719, 1983.

3169. Adams, W. C. and Schlegele, E. S. Ozone and high ventilation effects on pulmonary function and endurance performance. J. Appl. Physiol. 55: 805–812, 1983.

3170. Friedman, M., Gallo, J. M., Nicholls, H. P., and Bromberg, P. A. Changes in inert gas rebreathing parameters after ozone exposure in dogs. Am. Rev. Respir. Dis. 128: 851–856, 1983.

3171. Kulle, T. J., Kerr, H. D., Farrell, B. P., Sauder, L. R., and Bermel, M. S. Pulmonary function and bronchial reactivity in human subjects with exposure to ozone and respirable sulfuric acid aerosol. Am. Rev. Respir. Dis. 126: 996–1000, 1982.

3172. Johnson, K. G., Loftsgaarden, D. O., and Gideon, R. A. The effects of Mount St. Helens volcanic ash on the pulmonary function of 120 elementary school children. Am. Rev. Respir. Dis. 126: 1066–1069, 1982.

3173. Bethel, R. A., Epstein, J., Sheppard, D., Nadel, J. A., and Boushey, H. A. Sulfur dioxide-induced bronchoconstriction in freely breathing, exercising asthmatic subjects. Am. Rev. Respir. Dis. 128: 987–990, 1983.

3174. Lam, C., Kattan, M., Collins, A., and Kleinerman, J. Long-term sequelae of bronchiolitis induced by nitrogen dioxide in hamsters. Am. Rev. Respir. Dis. 128: 1020–1023, 1983.

3175. Bethel, R. A., Erle, D. J., Epstein, J., Sheppard, D., Nadel, J. A., and Boushey, H. A. Effect of exercise rate and route of inhalation on sulfur-dioxide-induced bronchoconstriction in asthmatic subjects. Am. Rev. Respir. Dis. 128: 592–596, 1983.

3176. Koenig, J. Q., Pierson, W. E., and Horike, M. The effects of inhaled sulfuric acid on pulmonary function in adolescent asthmatics. Am. Rev. Respir. Dis. 128: 221–225, 1983.

3177. Utell, M. J., Morrow, P. E., Speers, D., Darling, J., and Hyde, R. W. Airway responses to sulfate and sulfuric acid aerosols in asthmatics. Am. Rev. Respir. Dis. 128: 444–450, 1983.

3178. Gordon, R. E., Case, B. W., and Kleinerman, J. Acute NO_2 effects on penetration and transport of horseradish peroxidase in hamster respiratory epithelium. Am. Rev. Respir. Dis. 128: 528–533, 1983.

3179. Last, J. A., Gerriets, J. E., and Hyde, D. M. Synergistic effects on rat lungs of mixtures of oxidant air pollutants (ozone or nitrogen dioxide) and respirable aerosols. Am. Rev. Respir. Dis. 128: 539–544, 1983.

3180. Nambu, Z. and Yokoyama, E. Antioxidant system and ozone tolerance. Environ. Res. 32: 111–117, 1983.

3181. Sexton, K., Letz, R., and Spengler, J. D. Estimating human exposure to nitrogen dioxide: an indoor/outdoor modelling approach. Environ. Res. 32: 151–166, 1983.

3182. Vachon, L., Fitzgerald, M. X., Solliday, N. H., Gould, I. A., and Gaensler, E. A. Single-dose effect of marihuana smoke. N. Engl. J. Med. 288: 985–989, 1973.

3183. Linn, W. S., Shamoo, D. A., Spier, C. E., Valencia, L. M., Anzar, U. T., Venet, T. G., and Hackney, J. D. Respiratory effects of 0.75 ppm sulfur dioxide in exercising asthmatics: influence of upper respiratory diseases. Environ. Res. 30: 340–348, 1983.

3184. Tan, W. C., Cripps, E., Douglas, N., and Sudlow, M. F. Protective effect of drugs on bronchoconstriction induced by sulphur dioxide. Thorax 37: 671–676, 1982.

3185. Drazen, J. M., O'Cain, C. F., and Ingram, R. H. Jr. Experimental induction of chronic bronchitis in dogs. Am. Rev. Respir. Dis. 126: 75–79, 1982.

3186. Blackwelder, W. C., Alling, D. W., and Stuart-Harris, C. H. Association of excess mortality from chronic nonspecific lung disease with epidemics of influenza. Am. Rev. Respir. Dis. 125: 511–516, 1982.

3187. Kirkpatrick, M. B., Sheppard, D., Nadel, J. A., and Boushey, H. A. Effect of the oronasal breathing route on sulfur dioxide-induced bronchoconstriction in exercising asthmatic subjects. Am. Rev. Respir. Dis. 125: 627–631, 1982.

3188. Downs, J. B. and Olsen, G. N. Pulmonary function following adult respiratory distress syndrome. Chest 65: 92–93, 1974.

3189. Andersen, I., Molhave, L., and Proctor, D. F. Human response to controlled levels of combinations of sulfur dioxide and inert dust. Scand. J. Work Environ. Health 7: 1–7, 1981.

3190. Air pollution and chronic respiratory disease. I. Methods and material. Groupe Cooperatif PAARC. Bull. Eur. Physiopathol. Respir. 18: 87–99, 1982.

3191. Air pollution and chronic or repeated respiratory diseases. II. Results and discussion. Groupe Cooperatif PAARC. Bull. Eur. Physiopathol. Respir. 18: 101–116, 1982.

3192. Detels, R., Tashkin, D. P., Simmons, M. S., Carmichael, H. E. Jr., Sayre, J. W., Rokaw, S. N., and Coulson, A. H. The UCLA population studies of chronic obstructive respiratory disease. Chest 82: 630–638, 1982.

3193. Van der Lende, R., Kok, T., Peset, R., Quanjer, Ph. H., Schouten, J. P., and Orie, N. G. M. Longterm exposure to air pollution and decline in VC and FEV_1. Chest 80(Suppl.): 23S–26S, 1981.

3194. Mostardi, R. A., Ely, D. L., Woebkenberg, N. R., and Conlon, M. Air pollution and health effects in children residing in Akron, Ohio. Chest 80(Suppl.): 26S–27S, 1981.

3195. Detels, R., Sayre, J. W., Coulson, A. H., Rokaw, S. N., Masset, F. J. Jr., Tashkin, D. P., and Wu, M-M. Respiratory effect of longterm exposure to two mixes of air pollutants in Los Angeles county. Chest 80(Suppl.): 27S–29S, 1981.

3196. Cross, C. E., Hesterberg, T. W., Reiser, K. M., and Last, J. A. Ozone toxicity as a model of lung fibrosis. Chest 80(Suppl.): 52S–54S, 1981.

3197. Detels, R., Tashkin, D. P., Sayre, J. W., Rokaw, S. N., Coulson, A. H., Massey, F. J. Jr., and Wegman, D. H. The UCLA population studies of chronic obstructive respiratory disease. IX. A cohort study of changes in respiratory function associated with chronic exposure to photochemical oxidants in community air. (submitted for publication August 1984)

3198. Gorham, E., Martin, F. B., and Litzau, J. T. Acid rain: ionic correlations in the eastern United States, 1980–1981. Science 225: 407–409, 1984.

3199. Whittemore, A. S. Air pollution and respiratory disease. Annu. Rev. Public Health 2: 397–429, 1981.

3200. Ferris, B. G. Jr., chairman. Guidelines as to what constitutes an adverse respiratory health effect, with special reference to air pollution. Committee of the Scientific Assembly on Environmental and Occupational Health, American Thoracic Society. ATS News 10: 6–8, 1984.

3201. Ferris, B. G. Jr., Dockery, D. W., Ware, J. H., Speizer, F. E., and Spiro, R. III. The six-city study: examples of problems in analysis of data. Environ. Health Perspect. 52: 115–123, 1983.

3202. Avol, E. L., Linn, W. S., Venet, T. G., Shamoo, D. A., and Hackney, J. D. Comparative respiratory effects of ozone and ambient oxidant pollution exposure during heavy exercise. J. Air Pollut. Control Assoc. 34: 804–809, 1984.

3203. Bouhuys, A., Beck, G. J., and Schoenberg, J. B. Do present levels of air pollution outdoors affect respiratory health? Nature 276: 466–471, 1978.

3204. Stacy, R. W., Seal, E. Jr., House, D. E., Green, J., Roger, L. J., and Raggio, L. A survey of effects of gaseous and aerosol pollutants on pulmonary function of normal males. Arch. Environ. Health 38: 104–115, 1983.

3205. Niinimaa, V. Oronasal airway choice during running. Respir. Physiol. 53: 129–133, 1983.

3206. Pride, N. B. and Connellan, S. J. Introductory review. Eur. J. Respir. Dis. 63(Suppl. 118): 9–13, 1982.

3207. Hazucha, M. J., Ginsberg, J. F., McDonnell, W. F., Haak, E. D., Pimmel, R. L., House, D. E., and Bromberg, P. A. Changes in bronchial reactivity of asthmatics and normals following exposures to 0.1 ppm NO$_2$. In: Schneider, T. and Grant, L. (eds.). Air Pollution by Nitrogen Oxides. Elsevier Publishing Company, Amsterdam, 1982.

3208. Hazucha, M., Haak, E. D., Ketcham, B. T., and Knelson, J. H. The effects of ozone on the respiratory zone of the human lung. Bull. Int. Union Against Tuberculosis. Proceedings of the 24th Conference. 54(3–4): 417–418, 1979.

3209. Holland, W. W. and Reid, D. D. The urban factor in chronic bronchitis. Lancet i: 445–448, 1965.

3210. Hazucha, M. J., Ginsberg, J. F., McDonnell, W. F., Haak, E. D. Jr., Pimmel, R. L., Salaam, S. A., House, D. E., and Bromberg, P. A. Effects of 0.1 ppm nitrogen dioxide on airways of normal and asthmatic subjects. J. Appl. Physiol. 54: 730–739, 1983.

3211. Health Consequences of Sulfur Oxides: A Report from CHESS, 1970–1971. EPA-650/1-74-004. US Environmental Protection Agency, Washington, D.C., 1974.

3212. Ashby, E. and Anderson, M. The Politics of Clean Air. Monographs on Science, Technology, and Society. Oxford University Press, Oxford and New York, 1981.

3213. Bates, D. V., Knott, J. M. S., and Christie, R. V. Respiratory function in emphysema in relation to prognosis. Q. J. Med. 25: 137–142, 1956.

3214. Sexton, K., Letz, R., and Spengler, J. D. Estimating human exposure to nitrogen dioxide: an indoor/outdoor modeling approach. Environ. Res. 32: 151–166, 1983.

3215. Spengler, J. D., Duffy, C. P., Letz, R., Tibbitts, T. W., and Ferris, B. G. Jr. Nitrogen dioxide inside and outside 137 homes and implications for ambient air quality standards and health effects research. Environ. Sci. Technol. 17: 164–168, 1983.

3216. Utell, M. J., Morrow, P. E., and Hyde, R. W. Airway reactivity to sulfate and sulfuric acid aerosols in normal and asthmatic subjects. J. Air Pollut. Control Assoc. 34: 931–935, 1984.

3217. Hexter, A. C. and Goldsmith, J. R. Carbon monoxide: association of community air pollution with mortality. Science 172: 265–267, 1971.

3218. Douglas, J. W. B. and Waller, R. W. Air pollution and respiratory infections in children. Br. J. Prev. Soc. Med. 20: 1–8, 1966.

3219. Lunn, J. E., Knowelden, J., and Handyside, A. J. Patterns of respiratory illness in Sheffield infant schoolchildren. Br. J. Prev. Soc. Med. 21: 7–16, 1967.

3220. Lunn, J. E., Knowelden, J., and Roe, J. W. Patterns of respiratory illness in Sheffield junior schoolchildren. A follow-up study. Br. J. Prev. Soc. Med. 24: 223–228, 1970.

3221. Air Quality Criteria for Particulate Matter and Sulfur Oxides. Vol. III. EPA 600/8-82-029c. EPA, Washington, D.C., 1982.

3222. Roberts, G. H. and Scott, K. W. M. A necropsy study of pulmonary emphysema in Glasgow. Thorax 27: 28–32, 1972.

3223. Lawther, P. J., Waller, R. E., and Henderson, M. Air pollution and exacerbations of bronchitis. Thorax 25: 525–539, 1970.

3224. Zapletal, A., Jech, J., Kaspar, J., and Samanek, M. Flow volume curves as a method for detecting airway obstruction

in children from an air polluted area. Bull. Eur. Physiopathol. Respir. 13: 803–812, 1977.

3225. Neri, L. C., Mandel, J. S., Hewitt, D., and Jurkowski, D. Chronic obstructive pulmonary disease in two cities of contrasting air quality. Can. Med. Assoc. J. 113: 1043–1050, 1975.

3226. Lee, D. H. K. (ed.). Environmental Factors in Respiratory Disease. Fogarty International Center Proceedings No. 11. Sponsored by NIEHS and Fogarty Center. Academic Press, New York and London, 1972.

3227. Bischof, W. Ozone measurements in jet airliner cabin air. Water Air Soil Pollut. 2: 3–14, 1973.

3228. McDonnell, W. F., Horstmann, D. H., Hazucha, M. J., Seal, E. Jr., Haak, E. D., Salaam, S. A., and House, D. E. Pulmonary effects of ozone exposure during exercise: dose-response characteristics. J. Appl. Physiol. 54: 1345–1352, 1983.

3229. Thurlbeck, W. M. T. The pathobiology and epidemiology of human emphysema. In: Miller, F. J. and Menzel, D. B. (eds.). Fundamentals of extrapolation modeling of inhaled toxicants. Hemisphere Publishing Corp., New York, 1984.

3230. Chappie, M. and Lave, L. The health effects of air pollution: a reanalysis. J. Urban Econ. 12: 346–376, 1982.

3231. Tager, I. B., Weiss, S. T., Munoz, A., Rosner, B., and Speizer, F. E. Longitudinal study of the effects of maternal smoking on pulmonary function in children. N. Engl. J. Med. 309: 699–703, 1983.

3232. Potter, W. A., Olafsson, S., and Hyatt, R. E. Ventilatory mechanics and expiratory flow limitation during exercise in patients with obstructive lung disease. J. Clin. Invest. 50: 910–919, 1971.

3233. Catterall, J. R., Douglas, N. J., Calverley, P. M. A., Shapiro, C. M., Brezinova, V., Brash, H. M., and Flenley, D. C. Transient hypoxemia during sleep in chronic obstructive pulmonary disease is not a sleep apnea syndrome. Am. Rev. Respir. Dis. 128: 24–29, 1983.

3234. Davis, P. B., Del Rio, S., Muntz, J. A., and Dieckman, L. Sweat chloride concentration in adults with pulmonary diseases. Am. Rev. Respir. Dis. 128: 34–37, 1983.

3235. Hoop, B., Shih, V. E., and Kazemi, H. Relationship between central nervous system hydrogen ion regulation and amino acid metabolism in hypercapnia. Am. Rev. Respir. Dis. 128: 45–49, 1983.

3236. Shore, S. A., Huk, O., Mannix, S., and Martin, J. G. Effect of panting frequency on the plethysmographic determination of thoracic gas volume in chronic obstructive pulmonary disease. Am. Rev. Respir. Dis. 128: 54–59, 1983.

3237. Sourk, R. L. and Nugent, K. M. Bronchodilator testing: confidence intervals derived from placebo inhalations. Am. Rev. Respir. Dis. 128: 153–157, 1983.

3238. Kilbourn, J. P., Haas, H., Morris, J. F., and Samson, S. Hemophilus influenzae biotypes and chronic bronchitis. Am. Rev. Respir. Dis. 128: 1093–1094, 1983.

3239. Campbell, E. J. and Wald, M. S. Hypoxic injury to human alveolar macrophages accelerates release of previously bound neutrophil elastase. Am. Rev. Respir. Dis. 127: 631–635, 1983.

3240. Wright, J. L., Lawson, L., Pare, P. D., Hooper, R. O., Peretz, D. I., Nelems, J. M., Schulzer, M., and Hogg, J. C. The structure and function of the pulmonary vasculature in mild chronic obstructive pulmonary disease. Am. Rev. Respir. Dis. 128: 702–707, 1983.

3241. Rodenstein, D. O. and Stanescu, D. C. Absence of nasal air flow during pursed lips breathing. Am. Rev. Respir. Dis. 128: 716–718, 1983.

3242. Kauffmann, F., Kleisbauer, J-P., Cambon-de-Mouzon, A., Mercier, P., Constans, J., Blanc, M., Rouch, Y., and Feingold, N. Genetic markers in chronic air-flow limitation. Am. Rev. Respir. Dis. 127: 263–269, 1983.

3243. Powles, A. C. P., Tuxen, D. V., Mahood, C. B., Pugsley, S. O., and Campbell, E. J. M. The effect of intravenously administered almitrine, a peripheral chemoreceptor agonist, on patients with chronic air-flow obstruction. Am. Rev. Respir. Dis. 127: 284–289, 1973.

3244. Arnup, M. E., Mendella, L. A., and Anthonisen, N. R. Effects of cold air hyperpnea in patients with chronic obstructive lung disease. Am. Rev. Respir. Dis. 128: 236–239, 1983.

3245. Glauser, F. L. and Smith, W. R. Pulmonary interstitial fibrosis following near-drowning and exposure to short-term high oxygen concentrations. Chest 68: 373–375, 1975.

3246. Linhartova, A. and Anderson, A. E. Jr. Small airways in severe panlobular emphysema: Mural thickening and premature closure. Am. Rev. Respir. Dis. 127: 42–45, 1983.

3247. Sparrow, D., Rosner, B., Cohen, M., and Weiss, S. T. Alcohol consumption and pulmonary function. Am. Rev. Respir. Dis. 127: 735–738, 1983.

3248. Hodous, T. K., Petsonk, L., Boyles, C., Hankinson, J., and Amandus, H. Effects of added resistance to breathing during exercise in obstructive lung disease. Am. Rev. Respir. Dis. 128: 943–948, 1983.

3249. Ashutosh, K., Mead, G., and Dunsky, M. Early effects of oxygen administration and prognosis in chronic obstructive pulmonary disease and cor pulmonale. Am. Rev. Respir. Dis. 127: 399–404, 1983.

3250. Samet, J. M., Tager, I. B., and Speizer, F. E. The relationship between respiratory illness in childhood and chronic airflow obstruction in adulthood. Am. Rev. Respir. Dis. 127: 508–523, 1983.

3251. Jenkinson, S. G. and George, R. B. Serial pulmonary function studies in survivors of near drowning. Chest 77: 777–780, 1980.

3252. Kawakami, Y., Irie, T., Shida, A., and Yoshikawa, T. Familial factors affecting arterial blood gas values and respiratory chemosensitivity in chronic obstructive pulmonary disease. Am. Rev. Respir. Dis. 125: 420–425, 1982.

3253. Raffestin, B., Escourrou, P., Legrand, A., Duroux, P., and Lockhart, A. Circulatory transport of oxygen in patients with chronic airflow obstruction exercising maximally. Am. Rev. Respir. Dis. 125: 426–431, 1982.

3254. Raub, J. A., Mercer, R. R., Miller, F. J., Graham, J. A., and O'Neill, J. J. Dose response of elastase-induced emphysema in hamsters. Am. Rev. Respir. Dis. 125: 432–435, 1982.

3255. Tenney, S. M. and Mithoefer, J. C. The relationship of mixed venous oxygenation to oxygen transport: with special reference to adaptations to high altitude and pulmonary disease. Am. Rev. Respir. Dis. 125: 474–479, 1982.

3256. Salmon, R. B., Saidel, G. M., Inkley, S. R., and Niewoehner, D. E. Relationship of ventilation inhomogeneity to morphologic variables in excised human lungs. Am. Rev. Respir. Dis. 126: 686–690, 1982.

3257. Anthonisen, N. R. Hypoxemia and O_2 therapy. Am. Rev. Respir. Dis. 126: 729–733, 1982.

3258. Icochea, A., Cooper, B. S., and Kuhn, C. The effect of oxygen on cor pulmonale in experimental emphysema induced by elastase or elastase and beta-aminoproprionitrile in hamsters. Am. Resp. Dis. 126: 792–796, 1982.

3259. Konno, K., Arai, H., Motomiya, M., Nagai, H., Ito, M., Sato, H., and Satoh, K. A biochemical study on glycosaminoglycans (mucopolysaccharides) in emphysematous and in aged lungs. Am. Rev. Respir. Dis. 126: 797–801, 1982.

3260. Ramsdell, J. W., Nachtwey, F. J., and Moser, K. M. Bronchial hyperreactivity in chronic obstructive bronchitis. Am. Rev. Respir. Dis. 126: 829–832, 1982.

3261. Murciano, D., Aubier, M., Bussi, S., Derenne, J-P., Pariente, R., and Milic-Emili, J. Comparison of esophageal, tracheal, and mouth occlusion pressure in patients with chronic obstructive pulmonary disease during acute respiratory failure. Am. Rev. Respir. Dis. 126: 837–841, 1982.

3262. Lucey, E. C. and Clark, B. D. Differing susceptibility of young and adult hamster lungs to injury with pancreatic elastase. Am. Rev. Respir. Dis. 126: 877–881, 1982.

3263. Parot, S., Miara, B., Milic-Emili, J., and Gautier, H. Hypoxemia, hypercapnia, and breathing pattern in patients with chronic obstructive pulmonary disease. Am. Rev. Respir. Dis. 126: 882–886, 1982.

3264. Martorana, P. A., Wusten, B., Van Even, P., Gobel, H., and Schaper, J. A six-month study of the evolution of papain-induced emphysema in the dog. Am. Rev. Respir. Dis. 126: 898–903, 1982.

3265. Ries, A. L. and Moser, K. M. Predicting treadmill/walking speed from cycle ergometry exercise in chronic obstructive pulmonary disease. Am. Rev. Respir. Dis. 126: 924–927, 1982.

3266. Kimball, W. R., Leith, D. E., and Robins, A. G. Dynamic hyperinflation and ventilator dependence in chronic obstructive pulmonary disease. Am. Rev. Respir. Dis. 126: 991–995, 1982.

3267. Lupi-Herrera, E., Sandoval, J., Seoane, M., and Bialostozky, D. Behavior of the pulmonary circulation in chronic obstructive pulmonary disease. Am. Rev. Respir. Dis. 126: 509–514, 1982.

3268. Abboud, R. T., Yu, P., Chan-Yeung, M., and Tan, F. Lack of relationship between ABH secretor status and lung function in pulp mill workers. Am. Rev. Respir. Dis. 126: 1089–1091, 1982.

3269. Fleetham, J., West, P., Mezon, B., Conway, W., Roth, T., and Kryger, M. Sleep, arousals, and oxygen desaturation in chronic obstructive pulmonary disease. Am. Rev. Respir. Dis. 126: 429–433, 1982.

3270. Raaijmakers, J. A. M., Terpstra, G. K., Van Rozen, A. J., Witter, A., and Kreukniet, J. Muscarinic cholinergic receptors in peripheral lung tissue of normal subjects and of patients with chronic obstructive lung disease. Clin. Sci. 66: 585–590, 1983.

3271. Stradling, J. R., Nicholl, C. G., Cover, D., Davies, E. E., Hughes, J. M. B., and Pride, N. B. The effects of oral almitrine on pattern of breathing and gas exchange in patients with chronic obstructive pulmonary disease. Clin. Sci. 66: 435–442, 1984.

3272. Cooke, N. T., Wilson, S. H., and Freedman, S. Blood lactate and respiratory muscle fatigue in patients with chronic airways obstruction. Thorax 38: 184–187, 1983.

3273. Stanley, N. N., Galloway, J. M., Gordon, B., and Pauly, N. Increased respiratory chemosensitivity induced by infusing almitrine intravenously in healthy man. Thorax 38: 200–204, 1983.

3274. Sutinen, S., Lohela, P., Paakko, P., and Lahti, R. Accuracy of postmortem radiography of excised air-inflated human lungs in assessment of pulmonary emphysema. Thorax 37: 906–912, 1982.

3275. Sproule, B. J., Cox, D. W., Hsu, K., Salkie, M. L., and Herbert, F. A. Pulmonary function associated with the Mmalton deficient variant of alpha$_1$-antitrypsin. Am. Rev. Respir. Dis. 127: 237–240, 1983.

3276. Tabona, M. V. Z., Ambrosino, N., and Barnes, P. J. Endogenous opiates and the control of breathing in normal subjects and patients with chronic airflow obstruction. Thorax 37: 834–839, 1982.

3277. Huppert, F. Memory impairment associated with chronic hypoxia. Thorax 37: 858–860, 1982.

3278. Semple, P. D. and Macpherson, P. Radiological pituitary fossa changes in chronic bronchitis. Thorax 37: 512–515, 1982.

3279. Catterall, J. R., Douglas, N. J., Calverley, P. M. A., Shapiro, C. M., and Flenley, D. C. Arterial oxygenation during sleep in patients with right-to-left cardiac or intrapulmonary shunts. Thorax 38: 344–348, 1983.

3280. Turner-Stokes, L., Turton, C., Pope, F. M., and Green, M. Emphysema and cutis laxa. Thorax 38: 790–792, 1983.

3281. Hughes, J. A., Tobin, M. J., Bellamy, D., and Hutchison, D. C. S. Effects of ipratropium bromide and fenoterol aerosols in pulmonary emphysema. Thorax 37: 667–670, 1982.

3282. Heath, D. The human carotid body (editorial). Thorax 38: 561–564, 1983.

3283. Greening, A. P. and Lowrie, D. B. Extracellular release of hydrogen peroxide by human alveolar macrophages: the relationship to cigarette smoking and lower respiratory tract infections. Clin. Sci. 65: 661–664, 1983.

3284. Curzon, P. G. D., Martin, M. A., Cooke, N. J., and Muers, M. F. Effect of oral prednisolone on response to salbutamol and ipratropium bromide aerosols in patients with chronic airflow obstruction. Thorax 38: 601–604, 1983.

3285. Winter, J. H., Buckler, P. W., Bautista, A. P., Smith, F. W., Sharp, P. F., Bennett, B., and Douglas, A. S. Frequency of venous thrombosis in patients with an exacerbation of chronic obstructive lung disease. Thorax 38: 605–608, 1983.

3286. Semple, P. d'A., Watson, W. S., Beastall, G. H., and Hume, R. Endocrine and metabolic studies in unstable cor pulmonale. Thorax 38: 45–49, 1983.

3287. Campbell, J. L., Calverley, P. M. A., Lamb, D., and Flenley, D. C. The renal glomerulus in hypoxic cor pulmonale. Thorax 37: 607–611, 1982.

3288. Gomm, S. A., Keaney, N. P., Hunt, L. P., Allen, S. C., and Stretton, T. B. Dose-response comparison of ipratropium bromide from a metered-dose inhaler and by jet nebulisation. Thorax 38: 297–301, 1983.

3289. Waterhouse, J. C. and Howard, P. Breathlessness and portable oxygen in chronic obstructive airways disease. Thorax 38: 302–306, 1983.

3290. Nicotra, M. B., Rivera, M., and Awe, R. J. Antibiotic therapy of acute exacerbations of chronic bronchitis. Ann. Intern. Med. 97: 18–21, 1982.

3291. Brown, S. E., Linden, G. S., King, R. R., Blair, G. P., Stansbury, D. W., and Light, R. W. Effects of verapamil on pulmonary haemodynamics during hypoxaemia, at rest, and during exercise in patients with chronic obstructive pulmonary disease. Thorax 38: 840–844, 1983.

3292. Pardy, R. L., Rivington, R. N., Milic-Emili, J., and Mortola, J. P. Control of breathing in chronic obstructive pulmonary disease. Am. Rev. Respir. Dis. 125: 6–11, 1982.

3293. Guenard, H., Verhas, M., Todd-Prokopek, A., Solvignon, F., Crouzel, C., Manigne, P., and Soussaline, F. Effects of oxygen breathing on regional distribution of ventilation and perfusion in hypoxemic patients with chronic lung disease. Am. Rev. Respir. Dis. 125: 12–17, 1982.

3294. Buchser, E., Leuenberger, P., Chiolero, R., Perret, C., and Freeman, J. Reduced pulmonary capillary blood volume as a long-term sequel of ARDS. Chest 87: 608–611, 1985.

3295. Samet, J. M., Schrag, S. D., Howard, C. A., Key, C. R., and Pathak, D. R. Respiratory disease in a New Mexico population sample of Hispanic and non-Hispanic whites. Am. Rev. Respir. Dis. 125: 152–157, 1982.

3296. Vozeh, S., Kewitz, G., Perrouchoud, A., Tschan, M., Kopp, C., Heitz, M., and Follath, F. Theophylline serum concentration and therapeutic effect in severe acute bronchial obstruction: the optimal use of intravenously administered aminophylline. Am. Rev. Respir. Dis. 125: 181–184, 1982.

3297. Pang, J. A., Butland, R. J. A., Brooks, N., Cattell, M., and Geddes, D. M. Impaired lung uptake of propanolol in human pulmonary emphysema. Am. Rev. Respir. Dis. 125: 194–198, 1982.

3298. Goldstein, R. Response of the aging hamster lung to elastase injury. Am. Rev. Respir. Dis. 125: 295–298, 1982.

3299. Lucey, E. C., Snider, G. L., and Javaheri, S. Pulmonary ventilation and blood gas values in emphysematous hamsters. Am. Rev. Respir. Dis. 125: 299–303, 1982.

3300. Pak, C. C. F., Kradjan, W. A., Lakshminarayan, S., and Marini, J. J. Inhaled atropine sulfate: dose-response characteristics in adult patients with chronic airflow obstruction. Am. Rev. Respir. Dis. 125: 331–334, 1982.

3301. Murciano, D., Aubier, M., Viau, F., Bussi, S., Milic-Emili, J., Pariente, R., and Derenne, J-P. Effects of airway anesthesia on pattern of breathing and blood gases in patients with chronic obstructive pulmonary disease during acute respiratory failure. Am. Rev. Respir. Dis. 126: 113–117, 1982.

3302. Poe, R. H., Israel, R. H., Utell, M. J., and Hall, W. J. Chronic cough: bronchoscopy or pulmonary function testing? Am. Rev. Respir. Dis. 126: 160–162, 1982.

3303. Calverley, P. M. A., Leggett, R. J., McElderry, L., and Flenley, D. C. Cigarette smoking and secondary polycythemia in hypoxic cor pulmonale. Am. Rev. Respir. Dis. 125: 507–510, 1982.

3304. Petty, T. L., Silvers, G. W., and Stanford, R. E. Small airway dimension and size distribution in human lungs with an increased closing capacity. Am. Rev. Respir. Dis. 125: 535–539, 1982.

3305. Clement, J. and Van De Woestijne, K. P. Rapidly decreasing forced expiratory volume in one second or vital capacity and development of chronic airflow obstruction. Am. Rev. Respir. Dis. 125: 553–558, 1982.

3306. Horne, S. L., Tennent, R. K., and Cockcroft, D. W. A new anodal alpha$_1$-antitrypsin variant associated with emphysema: Pi Bsaskatoon. Am. Rev. Respir. Dis. 125: 594–600, 1982.

3307. Aldrich, T. K., Arora, N. S., and Rochester, D. F. The influence of airway obstruction and respiratory muscle strength on maximal voluntary ventilation in lung disease. Am. Rev. Respir. Dis. 126: 195–199, 1982.

3308. Delgado, H. R., Braun, S. R., Skatrud, J. B., Reddan, W.

3309. G., and Pegelow, D. F. Chest wall and abdominal motion during exercise in patients with chronic obstructive pulmonary disease. Am. Rev. Respir. Dis. 126: 200–205, 1982.

3309. Calverley, P. M. A., Brezinova, V., Douglas, N. J., Catterall, J. R., and Flenley, D. C. The effect of oxygenation on sleep quality in chronic bronchitis and emphysema. Am. Rev. Respir. Dis. 126: 206–210, 1982.

3310. Moore, L. G., Rohr, A. L., Maisenbach, J. K., and Reeves, J. T. Emphysema mortality is increased in Colorado residents at high altitude. Am. Rev. Respir. Dis. 126: 225–228, 1982.

3311. Cohen, A. B., Chenoweth, D. E., and Hugli, T. E. The release of elastase, myeloperoxidase, and lysozyme from human alveolar macrophages. Am. Rev. Respir. Dis. 126: 241–247, 1982.

3312. Bake, B., Larsson, S., and Mossberg, B. (eds.). Chronic bronchitis in non-smokers. Eur. J. Respir. Dis. 63(Suppl. 118): 1982.

3313. David, P., Denis, P., Nouvet, G., Pasquis, P., Lefrançois, R., and Morere, P. Fonction respiratoire et reflux gastro-oesophagien au cours de la bronchite chronique. Bull. Eur. Physiopathol. Respir. 18: 81–86, 1982.

3314. Parot, S., Saunier, C., Schrijen, F., Gautier, H., and Milic-Emili, J. Concomitant changes in function tests, breathing pattern and PaCO$_2$ in patients with chronic obstructive pulmonary disease. Bull. Eur. Physiopathol. Respir. 18: 145–151, 1982.

3315. Brundler, J. P., Lewis, C. M., and De Kock, M. A. Functional classification of chronic airflow limitation based on flow-volume and single-breath nitrogen washout criteria. Respiration 44: 1–9, 1983.

3316. Magnussen, H., Kluwig, M., Scheidt, M., Jorres, R., and Kesseler, K. Effect of breath-holding on expired gas concentrations of He and SF6 in healthy subjects and patients with obstructive lung disease. Bull. Eur. Physiopathol. Respir. 18: 255–259, 1982.

3317. Nenci, G. G., Berrettini, M., Todisco, T., Costantini, V., and Grasselli, S. Exhausted platelets in chronic obstructive pulmonary disease. Respiration 44: 71–76, 1983.

3318. Cutillo, A., Perondi, R., Turiel, M., Bigler, A. H., Watanabe, S., and Renzetti, A. D. Jr. Pulmonary resistance and dynamic compliance as functions of respiratory frequency. Respiration 44: 81–89, 1983.

3319. Marazzini, L., Cavestri, R., Mastropasqua, B., Banducci, S., Pelucchi, A., and Longhini, E. Pressure available for expiration in chronic airway disease. Respiration 44: 241–251, 1983.

3320. Rasche, B., Hochstrasser, K., Albrecht, G. J., and Ulmer, W. T. An elastase-specific inhibitor from human bronchial mucus. Pathogenesis in lung emphysema. Respiration 44: 397–402, 1983.

3321. Tobin, M. J., Jenouri, G., and Sackner, M. A. Effect of naloxone on breathing pattern in patients with chronic obstructive pulmonary disease with and without hypercapnia. Respiration 44: 419–424, 1983.

3322. Stradling, J. R., Barnes, P., and Pride, N. B. The effects of almitrine on the ventilatory response to hypoxia and hypercapnia in normal subjects. Clin. Sci. 63: 401–404, 1982.

3323. Lippmann, M. and Fein, A. Pulmonary embolism in the patient with chronic obstructive, pulmonary disease. Chest 79: 39–42, 1981.

3324. Dosman, J. A. and Cotton, D. J. Interpretation of tests of early lung dysfunction. Chest 79: 261–262, 1981.

3325. Gelb, A. F., Gobel, P. H., Fairshter, R., and Zamel, N. Predominant site of airway resistance in chronic obstructive pulmonary disease. Chest 79: 273–276, 1981.

3326. Casciari, R. J., Fairshter, R. D., Harrison, A., Morrison, J. T., Blackburn, C. M., and Wilson, A. F. Effects of breathing retraining in patients with chronic obstructive pulmonary disease. Chest 79: 393–398, 1981.

3327. Chester, E. H., Schwartz, H. J., and Fleming, G. M. Adverse effect of propanolol on airway function in nonasthmatic chronic obstructive lung disease. Chest 79: 540–544, 1981.

3328. DeMarco, F. J., Wynee, J. W., Block, A. J., Boysen, P. G., and Taasen, V. C. Oxygen desaturation during sleep as a determinant of the "blue and bloated" syndrome. Chest 79: 621–625, 1981.

3329. Stein, D. A., Bradley, B. L., and Miller, W. C. Mechanisms of oxygen effects on exercise in patients with chronic obstructive pulmonary disease. Chest 81: 6–10, 1982.

3330. Kawakami, Y., Terai, T., Yamamoto, H., and Murao, M. Exercise and oxygen inhalation in relation to prognosis of chronic pulmonary disease. Chest 81: 182–188, 1982.

3331. Fletcher, E. C. and Martin, R. J. Sexual dysfunction and erectile impotence in chronic obstructive pulmonary disease. Chest 81: 413–421, 1982.

3332. Sonne, L. J. and Davis, J. A. Increased exercise performance in patients with severe COPD following inspiratory resistive training. Chest 81: 436–439, 1982.

3333. Belman, M. J. and Kendregan, B. A. Physical training fails to improve ventilatory muscle endurance in patients with chronic obstructive pulmonary disease. Chest 81: 440–443, 1982.

3334. Martin, T. R., Lewis, S. W., and Albert, R. K. The prognosis of patients with chronic obstructive pulmonary disease after hospitalization for acute respiratory failure. Chest 82: 310–314, 1982.

3335. Cockcroft, D. W. and Horne, S. L. Localization of emphysema within the lung. Chest 82: 483–487, 1982.

3336. Eaton, M. L., MacDonald, F. M., Church, T. R., and Niewohner, D. E. Effects of theophylline on breathlessness and exercise tolerance in patients with chronic airflow obstruction. Chest 82: 538–542, 1982.

3337. Driver, A. G., McAlevy, M. T., and Smith, J. L. Nutritional assessment of patients with chronic obstructive pulmonary disease and acute respiratory failure. Chest 82: 568–571, 1982.

3338. Arand, D. L., McGinty, D. J., and Littner, M. R. Respiratory patterns associated with hemoglobin desaturation during sleep in chronic obstructive pulmonary disease. Chest 80: 183–190, 1981.

3339. Marini, J. J., Lakshminarayan, S., and Kradjan, W. A. Atropine and terbutaline aerosols in chronic bronchitis. Chest 80: 285–291, 1981.

3340. Bowen, J. H., Woodard, B. H., and Pratt, P. C. Bronchial collapse in obstructive lung disease. Chest 80: 510–513, 1981.

3341. Lalli, C. M. and Raju, L. Pregnancy and chronic obstructive pulmonary disease. Chest 80: 759–761, 1981.

3342. Opernbrier, D. R., Irwin, M. M., Rogers, R. M., Gottlieb, G. P., Dauber, J. H., Van Thiel, D. H., and Pennock, B. E. Nutritional status and lung function in patients with emphysema and chronic bronchitis. Chest 83: 17–22, 1983.

3343. Homma, H., Yamanaka, A., Tanimoto, S., Tamura, M., Chijimatsu, Y., Kira, S., and Izumi, T. Diffuse panbronchiolitis: a disease of the transitional zone of the lung. Chest 83: 63–69, 1983.

3344. Popio, K. A., Jackson, D. H. Jr., Utell, M. J., Swinburne, A. J., and Hyde, R. W. Inhalation challenge with carbachol and isoproterenol to predict bronchospastic response to propanolol in COPD. Chest 83: 175–179, 1983.

3345. Hughes, R. L. and Davison, R. Limitations of exercise reconditioning in COLD. Chest 83: 241–249, 1983.

3346. Ries, A. L., Fedullo, P. F., and Clausen, J. L. Rapid changes in arterial blood gas levels after exercise in pulmonary patients. Chest 83: 454–456, 1983.

3347. Wagener, J. S., Sobonya, R. E., Taussig, L. M., and Lemen, R. J. Unusual abnormalities in adolescent siblings with alpha₁-antitrypsin deficiency. Chest 83: 464–468, 1983.

3348. Dolly, F. R. and Block, A. J. Increased ventricular ectopy and sleep apnea following ethanol ingestion in COPD patients. Chest 83: 469–472, 1983.

3349. Melot, C., Naeije, R., Rothschild, T., Mertens, P., Mols, P., and Hallemans, R. Improvement in ventilation-perfusion matching by almitrine in COPD. Chest 83: 528–533, 1983.

3350. Hoidal, J. R. and Niewohner, D. E. Pathogenesis of emphysema. Chest 83: 679–685, 1983.

3351. Pardy, R. L. and Roussos, C. Endurance of hyperventilation in chronic airflow limitation. Chest 83: 744–750, 1983.

3352. Kinsman, R. A., Yaroush, R. A., Fernandez, E., Dirks, J. F., Schocket, M., and Fukuhara, J. Symptoms and experiences in chronic bronchitis and emphysema. Chest 83: 755–761, 1983.

3353. Mookherjee, S., Ashutosh, K., Smulyan, H., Vardan, S., and

3354. Warner, R. Arterial oxygenation and pulmonary function with saralasin in chronic lung disease. Chest 83: 842–847, 1983.

3354. Manier, G., Guenard, H., Castaing, Y., and Varene, N. Etude par les gaz inertes des echanges gazeux en heliox chez les malades atteints de BPCO. Bull. Eur. Physiopathol. Respir. 19: 401–406, 1983.

3355. Servera, E., Gimenez, M., Mohan-Kumar, T., Candina, R., and Bonassis, J. B. Oxygen uptake at maximal exercises in chronic airflow obstruction. Bull. Eur. Physiopathol. Respir. 19: 553–556, 1983.

3356. Gaultier, C., Boule, M., Tournier, G., and Girard, F. Effects of naloxone on the control of breathing in children with chronic obstructive pulmonary disease. Bull. Eur. Physiopathol. Respir. 19: 557–561, 1983.

3357. Higgins, M. W., Keller, J. B., Landis, J. R., Beaty, T. H., Burrows, B., Demets, D., Diem, J. E., Higgins, I. T. T., Lakatos, E., Lebowitz, M. D., Menkes, H., Speizer, F. E., Tager, I. B., and Weill, H. Risk of chronic obstructive pulmonary disease. Am. Rev. Respir. Dis. 130: 380–385, 1984.

3358. Lungarella, G., Fonzi, L., and Ermini, G. Abnormalities of bronchial cilia in patients with chronic bronchitis. Lung 161: 147–156, 1983.

3359. Berend, N. A correlation of lung structure with function. Lung 160: 115–130, 1982.

3360. Woodcock, A. A., Gross, E. R., Gellert, A., Shah, S., Johnson, M., and Geddes, D. M. Effects of dihydrocodeine, alcohol, and caffeine on breathlessness and exercise tolerance in patients with chronic obstructive lung disease and normal blood gases. N. Engl. J. Med. 305: 1611–1616, 1981.

3361. Laurent, P., Janoff, A., and Kagan, H. M. Cigarette smoke blocks cross-linking of elastin in vitro. Am. Rev. Respir. Dis. 127: 189–192, 1983.

3362. Dull, W. L., Alexander, M. R., Sadoul, P., and Woolson, R. F. The efficacy of isoproterenol inhalation for predicting the response to orally administered theophylline in chronic obstructive pulmonary disease. Am. Rev. Respir. Dis. 126: 656–659, 1982.

3363. Yernault, J-C., Paiva, M., Ravez, P., Van Muylem, A., Mertens, P., and Rozen, D. Effect of almitrine on the mechanics of breathing in normal man. Bull. Eur. Physiopathol. Respir. 18: 659–663, 1982.

3364. Bates, D. V. Perspectives on the Annual Aspen Lung Conference. Chest 85(Suppl.): 74S–75S, 1984.

3365. Laurent, G. J. and McAnulty, R. J. Protein metabolism during bleomycin-induced pulmonary fibrosis in rabbits. Am. Rev. Respir. Dis. 128: 82–88, 1983.

3366. Rotman, H. H., Lavelle, T. F., Dimcheff, D. G., Vandenbelt, R. J., and Weg, J. G. Long-term physiologic consequences of the adult respiratory distress syndrome. Chest 72: 190–192, 1977.

3367. Murphy, K. C., Atkins, C. J., Offer, R. C., Hogg, J. C., and Stein, H. B. Obliterative bronchiolitis in two rheumatoid arthritis patients treated with penicillamine. Arthritis Rheum. 24: 557–560, 1981.

3368. Pare, P. D., Brooks, L. A., Bates, J., Lawson, L. M., Nelems, J. M. B., Wright, J. L., and Hogg, J. C. Exponential analysis of the lung pressure-volume curve as a predictor of pulmonary emphysema. Am. Rev. Respir. Dis. 126: 54–61, 1982.

3369. The Health Consequences of Smoking Chronic Obstructive Lung Disease. A Report of the Surgeon General. DHHS (PHS) 84-50205. US Dept of Health and Human Services, Washington, D.C., 1984.

3370. Barnes, P. J., Basbaum, C. B., and Nadel, J. A. Autoradiographic localization of autonomic receptors in airway smooth muscle. Am. Rev. Respir. Dis. 127: 758–762, 1983.

3371. Sheppard, D., Rizk, N. W., Boushey, H. A., and Bethel, R. A. Mechanism of cough and bronchoconstriction induced by distilled water aerosol. Am. Rev. Respir. Dis. 127: 691–694, 1983.

3372. Thomson, N. C., Daniel, E. E., and Hargreave, F. E. Role of smooth muscle alpha₁-receptors in nonspecific bronchial responsiveness in asthma. Am. Rev. Respir. Dis. 126: 521–525, 1982.

3373. Weinberger, S. E., Weiss, S. T., Johnson, T. S., Von Gal, E., and Balsavich, L. Naloxone does not affect bronchoconstriction induced by isocapnic hyperpnea of subfreezing air. Am. Rev. Respir. Dis. 126: 468–471, 1982.

3374. Marom, Z., Shelhamer, J. H., Bach, M. K., Morton, D. R., and Kaliner, M. Slow-reacting substances, leukotrienes C₄ and D₄, increase the release of mucus from human airways in vitro. Am. Rev. Respir. Dis. 126: 449–451, 1982.

3375. Benumof, J. L. and Trousdale, F. R. Aminophylline does not inhibit canine hypoxic pulmonary vasoconstriction. Am. Rev. Respir. Dis. 126: 1017–1019, 1982.

3376. Burdon, J. G. W., Juniper, E. F., Killian, K. J., Hargreave, F. E., and Campbell, E. J. M. The perception of breathlessness in asthma. Am. Rev. Respir. Dis. 126: 825–828, 1982.

3377. Martin, J. G., Shore, S., and Engel, L. A. Effect of continuous positive airway pressure on respiratory mechanics and pattern of breathing in induced asthma. Am. Rev. Respir. Dis. 126: 812–817, 1982.

3378. Ben-Zvi, Z., Spohn, W. A., Young, S. H., and Kattan, M. Hypnosis for exercise-induced asthma. Am. Rev. Respir. Dis. 125: 392–395, 1982.

3379. Klein, J. J., Lefkowitz, M. S., Spector, S. L., and Cherniack, R. M. Relationship between serum theophylline levels and pulmonary function before and after inhaled beta-agonist in "stable" asthmatics. Am. Rev. Respir. Dis. 127: 413–416, 1983.

3380. Abraham, W. M., Delehunt, J. C., Yerger, L., and Marchette, B. Characterization of a late phase pulmonary response after antigen challenge in allergic sheep. Am. Rev. Respir. Dis. 128: 839–844, 1983.

3381. Pasquis, P., Tardif, C., and Nouvet, G. Reflux gastro-oesophagien et affections respiratoires. Bull. Eur. Physiopathol. Respir. 19: 645–658, 1983.

3382. Gillioz, F. and Orehek, J. Reponse bronchique au carbachol et à l'hyperventilation isocapnique dans l'asthme. Bull. Eur. Physiopathol. Respir. 19: 563–566, 1983.

3383. Newman, S. P. and Clarke, S. W. Therapeutic aerosols 1—physical and practical considerations (editorial). Thorax 38: 881–886, 1983.

3384. Cushley, M. J., Lewis, R. A., and Tattersfield, A. E. Comparison of three techniques of inhalation on the airway response to terbutaline. Thorax 38: 908–913, 1983.

3385. Al-Damluji, S., Thompson, P. J., Citron, K. M., and Turner-Warwick, M. Effect of naloxone on circadian rhythms in lung function. Thorax 38: 914–918, 1983.

3386. Nogrady, S. G. and Furnass, S. B. Ionisers in the management of bronchial asthma. Thorax 38: 919–922, 1983.

3387. Barnes, P. J. Calcium-channel blockers and asthma (editorial). Thorax 38: 481–485, 1983.

3388. Dehaut, P., Rachielle, A., Martin, R. R., and Malo, J. L. Histamine dose-response curves in asthma: reproducibility and sensitivity of different indices to assess response. Thorax 38: 516–522, 1983.

3389. O'Byrne, P. M., Morris, M., Roberts, R., and Hargreave, F. E. Inhibition of the bronchial response to respiratory heat exchange by increasing doses of terbutaline sulphate. Thorax 37: 913–917, 1982.

3390. Walters, E. H. and Davies, B. H. Dual effect of prostaglandin E₂ on normal airways smooth muscle in vivo. Thorax 37: 918–922, 1982.

3391. Mohsenin, V., Dubois, A. B., and Douglas, J. S. Effect of ascorbic acid on response to methacholine challenge in asthmatic subjects. Am. Rev. Respir. Dis. 127: 143–147, 1983.

3392. Sovijarvi, A. R. A., Poyhonen, L., Kellomaki, L., and Muittari, A. Effects of acute and long-term bronchodilator treatment on regional lung function in asthma assessed with krypton-81m and technetium-99m-labelled macroaggregates. Thorax 37: 516–520, 1982.

3393. Patakas, D., Argiropoulou, V., Louridas, G., and Tsara, V. Beta-blockers in bronchial asthma: effect of propranolol and pindolol on large and small airways. Thorax 38: 108–112, 1983.

3394. Aquilina, A. T. Comparison of airway reactivity induced by histamine, methacholine, and isocapnic hyperventilation in normal and asthmatic subjects. Thorax 38: 766–770, 1983.

3395. Morgan, D. J. R., Moodley, I., Phillips, M. J., and Davies, R. J. Plasma histamine in asthmatic and control subjects following exercise: influence of circulating basophils and different assay techniques. Thorax 38: 771–777, 1983.

3396. Wilson, N. M., Barnes, P. J., Vickers, H., and Silverman, M. Hyperventilation-induced asthma: evidence for two mechanisms. Thorax 37: 657–662, 1982.

3397. Patel, K. R., Berkin, K. E., and Kerr, J. W. Dose-response study of sodium cromoglycate in exercise-induced asthma. Thorax 37: 663–666, 1982.

3398. Dawson, K. P., Fergusson, D. M., West, J., Wynne, C., and Sadler, W. A. Acute asthma and antidiuretic hormone secretion. Thorax 38: 589–591, 1983.

3399. Clague, H., Ahmad, D., Chamberlain, M. J., Morgan, W. K. C., and Vinitski, S. Histamine bronchial challenge: effect on regional ventilation and aerosol deposition. Thorax 38: 668–675, 1983.

3400. Bateman, J. R. M., Pavia, D., Sheahan, N. F., Agnew, J. E., and Clarke, S. W. Impaired tracheobronchial clearance in patients with mild stable asthma. Thorax 38: 463–467, 1983.

3401. Tullett, W. M., Patel, K. R., Berkin, K. E., and Kerr, J. W. Effect of lignocaine, sodium cromoglycate, and ipratropium bromide in exercise-induced asthma. Thorax 37: 737–740, 1982.

3402. Griffin, M. P., McFadden, E. R. Jr., Ingram, R. H. Jr., and Pardee, S. Controlled-analysis of the effects of inhaled lignocaine in exercise-induced asthma. Thorax 37: 741–745, 1982.

3403. Anderson, P. B., Goude, A., and Peake, M. D. Comparison of salbutamol given by intermittent positive-pressure breathing and pressure-packed aerosol in chronic asthma. Thorax 37: 612–616, 1982.

3404. Ben-Dov, I., Bar-Yishay, E., and Godfrey, S. Exercise-induced asthma without respiratory heat loss. Thorax 37: 630–631, 1982.

3405. Smith, J. M. The recent history of the treatment of asthma: a personal view. Thorax 38: 244–253, 1983.

3406. Anderson, S. D., Schoeffel, R. E., and Finney, M. Evaluation of ultrasonically nebulised solutions for provocation testing in patients with asthma. Thorax 38: 284–291, 1983.

3407. Stableforth, D. Death from asthma (editorial). Thorax 38: 801–805, 1983.

3408. Williams, A. J., Baghat, M. S., Stableforth, D. E., Clayton, R. M., Shenoi, P. M., and Skinner, C. Dysphonia caused by inhaled steroids: recognition of a characteristic laryngeal abnormality. Thorax 38: 813–821, 1983.

3409. Catterall, J. R., Calverley, P. M. A., Power, J. T., Shapiro, C. M., Douglas, N. J., and Flenley, D. C. Ketotifen and nocturnal asthma. Thorax 38: 845–848, 1983.

3410. Ben-Dov, I., Gur, I., Bar-Yishay, E., and Godfrey, S. Refractory period following induced asthma: contributions of exercise and isocapnic hyperventilation. Thorax 38: 849–853, 1983.

3411. Salome, C. M., Schoeffel, R. E., Yan, K., and Woolcock, A. J. Effect of aerosol fenoterol on the severity of bronchial hyperreactivity in patients with asthma. Thorax 38: 854–858, 1983.

3412. Montplaisir, J., Walsh, J., and Malo, J. L. Nocturnal asthma: features of attacks, sleep and breathing patterns. Am. Rev. Respir. Dis. 125: 18–22, 1982.

3413. Tashkin, D. P., Conolly, M. E., Deutsch, R. I., Hui, K. K., Littner, M., Scarpace, P., and Abrass, I. Subsensitization of beta-adrenoreceptors in airways and lymphocytes of healthy and asthmatic subjects. Am. Rev. Respir. Dis. 125: 185–193, 1982.

3414. Korsgaard, J. Preventive measures in house-dust allergy. Am. Rev. Respir. Dis. 125: 80–84, 1982.

3415. O'Byrne, P. M., Ryan, G., Morris, M., McCormack, D., Jones, N. L., Morse, J. L. C., and Hargreave, F. E. Asthma induced by cold air and its relation to nonspecific bronchial responsiveness to methacholine. Am. Rev. Respir. Dis. 125: 281–285, 1982.

3416. Young, I. H., Corte, P., and Schoeffel, R. E. Pattern and time course of ventilation-perfusion inequality in exercise-induced asthma. Am. Rev. Respir. Dis. 125: 304–311, 1982.

3417. Martin, J., Aubier, M., and Engel, L. A. Effects of inspiratory loading on respiratory muscle activity during expiration. Am. Rev. Respir. Dis. 125: 352–358, 1982.

3418. Hudgel, D. W., Cooperson, D. M., and Kinsman, R. A. Recognition of added resistive loads in asthma: the importance of behavioral styles. Am. Rev. Respir. Dis. 126: 121–125, 1982.

3419. Ben-Dov, I., Bar-Yishay, E., and Godfrey, S. Refractory period after exercise-induced asthma unexplained by respiratory heat loss. Am. Rev. Respir. Dis. 125: 530–534, 1982.

3420. Corkey, C., Mindorff, C., Levison, H., and Newth, C. Comparison of three different preparations of disodium cromoglycate in the prevention of exercise-induced bronchospasm. Am. Rev. Respir. Dis. 125: 623–626, 1982.

3421. Neijens, H. J., Hofkamp, M., Degenhart, H. J., and Kerrebijn, K. F. Bronchial responsiveness as a function of inhaled histamine and the methods of measurement. Bull. Eur. Physiopathol. Respir. 18: 427–438, 1982.

3422. Verhamme, M., Demedts, M., and Van de Woestijne, K. P. Changes in single-breath washout curves during recovery from an asthmatic attack. Bull. Eur. Physiopathol. Respir. 18: 353–360, 1982.

3423. Crompton, G., Moren, F., and Simonsson, B. G. (eds.). Inhalation Therapy in the Management of Airway Obstruction. Eur. J. Respir. Dis. 63(Suppl. 119): 1982.

3424. Jones, A. W. Effects of temperature and humidity of inhaled air on the concentration of ethanol in a man's exhaled breath. Clin. Sci. 63: 441–445, 1982.

3425. Chow, O. K. W., So, S. Y., Lam, W. K., Yu, D. Y. C., and Yeung, C. Y. Effect of acupuncture on exercise-induced asthma. Lung 161: 321–326, 1983.

3426. Chapman, K. R. and Rebuck, A. S. Inspiratory and expiratory resistive loading as a model of dyspnea in asthma. Respiration 44: 425–432, 1983.

3427. Jolobe, O. M. P. Impaired atropine responsiveness in asthma: role of atopy. Respiration 44: 97–102, 1983.

3428. Orehek, J., Beaupre, A., Badier, M., Nicoli, M. M., and Delpierre, S. Perception of airway tone by asthmatic patients. Bull. Eur. Physiopathol. Respir. 18: 601–607, 1982.

3429. Higgs, C. M. B., Richardson, R. B., and Laszlo, G. The effect of regular inhaled salbutamol on the airway responsiveness of normal subjects. Clin. Sci. 63: 513–517, 1982.

3430. Anderson, H. R., Bailey, P. A., and Bland, J. The effect of birth month on asthma, eczema, hayfever, respiratory symptoms, lung function, and hospital admissions for asthma. Int. J. Epidemiol. 10: 45–51, 1981.

3431. Fairshter, R. D., Novey, H. S., and Wilson, A. F. Site and duration of bronchodilation in asthmatic patients after oral administration of terbutaline. Chest 79: 50–57, 1981.

3432. Christensson, P., Arborelius, M. Jr., and Lilja, B. Salbutamol inhalation in chronic asthma bronchiale: dose aerosol vs jet nebulizer. Chest 79: 416–419, 1981.

3433. Pierce, R. J., Payne, C. R., Williams, S. J., Denison, D. M., and Clark, T. J. H. Comparison of intravenous and inhaled terbutaline in the treatment of asthma. Chest 79: 506–511, 1981.

3434. Chen, W. Y., Brenner, A. M., Weiser, P. C., and Chai, H. Atropine and exercise-induced bronchoconstriction. Chest 79: 651–656, 1981.

3435. Bernstein, I. L., Chervinsky, P., and Falliers, C. J. Efficacy and safety of triamcinolone acetonide aerosol in chronic asthma. Chest 81: 20–26, 1982.

3436. Kassabian, J., Miller, K. D., and Lavietes, M. H. Respiratory center output and ventilatory timing in patients with acute airway (asthma) and alveolar (pneumonia) disease. Chest 81: 536–543, 1982.

3437. Reynolds, H. Y. Immunologic lung diseases (part 1). Chest 81: 626–631, 1982.

3438. Chen, W. Y. and Chai, H. Airway cooling and nocturnal asthma. Chest 81: 675–680, 1982.

3439. Tanaka, R. M., Santiago, S. M., Kuhn, G. J., Williams, R. E., and Klaustermeyer, W. B. Intravenous methylprednisolone in adults in status asthmaticus. Chest 82: 438–440, 1982.

3440. Larsson, K., Hjemdahl, P., and Martinsson, A. Sympathoadrenal reactivity in exercise-induced asthma. Chest 82: 560–567, 1982.

3441. Gong, H. Jr., Tashkin, D. P., and Calvarese, B. M. Alcohol-induced bronchospasm in an asthmatic patient. Chest 80: 167–173, 1981.

3442. Zamel, N., Hughes, D., Levison, H., Fairshter, R. D., and Gelb, A. F. Partial and complete maximum expiratory flow-volume curves in asthmatic patients with spontaneous bronchospasm. Chest 83: 35–39, 1983.

3443. Terral, C., Bourgouin-Karaouni, D., Jonquet, O., Godard, P., and Prefaut, C. Effets de l'helium-oxygene au cours des tests de provocation bronchique chez l'asthmatique. Bull. Eur. Physiopathol. Respir. 19: 51–58, 1983.

3444. Rachiele, A., Malo, J. L., Cartier, A., Pineau, L., Ghezzo, H., and Martin, R. R. Circadian variations of airway response to histamine in asthmatic subjects. Bull. Eur. Physiopathol. Respir. 19: 465–469, 1983.

3445. Wolf, B., Gaultier, C., Lopez, C., Boule, M., and Girard, F. Hypoxemia in attack free asthmatic children: relationship with lung volumes and lung mechanics. Bull. Eur. Physiopathol. Respir. 19: 471–476, 1983.

3446. Denjean, A., Matran, R., Mathieu, M., Cerrina, J., Duroux, P., and Lockhart, A. Bronchial response to hyperventilation of dry air at room temperature in normals and asthmatics. Bull. Eur. Physiopathol. Respir. 19: 477–482, 1983.

3447. Machiels, J. and Ferriere, A. Reponse bronchique à l'acetylcholine et au dermatophagoides pteronissimus chez les asthmatiques asymptomatiques. Bull. Eur. Physiopathol. Respir. 19: 483–488, 1983.

3448. Hillman, D. R. and Finucane, K. E. The effect of hyperinflation on lung elasticity in healthy subjects. Respir. Physiol. 54: 295–305, 1983.

3449. Lewis, F. H., Beals, T. F., Carey, T. E., Baker, S. R., and Mathews, K. P. Ultrastructural and functional studies of cilia from patients with asthma, aspirin intolerance, and nasal polyps. Chest 83: 487–490, 1983.

3450. Orenstein, D. M., Franklin, B. A., Doerschuk, C. F., Hellerstein, H. K., Germann, K. J., Horowitz, J. G., and Stern, R. C. Exercise conditioning and cardiopulmonary fitness in cystic fibrosis. Chest 80: 392–398, 1981.

3451. Loughlin, G. M., Cota, K. A., and Taussig, L. M. The relationship between flow transients and bronchial lability in cystic fibrosis. Chest 79: 206–210, 1981.

3452. Boucher, R. C., Knowles, M. R., Stutts, M. J., and Gatzy, J. T. Epithelial dysfunction in cystic fibrosis lung disease. Lung 161: 1–17, 1983.

3453. Guidotti, T. L., Line, B. R., and Luetzeler, J. Cystic fibrosis related lung disease in young adults with minimal impairment. Respiration 44: 351–359, 1983.

3454. Mygind, N., Nielsen, M. H., and Pedersen, M. (eds.). Kartagener's Syndrome and Abnormal Cilia. Eur. J. Respir. Dis. 64(Suppl. 127): 1983.

3455. Chao, J., Turner, J. A. P., and Sturgess, J. M. Genetic heterogeneity of dynein-deficiency in cilia from patients with respiratory disease. Am. Rev. Respir. Dis. 126: 302–305, 1982.

3456. Cropp, G. J., Pullano, T. P., Cerny, F. J., and Nathanson, I. T. Exercise tolerance and cardiorespiratory adjustments at peak work capacity in cystic fibrosis. Am. Rev. Respir. Dis. 126: 211–216, 1982.

3457. Cerny, F. J., Pullano, T. P., and Cropp, G. J. A. Cardiorespiratory adaptations to exercise in cystic fibrosis. Am. Rev. Respir. Dis. 126: 217–220, 1982.

3458. Redding, G. J., Restuccia, R., Cotton, E. K., and Brooks, J. G. Serial changes in pulmonary functions in children hospitalized with cystic fibrosis. Am. Rev. Respir. Dis. 126: 31–36, 1982.

3459. Pearson, M. G. and Ogilvie, C. Surgical treatment of emphysematous bullae: late outcome. Thorax 38: 134–137, 1983.

3460. Neville, E., Brewis, R., Yeates, W. K., and Burridge, A. Respiratory tract disease and obstructive azoospermia. Thorax 38: 929–933, 1983.

3461. Murphy, M. B., Reen, D. J., and Fitzgerald, M. X. Atopy, immunological changes, and respiratory function in bronchiectasis. Thorax 39: 179–184, 1984.

3462. O'Neill, S., Leahy, F., Pasterkamp, H., and Tal, A. The effects of chronic hyperinflation, nutritional status, and posture on respiratory muscle strength in cystic fibrosis. Am. Rev. Respir. Dis. 128: 1051–1054, 1983.

3463. Holden, W. E., Mulkey, D. D., and Kessler, S. Multiple peripheral lung cysts and hemoptysis in an otherwise asymptomatic adult. Am. Rev. Respir. Dis. 126: 930–932, 1982.

3464. Asher, M. I., Pardy, R. L., Coates, A. L., Thomas, E., and Macklem, P. T. The effects of inspiratory muscle training in patients with cystic fibrosis. Am. Rev. Respir. Dis. 126: 855–859, 1982.

3465. Belin, L., Jarvholm, B., Larsson, S., and Thiringer, G. (eds.). Chest Disease and the Working Environment. Eur. J. Respir. Dis. 61(Suppl. 107): 1980.

3466. Weitzenblum, E., Ehrhart, M., Rasaholinjanahary, J., and Hirth, C. Pulmonary hemodynamics in idiopathic pulmonary fibrosis and other interstitial pulmonary diseases. Respiration 44: 118–127, 1983.

3467. Keith, H. H., Holsclaw, D. S. Jr., and Dunsky, E. H. Pigeon breeder's disease in children. Chest 79: 107–110, 1981.

3468. Reyes, C. N., Wenzel, F. J., Lawton, B. R., and Emanuel, D. A. The pulmonary pathology of farmer's lung disease. Chest 81: 142–146, 1982.

3469. Reynolds, H. Y. Immunologic lung diseases (part 2). Chest 81: 745–751, 1982.

3470. Earis, J. E., Marsh, K., Pearson, M. G., and Ogilvie, C. M. The inspiratory "squawk" in extrinsic allergic alveolitis and other pulmonary fibroses. Thorax 37: 923–926, 1982.

3471. Van den Bosch, J. M. M., Van Toorn, D. W., and Wagenaar, S. S. Coffee worker's lung: reconsideration of a case report (letter to editor). Thorax 38: 720, 1983.

3472. Cuthbert, O. D. and Gordon, M. F. Ten year follow up of farmers with farmer's lung. Br. J. Ind. Med. 40: 173–176, 1983.

3473. Costabel, U., Matthys, H., and Ruehle, K.-H. Pulmonary arterial hypertension in extrinsic allergic alveolitis (EAA) (letter to editor). Am. Rev. Respir. Dis. 126: 184, 1982.

3474. Schuyler, M. R., Kleinerman, J., Pensky, J. R., Brandt, C., and Schmitt, D. Pulmonary response to repeated exposure to Micropolyspora faeni. Am. Rev. Respir. Dis. 128: 1071–1076, 1983.

3475. Campbell, J. A., Kryda, M. J., Treuhaft, M. W., Marx, J. J. Jr., and Roberts, R. C. Cheese worker's hypersensitivity pneumonitis. Am. Rev. Respir. Dis. 127: 495–496, 1983.

3476. Solal-Celigny, P., Laviolette, M., Hebert, J., and Cormier, Y. Immune reactions in the lungs of asymptomatic dairy farmers. Am. Rev. Respir. Dis. 126: 964–967, 1982.

3477. Bye, P. T. P., Anderson, S. D., Woolcock, A. J., Young, I. H., and Alison, J. A. Bicycle endurance performance of patients with interstitial lung disease breathing air and oxygen. Am. Rev. Respir. Dis. 126: 1005–1012, 1982.

3478. Asherson, R. A., Mackworth-Young, C. G., Boey, M. L., Hull, R. G., Saunders, A., Gharavi, A. E., and Hughes, G. R. V. Pulmonary hypertension in systemic lupus erythematosus. Br. Med. J. 287: 1024–1025, 1983.

3479. Chappell, T. R., Rubin, L. J., Marckham, R. V. Jr., and Firth, B. G. Independence of oxygen consumption and systemic oxygen transport in patients with either stable pulmonary hypertension or refractory left ventricular failure. Am. Rev. Respir. Dis. 128: 30–33, 1983.

3480. Horn, M., Ries, A., Neveu, C., and Moser, K. Restrictive ventilatory pattern in precapillary pulmonary hypertension. Am. Rev. Respir. Dis. 128: 163–165, 1983.

3481. D'Alonzo, G. E., Bower, J. S., Dehart, P., and Dantzker, D. R. The mechanisms of abnormal gas exchange in acute massive pulmonary embolism. Am. Rev. Respir. Dis. 128: 170–172, 1983.

3482. Pare, P. D., Warriner, B., Baile, E. M., and Hogg, J. C. Redistribution of pulmonary extravascular water with positive end-expiratory pressure in canine pulmonary edema. Am. Rev. Respir. Dis. 127: 590–593, 1983.

3483. Romaldini, H., Rodriguez-Roisin, R., Wagner, P. D., and West, J. B. Enhancement of hypoxic pulmonary vasoconstriction by almitrine in the dog. Am. Rev. Respir. Dis. 128: 288–293, 1983.

3484. Ahmed, T., Oliver, W. Jr., and Wanner, A. Variability of hypoxic pulmonary vasoconstriction in sheep. Am. Rev. Respir. Dis. 127: 59–62, 1983.

3485. Nakahara, K., Nanjo, S., Maeda, M., and Kawashima, Y. Dynamic insufficiency of lung lymph flow from the right lymph duct in dogs with acute filtration edema. Am. Rev. Respir. Dis. 127: 67–71, 1983.

3486. Coates, G., Powles, A. C. P., Morrison, S. C., Sutton, J. R., Webber, C. E., and Zylak, C. J. The effects of intravenous infusion of saline on lung density, lung volumes, nitrogen washout, computed tomographic scans, and chest radiographs in humans. Am. Rev. Respir. Dis. 127: 91–96, 1983.

3487. McDonnell, P. J., Toye, P. A., and Hutchins, G. M. Primary pulmonary hypertension and cirrhosis: are they related? Am. Rev. Respir. Dis. 127: 437–441, 1983.

3488. Tate, R. M., Vanbenthuysen, K. M., Shasby, D. M., McMurtry, I. F., and Repine, J. E. Oxygen-radical-mediated permeability edema and vasoconstriction in isolated perfused rabbit lungs. Am. Rev. Respir. Dis. 126: 802–806, 1982.

3489. Barie, P. S., Tahamont, M. V., and Malik, A. B. Prevention of increased pulmonary vascular permeability after pancreatitis by granulocyte depletion in sheep. Am. Rev. Respir. Dis. 126: 904–908, 1982.

3490. Xue, Q. F., Macnee, W., Flenley, D. C., Hannan, W. J., Adie, C. J., and Muir, A. L. Can right ventricular performance be assessed by equilibrium radionuclide ventriculography? Thorax 38: 486–493, 1983.

3491. Macnee, W., Xue, Q. F., Hannan, W. J., Flenley, D. C., Adie, C. J., and Muir, A. L. Assessment by radionuclide angiography of right and left ventricular function in chronic bronchitis and emphysema. Thorax 38: 494–500, 1983.

3492. Howard, P. Oxygen in the home (editorial). Thorax 38: 161–164, 1983.

3493. Westaby, S. Complement and the damaging effects of cardiopulmonary bypass (editorial). Thorax 38: 321–325, 1983.

3494. Chung, K. F., Keyes, S. J., Morgan, B. M., Jones, P. W., and Snashall, P. D. Mechanisms of airway narrowing in acute pulmonary oedema in dogs: influence of the vagus and lung volume. Clin. Sci. 65: 289–296, 1983.

3495. Rhodes, K. M., Evemy, K., Nariman, S., and Gibson, G. J. Relation between severity of mitral valve disease and results of routine lung function tests in non-smokers. Thorax 37: 751–755, 1982.

3496. Farber, H. W., Fairman, R. P., and Glauser, F. L. Talc granulomatosis: laboratory findings similar to sarcoidosis. Am. Rev. Respir. Dis. 125: 258–261, 1982.

3497. Luce, J. M., Robertson, H. T., Huang, T., Colley, P. S., Gronka, R., Nessly, M. L., and Cheney, F. W. The effects of expiratory positive airway pressure on the resolution of oleic acid-induced lung injury in dogs. Am. Rev. Respir. Dis. 125: 716–722, 1982.

3498. Ahmed, T., Oliver, W. Jr., Frank, B. L., Robinson, M. J., and Wanner, A. Hypoxic pulmonary vasoconstriction in conscious sheep. Am. Rev. Respir. Dis. 126: 291–297, 1982.

3499. Chetty, K. G., Brown, S. E., and Light, R. W. Identification of pulmonary hypertension in chronic obstructive pulmonary disease from routine chest radiographs. Am. Rev. Respir. Dis. 126: 338–341, 1982.

3500. Hawrylkiewicz, I., Izdebska-Makosa, Z., Grebska, E., and Zielinski, J. Pulmonary haemodynamics at rest and on exercise in patients with idiopathic pulmonary fibrosis. Bull. Eur. Physiopathol. Respir. 18: 403–410, 1982.

3501. Rolla, G., Bucca, C., Polizzi, S., Giachino, O., Maina, A., Arossa, W., and Spinaci, S. Site of airways obstruction after rapid saline infusion in healthy subjects. Respiration 44: 90–96, 1983.

3502. Weitzenblum, E., Ehrhart, M., Rasaholinjanahary, J., and Hirth, C. Pulmonary hemodynamics in idiopathic pulmonary fibrosis and other interstitial pulmonary diseases. Respiration 44: 118–127, 1983.

3503. Bertoli, L., Rizzato, G., Sala, G., Merlini, R., Cicero, S. L., and Pezzano, A. Echocardiographic and hemodynamic assessment of right heart impairment in chronic obstructive lung disease. Respiration 44: 282–288, 1983.

3504. Petrini, M. F., Phillips, M. S., Dwyer, T. M., and Norman, J. R. Reproducibility of rebreathing parameters in normal humans. Lung 161: 327–335, 1983.

3505. Hammer, S. P., Winterbauer, R. H., Bockus, D., Remington, F., Sale, G. E., and Meyers, J. D. Endothelial cell damage and tuboreticular structures in interstitial lung disease associated with collagen vascular disease and viral pneumonia. Am. Rev. Respir. Dis. 127: 77–84, 1983.

3506. Carlson, R. W., Schaeffer, R. C. Jr., Carpio, M., and Weil, M. H. Edema fluid and coagulation changes during fulminant pulmonary edema. Chest 79: 43–49, 1981.

3507. Fanta, C. H., Wright, T. C., and McFadden, E. R. Jr. Differentiation of recurrent pulmonary emboli from chronic obstructive lung disease as a cause of cor pulmonale. Chest 79: 92–95, 1981.

3508. Bunch, T. W., Tancredi, R. G., and Lie, J. T. Pulmonary hypertension in polymyositis. Chest 79: 105–107, 1981.

3509. Guenter, C. A. and Braun, T. E. Fat embolism syndrome. Chest 79: 143–145, 1981.

3510. Riedel, M., Stanek, V., Widimsky, J., and Prerovsky, I. Longterm follow-up of patients with pulmonary thromboembolism. Chest 81: 151–158, 1982.

3511. Fein, I. A. and Rackow, E. C. Neurogenic pulmonary edema. Chest 81: 318–320, 1982.

3512. Dantzker, D. R. and Bower, J. S. Alterations in gas exchange following pulmonary thromboembolism. Chest 81: 495–501, 1982.

3513. Schrijen, F. and Urtiaga, B. Pulmonary blood volume in chronic lung disease. Chest 81: 544–549, 1982.

3514. Iskandrian, A. S., Hakki, A-H., Kane, S. A., and Segal, B. L. Changes in pulmonary blood volume during upright exercise. Chest 82: 54–58, 1982.

3515. De Olazabal, J. R., Miller, M. J., Cook, W. R., and Mithoefer, J. C. Disordered breathing and hypoxia during sleep in coronary artery disease. Chest 82: 548–552, 1982.

3516. Louridas, G., Galanis, N., and Patakas, D. Vectorcardiographic and hemodynamic correlation in chronic obstructive pulmonary disease. Chest 82: 593–597, 1982.

3517. Melot, C., Naeije, R., Mols, P., Vandenbossche, J.-L., and Denolin, H. Effects of nifedipine on ventilation/perfusion matching in primary pulmonary hypertension. Chest 83: 203–207, 1983.

3518. Nery, L. E., Wasserman, K., French, W., Oren, A., and Davis, J. A. Contrasting cardiovascular and respiratory responses to exercise in mitral valve and chronic obstructive pulmonary diseases. Chest 83: 446–453, 1983.

3519. Sibbald, W. J., Warshawski, F. J., Short, A. K., Harris, J., Lefcoe, M. S., and Holliday, R. L. Clinical studies of measuring extravascular lung water by the thermal dye technique in critically ill patients. Chest 83: 725–731, 1983.

3520. Fernandez-Bonetti, P., Lupi-Herrera, E., Martinez-Guerra, M. L., Barrios, R., Seoane, M., and Sandoval, J. Peripheral airways obstruction in idiopathic pulmonary artery hypertension (primary). Chest 83: 732–737, 1983.

3521. Mojarad, M., Hamasaki, Y., and Said, S. I. Platelet-activating factor increases pulmonary microvascular permeability and induces pulmonary edema. Bull. Eur. Physiopathol. Respir. 19: 253–256, 1983.

3522. Weitzenblum, E., Zielinski, J., and Bishop, J. M. The diagnosis of "cor pulmonale" by non-invasive methods: a challenge for pulmonologists and cardiologists (editorial). Bull. Eur. Physiopathol. Respir. 19: 423–426, 1983.

3523. Camus, P., Degat, O. R., Justrabo, E., and Jeannin, L. D-Penicillamine-induced severe pneumonitis. Chest 81: 376–378, 1982.

3524. Fulmer, J. D. The interstitial lung diseases. Chest 82: 173–178, 1982.

3525. Fulmer, J. D. and Kaltreider, H. B. The pulmonary vasculitides. Chest 82: 615–624, 1982.

3526. Kinney, W. W. and Angelillo, V. A. Bronchiolitis in systemic lupus erythematosus. Chest 82: 646–649, 1982.

3527. Karam, G. H. and Fulmer, J. D. Giant cell arteritis presenting as interstitial lung disease. Chest 82: 781–784, 1982.

3528. Strumpf, I. J., Feld, M. K., Cornelius, M. J., Keogh, B. A., and Crystal, R. G. Safety of fiberoptic bronchoalveolar lavage in evaluation of interstitial lung disease. Chest 80: 268–271, 1981.

3529. Bradley, S. L., Dines, D. E., Banks, P. M., and Hill, R. W. The lung in immunoblastic lymphadenopathy. Chest 80: 312–318, 1981.

3530. Clee, M. D., Lamb, D., Urbaniak, S. J., and Clark, R. A. Progressive bronchocentric granulomatosis: case report. Thorax 37: 947–949, 1982.

3531. Jones, D. A., Pillai, D. K., Rathbone, B. J., and Cookson, J. B. Persisting "asthma" in tropical pulmonary eosinophilia. Thorax 38: 692–693, 1983.

3532. Barnes, N., Gray, B. J., Heaton, R., and Costello, J. F. Pulmonary eosinophilia in identical twins. Thorax 38: 318–319, 1983.

3533. McCann, B. G., Hart, G. J., Stokes, T. C., and Harrison, B. D. W. Obliterative bronchiolitis and upper-zone pulmonary consolidation in rheumatoid arthritis. Thorax 38: 73–74, 1983.

3534. Kullberg, F. C., Funahashi, A., and Siegesmund, K. A. Pulmonary eosinophilic granuloma: electron microscopic detection of X-bodies on lung lavage cell and transbronchoscopic lung biopsy in one patient. Ann. Intern. Med. 96: 188–189, 1982.

3535. Edwards, C., Penny, M., and Newman, J. Mycoplasma pneumonia, Stevens-Johnson syndrome, and chronic obliterative bronchitis. Thorax 38: 867–869, 1983.

3536. Robinson, R. G., Wehunt, W. D., Tsou, E., Koss, M. N., and Hochholzer, L. Bronchocentric granulomatosis: roentgenographic manifestations. Am. Rev. Respir. Dis. 125: 751–756, 1982.

3537. Baile, E. M., Wright, J. L., Pare, P. D., and Hogg, J. C. The effect of acute small airway inflammation on pulmonary function in dogs. Am. Rev. Respir. Dis. 126: 298–301, 1982.

3538. Weidemann, H. P., Bensinger, R. E., and Hudson, L. D. Bronchocentric granulomatosis with eye involvement. Am. Rev. Respir. Dis. 126: 347–350, 1982.

3539. Kaelin, R. M., Canter, D. M., Bernardo, J., Grant, M., and Snider, G. L. The role of macrophage-derived chemotattractant activities in the early inflammatory events of bleomycin-induced pulmonary injury. Am. Rev. Respir. Dis. 128: 132–137, 1983.

3540. Wesselius, L. J., Witztum, K. F., Taylor, A. T., Hartman, M. T., and Moser, K. M. Computer-assisted versus visual lung gallium-67 index in normal subjects and in patients with interstitial lung disorders. Am. Rev. Respir. Dis. 128: 1084–1089, 1983.

3541. Libby, D. M., Gibofsky, A., Fotino, M., Waters, S. J., and Smith, J. P. Immunogenetic and clinical findings in idiopathic pulmonary fibrosis. Am. Rev. Respir. Dis. 127: 618–622, 1983.

3542. Hakkinen, P. J., Schmoyer, R. L., and Witschi, H. P. Potentiation of butylated-hydroxytoluene-induced acute lung damage by oxygen. Am. Rev. Respir. Dis. 128: 648–651, 1983.

3543. Jakab, G. J., Astry, C. L., and Warr, G. A. Alveolitis induced by influenza virus. Am. Rev. Respir. Dis. 128: 730–739, 1983.

3544. Berend, N. Low temperature inhibits bleomycin lung toxicity in the rat. Am. Rev. Respir. Dis. 128: 304–306, 1983.

3545. Keogh, B. A., Bernardo, J., Hunninghake, G. W., Line, B. R., Price, D. L., and Crystal, R. G. Effect of intermittent high dose parenteral corticosteroids on the alveolitis of idiopathic pulmonary fibrosis. Am. Rev. Respir. Dis. 127: 18–22, 1983.

3546. Haschek, W. M., Reiser, K. M., Klein-Szanto, A. J. P., Kehrer, J. P., Smith, L. H., Last, J. A., and Witschi, H. P. Potentiation of butylated hydroxytoluene-induced acute lung damage by oxygen. Am. Rev. Respir. Dis. 127: 28–34, 1983.

3547. Luursema, P. B., Star-Kroesen, M. A., Van der Mark, Th. W., Sleyfer, D. T., Koops, H. S., and Peset, R. Bleomycin-induced changes in the carbon monoxide transfer factor of the lungs and its components. Am. Rev. Respir. Dis. 128: 880–883, 1983.

3548. Dimarco, A. F., Kelsen, S. G., Cherniack, N. S., and Gothe, B. Occlusion pressure and breathing pattern in patients with interstitial lung disease. Am. Rev. Respir. Dis. 127: 425–430, 1983.

3549. Martin, W. J. Jr. Nitrofurantoin: evidence for the oxidant injury of lung parenchymal cells. Am. Rev. Respir. Dis. 127: 482–486, 1983.

3550. Clark, J. G. and Kuhn, C. III. Bleomycin-induced pulmonary fibrosis in hamsters: effect of neutrophil depletion on lung collagen synthesis. Am. Rev. Respir. Dis. 126: 737–739, 1982.

3551. Ozaki, T., Nakayama, T., Ishimi, H., Kawano, T., Yasuoka, S., and Tsubura, E. Glucocorticoid receptors in bronchoalveolar cells from patients with idiopathic pulmonary fibrosis. Am. Rev. Respir. Dis. 126: 968–971, 1982.

3552. Rinaldo, J., Goldstein, R. H., and Snider, G. L. Modification of oxygen toxicity after lung injury by bleomycin in hamsters. Am. Rev. Respir. Dis. 126: 1030–1033, 1982.

3553. Tryka, A. F., Skornik, W. A., Godleski, J. J., and Brain, J.

D. Potentiation of bleomycin-induced lung injury by exposure to 70 per cent oxygen. Am. Rev. Respir. Dis. 126: 1074–1079, 1982.

3554. Lewis, L. D. Procarbazine associated alveolitis. Thorax 39: 206–207, 1984.

3555. Carmichael, D. J. S., Hamilton, D. V., Evans, D. B., Stovin, P. G. I., and Calne, R. Y. Interstitial pneumonitis secondary to azothioprine in a renal transplant patient. Thorax 38: 951–952, 1983.

3556. Edwards, C. W. and Carlile, A. The larger bronchi in cryptogenic fibrosing alveolitis: a morphometric study. Thorax 37: 828–833, 1982.

3557. Tukiainen, P., Taskinen, E., Holsti, P., Korhola, O., and Valle, M. Prognosis of cryptogenic fibrosing alveolitis. Thorax 38: 349–355, 1983.

3558. Last, J. A., Siefkin, A. D., and Reiser, K. M. Type I collagen content is increased in lungs of patients with adult respiratory distress syndrome. Thorax 38: 364–368, 1983.

3559. Fernandez-Segoviano, P., Esteban, A., and Martinez-Cabruja, R. Pulmonary vascular lesions in the toxic oil syndrome in Spain. Thorax 38: 724–729, 1983.

3560. Burdon, J. G. W., Killian, K. J., and Jones, N. L. Pattern of breathing during exercise in patients with interstitial lung disease. Thorax 38: 778–784, 1983.

3561. Brennan, N. J., Morris, A. J. R., and Green, M. Thoracoabdominal mechanics during tidal breathing in normal subjects and in emphysema and fibrosing alveolitis. Thorax 38: 62–66, 1983.

3562. Holgate, S. T., Haslam, P., and Turner-Warwick, M. The significance of antinuclear and DNA antibodies in cryptogenic fibrosing alveolitis. Thorax 38: 67–70, 1983.

3563. Fergusson, R. J., Davidson, N. M., Nuki, G., and Crompton, G. K. Dermatomyositis and rapidly progressive fibrosing alveolitis. Thorax 38: 71–72, 1983.

3564. Michael, J. R. and Rudin, M. L. Acute pulmonary disease caused by phenytoin. Ann. Intern. Med. 95: 452–454, 1981.

3565. Clague, H. W., Wallace, A. C., and Morgan, W. K. C. Pulmonary interstitial fibrosis associated with alveolar proteinosis. Thorax 38: 865–866, 1983.

3566. Riley, D. J., Kerr, J. S., Berg, R. A., Ianni, B. D., Pietra, G. G., Edelman, N. H., and Prockop, D. J. Beta-aminopropriprionitrile prevents bleomycin-induced pulmonary fibrosis in the hamster. Am. Rev. Respir. Dis. 125: 67–73, 1982.

3567. Evans, J. N., Kelley, J., Low, R. B., and Adler, K. B. Increased contractility of isolated lung parenchyma in an animal model of pulmonary fibrosis induced by bleomycin. Am. Rev. Respir. Dis. 125: 89–94, 1982.

3568. Golden, E. B., Warnock, M. L., Hulett, L. D. Jr., and Churg, A. M. Fly ash lung: a new pneumoconiosis? Am. Rev. Respir. Dis. 125: 108–112, 1982.

3569. Fahey, P. J., Utell, M. J., Mayewski, R. J., Wandtke, J. D., and Hyde, R. W. Early diagnosis of bleomycin pulmonary toxicity using bronchoalveolar lavage in dogs. Am. Rev. Respir. Dis. 126: 126–130, 1982.

3570. Divertie, M. B., Owen, C. A. Jr., Barham, S. S., and Ludwig, J. Accumulation of radionuclide-labeled platelets and fibrinogen in paraquat-damaged rat lungs. Am. Rev. Respir. Dis. 125: 574–578, 1982.

3571. Hakkinen, P. J., Whiteley, J. W., and Witschi, H. R. Hyperoxia, but not thoracic X-irradiation, potentiates bleomycin- and cyclophosphamide-induced lung damage in mice. Am. Rev. Respir. Dis. 126: 281–285, 1982.

3572. Renzi, G., Milic-Emili, J., and Grassino, A. E. The pattern of breathing in diffuse lung fibrosis. Bull. Eur. Physiopathol. Respir. 18: 461–472, 1982.

3573. Saunier, C. Fibroses pulmonaires interstitielles experimentales. Bull. Eur. Physiopathol. Respir. 18: 515–547, 1982.

3574. Rowen, A. J. and Reichel, J. Dermatomyositis with lung involvement, successfully treated with azathioprine. Respiration 44: 143–146, 1983.

3575. Valeyre, D., Perret, G., Amouroux, J., Saumon, G., Georges, R., Pre, J., and Battesti, J.-P. Diffuse interstitial pulmonary disease due to prolonged inhalation of hair spray. Lung 161: 19–26, 1983.

3576. Etoh, T., Shioya, S., Ohta, Y., Yamabayashi, H., and Hata, J. Role of alveolar macrophages in development of paraquat-induced lung injury. Lung 161: 47–55, 1983.

3577. Wise, R. A., Wigley, F., Newball, H. H., and Stevens, M. B. The effect of cold exposure on diffusing capacity in patients with Raynaud's phenomenon. Chest 81: 695–698, 1982.

3578. Williams, T., Eidus, L., and Thomas, P. Fibrosing alveolitis, bronchiolitis obliterans, and sulfasalazine therapy. Chest 81: 766–768, 1982.

3579. Rebuck, A. S., Braude, A. C., and Chamberlain, D. W. Arterial PCO_2 as an index of activity in fibrosing alveolitis. Chest 82: 757–760, 1982.

3580. Abraham, J. L. and Hertzberg, M. A. Inorganic particulates associated with desquamative interstitial pneumonia. Chest 80(Suppl.): 67S–70S, 1981.

3581. Lakshminarayan, S., Stanford, R. E., and Petty, T. L. Prognosis after recovery from adult respiratory distress syndrome. Am. Rev. Respir. Dis. 113: 7–16, 1976.

3582. Bondi, E. and Slater, S. Tolazamide-induced chronic eosinophilic pneumonia (letter to editor). Chest 80: 652, 1981.

3583. Nader, D. A. and Schillaci, R. F. Pulmonary infiltrates with eosinophilia due to naproxen. Chest 83: 280–282, 1983.

3584. Yernault, J. C. and Gibson, G. J. Interactions between lung and chest wall in restrictive ventilatory defects (editorial). Bull. Eur. Physiopathol. Respir. 18: 395–401, 1982.

3585. Harkleroad, L. E., Young, R. L., Savage, P. J., Jenkins, D. W., and Lordon, R. E. Pulmonary sarcoidosis: long-term follow-up of the effects of steroid therapy. Chest 82: 84–87, 1982.

3586. Matthews, J. I. and Hooper, R. G. Exercise testing in pulmonary sarcoidosis. Chest 83: 75–81, 1983.

3587. Deremee, R. A. The roentgenographic staging of sarcoidosis. Chest 83: 128–133, 1983.

3588. Du Bois, R. M., McAllister, W. A. C., and Branthwaite, M. A. Alveolar proteinosis: diagnosis and treatment over a 10-year period. Thorax 38: 360–363, 1983.

3589. Valeyre, D., Saumon, G., Bladier, D., Amouroux, J., Pre, J., Battesti, J.-P., and Georges, R. The relationships between noninvasive explorations in pulmonary sarcoidosis of recent origin, as shown in bronchoalveolar lavage, serum, and pulmonary function tests. Am. Rev. Respir. Dis. 126: 41–45, 1982.

3590. Mordelet-Dambrine, M. S., Stanislas-Leguern, G. M., Huchon, G. J., Baumann, F. C., Marsac, J. H., and Chretien, J. Elevation of the bronchoalveolar concentration of angiotensin I converting enzyme in sarcoidosis. Am. Rev. Respir. Dis. 126: 472–475, 1982.

3591. Fulmer, J. D. Bronchoalveolar lavage (editorial). Am. Rev. Respir. Dis. 126: 961–963, 1982.

3592. Rankin, J. A., Naegel, G. P., Schrader, C. E., Matthay, R. A., and Reynolds, H. Y. Air-space immunoglobulin production and levels in bronchoalveolar lavage fluid of normal subjects and patients with sarcoidosis. Am. Rev. Respir. Dis. 127: 442–448, 1983.

3593. Keogh, B. A., Hunninghake, G. W., Line, B. R., and Crystal, R. G. The alveolitis of pulmonary sarcoidosis. Am. Rev. Respir. Dis. 128: 256–265, 1983.

3594. Kass, I., et al. Evaluation of Impairment/Disability Secondary to Respiratory Disease. Official Statement of the American Thoracic Society. Am. Rev. Respir. Dis. 126: 945–951, 1982.

3595. Brooks, S. M., et al. Surveillance for Respiratory Hazards in the Occupational Setting. Official Statement of the American Thoracic Society. Am. Rev. Respir. Dis. 126: 952–956, 1982.

3596. Davis, J. M. G., Chapman, J., Collings, P., Douglas, A. N., Fernie, J., Lamb, D., and Ruckley, V. A. Variations in the histological patterns of the lesions of coal worker's pneumoconiosis in Britain and their relationship to lung dust content. Am. Rev. Respir. Dis. 128: 118–124, 1983.

3597. Harber, P., Schnur, R., Emery, J., Brooks, S., and Ploy-Song-Sang, Y. Statistical "biases" in respiratory disability determinations. Am. Rev. Respir. Dis. 128: 413–418, 1983.

3598. Martin, T. R., Wehner, A. P., and Butler, J. Pulmonary toxicity of Mt. St. Helens volcanic ash. Am. Rev. Respir. Dis. 128: 158–162, 1983.

3599. Churg, A. Nonasbestos pulmonary mineral fibers in the general population. Environ. Res. 31: 189–200, 1983.

3600. Manfreda, J., Sidwall, G., Maini, K., West, P., and Cherniack, R. M. Respiratory abnormalities in employees of the hard rock mining industry. Am. Rev. Respir. Dis. 126: 629–634, 1982.

3601. Nonoccupational Health Risks of Asbestiform Fibers. Committee of the Board on Toxicology and Environmental Health Hazards, Commission on Life Sciences, National Research Council. National Academy Press, Washington, D.C., 1984.

3602. Begin, R., Cantin, A., Drapeau, G., Lamoureux, G., Boctor, M., Masse, S., and Rola-Pleszczynski, M. Pulmonary uptake of gallium-67 in asbestos-exposed humans and sheep. Am. Rev. Respir. Dis. 127: 623–630, 1983.

3603. Becklake, M. R., Toyota, B., Stewart, M., Hanson, R., and Hanley, J. Lung structure as a risk factor in adverse pulmonary responses to asbestos exposure. Am. Rev. Respir. Dis. 128: 385–388, 1983.

3604. Gamble, J. F. and Jones, W. G. Respiratory effects of diesel exhaust in salt miners. Am. Rev. Respir. Dis. 128: 389–394, 1983.

3605. Churg, A. and Wood, P. Observations on the distribution of asbestos fibers in human lungs. Environ. Res. 31: 374–380, 1983.

3606. Oleru, U. G., Elegbeleye, O. O., Enu, C. C., and Olumide, Y. M. Pulmonary function and symptoms of Nigerian workers exposed to carbon black in dry cell battery and tire factories. Environ. Res. 30: 161–168, 1983.

3607. Goldstein, B., Rendall, R. E. G., and Webster, I. A comparison of the effects of exposure of baboons to crocidolite and fibrous-glass dusts. Environ. Res. 32: 344–359, 1983.

3608. Churg, A. Asbestos fiber content of the lungs in patients with and without asbestos airways disease. Am. Rev. Respir. Dis. 127: 470–473, 1983.

3609. Albelda, S. M., Epstein, D. M., Gefter, W. B., and Miller, W. T. Pleural thickening: its significance and relationship to asbestos dust exposure. Am. Rev. Respir. Dis. 126: 621–624, 1982.

3610. Begin, R., Masse, S., and Bureau, M. A. Morphologic features and function of the airways in early asbestosis in the sheep model. Am. Rev. Respir. Dis. 126: 870–876, 1982.

3611. De Vuyst, P., Jedwab, J., Dumortier, P., Vandermoten, G., Vande Weyer, R., and Yernault, J.-C. Asbestos bodies in bronchoalveolar lavage. Am. Rev. Respir. Dis. 126: 972–976, 1982.

3612. Mundie, T. G., Cordova-Salinas, M., Bray, V. J., and Ainsworth, S. K. Bioassays of smooth muscle contracting agents in cotton mill dust and bract extracts: arachidonic acid metabolites as possible mediators of the acute byssinotic reaction. Environ. Res. 32: 62–71, 1983.

3613. McKay, R. T. and Brooks, S. M. Effect of toluene diisocyanate on beta adrenergic receptor function. Am. Rev. Respir. Dis. 128: 50–53, 1983.

3614. Robbins, J., Greaves, I. A., and Eisen, E. A. Five-year longitudinal study of workers employed in a new toluene diisocyanate manufacturing plant (letter to editor). Am. Rev. Respir. Dis. 128: 327, 1983.

3615. Do Pico, G. A., Reddan, W., Anderson, S., Flaherty, D., and Smalley, E. Acute effects of grain dust exposure during a work shift. Am. Rev. Respir. Dis. 128: 399–404, 1983.

3616. Harkonen, H., Nordman, H., Korhonen, O., and Winblad, I. Long-term effects of exposure to sulfur dioxide. Am. Rev. Respir. Dis. 128: 890–893, 1983.

3617. Enterline, P. E., Marsh, G. M., and Esmen, N. A. Respiratory disease among workers exposed to man-made mineral fibers. Am. Rev. Respir. Dis. 128: 1–7, 1983.

3618. Kauffman, F., Drouet, D., Lellouch, J., and Brille, D. Twelve years spirometric changes among Paris area workers. Int. J. Epidemiol. 8: 201–212, 1979.

3619. Cotton, D. J., Graham, B. L., Li, K.-Y. R., Barnett, D. H., and Dosman, J. A. Effects of smoking and occupational exposure on peripheral airway function in young cereal grain workers. Am. Rev. Respir. Dis. 126: 660–665, 1982.

3620. Weill, H., Hughes, J. M., Hammad, Y. Y., Glindmeyer, H. W. III., Sharon, G., and Jones, R. N. Respiratory health in workers exposed to man-made vitreous fibers. Am. Rev. Respir. Dis. 128: 104–112, 1983.

3621. Douglas, A. N., Lamb, D., and Ruckley, V. A. Bronchial gland dimensions in coalminers: influence of smoking and dust exposure. Thorax 37: 760–764, 1982.

3622. Cockcroft, A., Berry, G., Cotes, J. E., and Lyons, J. P. Shape of small opacities and lung function in coalworkers. Thorax 37: 765–769, 1982.

3623. Seaton, A. Coal and the lung (editorial). Thorax 38: 241–243, 1983.

3624. Kennedy, M. C. S. Coal and the lung (letter to editor). Thorax 38: 877–880, 1983.

3625. Morgan, W. K. C. Coal and the lung (letter to editor). Thorax 38: 878, 1983.

3626. Cochrane, A. L. Coal and the lung (letter to editor). Thorax 38: 877–878, 1983.

3627. Seaton, A. Coal and the lung (letter to editor). Thorax 38: 878–879, 1983.

3628. Richman, S. L. Why change? A look at the current system of disability determination and worker's compensation for occupational lung disease. Ann. Intern. Med. 97: 908–914, 1982.

3629. Fernie, J. M., Douglas, A. N., Lamb, D., and Ruckley, V. A. Right ventricular hypertrophy in a group of coalworkers. Thorax 38: 436–442, 1983.

3630. Begin, R., Rola-Pleszczynski, M., Masse, S., Nadeau, D., and Grapeau, G. Assessment of progression of asbestosis in the sheep model by bronchoalveolar lavage and pulmonary function tests. Thorax 38: 449–457, 1983.

3631. Banks, D. E., Bauer, M. A., Castellan, R. M., and Lapp, N. L. Silicosis in surface coalmine drillers. Thorax 38: 275–278, 1983.

3632. Oldham, P. D. Pneumoconiosis in Cornish china clay workers. Br. J. Ind. Med. 40: 131–137, 1983.

3633. Finkelstein, M. M. Mortality among long-term employees of an Ontario asbestos-cement factory. Br. J. Ind. Med. 40: 138–144, 1983.

3634. Browne, K. and Smither, W. J. Asbestos-related mesothelioma: factors discriminating between pleural and peritoneal sites. Br. J. Ind. Med. 40: 145–152, 1983.

3635. Love, R. G. Lung function studies before and after a work shift. Br. J. Ind. Med. 40: 153–159, 1983.

3636. Cockcroft, A., Lyons, J. P., Andersson, N., and Saunders, M. J. Prevalence and relation to underground exposure of radiological irregular opacities in South Wales coal workers with pneumoconiosis. Br. J. Ind. Med. 40: 169–172, 1983.

3637. Cordes, L. G., Brink, E. W., Checko, P. J., Lentnek, A., Lyons, R. W., Hayes, P. S., Wu, T. C., Tharr, D. G., and Fraser, D. W. A cluster of acinetobacter pneumonia in foundry workers. Ann. Intern. Med. 95: 688–693, 1981.

3638. Rosenstock, L. Occupational Medicine: too long neglected (editorial). Ann. Intern. Med. 95: 774–776, 1981.

3639. Bernstein, L. Occupational asthma: coming of age (editorial). Ann. Intern. Med. 97: 125–127, 1982.

3640. Golden, E. B., Warnock, M. L., Hulett, L. D. Jr., and Churg, A. M. Fly ash lung: a new pneumoconiosis? Am. Rev. Respir. Dis. 125: 108–112, 1982.

3641. Malo, J.-L. and Zeiss, C. R. Occupational hypersensitivity pneumonitis after exposure to diphenylmethane diisocyanate. Am. Rev. Respir. Dis. 125: 113–116, 1982.

3642. Report of the Royal Commission on Matters of Health and Safety Arising from the Use of Asbestos in Ontario. Ontario Ministry of the Attorney General, 1984.

3643. McDonald, A. D., Fry, J. S., Woolley, A. J., and McDonald, J. Dust exposure and mortality in an American chrysotile textile plant. Br. J. Ind. Med. 40: 361–367, 1983.

3644. McDonald, A. D., Fry, J. S., Woolley, A. J., and McDonald, J. C. Dust exposure and mortality in an American factory using chrysotile, amosite, and crocidolite in mainly textile manufacture. Br. J. Ind. Med. 40: 368–374, 1983.

3645. Gylseth, B., Mowe, G., and Wannag, A. Fibre type and concentration in the lungs of workers in an asbestos cement factory. Br. J. Ind. Med. 40: 375–379, 1983.

3646. Marsh, G. M. Proportional mortality patterns among chemical plant workers exposed to formaldehyde. Br. J. Ind. Med. 39: 313–322, 1982.

3647. Corey, P., Hutcheon, M., Broder, I., and Mintz, S. Grain elevator workers show work-related pulmonary function changes and dose-effect relationships with dust exposure. Br. J. Ind. Med. 39: 330–337, 1982.

3648. McDermott, M., Bevan, M. M., Elmes, P. C., Allardice, J. T., and Bradley, A. C. Lung function and radiographic change in chrysotile workers in Swaziland. Br. J. Ind. Med. 39: 338–343, 1982.

3649. Acheson, E. D., Gardner, M. J., Pippard, E. C., and Grime,

L. P. Mortality of two groups of women who manufactured gas masks from chrysotile and crocidolite asbestos: a 40-year follow-up. Br. J. Ind. Med. 39: 344–348, 1982.

3650. Steele, R. H. and Thomson, K. J. Asbestos bodies in the lung: Southampton (UK) and Wellington (New Zealand). Br. J. Ind. Med. 39: 349–354, 1982.

3651. Lings, S. Pesticide lung: a pilot investigation of fruit-growers and farmers during the spraying season. Br. J. Ind. Med. 39: 370–376, 1982.

3652. Schoenberger, C. I., Hunninghake, G. W., Kawanami, O., Ferrans, V. J., and Crystal, R. G. Role of alveolar macrophages in asbestosis: modulation of neutrophil migration to the lung after acute asbestos exposure. Thorax 37: 803–809, 1982.

3653. Law, M. R., Ward, F. G., Hodson, M. E., and Heard, B. E. Evidence for longer survival of patients with pleural mesothelioma without asbestos exposure. Thorax 38: 744–746, 1983.

3654. Lee, W. R. Occupational medicine (editorial). Br. Med. J. 287: 241–242, 1983.

3655. Cookson, W. O. C., Musk, A. W., and Glancy, J. J. Pleural thickening and gas transfer in asbestosis. Thorax 38: 657–661, 1983.

3656. Berry, G. and Newhouse, M. L. Mortality of workers manufacturing friction materials using asbestos. Br. J. Ind. Med. 40: 1–7, 1983.

3657. Cotes, J. E., Gilson, J. C., McKerrow, C. B., and Oldham, P. D. A long-term follow-up of workers exposed to beryllium. Br. J. Ind. Med. 40: 13–21, 1983.

3658. Davies, D. and Cotton, R. Mica pneumoconiosis. Br. J. Ind. Med. 40: 22–27, 1983.

3659. Legg, S. J., Cotes, J. E., and Bevan, C. Lung mechanics in relation to radiographic category of coalworker's simple pneumoconiosis. Br. J. Ind. Med. 40: 28–33, 1983.

3660. Petronio, L. and Bivenzi, M. Byssinosis and serum IgE concentrations in textile workers in an Italian cotton mill. Br. J. Ind. Med. 40: 39–44, 1983.

3661. Morgan, A. and Holmes, A. Distribution and characteristics of amphibole asbestos fibres, measured with the light microscope, in the left lung of an insulation worker. Br. J. Ind. Med. 40: 45–50, 1983.

3662. Dechoux, J., Pivoteau, C., and Wantz, J. M. Troubles fonctionnels respiratoires des mineurs des houillieres du bassin de Lorraine à l'heure de la retraite. Bull. Eur. Physiopathol. Respir. 19: 385–391, 1983.

3663. Cockcroft, A., Wagner, J. C., Ryder, R., Seal, R. M. E., Lyons, J. P., and Andersson, N. Post-mortem study of emphysema in coalworkers and non-coalworkers. Lancet ii: 600–603, 1982.

3664. Belin, L., Wass, U., Audunsson, G., and Mathiasson, L. Amines: possible causative agents in the development of bronchial hyperreactivity in workers manufacturing polyurethanes from isocyanates. Br. J. Ind. Med. 40: 251–257, 1983.

3665. Leigh, J., Outhred, K. G., McKenzie, H. I., Glick, M., and Wiles, A. N. Quantified pathology of emphysema, pneumoconiosis, and chronic bronchitis in coal workers. Br. J. Ind. Med. 40: 258–263, 1983.

3666. Hwang, C.-Y. Size and shape of airborne asbestos fibres in mines and mills. Br. J. Ind. Med. 40: 273–279, 1983.

3667. Diem, J. E., Jones, R. N., Hendrick, D. J., Glindmeyer, H. W., Dharmarajan, V., Butcher, B. T., Salvaggio, J. E., and Weill, H. Five-year longitudinal study of workers employed in a new toluene diisocyanate manufacturing plant. Am. Rev. Respir. Dis. 126: 420–428, 1982.

3668. Epstein, P. E., Dauber, J. H., Rossman, M. D., and Daniele, R. P. Bronchoalveolar lavage in a patient with chronic berylliosis: evidence for hypersensitivity pneumonitis. Ann. Intern. Med. 97: 213–216, 1982.

3669. Morgan, W. K. C. Kaolin and the lung (editorial). Am. Rev. Respir. Dis. 127: 141–142, 1983.

3670. Lapedes, D. N. (ed. in chief). McGraw-Hill Dictionary of Scientific and Technical Terms. 2nd ed. McGraw-Hill, New York, 1978.

3671. Secker-Walker, R. H. and Ho, J. E. Regional lung function in asbestos workers: observations and speculations. Respiration 43: 8–22, 1982.

3672. Stark, P. Round atelectasis: another pulmonary pseudotumor. Am. Rev. Respir. Dis. 125: 248–250, 1982.

3673. Simpson, D. L., Goodman, M., Spector, S. L., and Petty, T. L. Long-term follow-up and bronchial reactivity testing in survivors of the adult respiratory distress syndrome. Am. Rev. Respir. Dis. 117: 449–454, 1978.

3674. Finkelstein, M. M. Asbestosis in long-term employees of an Ontario asbestos-cement factory. Am. Rev. Respir. Dis. 125: 496–501, 1982.

3675. Becklake, M. R. Astestos-related diseases of the lungs and pleura: current clinical issues (editorial). Am. Rev. Respir. Dis. 126: 187–194, 1982.

3676. Beck, G. J., Schachter, E. N., Maunder, L. R., and Schilling, R. S. F. A prospective study of chronic lung disease in cotton textile workers. Ann. Intern. Med. 97: 645–651, 1982.

3677. Epler, G. R. Byssinosis: defining cause and disability (editorial). Ann. Intern. Med. 97: 772–774, 1982.

3678. Russell, J. A., Gilberstadt, M. L., and Rohrbach, M. S. Constrictor effect of cotton bract extract on isolated canine airways. Am. Rev. Respir. Dis. 125: 727–733, 1982.

3679. Al-Zuhair, Y. S., Whitaker, C. J., and Cinkotai, F. F. Ventilatory function in workers exposed to tea and wood dust. Br. J. Ind. Med. 38: 339–345, 1981.

3680. Fox, A. J., Goldblatt, P., and Kinlen, L. J. A study of the mortality of Cornish tin miners. Br. J. Ind. Med. 38: 378–380, 1981.

3681. Wignall, B. K. and Fox, A. J. Mortality of female gas mask assemblers. Br. J. Ind. Med. 39: 34–38, 1982.

3682. McMillan, G. H. G. and Rossiter, C. E. Development of radiological and clinical evidence of parenchymal fibrosis in men with non-malignant asbestos-related pleural lesions. Br. J. Ind. Med. 39: 54–59, 1982.

3683. McMillan, G. H. G., Rossiter, C. E., and Deacon, R. Comparison of independent randomised reading of radiographs with direct progression scoring for assessing change in asbestos-related pulmonary and pleural lesions. Br. J. Ind. Med. 39: 60–61, 1982.

3684. Morgan, A. and Holmes, A. Concentrations and characteristics of amphibole fibres in the lungs of workers exposed to crocidolite in the British gas-mask factories, and elsewhere, during the second world war. Br. J. Ind. Med. 39: 62–69, 1982.

3685. Jones, R. N., Hughes, J. M., Lehrer, S. B., Butcher, B. T., Glindmeyer, H. W., Diem, J. E., Hammad, Y. Y., Salvaggio, J., and Weill, H. Lung function consequences of exposure and hypersensitivity in workers who process green coffee beans. Am. Rev. Respir. Dis. 125: 199–202, 1982.

3686. Ames, R. G., Attfield, M. D., Hankinson, J. L., Hearl, F. J., and Reger, R. B. Acute respiratory effects of exposure to diesel emissions in coal miners. Am. Rev. Respir. Dis. 125: 39–42, 1982.

3687. Sparrow, D., Bosse, R., Rosner, B., and Weiss, S. T. The effect of occupational exposure on pulmonary function: a longitudinal evaluation of fire fighters and nonfire fighters. Am. Rev. Respir. Dis. 125: 319–322, 1982.

3688. Occupation and bronchitis (editorial). Lancet i: 235–236, 1980.

3689. Zeiss, C. R., Wolkonsky, P., Chacon, R., Tuntland, P. A., Levitz, D., Prunzansky, J. J., and Patterson, R. Syndromes in workers exposed to trimellitic anhydride. Ann. Intern. Med. 98: 8–12, 1983.

3690. Kennedy, T., Rawlings, W. Jr., Baser, M., and Tockman, M. Pneumoconiosis in Georgia kaolin workers. Am. Rev. Respir. Dis. 127: 215–220, 1983.

3691. Sepulveda, M-J., Vallyathan, V., Attfield, M. D., Piacitelli, L., and Tucker, J. H. Pneumoconiosis and lung function in a group of kaolin workers. Am. Rev. Respir. Dis. 127: 231–235, 1983.

3692. Townshend, R. H. Acute cadmium pneumonitis: a 17-year follow-up. Br. J. Ind. Med. 39: 411–412, 1982.

3693. Williams, W. J. and Williams, W. R. Value of beryllium transformation tests in chronic beryllium disease and in potentially exposed workers. Thorax 38: 41–44, 1983.

3694. Soutar, C. A. and Gauld, S. Clinical studies of workers exposed to polyvinylchloride dust. Thorax 38: 834–839, 1983.

3695. Mason, G. R., Abraham, J. L., Hoffman, L., Cole, S., Lippmann, M., and Wasserman, K. Treatment of mixed-dust pneumoconiosis with whole lung lavage. Am. Rev. Respir. Dis. 126: 1102–1107, 1982.

3696. Sablonniere, B., Scharfman, A., Lafitte, J. J., Laine, A., Aerts, C., and Hayem, A. Enzymatic activities of bronchoalveolar lavages in coal workers pneumoconiosis. Lung 161: 219–228, 1983.

3697. Weill, H. Problem solving in occupational airways disorders (editorial). Chest 79: 1S–2S, 1981.

3698. Schilling, R. Worldwide problems of byssinosis. Chest 79: 3S–5S, 1981.

3699. Berry, G. and Molyneux, M. K. B. A mortality study of workers in Lancashire cotton mills. Chest 79: 11S–15S, 1981.

3700. Beck, G. J., Schachter, E. N., Maunder, L. R., and Bouhuys, A. The relation of lung function to subsequent employment status and mortality in cotton textile workers. Chest 79: 26S–30S, 1981.

3701. Jones, R. N., Hughes, J., Hammad, Y. Y., Glindmeyer, H. III, Butcher, B. T., Diem, J. E., and Weill, H. Respiratory health in cottonseed crushing mills. Chest 79: 30S–33S, 1981.

3702. Edwards, J. Mechanisms of disease induction. Chest 79: 38S–42S, 1981.

3703. Buck, M. G. and Bouhuys, A. A purified extract from cotton bracts induces airway constriction in humans. Chest 79: 43S–49S, 1981.

3704. Pratt, P. C. Comparative prevalence and severity of emphysema and bronchitis at autopsy in cotton mill workers vs controls. Chest 79: 49S–53S, 1981.

3705. Noweir, M. H. Studies on the etiology of byssinosis. Chest 79: 62S–67S, 1981.

3706. Rooke, G. B. The pathology of byssinosis. Chest 79: 67S–71S, 1981.

3707. Glindmeyer, H. III, Diem, J., Hughes, J., Jones, R. N., and Weill, H. Factors influencing the interpretation of FEV_1 declines across the working shift. Chest 79: 71S–73S, 1981.

3708. Boehlecke, B., Cocke, J., Bragg, K., Hancock, J., Petsonk, E., Piccirillo, R., and Merchant, J. Pulmonary function response to dust from standard and closed boll harvested cotton. Chest 79: 77S–81S, 1981.

3709. Castellan, R. M., Boehlecke, B. A., Petersen, M. R., Thedell, T. D., and Merchant, J. A. Pulmonary function and symptoms in herbal tea workers. Chest 79: 81S–85S, 1981.

3710. Battigelli, M. C., Berni, R. J., Sasser, P. E., and Symons, M. J. The relationship of acute respiratory response and chronic respiratory symptoms in byssinosis. Chest 79: 86S–90S, 1981.

3711. Boehlecke, B. A. and Merchant, J. A. The use of pulmonary function testing and questionnaires as epidemiologic tools in the study of occupational lung disease. Chest 79: 114S–122S, 1981.

3712. Imbus, H. R. Worker monitoring in byssinosis. Chest 79: 122S–123S, 1981.

3713. Rooke, G. B. Compensation for byssinosis in Great Britain. Chest 79: 124S–127S, 1981.

3714. Brown, T. C. Evaluating work relatedness of diseases. Chest 79: 127S–129S, 1981.

3715. Hughes, J. T. Jr. Diagnosing byssinosis: the medical controversy. Chest 79: 129S–130S, 1981.

3716. Perkel, G. Evaluating work relatedness of byssinosis for worker compensation purposes. Chest 79: 131S–132S, 1981.

3717. Stephenson, W. H. Administrative law problems with byssinosis. Chest 79: 132S–133S, 1981.

3718. Make, B., Miller, A., Epler, G., and Gee, J. B. L. Single breath diffusing capacity in the industrial setting. Chest 82: 351–356, 1982.

3719. Murphy, D. M. F., Metzger, L. F., Silage, D. A., and Fogarty, C. M. Effect of simple anthracite pneumoconiosis on lung mechanics. Chest 82: 744–750, 1982.

3720. Becklake, M. R., Thomas, D., Liddell, F. D. K., and McDonald, J. C. Follow-up respiratory measurements in Quebec chrysotile asbestos miners and millers. Scand. J. Work Environ. Health 8(Suppl.): 105–110, 1982.

3721. Saric, M., Gomzi, M., and Hrustic, O. Comparison of measured and predicted ventilatory volumes in selected groups of industrial workers. Scand. J. Work Environ. Health 8(Suppl.): 111–116, 1982.

3722. Kalliomaki, P.-L., Kalliomaki, K., Korhonen, O., Nordman, H., Rahkonen, E., and Vaaranen, V. Respiratory status of stainless steel and mild steel welders. Scand. J. Work Environ. Health 8(Suppl.): 117–121, 1982.

3723. Enterline, P. E. Epidemiologic basis for the asbestos standard. Environ. Health Perspect. 52: 93–97, 1983.

3724. Mintzer, R. A. and Cugell, D. W. The association of asbestos-induced pleural disease and rounded atelectasis. Chest 81: 457–460, 1982.

3725. Pearle, J. Exercise performance and functional impairment in asbestos-exposed workers. Chest 80: 701–705, 1981.

3726. Niemela, R. and Vainio, H. Formaldehyde exposure in work and the general environment. Scand. J. Work Environ. Health 7: 95–100, 1981.

3727. Gylseth, B., Mowe, G., Skaug, V., and Wannag, A. Inorganic fibers in lung tissue from patients with pleural plaques or malignant mesothelioma. Scand. J. Work Environ. Health 7: 109–113, 1981.

3728. Ulfvarson, U. Survey of air contaminants from welding. Scand. J. Work Environ. Health 7(Suppl. 2): 1981.

3729. Gylseth, B. and Baunan, R. Topographic and size distribution of asbestos bodies in exposed human lungs. Scand. J. Work Environ. Health 7: 190–195, 1981.

3730. Eduard, W. and Lie, A. Influence of fluoride recovery alumina on the work environment and the health of aluminum potroom workers. Scand. J. Work Environ. Health 7: 214–222, 1981.

3731. Kjuus, H., Istad, H., and Langard, S. Emphysema and occupational exposure to industrial pollutants. Scand. J. Work Environ. Health 7: 290–297, 1981.

3732. Pershagen, G., Wall, S., Taube, A., and Linnman, L. On the interaction between occupational arsenic exposure and smoking and its relationship to lung cancer. Scand. J. Work Environ. Health 7: 302–309, 1981.

3733. Belin, L., Hjorstberg, U., and Wass, U. Life-threatening pulmonary reaction to car paint containing a prepolymerized isocyanate (letter to editor). Scand. J. Work Environ. Health 7: 310–311, 1981.

3734. Simonsson, B. G. (ed.). Airway Hyperreactivity. Eur. J. Respir. Dis. 64(Suppl. 131): 1983.

3735. Nordman, H. (ed.). International Course on Occupational Respiratory Disease. Eur. J. Respir. Dis. 63(Suppl. 123): 1982.

3736. Frigas, E., Filley, W. V., and Reed, C. E. Asthma induced by dust from urea-formaldehyde foam insulating material. Chest 79: 706–707, 1981.

3737. Do Pico, G. A., Jacobs, S., Flaherty, D., and Rankin, J. Pulmonary reaction to durum wheat. Chest 81: 55–61, 1982.

3738. Cockcroft, D. W., Hoeppner, V. H., and Dolovich, J. Occupational asthma caused by cedar urea formaldehyde particle board. Chest 82: 49–53, 1982.

3739. Brooks, S. M., Edwards, J. J. Jr., Apol, A., and Edwards, F. H. An epidemiologic study of workers exposed to Western red cedar and other wood dusts. Chest 80: 30S–32S, 1981.

3740. Butler, J., Culver, B. H., and Robertson, H. T. Meat wrappers' asthma. Chest 80: 71S–73S, 1981.

3741. Epler, G. R. and Colby, T. V. The spectrum of bronchiolitis obliterans (editorial). Chest 83: 161–162, 1983.

3742. Seggev, J. S., Mason, U. G. III, Worthen, S., Stanford, R. E., and Fernandez, E. Bronchiolitis obliterans: report of three cases with detailed physiologic studies. Chest 83: 169–174, 1983.

3743. Cole, H. M., Benton, R. E., and Skalsky, H. L. Pulmonary fibrosis in an aluminum arc welder (letter to editor). Chest 83: 291–292, 1983.

3744. Parkes, W. R. Occupational Lung Disorders. Butterworth & Co., London, 1974.

3745. Lozano, F. M., Sanchez, J. F., Rodriguez, A. V., Avellaneda, J. L. C., and Berdugo, J. M. Pathophysiological disturbances in bagassosis and bagasse workers. Bull. Eur. Physiopathol. Respir. 18: 623–642, 1982.

3746. Mur, J. M., Cavelier, C., Meyer-Bisch, C., Pham, Q. T., and Masset, J. C. Etude de la fonction pulmonaire de soudeurs à l'arc. Respiration 44: 50–57, 1983.

3747. Brooks, S. M. Pulmonary manifestations of vinyl and polyvinyl chloride (letter to editor). Chest 81: 262, 1982.

3748. Vallyathan, V., Bergeron, W. N., Robichaux, P. A., and Craighead, J. E. Pulmonary fibrosis in an aluminum arc welder. Chest 81: 372–374, 1982.

3749. Soutar, C., Copland, L., Thornley, P., Hurley, F., Ottery, J., Adams, W., and Bennett, B. An epidemiologic study of respiratory diseases in workers exposed to polyvinylchloride dust. Chest 80: 60S, 1981.

3750. McKay, R. T., Brooks, S. M., and Johnson, C. Isocyanate-induced abnormality of beta-adrenergic receptor function. Chest 80: 61S–63S, 1981.

3751. Brody, A. R. and Hill, L. H. Deposition pattern and clearance pathways of inhaled chrysotile asbestos. Chest 80: 64S–66S, 1981.

3752. Davison, A. G., Haslam, P. L., Corrin, B., Coutts, I., Dewar, A., Riding, W. D., Studdy, P. R., and Newman-Taylor, A. J. Interstitial lung disease and asthma in hard-metal workers: bronchoalveolar lavage, ultrastructural, and analytical findings and results of bronchial provocation tests. Thorax 38: 119–128, 1983.

3753. Klein, J. J., van Haeringen, J. R., Sluiter, H. J., Holloway, R., and Peset, R. Pulmonary function after recovery from the adult respiratory distress syndrome. Chest 69: 350–355, 1976.

3754. Lockwood, P. Discriminant analysis of lung function test results in the selection of patients for bronchial carcinoma surgery. Respiration 44: 368–375, 1983.

3755. Nagasaki, F., Flehinger, B. J., and Martini, N. Complications of surgery in the treatment of carcinoma of the lung. Chest 82: 25–29, 1982.

3756. Dixon, G. F., Schonfeld, S. A., and Whitcomb, M. E. Two cases of interstitial infiltrates with hyperinflation. Chest 82: 625–629, 1982.

3757. Coy, P., Elwood, J. M., and Coldman, A. J. Clinical indicators of prognosis in unresected lung cancer. Chest 80: 453–458, 1981.

3758. Hillerdal, G., Karlen, E., and Aberg, T. Tobacco consumption and asbestos exposure in patients with lung cancer: a three year perspective. Br. J. Ind. Med. 40: 380–383, 1983.

3759. Coggon, D. and Acheson, E. D. Trends in lung cancer mortality (editorial). Thorax 38: 721–723, 1983.

3760. Pastorino, U., Valente, M., Bedini, V., Pagnoni, A., and Ravasi, G. Effect of chronic cardiopulmonary disease on survival after resection for stage Ia lung cancer. Thorax 37: 680–683, 1982.

3761. Belcher, J. R. Thirty years of surgery for carcinoma of the bronchus. Thorax 38: 428–432, 1983.

3762. Ives, J. C., Buffler, P. A., and Greenberg, S. D. Environmental associations and histopathologic patterns of carcinoma of the lung: the challenge and dilemma in epidemiologic studies. Am. Rev. Respir. Dis. 128: 195–209, 1983.

3763. Easton, P. A., Arnup, M. E., De La Rocha, A., Fleetham, J. A., and Anthonisen, N. R. Ventilatory control after pulmonary resection. Am. Rev. Respir. Dis. 128: 627–630, 1983.

3764. Huhti, E., Saloheimo, M., and Sutinen, S. The value of roentgenologic screening in lung cancer. Am. Rev. Respir. Dis. 128: 395–398, 1983.

3765. Ball, W. C. The effect of surgical treatment on the natural history of lung cancer (editorial). Am. Rev. Respir. Dis. 127: 1, 1983.

3766. Gimeno, F., Kraan, J. K., Orie, N. G. M., and Peset, R. Pulmonary gas transfer 20 years after pneumonectomy for pulmonary tuberculosis. Thorax 32: 80–83, 1977.

3767. Prefaut, C., Kienlen, J., Lloret, M. C., Chardon, G., and du Cailar, J. Les sequelles fonctionelles du syndrome de Mendelson. Myth ou realite? Poumon Coeur 33: 391–394, 1977.

3768. Gaultier, C., Boule, M., Tournier, G., and Girard, F. Effects of naloxone on the control of breathing in children with chronic obstructive pulmonary disease. Bull. Eur. Physiopathol. Respir. 19: 557–561, 1983.

3769. Light, R. B., Mink, S. N., Cooligan, T. G., and Wood, L. D. H. The physiology of recovery in experimental pneumococcal pneumonia. Clin. Invest. Med. 6: 147–151, 1983.

3770. Walters, E. H. Effect of inhibition of prostaglandin synthesis on induced bronchial hyperresponsiveness. Thorax 38: 195–199, 1983.

3771. Shure, D., Spragg, R. G., and Moser, K. M. Large cavitary dead space as an unusual cause of hypercapnic respiratory failure in pulmonary tuberculosis. Thorax 37: 550–551, 1982.

3772. Guntapalli, K. K., Sladen, A., and Klain, M. High-frequency jet ventilation: a case report. Thorax 37: 558–559, 1982.

3773. Milner, A. D. and Henry, R. L. Acute airways obstruction in children under 5 (editorial). Thorax 37: 641–645, 1982.

3774. Sawicka, E. H., Branthwaite, M. A., and Spencer, G. T. Respiratory failure after thoracoplasty: treatment by intermittent negative-pressure ventilation. Thorax 38: 433–435, 1983.

3775. Cooligan, T., Light, R. B., Wood, L. D. H., and Mink, S. N. Plasma volume expansion in canine pneumococcal pneumonia. Am. Rev. Respir. Dis. 126: 86–91, 1982.

3776. Ploysongsang, Y. and Schonfield, S. A. Pulmonary function studies in diffuse pulmonary North American blastomycosis. Am. Rev. Respir. Dis. 128: 1095–1098, 1983.

3777. Hammar, S. P., Winterbauer, R. H., Bockus, D., Remington, F., Sale, G. E., and Meyers, J. D. Endothelial cell damage and tubuloreticular structures in interstitial lung disease associated with collagen vascular disease and viral pneumonia. Am. Rev. Respir. Dis. 127: 77–84, 1983.

3778. Wagener, J. S., Minnich, L., Sobonya, R., Taussig, L. M., Ray, C. G., and Fulginiti, V. Parainfluenza type II infection in dogs. Am. Rev. Respir. Dis. 127: 771–775, 1983.

3779. Halperin, S. A., Eggleston, P. A., Hendley, J. O., Suratt, P. M., Groschel, D. H. M., and Gwaltney, J. M. Jr. Pathogenesis of lower respiratory tract symptoms in experimental rhinovirus infection. Am. Rev. Respir. Dis. 128: 806–810, 1983.

3780. Simila, S., Linna, O., Lanning, P., Heikkinen, E., and Ala-Houhala, M. Chronic lung damage caused by adenovirus type 7: a ten-year follow-up study. Chest 80: 127–131, 1981.

3781. Petro, W., Konietzko, N., and Maasen, W. Effects of surgery on airway mechanics in tracheal stenosis. Respiration 43: 424–431, 1982.

3782. Teja, K., Cooper, P. H., Squires, J. E., and Schnatterly, P. T. Pulmonary alveolar proteinosis in four siblings. N. Engl. J. Med. 305: 1390–1392, 1981.

3783. Folgering, H., Rutten, H., and Roumen, Y. Beta-blockade in the hyperventilation syndrome. A retrospective assessment of symptoms and complaints. Respiration 44: 19–25, 1983.

3784. Mohsenifar, Z., Tashkin, D. P., Wolfe, J. D., and Genovese, M. Abnormal responses of wasted ventilation fraction (VD/VT) during exercise in patients with pulmonary vascular abnormalities. Respiration 44: 44–49, 1983.

3785. Fairshter, R. D., Vaziri, N. D., and Gordon, S. Frequency and spectrum of pulmonary diseases in patients with chronic renal failure associated with spinal cord injury. Respiration 44: 58–62, 1983.

3786. Starke, I. D., Elkon, K. B., Harmer, C. L., Hughes, G. V. R., and Wiltshaw, E. Pulmonary involvement in angioimmunoblastic lymphadenopathy following autoimmune disease. Respiration 44: 136–142, 1983.

3787. Williams, A. J. and Fisher, H. K. Diffusing capacity in alcoholics (letter to editor). Chest 79: 123, 1981.

3788. Mohsenifar, Z., Tashkin, D. P., Carson, S. A., and Bellamy, P. E. Pulmonary function in patients with relapsing polychondritis. Chest 81: 711–717, 1982.

3789. Huseby, J. S. and Petersen, D. Pulmonary function in Klinefelter's syndrome. Chest 80: 31–33, 1981.

3790. Naeije, R., Hallemans, R., Mols, P., and Melot, C. Hypoxic pulmonary vasoconstriction in liver cirrhosis. Chest 80: 570–574, 1981.

3791. Tarlo, S. M., Broder, I., Prokipchuk, E. J., Peress, L., and Mintz, S. Association between celiac disease and lung disease. Chest 80: 715–718, 1981.

3792. Lonsdorfer, J., Bogui, P., Otayeck, A., Bursaux, E., Poyart, C., and Cabannes, R. Cardiorespiratory adjustments in chronic sickle cell anemia. Bull. Eur. Physiopathol. Respir. 19: 339–344, 1983.

3793. Heatley, R. V., Thomas, P., Prokipchuk, E. J., Gauldie, J., Sieniewicz, D. J., and Bienenstock, J. Pulmonary function abnormalities in patients with inflammatory bowel disease. Q. J. Med. 51(203): 241–250, 1982.

3794. Mansell, A., Levison, H., and Bailey, J. D. Maturation of lung function in children with hypopituitarism. Am. Rev. Respir. Dis. 127: 166–170, 1983.

3795. Proctor, D. F. "All that wheezes . . ." (editorial). Am. Rev. Respir. Dis. 127: 261–262, 1983.

3796. White, D. P., Miller, F., and Erickson, R. W. Sleep apnea and nocturnal hypoventilation after western equine encephalitis. Am. Rev. Respir. Dis. 127: 132–133, 1983.

3797. Nugent, K. M. and Pesanti, E. L. Macrophage function in pulmonary alveolar proteinosis. Am. Rev. Respir. Dis. 127: 780–781, 1983.

3798. Collett, P. W., Brancatisano, T., and Engel, L. A. Spasmodic croup in the adult. Am. Rev. Respir. Dis. 127: 500–504, 1983.

3799. Millman, R. P., Bevilacqua, J., Peterson, D. D., and Pack, A. I. Central sleep apnea in hypothyroidism. Am. Rev. Respir. Dis. 127: 504–507, 1983.

3800. Gustman, P., Yerger, L., and Wanner, A. Immediate cardiovascular effects of tension pneumothorax. Am. Rev. Respir. Dis. 127: 171–174, 1983.

3801. Weeden, D. and Smith, G. H. Surgical experience in the management of spontaneous pneumothorax, 1972–82. Thorax 38: 737–743, 1983.

3802. Yamazaki, S., Ogawa, J., Shozu, A., and Suzuki, Y. Pulmonary blood flow to rapidly reexpanded lung in spontaneous pneumothorax. Chest 81: 118–120, 1982.

3803. Hanning, C. D., Ledingham, E., and Ledingham, I. M. Late respiratory sequelae of blunt chest injury: a preliminary report. Thorax 36: 204–207, 1981.

3804. Wilson, M. M. G. and Jungner, G. Principles of screening for disease. Public Health Papers No. 34, 1968. World Health Organization, Geneva.

3805. Haynes, R. B., Sackett, D. L., Taylor, D. W., Gibson, E. S., and Johnson, A. L. Increased absenteeism from work after detection and labelling of hypertensive patients. N. Engl. J. Med. 299: 741–744, 1978.

3806. Spitzer, W. O. Task Force Report: the periodic health examination. Can. Med. Assoc. J. 121: 1193–1256, 1979.

3807. Glindmeyer, H. and Lissack, T. A network approach to National Respiratory Health Care. In: Rubin, M. (ed.). Computerization and Automation in Health Facilities. CRC Press, Boca Raton, 1983.

3808. Macklem, P. T., Chairman. Conference Report. Workshop on Screening Programs for Early Diagnosis of Airway Obstruction. Am. Rev. Respir. Dis. 109: 567–571, 1974.

3809. Townsend, M. C. and Belk, H. D. Development of a standardized pulmonary function evaluation program in industry. J. Occup. Med. 26: 657–661, 1984.

3810. Morris, J. N. Four cheers for prevention. Proc. R. Soc. Med. 66: 225–232, 1973.

3811. Reid, D. D., Hamilton, P. J. S., Keen, H., Brett, G. Z., Jarrett, R. J., and Rose, G. Cardiorespiratory disease and diabetes among middle-aged civil servants. Lancet i: 469–473, 1974.

3812. Colley, J. R. T. Diseases of the lung. Lancet ii: 1125–1127, 1974.

3813. Holland, W. W. Taking stock. Lancet ii: 1494–1497, 1974.

3814. Townsend, M. C. The effects of leaks in spirometers on measurements of pulmonary function—the implications of epidemiologic studies. J. Occup. Med. 26: 835–841, 1984.

3815. Eisen, E. A., Oliver, L. C., Christiani, D. C., Robins, J. M., and Wegman, D. H. Effects of spirometry standards in two occupational cohorts. Am. Rev. Respir. Dis. 132: 120–124, 1985.

3816. Love, R. G., Attfield, M. D., and Isles, K. D. Reproducibility of pulmonary function tests under laboratory and field conditions. Br. J. Ind. Med. 37: 63–69, 1980.

3817. Laszlo, G. Standardised lung function testing (editorial). Thorax 39: 881–886, 1984.

3818. Screening for adult respiratory disease. Official ATS statement. Am. Rev. Respir. Dis. 128: 768–773, 1983.

3819. Townsend, M. C., Du Chene, A. G., and Fallat, R. J. The effects of underrecorded forced expirations on spirometric lung function indices. Am. Rev. Respir. Dis. 126: 734–737, 1982.

3820. Mengesha, Y. A. and Mekonnen, Y. Spirometric lung function tests in normal non-smoking Ethiopian men and women. Thorax 40: 465–468, 1985.

3821. Dockery, D. W., Ware, J. H., Ferris, B. G. Jr., Glicksberg, D. S., Fay, M. E., Spiro, A. III, and Speizer, F. E. Distribution of forced expiratory volume in one second and forced vital capacity in healthy, white, adult never-smokers in six U.S. cities. Am. Rev. Respir. Dis. 131: 511–520, 1985.

3822. Martin, B. J. and Thomas, C. M. Variation among normal persons in short-term ventilatory capacity. Respiration 43: 23–28, 1982.

3823. Pagtakhan, R. D., Bjelland, J. C., Landau, L. I., Loughlin, G., Kaltenborn, W., Seeley, G., and Taussig, L. M. Sex differences in growth patterns of the airways and lung parenchyma in children. J. Appl. Physiol. 56: 1204–1210, 1984.

3824. Aitken, M. L., Schoene, R. B., Franklin, J., and Pierson, D. J. Pulmonary function in subjects at the extremes of stature. Am. Rev. Respir. Dis. 131: 166–168, 1985.

3825. Osmanliev, D. P., Davies, E. E., and Pride, N. B. Transit time analysis of the forced expiratory spirogram in male smokers. Bull. Eur. Physiopathol. Respir. 20: 285–293, 1984.

3826. Colin, A. and Said, E. How to cheat with the miniature Wright peak flow meter (letter to editor). Chest 86: 156, 1984.

3827. Wilson, S. H., Cooke, N. T., Edwards, R. H. T., and Spiro, S. G. Predicted normal values for maximal respiratory pressures in Caucasian adults and children. Thorax 39: 535–538, 1984.

3828. Wagener, J. S., Hibbert, M. E., and Landau, L. I. Maximal respiratory pressures in children. Am. Rev. Respir. Dis. 129: 873–875, 1984.

3829. Smyth, R. J., Chapman, K. R., and Rebuck, A. S. Maximal inspiratory and expiratory pressures in adolescents. Chest 86: 568–572, 1984.

3830. Teculescu, D. B. Density dependence of forced expiratory flows. Methodological aspects. Bull. Eur. Physiopathol. Respir. 21: 193–204, 1985.

3831. Burns, C. B. and Scheinhorn, D. J. Evaluation of the single-breath helium dilution total lung capacity in obstructive lung disease. Am. Rev. Respir. Dis. 130: 580–583, 1984.

3832. Miller, M. R., Grove, D. M., and Pincock, A. C. Time domain spirogram indices. Am. Rev. Respir. Dis. 132: 1041–1048, 1985.

3833. Huttemann, U. and Huckauf, H. Mechanical effects of the compressibility of alveolar gas in patients with chronic obstructive lung disease. Bull. Eur. Physiopathol. Respir. 7: 445–455, 1971.

3834. Rodenstein, D. O., Sopwith, T., Denison, D. M., and Stanescu, D. C. Reevaluation of the radiographic method for measurement of total lung capacity. Bull. Eur. Physiopathol. Respir. 21: 521–525, 1985.

3835. Chinn, D. J., Naruse, Y., and Cotes, J. E. Accuracy of gas analysis in lung function laboratories. Thorax 41: 133–137, 1986.

3836. Brown, R. and Slutsky, A. S. Frequency dependence of plethysmographic measurement of thoracic gas volume. J. Appl. Physiol. 57: 1865–1871, 1984.

3837. Sixt, R., Bake, B., and Oxhoj, H. The single-breath N2-test and spirometry in healthy non-smoking males. Eur. J. Respir. Dis. 65: 296–304, 1984.

3838. Degroodt, E. G., Quanjer, P. H., and Wise, M. E. Short and long term variability of indices from the single and multiple breath nitrogen test. Bull. Eur. Physiopathol. Respir. 20: 271–277, 1984.

3839. Hurst, T. S., Graham, B. L., and Cotton, D. J. Fast vs. slow exhalation before O_2 inhalation alters subsequent phase III slope. J. Appl. Physiol. 56: 52–56, 1984.

3840. Cormier, Y., Belanger, J., and Cote, A. Contribution of residual volume to the increased alveolar plateau with bronchoconstriction. Respiration 43: 174–178, 1982.

3841. Olofsson, J., Bake, B., Svardsudd, K., and Skoogh, B. -E. The single breath N2-test predicts the rate of decline in FEV_1. Eur. J. Respir. Dis. 69: 46–56, 1986.

3842. Beaty, T. H., Menkes, H. A., Cohen, B. H., and Newill, C. A. Risk factors associated with longitudinal change in pulmonary function. Am. Rev. Respir. Dis. 129: 660–667, 1984.

3843. Knudson, R. J. and Knudson, D. E. Frequency dependent phase and amplitude differences between simulated mouth and pleural pressures during panting. Chest 86: 589–591, 1984.

3844. Knudson, R. J., Bloom, J. W., Kaltenborn, W. T., Burrows, B., and Lebowitz, M. D. Assessment of air vs helium-oxygen flow-volume curves as an epidemiologic screening test. Chest 86: 419–423, 1984.

3845. Harf, A., Zidulka, A., and Chang, H. K. Nitrogen washout during tidal breathing with superimposed high-frequency chest wall oscillation. Am. Rev. Respir. Dis. 132: 350–353, 1985.

3846. Crawford, A. B. H., Makowska, M., Paiva, M., and Engel, L. A. Convection- and diffusion-dependent ventilation maldistribution in normal subjects. J. Appl. Physiol. 59: 838–846, 1985.

3847. Huang, S. Y., White, D. P., Douglas, N. J., Moore, L. G., McCullough, R. E., Weil, J. V., and Reeves, J. T. Respiratory function in normal Chinese: comparison with Caucasians. Respiration 46: 265–271, 1984.

3848. Sullivan, T. Y. and Yu, P-L. Reproducibility of CO_2 response curves with ten minutes separating each rebreathing test. Am. Rev. Respir. Dis. 129: 23–26, 1984.

3849. Gibellino, F., Osmanliev, D. P., Watson, A., and Pride, N. B. Increase in tracheal size with age. Am. Rev. Respir. Dis. 132: 784–787, 1985.

3850. Knudson, R. J., Schroter, R. C., Knudson, D. E., and Sugihara, S. Influence of airway geometry on expiratory flow limitation and density dependence. Respir. Physiol. 52: 113–123, 1983.

3851. Rodenstein, D. O., Goncette, L., and Stanescu, D. C. Extrathoracic airways changes during plethysmographic measurements of lung volume. Respir. Physiol. 52: 217–227, 1983.

3852. McCuaig, K. E., Vessal, S., Coppin, K., Wiggs, B. J. R., Dahlby, R., and Pare, P. D. Variability in measurements of pressure-volume curves in normal subjects. Am. Rev. Respir. Dis. 131: 656–658, 1985.

3853. Krell, W. S., Agrawal, K. P., and Hyatt, R. E. Quiet-breathing vs panting methods for determination of specific airway conductance. J. Appl. Physiol. 57: 1917–1922, 1984.

3854. Rozen, D., Bracamonte, M., and Sergysels, R. Comparison between plethysmographic and forced oscillation techniques in the assessment of airflow obstruction. Respiration 44: 197–203, 1983.

3855. Sepulveda, M.-J., Hankinson, J. L., Castellan, R. M., and Cocke, J. B. Cotton induced bronchoconstriction detected by a forced random noise oscillator. Br. J. Ind. Med. 41: 480–486, 1984.

3856. Cauberghs, M. and Van de Woestijne, K. P. Comparison of two forced oscillation techniques. Respiration 45: 22–25, 1984.

3857. Duiverman, E. J., Clement, J., Van de Woestijne, K. P., Neijens, H. J., Van den Bergh, A. C. M., and Kerrebijn, K. F. Forced oscillation technique. Reference values for resistance and reactance over a frequency spectrum of 2–26 Hz in healthy children aged 2.3–12.5 years. Bull. Eur. Physiopathol. Respir. 21: 171–178, 1985.

3858. James, P. N. E., Rees, P. J., Chowienczyk, P. J., and Cochrane, G. M. Assessment of changes in airway calibre using the body plethysmograph. Bull. Eur. Physiopathol. Respir. 21: 393–397, 1985.

3859. Teculescu, D. B. Conference report: transfer factor for the lung: time is come for standardization. Bull. Eur. Physiopathol. Respir. 21: 215–217, 1985.

3860. Chinn, D. J., Naruse, Y., and Cotes, J. E. Accuracy of gas analysis in lung function laboratories. Thorax 41: 158–159, 1986.

3861. Miller, A. and Thornton, J. C. Reference equations for the single-breath diffusing capacity (letter to editor). Am. Rev. Respir. Dis. 133: 1210, 1986.

3862. Paoletti, P., Viegi, G., Pistelli, G., Di Pede, F., Giuntini, C., Lebowitz, M. D., and Knudson, R. J. Reference equations for the single-breath diffusing capacity (letter to editor). Am. Rev. Respir. Dis. 133: 1211, 1986.

3863. Paoletti, P., Viegi, G., Pistelli, G., Di Pede, F., Fazzi, P., Polato, R., Saetta, M., Zambon, R., Carli, G., Giuntini, C., Lebowitz, M. D., and Knudson, R. J. Reference equations for the single-breath diffusing capacity. Am. Rev. Respir. Dis. 132: 806–813, 1985.

3864. Morris, A. H. and Crapo, R. O. Standardization of computation of single-breath transfer factor. Bull. Eur. Physiopathol. Respir. 21: 183–189, 1985.

3865. Petermann, W. Effect of low hemoglobin levels on the diffusing capacity of the lungs for CO. Respiration 47: 30–38, 1985.

3866. Felton, C., Rose, G. L., Cassidy, S. S., and Johnson, R. L. Jr. Comparison of lung diffusing capacity during rebreathing and during slow exhalation. Respir. Physiol. 43: 13–22, 1981.

3867. Leech, J. A., Martz, L., Liben, A., and Becklake, M. R. Diffusing capacity for carbon monoxide. Am. Rev. Respir. Dis. 132: 1127–1129, 1985.

3868. Cotes, J. E. Standardization of lung transfer factor (editorial). Bull. Eur. Physiopathol. Respir. 21: 123–124, 1985.

3869. Graham, B. L., Mink, J. T., and Cotton, D. J. Effect of breath-hold time on DLco(SB) in patients with airway obstruction. J. Appl. Physiol. 58: 1319–1325, 1985.

3870. Rubin, D. Z., Lewis, S. M., and Mittman, C. Factors affecting expired waveform for carbon monoxide. J. Appl. Physiol. 56: 708–715, 1984.

3871. Kanner, R. E. and Crapo, R. O. The relationship between alveolar oxygen tension and the single-breath carbon monoxide diffusing capacity. Am. Rev. Respir. Dis. 133: 676–678, 1986.

3872. Neville, E., Kendrick, A. H., and Gibson, G. J. A standardised method of estimating Kco on exercise. Thorax 39: 823–827, 1984.

3873. Kindig, N. B. and Hazlett, D. R. The effects of breathing pattern in the estimation of pulmonary diffusing capacity. Q. J. Exp. Physiol. 59: 311–329, 1974.

3874. Burchardi, H. and Stokke, T. Pulmonary diffusing capacity for carbon monoxide by rebreathing in mechanically ventilated patients. Bull. Eur. Physiopathol. Respir. 21: 263–273, 1985.

3875. Hlastala, M. P. Multiple inert gas elimination technique. J. Appl. Physiol. 56: 1–7, 1984.

3876. Wagner, P. D., Smith, C. M., Davies, N. J. H., McEvoy, R. D., and Gale, G. E. Estimation of ventilation-perfusion inequality by inert gas elimination without arterial sampling. J. Appl. Physiol. 59: 376–383, 1985.

3877. Burki, N. K. Arterial blood gas measurement (editorial). Chest 88: 3–4, 1985.

3878. Pennock, B. E. The determination of static lung volumes (letter to editor). Chest 87: 846, 1985.

3879. Schulzer, M., Chan-Yeung, M., and Tan, F. On the possible significance of the quadratic effect of age on lung-function measurements. Can. J. Stat. 10: 293–303, 1982.

3880. Altose, M. D., Crapo, R. O., and Wanner, A. (eds.). Determination of Static Lung Volumes. Report of the Section on Respiratory Pathophysiology. Chest 86: 471–474, 1984.

3881. Pimmel, R. L., Fullton, J. M., Ginsberg, J. F., Hazucha, M. J., Haak, E. D., McDonnell, W. F., and Bromberg, P. A. Correlation of airway resistance with forced random noise parameters. J. Appl. Physiol. 51: 33–39, 1981.

3882. Pimmel, R. L., Tsai, M. J., Winter, D. C., and Bromberg, P. A. Estimating central and peripheral respiratory resistance. J. Appl. Physiol. 45: 375–380, 1978.

3883. Graham, B. L., Mink, J. T., and Cotton, D. J. Overestimation of the single-breath carbon monoxide diffusing capacity in patients with air-flow obstruction. Am. Rev. Respir. Dis. 129: 403–408, 1984.

3884. Miller, A. C. and Pincock, A. C. Transit time analysis of spirograms (letter to editor). Bull. Eur. Physiopathol. Respir. 21: 113, 1985.

3885. Kawakami, Y., Shida, A., Yamamoto, H., and Yoshikawa, T. Pattern of genetic influences on pulmonary function. Chest 87: 507–511, 1985.

3886. Buist, A. S. Evaluation of lung function: concepts of normality. In: Simmons, D. H. (ed.). Pulmonology, Vol. 4. John Wiley & Sons, New York, 1982.

3887. Prefaut, Ch. and Engel, L. A. Vertical distribution of perfusion and inspired gas in supine man. Respir. Physiol. 43: 209–219, 1981.

3888. Paiva, M. and Engel, L. A. The anatomical basis for the sloping N2 plateau. Respir. Physiol. 44: 325–337, 1981.

3889. Richards, W., Azen, S. P., Weiss, J., Stocking, S., and Church, J. Los Angeles air pollution and asthma in children. Ann. Allergy 47: 348–354, 1981.

3890. Roger, L. J., Kehrl, H. R., Hazucha, M., and Horstman, D. H. Bronchoconstriction in asthmatics exposed to sulfur dioxide during repeated exercise. J. Appl. Physiol. 59: 784–791, 1985.

3891. Lauritzen, S. K. and Adams, W. C. Ozone inhalation effects consequent to continuous exercise in females: comparison to males. J. Appl. Physiol. 59: 1601–1606, 1985.

3892. Pearson, M. G., Chamberlain, M. J., Morgan, W. K. C., and Vinitski, S. Regional deposition of particles in the lung during cigarette smoking in humans. J. Appl. Physiol. 59: 1828–1833, 1985.

3893. Hogg, J. C., Wright, J. L., and Pare, P. D. Airways disease: evolution, pathology, and recognition. Med. J. Aust. 142: 605–607, 1985.

3894. Colebatch, H. J. H. and Greaves, I. A. Chronic airflow obstruction. Med. J. Aust. 142: 607–610, 1985.

3895. O'Byrne, P. M., Dolovich, M., Dirks, R., Roberts, R. S., and Newhouse, M. T. Lung epithelial permeability: relation to nonspecific airway responsiveness. J. Appl. Physiol. 57: 77–84, 1984.

3896. Hartiala, J., Mapp, C., Mitchell, R. A., Shields, R. L., and Gold, W. M. Cigarette smoke-induced bronchoconstriction in dogs: vagal and extravagal mechanisms. J. Appl. Physiol. 57: 1261–1270, 1984.

3897. Davis, C. S., Reid, N. W., Heidorn, K. C., and Ormrod, D. P. Final Report: oxidants assessment Ontario data base—phase 1 CSC J657. Environ. Can. April 1986.

3898. Korn, E. L. and Whittemore, A. S. Methods for analyzing panel studies of acute health effects of air pollution. Biometrics 35: 795–802, 1979.

3899. Samet, J. M., Speizer, F. E., Bishop, Y., Spengler, J. D., and Ferris, B. G. Jr. The relationship between air pollution and emergency room visits in an industrial community. J. Air. Pollut. Control Assoc. 31: 236–240, 1981.

3900. Weiss, S. T. Passive smoking and lung cancer (editorial). Am. Rev. Respir. Dis. 133: 1–3, 1986.

3901. Linn, W. S., Avol, E. L., Shamoo, D. A., Spier, C. E., Valencia, L. M., Venet, T. G., Fischer, D. A., and Hackney, J. D. A dose-response study of healthy, heavily exercising men exposed to ozone at concentrations near the ambient air quality standard. Toxicol. Ind. Health 2: 99–112, 1986.

3902. Tager, I. B. "Passive smoking" and respiratory health in children—sophistry or cause for concern? (editorial). Am. Rev. Respir. Dis. 133: 959–961, 1986.

3903. Burchfiel, C. M., Higgins, M. W., Keller, J. B., Howatt, W. F., Butler, W. J., and Higgins, I. T. T. Passive smoking in childhood. Am. Rev. Respir. Dis. 133: 966–973, 1986.

3904. Fera, T., Abboud, R. T., Richter, A., and Johal, S. S. Acute effect of smoking on elastaselike esterase activity and immunologic neutrophil elastase levels in bronchoalveolar lavage fluid. Am. Rev. Respir. Dis. 133: 568–573, 1986.

3905. Turner, J. A. McM., McNicol, M. W., and Sillett, R. W. Distribution of carboxyhaemoglobin concentrations in smokers and non-smokers. Thorax 41: 25–27, 1986.

3906. Peach, H., Shah, D., and Morris, R. W. Validity of smokers' information about present and past cigarette brands—implications for studies of the effects of falling tar yields of cigarettes on health. Thorax 41: 203–207, 1986.

3907. Abraham, W. M., Sielczak, M. W., Delehunt, J. C., Marchette, B., and Wanner, A. Impairment of tracheal mucociliary clearance but not ciliary beat frequency by a combination of low level ozone and sulfur dioxide in sheep. Eur. J. Respir. Dis. 68: 114–120, 1986.

3908. Portnoy, P. R. and Mullahy, J. Urban air quality and acute respiratory illness. J. Urban Economics 20: 21–38, 1986.

3909. Gammage, R. B. and Kaye, S. V. (eds.). Indoor Air and Human Health. Lewis Publishers, Chelsea, MI, 1985.

3910. Taylor, R. G. and Clarke, S. W. Bronchial reactivity to histamine in young male smokers. Eur. J. Respir. Dis. 66: 320–326, 1985.

3911. Bridges, R. B., Fu, M. C., and Rehm, S. R. Increased neutrophil myeloperoxidase activity associated with cigarette smoking. Eur. J. Respir. Dis. 67: 84–93, 1985.

3912. Eriksson, S., Lindell, S-E., and Wiberg, R. Effects of smoking and intermediate alpha 1–antitrypsin deficiency (PiMZ) on lung function. Eur. J. Respir. Dis. 67: 279–285, 1985.

3913. Horvath, S. M., Gliner, J. A., and Matsen-Twisdale, J. A. Pulmonary function and maximum exercise responses following acute ozone exposure. Aviat. Space Environ. Med. 50: 901–905, 1979.

3914. Hedenstrom, H., Malmberg, P., and Agarwal, K. Reference values for lung function tests in females. Regression equations with smoking variables. Bull. Eur. Physiopathol. Respir. 21: 551–557, 1985.

3915. Folinsbee, L. J., Bedi, J. F., and Horvath, S. M. Pulmonary function changes after 1 hr continuous heavy exercise in 0.21 ppm ozone. J. Appl. Physiol. 57: 984–988, 1984.

3916. Kulle, T. J., Sauder, L. R., Kerr, H. D., Farrell, B. P., Bermel, M. S., and Smith, D. M. Duration of pulmonary function adaptation to ozone in humans. Am. Ind. Hyg. Assoc. J. 43: 832–837, 1982.

3917. Folinsbee, L. J., Bedi, J. F., and Horvath, S. M. Pulmonary response to threshold levels of sulfur dioxide (1.0 ppm) and ozone (0.3 ppm). J. Appl. Physiol. 58: 1738–1787, 1985.

3918. Adams, W. C. and Schlelegle, E. S. Ozone and high ventilation effects on pulmonary function and endurance performance. J. Appl. Physiol. 55: 805–812, 1983.

3919. Schneider, T. and Grant, L. (eds.). Air Pollution by Nitrogen Oxides. Studies in Environmental Science 21. Proceedings of the US-Dutch International Symposium, Maastricht, The Netherlands, May 24–28, 1982. Elsevier Scientific Publishing, Amsterdam, Oxford, and New York, 1982.

3920. Guyatt, G. H. and Newhouse, M. T. Are active and passive smoking harmful? Chest 88: 445–451, 1985.

3921. Minty, B. D., Royston, D., and Jones, J. G. Some short-term effects of changing to lower yield cigarettes. Chest 88: 531–536, 1985.

3922. Linn, W. S., Fischer, D. A., Shamoo, D. A., Spier, C. E., Valencia, L. M., Anzar, U. T., and Hackney, J. D. Controlled exposures of volunteers with chronic obstructive pulmonary disease to sulfur dioxide. Environ. Res. 37: 445–451, 1985.

3923. Berkey, C. S., Ware, J. H., Dockery, D. W., and Ferris, B. G. Jr. Indoor air pollution and pulmonary function growth in preadolescent children. Am. J. Epidemiol. 123: 250–260, 1986.

3924. Dodge, R., Solomon, P., Moyers, J., and Hayes, C. A longitudinal study of children exposed to sulfur oxides. Am. J. Epidemiol. 121: 720–736, 1985.

3925. Chadha, T. S., Lang, E., Birch, S., and Sackner, M. A. Respiratory drive in nonsmokers and smokers assessed by passive tilt and mouth occlusion pressure. Chest 87: 6–10, 1985.

3926. Burki, N. K. Correction (letter to editor). Chest 88: 314–315, 1985.

3927. Linn, W. S., Solomon, J. C., Trim, S. C., Spier, C. E., Shamoo, D. A., Venet, T. G., Avol, E. L., and Hackney, J. D. Effects of exposure to 4 ppm nitrogen dioxide in healthy and asthmatic volunteers. Arch. Environ. Health 40: 234–239, 1985.

3928. Hatzakis, A., Katsouyyanni, K., Kalandidi, A., Day, N., and Trichopoulos, D. Short-term effects of air pollution on mortality in Athens. Int. J. Epidemiol. 15: 73–81, 1986.

3929. Linn, W. S., Avol, E. L., Shamoo, D. A., Venet, T. G., Anderson, K. R., Whynot, J. D., and Hackney, J. D. Asthmatics' responses to 6-hr sulfur dioxide exposures on two successive days. Arch. Environ. Health 39: 313–319, 1984.

3930. Schachter, E. N., Witek, T. J. Jr., Beck, G. J., Hosein, H. R., Colice, G., Leaderer, B. P., and Cain, W. Airway effects of low concentrations of sulfur dioxide: dose-response characteristics. Arch. Environ. Health 39: 34–42, 1984.

3931. Dodge, R., Solomon, P., Moyers, J., and Hayes, C. A longitudinal study of children exposed to sulfur oxides. Am. J. Epidemiol. 121: 720–736, 1985.

3932. McLeod, R., Mack, D. G., McLeod, E. G., Campbell, E. J., and Estes, R. G. Alveolar macrophage function and inflammatory stimuli in smokers with and without obstructive lung disease. Am. Rev. Respir. Dis. 131: 377–384, 1985.

3933. Medici, T. C., Unger, S., and Ruegger, M. Smoking pattern of smokers with and without tobacco-smoke-related lung diseases. Am. Rev. Respir. Dis. 131: 385–388, 1985.

3934. McDonnell, W. F. III, Horstmann, D. H., Abdul-Salaam, S., and House, D. E. Reproducibility of individual responses to ozone exposure. Am. Rev. Respir. Dis. 131: 36–40, 1985.

3935. Abboud, R. T., Fera, T., Richter, A., Tabona, M. Z., and Johal, S. Acute effect of smoking on the functional activity of alpha$_1$-protease inhibitor in bronchoalveolar lavage fluid. Am. Rev. Respir. Dis. 131: 79–85, 1985.

3936. Samet, J. M. Defining an adverse respiratory health effect (editorial). Am. Rev. Respir. Dis. 131: 487, 1985.

3937. Bethel, R. A., Sheppard, D., Geffroy, B., Tam, E., Nadel, J. A., and Boushey, H. A. Effect of 0.25 ppm sulfur dioxide on airway resistance in freely breathing, heavily exercising, asthmatic subjects. Am. Rev. Respir. Dis. 131: 659–661, 1985.

3938. American Thoracic Society. Guidelines as to what constitutes an adverse respiratory health effect, with special reference to epidemiologic studies of air pollution. Ferris, B. G. Jr., Chairman. Am. Rev. Respir. Dis. 131: 666–668, 1985.

3939. Castellan, R. M., Sanderson, W. T., and Petersen, M. R. Prevalence of radiographic appearance of pneumoconiosis in an unexposed blue collar population. Am. Rev. Respir. Dis. 131: 684–686, 1985.

3940. Kehrl, H. R., Hazucha, M. J., Solic, J. J., and Bromberg, P. A. Responses of subjects with chronic obstructive pulmonary disease after exposures to 0.3 ppm ozone. Am. Rev. Respir. Dis. 131: 719–724, 1985.

3941. Kulle, T. J., Sauder, L. R., Hebel, J. R., and Chatham, M. D. Ozone response relationships in healthy nonsmokers. Am. Rev. Respir. Dis. 132: 36–41, 1985.

3942. Chapman, R. S., Calafiore, D. C., and Hasselblad, V. Prevalence of persistent cough and phlegm, in young adults in relation to long-term ambient sulfur oxide exposure. Am. Rev. Respir. Dis. 132: 261–267, 1985.

3943. Rodenstein, D. O. and Stanescu, D. C. Pattern of inhalation of tobacco smoke in pipe, cigarette, and never smokers. Am. Rev. Respir. Dis. 132: 628–632, 1985.

3944. Lellouch, J., Claude, J. -R., Martin, J. -P., Orssaud, G., Zaoui, D., and Bieth, J. G. Smoking does not reduce the functional activity of serum alpha-1-proteinase inhibitor. Am. Rev. Respir. Dis. 132: 818–820, 1985.

3945. McDonnell, W. F. III, Chapman, R. S., Leigh, M. W., Strope, G. L., and Collier, A. M. Respiratory responses of vigorously exercising children to 0.12 ppm ozone exposure. Am. Rev. Respir. Dis. 132: 875–879, 1985.

3946. Kimmel, E. C., Winsett, D. W., and Diamond, L. Augmentation of elastase-induced emphysema by cigarette smoke. Am. Rev. Respir. Dis. 132: 885–893, 1985.

3947. Saetta, M., Ghezzo, H., Kim, W. D., King, M., Angus, G. E., Wang, N. -S., and Cosio, M. G. Loss of alveolar attachments in smokers. Am. Rev. Respir. Dis. 132: 894–900, 1985.

3948. Miller, M. R., Pincock, A. C., and Grove, D. M. Patterns of spirogram abnormality in individual smokers. Am. Rev. Respir. Dis. 132: 1034–1040, 1985.

3949. American Thoracic Society. Health effects of smoking on children. Am. Rev. Respir. Dis. 132: 1137–1138, 1985.

3950. Morgan, W. K. C. Prevalence of radiographic appearance of pneumoconiosis in an unexposed blue collar population (letter to editor). Am. Rev. Respir. Dis. 132: 1139, 1985.

3951. Ludwig, P. W., Schwartz, B. A., Hoidal, J. R., and Niewohner, D. E. Cigarette smoking causes accumulation of polymorphonuclear leukocytes in alveolar septum. Am. Rev. Respir. Dis. 131: 828–830, 1985.

3952. Taylor, R. G., Gross, E., Joyce, H., Holland, F., and Pride, N. B. Smoking, allergy, and the differential white blood cell count. Thorax 40: 17–22, 1985.

3953. Zamel, N. and Webster, P. M. Improved expiratory airflow dynamics with smoking cessation. Bull. Eur. Physiopathol. Respir. 20: 19–23, 1984.

3954. Knudson, R. J., Bloom, J. W., Knudson, D. E., and Kaltenborn, W. T. Subclinical effects of smoking. Chest 86: 20–29, 1984.

3955. Minty, B. D., Royston, D., Jones, J. G., and Hulands, G. H. The effect of nicotine on pulmonary epithelial permeability in man. Chest 86: 72–74, 1984.

3956. Sparrow, D., Glynn, R. J., Cohen, M., and Weiss, S. T. The relationship of the peripheral leukocyte count and cigarette smoking to pulmonary function among adult men. Chest 86: 383–386, 1984.

3957. Decramer, M., Demedts, M., and Van de Woestijne, K. P. Isocapnic hyperventilation with cold air in healthy nonsmokers, smokers and asthmatic subjects. Bull. Eur. Physiopathol. Respir. 20: 237–243, 1984.

3958. Groth, S., Lindell, S. E., Kabiraj, M. U., Bulow, K., Arborelius, M. Jr., and Simonsson, B. G. Bronchial reactivity and small airway dysfunction in subjects with intermediate

3959. alpha-antitrypsin deficiency. Bull. Eur. Physiopathol. Respir. 20: 279–284, 1984.

3959. Nocturnal Oxygen Therapy Trial Group. Continuous or nocturnal oxygen therapy in hypoxemic obstructive lung disease. Ann. Intern. Med. 93: 391–398, 1980.

3960. Emmett, P. C., Love, R. G., Hannan, W. J., Millar, A. M., and Soutar, C. A. The relationship between the pulmonary distribution of inhaled fine aerosols and tests of small airway function. Bull. Eur. Physiopathol. Respir. 20: 325–332, 1984.

3961. Malik, S. K., Behera, D., and Jindal, S. K. Reverse smoking and chronic obstructive lung disease. Br. J. Dis. Chest 77: 199–201, 1983.

3962. Chan-Yeung, M. and Buncio, D. Leukocyte count, smoking and lung function. Am. J. Med. 76: 31–37, 1984.

3963. Brunekreef, B., Fischer, P., Remijn, B., Van der Lende, R., Schouten, J., and Quanjer, P. Indoor air pollution and its effect on pulmonary function of adult non-smoking women: III. Passive smoking and pulmonary function. Int. J. Epidemiol. 14: 227–230, 1985.

3964. Vedal, S., Schenker, M. B., Samet, J. M., and Speizer, F. E. Risk factors for childhood respiratory disease. Am. Rev. Respir. Dis. 130: 187–192, 1984.

3965. Welty, C., Weiss, S. T., Tager, I. B., Munoz, A., Becker, C., Speizer, F. E., and Ingram, R. H. Jr. The relationship of airways responsiveness to cold air, cigarette smoking, and atopy to respiratory symptoms and pulmonary function in adults. Am. Rev. Respir. Dis. 130: 198–200, 1984.

3966. Huchon, G. J., Russell, J. A., Barritault, L. G., Lipavsky, A., and Murray, J. F. Chronic air-flow limitation does not increase respiratory epithelial permeability assessed by aerosolized solute, but smoking does. Am. Rev. Respir. Dis. 130: 457–460, 1984.

3967. Tashkin, D. P., Clark, V. A., Coulson, A. H., Simmons, M., Bourque, L. B., Reems, C., Detels, R., Sayre, J. W., and Rokaw, S.N. The UCLA population studies of chronic obstructive respiratory disease. VIII. Effects of smoking cessation on lung function: a prospective study of a free-living population. Am. Rev. Respir. Dis. 130: 707–715, 1984.

3968. McBride, M. J., Guyatt, A. R., Kirkham, A. J. T., and Cumming, G. Assessment of smoking behaviour and ventilation with cigarettes of differing nicotine yields. Clin. Sci. 67: 619–631, 1984.

3969. Buist, A. S., Vollmer, W. M., and Johnson, L. R. Does the single-breath N2 test identify the susceptible individual? Chest 85: 10S, 1984.

3970. O'Brien, T. G. and Sweeney, D. F. Interstitial viral pneumonitis complicated by severe respiratory failure. Chest 63: 314–322, 1973.

3971. Buist, A. S. Evaluation of lung function: tests of small airway function. In: Simmons, D. H. (ed.). Pulmonology. Vol. 3. John Wiley & Sons, New York, 1981.

3972. Adams, L., Lonsdale, D., Robinson, M., Rawbone, R., and Guz, A. Respiratory impairment induced by smoking in children in secondary schools. Br. Med. J. 288: 891–895, 1984.

3973. Sutton, S. R., Russell, M. A. H., Iyer, R., Feyerabend, C., and Saloojee, Y. Relationship between cigarette yields, puffing patterns, and smoke intake: evidence for tar compensation? Br. Med. J. 285: 600–602, 1982.

3974. Da Silva, A. M. T. and Hamosh, P. Effect of smoking a cigarette on the density dependence of maximal expiratory flow. Respiration 43: 258–262, 1982.

3975. Tager, I. B., Weiss, S. T., Munoz, A., Rosner, B., and Speizer, F. E. Longitudinal study of the effects of maternal smoking on pulmonary function in children. N. Engl. J. Med. 309: 699–703, 1983.

3976. Lumsden, A. B., McLean, A., and Lamb, D. Goblet and Clara cells of human distal airways: evidence for smoking induced changes in their numbers. Thorax 39: 844–849, 1984.

3977. Ando, M., Sugimoto, M., Nishi, R., Suga, M., Horio, S., Kohrogi, H., Shimazu, K., and Araki, S. Surface morphology and function of human pulmonary alveolar macrophages from smokers and non-smokers. Thorax 39: 850–856, 1984.

3978. Buczko, G. B., Day, A., Vanderdoelen, J. L., Boucher, R., and Zamel, N. Effects of cigarette smoking and short-term cessation on airway responsiveness to inhaled methacholine. Am. Rev. Respir. Dis. 129: 12–14, 1984.

3979. Buczko, G. B. and Zamel, N. Combined effect of cigarette smoking and allergic rhinitis on airway responsiveness to inhaled methacholine. Am. Rev. Respir. Dis. 129: 15–16, 1984.

3980. Kennedy, S. M., Elwood, R. K., Wiggs, B. J. R., Pare, P. D., and Hogg, J. C. Increased airway mucosal permeability in smokers. Am. Rev. Respir. Dis. 129: 143–148, 1984.

3981. Galdston, M., Levytska, V., Schwartz, M., and Magnusson, B. Ceruloplasmin. Am. Rev. Respir. Dis. 129: 258–263, 1984.

3982. Ware, J. H., Dockery, D. W., Spiro, A., III, Speizer, F. E., and Ferris, B. G. Jr. Passive smoking, gas cooking, and respiratory health of children living in six cities. Am. Rev. Respir. Dis. 129: 366–374, 1984.

3983. Brambilla, I., Arlati, S., Micallef, E., Sacerdoti, C., and Rolo, J. A portable oxygen system corrects hypoxemia without significantly increasing metabolic demands. Am. Rev. Respir. Dis. 131: 51–53, 1985.

3984. Tashkin, D. P., Clark, V. A., Simmons, M., Reems, C., Coulson, A. H., Bourque, L. B., Sayre, J. W., Detels, R., and Rokaw, S. The UCLA population studies of chronic obstructive respiratory disease. VII. Relationship between parental smoking and children's lung function. Am. Rev. Respir. Dis. 129: 891–897, 1984.

3985. Niederman, M. S., Fritts, L. L., Merrill, W. W., Fick, R. B., Matthay, R. A., Reynolds, H. Y., and Gee, J. B. L. Demonstration of a free elastolytic metalloenzyme in human lung lavage fluid and its relationship to alpha$_1$-antiprotease. Am. Rev. Respir. Dis. 129: 943–947, 1984.

3986. Susuki, S., Sasaki, H., and Takishima, T. Effects of smoking on dynamic compliance and respiratory resistance. Arch. Environ. Health 38: 133–137, 1983.

3987. Taylor, R. G., Woodman, G., and Clarke, S. W. Plasma nicotine concentration and the white blood cell count in smokers. Thorax 41: 407–408, 1986.

3988. Environmental Tobacco Smoke. National Academy Press, Washington, D.C., 1986.

3989. The Health Consequences of Involuntary Smoking. US Dept of Health and Human Services, 1986.

3990. Lee, S. D., Schneider, T., Grant, L. D., and Verkerk, P. J. (eds.). Aerosols. Lewis Publishers, Chelsea, MI, 1986.

3991. Bates, D. V. and Sizto, R. A study of hospital admissions and air pollutants in southern Ontario. In: Lee, S. D., Schneider, T., Grant, L. D., and Verkerk, P. J. (eds.). Aerosols. Lewis Publishers, Chelsea, MI, 1986.

3992. Adams, W. C., Savin, W. M., and Christo, A. E. Detection of ozone toxicity during continuous exercise via the effective dose concept. J. Appl. Physiol. 51: 415–422, 1981.

3993. Silverman, F. Asthma and respiratory irritants (ozone). Environ. Health Perspect. 29: 131–136, 1979.

3994. Holguin, A. H., Buffler, P. A., Contant, M. P. H. Jr., Stock, T. H., Kotchmar, D., Hsi, B. P., Jenkins, D. E., Gehan, B. M., Noel, L. M., and Mei, M. The effects of ozone on asthmatics in the Houston area. Manuscript for Proceedings of APCA Specialty Conference on the Evaluation of Scientific Data Basis for Ozone/Oxidant Standards, 1985.

3995. Ernst, P., Thomas, D., and Becklake, M. R. Respiratory survey of North American Indian children living in proximity to an aluminum smelter. Am. Rev. Respir. Dis. 133: 307–312, 1986.

3996. Teculescu, D. B., Pham, Q. T., and Hannhart, B. Tests of small airway dysfunction: their correlation with the "conventional" lung function tests. Eur. J. Respir. Dis. 69: 175–187, 1986.

3997. Stradling, J. R., Barnes, P., and Pride, N. B. The effects of almitrine on the ventilatory response to hypoxia and hypercapnia in normal subjects. Clin. Sci. 63: 401–404, 1982.

3998. Bande, J., Clement, J., and Van de Woestijne, K. P. The influence of smoking habits and body weight on vital capacity and FEV$_1$ in male Air Force personnel: a longitudinal and cross-sectional analysis. Am. Rev. Respir. Dis. 122: 781–790, 1980.

3999. Tager, I. B., Munoz, A., Rosner, B., Weiss, S. T., Carey, V., and Speizer, F. E. Effect of cigarette smoking on the pulmonary function of children and adolescents. Am. Rev. Respir. Dis. 131: 752–759, 1985.

4000. Barter, S. J., Cunningham, D. A., Lavender, J. P., Gibellino, F., Connelan, S. J., and Pride, N. B. Abnormal ventilation scans in middle-aged smokers. Am. Rev. Respir. Dis. 132: 148–151, 1985.

4001. Taylor, R. G., Joyce, H., Gross, E., Holland, F., and Pride, N. B. Bronchial reactivity to inhaled histamine and annual rate of decline in FEV1 in male smokers and ex-smokers. Thorax 40: 9–16, 1985.

4002. Petty, T. L. Who need home oxygen? (editorial). Am. Rev. Respir. Dis. 131: 930–931, 1985.

4003. Prior, J. G., Powlson, M., Cochrane, G. M., and Wolff, C. B. Ventilatory changes during exercise and arterial PCO_2 oscillations in chronic airway obstruction patients. J. Appl. Physiol. 58: 1942–1948, 1985.

4004. Dal Nogare, A. R. and Rubin, L. J. The effects of hydralazine on exercise capacity in pulmonary hypertension secondary to chronic obstructive pulmonary disease. Am. Rev. Respir. Dis. 133: 385–369, 1986.

4005. Morrison, D. A., Henry, R., and Goldman, S. Preliminary study of the effects of low flow oxygen on oxygen delivery and right ventricular function in chronic lung disease. Am. Rev. Respir. Dis. 133: 390–395, 1986.

4006. Raff, H. and Levy, S. A. Renin-angiotensin II-aldosterone and ACTH-cortisol control during acute hypoxemia and exercise in patients with chronic obstructive pulmonary disease. Am. Rev. Respir. Dis. 133: 396–399, 1986.

4007. Levine, S., Weiser, P., and Gillen, J. Evaluation of a respiratory muscle endurance training program in the rehabilitation of patients with chronic obstructive pulmonary disease. Am. Rev. Respir. Dis. 133: 400–406, 1986.

4008. Bergin, C., Muller, N., Nichols, D. M., Lillington, G., Hogg, J. C., Mullen, B., Grymaloski, M. R., Osborne, S., and Pare, P. D. The diagnosis of emphysema. Am. Rev. Respir. Dis. 133: 541–546, 1986.

4009. Tatsumi, K., Kimura, H., Kunimoto, F., Okita, S., Tojima, H., Yuguchi, Y., Kuriyama, T., Watanabe, S., and Honda, Y. Effect of chlormadinone acetate on ventilatory control in patients with chronic obstructive pulmonary disease. Am. Rev. Respir. Dis. 133: 552–557, 1986.

4010. Greentree, L. B. Home oxygen therapy. Am. Rev. Respir. Dis. 131: 932–933, 1985.

4011. Colebatch, H. J. H. and Greaves, I. A. Chronic airflow obstruction. Med. J. Aust. 142: 607–610, 1985.

4012. Brown, S. E., King, R. R., Temerlin, S. M., Stansbury, D. W., Mahutte, C. K., and Light, R. W. Exercise performance with added dead space in chronic airflow obstruction. J. Appl. Physiol. 56: 1020–1026, 1984.

4013. Brown, R. and Slutsky, A. S. Frequency dependence of plethysmographic measurement of thoracic gas volume. J. Appl. Physiol. 57: 1865–1871, 1984.

4014. Williams, B. T. and Nicholl, J. P. Prevalence of hypoxaemic chronic obstructive lung disease with reference to long-term oxygen therapy. Lancet 2: 369–372, 1985.

4015. Anthonisen, N. R., Wright, E. C., Hodgkin, J. E., and the IPPB Trial Group. Prognosis in chronic obstructive pulmonary disease. Am. Rev. Respir. Dis. 133: 14–20, 1986.

4016. Anthonisen, N. R., Wright, E. C., and the IPPB Trial Group. Bronchodilator response in chronic obstructive pulmonary disease. Am. Rev. Respir. Dis. 133: 814–819, 1986.

4017. Wright, J. L., Wiggs, B., Pare, P. D., and Hogg, J. C. Ranking the severity of emphysema on whole lung slices. Am. Rev. Respir. Dis. 133: 930–931, 1986.

4018. Snider, G. L. Chronic obstructive pulmonary disease—a continuing challenge. Am. Rev. Respir. Dis. 133: 942–944, 1986.

4019. Cosio, M. G., Shiner, R. J., Saetta, M., Wang, N. -S., King, M., Ghezzo, H., and Angus, E. Alveolar fenestrae in smokers. Am. Rev. Respir. Dis. 133: 126–131, 1986.

4020. Petty, T. L., Silvers, G. W., and Stanford, R. E. Radial traction and small airways disease in excised human lungs. Am. Rev. Respir. Dis. 133: 132–135, 1986.

4021. Postma, D. S., Steenhuis, E. J., Van der Weele, L. Th., and Sluiter, H. J. Severe chronic airflow obstruction: can corticosteroids slow down progression? Eur. J. Respir. Dis. 67: 56–64, 1985.

4022. Flenley, D. C. Short review: inspiratory muscle training (editorial). Eur. J. Respir. Dis. 67: 153–158, 1985.

4023. Jones, D. T., Thomson, R. J., and Sears, M. R. Physical exercise and resistive breathing training in severe chronic airways obstruction—are they effective? Eur. J. Respir. Dis. 67: 159–166, 1985.

4024. Madsen, F., Secher, N. H., Kay, L., Kok-Jensen, A., and Rube, N. Inspiratory resistance versus general physical training in patients with chronic obstructive pulmonary disease. Eur. J. Respir. Dis. 67: 167–176, 1985.

4025. Pavia, D., Agnew, J. E., Glassman, J. M., Sutton, P. P., Lopez-Vidriero, M. T., Soyka, J. P., and Clarke, S. W. Effects of iodopropylidene glycerol on tracheobronchial clearance in stable, chronic bronchitic patients. Eur. J. Respir. Dis. 67: 177–184, 1985.

4026. Bratel, T., Hedenstierna, G., Nyquist, O., and Ripe, E. The effect of a new calcium antagonist, felodipine, on pulmonary hypertension and gas exchange in chronic obstructive lung disease. Eur. J. Respir. Dis. 67: 244–253, 1985.

4027. Castaing, Y., Manier, G., and Guenard, H. Effect of 26 per cent oxygen breathing on ventilation and perfusion distribution in patients with COLD. Bull. Eur. Physiopathol. Respir. 21: 17–23, 1985.

4028. Wilson, D. K., Kaplan, R. M., Timms, R. M., and Dawson, A. Acute effects of oxygen treatment upon information processing in hypoxemic COPD patients. Chest 88: 239–243, 1985.

4029. Charpin, D., Badier, M., and Orehek, J. Dose-response curves to inhaled carbachol in asthma and chronic bronchitis. Bull. Eur. Physiopathol. Respir. 21: 417–420, 1985.

4030. De Backer, W., Vermeire, P., Bogaert, E., Janssens, E., and Van Maele, R. Almitrine has no effect on gas exchange after bilateral carotid body resection in severe chronic airflow obstruction. Bull. Eur. Physiopathol. Respir. 21: 427–432, 1985.

4031. Cockcroft, A., Beaumont, A., Adams, L., and Guz, A. Arterial oxygen desaturation during treadmill and bicycle exercise in patients with chronic obstructive airways disease. Clin. Sci. 68: 327–332, 1985.

4032. Light, R. W., Merrill, E. J., Despars, J. A., Gordon, G. H., and Mutalipassi, L. R. Prevalence of depression and anxiety in patients with COPD. Chest 87: 35–38, 1985.

4033. Marthan, R., Castaing, Y., Manier, G., and Guenard, H. Gas exchange alterations in patients with chronic obstructive lung disease. Chest 87: 470–475, 1985.

4034. Mohensifar, Z., Rosenberg, N., Goldberg, H. S., and Koerner, S. K. Mechanical vibration and conventional chest physiotherapy in outpatients with stable chronic obstructive lung disease. Chest 87: 483–485, 1985.

4035. Swidwa, D. M., Montenegro, H. D., Goldman, M. D., Lutchen, K. R., and Saidel, G. M. Helium-oxygen breathing in severe chronic obstructive pulmonary disease. Chest 87: 790–795, 1985.

4036. Zack, M. B. and Palange, A. V. Oxygen supplemented exercise of ventilatory and nonventilatory muscles in pulmonary rehabilitation. Chest 88: 669–675, 1985.

4037. Strain, D. S., Kinasewitz, G. T., Franco, D. P., and George, R. B. Effect of steroid therapy on exercise performance in patients with irreversible chronic obstructive pulmonary disease. Chest 88: 718–721, 1985.

4038. Ploysongsang, Y. and Wiltse, D. W. Effects of breathing pattern and oxygen upon the alveolar arterial oxygen pressure difference in lung disease. Respiration 47: 39–47, 1985.

4039. Delaunois, L., Delwiche, J. P., and Lulling, J. Effect of medroxyprogesterone on ventilatory control and pulmonary gas exchange in chronic obstructive patients. Respiration 47: 107–113, 1985.

4040. Kawakami, Y., Yoshikawa, T., Yamamoto, H., and Nishimura, M. Involvement of respiratory perception in the resistive load compensation. Respiration 47: 247–252, 1985.

4041. Keller, R., Ragaz, A., and Borer, P. Predictors of early mortality in patients with long-term oxygen home therapy. Respiration 48: 216–221, 1985.

4042. Krzyzanowski, M. and Wysocki, M. The relation of thirteen-year mortality to ventilatory impairment and other respiratory symptoms: the Cracow study. Int. J. Epidemiol. 15: 56–64, 1986.

4043. Ware, J. H. Linear models for the analysis of longitudinal studies. Am. Stat. 39: 95–101, 1985.

4044. Albert, R. K., Muramoto, A., Caldwell, J., Koepsell, T., and Butler, J. Increases in intrathoracic pressure do not explain

the rise in left ventricular end-diastolic pressure that occurs during exercise in patients with chronic obstructive pulmonary disease. Am. Rev. Respir. Dis. 132: 623–627, 1985.

4045. Dodd, D. S., Brancatisano, T. P., and Engel, L. A. Effect of abdominal strapping on chest wall mechanics during exercise in patients with severe chronic air-flow obstruction. Am. Rev. Respir. Dis. 131: 816–821, 1985.

4046. Fleury, B., Murciano, D., Talamo, C., Aubier, M., Pariente, R., and Milic-Emili, J. Work of breathing in patients with chronic obstructive pulmonary disease in acute respiratory failure. Am. Rev. Respir. Dis. 131: 822–827, 1985.

4047. Oliven, A., Cherniack, N. S., Deal, E. C., and Kelsen, S. G. The effects of acute bronchoconstriction on respiratory activity in patients with chronic obstructive pulmonary disease. Am. Rev. Respir. Dis. 131: 236–241, 1985.

4048. Pare, P. D., Brooks, L. A., Coppin, C. A., Wright, J. L., Kennedy, S., Dahlby, R., Mink, S., and Hogg, J. C. Density-dependence of maximal expiratory flow and its correlation with small airway disease in smokers. Am. Rev. Respir. Dis. 131: 521–526, 1985.

4049. Weiss, S. T., Tager, I. B., Munoz, A., and Speizer, F. E. The relationship of respiratory infections in early childhood to the occurrence of increased levels of bronchial responsiveness and atopy. Am. Rev. Respir. Dis. 131: 573–578, 1985.

4050. Mullen, J. B. M., Wright, J. L., Wiggs, B. R., Pare, P. D., and Hogg, J. C. Reassessment of inflammation of airways in chronic bronchitis. Br. Med. J. 291: 1235–1239, 1985.

4051. Yan, K., Salome, C. M., and Woolcock, A. J. Prevalence and nature of bronchial hyperresponsiveness in subjects with chronic obstructive pulmonary disease. Am. Rev. Respir. Dis. 132: 25–29, 1985.

4052. Rochester, D. F. and Braun, N. M. T. Determinants of maximal inspiratory pressure in chronic obstructive pulmonary disease. Am. Rev. Respir. Dis. 132: 42–47, 1985.

4053. Menkes, H. A., Beaty, T. H., Cohen, B. H., and Weinmann, G. Nitrogen washout and mortality. Am. Rev. Respir. Dis. 132: 115–119, 1985.

4054. Lertzmann, M. M. and Cherniack, R. M. Rehabilitation of patients with chronic obstructive pulmonary disease. Am. Rev. Respir. Dis. 114: 1145–1165, 1976.

4055. Ward, M. E. and Stubbing, D. G. Effect of chronic lung disease on the perception of added inspiratory loads. Am. Rev. Respir. Dis. 132: 652–656, 1985.

4056. Ries, A. L., Farrow, J. T., and Clausen, J. L. Accuracy of two ear oximeters at rest and during exercise in pulmonary patients. Am. Rev. Respir. Dis. 132: 685–689, 1985.

4057. Peslin, R., Divivier, C., Gallina, C., and Cervantes, P. Upper airway artifact in respiratory impedance measurements. Am. Rev. Respir. Dis. 132: 712–714, 1985.

4058. Eliasson, O. and De Graff, A. C. Jr. The use of criteria for reversibility and obstruction to define patient groups for bronchodilator trials. Am. Rev. Respir. Dis. 132: 858–864, 1985.

4059. Nagai, A., West, W. W., Paul, J. L., and Thurlbeck, W. M. The National Institutes of Health intermittent positive-pressure breathing trial: pathology studies. I. Interrelationship between morphologic lesions. Am. Rev. Respir. Dis. 132: 937–945, 1985.

4060. Nagai, A., West, W. W., and Thurlbeck, W. M. The National Institutes of Health intermittent positive-pressure breathing trial: pathology studies. II. Correlation between morphologic findings, clinical findings, and evidence of expiratory air-flow obstruction. Am. Rev. Respir. Dis. 132: 946–953, 1985.

4061. Gottfried, S. B., Redline, S., and Altose, M. D. Respiratory sensation in chronic obstructive pulmonary disease. Am. Rev. Respir. Dis. 132: 954–959, 1985.

4062. Muramoto, A., Caldwell, J., Albert, R. K., Lakshminarayan, S., and Butler, J. Nifedipine dilates the pulmonary vasculature without producing symptomatic systemic hypotension in upright resting and exercising patients with pulmonary hypertension secondary to chronic obstructive pulmonary disease. Am. Rev. Respir. Dis. 132: 963–966, 1985.

4063. Vollmer, W. M., Johnson, L. R., and Buist, A. S. Relationship of response to a bronchodilator and decline in forced expiratory volume in one second in population studies. Am. Rev. Respir. Dis. 132: 1186–1193, 1985.

4064. Dillard, T. A., Piantadosi, S., and Rajagopal, K. R. Prediction of ventilation at maximal exercise in chronic air-flow obstruction. Am. Rev. Respir. Dis. 132: 230–235, 1985.

4065. Bye, P. T. P., Esau, S. A., Levy, R. D., Shiner, R. J., Macklem, P. T., Martin, J. G., and Pardy, R. L. Ventilatory muscle function during exercise in air and oxygen in patients with chronic air-flow obstruction. Am. Rev. Respir. Dis. 132: 236–240, 1985.

4066. Wilson, D. O., Rogers, R. M., and Hoffman, R. M. Nutrition and chronic lung disease. Am. Rev. Respir. Dis. 132: 1347–1365, 1985.

4067. Campbell, A. H., Barter, C. E., O'Connell, J. M., and Huggins, R. Factors affecting the decline of ventilatory function in chronic bronchitis. Thorax 40: 741–748, 1985.

4068. Fennerty, A. G., Banks, J., Bevan, C., and Smith, A. P. Role of airway receptors in the breathing pattern of patients with chronic obstructive lung disease. Thorax 40: 268–271, 1985.

4069. Janoff, A. Elastases and emphysema. Am. Rev. Respir. Dis. 132: 417–433, 1985.

4070. Ramsdale, E. H., Roberts, R. S., Morris, M. M., and Hargreave, F. E. Differences in responsiveness to hyperventilation and methacholine in asthma and chronic bronchitis. Thorax 40: 422–426, 1985.

4071. Swinburn, C. R., Wakefield, J. M., and Jones, P. W. Performance, ventilation, and oxygen consumption in three different types of exercise test in patients with chronic obstructive lung disease. Thorax 40: 581–586, 1985.

4072. Matthay, R. A. and Loke, J. Noninvasive assessment of cardiovascular performance in interstitial and chronic obstructive lung disease (editorial). Chest 85: 299–300, 1984.

4073. Braun, S. R., Dixon, R. M., Keim, N. L., Luby, M., Anderegg, A., and Shrago, E. S. Predictive clinical value of nutritional assessment factors in COPD. Chest 85: 353–357, 1984.

4074. Rochester, D. F. and Esau, S. A. Malnutrition and the respiratory system. Chest 85: 411–415, 1984.

4075. Healy, F., Wilson, A. F., and Fairshter, R. D. Physiologic correlates of airway collapse in chronic airflow obstruction. Chest 85: 476–481, 1984.

4076. Piquet, J., Harf, A., Lorino, H., Atlan, G., and Bignon, J. Lung volume measurement by plethysmography in chronic obstructive pulmonary disease. Influence of the panting pattern. Bull. Physiopathol. Respir. 20: 31–36, 1984.

4077. Weitzenblum, E. and Jezek, V. Evolution of pulmonary hypertension in chronic respiratory diseases. Bull. Physiopathol. Respir. 20: 73–81, 1984.

4078. Howard, P. Almitrine bismesylate (Vectarion) (editorial). Bull. Physiopathol. Respir. 20: 99–103, 1984.

4079. Lauque, D., Aug, F., Puchelle, E., Karcher, G., Tournier, J. M., Bertrand, A., Polu, J. M., and Sadoul, P. Efficiency of mucociliary clearance and cough in bronchitis. Bull. Physiopathol. Respir. 20: 145–149, 1984.

4080. Kauffmann, F. Genetics of chronic obstructive pulmonary diseases. Searching for their heterogeneity. Bull. Physiopathol. Respir. 20: 163–210, 1984.

4081. Weiss, S. T. and Speizer, F. E. Increased levels of airways responsiveness as a risk factor for development of chronic obstructive lung disease (editorial). Chest 86: 3–4, 1984.

4082. Knudson, R. J., Bloom, J. W., Knudson, D. E., and Kaltenborn, W. T. Subclinical effects of smoking. Chest 86: 20–29, 1984.

4083. Kanner, R. E. The relationship between airways responsiveness and chronic airflow limitation. Chest 86: 54–57, 1984.

4084. Nietrzeba, R. M., Elliott, C. G., Adams, T. D., Yeh, M. P., and Yanowitz, F. G. Effects of aminophylline upon the exercise performance of patients with stable chronic airflow obstruction. Bull. Eur. Physiopathol. Respir. 20: 361–367, 1984.

4085. Braun, S. R., Keim, N. L., Dixon, R. M., Clagnaz, P., Anderegg, A., and Shrago, E. S. The prevalence and determinants of nutritional changes in chronic obstructive pulmonary disease. Chest 86: 558–563, 1984.

4086. Pineda, H., Haas, F., Axen, K., and Haas, A. Accuracy of pulmonary function tests in predicting exercise tolerance in chronic obstructive pulmonary disease. Chest 86: 564–567, 1984.

4087. Miller, W. C., Heard, J. G., and Unger, K. M. Enlarged

4088. Jederlinic, P., Muspratt, J. A., and Miller, M. J. Inspiratory muscle training in clinical practice. Chest 86: 870–873, 1984.

4089. Thurlbeck, W. M. and Simon, G. Radiographic appearance of the chest in emphysema. Am. J. Roentgenol. 130: 429–440, 1978.

4090. Kaplan, R. M., Atkins, C. J., and Timms, R. Validity of a quality of well-being scale as an outcome measure in chronic obstructive pulmonary disease. J. Chron. Dis. 37: 85–93, 1984.

4091. Woodbury, M. A., Manton, K. G., and Stallard, E. Longitudinal models for chronic disease risk: and evaluation of logistic multiple regression and alternatives. Int. J. Epidemiol. 10: 187–197, 1981.

4092. Torzillo, P. J., Waterford, J. E., Hollows, F. C., and Jones, D. L. Respiratory disease amongst aborigines in the Pilbara. Int. J. Epidemiol. 12: 105–106, 1983.

4093. Schulzer, M., Enarson, D. A., and Chan-Yeung, M. Analyzing cross-sectional and longitudinal lung-function measurements: the effects of age. Can. J. Stat. 13: 7–15, 1985.

4094. Cook, N. R. and Ware, J. H. Design and analysis for longitudinal research. Annu. Rev. Public Health 4: 1–23, 1983.

4095. Woolcock, A. J. Perspective: the search for words to describe the bad blowers. Chest 85: 73S–74S, 1984.

4096. Brown, S. E., Pakron, F. J., Milne, N., Linden, G. S., Stansbury, D. W., Fischer, C. E., and Light, R. W. Effects of digoxin on exercise capacity and right ventricular function during exercise in chronic airflow obstruction. Chest 85: 187–191, 1984.

4097. Santiago, T. V., Sheft, S. A., Khan, A. U., and Edelman, N. H. Effect of naloxone on the respiratory responses to hypoxia in chronic obstructive pulmonary disease. Am. Rev. Respir. Dis. 130: 183–186, 1984.

4098. Fantone, J. C. and Ward, P. A. Mechanisms of lung parenchymal injury. Am. Rev. Respir. Dis. 130: 484–491, 1984.

4099. Burns, C. B. and Scheinhorn, D. J. Evaluation of the single-breath helium dilution total lung capacity in obstructive lung disease. Am. Rev. Respir. Dis. 130: 580–583, 1984.

4100. Sackner, M. A., Gonzalez, H., Rodriguez, M., Belsito, A., Sackner, D. R., and Grenvik, S. Assessment of asynchronous and paradoxic motion between rib cage and abdomen in normal subjects and in patients with chronic obstructive pulmonary disease. Am. Rev. Respir. Dis. 130: 588–593, 1984.

4101. Keller, C. A., Shepard, J. W. Jr., Chun, D. S., Dolan, G. F., Vasquez, P., and Minh, V. -D. Effects of hydralazine on hemodynamics, ventilation, and gas exchange in patients with chronic obstructive pulmonary disease and pulmonary hypertension. Am. Rev. Respir. Dis. 130: 606–611, 1984.

4102. Melot, C., Hallemans, R., Naeije, R., Mols, P., and Lejeune, P. Deleterious effect of nifedipine on pulmonary gas exchange in chronic obstructive pulmonary disease. Am. Rev. Respir. Dis. 130: 612–616, 1984.

4103. Hale, K. A., Ewing, S. L., Gosnell, B. A., and Niewohner, D. E. Lung disease in long-term cigarette smokers with and without chronic air-flow obstruction. Am. Rev. Respir. Dis. 130: 716–721, 1984.

4104. Mahler, D. A., Brent, B. N., Loke, J., Zaret, B. L., and Matthay, R. A. Right ventricular performance and central circulatory hemodynamics during upright exercise in patients with chronic obstructive pulmonary disease. Am. Rev. Respir. Dis. 130: 722–729, 1984.

4105. Loveridge, B., West, P., Anthonisen, N. R., and Kryger, M. H. Breathing patterns in patients with chronic obstructive pulmonary disease. Am. Rev. Respir. Dis. 130: 730–733, 1984.

4106. Snider, G. L. Conference summary. Chest 85: 84S–89S, 1984.

4107. Catford, J. C. and Ford, S. On the state of the public ill health: premature mortality in the United Kingdom and Europe. Br. Med. J. 289: 1668–1670, 1984.

4108. Tager, I. B. Surveillance techniques for respiratory illness. Arch. Environ. Health 31: 25–28, 1976.

4109. Buist, A. S. The relative contributions of nature and nurture in chronic obstructive pulmonary disease. West. J. Med. 131: 114–121, 1979.

4110. Kawakami, Y., Kishi, F., Yamamoto, H., and Miyamoto, K. Relation of oxygen delivery, mixed venous oxygenation, and pulmonary hemodynamics to prognosis in chronic obstructive pulmonary disease. N. Engl. J. Med. 308: 1045–1049, 1983.

4111. Mitchell, R. S., Webb, N. C., and Filley, G. F. Chronic obstructive bronchopulmonary disease. III. factors influencing prognosis. Am. Rev. Respir. Dis. 89: 878–896, 1964.

4112. Allegra, L., Bonsignore, G., Cresci, F., Fumagalli, G., Mandelli, V., Morpurgo, M., Panuccio, P., Pasargiklian, M., Rampulla, C., and Viroli, L. Classification of respiratory functional impairment in chronic obstructive pulmonary disease. Respiration 45: 175–184, 1984.

4113. Severa, E. and Gimenez, M. Vo_{2max} during progressive and constant bicycle exercise in patients with chronic obstructive lung disease. Respiration 45: 197–206, 1984.

4114. Ambrosino, N., Paggiaro, P. L., Roselli, M. G., and Contini, V. Failure of resistive breathing training to improve pulmonary function tests in patients with chronic obstructive pulmonary disease. Respiration 45: 455–459, 1984.

4115. Patakas, D., Sproule, B., Jones, D., Phillipow, L., and Ziutas, G. Cerebral blood flow, oxygen, carbon dioxide tensions, and blood bicarbonate in controlling drive and timing in patients with chronic obstructive pulmonary diseases. Respiration 46: 45–51, 1984.

4116. Higgins, M. W., Keller, J. B., Landis, J. R., Beaty, T. H., Burrows, B., Demets, D., Diem, J. E., Higgins, I. T. T., Lakatos, E., Lebowitz, M. D., Menkes, H., Speizer, F. E., Tager, I. B., and Weill, H. Risk of chronic obstructive pulmonary disease. Am. Rev. Respir. Dis. 130: 380–385, 1984.

4117. Lungarella, G., Fonzi, L., and Ermini, G. Abnormalities of bronchial cilia in patients with chronic bronchitis. Lung 161: 147–156, 1983.

4118. Woodcock, A. A., Gross, E. R., Gellert, A., Shah, S., Johnson, M., and Geddes, D. M. Effects of dihydrocodeine, alcohol, and caffeine on breathlessness and exercise tolerance in patients with chronic obstructive lung disease and normal blood gases. N. E. J. Med. 305: 1611–1616, 1981.

4119. Snider, G. L. A perspective on emphysema. Clin. Chest Med. 4: 329–336, 1983.

4120. Fletcher, C. M. and Pride, N. B. Definitions of emphysema, chronic bronchitis, asthma, and airflow obstruction: 25 years on from the Ciba symposium (editorial). Thorax 39: 81–85, 1984.

4121. Gilmartin, J. J. and Gibson, G. J. Abnormalities of chest wall motion in patients with chronic airflow obstruction. Thorax 39: 264–271, 1984.

4122. Pandey, M. R. Prevalence of chronic bronchitis in a rural community of the hill region of Nepal. Thorax 39: 331–336, 1984.

4123. Pandey, M. R. Domestic smoke pollution and chronic bronchitis in a rural community of the hill region of Nepal. Thorax 39: 337–339, 1984.

4124. Ramsdale, E. H., Morris, M. M., Roberts, R. S., and Hargreave, F. E. Bronchial responsiveness to methacholine in chronic bronchitis: relationship to airflow obstruction and cold air responsiveness. Thorax 39: 912–918, 1984.

4125. Macklem, P. T. Hyperinflation (editorial). Am. Rev. Respir. Dis. 129: 1–2, 1984.

4126. Fleetham, J. A., Arnup, M. E., and Anthonisen, N. R. Familial aspects of ventilatory control in patients with chronic obstructive pulmonary disease. Am. Rev. Respir. Dis. 129: 3–7, 1984.

4127. Dodd, D. S., Brancatisano, T., and Engel, L. A. Chest wall mechanics during exercise in patients with severe chronic air-flow obstruction. Am. Rev. Respir. Dis. 129: 33–38, 1984.

4128. Marini, J. J., Tyler, M. L., Hudson, L. D., Davis, B. S., and Huseby, J. S. Influence of head-dependent positions on lung volume and oxygen saturation in chronic air-flow obstruction. Am. Rev. Respir. Dis. 129: 101–105, 1984.

4129. Snider, G. L., Lucey, E. C., Christensen, T. G., Stone, P. J., Calore, J. D., Catanese, A., and Franzblau, C. Emphysema and bronchial secretory cell metaplasia induced in hamsters by human neutrophil products. Am. Rev. Respir. Dis. 129: 155–160, 1984.

4130. Jones, N. L. and Berman, L. B. Gas exchange in chronic airflow obstruction. Exercise Testing in the Dyspneic Patient. Am. Rev. Respir. Dis. 129(2)(Pt. 2)(Suppl.): S81–S83, 1984.

4131. Tuxen, D. V., Powles, A. C. P., Mathur, P. N., Pugsley, S. O., and Campbell, E. J. M. Detrimental effects of hydralazine in patients with chronic air-flow obstruction and pulmonary hypertension. Am. Rev. Respir. Dis. 129: 388–395, 1984.

4132. Aoki, T., Inoue, H., Sasaki, H., Shimura, S., Maeda, S., Tomioka, M., Takashima, T., and Niwa, T. Relation between selective alveolo-bronchograms and pulmonary function tests in patients with chronic obstructive pulmonary disease. Am. Rev. Respir. Dis. 129: 465–472, 1984.

4133. Wilson, S. H., Cooke, N. T., Moxham, J., and Spiro, S. G. Sternomastoid muscle function and fatigue in normal subjects and in patients with chronic obstructive pulmonary disease. Am. Rev. Respir. Dis. 129: 460–464, 1984.

4134. Gross, N. J. and Skorodin, M. S. Anticholinergic, antimuscarinic bronchodilators. Am. Rev. Respir. Dis. 129: 856–870, 1984.

4135. Wright, J. L., Pare, P. D., Kennedy, S., Wiggs, B., and Hogg, J. C. The detection of small airways disease. Am. Rev. Respir. Dis. 129: 989–994, 1984.

4136. Petty, T. L., Silvers, G. W., and Stanford, R. E. Small airway disease is associated with elastic recoil changes in excised human lungs. Am. Rev. Respir. Dis. 130: 42–45, 1984.

4137. Murciano, D., Aubier, M., Viau, F., Bussi, S., Milic-Emili, J., Pariente, R., and Derenne, J. -P. Effects of airway anesthesia on pattern of breathing and blood gases in patients with chronic obstructive pulmonary disease during acute respiratory failure. Am. Rev. Respir. Dis. 126: 113–117, 1982.

4138. Pardy, R. L., Rivington, R. N., Milic-Emili, J., and Mortola, J. P. Control of breathing in chronic obstructive pulmonary disease. Am. Rev. Respir. Dis. 125: 6–11, 1982.

4139. Powles, A. C. P., Tuxen, D. V., Mahood, C. B., Pugsley, S. O., and Campbell, E. J. M. The effect of intravenously administered almitrine, a peripheral chemoreceptor agonist, on patients with chronic air-flow obstruction. Am. Rev. Respir. Dis. 127: 284–289, 1973.

4140. Stradling, J. R., Nicholl, C. G., Cover, D., Davies, E. E., Hughes, J. M. B., and Pride, N. B. The effects of oral almitrine on pattern of breathing and gas exchange in patients with chronic obstructive pulmonary disease. Clin. Sci. 66: 435–442, 1984.

4141. Marazzini, L., Cavestri, R., Mastropasqua, B., Banducci, S., Pelucchi, A., and Longhini, E. Pressure available for expiration in chronic airway disease. Respiration 44: 241–251, 1983.

4142. Tobin, M. J., Jenouri, G., and Sackner, M. A. Effect of naloxone on breathing pattern in patients with chronic obstructive pulmonary disease with and without hypercapnia. Respiration 44: 419–424, 1983.

4143. Bahous, R. G., Carter, A., Ouimet, G., Pineau, L., and Malo, J. -L. Nonallergic bronchial hyperexcitability in chronic bronchitis. Am. Rev. Respir. Dis. 129: 216–220, 1984.

4144. Greaves, I. A. and Colebatch, H. J. H. Observations on the pathogenesis of chronic airflow obstruction in smokers: implications for the detection of "early" lung disease (editorial). Thorax 41: 81–87, 1986.

4145. Sackner, M. A., Gonzalez, H. F., Jenouri, G., and Rodriguez, M. Effects of abdominal and thoracic breathing on breathing pattern components in normal subjects and in patients with chronic obstructive pulmonary disease. Am. Rev. Respir. Dis. 130: 584–587, 1984.

4146. Hughes, J. A., Gray, B. J., and Hutchison, D. C. S. Changes in transcutaneous oxygen tension during exercise in pulmonary emphysema. Thorax 39: 424–431, 1984.

4147. Baile, E. M., Dahlby, R. W., Wiggs, B. R., and Pare, P. D. Role of tracheal and bronchial circulation in respiratory heat exchange. J. Appl. Physiol. 58: 217–222, 1985.

4148. McFadden, E. R. Jr., Pichurko, B. M., Bowman, H. F., Ingenito, E., Burns, S., Dowling, N., and Solway, J. Thermal mapping of the airways in humans. J. Appl. Physiol. 58: 564–570, 1985.

4149. Anthonisen, N. R. Hypoxemia and O_2 therapy. Am. Rev. Respir. Dis. 126: 729–733, 1982.

4150. Long, W. M., Sprung, C. L., El Fawal, H., Yerger, L. D., Eyre, P., Abraham, W. M., and Wanner, A. Effects of histamine on bronchial artery blood flow and bronchomotor tone. J. Appl. Physiol. 59: 254–261, 1985.

4151. Gavriely, N., Palti, Y., Alroy, G., and Grotberg, J. B. Measurement and theory of wheezing breath sounds. J. Appl. Physiol. 57: 481–492, 1984.

4152. Fuller, R. W., Dixon, C. M. S., Dollery, C. T., and Barnes, P. J. Prostaglandin D$_2$ potentiates airway responsiveness to histamine and methacholine. Am. Rev. Respir. Dis. 133: 252–254, 1986.

4153. Marks, J., Pasterkamp, H., Tal, A., and Leahy, F. Relationship between respiratory muscle strength, nutritional status, and lung volume in cystic fibrosis and asthma. Am. Rev. Respir. Dis. 133: 414–417, 1986.

4154. Hillman, D. R., Prentice, L., and Finucane, K. E. The pattern of breathing in acute severe asthma. Am. Rev. Respir. Dis. 133: 587–592, 1986.

4155. McFadden, E. R. Jr., Critical appraisal of the therapy of asthma—an idea whose time has come (editorial). Am. Rev. Respir. Dis. 133: 723–724, 1986.

4156. Gross, N. J. COPD: A disease of reversible air-flow obstruction (editorial). Am. Rev. Respir. Dis. 133: 725–726, 1986.

4157. Karpel, J. P., Appel, D., Breidbart, D., and Fusco, M. J. A comparison of atropine sulfate and metaproterenol sulfate in the emergency treatment of asthma. Am. Rev. Respir. Dis. 133: 727–729, 1986.

4158. Dodge, R., Cline, M. G., and Burrows, B. Comparisons of asthma, emphysema, and chronic bronchitis diagnoses in a general population sample. Am. Rev. Respir. Dis. 133: 981–986, 1986.

4159. Collett, P. W., Brancatisano, A. P., and Engel, L. A. Upper airway dimensions and movements in bronchial asthma. Am. Rev. Respir. Dis. 133: 1143–1149, 1986.

4160. Togias, A. G., Naclerio, R. M., Peters, S. P., Nimmagadda, I., Proud, D., Kagey-Sobotka, A., Adkinson, N. F. Jr., Norman, P. S., and Lichtenstein, L. M. Am. Rev. Respir. Dis. 133: 1133–1137, 1986.

4161. Moreno, R. H., Hogg, J. C., and Pare, P. D. Mechanics of airway narrowing. Am. Rev. Respir. Dis. 133: 1171–1180, 1986.

4162. Ayres, J. G. Seasonal pattern of acute bronchitis in general practice in the United Kingdom, 1976–83. Thorax 41: 106–110, 1986.

4163. Ayres, J. G. Trends in asthma and hay fever in general practice in the United Kingdom 1976–83. Thorax 41: 111–116, 1986.

4164. Gaillard, R. C., Bachman, M., Rochat, T., Egger, D., De Haller, R., and Junod, A. F. Exercise induced asthma and endogenous opioids. Thorax 41: 350–354, 1986.

4165. Luksza, A. R., Smith, P., Coakley, J., Gordan, I. J., and Atherton, S. T. Acute severe asthma treated by mechanical ventilation: 10 years' experience from a district general hospital. Thorax 41: 459–463, 1986.

4166. Higgins, B., Greening, A. P., and Crompton, G. K. Assisted ventilation in severe acute asthma. Thorax 41: 464–467, 1986.

4167. Godfrey, S. Controversies in the pathogenesis of exercise-induced asthma. Eur. J. Respir. Dis. 68: 81–88, 1986.

4168. Poppius, H., Sovijarvi, A., and Tammilehto, L. Lack of protective effect of high-dose ipratropium on bronchoconstriction following exercise with cold air breathing in patients with mild asthma. Eur. J. Respir. Dis. 68: 319–325, 1986.

4169. Halfon, N. and Newacheck, P. W. Trends in hospitalization for acute childhood asthma, 1970–84. Am. J. Public Health 76: 1308–1311, 1986.

4170. Bates, D. V. and Baker-Anderson, M. Asthma mortality and morbidity in Canada. J. Allergy Clin. Immunol. 80: 395–397, 1987.

4171. Nery, L. E., Wasserman, K., Andrews, J. D., Huntsman, D. J., Hansen, J. E., and Whipp, B. J. Ventilatory and gas exchange kinetics during exercise in chronic airways obstruction. J. Appl. Physiol. 53: 1594–1602, 1982.

4172. Boner, A. L., Niero, E., Grigolini, C., Valletta, E. A., Biancotto, R., and Gaburro, D. Inhibition of exercise-induced asthma by three forms of sodium cromoglycate. Eur. J. Respir. Dis. 66: 21–24, 1985.

4173. Anderson, S. D., Schoeffel, R. E., Black, J. L., and Daviskas, E. Airway cooling as the stimulus to exercise-induced asthma—a re-evaluation. Eur. J. Respir. Dis. 67: 20–30, 1985.

4174. Madsen, F., H-Rathlou, N. H., Frolund, L., Svendsen, U. G., and Weeke, B. Short and long term reproducibility of responsiveness to inhaled histamine: Rt compared to FEV$_1$ as measurement of response to challenge. Eur. J. Respir. Dis. 67: 193–203, 1985.

4175. Lofdahl, C. -G. and Barnes, P. J. Calcium channel blockade and asthma—the current position (editorial). Eur. J. Respir. Dis. 67: 233–237, 1985.

4176. Ozenne, G., Moore, N. D., Leprevost, A., Tardif, C., Boismare, F., Pasquis, P., and Lemercier, J. -P. Nifedipine in chronic bronchial asthma: a randomized double-blind cross-over trial against placebo. Eur. J. Respir. Dis. 67: 238–243, 1985.

4177. Bahous, J., Cartier, A., and Malo, J. L. Monitoring of peak expiratory flow rates in subjects with mild airway hyperexcitability. Bull. Eur. Physiopathol. Respir. 21: 25–30, 1985.

4178. Olofsson, J., Bake, B., Blomqvist, N., and Skoogh, B. E. Effect of increasing bronchodilation on the single breath nitrogen test. Bull. Eur. Physiopathol. Respir. 21: 31–36, 1985.

4179. Shelhamer, J. H. and Kaliner, M. A. Respiratory mucus production in asthma (editorial). Bull. Eur. Physiopathol. Respir. 21: 301–307, 1985.

4180. Lockhart, A., Regnard, J., Dessanges, J. F., Florentin, D., and Lurie, A. Exercise- and hyperventilation-induced asthma. Bull. Eur. Physiopathol. Respir. 21: 399–409, 1985.

4181. Flint, K. C., Leung, K. B. P., Pearce, F. L., Hudspith, B. N., Brostoff, J., and Johnson, N. McI. Human mast cells recovered by bronchoalveolar lavage: their morphology, histamine release and the effects of sodium cromoglycate. Clin. Sci. 68: 427–432, 1985.

4182. Twort, C. H. C., Neild, J. E., and Cameron, I. R. The effect of verapamil and inspired CO$_2$ on the bronchoconstriction provoked by hyperventilation in normal humans. Clin. Sci. 69: 361–364, 1985.

4183. Gelb, A. F., Tashkin, D. P., Epstein, J. D., Gong, H. Jr., and Zamel, N. Exercise-induced bronchodilation in asthma. Chest 87: 196–201, 1985.

4184. Bellia, V., Cibella, F., Migliara, G., Peralta, G., and Bonsignore, G. Characteristics and prognostic value of morning dipping of peak expiratory flow rate in stable asthmatic subjects. Chest 88: 89–93, 1985.

4185. Corte, P. and Young, I. H. Ventilation-perfusion relationships in symptomatic asthma. Chest 88: 167–175, 1985.

4186. Baughman, R. P. and Loudon, R. G. Lung sound analysis for continuous evaluation of airflow obstruction in asthma. Chest 88: 364–368, 1985.

4187. Martinsson, A., Larsson, K., and Hjemdahl, P. Reduced beta$_2$-adrenoreceptor responsiveness in exercise-induced asthma. Chest 88: 594–600, 1985.

4188. Deychakiwsky, Y. A., Deal, E. C. Jr., and Saidel, G. M. Ventilatory inhomogeneity associated with acute bronchoconstriction in asthmatic patients. Respiration 47: 201–208, 1985.

4189. Bonnel, A. M., Mathiot, M. J., and Grimaud, C. Inspiratory and expiratory resistive load detection in normal and asthmatic subjects. Respiration 48: 12–23, 1985.

4190. Aitken, M. L. and Marini, J. J. Effect of heat delivery and extraction on airway conductance in normal and in asthmatic subjects. Am. Rev. Respir. Dis. 131: 357–361, 1985.

4191. Phillips, Y. Y., Jaeger, J. J., Laube, B. L., and Rosenthal, R. R. Eucapnic voluntary hyperventilation of compressed gas mixture. Am. Rev. Respir. Dis. 131: 31–35, 1985.

4192. Laitinen, L. A., Heino, M., Laitinen, A., Kava, T., and Haahtela, T. Damage of the airway epithelium and bronchial reactivity in patients with asthma. Am. Rev. Respir. Dis. 131: 599–606, 1985.

4193. Marsh, W. R., Irvin, C. G., Murphy, K. R., Behrens, B. L., and Larsen, G. L. Increases in airway reactivity to histamine and inflammatory cells in bronchoalveolar lavage after the late asthmatic response in an animal model. Am. Rev. Respir. Dis. 131: 875–879, 1985.

4194. Eschenbacher, W. L. and Sheppard, D. Respiratory heat loss is not the sole stimulus for bronchoconstriction induced by isocapnic hyperpnea with dry air. Am. Rev. Respir. Dis. 131: 894–901, 1985.

4195. Hulbert, W. M., McLean, T., and Hogg, J. C. The effect of acute airway inflammation on bronchial reactivity in guinea pigs. Am. Rev. Respir. Dis. 132: 7–11, 1985.

4196. NHLBI Workshop Summary. Summary and recommendations of a workshop on the investigative use of fiberoptic bronchoscopy and bronchoalveolar lavage in asthmatics. Am. Rev. Respir. Dis. 132: 180–182, 1985.

4197. Malo, J.-L., Cartier, A., Pineau, L., Gagnon, G., and Martin, R. R. Slope of the dose-response curve to inhaled histamine and methacholine and PC20 in subjects with symptoms of airway hyperexcitability and in normal subjects. Am. Rev. Respir. Dis. 132: 644–647, 1985.

4198. Shindoh, C., Sekizawa, K., Hida, W., Sasaki, H., and Takishima, T. Upper airway response during bronchoprovocation and asthma attack. Am. Rev. Respir. Dis. 132: 671–678, 1985.

4199. Malo, J.-L., Gauthier, R., Lemire, I., Cartier, A., Ghezzo, H., and Martin, R. R. Kinetics of the recovery of airway response caused by inhaled histamine. Am. Rev. Respir. Dis. 132: 848–852, 1985.

4200. Solway, J., Pichurko, B. M., Ingenito, E. P., McFadden, E. R. Jr., Fanta, C. H., Ingram, R. H. Jr., and Drazen, J. M. Breathing pattern affects airway wall temperature during cold air hyperpnea in humans. Am. Rev. Respir. Dis. 132: 853–857, 1985.

4201. Tullett, W. M., Tan, K. M., Wall, R. T., and Patel, K. R. Dose-response effect of sodium cromoglycate pressurised aerosol in exercise induced asthma. Thorax 40: 41–44, 1985.

4202. Pavia, D., Bateman, J. R. M., Sheahan, N. F., Agnew, J. E., and Clarke, S. W. Tracheobronchial mucociliary clearance in asthma: impairment during remission. Thorax 40: 171–175, 1985.

4203. Roberts, J. A., Rodger, I. W., and Thomson, N. C. Airway responsiveness to histamine in man: effect of atropine on in vivo and in vitro comparison. Thorax 40: 261–267, 1985.

4204. Lee, T. H. and Anderson, S. D. Heterogeneity of mechanisms in exercise induced asthma (editorial). Thorax 40: 481–487, 1985.

4205. Burton, G. H., Seed, W. A., and Vernon, P. Computer analysis of ventilation-perfusion scans for detection and assessment of lung disease. Thorax 40: 519–525, 1985.

4206. Hahn, A. G., Nogrady, S. G., Burton, G. R., and Morton, A. R. Absence of refractoriness in asthmatic subjects after exercise with warm, humid inspirate. Thorax 40: 418–421, 1985.

4207. Black, J. L., Schoeffel, R. E., Sundrum, R., Berend, N., and Anderson, S. D. Increased responsiveness to methacholine and histamine after challenge with ultrasonically nebulised water in asthmatic subjects. Thorax 40: 427–432, 1985.

4208. Wilson, N. M., Charette, L., Thomson, A. H., and Silverman, M. Gastro-oesophageal reflux and childhood asthma: the acid test. Thorax 40: 592–597, 1985.

4209. Reed, S., Diggle, S., Cushley, M. J., Sleet, R. A., and Tattersfield, A. E. Assessment and management of asthma in an accident and emergency department. Thorax 40: 897–902, 1985.

4210. Schachter, E. N., Doyle, C. A., and Beck, G. J. A prospective study of asthma in a rural community. Chest 85: 623–630, 1984.

4211. Hodgson, W. C., Cotton, D. J., Werner, G. D., Cockcroft, D. W., and Dosman, J. A. Relationship between bronchial response to respiratory heat exchange and nonspecific airways reactivity in asthmatic patients. Chest 85: 465–479, 1984.

4212. Lakin, R. C., Metzger, W. J., and Haughey, B. H. Upper airway obstruction presenting as exercise-induced asthma. Chest 86: 499–501, 1984.

4213. Chadha, T. S., Birch, S., Allegra, L., and Sackner, M. A. Effects of ultrasonically nebulized distilled water on respiratory resistance and breathing pattern in normals and asthmatics. Bull. Eur. Physiopathol. Respir. 20: 257–262, 1984.

4214. Heaton, R. W., Henderson, A. F., and Costello, J. F. Cold air as a bronchial provocation technique. Chest 86: 810–814, 1984.

4215. Arnold, A. G., Lane, D. J., and Zapata, E. Acute severe asthma: factors that influence hospital referral by the general practitioner and self-referral by the patient. Br. J. Dis. Chest 77: 51–59, 1983.

4216. Cockcroft, D. W., Murdock, K. Y., and Berscheid, B. A. Relationship between atopy and bronchial responsiveness to histamine in a random population. Ann. Allergy 53: 26–29, 1984.

4217. Cockcroft, D. W. and Berscheid, B. A. Measurement of responsiveness to inhaled histamine: comparison of FEV$_1$ and SGaw. Ann. Allergy 51: 374–377, 1983.

4218. Dantzler, B. S., Martin, B. G., and Nelson, H. S. The effect of positive and negative air ions on bronchial asthma. Ann. Allergy 51: 362–366, 1983.

4219. Wagner, C. J., Danziger, R. E., and Nelson, H. S. Relation between positive small air ion weather fronts and pulmonary function in patients with bronchial asthma. Ann. Allergy 51: 430–435, 1983.

4220. Mitchell, E. A. and Cutler, D. R. Paediatric admissions to Auckland Hospital for asthma from 1970–1980. N. Z. Med. J. 97: 67–70, 1984.

4221. Krop, H. D., Block, A. J., and Cohen, E. Neuropsychologic effects of continuous oxygen therapy in chronic obstructive pulmonary disease. Chest 64: 317–322, 1973.

4222. Stewart, B. N., Hood, C. I., and Block, A. J. Long-term results of continuous oxygen therapy at sea level. Chest 68: 486–492, 1975.

4223. Sobonya, R. E. Quantitative structural alterations in long-standing allergic asthma. Am. Rev. Respir. Dis. 130: 289–292, 1984.

4224. Hahn, A., Anderson, S. D., Morton, A. R., Black, J. L., and Fitch, K. D. A reinterpretation of the effect of temperature and water content of the inspired air in exercise-induced asthma. Am. Rev. Respir. Dis. 130: 575–579, 1984.

4225. Aubas, P., Cosso, B., Godard, Ph., Michel, F. B., and Clot, J. Decreased suppressor cell activity of alveolar macrophages in bronchial asthma. Am. Rev. Respir. Dis. 130: 875–878, 1984.

4226. Pichurko, B. M., McFadden, E. R. Jr., Bowman, H. F., Solway, J., Burns, S., and Dowling, N. Influence of cromolyn sodium on airway temperature in normal subjects. Am. Rev. Respir. Dis. 130: 1002–1005, 1984.

4227. Martin, A. J., McLellan, L. A., Landau, L. I., and Phelan, P. D. The natural history of childhood asthma to adult life. Br. Med. J. 280: 1397–1400, 1980.

4228. Martin, A. J., Landau, L. I., and Phelan, P. D. The effect on growth of childhood asthma. Acta Paediatr. Scand. 70: 683–688, 1981.

4229. Robertson, C. E., Steedman, D., Sinclair, C. J., Brown, D., and Malcolm-Smith, N. Use of ether in life-threatening acute severe asthma. Lancet I: 187–188, 1985.

4230. Pearce, J. L. and Wesley, H. M. M. Children with asthma: will nebulised salbutamol reduce hospital admissions? Br. Med. J. 290: 595–597, 1985.

4231. Anderson, H. R. Increase in hospitalisation for childhood asthma. Arch. Dis. Child. 53: 295–300, 1978.

4232. Anderson, H. R., Bailey, P., and West, S. Trends in the hospital care of acute childhood asthma 1970–8: a regional study. Br. Med. J. 281: 1191–1194, 1980.

4233. Bellia, V., Cibella, F., Coppola, P., Greco, V., Insalaco, G., Milone, F., Oddo, S., and Peralta, G. Variability of peak expiratory flow rate as a prognostic index in asymptomatic asthma. Respiration 46: 328–333, 1984.

4234. Khot, A. and Burn, R. Seasonal variation and time trends of deaths from asthma in England and Wales 1960–82. Br. Med. J. 289: 233–235, 1984.

4235. Khot, A., Burn, R., Evans, N., Lenney, C., and Lenney, W. Seasonal variation and time trends in childhood asthma in England and Wales 1975–81. Br. Med. J. 289: 235–237, 1984.

4236. Degaute, J.-P., Domenighetti, G., Naeije, R., Vincent, J.-L., Treyvaud, D., and Perret, Ch. Oxygen delivery in acute exacerbations of chronic obstructive pulmonary disease. Am. Rev. Respir. Dis. 124: 26–30, 1981.

4237. Kraman, S. S. The forced expiratory wheeze. Respiration 44: 189–196, 1983.

4238. Martin, J. G., Habib, M., and Engel, L. A. Inspiratory muscle activity during induced hyperinflation. Respir. Physiol. 39: 303–313, 1980.

4239. Goldstein, I. F. and Currie, B. Seasonal patterns of asthma: a clue to etiology. Environ. Res. 33: 201–215, 1984.

4240. Hida, W., Arai, M., Shindoh, C., Liu, Y.-N., Sasaki, H., and Takashima, T. Effect of inspiratory flow rate on bronchomotor tone in normal and asthmatic subjects. Thorax 39: 86–92, 1984.

4241. Sakula, A. Sir John Floyer's "A Treatise of the Asthma" (1698). Thorax 39: 248–254, 1984.

4242. Accuracy of Death Certificates in Bronchial Asthma. Subcommittee Report to BTA Research Committee. Thorax 39: 505–509, 1984.

4243. Lipin, I., Gur, I., Amitai, Y., Amirav, I., and Godfrey, S. Effect of positive ionisation of inspired air on the response of asthmatic children to exercise. Thorax 39: 594–596, 1984.

4244. Fuller, R. W. and Collier, J. G. Sodium cromoglycate and atropine block the fall in FEV_1 but not the cough induced by hypotonic mist. Thorax 39: 766–770, 1984.

4245. Pedersen, O. F., Thiessen, B., Naeraa, N., Lyager, S., and Hilberg, C. Factors determining residual volume in normal and asthmatic subjects. Eur. J. Respir. Dis. 65: 99–105, 1984.

4246. Jonsson, E. and Mossberg, B. Impairment of ventilatory function by supine posture in asthma. Eur. J. Respir. Dis. 65: 496–503, 1984.

4247. Clark, T. J. H. and Godfrey, S. (eds.). Asthma. 2nd ed. Chapman and Hall, London, 1983.

4248. Hogg, J. C. and Eggleston, P. A. Is asthma an epithelial disease? (editorial). Am. Rev. Respir. Dis. 129: 207–208, 1984.

4249. Darioli, R. and Perret, C. Mechanical controlled hypoventilation in status asthmaticus. Am. Rev. Respir. Dis. 129: 385–387, 1984.

4250. Lee, T. H., Nagakura, T., Cromwell, O., Brown, M. J., Causon, R., and Kay, A. B. Neutrophil chemotactic activity and histamine in atopic and nonatopic subjects after exercise-induced asthma. Am. Rev. Respir. Dis. 129: 409–412, 1984.

4251. Weiss, S. T., Tager, I. B., Weiss, J. W., Munoz, A., Speizer, F. E., and Ingram, R. H. Airways responsiveness in a population sample of adults and children. Am. Rev. Respir. Dis. 129: 898–902, 1984.

4252. Tomioka, M., Ida, S., Shindoh, Y., Ishihara, T., and Takashima, T. Mast cells in bronchoalveolar lumen of patients with bronchial asthma. Am. Rev. Respir. Dis. 129: 1000–1005, 1984.

4253. Sotomayor, H., Badier, M., Vervloet, D., and Orehek, J. Seasonal increase of carbachol airway responsiveness in patients allergic to grass pollen. Am. Rev. Respir. Dis. 130: 56–58, 1984.

4254. Woolcock, A. J., Salome, C. M., and Yan, K. The shape of the dose-response curve to histamine in asthmatic and normal subjects. Am. Rev. Respir. Dis. 130: 71–75, 1984.

4255. Ten Velde, G. P. M. and Kreukniet, J. The histamine inhalation provocation test and its reproducibility. Respiration 45: 131–138, 1984.

4256. Sears, M. R., Rea, H. H., Rothwell, R. P. G., O'Donnell, T. V., Holst, P. E., Gillies, A. J. D., and Beaglehole, R. Asthma mortality: a comparison between New Zealand and England. Br. Med. J. 293: 1342–1345, 1986.

4257. Pantin, C. F. A., Stead, R. J., Hodson, M. E., and Batten, J. C. Prednisolone in the treatment of airflow obstruction in adults with cystic fibrosis. Thorax 41: 34–38, 1986.

4258. Cormier, Y., Belanger, J., and Laviolette, M. Persistent bronchoalveolar lymphocytosis in asymptomatic farmers. Am. Rev. Respir. Dis. 133: 843–847, 1986.

4259. Soda, K., Ando, M., Shimazu, K., Sakata, T., Yoshida, K., and Araki, S. Different classes of antibody activities to Trichosporon cutaneum antigen in summer-type hypersensitivity pneumonitis by enzyme-linked immunosorbent assay. Am. Rev. Respir. Dis. 133: 83–87, 1986.

4260. Anttinen, H., Terho, E. O., Myllyla, R., and Savolainen, E. -R. Two serum markers of collagen biosynthesis as possible indicators of irreversible pulmonary impairment in farmer's lung. Am. Rev. Respir. Dis. 133: 88–93, 1986.

4261. Armstrong, P. J., Derksen, F. J., Slocombe, R. F., and Robinson, N. E. Airway responses to aerosolized methacholine and citric acid in ponies with recurrent airway obstruction (heaves). Am. Rev. Respir. Dis. 133: 357–361, 1986.

4262. Cormier, Y., Belanger, J., Tardif, A., Leblanc, P., and Laviolette, M. Relationships between radiographic change, pulmonary function, and bronchoalveolar lavage in farmer's lung disease. Thorax 41: 28–33, 1986.

4263. Heller, R. F., Hayward, D. M., and Farebrother, M. T. B. Lung function of farmers in England and Wales. Thorax 41: 117–121, 1986.

4264. Wiessmann, K. -J. and Baur, X. Occupational lung disease following long-term inhalation of pancreatic extracts. Eur. J. Respir. Dis. 66: 13–20, 1985.

4265. Hodgson, M. J., Morey, P. R., Attfield, M., Sorenson, W., Fink, J. N., Rhodes, W. W., and Visvesvara, G. S. Pulmonary disease associated with cafeteria flooding. Arch. Environ. Health 40: 96–101, 1985.

4266. Hida, W., Konishi, Y., Kikuchi, R., Shibata, H., Fuyuki, T., Sekizawa, K., Sasaki, H., and Takashima, T. Airway responsiveness after antigen inhalation challenge in hypersensitive pneumonia. Respiration 47: 11–20, 1985.

4267. Monkare, S., Ikonen, M., and Haahtela, T. Radiologic findings in farmer's lung: prognosis and correlation to lung function. Chest 87: 460–466, 1985.

4268. Epler, G. R., Colby, T. V., McLoud, T. C., Carrington, C. B., and Gaensler, E. A. Bronchiolitis obliterans organising pneumonia. N. Engl. J. Med. 312: 152–158, 1985.

4269. Lungarella, G., De Santi, M. M., Palatresi, R., and Tosi, P. Ultrastructural observations on basal apparatus of respiratory cilia in immotile cilia syndrome. Eur. J. Respir. Dis. 66: 165–172, 1985.

4270. Afzelius, B. A., Gargani, G., and Romano, C. Abnormal length of cilia as a possible cause of defective mucociliary clearance. Eur. J. Respir. Dis. 66: 173–180, 1985.

4271. Cotton, D. J., Graham, B. L., Mink, J. T., and Habbick, B. F. Reduction of the single breath diffusing capacity in cystic fibrosis. Chest 87: 217–221, 1985.

4272. Stokes, D. C., Wohl, M. E. B., Khaw, K. T., and Strieder, D. J. Postural hypoxemia in cystic fibrosis. Chest 87: 785–789, 1985.

4273. Bruce, M. C., Poncz, L., Klinger, J. D., Stern, R. C., Tomashefski, J. F. Jr., and Dearborn, D. G. Biochemical and pathologic evidence for proteolytic destruction of lung connective tissue in cystic fibrosis. Am. Rev. Respir. Dis. 132: 529–535, 1985.

4274. Szeinberg, A., England, S., Mindorff, C., Frase, I. M., and Levison, H. Maximal inspiratory and expiratory pressures are reduced in hyperinflated, malnourished, young adult male patients with cystic fibrosis. Am. Rev. Respir. Dis. 132: 766–769, 1985.

4275. Geggel, R. L., Dozor, A. J., Fyler, D. C., and Reid, L. M. Effect of vasodilators at rest and during exercise in young adults with cystic fibrosis and chronic cor pulmonale. Am. Rev. Respir. Dis. 131: 531–536, 1985.

4276. Hunt, B. and Geddes, D. M. Newly diagnosed cystic fibrosis in middle and later life. Thorax 40: 23–26, 1985.

4277. Davis, P. B., Hubbard, V. S., and Garvin, A. J. Bronchiectasis and oligospermia: two families. Thorax 40: 376–379, 1985.

4278. Greenstone, M., Rutman, A., Pavia, D., Lawrence, D., and Cole, P. J. Normal axonemal structure and function in Kartagener's syndrome: an explicable paradox. Thorax 40: 956–957, 1985.

4279. Costabel, U., Bross, K. J., Ruhle, K. H., Lohr, G. W., and Matthys, H. Ia-like antigens on T-cells and their subpopulations in pulmonary sarcoidosis and in hypersensitivity pneumonitis. Am. Rev. Respir. Dis. 131: 337–342, 1985.

4280. Kopp, W. C., Dierks, S. E., Butler, J. E., Upadrashta, B. S., and Richerson, H. B. Cyclosporine immunomodulation in a rabbit model of chronic hypersensitivity pneumonitis. Am. Rev. Respir. Dis. 132: 1027–1033, 1985.

4281. Anderson, K., McSharry, C. P., and Boyd, G. Radiographic changes in humidifier fever. Thorax 40: 312–313, 1985.

4282. Hendrick, D. J. Contaminated humidifiers and the lung (editorial). Thorax 40: 244–247, 1985.

4283. Semenzato, G., Chilosi, M., Ossi, E., Trentin, L., Pizzolo, G., Cipriani, A., Agostoni, C., Zambello, R., Marcer, G., and Gasparotto, G. Bronchoalveolar lavage and lung histology. Am. Rev. Respir. Dis. 132: 400–404, 1985.

4284. Bahous, J., Cartier, A., Pineau, L., Bernard, C., Ghezzo, H., Martin, R. R., and Malo, J. L. Pulmonary function tests and airway responsiveness to methacholine in chronic bronchiectasis of the adult. Bull. Eur. Physiopathol. Respir. 20: 375–380, 1984.

4285. Morgan, M. D. L. and Strickland, B. Computed tomography in the assessment of bullous lung disease. Br. J. Dis. Chest 78: 10–25, 1984.

4286. Kawai, T., Tamura, M., and Murao, M. Summer-type hypersensitivity pneumonitis. Chest 85: 311–317, 1984.

4287. Lenhart, S. W. and Olenchock, S. A. Sources of respiratory insult in the poultry processing industry. Am. J. Ind. Med. 6: 89–96, 1984.

4288. Edwards, J. H. Microbial and immunological investigations and remedial action after an outbreak of humidifier fever. Br. J. Ind. Med. 37: 55–62, 1980.

4289. Harries, M. G., Burge, P. S., and O'Brien, I. M. Occupational type bronchial provocation tests: testing with soluble antigens by inhalation. Br. J. Ind. Med. 37: 248–252, 1980.

4290. Shimazu, K., Ando, M., Sakata, T., Yoshida, K., and Araki, S. Hypersensitivity pneumonitis induced by Trichosporon cutaneum. Am. Rev. Respir. Dis. 130: 407–411, 1984.

4291. Keller, R. H., Swartz, S., Schlueter, D. P., Bar-Sela, S., and Fink, J. N. Immunoregulation in hypersensitivity pneumonitis: phenotypic and functional studies of bronchoalveolar lavage lymphocytes. Am. Rev. Respir. Dis. 130: 766–771, 1984.

4292. Schuyler, M. R. and Schmitt, D. Experimental hypersensitivity pneumonitis: lack of tolerance. Am. Rev. Respir. Dis. 130: 772–777, 1984.

4293. Cormier, Y., Belanger, J., Beaudoin, J., Laviolette, M., Beaudoin, R., and Hebert, J. Abnormal bronchoalveolar lavage in asymptomatic dairy farmers. Am. Rev. Respir. Dis. 130: 1046–1049, 1984.

4294. Huuskonen, M. S., Husman, K., Jarvisalo, J., Korhonen, O., Kotimaa, M., Kuusela, T., Nordman, H., Zitting, A., and Mantyjarvi, R. Extrinsic allergic alveolitis in the tobacco industry. Br. J. Ind. Med. 41: 77–83, 1984.

4295. Harries, M. G., Heard, B., and Geddes, D. Extrinsic allergic bronchiolitis in a bird fancier. Br. J. Ind. Med. 41: 220–223, 1984.

4296. Cantin, A., Begin, R., Boileau, R., Drapeau, G., and Rola-Pleszczynski, M. Features of bronchoalveolar lavage differentiating hypersensitivity pneumonitis and pulmonary sarcoidosis at time of initial presentation. Clin. Invest. Med. 7: 89–94, 1984.

4297. Bauer, X. and Dexheimer, E. Hypersensitivity pneumonitis concomitant with acute airway obstruction after exposure to hay dust. Respiration 46: 354–361, 1984.

4298. Michael, J. R., Kennedy, T. P., Fitzpatrick, S., and Rosenstein, B. J. Nifedipine inhibits hypoxic pulmonary vasoconstriction during rest and exercise in patients with cystic fibrosis and cor pulmonale. Am. Rev. Respir. Dis. 130: 516–519, 1984.

4299. Canny, G. J., De Souza, M. E., Gilday, D. L., and Newth, C. J. L. Radionuclide assessment of cardiac performance in cystic fibrosis. Am. Rev. Respir. Dis. 130: 822–826, 1984.

4300. Benson, L. N., Newth, C. J. L., Desouza, M., Lobraico, R., Kartodihardjo, W., Corkey, C., Gilday, D., and Olley, P. M. Radionuclide assessment of right and left ventricular function during bicycle exercise in young patients with cystic fibrosis. Am. Rev. Respir. Dis. 130: 987–992, 1984.

4301. Davis, P. B. Cystic fibrosis: clinical manifestations in older patients. Clin. Notes Respir. Dis. 21: 3–12, 1983.

4302. Holzer, F. J., Olinsky, A., and Phelan, P. D. Variability of airways hyper-reactivity and allergy in cystic fibrosis. Arch. Dis. Child. 56: 455–459, 1981.

4303. Hughes, J. A., Macarthur, A. M., Hutchison, D. C. S., and Hugh-Jones, P. Long term changes in lung function after surgical treatment of bullous emphysema in smokers and ex-smokers. Thorax 39: 140–142, 1984.

4304. Whyte, K. F. and Williams, G. R. Bronchiectasis after mycoplasma pneumonia. Thorax 39: 390–391, 1984.

4305. Stockley, R. A., Hill, S. L., Morrison, H. M., and Starkie, C. M. Elastolytic activity of sputum and its relation to purulence and to lung function in patients with bronchiectasis. Thorax 39: 408–413, 1984.

4306. Murphy, M. B., Reen, D. J., and Fitzgerald, M. X. Atopy,

immunological changes, and respiratory function in bronchiectasis. Thorax 39: 179–184, 1984.

4307. De Boeck, C. and Zinman, R. Cough versus chest physiotherapy. Am. Rev. Respir. Dis. 129: 182–184, 1984.

4308. Wall, M. A., Misley, M. C., and Dickerson, D. Partial expiratory flow-volume curves in young children. Am. Rev. Respir. Dis. 129: 557–562, 1984.

4309. Davis, P. B. Autonomic and airway reactivity in obligate heterozygotes for cystic fibrosis. Am. Rev. Respir. Dis. 129: 911–914, 1984.

4310. Fergusson, R. J., Milne, L. J. R., and Crompton, G. K. Penicillium allergic alveolitis: faulty installation of central heating. Thorax 39: 294–298, 1984.

4311. Terho, E. O., Heinonen, O. P., Mantyjarvi, R. A., and Vohlonen, I. Familial aggregation of symptoms of farmer's lung. Scand. J. Work Environ. Health 10: 57–58, 1984.

4312. Chiron, C., Gaultier, C., Boule, M., Grimfeld, A., and Girard, F. Lung function in children with hypersensitivity pneumonitis. Eur. J. Respir. Dis. 65: 79–91, 1984.

4313. Mootoosamy, I. M., Reznek, R. H., Osman, J., Rees, R. S. O., and Green, M. Assessment of bronchiectasis by computed tomography. Thorax 40: 920–924, 1985.

4314. Anthonisen, N. R., Manfreda, J., Warren, C. P. W., Hershfield, E. S., Harding, G. K. M., and Nelson, N. A. Antibiotic therapy in exacerbations of chronic obstructive pulmonary disease. Ann. Intern. Med. 106: 196–204, 1987.

4315. Apthorp, G. H. and Bates, D. V. Report of a case of pulmonary telangiectasia. Thorax 12: 63–65, 1957.

4316. Gluskowski, J., Jedrzejewska-Makowska, M., Hawrylkiewicz, I., Vertun, B., and Zielinski, J. Effects of prolonged oxygen therapy on pulmonary hypertension and blood viscosity in patients with advanced cor pulmonale. Respiration 44: 177–183, 1983.

4317. Jardin, F., Gueret, P., Prost, J.-F., Farcot, J.-C., Ozier, Y., and Bourdarias, J.-P. Two-dimensional echocardiographic assessment of left ventricular function in chronic obstructive pulmonary disease. Am. Rev. Respir. Dis. 129: 135–142, 1984.

4318. Loyd, J. E., Primm, R. K., and Newman, J. H. Familial primary pulmonary hypertension: clinical patterns. Am. Rev. Respir. Dis. 129: 194–197, 1984.

4319. Weber, K. T., Wilson, J. R., Janicki, J. S., and Likoff, M. J. Exercise testing in the evaluation of the patient with chronic cardiac failure. Exercise Testing in the Dyspneic Patient. Am. Rev. Respir. Dis. 129(2)(Pt. 2)(Suppl.): S60–S62, 1984.

4320. Rubin, S. A. and Brown, H. V. Ventilation and gas exchange during exercise in severe chronic heart failure. Exercise Testing in the Dyspneic Patient. Am. Rev. Respir. Dis. 129(2)(Pt. 2)(Suppl.): S63–S64, 1984.

4321. Janicki, J. S., Weber, K. T., Likoff, M. J., and Fishman, A. P. Exercise testing to evaluate patients with pulmonary vascular disease. Exercise Testing in the Dyspneic Patient. Am. Rev. Respir. Dis. 129(2)(Pt. 2)(Suppl.): S93–S95, 1984.

4322. Tuxen, D. V., Powles, A. C. P., Mathur, P. N., Pugsley, S. O., and Campbell, E. J. M. Detrimental effects of hydralazine in patients with chronic air-flow obstruction and pulmonary hypertension. Am. Rev. Respir. Dis. 129: 388–395, 1984.

4323. Kennedy, T. P., Michael, J. R., Huang, C.-K., Kallman, C. H., Zahka, K., Schlott, W., and Summer, W. Nifedipine inhibits hypoxic pulmonary vasoconstriction during rest and exercise in patients with chronic obstructive pulmonary disease. Am. Rev. Respir. Dis. 129: 544–551, 1984.

4324. Fein, A. M., Goldberg, S. K., Walkenstein, M. D., Dershaw, B., Braitman, L., and Lippmann, M. L. Is pulmonary artery catheterization necessary for the diagnosis of pulmonary edema? Am. Rev. Respir. Dis. 129: 1006–1009, 1984.

4325. Stanbrook, H. S., Morris, K. G., and McMurtry, I. F. Prevention and reversal of hypoxic pulmonary hypertension by calcium antagonists. Am. Rev. Respir. Dis. 130: 81–85, 1984.

4326. Darmanata, J. I., van Zandwijk, N., Duren, D. R., van Royen, E. A., Mooi, W. J., Plomp, T. A., Jansen, H. M., and Durrer, D. Amiodarone pneumonitis: three further cases with a review of published reports. Thorax 39: 57–64, 1984.

4327. Wollmer, P., Rhodes, C. G., and Hughes, J. M. B. Regional extravascular density and fractional blood volume of the lung in interstitial disease. Thorax 39: 286–293, 1984.

4328. Durand, D. V., Dellinger, A., Guerin, C., Guerin, J. C., and Levrat, R. Pleural sarcoidosis: one case presenting with an eosinophilic effusion. Thorax 39: 468–469, 1984.

4329. Lewis, L. D. Procarbazine associated alveolitis. Thorax 39: 206–207, 1984.

4330. Wright, P. H., Buxton-Thomas, M., Kreel, L., and Steel, S. J. Cryptogenic fibrosing alveolitis: pattern of disease in the lung. Thorax 39: 857–861, 1984.

4331. Hendy, M. S., Williams, P. S., and Ackrill, P. Recovery from severe pulmonary damage due to paraquat administered intravenously and orally. Thorax 39: 874–875, 1984.

4332. Jacobs, P., Bonnyns, M., Depierreux, M., Duchateau, J., and Sergysels, R. Rapidly fatal bronchiolitis obliterans with circulating antinuclear and rheumatoid factors. Eur. J. Respir. Dis. 65: 384–388, 1984.

4333. Schoenberger, C. I., Rennard, S. I., Bitterman, P. B., Fukuda, Y., Ferrans, V. J., and Crystal, R. G. Paraquat-induced pulmonary fibrosis. Am. Rev. Respir. Dis. 129: 168–173, 1984.

4334. Low, R. B., Woodcock-Mitchell, J., Evans, J. N., and Adler, K. B. Actin content of normal and of bleomycin-fibrotic rat lung. Am. Rev. Respir. Dis. 129: 311–316, 1984.

4335. Schiavi, E. A., Roncoroni, A. J., and Puy, R. J. M. Isolated bilateral diaphragmatic paresis with interstitial lung disease: an unusual presentation of dermatomyositis. Am. Rev. Respir. Dis. 129: 337–339, 1984.

4336. Deremee, R. A. The alveolitis of pulmonary sarcoidosis (letter to editor). Am. Rev. Respir. Dis. 129: 343, 1984.

4337. Keogh, B. A., Lakatos, E., Price, D., and Crystal, R. G. Importance of the lower respiratory tract in oxygen transfer. Exercise Testing in the Dyspneic Patient. Am. Rev. Respir. Dis. 129(2)(Pt. 2)(Suppl.): S76–S80, 1984.

4338. Powers, M. A., Askin, F. B., and Cresson, D. H. Pulmonary eosinophilic granuloma: 25-year follow-up. Am. Rev. Respir. Dis. 129: 503–507, 1984.

4339. Ceuppens, J. L., Lacquet, L. M., Marien, G., Demedts, M., Van Den Eeckhout, A., and Stevens, E. Alveolar T-cell subsets in pulmonary sarcoidosis. Am. Rev. Respir. Dis. 129: 563–568, 1984.

4340. Skillrud, D. M. and Martin, W. J. II. Paraquat-induced injury of type II alveolar cells. Am. Rev. Respir. Dis. 129: 995–999, 1984.

4341. Hillerdal, G., Nou, E., Osterman, K., and Schmekel, B. Sarcoidosis: epidemiology and prognosis. Am. Rev. Respir. Dis. 130: 29–32, 1984.

4342. Martin, W. J. II. Neutrophils kill pulmonary endothelial cells by a hydrogen-peroxide-dependent pathway. Am. Rev. Respir. Dis. 130: 209–213, 1984.

4343. Mustafa, K. Y., Nour, M. M., Shuhaiber, H., and Yousof, A. M. Pulmonary function before and sequentially after valve replacement surgery with correlation to preoperative hemodynamic data. Am. Rev. Respir. Dis. 130: 400–406, 1984.

4344. Dantzker, D. R., D'Alonzo, G. E., Bower, J. S., Popat, K., and Crevey, B. J. Pulmonary gas exchange during exercise in patients with chronic obliterative pulmonary hypertension. Am. Rev. Respir. Dis. 130: 412–416, 1984.

4345. Arms, R. A., Dines, D. E., and Tinstman, T. C. Aspiration pneumonia. Chest 65: 136–139, 1974.

4346. Keller, C. A., Shepard, J. W. Jr., Chun, D. S., Dolan, S. F., Vasquez, P., and Minh, V.-D. Effects of hydralazine on hemodynamics, ventilation, and gas exchange in patients with chronic obstructive pulmonary disease and pulmonary hypertension. Am. Rev. Respir. Dis. 130: 606–611, 1984.

4347. Melot, C., Hallemans, R., Naeije, R., Mols, P., and Lejeune, P. Deleterious effect of nifedipine on pulmonary gas exchange in chronic obstructive pulmonary disease. Am. Rev. Respir. Dis. 130: 612–616, 1984.

4348. Mahler, D. A., Brent, B. N., Loke, J., Zaret, B. L., and Matthay, R. A. Right ventricular performance and central circulatory hemodynamics during upright exercise in patients with chronic obstructive pulmonary disease. Am. Rev. Respir. Dis. 130: 722–729, 1984.

4349. Colice, G. L., Matthay, M. A., Bass, E., and Matthay, R. A. Neurogenic pulmonary oedema. Am. Rev. Respir. Dis. 130: 941–948, 1984.

4350. Lockhart, A. and Reeves, J. T. Plexogenic pulmonary hypertension of unknown origin. What's new? (editorial). Clin. Sci. 67: 1–5, 1984.

4351. Corris, P. A. and Gibson, G. J. Asthma presenting as cor pulmonale. Br. Med. J. 288: 389–390, 1984.

4352. Burghuber, O., Bergmann, H., Silberbauer, K., and Hofer, R. Right ventricular performance in chronic air flow obstruction. Respiration 45: 124–130, 1984.

4353. Rasanen, J., Nikki, P., and Heikkila, J. Acute myocardial infarction complicated by respiratory failure. Chest 85: 21–28, 1984.

4354. Farber, M. O., Weinberger, M. H., Robertson, G. L., Fineberg, N. S., and Manfredi, F. Hormonal abnormalities affecting sodium and water balance in acute respiratory failure due to chronic obstructive lung disease. Chest 85: 49–54, 1984.

4355. Zema, M. J., Masters, A. P., and Margouleff, D. Dyspnea: the heart or the lungs? Chest 85: 59–64, 1984.

4356. Lupi-Herrera, E., Seoane, M., and Verdejo, J. Hemodynamic effect of hydralazine in advanced, stable, chronic obstructive pulmonary disease with cor pulmonale. Chest 85: 156–163, 1984.

4357. Brown, S. E., Pakron, F. J., Milne, N., Linden, G. S., Stansbury, D. W., Fischer, C. E., and Light, R. W. Effects of digoxin on exercise capacity and right ventricular function during exercise in chronic airflow obstruction. Chest 85: 187–191, 1984.

4358. Kehrer, J. P., Klein-Szanto, A. J. P., Sorensen, E. M. B., Pearlman, R., and Rosner, M. H. Enhanced acute lung damage following corticosteroid treatment. Am. Rev. Respir. Dis. 130: 256–261, 1984.

4359. Mordelet-Dambrine, M., Arnoux, A., Stanislas-Leguern, G., Sandron, D., Chretien, J., and Huchon, G. Processing of lung lavage fluid causes variability in bronchoalveolar cell count. Am. Rev. Respir. Dis. 130: 305–306, 1984.

4360. Saltini, C., Hance, A. J., Ferrans, V. J., Basset, F., Bitterman, P. B., and Crystal, R. G. Accurate quantification of cells recovered by bronchoalveolar lavage. Am. Rev. Respir. Dis. 130: 650–658, 1984.

4361. Braude, A. C., Cohen, R., Rahmani, R., Hornstein, A., Klein, M., Meindok, H. O., Chamberlain, D. W., and Rebuck, A. S. An in vitro gallium-67 lung index for the evaluation of sarcoidosis. Am. Rev. Respir. Dis. 130: 783–785, 1984.

4362. Goto, T., Befus, D., Low, R., and Bienenstock, J. Mast cell heterogeneity and hyperplasia in bleomycin-induced pulmonary fibrosis of rats. Am. Rev. Respir. Dis. 130: 797–802, 1984.

4363. Smith, L. J. Lung damage induced by butylated hydroxytoluene in mice. Am. Rev. Respir. Dis. 130: 895–904, 1984.

4364. Van Barneveld, P. W. C., Van Der Mark, Th. W., Sleijer, D. Th., Mulder, N. H., Koops, H. S., Sluiter, H. J., and Peset, R. Predictive factors for bleomycin-induced pneumonitis. Am. Rev. Respir. Dis. 130: 1078–1081, 1984.

4365. Moseley, P. L., Shasby, D. M., Brady, M., and Hunninghake, G. W. Lung parenchymal injury induced by bleomycin. Am. Rev. Respir. Dis. 130: 1082–1086, 1984.

4366. Burke, D. A., Stoddart, J. C., Ward, M. K., and Simpson, C. G. B. Fatal pulmonary fibrosis occuring during treatment with cyclophosphamide. Br. Med. J. 285: 696, 1982.

4367. Argyropoulou, P. K., Patakas, D. A., and Louridas, G. E. Airway function in stage I and stage II pulmonary sarcoidosis. Respiration 46: 17–25, 1984.

4368. Gluskowski, J., Hawrulkiewicz, I., Zych, D., Wojttczak, A., and Zielinski, J. Pulmonary haemodynamics at rest and during exercise in patients with sarcoidosis. Respiration 46: 26–32, 1984.

4369. Ploysongsang, Y. and Foad, B. S. I. Lung function tests in connective tissue diseases associated with Raynaud's phenomenon. Respiration 46: 222–230, 1984.

4370. Constantopoulos, S. H., Drosos, A. A., Maddison, P. J., and Moutsopoulos, H. M. Xerotrachea and interstitial lung disease in primary Sjogren's syndrome. Respiration 46: 310–314, 1984.

4371. Risk, C., Epler, G. R., and Gaensler, E. A. Exercise alveolar-arterial oxygen pressure difference in interstitial lung disease. Chest 85: 69–74, 1984.

4372. Rounds, S. and Hill, N. S. Pulmonary hypertensive diseases. Chest 85: 397–405, 1984.

4373. Matthay, R. A. and Loke, J. Noninvasive assessment of cardiovascular performance in interstitial and chronic obstructive lung disease (editorial). Chest 85: 299–300, 1984.

4374. Baughman, R. P., Gerson, M., and Bosken, C. H. Right and left ventricular function at rest and with exercise in patients with sarcoidosis. Chest 85: 301–306, 1984.

4375. D'Alonzo, G. E., Bower, J. S., and Dantzker, D. R. Differentiation of patients with primary and thromboembolic pulmonary hypertension. Chest 85: 457–461, 1984.

4376. Maeda, H., Monden, Y., Nakahara, K., Miyoshi, S., and Kawashima, Y. Pulmonary arteriovenous fistula showing a fall in shunt fraction during exercise. Chest 85: 575–577, 1984.

4377. Theodore, J., Jamieson, S. W., Burke, C. M., Reitz, B. A., Stinson, E. B., Van Kessel, A., Dawkins, K. D., Herran, J. J., Oyer, P. E., Hunt, S. A., Shumway, N. E., and Robin, E. D. Physiologic aspects of human heart-lung transplantation. Chest 86: 349–357, 1984.

4378. Morpurgo, M., Saviotti, M., Dickele, M. C., Casazza, F., Torbicki, J., Weitzenblum, E., and Zielinski, J. Echocardiographic aspects of pulmonary arterial hypertension in chronic lung disease. Bull. Eur. Physiopathol. Respir. 20: 251–255, 1984.

4379. Padmanabhan, K. and Dhar, S. R. Irreversible hypercapnia secondary to embolic occlusion of the pulmonary artery. Chest 86: 927–928, 1984.

4380. Estenne, M. and Yernault, J.-C. The mechanism of CO_2 retention in cardiac pulmonary edema. Chest 86: 936–938, 1984.

4381. Williams, I. P., Boyd, M. J., Humbertstone, A. M., Wilson, A. G., and Millard, F. J. C. Pulmonary arterial hypertension and emphysema. Br. J. Dis. Chest 78: 211–216, 1984.

4382. Konig, G., Luderschmidt, C., Hammer, C., Adelmann-Grill, B. C., Braun-Falco, O., and Fruhmann, G. Lung involvement in scleroderma. Chest 85: 318–324, 1984.

4383. Leech, J. A., Gallastegui, J., and Swiryn, S. Pulmonary toxicity of amiodarone. Chest 85: 444–445, 1984.

4384. Ettensohn, D. B., Roberts, N. J. Jr., and Condemi, J. J. Bronchoalveolar lavage in gold lung. Chest 85: 569–570, 1984.

4385. Abe, S., Munakata, M., Nishimura, M., Tsuneta, Y., Terai, T., Nakano, I., Ohsaki, Y., and Kawakami, Y. Gallium-67 scintigraphy, bronchoalveolar lavage, and pathologic changes in patients with pulmonary sarcoidosis. Chest 85: 650–655, 1984.

4386. Lahdensuo, A., Mattila, J., and Vilppula, A. Bronchiolitis in rheumatoid arthritis. Chest 85: 705–708, 1984.

4387. Whitcomb, M. E. and Dixon, G. F. Gallium scanning, bronchoalveolar lavage, and the national debt (editorial). Chest 85: 719–721, 1984.

4388. Dalmasso, F., Guarene, M. M., Spagnolo, R., Benedetto, G., and Righini, G. A computer system for timing and acoustical analysis of crackles: a study in cryptogenic fibrosing alveolitis. Bull. Physiopathol. Respir. 20: 139–144, 1984.

4389. Kallenberg, C. G. M., Jansen, H. M., Elema, J. D., and The, T. H. Steroid-responsive interstitial pulmonary disease in systemic sclerosis. Chest 86: 489–492, 1984.

4390. Dreis, D. F., Winterbauer, R. H., Van Norman, G. A., Sullivan, S. L., and Hammar, S. P. Cephalosporin-induced interstitial pneumonitis. Chest 86: 138–140, 1984.

4391. Dusser, D., Modelet-Dambrine, M., Collignon, M. A., Barritault, L., Chretien, J., and Huchon, G. Assessment of pulmonary epithelial permeability by clearance of an aerosolized solute and bronchoalveolar lavage in interstitial lung disease. Bull. Eur. Physiopathol. Respir. 20: 223–227, 1984.

4392. Escribano, P. M., Alarcos, J. M. F. S., Dominguez-Lozano, M. J., Diaz de Atauri, J., Barbosa-Ayucar, C., Cantalapiedra, J. A., and Encuentra, A. L. Lung function testing at various stages of the toxic oil syndrome. Bull. Eur. Physiopathol. Respir. 20: 307–312, 1984.

4393. Kudenchuk, P. J., Pierson, D. J., Greene, H. L., Graham, E. L., Sears, G. K., and Trobaugh, G. B. Prospective evaluation of amiodarone pulmonary toxicity. Chest 86: 541–548, 1984.

4394. Glazer, H. S., Levitt, R. G., and Shackelford, G. D. Peripheral pulmonary infiltrates in sarcoidosis. Chest 86: 741–744, 1984.

4395. Hodson, M. E., Haslam, P. L., Spiro, S. G., and Turner-Warwick, M. Digital vasculitis in patients with cryptogenic fibrosing alveolitis. Br. J. Dis. Chest 78: 140–148, 1984.

4396. Fahey, P. J., Utell, M. J., Condemi, J. J., Green, R., and Hyde, R. W. Raynaud's phenomenon of the lung. Am. J. Med. 76: 263–269, 1984.

4397. Barst, R. J., Stalcup, S. A., Steeg, C. N., Hall, J. C., Frosolonio, M. F., Cato, A. E., and Mellins, R. B. Relation of arachidonate metabolites to abnormal control of the pulmonary circulation in a child. Am. Rev. Respir. Dis. 131: 171–177, 1985.

4398. Sibbald, W. J., Short, A. I. K., Driedger, A. A., and Wells, G. A. The immediate effects of isosorbide dinitrate on right ventricular function in patients with acute hypoxemic respiratory failure. Am. Rev. Respir. Dis. 131: 862–868, 1985.

4399. Manier, G., Castaing, Y., and Guenard, H. Determinants of hypoxemia during the acute phase of pulmonary embolism in humans. Am. Rev. Respir. Dis. 132: 332–338, 1985.

4400. Bradley, C. A., Fleetham, J. A., and Anthonisen, N. R. Ventilatory control in patients with hypoxemia due to obstructive lung disease. Am. Rev. Respir. Dis. 120: 21–30, 1979.

4401. Grover, R. F. The politics of the pulmonary circulation (editorial). Am. Rev. Respir. Dis. 132: 1152–1154, 1985.

4402. Estenne, M., Yernault, J.-C., De Smet, J.-M., and De Troyer, A. Phrenic and diaphragm function after coronary artery bypass grafting. Thorax 40: 293–299, 1985.

4403. MacNee, W., Buist, T. A. S., Finlayson, N. D. C., Lamb, D., Miller, H. C., Muir, A. L., and Douglas, A. C. Multiple microscopic pulmonary arteriovenous connections in the lungs presenting as cyanosis. Thorax 40: 316–318, 1985.

4404. Burton, G. H., Seed, W. A., and Vernon, P. Computer analysis of ventilation-perfusion scans for detection and assessment of lung disease. Thorax 40: 519–525, 1985.

4405. Large, S. R., Heywood, L. J., Flower, C. D., Cory-Pearce, R., Wallwork, J., and English, T. A. H. Incidence and aetiology of a raised hemidiaphragm after cardiopulmonary bypass. Thorax 40: 444–447, 1985.

4406. Flint, K. C., Johnson, N. McI., Mannhire, A., Dawson, P., George, S., and Ell, P. J. Comparison of intravenous digital subtraction angiography with radionuclide ventilation-perfusion lung scanning in patients with suspected pulmonary embolism. Thorax 40: 576–580, 1985.

4407. Demedts, M., Auwerx, J., Goddeeris, P., Bouillon, R., Gyselen, A., and Lauweryns, J. The inherited association of interstitial lung disease, hypocalciuric hypercalcemia, and defective granulocyte function. Am. Rev. Respir. Dis. 131: 470–475, 1985.

4408. Chandler, D. B. and Fulmer, J. D. The effect of deferoxamine on bleomycin-induced lung fibrosis in the hamster. Am. Rev. Respir. Dis. 131: 596–598, 1985.

4409. Rossi, G. A., Bitterman, P. B., Rennard, S. I., Ferrans, V. J., and Crystal, R. G. Evidence for chronic inflammation as a component of the interstitial lung disease associated with progressive systemic sclerosis. Am. Rev. Respir. Dis. 131: 612–617, 1985.

4410. Jacobs, M. P., Baughman, R. P., Hughes, J., and Fernandez-Ulloa, M. Radioaerosol lung clearance in patients with active pulmonary sarcoidosis. Am. Rev. Respir. Dis. 131: 687–689, 1985.

4411. Yousem, S. A., Colby, T. V., and Carrington, C. B. Lung biopsy in rheumatoid arthritis. Am. Rev. Respir. Dis. 131: 770–777, 1985.

4412. Hollinger, W. M., Staton, G. W. Jr., Fajman, W. A., Gilman, M. J., Pine, J. R., and Check, I. J. Prediction of therapeutic response in steroid-treated pulmonary sarcoidosis. Am. Rev. Respir. Dis. 132: 65–69, 1985.

4413. Berend, N., Feldsien, D., Cederbaums, D., and Cherniack, R. M. Structure-function correlation of early stages of lung injury induced by intratracheal bleomycin in the rabbit. Am. Rev. Respir. Dis. 132: 582–589, 1985.

4414. Tryka, A. F., Sweeney, T. D., Brain, J. D., and Godleski, J. J. Short-term regional clearance of an inhaled submicrometric aerosol in pulmonary fibrosis. Am. Rev. Respir. Dis. 132: 606–611, 1985.

4415. Oliven, A., Cherniack, N. S., Deal, E. C., and Kelsen, S.

G. The effects of acute bronchoconstriction on respiratory activity in patients with chronic obstructive pulmonary disease. Am. Rev. Respir. Dis. 131: 236–241, 1985.

4416. Delacroix, D. L., Marchandise, F. X., Francis, C., and Sibille, Y. Alpha-2-macroglobulin, monomeric and polymeric immunoglobulin A, and immunoglobulin M in bronchoalveolar lavage. Am. Rev. Respir. Dis. 132: 829–835, 1985.

4417. Vaccaro, C. A., Brody, J. S., and Snider, G. L. Alveolar wall basement membranes in bleomycin-induced pulmonary fibrosis. Am. Rev. Respir. Dis. 132: 905–912, 1985.

4418. Bauer, W., Gorny, M. K., Baumann, H. R., and Morell, A. T-lymphocyte subsets and immunoglobulin concentrations in bronchoalveolar lavage of patients with sarcoidosis and high and low intensity alveolitis. Am. Rev. Respir. Dis. 132: 1060–1065, 1985.

4419. Thompson, P. J., Dhillon, D. P., Ledingham, J., and Turner-Warwick M. Shrinking lungs, diaphragmatic dysfunction, and systemic lupus erythematosus. Am. Rev. Respir. Dis. 132: 926–928, 1985.

4420. Burki, N. K. Detection of added respiratory loads in patients with restrictive lung disease. Am. Rev. Respir. Dis. 132: 1210–1213, 1985.

4421. Campbell, D. A., Poulter, L. W., and Du Bois, R. M. Immunocompetent cells in bronchoalveolar lavage reflect the cell populations in transbronchial biopsies in pulmonary sarcoidosis. Am. Rev. Respir. Dis. 132: 1300–1306, 1985.

4422. Olafsson, M., Simonsson, B. G., and Hansson, S.-B. Bronchial reactivity in patients with recent pulmonary sarcoidosis. Thorax 40: 51–53, 1985.

4423. Greening, A. P., Nunn, P., Dobson, N., Rudolf, M., and Rees, A. D. M. Pulmonary sarcoidosis: alterations in bronchoalveolar lymphocytes and T cell subsets. Thorax 40: 278–283, 1985.

4424. Cohen, R. D., Bunting, P. S., Meindock, H. O., Chamberlain, D. W., and Rebuck, A. S. Does serum angiotensin converting enzyme reflect intensity of alveolitis in sarcoidosis? Thorax 40: 497–500, 1985.

4425. Lin, Y. H., Haslam, P. L., and Turner-Warwick, M. Chronic pulmonary sarcoidosis: relationship between lung lavage cell counts, chest radiograph, and results of standard lung function tests. Thorax 40: 501–507, 1985.

4426. Laviolette, M. Lymphocyte fluctuation in bronchoalveolar lavage fluid in normal volunteers. Thorax 40: 651–656, 1985.

4427. Campbell, D. A., Poulter, L. W., Janossy, G., and Du Bois, R. M. Immunohistological analysis of lung tissue from patients with cryptogenic fibrosing alveolitis suggesting local expression of immune hypersensitivity. Thorax 40: 405–411, 1985.

4428. Venn, G. E., Kay, P. H., Midwood, C. J., and Goldstraw, P. Open lung biopsy in patients with diffuse pulmonary shadowing. Thorax 40: 931–935, 1985.

4429. King, T. K. C. and Briscoe, W. A. Treatment of hypoxia with 24 per cent oxygen. Am. Rev. Respir. Dis. 108: 19–29, 1973.

4430. Neuhold, A., Miczoch, J., Grabner, G., and Kotscher, E. Long term follow up of radiological signs of pulmonary hypertension in correlation with haemodynamic changes. Bull. Eur. Physiopathol. Respir. 21: 7–10, 1985.

4431. Midgren, B., White, T., Petersson, K., Bryhn, M., Airikkala, P., and Elmqvist, D. Nocturnal hypoxaemia and cor pulmonale in severe chronic lung disease. Bull. Eur. Physiopathol. Respir. 21: 527–533, 1985.

4432. Theodore, J., Robin, E. D., Burke, C. M., Jamieson, S. W., Van Kessel, A., Rubin, D., Stinson, E. B., and Shumway, N. E. Impact of profound reductions of PaO_2 on O_2 transport and utilization in congenital heart disease. Chest 87: 293–302, 1985.

4433. Brundin, A. Arterial blood gases in respiratory insufficiency in the clinically stable state and during acute exacerbations of respiratory failure. Scand. J. Respir. Dis. 55: 181–190, 1974.

4434. Sibbald, W. J., Short, A. K., Warshawski, F. J., Cunningham, D. G., and Cheung, H. Thermal dye measurements of extravascular lung water in critically ill patients. Chest 87: 585–592, 1985.

4435. Mason, G. R., Effros, R. M., Uszler, J. M., and Mena, I. Small solute clearance from the lungs of patients with cardiogenic and noncardiogenic pulmonary edema. Chest 88: 327–334, 1985.

4436. Halperin, B. D., Feeley, T. W., Mihm, F. G., Chiles, C., Guthaner, D. F., and Blank, N. E. Evaluation of the portable chest roentgenogram for quantitating extravascular lung water in critically ill adults. Chest 88: 649–652, 1985.

4437. Stahl, M. G., Bonekat, H. W., and Shigeoka, J. W. Concomitant pulmonary thromboembolism and metallic mercury embolism. Chest 88: 787–789, 1985.

4438. Hull, R. D., Hirsh, J., Carter, C. J., Raskob, G. E., Gill, G. J., Jay, R. M., Leclerc, J. R., David, M., and Coates, G. Diagnostic value of ventilation-perfusion lung scanning in patients with suspected pulmonary embolism. Chest 88: 819–828, 1985.

4439. Huet, Y., Lemaire, F., Brun-Buisson, C., Knaus, W. A., Teisseire, B., Payen, D., and Mathieu, D. Hypoxemia in acute pulmonary embolism. Chest 88: 829–836, 1985.

4440. Soroldoni, M., Ferrarini, F., Biffi, E., Pozzi, M., Gatto, R., and Longhini, E. M-mode subxiphoid echocardiography in assessing pulmonary hypertension. Respiration 47: 164–170, 1985.

4441. Glassroth, J., Woodford, D. W., Carrington, C. B., and Gaensler, E. A. Pulmonary veno-occlusive disease in the middle-aged. Respiration 47: 309–321, 1985.

4442. Macnee, W., Morgan, A. D., Wathen, C. G., Muir, A. L., and Flenley, D. C. Right ventricular performance during exercise in chronic obstructive pulmonary disease. Respiration 48: 206–215, 1985.

4443. Van Der Elst, A. M. C. and Van Der Werf, T. Some circulatory aspects of the oxygen transport in patients with emphysema. Respiration 48: 310–320, 1985.

4444. Reihman, D. H., Farber, M. O., Weinberger, M. H., Henry, D. P., Fineberg, N. S., Dowdeswell, I. R. G., Burt, R. W., and Manfredi, F. Effect of hypoxemia on sodium and water excretion in chronic obstructive lung disease. Am. J. Med. 78: 87–94, 1985.

4445. Shuck, J. W., Oetgen, W. J., and Tesar, J. T. Pulmonary vascular response during Raynaud's phenomenon in progressive systemic sclerosis. Am. J. Med. 78: 221–227, 1985.

4446. Case records of the Massachusetts General Hospital. Case 19-1985. N. Engl. J. Med. 312: 1242–1251, 1985.

4447. Blom-Bulow, B., Jonson, B., and Brauer, K. Lung function in progressive systemic sclerosis is dominated by poorly compliant lungs and stiff airways. Eur. J. Respir. Dis. 66: 1–8, 1985.

4448. Sorensen, P. G., Rossing, and Rorth, M. Carbon monoxide diffusing capacity: a reliable indicator of bleomycin-induced pulmonary toxicity. Eur. J. Respir. Dis. 66: 333–340, 1985.

4449. Barzo, P. Familial idiopathic fibrosing alveolitis. Eur. J. Respir. Dis. 66: 350–352, 1985.

4450. Ishizaki, T., Miyabo, S., Koshino, T., Fujimura, M., Ueda, M., Sato, H., and Kitigawa, M. Lymphoid interstitial pneumonia: findings at bronchoalveolar lavage. Eur. J. Respir. Dis. 67: 128–132, 1985.

4451. Lamberto, C., Saumon, G., Loiseau, P., Battesti, J. P., and Georges, R. Respiratory function in recent pulmonary sarcoidosis with special reference to small airways. Bull. Eur. Physiopathol. Respir. 21: 309–315, 1985.

4452. Addleman, M., Logan, A., and Grossman, R. E. Monitoring intrapulmonary hemorrhage in Goodpasture's syndrome. Chest 87: 119–120, 1985.

4453. Derderian, S. S., Tellis, C. J., Abbrecht, P. H., Welton, R. C., and Rajagopal, K. R. Pulmonary involvement in mixed connective tissue disease. Chest 88: 45–48, 1985.

4454. Yousem, S. A., Lifson, J. D., and Colby, T. V. Chemotherapy-induced eosinophilic pneumonia. Chest 88: 103–106, 1985.

4455. Standertskjold-Nordenstam, C. G., Wandtke, J. C., Hood, W. B. Jr., Zugibe, F. T., and Butler, L. Amiodarone pulmonary toxicity. Chest 88: 143–145, 1985.

4456. Constantopoulos, S. H., Papadimitriou, C. S., and Moutsopoulos, H. M. Respiratory manifestations in primary Sjogren's syndrome. Chest 88: 226–229, 1985.

4457. Miller, L. R., Greenberg, S. D., and McLarty, J. W. Lupus lung. Chest 88: 265–269, 1985.

4458. Gilson, A. J. and Sahn, S. A. Reactivation of bleomycin lung toxicity following oxygen administration. Chest 88: 304–306, 1985.

4459. De La Cruz, J. L., Oteo, L. A., Lopez, C., Curto, L. M., Burgaleta, C., Campos, A., and Sueiro, A. Toxic-oil syndrome. Chest 88: 398–402, 1985.

4460. Spratling, L., Tenholder, M. F., Underwood, G. H., Feaster, B. L., and Requa, R. K. Daily vs alternate day prednisone therapy for stage II sarcoidosis. Chest 88: 687–690, 1985.

4461. Rossi, G. A., Di Negro, G. B., Balzano, E., Cerri, E., Sacco, O., Balbi, B., Venturini, A., Ramoino, R., and Ravazzoni, C. Suppression of the alveolitis in pulmonary sarcoidosis by oral corticosteroids. Lung 163: 83–93, 1985.

4462. Cazzadori, A., Braggio, P., and Bontempini, L. Salazopyrin-induced eosinophilic pneumonia. Respiration 47: 158–160, 1985.

4463. Wasicek, C. A., Reichlin, M., Montes, M., and Raghu, G. Polymyositis and interstitial lung disease in a patient with anti-Jo1 prototype. Am. J. Med. 76: 538–544, 1984.

4464. Kelley, M. A., Panettieri, R. A. Jr., and Krupinski, A. V. Resting single-breath diffusing capacity as a screening test for exercise-induced hypoxemia. Am. J. Med. 80: 807–812, 1986.

4465. Lloyd, T. C. Jr. Effect on breathing of acute pressure rise in pulmonary artery and right ventricle. J. Appl. Physiol. 57: 110–116, 1984.

4466. Kikuchi, R., Sekizawa, K., Sasaki, H., Hirose, Y., Matsumoto, N., Takishima, T., and Hildebrandt, J. Effects of pulmonary congestion on airway reactivity to histamine aerosol in dogs. J. Appl. Physiol. 57: 1640–1647, 1984.

4467. Gee, M. H., Perkowski, S. Z., Tahamont, M. V., Flynn, J. T., and Wasserman, M. A. Thromboxane as a mediator of pulmonary dysfunction during intravascular complement activation in sheep. Am. Rev. Respir. Dis. 133: 269–273, 1986.

4468. Burki, N. The dead space to tidal volume ratio in the diagnosis of pulmonary embolism. Am. Rev. Respir. Dis. 133: 679–685, 1986.

4469. Voelkel, N. F. Mechanisms of hypoxic pulmonary vasoconstriction. Am. Rev. Respir. Dis. 133: 1186–1195, 1986.

4470. Serra, J., Soulen, R., Moore, R., and McNicholas, K. Interrupted aortic arch associated with Pourfour du Petit syndrome. Thorax 41: 217–218, 1986.

4471. Gallagher, C. G. and Younes, M. Breathing pattern during and after maximal exercise in patients with chronic obstructive lung disease, interstitial lung disease, and cardiac disease, and in normal subjects. Am. Rev. Respir. Dis. 133: 581–586, 1986.

4472. Rhind, G. B., MacNee, W., and Flenley, D. C. Disodium cromoglycate fails to prevent the rise in pulmonary artery pressure in hypoxic chronic bronchitis and emphysema. Eur. J. Respir. Dis. 68: 58–63, 1986.

4473. Widimsky, J. Vasodilatory treatment of pulmonary hypertension. Eur. J. Respir. Dis. 68: 161–166, 1986.

4474. Bratel, T., Hedenstierna, G., Nyquist, O., and Ripe, E. Long-term treatment with a new calcium antagonist, felodipine, in chronic obstructive lung disease. Eur. J. Respir. Dis. 68: 351–361, 1986.

4475. Watters, L. C., King, T. E., Schwarz, M. I., Waldron, J. A., Stanford, R. E., and Cherniack, R. M. A clinical, radiographic, and physiologic scoring system for the longitudinal assessment of patients with idiopathic pulmonary fibrosis. Am. Rev. Respir. Dis. 133: 97–103, 1986.

4476. Martin, R. R., Lawrence, E. C., Teague, R. B., Gottlieb, M. S., and Putman, M. Chemiluminescence of lung macrophages and blood leukocytes in sarcoidosis. Am. Rev. Respir. Dis. 133: 298–301, 1986.

4477. Chapman, H. A., Allen, C. L., and Stone, O. L. Abnormalities in pathways of alveolar fibrin turnover among patients with interstitial lung disease. Am. Rev. Respir. Dis. 133: 437–443, 1986.

4478. Garcia, J. G. N., Wolven, R. G., Garcia, P. L., and Keogh, B. A. Assessment of interlobar variation of bronchoalveolar lavage cellular differentials in interstitial lung diseases. Am. Rev. Respir. Dis. 133: 444–449, 1986.

4479. Garcia, J. G. N., Parhami, N., Killam, D., Garcia, P. L., and Keogh, B. A. Bronchoalveolar lavage fluid evaluation in rheumatoid arthritis. Am. Rev. Respir. Dis. 133: 450–454, 1986.

4480. Wallaert, B., Hatron, P.-Y., Grosbois, J.-M., Tonnel, A.-B.,

Devulder, B., and Voisin, C. Subclinical pulmonary involvement in collagen-vascular diseases assessed by bronchoalveolar lavage. Am. Rev. Respir. Dis. 133: 574–580, 1986.

4481. Paradis, I. L., Dauber, J. H., and Rabin, B. S. Lymphocyte phenotypes in bronchoalveolar lavage and lung tissue in sarcoidosis and idiopathic fibrosis. Am. Rev. Respir. Dis. 133: 855–860, 1986.

4482. Adler, K. B., Callahan, L. M., and Evans, J. N. Cellular alterations in the alveolar wall in bleomycin-induced pulmonary fibrosis in rats. Am. Rev. Respir. Dis. 133: 1043–1048, 1986.

4483. Flint, K. C., Leung, K. P. B., Hudspith, B. N., Brostoff, J., Pearce, F. L., Geraint-James, D., and Johnson, N. McI. Bronchoalveolar mast cells in sarcoidosis: increased numbers and accentuation of mediator release. Thorax 41: 94–99, 1986.

4484. Liu, F. L.-W., Cohen, R. D., Downar, E., Butany, J. W., Edelson, J. D., and Rebuck, A. S. Amiodarone pulmonary toxicity: functional and ultrastructural evaluation. Thorax 41: 100–105, 1986.

4485. Miller, W. C., Heard, J. G., Unger, K. M., and Suich, D. M. Anatomical lung shunting in pulmonary fibrosis. Thorax 41: 208–209, 1986.

4486. Goldstein, D. S. and Williams, M. H. Rate of improvement of pulmonary function in sarcoidosis during treatment with corticosteroids. Thorax 41: 473–474, 1986.

4487. Rizzato, G. Recent advances in sarcoidosis. Eur. J. Respir. Dis. 68: 1–6, 1986.

4488. Jernudd-Wilhelmsson, Y., Hornblad, Y., and Hedenstierna, G. Ventilation-perfusion relationships in interstitial lung disease. Eur. J. Respir. Dis. 68: 39–49, 1986.

4489. Cooper, J. A. D., White, D. A., and Matthay, R. A. Drug-induced pulmonary disease: Part 2. Noncytotoxic drugs. Am. Rev. Respir. Dis. 133: 488–505, 1986.

4490. Wallaert, B., Ramon, Ph., Fournier, E. C., Hatron, P. Y., Muir, J. F., Tonnel, A. B., and Voisin, C. High-dose methylprednisolone pulse therapy in sarcoidosis. Eur. J. Respir. Dis. 68: 256–262, 1986.

4491. Luisetti, M., Fiocca, R., Pozzi, E., De Rose, V., Magrini, U., and Grassi, C. The Hermansky-Pudlak syndrome. A case with macrophage-neutrophil alveolitis. Eur. J. Respir. Dis. 68: 301–305, 1986.

4492. Dhillon, D. P., Haslam, P. L., Townsend, P. J., Primett, Z., Collins, J. V., and Turner-Warwick, M. Bronchoalveolar lavage in patients with interstitial lung diseases: side effects and factors affecting fluid recovery. Eur. J. Respir. Dis. 68: 342–350, 1986.

4493. Bloom, J. W., Sugihara, S., Garfield, M. D., Abraham, T. A., and Knudson, R. J. Characteristics of individuals with accelerated declines in lung function. Chest 85: 18S–19S, 1984.

4494. Bass, H., Heckscher, T., and Anthonisen, N. R. Regional pulmonary gas exchange in patients with pulmonary embolism. Clin. Sci. 33: 355–364, 1967.

4495. Singh, H., Ebejer, M. J., Higgins, D. A., Henderson, A. H., and Campbell, I. A. Acute haemodynamic effects of nifedipine at rest and during maximal exercise in patients with chronic cor pulmonale. Thorax 40: 910–914, 1985.

4496. Ardesty, J. and Wolf, K. Risk from exposure to asbestos. Science 234: 923, 1986.

4497. Brodeur, P. Outrageous Misconduct: The Asbestos Industry on Trial. Pantheon Books, New York, 1985.

4498. Bates, D. V., Grymaloski, M., and English, R. A. A case of silicosis. B. C. Med. J. 24: 66–68, 1982.

4499. Cockcroft, A., Wagner, J. C., Ryder, R., Seal, R. M. E., Lyons, J. P., and Anderson, N. Post-mortem study of emphysema in coalworkers and non-coalworkers. Lancet 2: 600–603, 1982.

4500. Morgan, A. and Holmes, A. The distribution and characteristics of asbestos fibers in the lungs of Finnish anthophyllite mine-workers. Environ. Res. 33: 62–75, 1984.

4501. Holness, D. L., Taraschuk, I. G., and Pelmear, P. L. Effect of dust exposure in Ontario cotton textile mills. J. Occup. Med. 25: 26–29, 1983.

4502. Broder, I., Davies, G., Hutcheon, M., Leznoff, A., Mintz, S., Thomas, P., and Corey, P. Variables of pulmonary allergy and inflammation in grain elevator workers. J. Occup. Med. 25: 43–47, 1983.

4503. Eisenbud, M. and Lisson, J. Epidemiological aspects of beryllium-induced nonmalignant lung disease: a 30-year update. J. Occup. Med. 25: 196–202, 1983.

4504. McMillan, G. H. G. The health of welders in naval dockyards. J. Occup. Med. 25: 727–730, 1983.

4505. Greaves, I. A., Wegman, D. H., Smith, T. J., and Spiegelman, D. L. Respiratory effects of two types of solder flux used in the electronics industry. J. Occup. Med. 26: 81–85, 1984.

4506. Kleinman, G. D. Occupational health and safety—the Swedish model. J. Occup. Med. 26: 901–905, 1984.

4507. Main, D. M. and Hogan, T. J. Health effects of low-level exposure to formaldehyde. J. Occup. Med. 25: 896–900, 1983.

4508. Townsend, M. C. and Belk, H. D. Development of a standardised pulmonary function evaluation program in industry. J. Occup. Med. 26: 657–661, 1984.

4509. McGrath, K. G., Roach, D., Zeiss, C. R., and Patterson, R. Four-year evaluation of workers exposed to trimellitic anhydride. J. Occup. Med. 26: 671–675, 1984.

4510. Moscato, G., Biscaldi, G. P., Brunetti, G., Pugliese, F., and Candura, F. Occupational asthma caused by styrene (letter to editor). J. Occup. Med. 26: 552, 1984.

4511. Levy, B. S., Hoffman, L., and Gottsegen, S. Boilermaker's bronchitis: respiratory tract irritation associated with vanadium pentoxide exposure during oil-to-coal conversion of a power plant. J. Occup. Med. 26: 567–570, 1984.

4512. Cooper, W. C. and Sargent, E. N. A 26-year radiographic follow-up of workers in a diatomite mine and mill. J. Occup. Med. 26: 456–460, 1984.

4513. Jones, R. N., Diem, J. E., Ziskind, M. M., Rodriguez, M., and Weill, H. Radiographic evidence of asbestos effects in American marine engineers. J. Occup. Med. 26: 281–284, 1984.

4514. Holness, D. L., Broder, I., Corey, P. N., Booth, N., Mozzon, D., Nazar, M. A., and Guirguis, S. Respiratory variables and exposure-effect relationships in isocyanate-exposed workers. J. Occup. Med. 26: 449–455, 1984.

4515. Baur, X., Dewair, M., and Rommelt, H. Acute airway obstruction followed by hypersensitivity pneumonitis in an isocyanate (MDI) worker. J. Occup. Med. 26: 285–287, 1984.

4516. Altekruse, E. B., Chaudhary, B. A., Pearson, M. G., and Morgan, W. K. C. Kaolin dust concentrations and pneumoconiosis at a kaolin mine. Thorax 39: 436–441, 1984.

4517. Hayden, S. P., Pincock, A. C., Hayden, J., Tyler, L. E., Cross, K. W., and Bishop, J. M. Respiratory symptoms and pulmonary function of welders in the engineering industry. Thorax 39: 442–447, 1984.

4518. Burge, P. S., Hendy, M., and Hodgson, E. S. Occupational asthma, rhinitis, and dermatitis due to tetrazene in a detonator manufacturer. Thorax 39: 470–471, 1984.

4519. McGavin, C. R. and Sheers, G. Diffuse pleural thickening in asbestos workers: disability and lung function abnormalities. Thorax 39: 604–607, 1984.

4520. Malo, J.-L., Gagnon, G., and Cartier, A. Occupational asthma due to heated freon. Thorax 39: 628–629, 1984.

4521. Field, G. B. Pulmonary function in aluminium smelters. Thorax 39: 743–751, 1984.

4522. Hillerdal, G. Asbestos related pleuropulmonary lesions and the erythrocyte sedimentation rate. Thorax 39: 752–758, 1984.

4523. Davis, J. M. G. The pathology of asbestos related disease. Thorax 39: 801–808, 1984.

4524. Schachter, E. N., Maunder, L. R., and Beck, G. J. The pattern of lung function abnormalities in cotton textile workers. Am. Rev. Respir. Dis. 129: 523–527, 1984.

4525. Ruckley, V. A., Gauld, S. J., Chapman, J. S., Davis, J. M. G., Douglas, A. N., Fernie, J. M., Jacobsen, M., and Lamb, D. Emphysema and dust exposure in a group of coal workers. Am. Rev. Respir. Dis. 129: 528–532, 1984.

4526. Finkelstein, M. M. and Vingilis, J. J. Radiographic abnormalities among asbestos-cement workers. Am. Rev. Respir. Dis. 129: 17–22, 1984.

4527. Nagy, L. and Orosz, M. Occupational asthma due to hexachlorophene. Thorax 39: 630–631, 1984.

4528. McKay, R. T. and Brooks, S. M. Hyperreactive airway smooth muscle responsiveness after inhalation of toluene diisocyanate vapors. Am. Rev. Respir. Dis. 129: 296–300, 1984.

4529. Warheit, D. B., Chang, L. Y., Hill, L. H., Hook, G. E. R., Crapo, J. D., and Brody, A. R. Pulmonary macrophage accumulation and asbestos-induced lesions at sites of fiber deposition. Am. Rev. Respir. Dis. 129: 301–310, 1984.

4530. Becklake, M. R. Organic or functional impairment. Exercise Testing in the Dyspneic Patient. Am. Rev. Respir. Dis. 129(2)(Pt. 2)(Suppl.): S96–S100, 1984.

4531. Murphy, R. L. H. Jr., Gaensler, E. A., Holford, S. K., Del Bono, E. A., and Epler, G. Crackles in the early detection of asbestosis. Am. Rev. Respir. Dis. 129: 375–379, 1984.

4532. Funahashi, A., Schlueter, D. P., Pintar, K., Siegesmund, K. A., Mandel, G. S., and Mandel, N. S. Pneumoconiosis in workers exposed to silicon carbide. Am. Rev. Respir. Dis. 129: 635–640, 1984.

4533. Beck, G. J., Schachter, E. N., and Maunder, L. R. The relationship of respiratory symptoms and lung function loss in cotton textile workers. Am. Rev. Respir. Dis. 130: 6–11, 1984.

4534. Demedts, M., Gheysens, B., Nagels, J., Verbeken, E., Lauweryns, J., Van Den Eeckhout, A., Lahaye, D., and Gyselen, A. Cobalt lung in diamond polishers. Am. Rev. Respir. Dis. 130: 130–135, 1984.

4535. Morgan, A. and Holmes, A. Concentrations and dimensions of coated and uncoated asbestos fibres in the human lung. Br. J. Ind. Med. 37: 25–32, 1980.

4536. Jones, R. N., Butcher, B. T., Hammad, Y. Y., Diem, J. E., Glindmeyer, H. W. III, Lehrer, S. B., Hughes, J. M., and Weill, H. Interaction of atopy and exposure to cotton dust in the bronchoconstrictor response. Br. J. Ind. Med. 37: 141–146, 1980.

4537. Chivers, C. P., Lawrence-Jones, C., and Paddle, G. M. Lung function in workers exposed to polyvinyl chloride dust. Br. J. Ind. Med. 37: 147–151, 1980.

4538. Glover, J. R., Bevan, C., Cotes, J. E., Elwood, P. C., Hodges, N. G., Kell, R. L., Lowe, C. R., McDermott, M., and Oldham, P. D. Effects of exposure to slate dust in North Wales. Br. J. Ind. Med. 37: 152–162, 1980.

4539. Cochrane, A. L. and Moore, F. A 20-year follow-up of men aged 55–64 including coal-miners and foundry workers in Staveley, Derbyshire. Br. J. Ind. Med. 37: 226–229, 1980.

4540. Cherry, N., Waldron, H. A., Wells, G. G., Wilkinson, R. T., Wilson, H. K., and Jones, S. An investigation of the acute behavioural effects of styrene on factory workers. Br. J. Ind. Med. 37: 234–240, 1980.

4541. Lees, R. E. M. Changes in lung function after exposure to vanadium compounds in fuel oil ash. Br. J. Ind. Med. 37: 253–256, 1980.

4542. Liddell, F. D. K. and McDonald, J. C. Radiological findings as predictors of mortality in Quebec asbestos workers. Br. J. Ind. Med. 37: 257–267, 1980.

4543. McMillan, G. H. G., Pethybridge, R. J., and Sheers, G. Effect of smoking on attack rates of pulmonary and pleural lesions related to exposure to asbestos dust. Br. J. Ind. Med. 37: 268–272, 1980.

4544. Ophus, E. M., Mowe, G., Osen, K. K., and Gylseth, B. Scanning electron microscopy and x-ray microanalysis of mineral deposits in lungs of a patient with pleural mesothelioma. Br. J. Ind. Med. 37: 375–381, 1980.

4545. Noweir, M. H., Moselhi, M., and Amine, E. K. Role of family susceptibility, occupational and family histories and individuals' blood groups in the development of silicosis. Br. J. Ind. Med. 37: 399–404, 1980.

4546. Kiviluto, M. Observations on the lungs of vanadium workers. Br. J. Ind. Med. 37: 363–366, 1980.

4547. Glassroth, J. L., Bernardo, J., Lucey, E. C., Center, D. M., Jung-Legg, Y., and Snider, G. L. Interstitial pulmonary fibrosis induced in hamsters by intratracheally administered chrysotile asbestos. Am. Rev. Respir. Dis. 130: 242–248, 1984.

4548. Lapenas, D., Gale, P., Kennedy, T., Rawlings, W. Jr., and Dietrich, P. Kaolin pneumoconiosis. Am. Rev. Respir. Dis. 130: 282–288, 1984.

4549. Weiss, W. Cigarette smoke, asbestos, and small irregular opacities. Am. Rev. Respir. Dis. 130: 293–301, 1984.

4550. Miller, R. R., Churg, A. M., Hutcheon, M., and Lam, S.

Pulmonary alveolar proteinosis and aluminum dust exposure. Am. Rev. Respir. Dis. 130: 312–315, 1984.

4551. Park, T., DiBenedotto, R., Morgan, K., Colmers, R., and Sherman, E. Diffuse endobronchial polyposis following a titanium tetrachloride inhalation injury. Am. Rev. Respir. Dis. 130: 315–317, 1984.

4552. Hargreave, F. E., Ramsdale, E. H., and Pugsley, S. O. Occupational asthma without bronchial hyperresponsiveness. Am. Rev. Respir. Dis. 130: 513–515, 1984.

4553. Dopico, G. A., Reddan, W., Tsiatis, A., Peters, M. E., and Rankin, J. Epidemiologic study of clinical and physiologic parameters in grain handlers of northern United States. Am. Rev. Respir. Dis. 130: 759–765, 1984.

4554. Chan-Yeung, M., Vedal, S., Kus, J., Maclean, L., Enarson, D., and Tse, K. S. Symptoms, pulmonary function, and bronchial hyperreactivity in Western red cedar workers compared with those in office workers. Am. Rev. Respir. Dis. 130: 1038–1041, 1984.

4555. Cloutier, M. M., Lesniak, K. M., Russell, J. A., and Rohrbach, M. S. Effect of cotton bracts extract on canine tracheal epithelium and shunt pathway. Am. Rev. Respir. Dis. 130: 1087–1090, 1984.

4556. Dolovich, J., Evans, S. L., and Nieboer, E. Occupational asthma from nickel sensitivity: I. Human serum albumin in the antigenic determinant. Br. J. Ind. Med. 41: 51–55, 1984.

4557. Douglas, J. S. and Duncan, P. G. Characterisation of textile dust extracts: I. Histamine release in vitro. Br. J. Ind. Med. 41: 64–69, 1984.

4558. Douglas, J. S., Duncan, P. G., and Zuskin, E. Characterisation of textile dust extracts: II. Bronchoconstriction in man. Br. J. Ind. Med. 41: 70–76, 1984.

4559. Tukainen, P., Nickels, J., Taskinen, E., and Nyberg, M. Pulmonary granulomatous reaction: talc pneumoconiosis or chronic sarcoidosis? Br. J. Ind. Med. 41: 84–87, 1984.

4560. Zuskin, E. and Skuric, Z. Respiratory function in tea workers. Br. J. Ind. Med. 41: 88–93, 1984.

4561. Broder, I., Hutcheon, M. A., Mintz, S., Davies, G., Leznoff, A., Thomas, P., and Corey, P. Changes in respiratory variables of grain handlers and civic workers during their initial months of employment. Br. J. Ind. Med. 41: 94–99, 1984.

4562. Peters, J. M., Smith, T. J., Bernstein, L., Wright, W. E., and Hammond, S. K. Pulmonary effects of exposures in silicon carbide manufacturing. Br. J. Ind. Med. 41: 109–115, 1984.

4563. McDonald, A. D., Fry, A. J., Woolley, A. J., and McDonald, J. C. Dust exposure and mortality in an American chrysotile asbestos friction products plant. Br. J. Ind. Med. 41: 151–157, 1984.

4564. McDowell, M. E. A mortality study of cement workers. Br. J. Ind. Med. 41: 179–182, 1984.

4565. Noweir, M. H., Abdel-Kader, H. M., and Omran, F. Role of histamine in the aetiology of byssinosis. I. Blood histamine concentrations in workers exposed to cotton and flax dusts. Br. J. Ind. Med. 41: 203–208, 1984.

4566. Noweir, M. H., Abdel-Kader, H. M., and Makar, A. Role of histamine in the aetiology of byssinosis. II. Lung histamine concentrations in guinea pigs chronically exposed to cotton and flax dusts. Br. J. Ind. Med. 41: 209–213, 1984.

4567. Pham, Q. T., Mur, J., Chau, N., Gabiano, M., Henquel, J. C., and Teculescu, D. Prognostic value of acetylcholine challenge test: a prospective study. Br. J. Ind. Med. 41: 267–271, 1984.

4568. Lloyd, M. H., Gauld, S., Copland, L., and Soutar, C. A. Epidemiological study of the lung function of workers at a factory manufacturing polyvinylchloride. Br. J. Ind. Med. 41: 328–333, 1984.

4569. Robertson, A., Dodgson, J., Collings, P., and Seaton, A. Exposure to oxides of nitrogen: respiratory symptoms and lung function in British coalminers. Br. J. Ind. Med. 41: 214–219, 1984.

4570. Soutar, C. A. and Collins, H. P. R. Classification of progressive massive fibrosis of coalminers by type of radiographic appearance. Br. J. Ind. Med. 41: 334–339, 1984.

4571. Begin, R., Boctor, M., Bergeron, D., Cantin, A., Berthiaume, Y., Peloquin, S., Bisson, G., and Lamourreux, G. Radiographic assessment of pleuropulmonary disease in asbestos workers: posteroanterior, four view films, and computed tomograms of the thorax. Br. J. Ind. Med. 41: 373–383, 1984.

4572. Jaurand, M. C., Gaudichet, A., Halpern, S., and Bignon, J. In vitro biodegradation of chrysotile fibers by alveolar macrophages and mesothelial cells in culture: comparison with a pH effect. Br. J. Ind. Med. 41: 389–395, 1984.

4573. Courtney, D. and Merrett, J. D. Respiratory symptoms and lung function in a group of solderers. Br. J. Ind. Med. 41: 346–351, 1984.

4574. Harvey, G., Page, M., and Dumas, L. Binding of environmental carcinogens to asbestos and mineral fibers. Br. J. Ind. Med. 41: 396–400, 1984.

4575. Prichard, M. G., Ryan, G., and Musk, A. W. Wheat flour sensitization and airways disease in urban bakers. Br. J. Ind. Med. 41: 450–454, 1984.

4576. Sepulveda, M.-J., Castellan, R. M., Hankinson, J. L., and Cocke, J. B. Acute lung function response to cotton dust in atopic and non-atopic individuals. Br. J. Ind. Med. 41: 487–491, 1984.

4577. Churg, A. and Wright, J. Small airways disease induced by asbestos and nonasbestos mineral dusts. Chest 85: 36S–38S, 1984.

4578. Saracci, R., Simonato, L., Acheson, E. D., Andersen, A., Bertazzi, P. A., Claude, J., Charnmay, N., Esteve, J., Frentzel-Beyme, R. R., Gardner, M. J., Jensen, O. M., Maasing, R., Olsen, J. H., Teppo, L., Westerholm, P., and Zocchetti, C. Mortality and incidence of cancer in workers in the man made vitreous fibres producing industry: an international investigation at 13 European plants. Br. J. Ind. Med. 41: 425–436, 1984.

4579. Lien, D. C., Todoruk, D. N., Rajani, H. R., Cook, D. A., and Herbert, F. A. Accidental inhalation of mercury vapour: respiratory and toxicologic consequences. Can. Med. Assoc. J. 129: 591–595, 1983.

4580. Tallroth, K. and Kiviranta, K. Round atelectasis. Respiration 45: 71–77, 1984.

4581. Cohen, B. M., Adasczik, A., and Cohen, E. M. Small airways changes in workers exposed to asbestos. Respiration 45: 296–302, 1984.

4582. Mur, J.-M., Chau, N., Pham, Q. T., Meyer-Bisch, C., and Cavelier, C. Reduction of pulmonary function indices: comparison of two hierarchical methods. Respiration 46: 61–68, 1984.

4583. Mandi, A., Galgoczy, G., Galambos, E., Nemeth, L., and Dombos, K. Changes in clinical status and lung functions of patients with chronic respiratory disease over 10 years. Respiration 46: 151–159, 1984.

4584. Edwards, J. H., Al Zubaidy, T. S., Altikriti, R., and Bunny, H. Byssinosis: inhalation challenge with polyphenol. Chest 85: 215–217, 1984.

4585. Jones, R. N. Cotton and chronic lung disease (editorial). Chest 85: 587–589, 1984.

4586. Tabona, M., Chan-Yeung, M., Enarson, D., MacLean, L., Dorken, E., and Schulzer, M. Host factors affecting longitudinal decline in lung spirometry among grain elevator workers. Chest 85: 782–786, 1984.

4587. Geremia, G. and Mintzner, R. A. An unusual case of rounded atelectasis. Chest 86: 485–486, 1984.

4588. Cullen, M. R. Respiratory diseases from hard metal exposure (editorial). Chest 86: 513–514, 1984.

4589. Sprince, N. L., Chamberlin, R. I., Hales, C. A., Weber, A. L., and Kazemi, H. Respiratory disease in tungsten carbide production workers. Chest 86: 549–557, 1984.

4590. Epstein, D. M. Pleural plaques: a marker for respiratory tract malignancy? (editorial). Chest 86: 660, 1984.

4591. Wain, S. L., Roggli, V. L., and Foster, W. L. Jr. Parietal pleural plaques, asbestos bodies, and neoplasia. Chest 86: 707–713, 1984.

4592. Barnhart, S. and Rosenstock, L. Cadmium chemical pneumonitis. Chest 86: 789–791, 1984.

4593. Siracusa, A., Cicioni, C., Volpi, R., Canalicchi, P., Brugnami, G., Comodi, A. R., and Abbritti, G. Lung function among asbestos cement factory workers: cross-sectional and longitudinal study. Am. J. Ind. Med. 5: 315–325, 1984.

4594. Ohlson, C.-G., Rydman, T., Sundell, L., Bodin, L., and Hogstedt, C. Decreased lung function in long-term asbestos cement workers: a cross-sectional study. Am. J. Ind. Med. 5: 359–366, 1984.

4595. Donham, K. J., Zavala, D. C., and Merchant, J. Acute effects of the work environment on pulmonary functions of swine confinement workers. Am. J. Ind. Med. 5: 367–375, 1984.

4596. Coutts, I. I., Lozewicz, S., Dally, M. B., Newman-Taylor, A. J., Burge, P. S., Flind, A. C., and Rogers, D. J. H. Respiratory symptoms related to work in a factory manufacturing cimetidine tablets. Br. Med. J. 288: 1418, 1984.

4597. Macfarlane, J. T. Prognosis in sarcoidosis (editorial). Br. Med. J. 288: 1557–1558, 1984.

4598. Samuel, H. D. International occupational health standards: an American perspective. Am. J. Ind. Med. 6: 67–73, 1984.

4599. Aubier, M., Murciano, D., Milic-Emili, J., Touaty, E., Daghfous, J., Pariente, R., and Derenne, J. P. Effects of the administration of O_2 on ventilation and blood gases in patients with chronic obstructive pulmonary disease during acute respiratory failure. Am. Rev. Respir. Dis. 122: 747–754, 1980.

4600. Fournier-Massey, G., Wong, G., and Hall, T. C. Retired and former asbestos workers in Hawaii. Am. J. Ind. Med. 6: 139–153, 1984.

4601. Noweir, M. H., Noweir, K. H., Osman, H. A., and Moselhi, M. An environmental and medical study of byssinosis and other respiratory conditions in the cotton textile industry in Egypt. Am. J. Ind. Med. 6: 173–183, 1984.

4602. Corn, M. Air-sampling strategies in the work environment (editorial). Am. J. Ind. Med. 6: 251–252, 1984.

4603. Brody, J., Miller, A., and Langer, A. M. Pneumoconiosis associated with exposure to glass and abrasive particles. Am. J. Ind. Med. 6: 339–345, 1984.

4604. Hagmar, L., Bellander, T., Ranstam, J., and Skerfving, S. Piperazine-induced airway symptoms: exposure-response relationships and selection in an occupational setting. Am. J. Ind. Med. 6: 347–357, 1984.

4605. Worth, G. Emphysema in coal workers (editorial). Am. J. Ind. Med. 6: 401–403, 1984.

4606. Ng, T. P., Chan, S.-L., and Lam, K.-P. Radiological progression and lung function in siliosis: a ten year follow up study. Br. Med. J. 295: 164–168, 1987.

4607. Nunn, J. F., Milledge, J. S., and Singaraya, J. Survival of patients ventilated in an intensive therapy unit. Br. Med. J. 1: 1525–1527, 1979.

4608. Asmundsson, T. and Kilburn, K. H. Survival after acute respiratory failure. Ann. Intern. Med. 80: 54–57, 1974.

4609. Attfield, M., Reger, R., and Glenn, R. The incidence and progression of pneumoconiosis over nine years in U.S. coalminers: I. Principal findings. Am. J. Ind. Med. 6: 407–415, 1984.

4610. Attfield, M., Reger, R., and Glenn, R. The incidence and progression of pneumoconiosis over nine years in U.S. coalminers: II. Relationship with dust exposure and other potential causative factors. Am. J. Ind. Med. 6: 417–425, 1984.

4611. Boden, L. I. and Gold, M. The accuracy of self-reported regulatory data: the case of coal mine dust. Am. J. Ind. Med. 6: 427–440, 1984.

4612. Cockcroft, D. W. Acquired persistent increase in nonspecific bronchial reactivity associated with isocyanate exposure. Ann. Allergy 48: 93–95, 1982.

4613. Hendrick, D. J. Bronchopulmonary disease in the workplace. Challenge testing with occupational agents. Ann. Allergy 51: 179–184, 1983.

4614. Dodd, K. T. and Gross, D. R. Ammonia inhalation toxicity in cats: a study of acute and chronic respiratory dysfunction. Arch. Environ. Health 35: 6–14, 1980.

4615. Burge, P. S., Harries, M. G., Lam, W. K., O'Brien, I. M., and Patchett, P. A. Occupational asthma due to formaldehyde. Thorax 40: 255–260, 1985.

4616. Gellert, A. R., Langford, J. A., Winter, R. J. D., Uthayakumar, S., Sinha, G., and Rudd, R. M. Asbestosis: assessment by bronchoalveolar lavage and measurement of pulmonary epithelial permeability. Thorax 40: 508–514, 1985.

4617. Gellert, A. R., Lewis, C. A., Langford, J. A., Tolfree, S. E. J., and Rudd, R. W. Regional distribution of pulmonary epithelial permeability in normal subjects and patients with asbestosis. Thorax 40: 734–740, 1985.

4618. Cowie, H., Lloyd, M. H., and Soutar, C. A. Study of lung function data by principal components analysis. Thorax 40: 438–443, 1985.

4619. Lozewicz, S., Davison, A. G., Hopkirk, A., Burge, P. S., Boldy, D., Riordan, J. F., McGivern, D. V., Platts, B. W., Davies, D., and Newman-Taylor, A. J. Occupational asthma due to methyl methacrylate and cyanoacrylates. Thorax 40: 836–839, 1985.

4620. Dernevik, L. Exogenous particles in lymph nodes in patients with shrinking pleuritis with atelectasis. Thorax 40: 948–951, 1985.

4621. Oleru, U. G. Pulmonary function of exposed and control workers in a Nigerian nonsoapy detergent factory. Arch. Environ. Health 39: 101–106, 1984.

4622. Bascom, R., Kennedy, T. P., Levitz, D., and Zeiss, C. R. Specific bronchoalveolar lavage IgG antibody in hypersensitivity pneumonitis from diphenylmethane diisocyanate. Am. Rev. Respir. Dis. 131: 463–465, 1985.

4623. Churg, A., Wright, J. L., Wiggs, B., Pare, P. D., and Lazar, N. Small airways disease and mineral dust exposure. Am. Rev. Respir. Dis. 131: 139–143, 1985.

4624. Lemaire, I. Characterization of the bronchoalveolar cellular response in experimental asbestosis. Am. Rev. Respir. Dis. 131: 144–149, 1985.

4625. Baser, M. E., Tockman, M. S., and Kennedy, T. P. Pulmonary function and respiratory symptoms in polyvinylchloride fabrication workers. Am. Rev. Respir. Dis. 131: 203–208, 1985.

4626. Rylander, R., Haglino, P., and Lundholm, M. Endotoxin in cotton dust and respiratory function decrement among cotton workers in an experimental cardroom. Am. Rev. Respir. Dis. 131: 209–213, 1985.

4627. Oliver, L. C., Eisen, E. A., Greene, R. E., and Sprince, N. L. Asbestos-related disease in railroad workers. Am. Rev. Respir. Dis. 131: 499–504, 1985.

4628. Yach, D., Myers, J., Bradshaw, D., and Benatar, S. R. A respiratory epidemiologic survey of grain mill workers in Cape Town, South Africa. Am. Rev. Respir. Dis. 131: 505–510, 1985.

4629. Kouzan, S., Brody, A. R., Nettesheim, P., and Eling, T. Production of arachidonic acid metabolites by macrophages exposed in vitro to asbestos, carbonyl iron particles, or calcium ionophore. Am. Rev. Respir. Dis. 131: 624–632, 1985.

4630. Dodson, R. F., Williams, M. G. Jr., O'Sullivan, M. F., Corn, C. J., Greenberg, S. D., and Hurst, G. A. A comparison of the feruginous body and uncoated fiber content in the lungs of former asbestos workers. Am. Rev. Respir. Dis. 132: 143–147, 1985.

4631. Christman, J. W., Emerson, R. J., Graham, W. G. B., and Davis, G. S. Mineral dust and cell recovery from the bronchoalveolar lavage of healthy Vermont granite workers. Am. Rev. Respir. Dis. 132: 393–399, 1985.

4632. Sue, D. Y., Oren, A., Hansen, J. E., and Wasserman, K. Lung function and exercise performance in smoking and nonsmoking asbestos-exposed workers. Am. Rev. Respir. Dis. 132: 612–618, 1985.

4633. Enarson, D. A., Vedal, S., and Chan-Yeung, M. Rapid decline in FEV_1 in grain handlers. Am. Rev. Respir. Dis. 132: 814–817, 1985.

4634. Gellert, A. R., Macey, M. G., Uthayakumar, S., Newland, A. C., and Rudd, R. M. Lymphocyte subpopulations in bronchoalveolar lavage fluid in asbestos workers. Am. Rev. Respir. Dis. 132: 824–828, 1985.

4635. Gordon, T., Sheppard, D., McDonald, D. M., Distefano, S., and Scypinski, L. Airway hyperresponsiveness and inflammation induced by toluene diisocyanate in guinea pigs. Am. Rev. Respir. Dis. 132: 1106–1112, 1985.

4636. Townsend, M. C., Enterline, P. E., Sussman, N. B., Bonney, T. B., and Rippey, L. L. Pulmonary function in relation to total dust exposure at a bauxite refinery and alumina-based chemical products plant. Am. Rev. Respir. Dis. 132: 1174–1180, 1985.

4637. Kennedy, S. M., Wright, J. L., Mullen, J. B., Pare, P. D., and Hogg, J. C. Pulmonary function and peripheral airway disease in patients with mineral dust or fume exposure. Am. Rev. Respir. Dis. 132: 1294–1299, 1985.

4638. Ames, R. G., Reger, R. B., and Hall, D. S. Chronic respiratory effects of exposure to diesel emissions in coal mines. Arch. Environ. Health 39: 389–394, 1984.

4639. Enarson, D. A., Maclean, S., Dybuncio, A., Chan-Yeung, M., Grzybowski, S., Johnson, A., Block, G., and Schragg, K. Respiratory health at a pulpmill in British Columbia. Arch. Environ. Health 39: 325–330, 1984.

4640. Attfield, M. D. Longitudinal decline in FEV_1 in United States coalminers. Thorax 40: 132–137, 1985.

4641. Yeung, M. and Grzybowski, S. Prognosis in occupational asthma (editorial). Thorax 40: 241–243, 1985.

4642. Warren, P. M., Millar, J. S., Flenley, D. C., and Avery, A. Respiratory failure revisited: acute exacerbations of chronic bronchitis between 1961–63 and 1970–76. Lancet i: 467–471, 1980.

4643. Dernevik, L., Bjorkander, J., Hanson, L. A., Larsson, S., Soderstrom, T., and William-Olsson, G. Immunological abnormalities in shrinking pleuritis with atelectasis. Eur. J. Respir. Dis. 66: 128–134, 1985.

4644. Simonsson, B. G., Sjoberg, A., Rolf, C., and Haeger-Aronsen, B. Acute and long-term airway hyperreactivity in aluminum-salt exposed workers with nocturnal asthma. Eur. J. Respir. Dis. 66: 105–118, 1985.

4645. Rasmussen, F. V. Occupational dust exposure and smoking. Different effects on forced expiration and slope of the alveolar plateau. Eur. J. Respir. Dis. 66: 119–127, 1985.

4646. Stjernberg, N., Eklund, A., Nystrom, L., Rosenhall, L., Emmelin, A., and Stromqvist, L.-H. Prevalence of bronchial asthma and chronic bronchitis in a community in northern Sweden; relation to environmental and occupational exposure to sulphur dioxide. Eur. J. Respir. Dis. 67: 41–49, 1985.

4647. Hurley, J. F. Longitudinal studies of lung function in occupational groups: can we trust the answers? Bull. Eur. Physiopathol. Respir. 21: 1A–13A, 1985.

4648. Bucca, C., Avolio, G., Rolla, G., Maina, A., Bugiani, M., Arossa, W., Spinaci, S., and Cacciabue, M. A long term follow-up of patients with silicosis. Bull. Eur. Physiopathol. Respir. 21: 8A–9A, 1985.

4649. Pham, Q. T., Mur, J. R., Chau, N., Teculescu, D. B., and Henquel, J. C. A longitudinal study of respiratory symptoms and lung function in French iron miners. Bull. Eur. Physiopathol. Respir. 21: 11A, 1985.

4650. Fabbri, L. M., Di Giacomo, R., Dal Vecchio, L., Zocca, E., De Marzo, N., Maestrelli, P., and Mapp, C. E. Prednisone, indomethacin and airway responsiveness in toluene diisocyanate sensitized subjects. Bull. Eur. Physiopathol. Respir. 21: 421–426, 1985.

4651. Gee, J. B. L. (ed.). Occupational Lung Disease. Churchill-Livingstone, New York, 1984.

4652. Schachter, E. N., Zuskin, E., Buck, M. G., Witek, T. J., Beck, G. J., and Tyler, D. Airway reactivity and cotton bract-induced bronchial obstruction. Chest 87: 51–55, 1985.

4653. Enarson, D. A., Chan-Yeung, M., Tabona, M., Kus, J., Vedal, S., and Lam, S. Predictors of bronchial hyperexcitability in grainhandlers. Chest 87: 452–455, 1985.

4654. Kilburn, K. H., Warshaw, R., and Thornton, J. C. Asbestosis, pulmonary symptoms and functional impairment in shipyard workers. Chest 88: 254–259, 1985.

4655. Chan-Yeung, M., Lam, S., and Enarson, D. Pulmonary function measurement in the industrial setting. Chest 88: 270–275, 1985.

4656. Lilis, R., Miller, A., and Lerman, Y. Acute mercury poisoning with severe chronic pulmonary manifestations. Chest 88: 306–309, 1985.

4657. Sinner, W. N. Rounded atelectasis or pleuroma? (letter to editor). Chest 88: 312–313, 1985.

4658. Brooks, S. M., Weiss, M. A., and Bernstein, I. L. Reactive airways dysfunction syndrome (RADS). Chest 88: 376–384, 1985.

4659. Becklake, M. R. Chronic airflow limitation: its relationship to work in dusty occupations. Chest 88: 608–617, 1985.

4660. Gellert, A. R., Perry, D., Langford, J. A., Riches, P. G., and Rudd, R. M. Asbestosis: Bronchoalveolar lavage fluid proteins and their relationship to pulmonary epithelial permeability. Chest 88: 730–735, 1985.

4661. Gheysens, B., Auwerx, J., Van Den Eeckhout, A., and Demedts, M. Cobalt-induced bronchial asthma in diamond polishers. Chest 88: 740–744, 1985.

4662. Constantinopoulos, S. H., Goudevenos, J. A., Saratzis, N., Langer, A. M., Selikoff, I. J., and Moutsopoulos, H. M. Metsovo lung: pleural calcification and restrictive lung function in northwestern Greece. Environmental exposure to mineral fiber as etiology. Environ. Res. 38: 319–331, 1985.

4663. Copes, R., Thomas, D., and Becklake, M. R. Temporal patterns of exposure and nonmalignant pulmonary abnormality in Quebec chrysotile workers. Arch. Environ. Health 40: 80–87, 1985.

4664. Kilburn, K. H., Warshaw, R., Boylen, C. T., Johnson, S.-J. S., Seidman, B., Sinclair, R., and Takaro, T. Jr. Pulmonary and neurobehavioral effects of formaldehyde exposure. Arch. Environ. Health 40: 254–260, 1985.

4665. Kilburn, K. H., Warshaw, R. H., Einstein, K., and Bernstein, J. Airway disease in non-smoking asbestos workers. Arch. Environ. Health 40: 293–295, 1985.

4666. Hendy, M. S., Beattie, B. E., and Burge, P. S. Occupational asthma due to an emulsified oil mist. Br. J. Ind. Med. 42: 51–54, 1985.

4667. Douglas, D. B., Douglas, R. B., Oakes, D., and Scott, G. Pulmonary function of London firemen. Br. J. Ind. Med. 42: 55–58, 1985.

4668. Watt, S. J. Effect of commercial diving on ventilatory function. Br. J. Ind. Med. 42: 59–62, 1985.

4669. Johnson, A., Chan-Yeung, M., Maclean, L., Atkins, E., Dybuncio, A., Cheng, F., and Enarson, D. Respiratory abnormalities among workers in an iron and steel foundry. Br. J. Ind. Med. 42: 94–100, 1985.

4670. Low, I. and Mitchell, C. Respiratory disease in foundry workers. Br. J. Ind. Med. 42: 101–105, 1985.

4671. Jamison, J. P., Langlands, J. H. M., and Bodel, C. C. Ventilatory responses of normal subjects to flax dust inhalation: the protective effect of autoclaving the flax. Br. J. Ind. Med. 42: 196–201, 1985.

4672. McCarthy, P. E., Cockcroft, A. E., and McDermott, M. Lung function after exposure to barley dust. Br. J. Ind. Med. 42: 106–110, 1985.

4673. Liddell, F. D. K. and Hanley, J. A. Relations between asbestos exposure and lung cancer SMRs in occupational cohort studies. Br. J. Ind. Med. 42: 389–396, 1985.

4674. Ohlson, C.-G. and Hogstedt, C. Lung cancer among asbestos cement workers. A Swedish cohort study and a review. Br. J. Ind. Med. 42: 397–402, 1985.

4675. Zuskin, E., Kanceljak, B., Skuric, Z., and Butkovic, D. Bronchial reactivity in green coffee exposure. Br. J. Ind. Med. 42: 415–420, 1985.

4676. Venables, K. M., Dally, M. B., Burge, P. S., Pickering, C. A. C., and Newman Taylor, A. J. Occupational asthma in a steel coating plant. Br. J. Ind. Med. 42: 517–524, 1985.

4677. Wright, J. L. and Churg, A. Severe diffuse small airways abnormalities in long term chrysotile asbestos miners. Br. J. Ind. Med. 42: 556–559, 1985.

4678. Ohlson, C.-G., Bodin, L., Rydman, T., and Hogstedt, C. Ventilatory decrements in former asbestos cement workers: a four year follow up. Br. J. Ind. Med. 42: 612–616, 1985.

4679. Minty, B. D., Royston, D., Jones, J. G., Smith, D. J., Searing, C. S. M., and Beeley, M. Changes in permeability of the alveolar-capillary barrier in firefighters. Br. J. Ind. Med. 42: 631–634, 1985.

4680. Ng, T. P., Tsin, T. W., and O'Kelly, F. J. An outbreak of illness after occupational exposure to ozone and acid chlorides. Br. J. Ind. Med. 42: 686–690, 1985.

4681. Miller, B. G. and Jacobsen, M. Dust exposure, pneumoconiosis, and mortality of coalminers. Br. J. Ind. Med. 42: 723–733, 1985.

4682. Maclaren, W. M. and Soutar, C. A. Progressive massive fibrosis and simple pneumoconiosis in ex-miners. Br. J. Ind. Med. 42: 734–740, 1985.

4683. Ng, T. P., Allan, W. G. L., Tsin, T. W., and O'Kelly, F. J. Silicosis in jade workers. Br. J. Ind. Med. 42: 761–764, 1985.

4684. Garabrant, D. H., Bernstein, L., Peters, J. M., Smith, T. J., and Wright, W. E. Respiratory effects of borax dust. Br. J. Ind. Med. 42: 831–837, 1985.

4685. Eisen, E. A., Wegman, D. H., and Smith, T. J. Across-shift changes in the pulmonary function of meat-wrappers and other workers in the retail food industry. Scand. J. Work Environ. Health 11: 21–26, 1985.

4686. Sjogren, B. and Ulfvarson, U. Respiratory symptoms and pulmonary function among welders working with aluminum, stainless steel and railroad tracks. Scand. J. Work Environ. Health 11: 27–32, 1985.

4687. Skulberg, K. R., Gylseth, B., Skaug, V., and Hanoa, R. Mica pneumoconiosis—a literature review. Scand. J. Work Environ. Health 11: 65–74, 1985.

4688. Koskinen, H. Symptoms and clinical findings in patients with silicosis. Scand. J. Work Environ. Health 11: 101–106, 1985.

4689. Gylseth, B., Churg, A., Davis, J. M. G., Johnson, N., Morgan, A., Mowe, G., Rogers, A., and Roggli, V. Analysis of asbestos fibers and asbestos bodies in tissue samples from human lung. Scand. J. Work Environ. Health 11: 107–110, 1985.

4690. Mohensifar, Z., Brown, H. V., and Koerner, S. K. Effect of breathing pattern on dead space ventilation VD/VT during exercise. Respiration 47: 232–236, 1985.

4691. Hurley, J. F. and Soutar, C. A. Can exposure to coalmine dust cause a severe impairment of lung function? Br. J. Ind. Med. 43: 150–157, 1986.

4692. Adams, T. In: Stevenson, B. (ed.). The Home Book of Quotations. 9th Ed. Dodd, Mead and Co., New York, 1964 (see page 598).

4693. Hughes, J. M. and Weill, H. Asbestos exposure—quantitative assessment of risk. Am. Rev. Respir. Dis. 133: 5–13, 1986.

4694. De Vuyst, P., Weyer, R. V., De Coster, A., Marchandise, F. X., Dumortier, P., Ketelbant, P., Jedwab, J., and Yernault, J. C. Dental technician's pneumoconiosis. Am. Rev. Respir. Dis. 133: 316–320, 1986.

4695. McFadden, D., Wright, J. L., Wiggs, B., and Churg, A. Smoking inhibits asbestos clearance. Am. Rev. Respir. Dis. 133: 372–374, 1986.

4696. Buist, A. S., Vollmer, W. M., Johnson, L. R., Bernstein, R. S., and McCamant, L. E. A four-year prospective study of the respiratory effects of volcanic ash from Mt. St. Helens. Am. Rev. Respir. Dis. 133: 526–534, 1986.

4697. Hendrick, D. J., Fabbri, L. M., Hughes, J. M., Banks, D. E., Barkman, H. W., Jr., Connolly, M. J., Jones, R. N., and Weill, H. Modification of the methacholine inhalation test and its epidemiologic use in polyurethane workers. Am. Rev. Respir. Dis. 133: 600–604, 1986.

4698. Chan-Yeung, M. and Lam, S. Occupational asthma. Am. Rev. Respir. Dis. 133: 686–703, 1986.

4699. Oliver, L. C., Eisen, E. A., and Sprince, N. L. A comparison of two definitions of abnormality on pulmonary outcome in epidemiologic studies. Am. Rev. Respir. Dis. 133: 825–829, 1986.

4700. Rom, W. N., Wood, S. D., White, G. L., Bang, K. M., and Reading, J. C. Longitudinal evaluation of pulmonary function in copper smelter workers exposed to sulfur dioxide. Am. Rev. Respir. Dis. 133: 830–833, 1986.

4701. Xaubet, A., Rodriguez-Roisin, R., Bombi, J. A., Marin, A., Roca, J., and Agusti-Vidal, A. Correlation of bronchoalveolar lavage and clinical and functional findings in asbestosis. Am. Rev. Respir. Dis. 133: 848–854, 1986.

4702. Cookson, W., De Klerk, N., Musk, A. W., Glancy, J. J., Armstrong, B., and Hobbs, M. The natural history of asbestosis in former crocidolite workers of Wittenoom Gorge. Am. Rev. Respir. Dis. 133: 994–998, 1986.

4703. Mundie, T. G. and Ainsworth, S. K. Etiopathogenic mechanisms of bronchoconstriction in byssinosis—a review. Am. Rev. Respir. Dis. 133: 1181–1185, 1986.

4704. Lee, W. R. and Stretton, T. B. Byssinosis: a disease or a symptom? (editorial). Thorax 41: 1–4, 1986.

4705. Honeybourne, D. and Pickering, C. A. C. Physiological evidence that emphysema is not a feature of byssinosis. Thorax 41: 6–11, 1986.

4706. Blainey, A. D., Ollier, S., Cundell, D., Smith, R. E., and Davies, R. J. Occupational asthma in a hairdressing salon. Thorax 41: 42–50, 1986.

4707. Wagner, J. C. and Pooley, F. D. Mineral fibres and mesothelioma (editorial). Thorax 41: 161–166, 1986.

4708. Davis, J. M. G., Gylseth, B., and Morgan, A. Assessment of mineral fibres from human lung tissue. Thorax 41: 167–175, 1986.

4709. Wagner, J. C., Pooley, F. D., Gibbs, A., Lyons, J., Sheers, G., and Moncrieff, C. B. Inhalation of china stone and china clay dusts: relationship between the mineralogy of dust retained in the lungs and pathological changes. Thorax 41: 190–196, 1986.

4710. Calhoun, W. J., Christman, J. W., Ershler, W. B., Graham, W. G. B., and Davis, G. S. Raised immunoglobulin concentrations in bronchoalveolar lavage fluid of healthy granite workers. Thorax 41: 266–273, 1986.

4711. Paggiaro, P. L., Innocenti, A., Bacci, E., Rossi, O., and Talini, D. Specific bronchial reactivity to toluene diisocyanate: relationship with baseline clinical findings. Thorax 41: 279–282, 1986.

4712. Mapp, C. E., Dal Vecchio, L., Boschetto, P., De Marzo, N., and Fabbri, L. M. Toluene diisocyanate-induced asthma without airway hyperresponsiveness. Eur. J. Respir. Dis. 68: 89–95, 1986.

4713. De Vuyst, P., Dumortier, P., Rickaert, F., Van De Weyer, R., Lenclud, C., and Yernault, J. C. Occupational lung fibrosis in an aluminium polisher. Eur. J. Respir. Dis. 68: 131–140, 1986.

4714. Hillerdal, G. Endemic pleural plaques (editorial). Eur. J. Respir. Dis. 69: 1–3, 1986.

4715. Boutin, C., Viallat, J. R., Steinbauer, J., Massey, D. G., Charpin, D., and Mouries, J. C. Bilateral pleural plaques in Corsica: a non-occupational asbestos exposure marker. Eur. J. Respir. Dis. 69: 4–9, 1986.

4716. Svenes, K. B., Borgersen, A., Haaveresen, O., and Holten, K. Parietal pleural plaques: a comparison between autopsy and x-ray findings. Eur. J. Respir. Dis. 69: 10–15, 1986.

4717. Lutsky, I. I., Baum, G. L., Teichtahl, H., Mazar, A., Aizer, F., and Bar-Sela, S. Respiratory disease in animal house workers. Eur. J. Respir. Dis. 69: 29–35, 1986.

4718. Bergin, C. J., Muller, N. L., Vedal, S., and Chan-Yeung, M. CT in silicosis: Correlation with plain films and pulmonary function tests. Am. J. Radiol. 146: 477–483, 1986.

4719. Bates, D. V. Asbestos: promotion or prohibition? (editorial). Can. Med. Assoc. J. 136: 107–109, 1987.

4720. Pham, Q. T., Meyer-Bisch, C., Mur, J. M., Teculescu, D., Gaertner, M., St-Eve, P., and Massin, N. Etude de l'évolution clinique et fonctionelle respiratoire sur 5 ans, d'ouvriers exposés à de faibles teneurs de diisocyanate de diphenylmethane (MDI). Arch. Mal. Prof. 47: 311–320, 1986.

4721. Cowie, H., Lloyd, M. H., and Soutar, C. A. Study of lung function data by principal components analysis. Thorax 40: 438–443, 1985.

4722. Scano, G., Garcia-Herreros, P., Stendardi, D., Degre, S., De Coster, A., and Sergysels, R. Cardiopulmonary adaptation to exercise in coal miners. Arch. Environ. Health 35: 360–366, 1980.

4723. Gottlieb, L. S. and Balchum, O. J. Course of chronic obstructive pulmonary disease following first onset of respiratory failure. Chest 63: 5–8, 1973.

4724. Handa, R. Graphite pneumoconiosis: a review of etiologic and epidemiologic aspects. Scand. J. Work Environ. Health 9: 303–314, 1984.

4725. Gellert, A. R., Langford, J. A., Winter, R. J. D., Uthayakumar, S., Sinha, G., and Rudd, R. M. Asbestosis: assessment by bronchoalveolar lavage and measurement of pulmonary epithelial permeability. Thorax 40: 508–514, 1985.

4726. Pratt, P. C., Vollmer, R. T., and Miller, J. A. Epidemiology of pulmonary lesions in nontextile and cotton textile workers: a retrospective autopsy analysis. Arch. Environ. Health 35: 133–138, 1980.

4727. Chan-Yeung, M., Schulzer, M., Maclean, L., Dorken, E., Tan, F., Lam, S., Enarson, D., and Grzybowski, S. A follow-up study of the grain elevator workers in the port of Vancouver. Arch. Environ. Health 36: 75–81, 1981.

4728. Nagy, L. and Orosz, M. Occupational asthma due to hexachlorophene. Thorax 39: 630–631, 1984.

4729. Fowler, A. A., Hamman, R. F., Zerbe, G. O., Benson, K. N., and Hyers, T. M. Adult respiratory distress syndrome. Am. Rev. Respir. Dis. 132: 472–478, 1985.

4730. Montgomery, A. B., Stager, M. A., Carrico, C. J., and Hudson, L. D. Causes of mortality in patients with the adult respiratory distress syndrome. Am. Rev. Respir. Dis. 132: 485–489, 1985.

4731. Edwards, M. J., Metcalfe, J., Dunham, M. J., and Paul, M.

S. Accelerated respiratory response to moderate exercise in late pregnancy. Respir. Physiol. 45: 229–241, 1981.

4732. Cluff, R. A. Chronic hyperventilation and its treatment by physiotherapy: discussion paper. J. R. Soc. Med. 77: 855–861, 1984.

4733. Prichard, M. G. and Musk, A. W. Adverse effect of pregnancy on familial fibrosing alveolitis. Thorax 39: 319–320, 1984.

4734. Wardle, E. N. Shock lungs: the post-traumatic respiratory distress syndrome. Q. J. Med. 53: 317–329, 1984.

4735. Whipp, B. J. and Davis, J. A. The ventilatory stress of exercise in obesity. Exercise Testing in the Dyspneic Patient. Am. Rev. Respir. Dis. 129(2)(Pt. 2)(Suppl.): S90–S92, 1984.

4736. Burki, N.K. and Baker, R. W. Ventilatory regulation in eucapnic morbid obesity. Am. Rev. Respir. Dis. 129: 538–543, 1984.

4737. Franco, D. P., Kinasewitz, G. T., Markham, R. V., Tucker, W. Y., and George, R. B. Postural hypoxemia in the post-pneumonectomy patient. Am. Rev. Respir. Dis. 129: 1021–1022, 1984.

4738. Townsend, M. C. Spirometric forced expiratory volumes measured in standing versus the sitting posture. Am. Rev. Respir. Dis. 130: 123–124, 1984.

4739. Liberatore, S. M., Pistelli, R., Patalano, F., Moneta, E., Incalzi, R. A., and Ciappi, G. Respiratory function during pregnancy. Respiration 46: 145–150, 1984.

4740. Rankin, J. A., Snyder, P. E., Schachter, A. N., and Matthay, R. A. Bronchoalveolar lavage: its safety in subjects with mild asthma. Chest 85: 723–728, 1984.

4741. Matsushima, Y., Jones, R. L., King, E. G., Moysa, G., and Alton, J. D. M. Alterations in pulmonary mechanics and gas exchange during routine fiberoptic bronchoscopy. Chest 86: 184–188, 1984.

4742. Matuschak, G. M., Owebs, G. R., Rogers, R. M., and Tibbals, S. C. Progressive intrapartum respiratory insufficiency due to pulmonary alveolar proteinosis. Chest 86: 496–499, 1984.

4743. Berry, D. T. R., Webb, W. B., and Block, A. J. Sleep apnea syndrome. Chest 86: 529–531, 1984.

4744. Littner, M., Young, E., McGinty, D., Beahm, E., Riege, W., and Sowers, J. Awake abnormalities of control of breathing and of the upper airway. Chest 86: 573–579, 1984.

4745. Hendy, M. S., Bateman, J. R. M., and Stableforth, D. E. The influence of transbronchial lung biopsy and bronchoalveolar lavage on arterial blood gas changes occurring in patients with diffuse interstitial lung disease. Br. J. Dis. Chest 78: 363–368, 1984.

4746. Rodenstein, D. O., Mercenier, C., and Stanescu, D. C. Influence of the respiratory route on the resting breathing pattern in humans. Am. Rev. Respir. Dis. 131: 163–166, 1985.

4747. Jones, N. L., Makrides, L., Hitchcock, C., Chypchar, T., and McCartney, N. Normal standards for an incremental progressive cycle ergometer test. Am. Rev. Respir. Dis. 131: 700–708, 1985.

4748. Catterall, J. R., Calverley, P. M. A., Shapiro, C. M., Flenley, D. C., and Douglas, N. J. Breathing and oxygenation during sleep are similar in normal men and normal women. Am. Rev. Respir. Dis. 132: 86–88, 1985.

4749. Kawakami, Y., Yamamoto, H., Yoshikawa, T., and Shida, A. Age-related variation of respiratory chemosensitivity in monozygotic twins. Am. Rev. Respir. Dis. 132: 89–92, 1985.

4750. NHLBI Workshop Summary. Summary and recommendations of a workshop on the investigative use of fiberoptic bronchoscopy and bronchoalveolar lavage in asthmatics. Am. Rev. Respir. Dis. 132: 180–182, 1985.

4751. Martin, T. R., Raghu, G., Maunder, R. J., and Springmeyer, S. C. The effects of chronic bronchitis and chronic air-flow obstruction on lung cell populations recovered by bronchoalveolar lavage. Am. Rev. Respir. Dis. 132: 254–260, 1985.

4752. Moore, F. D., Lyons, J. H., Pierce, E. C., Morgan, A. P., Drinker, P. A., MacArthur, J. P., and Dammin, G. J. Post-Traumatic Respiratory Insufficiency. W. B. Saunders, Philadelphia, 1969.

4753. Ingram, R. H. Adult respiratory distress syndrome. Harrison's Principles of Internal Medicine. 10th ed. McGraw-Hill, New York, 1987.

4754. Colebatch, H. J. H., Greaves, I. A., and Ng, C. K. Y.

Pulmonary distensibility and ventilatory function in smokers. Bull. Eur. Physiopathol. Respir. 21: 439–447, 1985.

4755. Makrides, L., Heigenhauser, G. J. F., McCartney, N., and Jones, N. L. Maximal short term exercise capacity in healthy subjects aged 15–70 years. Clin. Sci. 69: 197–205, 1985.

4756. Kawakami, Y., Shida, A., Yamamoto, H., and Yoshikawa, T. Pattern of genetic influences on pulmonary function. Chest 87: 507–511, 1985.

4757. Edde, R. R. and Burtis, B. B. Lung injury in anaphylactoid shock. Chest 63: 636–638, 1973.

4758. Jones, J. B., Wilhoit, S. C., Findley, L. J., and Suratt, P. M. Oxyhemoglobin saturation during sleep in subjects with and without the obesity-hypoventilation syndrome. Chest 88: 9–15, 1985.

4759. Neagley, S. R. and Zwillich, C. W. The effect of positional changes on oxygenation in patients with pleural effusions. Chest 88: 714–717, 1985.

4760. Lopata, M., O'Connor, T. D., and Onal, E. Effects of position on respiratory muscle function during CO_2 rebreathing. Respiration 47: 98–106, 1985.

4761. Hurewitz, A. N., Susskind, H., and Harold, W. H. Obesity alters regional ventilation in lateral decubitus position. J. Appl. Physiol. 59: 774–783, 1985.

4762. Menitove, S. M., Rapoport, D. M., Epstein, H., Sorkin, B., and Goldring, R. M. CO_2 rebreathing and exercise ventilatory responses in humans. J. Appl. Physiol. 56: 1039–1044, 1984.

4763. Suratt, P. M., Wilhoit, S. C., Hsiao, H. S., Atkinson, R. L., and Rochester, D. F. Compliance of chest wall in obese subjects. J. Appl. Physiol. 57: 403–407, 1984.

4764. Sharp, J. T., Druz, W. S., and Kondragunta, V. K. Diaphragmatic responses to body position changes in obese patients with obstructive sleep apnea. Am. Rev. Respir. Dis. 133: 32–37, 1986.

4765. Brownell, L. G., West, P., and Kryger, M. H. Breathing during sleep in normal pregnant women. Am. Rev. Respir. Dis. 133: 38–41, 1986.

4766. Light, R. W., Stansbury, D. W., and Brown, S. E. The relationship between pleural pressures and changes in pulmonary function after therapeutic thoracentesis. Am. Rev. Respir. Dis. 133: 658–661, 1986.

4767. Minh, V.-D., Chun, D., Fairshter, R. D., Vasquez, P., Wilson, A. F., and Dolan, G. F. Supine change in arterial oxygenation in patients with chronic obstructive pulmonary disease. Am. Rev. Respir. Dis. 133: 820–824, 1986.

4768. Simpson, F. G., Arnold, A. G., Purvis, A., Belfield, P. W., Muers, M. F., and Cooke, N. J. Postal survey of bronchoscopic practice by physicians in the United Kingdom. Thorax 41: 311–317, 1986.

4769. Holden, W. E., Carr, W. A., and Beals, R. K. Position dependence of pulmonary function in a patient with lordoscoliosis. Eur. J. Respir. Dis. 68: 146–150, 1986.

4770. Petty, T. L. and Ashbaugh, D. G. The adult respiratory distress syndrome. Chest 60: 233–239, 1971.

4771. Laros, C. D. Lung function data on 123 persons followed up for 20 years after total pneumonectomy. Respiration 43: 81–87, 1982.

4772. Teja, K., Cooper, P. H., Squires, J. E., and Schnatterly, P. T. Pulmonary alveolar proteinosis in four siblings. N. Engl. J. Med. 305: 1390–1392, 1981.

4773. Harrison, R. N. and Tattersfield, A. E. Airway response to inhaled salbutamol in hyperthyroid and hypothyroid patients before and after treatment. Thorax 39: 34–39, 1984.

4774. Williams, J. G., Morris, A. I., Hayter, R. C., and Ogilvie, C. M. Respiratory responses of diabetics to hypoxia, hypercapnia, and exercise. Thorax 39: 529–534, 1984.

4775. Wood, J. R., Bellamy, D., Child, A. H., and Citron, K. M. Pulmonary disease in patients with Marfan syndrome. Thorax 39: 780–784, 1984.

4776. Wyatt, S. E., Nunn, P., Hows, J. M., Yin, J., Hayes, M. C., Catovsky, D., Gordon-Smith, E. C., Hughes, J. M. B., Goldman, J. M., and Galton, D. Airways obstruction associated with graft versus host disease after bone marrow transplantation. Thorax 39: 887–894, 1984.

4777. Gaultier, C. L., Beaufils, F., Boule, M., Bompard, Y., and Devictor, D. Lung functional follow-up in children after severe viral infections. Eur. J. Respir. Dis. 65: 460–467, 1984.

4778. Jacobs, P., Bonnyns, M., Depierreux, M., Duchateau, J., and Sergysels, R. Rapidly fatal bronchiolitis obliterans with circulating antinuclear and rheumatoid factors. Eur. J. Respir. Dis. 65: 384–388, 1984.

4779. Salkin, D. Emotional laryngeal wheezing: a new syndrome (letter to editor). Am. Rev. Respir. Dis. 129: 199, 1984.

4780. Woodson, R. D. Hemoglobin concentration and exercise capacity. Exercise Testing in the Dyspneic Patient. Am. Rev. Respir. Dis. 129(2)(Pt. 2)(Suppl.): S72–S75, 1984.

4781. Garcia-Szabo, R. R. and Malik, A. B. Pancreatitis-induced increase in lung vascular permeability. Am. Rev. Respir. Dis. 129: 580–583, 1984.

4782. Ralph, D. D., Springmeyer, S. C., Sullivan, K. M., Hackman, R. C., Storb, R., and Thomas, E. D. Rapidly progressive air-flow obstruction in marrow transplant recipients. Am. Rev. Respir. Dis. 129: 641–644, 1984.

4783. Allen, C. J. and Newhouse, M. T. Gastroesophageal reflux and chronic respiratory disease. Am. Rev. Respir. Dis. 129: 645–647, 1984.

4784. Romaldini, H., Rodriquez-Roisin, R., Lopez, F. A., Ziegler, T. W., Bencowitz, H. Z., and Wagner, P. D. The mechanisms of arterial hypoxemia during hemodialysis. Am. Rev. Respir. Dis. 129: 780–784, 1984.

4785. Smith, T. P., Kinasewitz, G. T., Tucker, W. Y., Spillers, W. P., and George, R. B. Exercise capacity as a predictor of post-thoracotomy morbidity. Am. Rev. Respir. Dis. 129: 730–734, 1984.

4786. Reynolds, R. J. III, Penn, R. L., Grafton, W. D., and George, R. B. Tissue morphology of histoplasma capsulatum in acute histoplasmosis. Am. Rev. Respir. Dis. 130: 317–320, 1984.

4787. Engelberg, L. A., Lerner, C. W., and Tapper, M. L. Clinical features of pneumocystis pneumonia in the acquired immune deficiency syndrome. Am. Rev. Respir. Dis. 130: 689–694, 1984.

4788. Hoffstein, V. and Zamel, N. Tracheal stenosis measured by the acoustic reflection technique. Am. Rev. Respir. Dis. 130: 472–475, 1984.

4789. Schnapf, B. M., Banks, R. A., Silverstain, J. H., Rodenbloom, A. L., Chesrown, S. E., and Loughlin, G. M. Pulmonary function in insulin-dependent diabetes mellitus with limited joint mobility. Am. Rev. Respir. Dis. 130: 930–932, 1984.

4790. Mink, S. N., Coalson, J. J., Whitley, L., Greville, H., and Jadue, C. Pulmonary function tests in the detection of small airway obstruction in a canine model of bronchiolitis obliterans. Am. Rev. Respir. Dis. 130: 1125–1133, 1984.

4791. Jenkins, C. R. and Breslin, A. B. X. Upper respiratory tract infections and airway reactivity in normal and asthmatic subjects. Am. Rev. Respir. Dis. 130: 879–883, 1984.

4792. Vered, M., Schutzbank, T., and Janoff, A. Inhibitors of human neutrophil elastase in extracts of *Streptococcus pneumoniae*. Am. Rev. Respir. Dis. 130: 1118–1124, 1984.

4793. Key, M. What it is like to lose a lung. Br. Med. J. 290: 142–143, 1985.

4794. Bagg, L. R. The 12-min walking distance; its use in the pre-operative assessment of patients with bronchial carcinoma before lung resection. Respiration 46: 342–345, 1984.

4795. Mackay, D., Cooper, R. A., Bradbury, S., Gawkrodger, D. J., Prowse, K., and Van't Hoff, W. Sleep apnoea in myxoedema. J. R. Coll. Physicians (Lond.) 18: 248–252, 1984.

4796. McGregor, C. G. A., Herrick, M. J., Hardy, I., and Higenbottam, T. Variable intrathoracic airways obstruction masquerading as asthma. Br. Med. J. 287: 1457–1458, 1983.

4797. Kahn, A. and Beumer, H. M. Primary pulmonary amyloidosis. Respiration 45: 78–80, 1984.

4798. Sebert, P., Bellet, M., Girin, E., Cledes, J., and Barthelemy, L. Ventilatory and occlusion pressure responses to hypercapnia in patients with chronic renal failure. Respiration 45: 191–196, 1984.

4799. Dishner, W., Cordasco, E. M., Blackburn, J., Demeter, S., Levin, H., and Carey, W. D. Pulmonary lymphangiomyomatosis. Chest 85: 796–799, 1984.

4800. Burke, C. M., Theodore, J., Dawkins, K. D., Yousem, S. A., Blank, N., Billingham, M. E., Van Kessel, A., Jamieson, S. W., Oyer, P. E., Baldwin, J. C., Stinson, E. B., Shumway, N. E., and Robin, E. D. Post-transplant obliterative bronchiolitis and other late lung sequelae in human heart-lung transplantation. Chest 86: 824–829, 1984.

4801. Ricketti, A. J., Greenberger, P. A., Mintzer, R. A., and Patterson, R. Allergic bronchopulmonary aspergillosis. Chest 86: 773–778, 1984.

4802. Schoonover, G. A., Olsen, G. N., McLain, W. C. III, Habibian, M. R., and Spurrier, P. Lateral position test and quantitative lung scan in the preoperative evaluation for lung resection. Chest 86: 854–859, 1984.

4803. Whittaker, J. S., Pickering, C. A. C., Heath, D., and Smith, P. Pulmonary capillary haemangiomatosis. Diagn. Histopathol. 6: 77–84, 1983.

4804. Wagenvoort, C. A., Beetstra, A., and Spijker, J. Capillary haemangiomatosis of the lungs. Histopathology 2: 401–406, 1978.

4805. Williams, A. J., Cayton, R. M., Harding, L. K., Mostafa, A. B., and Matthews, H. R. Quantitative lung scintigrams and lung function in the selection of patients for pneumonectomy. Br. J. Dis. Chest 78: 105–112, 1984.

4806. Claypool, W. D., Rogers, R. M., and Matuschak, G. M. Update on the clinical diagnosis, management, and pathogenesis of pulmonary alveolar proteinosis. Chest 85: 550–558, 1984.

4807. Calhoun, W. J. and Davis, G. S. Variable tracheal stenosis related to body position. Chest 86: 87–89, 1984.

4808. Rodrigues, J. F., York, E. L., and Nair, C. P. V. Upper airway obstruction in Guillain-Barré syndrome. Chest 86: 147–148, 1984.

4809. Matuschak, G. M., Owebs, G. R., Rogers, R. M., and Tibbals, S. C. Progressive intrapartum respiratory insufficiency due to pulmonary alveolar proteinosis. Chest 86: 496–499, 1984.

4810. Lakin, R. C., Metzger, W. J., and Haughey, B. H. Upper airway obstruction presenting as exercise-induced asthma. Chest 86: 499–501, 1984.

4811. Winchester, J. F. Peritoneal dialysis and pulmonary function (editorial). Chest 86: 806–807, 1984.

4812. Singh, S., Dale, A., Morgan, B., and Sahebjami, H. Serial studies of pulmonary function in continuous ambulatory peritoneal dialysis. Chest 86: 874–877, 1984.

4813. Wright, P. H., Buxton-Thomas, M., Keeling, P. W. N., and Kreel, L. Adult idiopathic pulmonary haemosiderosis: a comparison of lung function changes and the distribution of pulmonary disease in patients with and without coeliac disease. Br. J. Dis. Chest 77: 282–292, 1983.

4814. Couriel, J. M., Hibbert, M., and Olinsky, A. Assessment of proximal airway obstruction in children by analysis of flow-volume loops. Br. J. Dis. Chest 78: 36–45, 1984.

4815. Chawla, S. S., Upadhyay, B. K., and MacDonnell, K. F. Laryngeal spasm mimicking bronchial asthma. Ann. Allergy 53: 319–321, 1984.

4816. Pitchenik, A. E. and Rubinson, H. A. The radiographic appearance of tuberculosis in patients with the acquired immune deficiency syndrome (AIDS) and pre-AIDS. Am. Rev. Respir. Dis. 131: 393–396, 1985.

4817. Lampron, N., Lemaire, F., Teisseire, B., Harf, A., Palot, M., Matamis, D., and Lorino, A. M. Mechanical ventilation with 100 per cent oxygen does not increase intrapulmonary shunt in patients with severe bacterial pneumonia. Am. Rev. Respir. Dis. 131: 409–413, 1985.

4818. Vered, M., Dearing, R., and Janoff, A. A new elastase inhibitor from streptococcus pneumoniae protects against acute lung injury induced by neutrophil granules. Am. Rev. Respir. Dis. 131: 131–133, 1985.

4819. Andreadis, N. and Petty, T. L. Adult respiratory distress syndrome: problems and progress. Am. Rev. Respir. Dis. 132: 1344–1346, 1985.

4820. Gaultier, C., Boule, M., Tournier, G., and Girard, F. Inspiratory force reserve of the respiratory muscles in children with chronic obstructive pulmonary disease. Am. Rev. Respir. Dis. 131: 811–815, 1985.

4821. Rinaldo, J. and Borovetz, H. Deterioration of oxygenation and abnormal lung microvascular permeability during resolution of leukopenia in patients with diffuse lung injury. Am. Rev. Respir. Dis. 131: 579–583, 1985.

4822. Kline, L. R., Dise, C. A., Ferro, T. J., and Hansen-Flaschen,

J. H. Diagnosis of pulmonary amyloidosis by transbronchial biopsy. Am. Rev. Respir. Dis. 132: 191–194, 1985.

4823. Robinson, R. W., White, D. P., and Zwillich, C. W. Moderate alcohol ingestion increases upper airway resistance in normal subjects. Am. Rev. Respir. Dis. 132: 1238–1241, 1985.

4824. Yamaki, S., Horiuchi, T., and Takahashi, T. Pulmonary changes in congenital heart disease with Down's syndrome: their significance as a cause of postoperative respiratory failure. Thorax 40: 380–386, 1985.

4825. Road, J. D., Jacques, J., and Sparling, J. R. Diffuse alveolar septal amyloidosis presenting with recurrent hemoptysis and medial dissection of pulmonary arteries. Am. Rev. Respir. Dis. 132: 1368–1370, 1985.

4826. Neilly, J. B., Winter, J. H., and Stevenson, R. D. Progressive tracheobronchial polychondritis: need for early diagnosis. Thorax 40: 78–79, 1985.

4827. Millar, A. B., O'Reilly, A. P., Clarke, S. W., and Hetzel, M. R. Amyloidosis of the respiratory tract treated by laser therapy. Thorax 40: 544–545, 1985.

4828. Cordonnier, C., Bernaudin, J. -F., Fleury, J., Feuilhade, M., Haioun, C., Payen, D., Huet, Y., Atassi, K., and Vernant, J.-P. Diagnostic yield of bronchoalveolar lavage in pneumonitis occurring after allogeneic bone marrow transplantation. Am. Rev. Respir. Dis. 132: 1118–1123, 1985.

4829. Breuer, R., Simpson, G. T., Rubinow, A., Skinner, M., and Cohen, A. S. Tracheobronchial amyloidosis: treatment by carbon dioxide laser photoresection. Thorax 40: 870–871, 1985.

4830. Mascie-Taylor, B. H., Wardman, A. G., Madden, C. A., and Page, R. L. A case of alveolar microlithiasis: observation over 22 years and recovery of material by lavage. Thorax 40: 952–953, 1985.

4831. Magee, F., Wright, J. L., Klay, J. M., Peretz, D., Donevan, R., and Churg, A. Pulmonary capillary hemangiomatosis. Am. Rev. Respir. Dis. 132: 922–925, 1985.

4832. Hills, B. A. The pleural interface (editorial). Thorax 40: 1–8, 1985.

4833. Hirschler-Schulte, C. J. W., Hylkema, B. S., and Meyer, R. W. Mechanical ventilation for acute postoperative respiratory failure after surgery for bronchial carcinoma. Thorax 40: 387–390, 1985.

4834. Dernevik, L. and Gatzinsky, P. Long term results of operation for shrinking pleuritis with atelectasis. Thorax 40: 448–452, 1985.

4835. Rosen, M. J., Tow, T. W. Y., Teirstein, A. S., Chuang, M. T., Marchevsky, A., and Bottone, E. J. Diagnosis of pulmonary complications of the acquired immune deficiency syndrome. Thorax 40: 571–575, 1985.

4836. Banks, J., Bevan, C., Fennerty, A., Ebden, P., Walters, E. H., and Smith, A. P. Association between rise in antibodies and increase in airway sensitivity after intramuscular injection of killed influenza virus in asthmatic patients. Eur. J. Respir. Dis. 66: 268–272, 1985.

4837. Hopewell, P. C. and Luce, J. M. Pulmonary involvement in the acquired immunodeficiency syndrome. Chest 87: 104–112, 1985.

4838. Luna, C. M., Gene, R., Jolly, E. C., Nahmod, N., Defranchi, H. A., Patino, G., and Elsner, B. Pulmonary lymphangiomyomatosis associated with tuberous sclerosis. Chest 88: 473–475, 1985.

4839. Gerrard, C. S., Levandowski, R. A., Gerrity, T. R., Yeates, D. B., and Klein, E. The effects of acute respiratory virus infection upon tracheal mucous transport. Arch. Environ. Health 40: 322–325, 1985.

4840. Brundler, H., Chen, S., and Perruchoud, A. P. Right heart catheterization in the pre-operative evaluation of patients with lung cancer. Respiration 48: 261–268, 1985.

4841. Montserrat, J. M., Cochrane, G. M., Wolf, C., Picado, C., Roca, J., and Vidal, A. A. Ventilatory control in diabetes mellitus. Eur. J. Respir. Dis. 67: 112–117, 1985.

4842. Bogaard, J. M., Pauw, K. H., Stam, H., and Versprille, A. Interpretation of changes in spirographic and flow-volume variables after operative treatment in bilateral vocal cord paralysis. Bull. Physiopathol. Respir. 21: 131–135, 1985.

4843. Vincken, W. and Cosio, M. G. Flow oscillations on the flow-volume loop: a nonspecific indicator of upper airway dysfunction. Bull. Eur. Physiopathol. Respir. 21: 559–567, 1985.

4844. Bush, A., Miller, J., Peacock, A. J., Sopwith, T., Gabriel, R., and Denison, D. Some observations on the role of the abdomen in breathing in patients on peritoneal dialysis. Clin. Sci. 68: 401–406, 1985.

4845. Karbowitz, S. R., Edelman, L. B., Nath, S., Dwek, J. H., and Rammohan, G. Spectrum of advanced upper airway obstruction due to goiters. Chest 87: 18–21, 1985.

4846. Krowka, M. J., Rosenow, E. C., and Hoagland, H. C. Pulmonary complications of bone marrow transplantation. Chest 87: 237–246, 1985.

4847. Wallaert, B., Colombel, J. F., Tonnel, A. B., Bonniere, Ph., Cortot, A., Paris, J. C., and Voisin, C. Evidence of lymphocytic alveolitis in Crohn's disease. Chest 87: 363–367, 1985.

4848. Ostrow, D., Buskard, N., Hill, R. S., Vickars, L., and Churg, A. Bronchiolitis obliterans complicating bone marrow transplantation. Chest 87: 828–830, 1985.

4849. Dorinsky, P. M., Davis, W. B., Lucas, J. G., Weiland, J. E., and Gadek, J. E. Adult bronchiolitis. Chest 88: 58–83, 1985.

4850. Miller, A., Brown, L. K., and Teirstein, A. S. Stenosis of main bronchi mimicking fixed upper airway obstruction in sarcoidosis. Chest 88: 244–248, 1985.

4851. Rodriguez, J. L., Askanazi, J., Weissman, C., Hensle, T. W., Rosenbaum, S. H., and Kinney, J. M. Ventilatory and metabolic effects of glucose infusions. Chest 88: 512–518, 1985.

4852. Petermann, W. Effect of low hemoglobin levels on the diffusing capacity of the lungs for CO. Respiration 47: 30–38, 1985.

4853. Hunt, J. M., Chappell, T. R., Henrich, W. L., and Rubin, L. J. Gas exchange during dialysis. Am. J. Med. 77: 255–260, 1984.

4854. Chediak, J., Chausow, A., Solarski, A., and Telfer, M. C. Pulmonary function in hemophiliac patients treated with commercial factor VIII concentrates. Am. J. Med. 77: 293–296, 1984.

4855. Epler, G. R., Colby, T. V., McLoud, T. C., Carrington, C. B., and Gaensler, E. A. Bronchiolitis obliterans organizing pneumonia. N. Engl. J. Med. 312: 152–158, 1985.

4856. Case records of the Massachusetts General Hospital. Case 50-1985. N. Engl. J. Med. 313: 1530–1537, 1985.

4857. Irwin, R. S., Pratter, M. R., Stivers, D. H., and Braverman, L. E. Airway reactivity and lung function in triiodothyronine-induced thyrotoxicosis. J. Appl. Physiol. 58: 1485–1488, 1985.

4858. Zwart, A., Kwant, G., Oeseburg, B., and Zijlstra, W. G. Human whole-blood oxygen affinity effect of carbon monoxide. J. Appl. Physiol. 57: 14–20, 1984.

4859. Stamenovic, D. Mechanical properties of pleural membrane. J. Appl. Physiol. 57: 1189–1194, 1984.

4860. Ware, J. H., Ferris, B. G. Jr., Dockery, D. W., Spengler, J. D., Stram, D. O., and Speizer, F. E. Effects of ambient sulfur oxides and suspended particulates on respiratory health of preadolescent children. Am. Rev. Respir. Dis. 133: 834–842, 1986.

4861. Krell, W. S., Staats, B. A., and Hyatt, R. E. Pulmonary function in relapsing polychondritis. Am. Rev. Respir. Dis. 133: 1120–1123, 1986.

4862. Veneskoski, T. and Sovijarvi, A. R. A. Prediction of ventilatory function after subtotal lung resection using preoperative dynamic spirometry and radiospirometry. Eur. J. Respir. Dis. 68: 167–172, 1986.

4863. Reinders Folmer, S. C. C., Danner, S. A., Bakker, A. J., Lange, J. M. A., Van Steenwijk, R. P., Alberts, Chr., Van Keulen, P. H. J., and Van Der Schoot, J. B. Gallium-67 lung scintigraphy in patients with acquired immune deficiency syndrome (AIDS). Eur. J. Respir. Dis. 68: 313–318, 1986.

4864. Herbert, A. Pathogenesis of pleurisy, pleural fibrosis, and mesothelial proliferation. Thorax 41: 176–189, 1986.

4865. Lyons, D. J., Howard, S. V., Milledge, J. S., and Peters, T. J. Contribution of ethanol and cigarette smoking to pulmonary dysfunction in chronic alcoholics. Thorax 41: 197–202, 1986.

4866. Mitchell, I. M., Saunders, N. R., Maher, O., Lennox, S. C., and Walker, D. R. Surgical treatment of idiopathic mediastinal fibrosis: report of five cases. Thorax 41: 210–214, 1986.

4867. Barker, D. J. P. and Osmond, C. Childhood respiratory

infection and adult chronic bronchitis in England and Wales. Br. Med. J. 293: 1271–1275, 1986.

4868. Vincken, W., Dollfuss, R. E., and Cosio, M. G. Upper airway dysfunction detected by respiratory flow oscillations. Eur. J. Respir. Dis. 68: 50–57, 1986.

4869. Meelem, H., Boye, N. P., Arnkvaern, R., and Fjeld, N. Bj. Stenotic tuberculous tracheitis treated with resection and anastomosis. Eur. J. Respir. Dis. 68: 224–225, 1986.

4870. Seggev, J., Shapiro, M. S., Levin, S., and Schey, G. Alveolar hypoventilation and daytime hypersomnia in acromegaly. Eur. J. Respir. Dis. 68: 381–383, 1986.

4871. Brandi, G. Frictional forces at the surface of the lung. Bull. Physiopathol. Respir. 8: 323–336, 1972.

4872. Packe, G. E., Edwards, C. W., and Cayton, R. M. Non-Hodgkin's lymphoma of the bronchial mucosa presenting with reversible airflow obstruction. Thorax 40: 954–955, 1985.

4873. Burki, N. K. and Diamond, L. A simple technique for cold air and exercise challenge to assess bronchial reactivity: the effects of acute coryzal rhinitis on airway reactivity. Ann. Allergy 52: 272–275, 1984.

4874. Bjure, J., Grimby, G., Kasalicky, J., Limdh, M., and Nachemson, A. Respiratory impairment and airway closure in patients with untreated idiopathic scoliosis. Thorax 25: 451–458, 1970.

4875. Boulding, K. E. Science: our common heritage. Science 297: 831–836, 1980.

4876. Littler, W. A., Brown, I. K., and Roaf, R. Regional lung function in scoliosis. Thorax 27: 420–428, 1972.

4877. Bake, B., Bjure, J., Kasalichy, J., and Nachemson, A. Regional pulmonary ventilation and perfusion distribution in patients with untreated idiopathic scoliosis. Thorax 27: 703–712, 1972.

4878. Grimby, G., Fugl-Meyer, A. R., and Blomstrand, A. Partitioning of the contributions of rib cage and abdomen to ventilation in ankylosing spondylitis. Thorax 29: 179–184, 1974.

4879. Stewart, R. M., Ridyard, J. B., and Pearson, J. D. Regional lung function in ankylosing spondylitis. Thorax 31: 433–437, 1976.

4880. Shneerson, J. M., Venco, A., and Prime, F. J. A study of pulmonary artery pressure, electrocardiography, and mechanocardiography in thoracic scoliosis. Thorax 32: 700–705, 1977.

4881. Rom, W. N. and Miller, A. Unexpected longevity in patients with severe kyphoscoliosis. Thorax 33: 106–110, 1978.

4882. Shneerson, J. M. The cardiorespiratory response to exercise in thoracic scoliosis. Thorax 33: 457–463, 1978.

4883. Shneerson, J. M. Pulmonary artery pressure in thoracic scoliosis during and after exercise while breathing air and pure oxygen. Thorax 33: 747–754, 1978.

4884. Shneerson, J. M. and Edgar, M. A. Cardiac and respiratory function before and after spinal fusion in adolescent idiopathic scoliosis. Thorax 34: 658–661, 1979.

4885. Shneerson, J. M. Cardiac and respiratory responses to exercise in adolescent idiopathic scoliosis. Thorax 35: 347–350, 1980.

4886. Davies, D. Ankylosing spondylitis and lung fibrosis. Q. J. Med. 41: 395–417, 1972.

4887. Kafer, E. and Donnelly, P. Reproducibility of data on steady-state gas exchange and indices of maldistribution of ventilation and blood flow. Chest 71: 758–761, 1977.

4888. Buhain, W. J., Rammohan, G., and Berger, H. W. Pulmonary function in myositis ossificans progressiva. Am. Rev. Respir. Dis. 110: 293–300, 1974.

4889. Kafer, E. R. Idiopathic scoliosis. J. Clin. Invest. 58: 825–833, 1976.

4890. Kafer, E. Idiopathic scoliosis. J. Clin. Invest. 55: 1153–1163, 1975.

4891. Kafer, E. Respiratory and cardiovascular functions in scoliosis. Bull. Europ. Physiopathol. Respir. 13: 299–321, 1977.

4892. Gimenez, M., Uffholtz, H., and Schrijen, F. Responses ventilatoires et cardio-respiratoires des restrictifs à l'exercise musculaire. Bull. Eur. Physiopathol. Respir. 13: 355–367, 1977.

4893. Repo, U. K., Kentala, E., Koistinen, J., Lehtipuu, A.-L., Miettinen, A., Pyrhonen, S., Tiilikainen, A., and Vuornos,

T. Pulmonary apical fibrocystic disease. Eur. J. Respir. Dis. 62: 46–55, 1981.

4894. Kentala, E., Repo, U. K., Lehtipuu, A.-L., and Vuornos, T. HLA-antigens and pulmonary upper lobe fibrocystic changes with and without ankylosing spondylitis. Scand. J. Respir. Dis. 59: 8–12, 1978.

4895. Lonsdorfer, J., Meunier-Carus, J., and Lampert, E. Recherche des indices fonctionnels de gravité dans les scolioses dorsales sévères. Poumon Coeur 30: 27–34, 1974.

4896. Josenhans, W. T., Wang, C. S., Josenhans, G., and Woodbury, J. F. L. Diaphragmatic contribution to ventilation in patients with ankylosing spondylitis. Respiration 28: 331–346, 1971.

4897. Secker-Walker, R. H., Ho, J. E., and Gill, I. S. Observations on regional ventilation and perfusion in kyphoscoliosis. Respiration 38: 194–203, 1979.

4898. Bergofsky, E. Respiratory failure in disorders of the thoracic cage. Am. Rev. Respir. Dis. 119: 643–669, 1979.

4899. Jones, R. S., Kennedy, J. D., Hasham, F., Owen, R., and Taylor, J. F. Mechanical efficiency of the thoracic cage in scoliosis. Thorax 36: 456–461, 1981.

4900. Olgiati, R., Levine, D., Smith, J. P., Briscoe, W. A., and King, T. K. C. Diffusing capacity in idiopathic scoliosis and its interpretation regarding alveolar development. Am. Rev. Respir. Dis. 126: 229–234, 1982.

4901. Iozzo, A., Cosentino, P., Ghai, P. C., and Garbagni, R. Alveolar-arterial gradients and small airways in kyphoscoliosis. Respiration 44: 314–320, 1983.

4902. Sehnal, E., Haber, P., and Lack, W. Entwicklung der Lungenfunktion und der körperlichen Leistungsfahigkeit bei Patienten mit idiopathischer Skoliose nach dorsaler Spondylodese mit dem Harrington-Instrumentarium (natürlicher Verlauf). Respiration 44: 376–381, 1983.

4903. Boffa, P., Stovin, P., and Shneerson, J. Lung developmental abnormalities in severe scoliosis. Thorax 39: 681–682, 1984.

4904. Smyth, R. J., Chapman, K. R., Wright, T. A., Crawford, J. S., and Rebuck, A. S. Pulmonary function in adolescents with mild idiopathic scoliosis. Thorax 39: 901–904, 1984.

4905. Fulkerson, W. J., Wilkins, J. K., Esbehshade, A. M., Eskind, J. B., and Newman, J. H. Life threatening hypoventilation in kyphoscoliosis: successful treatment with a molded body brace-ventilator. Am. Rev. Respir. Dis. 129: 185–187, 1984.

4906. Hoeppner, V. H., Cockcroft, D. W., Dosman, J. A., and Cotton, D. J. Nighttime ventilation improves respiratory failure in secondary kyphoscoliosis. Am. Rev. Respir. Dis. 129: 240–243, 1984.

4907. Cooper, D. M., Rojas, J. V., Mellins, R. B., Keim, H. A., and Mansell, A. L. Respiratory mechanics in adolescents with idiopathic scoliosis. Am. Rev. Respir. Dis. 130: 16–22, 1984.

4908. Lisboa, C., Moreno, R., Fava, M., Ferreti, R., and Cruz, E. Inspiratory muscle function in patients with severe kyphoscoliosis. Am. Rev. Respir. Dis. 132: 48–52, 1985.

4909. Elliott, C. G., Hill, T. R., Adams, T. E., Crapo, R. O., Nietrzeba, R. M., and Gardner, R. M. Exercise performance of subjects with ankylosing spondylitis and limited chest expansion. Bull. Eur. Physiopathol. Respir. 21: 363–368, 1985.

4910. Sinha, R. and Bergofsky, E. Prolonged alteration of lung mechanics in kyphoscoliosis by positive pressure inflation. Am. Rev. Respir. Dis. 106: 47–57, 1972.

4911. Hauge, B. N. Diaphragmatic movement and spirometric volume in patients with ankylosing spondylitis. Scand. J. Respir. Dis. 54: 38–44, 1973.

4912. Sawicka, E. H., Branthwaite, M. A., and Spencer, G. T. Respiratory failure after thoracoplasty: treatment by intermittent negative-pressure ventilation. Thorax 38: 433–435, 1983.

4913. DeTroyer, A. and Sampson, M. G. Activation of the parasternal intercostals during breathing efforts in human subjects. J. Appl. Physiol. 52: 524–529, 1982.

4914. Raper, A. J., Thompson, W. T. Jr., Shapiro, W., and Patterson, J. L. Jr. Scalene and sternomastoid muscle function. J. Appl. Physiol. 21: 497–502, 1966.

4915. DeTroyer, A. and Kelly, S. Chest wall mechanics in dogs with acute diaphragm paralysis. J. Appl. Physiol. 53: 373–379, 1982.

4916. DeTroyer, A. and Estenne, M. Coordination between ribcage muscles and diaphragm during quiet breathing in humans. J. Appl. Physiol. 57: 899–906, 1984.

4917. James, W. S., Minh, V., Minteer, M., and Moser, K. Cervical accessory respiratory muscle function in a patient with a high cervical cord lesion. Chest 71: 59–64, 1977.

4918. DeTroyer, A., Sampson, M., Sigrist, S., and Macklem, P. T. The diaphragm: two muscles. Science 213: 237–238, 1981.

4919. Loring, S. H. and Mead, J. Action of the diaphragm on the ribcage inferred from a force-balance analysis. J. Appl. Physiol. 53: 756–760, 1982.

4920. Gordon, A. M., Huxley, A. F., and Julian, F. J. The variation in isometric tension with sarcomere length in vertebrate muscle fibres. J. Physiol. (Lond.) 184: 170–192, 1965.

4921. McCully, K. K. and Faulkner, J. A. Length-tension relationship of mammalian diaphragm muscles. J. Appl. Physiol. 54: 1681–1686, 1983.

4922. Farkas, G. A., Decramer, M., Rochester, D. F., and DeTroyer, A. Contractile properties of intercostal muscles and their functional significance. J. Appl. Physiol. 59: 528–535, 1985.

4923. Road, J., Newman, S., Derenne, J. P., and Grassino, A. In vivo length-force relationship of canine diaphragm. J. Appl. Physiol. 60: 63–70, 1986.

4924. Braun, N. M. T., Arora, N. S., and Rochester, D. F. Force-length relationship of the normal human diaphragm. J. Appl. Physiol. 53: 405–412, 1982.

4925. Decramer, M. and DeTroyer, A. Respiratory changes in parasternal intercostal length. J. Appl. Physiol. 57: 1254–1260, 1984.

4926. Faulkner, J. A., Maxwell, L. C., Ruff, G. L., and White, T. P. The diaphragm as a muscle. Am. Rev. Respir. Dis. 119 (Part 2 Suppl.): 89–92, 1979.

4927. Lieberman, D. A., Faulkner, J. A., Craig, A. B. Jr., and Maxwell, L. C. Performance and histochemical composition of guinea pig and human diaphragm. J. Appl. Physiol. 34: 233–237, 1973.

4928. Keens, T. G., Bryan, A. C., Levison, H., and Ianuzzo, C. D. Developmental pattern of muscle fiber types in human ventilatory muscles. J. Appl. Physiol. 44: 909–913, 1978.

4929. Comtois, A., Gorczyca, W., and Grassino, A. Anatomy of diaphragmatic circulation. J. Appl. Physiol. 62: 238–244, 1987.

4930. Rochester, D. F. and Briscoe, A. M. Metabolism of the working diaphragm. Am. Rev. Respir. Dis. 119(Suppl.): 101–106, 1979.

4931. Roussos, C. S. and Macklem, P. T. Diaphragmatic fatigue in man. J. Appl. Physiol. 43: 189–197, 1977.

4932. Cohen, C. A., Zagelbaum, G., Gross, D., Roussos, Ch., and Macklem, P. T. Clinical manifestations of inspiratory muscle fatigue. Am. J. Med. 73: 308–316, 1982.

4933. Farkas, G. A., Decramer, M., Rochester, D. F., and DeTroyer, A. Contractile properties of intercostal muscles and their functional significance. J. Appl. Physiol. 59: 528–535, 1985.

4934. DeTroyer, A., Borenstein, S., and Cordier, R. Analysis of lung volume restriction in patients with respiratory muscle weakness. Thorax 35: 603–610, 1980.

4935. Gibson, G. J., Pride, N. B., Newsom-Davis, J., and Loh, L. C. Pulmonary mechanics in patients with respiratory muscle weakness. Am. Rev. Respir. Dis. 115: 389–395, 1977.

4936. DeTroyer, A. and Bastenier-Geens, J. Effects of neuromuscular blockade on respiratory mechanics in conscious man. J. Appl. Physiol. 47: 1162–1168, 1979.

4937. Ferris, B. G. Jr., Whittenberger, J. L., and Affeldt, J. E. Pulmonary function in convalescent poliomyelitic patients. N. Engl. J. Med. 246: 919–923, 1952.

4938. Affeldt, J. E., Whittenberger, J. L., Mead, J., and Ferris, B. G. Jr. Pulmonary function in convalescent poliomyelitis patients. N. Engl. J. Med. 247: 43–47, 1952.

4939. Kreitzer, S. M., Saunders, N. A., Tyler, H. R., and Ingram, R. H. Respiratory muscle function in amyotrophic lateral sclerosis. Am. Rev. Respir. Dis. 117: 437–447, 1978.

4940. Rahn, H., Otis, A. B., Chadwick, L. E., and Fenn, W. O. The pressure-volume diagram of the thorax and lung. Am. J. Physiol. 146: 161–178, 1946.

4941. Serisier, D. E., Mastaglia, F. L., and Gibson, G. J. Respiratory muscle function and ventilatory control. I. In patients with motor neuron disease. II. In patients with myotonic dystrophy. Q. J. Med. 202: 205–226, 1982.

4942. Hapke, E. J., Meek, J. C., and Jacobs, J. Pulmonary function in progressive muscular dystrophy. Chest 61: 41–47, 1972.

4943. DeTroyer, A. and Borenstein, S. Acute changes in respiratory mechanics after pyridostigmine injection in patients with myasthenia gravis. Am. Rev. Respir. Dis. 121: 629–638, 1980.

4944. Black, L. F. and Hyatt, R. E. Maximal respiratory pressures: normal values and relationship to age and sex. Am. Rev. Respir. Dis. 99: 696–702, 1969.

4945. Ringqvist, T. The ventilatory capacity in healthy subjects: an analysis of causal factors with special reference to the respiratory forces. Scand. J. Clin. Lab. Invest. 18(Suppl. 88): 1–179, 1966.

4946. Lewis, M. I., Sieck, G. C., Fournier, M., and Belman, M. J. Effect of nutritional deprivation on diaphragm contractility and muscle fiber size. J. Appl. Physiol. 60: 596–603, 1986.

4947. Black, L. F. and Hyatt, R. E. Maximal static respiratory pressures in generalized neuromuscular disease. Am. Rev. Respir. Dis. 103: 641–649, 1971.

4948. Fromm, G. B., Wisdom, D. J., and Block, A. J. Amyotrophic lateral sclerosis presenting with respiratory failure. Chest 71: 612–614, 1977.

4949. DeTroyer, A. and Estenne, M. Limitations of measurement of transdiaphragmatic pressure in detecting diaphragmatic weakness. Thorax 36: 169–174, 1981.

4950. Laporta, D. and Grassino, A. Assessment of transdiaphragmatic pressure in humans. J. Appl. Physiol. 58: 1469–1476, 1985.

4951. Miller, J. M., Moxham, J., and Green, M. The maximal sniff in the assessment of diaphragm function in man. Clin. Sci. 69: 91–96, 1985.

4952. Davis, J. N. Phrenic nerve conduction in man. J. Neurol. Neurosurg. Psychiatry 30: 420–426, 1967.

4953. Alexander, C. Diaphragm movements and the diagnosis of diaphragmatic paralysis. Radiology 17: 79–83, 1966.

4954. Nickerson, B. G. and Keens, T. G. Measuring ventilatory muscle endurance in humans as sustainable inspiratory pressure. J. Appl. Physiol. 52: 768–772, 1982.

4955. Belman, M. J. and Sieck, G. C. The ventilatory muscles, fatigue, endurance and training. Chest 82: 761–766, 1982.

4956. Begin, R., Bureau, M. A., Lupien, L., and Lemieux, B. Control of breathing in Duchenne's muscular dystrophy. Am. J. Med. 69: 227–234, 1980.

4957. Martyn, J. B., Moreno, R. H., Pare, P. D., and Pardy, R. L. Measurement of inspiratory muscle performance with incremental threshold loading. Am. Rev. Respir. Dis. 135: 919–923, 1987.

4958. Fallat, R. J., Jewitt, B., Bass, M., Kamm, B., and Norris, F. H. Spirometry in amyotrophic lateral sclerosis. Arch. Neurol. 36: 74–80, 1979.

4959. Civak, E. D. and Streib, E. W. Management of hypoventilation in motorneuron disease presenting with respiratory insufficiency. Ann. Neurol. 7: 188–191, 1980.

4960. Parhad, I. M., Clark, A. W., Barron, K. D., and Staunton, S. B. Diaphragmatic paralysis in motorneuron disease. Neurology 28: 18–22, 1978.

4961. Nakano, K. K., Bass, H., Tyler, R., and Carmel, R. J. Amyotrophic lateral sclerosis: a study of pulmonary function. Dis. Nerv. Syst. 37: 32–35, 1976.

4962. Miller, R. D., Mulder, D. W., Fowler, W. S., and Olsen, A. M. Exertional dyspnea: a primary complaint in unusual cases of progressive muscular atrophy and amyotrophic lateral sclerosis. Ann. Intern. Med. 46: 119–125, 1957.

4963. Haas, H., Johnson, L. R., Gill, T. H., and Armentrout, T. S. Diaphragm paralysis and ventilatory failure in chronic spinal muscular atrophy. Am. Rev. Respir. Dis. 123: 465–467, 1981.

4964. Brach, B. B. Expiratory flow patterns in amyotrophic lateral sclerosis. Chest 75: 648–649, 1979.

4965. Ferris, B. G. Jr., Warren, A., and Beals, C. A. The vital capacity as a measure of the spontaneous breathing ability in poliomyelitis. N. Engl. J. Med. 252: 618–621, 1955.

4966. Lucas, D. S. and Plum, F. Pulmonary function in patients convalescing from acute poliomyelitis with respiratory paralysis. Am. J. Med. 12: 388–396, 1952.

4967. Faerber, I., Liebert, P. B., and Suskind, M. Loss of functional residual capacity in poliomyelitis. J. Appl. Physiol. 17: 289–292, 1962.

4968. Lane, D. J., Hazleman, B., and Nichols, P. J. R. Late onset respiratory failure in patients with previous poliomyelitis. Q. J. Med. 172: 551–568, 1974.

4969. Campbell, A. M. G., Williams, E. R., and Pearce, J. Late motor neuron degeneration following poliomyelitis. Neurology 19: 1101–1106, 1969.

4970. Caro, C. G., Butler, J., and Dubois, A. B. Some effects of restriction of chest cage expansion on pulmonary function in man: an experimental study. J. Clin. Invest. 39: 573–583, 1960.

4971. Fugl-Meyer, A. R. Effects of respiratory paralysis in tetraplegic and paraplegic patients. Scand. J. Rehab. Med. 3: 141–150, 1971.

4972. DeTroyer, A. and Heilporn, A. Respiratory muscles in quadriplegia. The respiratory function of the intercostal muscles. Am. Rev. Respir. Dis. 122: 591–600, 1980.

4973. Roussel, P., Degand., P., Lamblin, G., Laine, A., and Lafitte, J. J. Review: biochemical definition of human tracheobronchial mucus. Lung 154: 241–260, 1978.

4974. Kreitzer, S., Feldman, N., Sanders, N., and Ingram, R. H. Bilateral diaphragmatic paralysis with hypercapnic respiratory failure. Am. J. Med. 65: 89–95, 1978.

4975. Newsom-Davies, J., Goldman, M., Loh, L., and Casson, M. Diaphragmatic function and alveolar hypoventilation. Q. J. Med. 45: 87–100, 1976.

4976. McCredie, M., Lovejoy, F. W., and Kaltreider, L. N. Pulmonary function and diaphragmatic paralysis. Thorax 17: 213–217, 1962.

4977. D'Angelo, E., Sant'Ambrogio, G., and Agostoni, E. Effect of diaphragm activity or paralysis on distribution of pleural pressure. J. Appl. Physiol. 37: 311–315, 1974.

4978. Clague, H. W. and Hall, D. R. Effect of posture on lung volume: airway closure and gas exchange in hemidiaphragmatic paralysis. Thorax 34: 523–526, 1979.

4979. Camfferman, F., Bogaard, J. M., Van Der Meche, F. G. A., and Hilvèring, C. Idiopathic bilateral diaphragmatic paralysis. Eur. J. Respir. Dis. 66: 65–71, 1985.

4980. Arborelius, M. Jr., Lilja, B., and Senyk, J. Regional and total lung function studies in patients with hemidiaphragmatic paralysis. Respiration 32: 253–264, 1975.

4981. Chandler, K. W., Razas, C. J., Kory, R. C., and Goldman, A. L. Bilateral diaphragmatic paralysis complicating local cardiac hypothermia during open heart surgery. Am. J. Med. 77: 243–249, 1984.

4982. Amis, T. C., Ciofetta, G., Hughes, J. M. B., and Loh, L. Regional lung function in bilateral diaphragmatic paralysis. Clin. Sci. 59: 485–492, 1980.

4983. Easton, P. A., Fleetham, J. A., De La Rocha, A., and Anthonisen, N. R. Respiratory function after paralysis of the right hemidiaphragm. Am. Rev. Respir. Dis. 127: 125–128, 1983.

4984. Riley, E. A. Idiopathic diaphragmatic paralysis. Am. J. Med. 32: 404–416, 1962.

4985. Dutt, A. K. Diaphragmatic paralysis caused by herpes zoster. Am. Rev. Respir. Dis. 101: 755–758, 1970.

4986. Wheeler, W. E., Rubis, L. J., Jones, C. W., and Harrah, J. D. Etiology and prevention of topical cardiac hypothermia-induced phrenic nerve injury and left lower lobe atelectasis during cardiac surgery. Chest 88: 680–683, 1985.

4987. Derveaux, L. and Lacquet, L. M. Hemidiaphragmatic paresis after cervical herpes zoster. Thorax 37: 870–871, 1982.

4988. Loh, L., Goldman, M., and Newsom-Davis, J. The assessment of diaphragm function. Medicine 56: 165–169, 1982.

4989. Higenbottam, T., Allen, D., Loh, L., and Clark, T. J. H. Abdominal wall movement in normals and patients with hemidiaphragmatic and bilateral diaphragmatic palsy. Thorax 32: 589–595, 1977.

4990. Sandham, J. D., Shaw, D. T., and Guenter, C. A. Acute supine respiratory failure due to bilateral diaphragmatic paralysis. Chest 72: 96–98, 1977.

4991. Lisboa, C., Pare, P. D., Pertuze, J., Contreras, G., Moreno, R., Guillemi, S., and Clues, E. Inspiratory muscle function in unilateral diaphragmatic paralysis. Am. Rev. Respir. Dis. 134: 488–492, 1986.

4992. Spitzer, S. A., Korczym, A. D., and Kalaci, J. Transient bilateral diaphragmatic paralysis. Chest 64: 355–357, 1973.

4993. Comroe, J. H., Wood, F. C., Kay, C. F., and Spoont, F. M. Motor neuritis after tetanus antitoxin with involvement of the muscles of respiration. Am. J. Med. 10: 786–789, 1951.

4994. Mixsell, H. R. and Giddings, E. Certain aspects of post diphtheritic diaphragmatic paralysis: report of 8 fatal cases in 4,259 cases of diphtheria. J.A.M.A. 77: 590–594, 1921.

4995. Moore, P. and James, O. Guillain-Barré syndrome: incidence, management and outcome of major complications. Crit. Care Med. 37: 479–491, 1968.

4996. Danon, J., Druz, W. S., Goldberg, N. B., and Sharp, J. T. Function of the isolated paced diaphragm and the cervical accessory muscles in C1 quadriplegics. Am. Rev. Respir. Dis. 119: 909–919, 1979.

4997. Ford, G. T., Whitelaw, W. A., Rosenal, W. T., Cruse, P. J., and Guenter, C. A. Diaphragm function after abdominal surgery in humans. Am. Rev. Respir. Dis. 127: 431–436, 1983.

4998. Road, J. D., Burgess, K. R., Whitelaw, W. A., and Ford, G. T. Diaphragm function and respiratory response after upper abdominal surgery in dogs. J. Appl. Physiol. 57: 576–582, 1984.

4999. Spiteri, M. A., Mier, A. K., Brophy, C. J., Pantin, C. F. A., and Green, M. Bilateral diaphragm weakness. Thorax 40: 631–632, 1985.

5000. Graham, A. N., Martin, P. D., and Haas, L. F. Neuralgic amyotrophy with bilateral diaphragmatic palsy. Thorax 40: 635–636, 1985.

5001. Cooper, C. B., Trend, P. St. J., and Wiles, C. M. Severe diaphragm weakness in multiple sclerosis. Thorax 40: 633–634, 1985.

5002. Gracey, D. R., McMichan, J. C., Divertie, M. B., and Howard, F. M. Respiratory failure in Guillain-Barré syndrome. Mayo Clin. Proc. 57: 742–746, 1982.

5003. Havard, C. W. H. Progress in myasthenia gravis. Br. Med. J. 2: 1008–1011, 1977.

5004. Flacke, W. Treatment of myasthenia gravis. N. Engl. J. Med. 288: 27–31, 1973.

5005. Seybold, M. E. Myasthenia gravis, a clinical and basic science review. J.A.M.A. 250: 2516–2521, 1983.

5006. Fluck, D. C. Chest movements in hemiplegia. Clin. Sci. 31: 382–388, 1966.

5007. Gracey, D. R., Divertie, M. B., Howard, F. M., and Payne, W. S. Postoperative respiratory care after trans-sternal thymectomy in myasthenia gravis. Chest 86: 67–71, 1984.

5008. Dau, P. C. Respiratory failure in myasthenia gravis: use of plasmapheresis. Chest 85: 721–722, 1984.

5009. Gracey, D. R., Howard, F. M., and Divertie, M. B. Plasmapheresis in the treatment of ventilator-dependent myasthenia gravis patients. Chest 85: 739–743, 1984.

5010. Gutmann, L. and Pratt, L. Pathophysiologic aspects of human botulism. Arch. Neurol. 33: 175–179, 1976.

5011. Cherington, M. Botulism. Arch. Neurol. 30: 432–437, 1974.

5012. Dau, P. C. Response to plasmapheresis and immunosuppressive drug therapy in 60 myasthenia gravis patients. Ann. N.Y. Acad. Sci. 377: 700–708, 1981.

5013. Lewis, S. W., Pierson, D. J., Cary, J. M., and Hudson, L. D. Prolonged respiratory paralysis in wound botulism. Chest 75: 59–61, 1979.

5014. Buchsbaum, H. D., Martin, W. A., and Turino, G. M. Chronic alveolar hypoventilation due to muscular dystrophy. Neurology 18: 319–327, 1968.

5015. Inkley, S. R., Alderberg, F. C., and Vignos, P. C. Pulmonary function in Duchenne muscular dystrophy related to stage of disease. Am. J. Med. 56: 297–306, 1974.

5016. Kilburn, K. H., Eagan, J. T., Sieker, H. O., and Heyman, A. Cardiopulmonary insufficiency in myotonic and progressive muscular dystrophy. N. Engl. J. Med. 261: 1089–1096, 1959.

5017. Hapke, E. J., Meek, J. C., and Jacobs, J. Pulmonary function in progressive muscular dystrophy. Chest 61: 41–47, 1972.

5018. Bach, J., Alba, A., Pilkington, L. A., and Lee, M. Long-term rehabilitation in advanced stage of childhood onset, rapidly progressive muscular dystrophy. Arch. Phys. Med. Rehabil. 62: 328–331, 1981.

5019. Curran, F. J. Night ventilation by body respirators for patients in chronic respiratory failure due to late stage Duchenne muscular dystrophy. Arch. Phys. Med. Rehabil. 62: 270–274, 1981.

5020. Garay, S. M., Turino, G. M., and Goldring, R. M. Sustained reversal of chronic hypercapnia in patients with alveolar hypoventilation syndromes. Am. J. Med. 70: 269–274, 1981.

5021. Coccagna, G., Mantovani, M., Parchi, C., Mironi, F., and Lugaresi, E. Alveolar hypoventilation and hypersomnia in myotonic dystrophy. J. Neurol. Neurosurg. Psychiatry 38: 977–984, 1975.

5022. Begin, R., Bureau, M. A., Lupien, L., and Lemieux, B. Control and modulation of respiration in Steinert's myotonic dystrophy. Am. Rev. Respir. Dis. 121: 281–289, 1980.

5023. Weng, T. R., Schultz, G. E., Chang, G. H., and Nigro, M. A. Pulmonary function and ventilatory response to chemical stimuli in familial myopathy. Chest 88: 488–495, 1985.

5024. DeTroyer, A., De Beyl, D. Z., and Thirion, M. Function of the respiratory muscles in acute hemiplegia. Am. Rev. Respir. Dis. 123: 631–632, 1981.

5025. Riley, D. J., Santiago, T., Daniele, R. P., Schall, B., and Edelman, N. H. Blunted respiratory drive in congenital myopathy. Am. J. Med. 63: 459–466, 1977.

5026. Carroll, J. E., Zwillich, C., Weil, J. V., and Brooke, M. H. Depressed ventilatory response in oculocraniosomatic neuromuscular disease. Neurology 26: 140–146, 1976.

5027. Estenne, M., Borenstein, S., and DeTroyer, A. Respiratory muscle dysfunction in myotonia congenita. Am. Rev. Respir. Dis. 130: 681–684, 1984.

5028. Rosenow, E. C. and Engel, A. G. Acid maltase deficiency in adults presenting as respiratory failure. Am. J. Med. 64: 485–491, 1978.

5029. Margolis, M. L. and Hill, A. R. Acid maltase deficiency in an adult. Am. Rev. Respir. Dis. 134: 328–331, 1986.

5030. Trend, P. J., Wiles, C. M., Spencer, G. T., Morgen-Hughes, J. A., Lake, B. D., and Patrick, A. D. Acid maltase deficiency in adults; diagnosis and management in 5 cases. Brain 108: 845–860, 1985.

5031. Edmondson, R. S. and Flowers, M. W. Intensive care in tetanus: management, complications, and mortality in 100 cases. Br. Med. J. 1: 1401–1404, 1979.

5032. Kloetzel, K. Studies on the cause of death in tetanus. Dis. Chest 45: 63–71, 1964.

5033. Femi-Pearse, D. Blood gas tensions, acid-base status, and spirometry in tetanus. Am. Rev. Respir. Dis. 110: 390–394, 1974.

5034. DeCramer, M., Demedts, M., Rochette, F., and Billiet, L. Maximal transrespiratory pressures in obstructive lung disease. Bull. Eur. Physiopathol. Respir. 16: 479–490, 1980.

5035. Martin, R. J., Sufit, R. L., Ringel, S. P., Hudgel, D. W., and Hill, P. L. Respiratory improvement by muscle training in adult onset acid maltase deficiency. Muscle Nerve 6: 201–203, 1983.

5036. Gibson, G. J., Clark, E., and Pride, N. B. Static transdiaphragmatic pressures in normal subjects and in patients with chronic hyperinflation. Am. Rev. Respir. Dis. 124: 685–689, 1981.

5037. Farkas, G. A. and Roussos, Ch. Diaphragm in emphysematous hamsters: sarcomere adaptability. J. Appl. Physiol. 54: 1635–1640, 1983.

5038. Hughes, R. L., Katz, H., Sahgal, V., Campbell, J. A., Hartz, R., and Shields, T. W. Fiber size and energy metabolites in five separate muscles from patients with chronic obstructive lung disease. Respiration 44: 321–328, 1983.

5039. Sanchez, J., Medrano, G., Debesse, B., Riquet, M., and Derenne, J. P. Muscle fiber types in costal and crural diaphragm in normal men and in patients with moderate chronic respiratory disease. Bull. Eur. Physiopathol. Respir. 21: 351–356, 1985.

5040. Campbell, J. A., Hughes, R. L., Sahgal, V., Frederiksen, J., and Shields, T. W. Alterations in intercostal muscle morphology and biochemistry in patients with obstructive lung disease. Am. Rev. Respir. Dis. 122: 679–686, 1980.

5041. Malo. J-L. Assessment of airway excitability in epidemiologic surveys (editorial). Chest 87: 413, 1985.

5042. Farkas, G. A. and Rochester, D. F. Contractile characteristics and operating lengths of canine inspiratory muscles. J. Appl. Physiol. 61: 220–226, 1986.

5043. Sharp, J. T., Danon, J., Druz, W. S., Goldberg, N. B., Fishman, H., and Macknack, W. Respiratory muscle function in patients with chronic obstructive pulmonary disease: its relationship to disability and to respiratory therapy. Am. Rev. Respir. Dis. 110: 154–167, 1974.

5044. Sharp, J. T., Goldberg, N. B., Druz, W. S., Fishman, H. C., and Danon, J. Thoraco-abdominal motion in chronic obstructive lung disease. Am. Rev. Respir. Dis. 115: 47–56, 1977.

5045. Sackett, D. L. Clinical diagnosis and the clinical laboratory. Clin. Invest. Med. 1: 37–43, 1978.

5046. Martin, J. G., Habib, M., and Engel, L. A. Inspiratory muscle activity during induced hyperinflation. Respir. Physiol. 39: 303–313, 1980.

5047. Martin, J. G., Powell, E., Shore, S., Emrick, J., and Engel, L. A. The role of respiratory muscles in the hyperinflation of bronchial asthma. Am. Rev. Respir. Dis. 121: 441–447, 1980.

5048. Melzer, E. and Souhrada, J. F. Decrease of respiratory muscle strength and static lung volumes in obese asthmatics. Am. Rev. Respir. Dis. 121: 17–22, 1980.

5049. McDonald, A. D., McDonald, J. C., and Pooley, F. D. Mineral fibre content of the lung in mesothelial tumours in North America. Ann. Occup. Hyg. 26: 417–422, 1982.

5050. Burrows, B., Lebowitz, M. D., Camilli, A. E., and Knudson, R. J. Longitudinal changes in forced expiratory volume in one second in adults. Am. Rev. Respir. Dis. 133: 974–980, 1986.

5051. McKenzie, D. K. and Gandevia, S. C. Strength and endurance of inspiratory, expiratory and limb muscles in asthma. Am. Rev. Respir. Dis. 134: 999–1004, 1986.

5052. Siconolfi, S. F., Garber, C. E., Lasater, T. M., and Carleton, R. A. A simple valid step test for estimating maximal oxygen uptake in epidemiological studies. Am. J. Epidemiol. 121: 382–390, 1985.

5053. DeTroyer, A., Estenne, M., and Yernault, J. C. Disturbances of respiratory muscle function in patients with mitral valve disease. Am. J. Med. 69: 867–873, 1980.

5054. Siconolfi, S. F., Lasater, T. M., Snow, R. C. K., and Carleton, R. A. Self-reported physical activity compared with maximal oxygen uptake. Am. J. Epidemiol. 122: 101–105, 1985.

5055. Chausow, A. M., Kane, T., Levinson, D., and Szidon, J. P. Reversible hypercapnic respiratory insufficiency in scleroderma caused by respiratory muscle weakness. Am. Rev. Respir. Dis. 130: 142–144, 1984.

5056. Venables, K. M., Burge, P. S., Davison, A. G., and Taylor, A. J. N. Peak flow rate records in surveys: reproducibility of observer's reports. Thorax 39: 828–832, 1984.

5057. Cramer, D., Peacock, A., and Denison, D. Temperature corrections in routine spirometry. Thorax 39: 771–774, 1984.

5058. Martens, J., Demedts, M. T., Van Meenen, M. T., and Dequerker, J. Respiratory muscle dysfunction in systemic lupus erythematosus. Chest 84: 170–175, 1983.

5059. Bohan, A., Peter, J. B., Bowman, R. L., and Pearson, C. M. A computer assisted analysis of 153 patients with polymyositis and dermatomyositis. Medicine 56: 255–286, 1977.

5060. Matamis, D., Lemaire, F., Harf, A., Teisseire, B., and Brun-Buisson, C. Redistribution of pulmonary blood flow induced by positive end-expiratory pressure and dopamine infusion in acute respiratory failure. Am. Rev. Respir. Dis. 129: 39–44, 1984.

5061. Dantzker, D. R., Brook, C. J., Dehart, P., Lynch, J. P., and Weg, J. G. Ventilation-perfusion distributions in the adult respiratory distress syndrome. Am. Rev. Respir. Dis. 120: 1039–1052, 1979.

5062. Newsom-Davis, J., Loh, L., and Casson, M. The effects of diaphragmatic paralysis on the release and time components of individual breaths in man. In: Duron, B. (ed.). Respiratory Centres and Afferent Systems. Inserm, Paris, 1976.

5063. Arora, N. S. and Rochester, D. F. Respiratory muscle strength and maximal ventilation in undernourished patients. Am. Rev. Respir. Dis. 126: 5–8, 1982.

5064. Arora, N. S. and Rochester, D. F. The effect of body weight and muscularity on human diaphragm muscle mass, thickness and area. J. Appl. Physiol. 52: 64–70, 1982.

5065. Newman, J. H., Neff, T. A., and Ziporin, P. Acute respiratory failure associated with hypophosphatemia. N. Engl. J. Med. 296: 1101–1103, 1977.

5066. Fitts, R. H. and Halloszy, J. A. Lactate and contractile force in frog muscle during development of fatigue and recovery. Am. J. Physiol. 231: 430–433, 1976.

5067. Scherrer, J. and Monod, H. Le travail musculaire local et la fatigue chez l'homme. J. Physiol. (Paris) 52: 419–510, 1960.

5068. Aubier, M., Murciano, D., Lecocguic, Y., Viires, N., Jacquens, Y., Squara, P., and Pariente, R. Effect of hypophosphatemia on diaphragmatic contractility in patients with acute respiratory failure. N. Engl. J. Med. 313: 420–424, 1985.

5069. Lentz, R. D., Brown, D. M., and Kjellstrand, C. Treatment of severe hypophosphatemia. Ann. Intern. Med. 89: 941–944, 1978.

5070. Dhingra, S., Solven, F., Wilson, A., and McCarthy, D. S. Hypomagnesia and respiratory muscle power. Am. Rev. Respir. Dis. 129: 497–498, 1984.

5071. Juan, G., Calverley, P., Talamo, C., Schnader, J., and Roussos, Ch. Effect of carbon dioxide on diaphragmatic function in human beings. N. Engl. J. Med. 310: 874–879, 1984.

5072. Aubier, M., Viires, N., Piquet, J., Murciano, D., Blanchet, F., Marty, C., Gherardi, R., and Pariente, R. Effect of hypocalcemia on diaphragmatic strength generation. J. Appl. Physiol. 58: 2054–2061, 1985.

5073. Howell, S., Fitzgerald, R. S., and Roussos, Ch. Effects of uncompensated metabolic acidosis on canine diaphragm. J. Appl. Physiol. 59: 1376–1382, 1985.

5074. Bellemare, F. and Grassino, A. Effect of pressure and timing of contraction on human diaphragm fatigue. J. Appl. Physiol. 53: 1196–1206, 1982.

5075. Grassino, A. and Macklem, P. T. Respiratory muscle fatigue and ventilatory failure. Ann. Rev. Med. 35: 625–647, 1984.

5076. Pardy, R. L. and Roussos, Ch. Endurance of hyperventilation in chronic airflow limitation. Chest 83: 744–750, 1983.

5077. Glenn, W. W. L., Holcomb, W. G., Albert, B. E. E., McLaughlin, J., O'Hare, J. M., Hogan, J. F., and Yasuda, R. Total ventilatory support in a quadriplegic patient with radio frequency electrophrenic respiration. N. Engl. J. Med. 286: 513–516, 1972.

5078. Glenn, W. W. L., Hogan, J. F., Loke, J. S., Ciesielski, T. E., Phelps, M. L., and Rowedder, R. Ventilatory support by pacing of the conditioned diaphragm in quadriplegia. N. Engl. J. Med. 310: 1150–1155, 1984.

5079. Splaingard, M. L., Frates, R. C., Jefferson, L. S., Rosen, C. L., and Harrison, G. M. Home negative pressure ventilation: report of 20 years of experience in patients with neuromuscular disease. Arch. Phys. Med. Rehabil. 66: 239–242, 1985.

5080. Splaingard, M. L., Frates, R. C., Harrison, G. M., Carter, R. E., and Jefferson, L. S. Home positive pressure ventilation. Chest 84: 376–382, 1983.

5081. Ellis, E. R., Bye, P. T. P., Bruderer, J. W., and Sullivan, C. E. Treatment of respiratory failure during sleep in patients with neuromuscular disease. Am. Rev. Respir. Dis. 135: 148–152, 1987.

5082. Meignan, M., George, C., and Lemaire, F. Eau pulmonaire extravasculaire au cours du syndrome de detrusse respiratoire aigue de l'adulte. Bull. Eur. Physiopathol. Respir. 14: 617–628, 1978.

5083. Riley, D. J., Santiago, T. V., Daniele, R. P., Schall, B., and Edelman, M. H. Blunted respiratory drive in congenital myopathy. Am. J. Med. 63: 459–466, 1977.

5084. Sibbald, W. J., Short, A. K., Warshawski, F. J., Cunningham, D. G., and Cheung, H. Thermal dye measurements of extravascular lung water in critically ill patients. Chest 87: 585–592, 1985.

5085. Hill, N. S. Clinical applications of body ventilators. Chest 99: 897–905, 1986.

5086. Martin, R. J., Sufit, R. L., Ringel, S. P., Hudgel, D. W., and Hill, P. L. Respiratory improvement by muscle training in adult onset acid maltase deficiency. Muscle Nerve 6: 201–203, 1983.

5087. Shennib, H., Chiu, C.-J., Mulder, D. S., Richards, G. K., and Prentis, J. Pulmonary bacterial clearance and alveolar macrophage function in septic shock lung. Am. Rev. Respir. Dis. 130: 444–449, 1984.

5088. Ralph, D. D., Robertson, H. T., Weaver, L. J., Hlastala,

M. P., Carrico, C. J., and Hudson, L. D. Distribution of ventilation and perfusion during positive end-expiratory pressure in the adult respiratory distress syndrome. Am. Rev. Respir. Dis. 131: 54–60, 1985.

5089. Oldham, P. D. A note on the analysis of repeated measurements of the same subjects. J. Chron. Dis. 15: 969–977, 1962.

5090. Storr, J., Barrell, E., and Lenney, W. Asthma in primary schools. Br. Med. J. 295: 251–252, 1987.

5091. Chen, H., Dukes, R., and Martin, B. J. Inspiratory muscle training in patients with chronic obstructive pulmonary disease. Am. Rev. Respir. Dis. 131: 251–255, 1985.

5092. Nochomovitz, M. L., Hopkins, M., Brodkey, J., Montenegro, H., Mortimer, J. T., and Cherniack, N. S. Conditioning of the diaphragm with phrenic nerve stimulation after prolonged disuse. Am. Rev. Respir. Dis. 130: 685–688, 1984.

5093. Pershagen, G., Hrubec, Z., Lorich, U., and Ronnqvist, P. Acute respiratory symptoms in patients with chronic obstructive pulmonary disease and in other subjects living near a coal-fired plant. Arch. Environ. Health 39: 27–33, 1984.

5094. Hodgkin, J. E., Abbey, D. E., Euler, G. L., and Magie, A. R. COPD prevalence in nonsmokers in high and low photochemical air pollution areas. Chest 86: 830–838, 1984.

5095. Melia, R. J. W., Florey, C. duV., Morris, R. W., Goldstein, B. D., Clark, D., and John, H. H. Childhood respiratory illness and the home environment. I. Relations between nitrogen dioxide, temperature and relative humidity. Int. J. Epidemiol. 11: 155–163, 1982.

5096. Melia, R. J. W., Florey, C. du V., Morris, R. W., Goldstein, B. D., John, H. H., Clark, D., Craighead, I. B., and MacKinlay, J. C. Childhood respiratory illness and the home environment. II. Association between respiratory illness and nitrogen dioxide, temperature and relative humidity. Int. J. Epidemiol. 11: 164–169, 1982.

5097. Wedzicha, J. A., Cotter, F. E., Wallis, P. J. W., Newland, A. C., and Empey, D. W. Gas transfer for carbon monoxide in polycythemia secondary to hypoxic lung disease. Clin. Sci. 68: 57–62, 1985.

5098. Burrows, B., Lebowitz, M. D., Camilli, A. E., and Knudson, R. J. Longitudinal changes in forced expiratory volume in one second in adults. Am. Rev. Respir. Dis. 133: 974–980, 1986.

5099. Packe, G. E. and Ayres, J. G. Asthma outbreak during a thunderstorm. Lancet ii: 199–204, 1985.

5100. De Monchy, J. G. R., Kauffman, H. K., Venge, P., Koeter, G. H., Jansen, H. M., Sluiter, H. J., and De Vries, K. Bronchoalveolar eosinophilia during allergen-induced late asthmatic reactions. Am. Rev. Respir. Dis. 131: 373–376, 1985.

5101. Hughes, J. M., Jones, R. N., Gilson, J. C., Hammad, Y. Y., Samimi, B., Hendrick, D. J., Turner-Warwick, M., and Weill, H. Determinants of progression in sandblasters' silicosis. Ann. Occup. Hyg. 26: 701–712, 1982.

5102. Burge, P. S., Finnegan, M., Horsfield, N., Emery, D., Austwick, P., Davies, P. S., and Pickering, C. A. C. Occupational asthma in a factory with a contaminated humidifier. Thorax 40: 248–254, 1985.

5103. Stover, D. E., White, D. A., Romano, P. A., Gellene, R. A., and Robeson, W. A. Spectrum of pulmonary diseases associated with the acquired immune deficiency syndrome. Am. J. Med. 78: 429–437, 1985.

5104. Douglas, N. J., Campbell, I. W., Ewing, D. J., Clarke, B. F., and Flenley, D. C. Reduced airway vagal tone in diabetic patients with autonomic neuropathy. Clin. Sci. 61: 581–584, 1981.

5105. Afzelius, B. A. A human syndrome caused by immobile cilia. Science 193: 317–319, 1979.

5106. Bach, B. A., Sherman, L., Benacerraf, B., and Greene, M. I. Mechanisms of regulation of cell mediated immunity: II. Induction and suppression of a delayed-type hypersensitivity by azobenzene-arsonate-coupled syngeneic cells. J. Immunol. 127: 1460–1468, 1978.

5107. Bachman, A. L., Hewitt, W. R., and Beekley, H. C. Bronchiectasis; a bronchographic study of sixty cases of pneumonia. Arch. Intern. Med. 91: 78–96, 1953.

5108. Barrowcliff, D. F. and Arblaster, P. G. Farmer's lung: a study of an early acute fatal case. Thorax 23: 490–500, 1968.

5109. Becroft, D. M. O. Bronchiolitis obliterans, bronchiectasis, and other sequelae of adenovirus type 21 infection in young children. J. Clin. Pathol. 24: 72–82, 1971.

5110. Bienenstock, J., Johnson, M., and Perry, D. Y. W. Bronchial lymphoid tissue. Lab. Invest. 28: 686–693, 1973.

5111. Blumenthal, M. N. and Bach, F. H. Immunogenetics of atopic disease. In: Elliott, M. Jr., Reed, C. E., and Ellis, E. F. (eds.). Allergy: Principles and Practice. C. V. Mosby, St. Louis and Toronto, 1983.

5112. Borros, D. L. Granulomatous inflammation. Prog. Allergy 24: 183–267, 1978.

5113. Borros, D. L. Hypersensitivity granulomas. In: Elliott, M. Jr., Reed, C. E., and Ellis, E. F. (eds.). Allergy: Principles and Practice. C. V. Mosby, St. Louis and Toronto, 1983.

5114. Boucher, R. C., Bromberg, P. A., and Gatzy, J. T. Airway mucosal permeability. Airway Reactivity. Symposium Proceedings, Astra Pharmaceuticals (Canada), Mississauga, Ontario, 1980.

5115. Bowden, D. H. and Adamson, I. Y. R. Pulmonary interstitial cell as an immediate precursor of the alveolar macrophage. Am. J. Pathol. 68: 521–536, 1972.

5116. Brain, J. D., Godleski, J. J., and Syroken, S. P. Respiratory Defense Mechanisms. Part II. Marcel Dekker, New York, 1977.

5117. Brunstetter, M., Hardy, J. A., Schiff, R., Lewis, J. P., and Cross, C. E. The origin of the pulmonary alveolar macrophage. Arch. Intern. Med. 127: 1064–1068, 1971.

5118. Buist, A. S. and Ducic, S. Smoking: evaluation of studies which have demonstrated pulmonary function changes. In: Macklem, P. T. and Permutt, S. (eds.). The Lung in Transition between Health and Disease. Marcel Dekker, New York and Basel, 1979.

5119. Butler, J., Caro, C., Alkaler, R., and Dubois, B. Physiological factors affecting airway resistance in normal subjects and in patients with obstructive airways disease. J. Clin. Invest. 39: 584–591, 1960.

5120. Callerame, M. L., Condemi, J. J., Bohrod, M. G., and Vaughan, J. H. Immunologic reactions of bronchial tissues in asthma. N. Engl. J. Med. 284: 459–464, 1971.

5121. Castleman, W. L. Alterations in pulmonary ultrastructure and morphometric parameters induced by parainfluenza (Sendai) virus in rats during postnatal growth. Am. J. Pathol. 114: 322–335, 1984.

5122. Caul, E. O., Waller, D. K., Clark, S. K. R., and Corner, B. D. A comparison of influenza and respiratory syncytial virus infections among infants admitted to hospital with acute respiratory infections. J. Hyg. (Lond.) 77: 383–392, 1976.

5123. Church, M. K. Biochemical basis of pulmonary and antiallergic drugs. In: Devlin, J. P. (ed.). Pulmonary and Antiallergic Drugs. John Wiley & Sons, New York, 1985.

5124. Porter, R. and Birch, J. (eds.). Identification of Asthma. Ciba Foundation Symposium. Churchill-Livingstone, Edinburgh and London, 1971.

5125. CIBA Guest Symposium Report. Terminology, definition and classification of chronic pulmonary emphysema and related conditions. Thorax 14: 286–299, 1959.

5126. Claman, H. N., Miller, S. D., Sy, M., and Moorehead, J. W. Suppressive mechanisms involving sensitization and tolerance in contact allergy. Immunol. Rev. 50: 105–132, 1980.

5127. Cockcroft, D. W., Killian, D. W., Mellen, J. A., and Hargreave, F. E. Bronchial reactivity to inhaled histamine: a method and clinical survey. Clin. Allergy 7: 235–243, 1977.

5128. Cohen, R. C. and Prentice, A. I. D. Metaplastic cells in sputum of patients with pulmonary eosinophilia. Tubercle 40: 44–46, 1959.

5129. Corry, D., Padmakar, K., and Lipscomb, M. F. The migration of macrophages into hilar lymph nodes. Am. J. Pathol. 115: 321–329, 1984.

5130. Curschmann, H. Ueber Bronchiolitis exsudativa und ihr Verhältniss zum Asthma Nervosum. Dtsch. Arch. Klin. Med. 32: 1–34, 1882.

5131. Dayman, H. Mechanics of airflow in health and emphysema. J. Clin. Invest. 30: 1175–1190, 1951.

5132. De Vries, K., Booij-Noord, H., Goei, A. T., Grobler, N. J., Sluiter, H. J., Tammeling, G. J., and Orie, N. G. M. In: Orie, N. G. M. and Sluiter, H. J. (eds.). Bronchitis II. An international symposium. Royal Van Gorcum, The Netherlands, 1964.

5133. Deal, E. C., McFadden, E. R., Jr., Ingram, R. H., Jr., Strauss, J. H., and Jaeger, J. J. Role of respiratory heat exchange in production of exercise-induced asthma. J. Appl. Physiol. 46: 467–475, 1979.

5134. Dickie, H. A. and Rankin, J. Farmer's lung: an acute granulomatous interstitial pneumonitis occurring in agricultural workers. J.A.M.A. 167: 1069–1076, 1958.

5135. Dines, D. D. Acute bronchiolitis as a cause of chronic obstructive lung disease in adults. Lancet i: 281–282, 1967.

5136. Downham, M. A., McQuillin, J., and Gardner, P. S. Diagnosis and significance of para-influenza virus infections in children. Arch. Dis. Child. 49: 8–15, 1974.

5137. Dunnill, M. S. The pathology of asthma, with special reference to changes in the bronchial mucosa. J. Clin. Pathol. 13: 27–33, 1960.

5138. Dunnill, M. S. In: Porter, R. and Birch, J. (eds.). Identification of asthma. Ciba Foundation Symposium. Churchill-Livingstone, Edinburgh and London, 1971.

5139. Eliason, R., Mosberg, B., Camner, P., and Afzelius, B. A. Immobile cilia, chronic airway infection and male sterility. N. Engl. J. Med. 277: 1–6, 1977.

5140. St. Engle, S. and Newns, G. H. Proliferative neuro-bronchiolitis. Arch. Dis. Child. 15: 219–226, 1940.

5141. Epler, G. R., Snider, G. L., Gaensler, E. A., Cathcart, E. S., Fitzgerald, M. X., and Carrington, C. B. Bronchiolitis and bronchitis in connective tissue disease: a possible relationship to the use of penicillamine. J.A.M.A. 242: 528–532, 1979.

5142. Esterly, J. R. and Oppenheimer, E. H. Observations in cystic fibrosis of the pancreas. Johns Hopkins Med. J. 122: 94–101, 1968.

5143. Esterly, J. R. and Oppenheimer, E. H. Cystic fibrosis of the pancreas: structural changes in peripheral airways. Thorax 23: 670–675, 1968.

5144. Fink, J. N., Banaszak, E. F., Theide, W. H., and Barboriak, J. J. Interstitial pneumonitis due to hypersensitivity to an organism contaminating a heating system. Ann. Intern. Med. 74: 80–83, 1971.

5145. Florey, H. W. General Pathology. Lloyd Luke Medical Books, London, 1962.

5146. Fox, B., Bull, T. B., Makay, A. R., and Rawbone, R. Significance of ultrastructural abnormalities in human cilia. Chest 80: 796–799, 1981.

5147. Foy, H. M., Cooney, M. K., Hall, C. E., Bore, E., and Maletzsky, A. J. Isolation of mumps virus from children with acute lower respiratory tract disease. Am. J. Epidemiol. 94: 467–472, 1971.

5148. Fry, D. Theoretical considerations of the bronchial pressure-flow-volume relationship with particular reference to the maximum expiratory flow volume curves. Phys. Med. Biol. 3: 174–194, 1959.

5149. Gadard, P., Klott, J., Jonquet, O., Bousquet, J., and Michel, F. B. Lymphocyte subpopulations, bronchoalveolar lavage in patients with sarcoidosis and hypersensitivity pneumonitis. Chest 80: 447–452, 1981.

5150. Gerrity, T. R., Lee, T. S., Haas, F. J., Marenelli, A., Werner, P., and Lourenco, R. V. Calculated deposition of inhaled particles in the airway generations of normal subjects. J. Appl. Physiol. 47: 867–873, 1979.

5151. Gleich, G. J., Frigas, E., Loegering, D. A., Wassom, D. L., and Steinmuller, D. Cytotoxic properties of eosinophil major basic protein. J. Immunol. 123: 2925–2927, 1979.

5152. Godleski, J. J. and Brain, J. D. The origin of the alveolar macrophage in mouse radiation shimmers. J. Exp. Med. 136: 630–643, 1972.

5153. Gold, R., Wilt, J. C., Adhikari, P. K., and MacPherson, R. I. Adenoviral pneumonia and its complications in infancy and childhood. J. Can. Assoc. Radiol. 20: 218–224, 1969.

5154. Greene, M. I. and Benacerraf, B. Studies on antigen specific cell immunity and suppression. Immunol. Rev. 50: 163–186, 1980.

5155. Guerzon, G. M., Pare, P. D., Michoud, M. C., and Hogg, J. C. The number and distribution of mast cells in monkey lungs. Am. Rev. Respir. Dis. 119: 59–66, 1979.

5156. Gurwitz, D., Mindorf, C. and Levison, H. Increased incidence of bronchial reactivity in children with a history of bronchiolitis. J. Pediatr. 98: 551–558, 1981.

5157. Hers, J. F. P. and Mulder, J. Broad aspects of pathology and pathogenesis of human influenza. Am. Rev. Respir. Dis. 83(Suppl.): 84–97, 1961.

5158. Hirata, T., Nagai, S., Ohshima, S., and Izumi, T. Comparative study of T-cell subsets in BAL fluid in patients with hypersensitivity pneumonitis and sarcoidosis (abstract). Chest 82: 232, 1982.

5159. Hogg, J. C., Hulbert, W. C., Armour, C., and Pare, P. D. Asthma: Immunopharmacology and Treatment. Third International Symposium. Academic Press, London, New York, and Toronto, 1984.

5160. Hogg, J. C., Macklem, P. T., and Thurlbeck, W. M. Site and nature of airway obstruction in chronic obstructive lung disease. N. Engl. J. Med. 278: 1355–1360, 1968.

5161. Hogg, J. C., Williams, J., Richardson, J. B., Macklem, P. T., and Thurlbeck, W. M. Age as a factor in the distribution of lower airway conductance and in the pathologic anatomy of obstructive lung disease. N. Engl. J. Med. 282: 1283–1287, 1970.

5162. Holt, L. E. Diseases of Infancy and Childhood. Appleton and Company, New York, 1897.

5163. Horsfield, K. and Cumming, G. Morphology of the bronchial tree in man. J. Appl. Physiol. 24: 373–383, 1968.

5164. Horsfield, K., Dart, G., Olson, D. E., Filley, G. F., and Cumming, G. Models of human bronchial tree. J. Appl. Physiol. 31: 207–217, 1971.

5165. Houston, J. C., DeNevasquez, S., and Trounce, J. R. A clinical and pathologic study of fatal cases of status asthmaticus. Thorax 8: 207–213, 1953.

5166. Huchon, G. J., Little, J. W., and Murray, J. F. Assessment of alveolar-capillary membrane permeability of dogs by aerosolization. J. Appl. Physiol. 51: 955–972, 1981.

5167. Hulbert, W. C., Forster, B. B., Laird, W., Pihl, C. E., and Walker, D. C. An improved method of fixation of the respiratory epithelial surface with mucus and surfactant layers. Lab. Invest. 47: 354–363, 1982.

5168. Hulbert, W. C., Walker, D. C., Jackson, A., and Hogg, J. C. Airway permeability to horseradish peroxidase in guinea pigs: the repair phase after injury by cigarette smoke. Am. Rev. Respir. Dis. 123: 320–326, 1981.

5169. Hunninghake, G. W., Gaudec, J. E., Kawamami, O., Feranz, V. J., and Crystal, R. G. Inflammatory and immune processes in the human lung in health and disease: evaluation by bronchoalveolar lavage. Am. J. Pathol. 97: 149–206, 1979.

5170. Ishizaka, K. and Ishizaka, T. Biological function of gamma E antibodies and mechanisms of reaginic hypersensitivity. Clin. Exp. Immunol. 6: 24–42, 1970.

5171. Jacobs, J. W., Peacock, D. B., Cornber, B. D., Caul, E. O., and Clark, S. K. R. Respiratory, syncytial and other viruses associated with respiratory tract disease in infants. Lancet i: 871–876, 1971.

5172. Jeffries, E., Pare, P. D., and Hogg, J. C. Measurements of airway edema in allergic bronchoconstriction in the guinea pig. Am. Rev. Respir. Dis. 123: 687–688, 1981.

5173. Jones, J. G., Minty, B. D., Lawler, P., Hulands, G., Crawley, J. C. W., and Veall, N. Increased alveolar epithelial permeability in cigarette smokers. Lancet i: 66–68, 1980.

5174. Joubert, J. R., Ascah, K., Moroz, L. A., and Hogg, J. C. Acute hypersensitivity pneumonitis in the rabbit: an animal model with horseradish peroxidase as antigen. Am. Rev. Respir. Dis. 113: 503–513, 1976.

5175. Kawanami, O., Basset, F., Barrios, R., Lacronique, J., Ferrans, V., and Crystal, R. G. Hypersensitivity pneumonitis in man: light and electron microscopic studies of 18 lung biopsies. Am. J. Pathol. 110: 275–289, 1983.

5176. Laennec, R. T. H. A Treatise on the Diseases of the Chest. Translated by J. Forbes. T & G Underwood, London, 1821.

5177. Lander, F. P. L. Bronchiectasis and atelectasis; temporary and permanent changes. Thorax 1: 198–210, 1946.

5178. Levine, B. B., Stember, R. H., and Fotino, M. Ragweed fever, genetic control and linkage to HLA haptotypes. Science 178: 1201–1203, 1972.

5179. Liebow, A. A. Pulmonary emphysema with special reference to vascular changes. Am. Rev. Respir. Dis. 80: 67–93, 1959.

5180. Liebow, A., Hales, M. R., and Lindskog, G. E. Enlargement of the bronchial arteries and their anastomoses with the pulmonary artery in bronchiectasis. Am. J. Pathol. 25: 211–231, 1949.

5181. Lindsay, M. I. Jr., Herrmann, E. C. Jr., Morrow, G. W. Jr., and Brown, A. L. Hong Kong influenza: clinical, microbiologic and pathologic features in 127 cases. J.A.M.A. 214: 1825–1832, 1970.

5182. Macleod, W. N. Abnormal transradiancy of one lung. Thorax 9: 147–153, 1954.

5183. Macklem, P. T., Fraser, R. G., and Brown, W. G. Bronchial pressure measurements in emphysema and bronchitis. J. Clin. Invest. 44: 897–905, 1965.

5184. Macklem, P. T. and Mead, J. The resistance of central and peripheral airways measured by a retrograde catheter. J. Appl. Physiol. 22: 395–402, 1967.

5185. Macklem, P. T., Proctor, D. F., and Hogg, J. C. The stability of the peripheral airways. Respir. Physiol. 8: 191–203, 1970.

5186. Mallory, T. B. The pathogenesis of bronchiectasis. N. Engl. J. Med. 237: 795–798, 1947.

5187. Man, S. F. P., Hulbert, W. C., Park, D. S. K., Thomson, A. B. R., and Hogg, J. C. Asymmetry of canine tracheal epithelium: osmotically-induced changes. J. Appl. Physiol. 57: 1338–1346, 1984.

5188. McLelland, L., Hilleman, M. R., Hamparian, V. V., Ketler, A., Riley, C. M., Cornfield, D., and Stokes, J. Jr. Stages of acute respiratory illness caused by respiratory syncytial virus. N. Engl. J. Med. 264: 1169–1175, 1961.

5189. McDermott, M. R., Befus, A. D., and Bienenstock, J. The structural basis of immunity in the respiratory tract. Int. Rev. Exp. Pathol. 23: 47–112, 1982.

5190. McLean, K. H. The pathology of acute bronchiolitis—a study of its evolution. Part I. The exudative phase. Aust. Ann. Med. 5: 254–267, 1956.

5191. McLean, K. H. The pathology of acute bronchiolitis—a study of its evolution. Part II. The repair phase. Aust. Ann. Med. 6: 29–43, 1957.

5192. Mead, J., Takishima, T., and Leith, D. Stress distribution in lungs: a model of pulmonary elasticity. J. Appl. Physiol. 28: 596–608, 1970.

5193. Mead, J., Turner, J. M., Macklem, P. T., and Little, J. B. The significance of the relationship between lung recoil and maximum expiratory flow. J. Appl. Physiol. 22: 95–108, 1967.

5194. Menkes, H. A., Permutt, S., and Cohen, B. H. Patterns of pulmonary function abnormalities in high risk groups. In: Macklem, P. T. and Permutt, S. (eds.). The Lung in the Transition between Health and Disease. Marcel Dekker, New York and Basel, 1979.

5195. Meyer, E. C., Dominguez, E. A. M., and Bensch, C. G. Pulmonary lymphatic and blood absorption of albumin from alveoli; a quantitative comparison. Lab. Invest. 20: 1–8, 1969.

5196. Miller, W. S. The distribution of lymphoid tissue in the lung. Anat. Rec. 5: 99–119, 1911.

5197. Morrow, P. E., Gibb, E. R., and Gazioglu, K. M. A study of particulate disappearance from the human lungs. Am. Rev. Respir. Dis. 96: 1209–1221, 1967.

5198. Nadel, J. A. Structure and function relationships in the airways. Med. Thoracalis 22: 231–243, 1965.

5199. Nagashi, C. Functional Anatomy and Histology of the Lung. University Park Press, Baltimore and London, 1972.

5200. Naylor, B. The shedding of the mucosa of the bronchial tree in asthma. Thorax 17: 69–72, 1962.

5201. Niewohner, D. E. and Kleinerman, J. Morphologic basis of pulmonary resistance in the human lung and effects of aging. J. Appl. Physiol. 36: 412–418, 1974.

5202. O'Reilly, J. F. Adult bronchiolitis in para-influenza type II. Postgrad. Med. J. 56: 787–788, 1980.

5203. Parish, W. E. Farmer's lung. Part I. An immunologic study of some antigenic components of mouldy foodstuffs. Thorax 18: 83–89, 1963.

5204. Patterson, R., Tomita, M., Oh, S. A., Suszko, I. M., and Pruzansky, J. J. Respiratory mast cells and basophil cells. I. Evidence that they are secreted into the bronchial lumen; morphology, degranulation and histamine release. Clin. Exp. Immunol. 16: 223–234, 1974.

5205. Pepys, J., Jenkins, P. A., Festenstein, G. N., Gregory, P. H., Lacey, M. E., and Skinner, F. A. Farmer's lung: thermophilic actinomycetes as a source of "farmer's lung" hay antigen. Lancet ii: 607–611, 1963.

5206. Petty, T. L., Silvers, G. W., Stanford, R. E., Baird, M. D., and Mitchell, R. S. Small airways pathology is related to increased closing capacity and abnormal slope of phase III in excised human lung. Am. Rev. Respir. Dis. 121: 449–456, 1980.

5207. Pickering, C. A., Moore, W. K. S., Lacey, J., Holford-Stevens, V., and Pepys, J. Investigation of respiratory disease associated with an air-conditioning system. Clin. Allergy 6: 109–118, 1976.

5208. Reid, L. Reduction in the bronchial subdivisions in bronchiectasis. Thorax 5: 233–247, 1950.

5209. Reid, L. and Simon, G. Unilateral lung transradiancy. Thorax 17: 230–239, 1962.

5210. Reynolds, H. Y., Fulmer, J. D., Kazmierowski, J. A., Roberts, W. C., Frank, M. M., and Crystal, R. G. Analysis of cellular and protein content of bronchoalveolar lavage fluid from patients with idiopathic pulmonary fibrosis and chronic hypersensitivity pneumonitis. J. Clin. Invest. 59: 165–175, 1977.

5211. Richardson, J. B. and Beland, J. Nonadrenergic inhibitory nervous system in human airways. J. Appl. Physiol. 41: 764–771, 1976.

5212. Richerson, H. B., Cheng, H. F., and Bauserman, S. C. Acute experimental hypersensitivity pneumonitis in rabbits. Am. Rev. Respir. Dis. 104: 568–575, 1971.

5213. Rigler, L. and Koucky, R. Roentgen studies of pathological physiology of bronchial asthma. Am. J. Roentgenol. 39: 353–362, 1938.

5214. Roser, B. The origins, kinetics and fate of macrophage populations. J. Reticuloendothel. Soc. 8: 139–161, 1970.

5215. Saltos, N., Sanders, N. A., Bhagwandeen, S. B., and Jarvie, B. Hypersensitivity pneumonitis in a mouldy house. Med. J. Aust. 2: 244–246, 1982.

5216. Salvaggio, J. E. and Laskowitz, S. The comparison of immunological responses of normal and atopic individuals to potential precipitated protein antigen. Int. Rev. Exp. Pathol. 26: 264–268, 1965.

5217. Salvato, G. Mast cells in bronchial connective tissues of man: their modification in asthma and after treatment with histamine liberator 48/80. Int. Arch. Allergy 18: 348–358, 1961.

5218. Salvato, G. Asthma and mast cells of bronchial connective tissue. Experientia 18: 330–331, 1962.

5219. Sanerkin, N. G. and Evans, D. M. D. The sputum in bronchial asthma: pathognomic patterns. J. Pathol. Bacteriol. 89: 535–541, 1965.

5220. Satir, P. How cilia move. Sci. Am. 231: 44–63, 1974.

5221. Schellenberg, R. R. Pathophysiology of allergic diseases. In: Devlin, J. P. (ed.). Pulmonary and Antiallergic Drugs. John Wiley & Sons, New York, 1985.

5222. Seal, R. M. E., Hapke, E. J., Thomas, G. O., Meek, J. C., and Hayes, M. The pathology of the acute and chronic stages of farmer's lung. Thorax 23: 469–489, 1968.

5223. Simami, A. S., Inoue, S., and Hogg, J. C. Penetration of respiratory epithelium of guinea pigs following exposure to cigarette smoke. Lab. Invest. 31: 75–81, 1974.

5224. Spencer, H. Pathology of the Lung, Vol. 1. Pergamon Press, Oxford, 1977.

5225. Stokes, G. M., Milner, A. D., Hodges, I. G., and Groggins, R. C. Lung function abnormalities after acute bronchiolitis. J. Pediatr. 98: 871–874, 1981.

5226. Sutinen, S., Reijula, K., Huhti, E., and Karkola, P. Extrinsic allergic bronchiolo-alveolitis: serology and biopsy findings. Eur. J. Respir. Dis. 64: 271–282, 1983.

5227. Swyer, P. R. and James, G. Case of unilateral pulmonary emphysema. Thorax 8: 133–136, 1953.

5228. Szentivanyi, A. The beta adrenergic theory of the atopic abnormality in bronchial asthma. J. Allergy 42: 203–232, 1968.

5229. Tada, T. Regulation of reaginic antibody formation in animals. Prog. Allergy 19: 122–194, 1975.

5230. Tannenberg, J. and Pinner, M. J. Atelectasis and bronchiectasis. J. Thorac. Surg. 11: 571–616, 1942.

5231. Thorsby, E., Engeset, A., and Lie, S. O. HLA antigens and susceptibility to diseases. Tissue Antigens 1: 147–152, 1971.

5232. Totten, R. S., Reid, D. H., Davis, H. D., and Moran, T. J.

Farmer's lung: report of two cases in which lung biopsies were performed. Am. J. Med. 25: 803–809, 1958.

5233. Turner-Warwick, M. Extrinsic allergic bronchiolo-alveolitis. Current Topics in Immunology Series. No. 10. Immunology of the Lung. Edward Arnold, London, 1978, pp. 165–190.

5234. Van Brabandt, H., Caubergh, S. M., Verbeken, P., Moerman, P., Lauweryns, J. M., and Van de Woestijne, K. P. Partitioning of impedance in excised human and canine lungs. J. Appl. Physiol. 55: 1733–1742, 1983.

5235. Vracko, R. V. Basal lamina layering in diabetes mellitus: evidence for accelerated rate of cell death and cell regeneration. Diabetes 23: 94–104, 1974.

5236. Vracko, R. V. and Benditt, E. P. Manifestations of diabetes mellitus: their possible relationships to an underlying cell defect. Am. J. Pathol. 75: 204–224, 1974.

5237. Warren, K. S. Granulomatous inflammation. In: Lepow, I. H. and Ward, P. A. (eds.). Inflammation: Mechanisms and Control. Academic Press, New York, 1972.

5238. Warte, D., Steele, R., Ross, I., Wakefield, J., McKay, J., and Wallace, J. Cilia and sperm tail abnormalities in Polynesian bronchiectatics. Lancet ii: 132–133, 1978.

5239. Weibel, E. R. Morphometry of the Human Lung. Springer, Heidelberg and Academic Press, New York, 1963.

5240. Weibel, E. R. Structure and Function of the Mammalian Respiratory System. Harvard University Press, Cambridge, 1984.

5241. Wenman, W. M., Pagtiakhan, R. D., Reed, M. H., Chernick, V., and Albritton, W. Adenovirus bronchiolitis in Manitoba: epidemiologic, clinical and radiologic features. Chest 81: 605–609, 1982.

5242. Wensel, F. J., Emmanuel, D. A., Lawton, B. R., and Magnen, G. E. Isolation of the causative agent of farmer's lung. Ann. Allergy 22: 533–540, 1964.

5243. Whitwell, F. A study of the pathology and pathogenesis of bronchiectasis. Thorax 7: 213–239, 1952.

5244. Winternitz, M. C., Smith, G. H., and McNamara, F. P. The effect of intrabronchial insufflation of acid. J. Exp. Med. 32: 199–217, 1920.

5245. Wohl, M. E. B. and Chernick, V. Bronchiolitis: state of the art. Am. Rev. Respir. Dis. 118: 759–786, 1978.

5246. Zweifach, E. W., Grant, L., and McCluskey, R. T. (eds.). The Inflammatory Process, Vols. I, II, and III. 2nd ed. Academic Press, New York, 1974.

5247. Zweiman, B. and Levinson, A. I. Cell-mediated immunity. In: Elliot, M. Jr., Reed, C. E., and Ellis, E. F. (eds.). Allergy: Principles and Practice. C. V. Mosby Co., St. Louis, 1983.

5248. Penketh, A., Higenbottam, T., Hakim, M., and Wallwork, J. Heart and lung transplantation in patients with end stage lung disease. Br. Med. J. 295: 311–314, 1987.

5249. DeTroyer, A., Kelly, S., Macklem, P. T., and Zin, W. A. Mechanics of intercostal space and actions of external and internal intercostal muscles. J. Clin. Invest. 75: 850–857, 1985.

5250. Wanner, A. State of the art. Clinical aspects of mucociliary transport. Am. Rev. Respir. Dis. 116: 73–125, 1977.

5251. Pavia, D., Bateman, J. R. M., Sheahan, N. F., Agnew, J. E., Newman, S. P., and Clarke, S. W. Techniques for measuring lung mucociliary clearance. Eur. J. Respir. Dis. 61(Suppl. 110): 157–168, 1980.

5252. Millar, A. B., Agnew, J. E., Newman, S. P., Lopez-Vidriero, M. T., Pavia, D., and Clarke, S. W. Comparison of nasal and tracheobronchial clearance by similar techniques in normal subjects. Thorax 41: 783–786, 1986.

5253. Puchelle, E., Zahm, J. M., and Bertrand, A. Influence of age on bronchial mucociliary transport. Scand. J. Respir. Dis. 60: 307–313, 1979.

5254. Vastag, E., Mattys, H., Zsamboki, G., Kohler, D., and Daikeler, G. Mucociliary clearance in smokers. Eur. J. Respir. Dis. 68: 107–113, 1986.

5255. Whaley, S. L., Muggenburg, B. A., Seiler, F. A., and Wolff, R. K. Effects of aging on tracheal mucociliary clearance in beagle dogs. J. Appl. Physiol. 62: 1331–1334, 1987.

5256. Landa, J. F., Hirsch, J. A., and Lebeaux, M. I. Effects of topical and general anesthetic agents on tracheal mucous velocity of sheep. J. Appl. Physiol. 38: 946–948, 1975.

5257. Forbes, A. R. and Horrigan, R. W. Mucociliary flow in the trachea during anesthesia with enflurane, ether, nitrous oxide, and morphine. Anesthesiology 46: 319–321, 1977.

5258. Yeates, D. B., Sturgess, J. M., Kahn, S. R., Levison, H., and Aspin, N. Mucociliary transport in trachea of patients with cystic fibrosis. Arch. Dis. Child. 51: 28–33, 1976.

5259. Pavia, D., Sutton, P. P., Lopez-Vidriero, M. T., Agnew, J. E., and Clarke, S. W. Drug effects on mucociliary function. Eur. J. Respir. Dis. 64(Suppl. 128): 304–317, 1983.

5260. Matthys, H. Mucociliary clearance measurements in patients. Excerpta Medica (Asia Pacific Congress Series) 33: 31–39, 1984.

5261. Wolff, R. K. Effects of airborne pollutants on mucociliary clearance. Environ. Health Perspect. 66: 223–237, 1986.

5262. Foster, W. M., Langenback, E. G., and Bergofsky, E. H. Dissociation in the mucociliary function of central and peripheral airways of asymptomatic smokers. Am. Rev. Respir. Dis. 132: 633–639, 1985.

5263. Agnew, J. E., Lopez-Vidriero, M. T., Pavia, D., and Clarke, S. W. Functional small airways defence in symptomless cigarette smokers. Thorax 41: 524–530, 1986.

5264. Agnew, J. E., Bateman, J. R. M., Pavia, D., and Clarke, S. W. Peripheral airways mucus clearance in stable asthma is improved by oral corticosteroid therapy. Bull. Eur. Physiopathol. 20: 295–301, 1984.

5265. Wanner, A., Zarzecki, S., Hirsch, J., and Epstein, S. Tracheal mucous transport in experimental canine asthma. J. Appl. Physiol. 39: 950–957, 1975.

5266. Sutton, P. P., Parker, R. A., Webber, B. A., Newman, S. P., Garland, N., Lopez-Vidriero, M. T., Pavia, D., and Clarke, S. W. Assessment of the forced expiration technique, postural drainage and directed coughing in chest physiotherapy. Eur. J. Respir. Dis. 64: 62–68, 1983.

5267. DeBoeck, C. and Zinman, R. Cough versus chest physiotherapy. A comparison of the acute effects on pulmonary function in patients with cystic fibrosis. Am. Rev. Respir. Dis. 129: 182–184, 1984.

5268. Pirsig, R. M. Zen and the Art of Motorcycle Maintenance. Bantam Books, Toronto, New York, and London, 1974.

5269. Rechtscaffen, A. and Kales, A. (eds.). A Manual of Standardized Terminology, Techniques, and Scoring Systems for Sleep Stages of Human Subjects. National Institute of Neurological Disease and Blindness, Washington, D.C. NIH Publication No. 204, 1968.

5270. Phillipson, E. A. Control of breathing during sleep. Am. Rev. Respir. Dis. 118: 909–939, 1978.

5271. Phillipson, E. A. and Sullivan, C. E. Arousal: the forgotten response to respiratory stimuli. Am. Rev. Respir. Dis. 118: 807–809, 1978.

5272. Robin, E. D., White, R. D., Crump, C. H., and Travis, D. M. Alveolar gas tensions, pulmonary ventilation and blood pH during physiologic sleep in normal subjects. J. Clin. Invest. 37: 981–989, 1958.

5273. Douglas, N. J., White, D. P., Pickett, C. K., Weil, J. V., and Zwillich, C. W. Respiration during sleep in normal man. Thorax 37: 840–844, 1982.

5274. Gothe, B., Altose, M. D., Goldman, M. D., and Cherniack, N. S. Effect of quiet sleep on resting and CO_2 stimulated breathing in humans. J. Appl. Physiol. 50: 724–730, 1981.

5275. Douglas, N. J., White, D. P., Weil, J. V., Pickett, C. K., and Zwillich, C. W. Hypercapnic ventilatory response in sleeping adults. Am. Rev. Respir. Dis. 126: 758–762, 1982.

5276. Gothe, B., Goldman, M. D., Cherniack, N. S., and Mantey, P. Effect of progressive hypoxia on breathing during sleep. Am. Rev. Respir. Dis. 126: 97–102, 1982.

5277. Douglas, N. J., White, D. P., Weil, J. V., Pickett, C. K., Martin, R. J., Hudgel, D. W., and Zwillich, C. W. Hypoxic ventilatory response decreases during sleep in normal men. Am. Rev. Respir. Dis. 125: 286–289, 1982.

5278. Phillipson, E. A., Kozar, L. F., Rebuck, A. S., and Murphy, E. Ventilatory and waking responses to CO_2 in sleeping dogs. Am. Rev. Respir. Dis. 115: 251–259, 1977.

5279. Phillipson, E. A., Sullivan, C. E., Read, D. J. C., Murphy, E., and Kozar, L. F. Ventilatory and waking responses to hypoxia in sleeping dogs. J. Appl. Physiol. 44: 512–520, 1978.

5280. Phillipson, E. A., Kozar, L. F., and Murphy, E. Respiratory load compensation in awake and sleeping dogs. J. Appl. Physiol. 40: 895–902, 1976.

5281. Sullivan, C. E., Murphy, E., Kozar, L. F., and Phillipson, E. A. Waking and ventilatory responses to laryngeal stimulation in sleeping dogs. J. Appl. Physiol. 45: 681–689, 1978.

5282. Sullivan, C. E., Kozar, L. F., Murphy, E., and Phillipson, E. A. Arousal, ventilatory, and airway responses to bronchopulmonary stimulation in sleeping dogs. J. Appl. Physiol. 47: 17–25, 1979.

5283. Berthon-Jones, M. and Sullivan, C. E. Ventilatory and arousal responses to hypoxia in sleeping humans. Am. Rev. Respir. Dis. 125: 632–639, 1982.

5284. Tusiewicz, K., Moldofsky, H., Bryan, A. C., and Bryan, M. H. Mechanics of the rib cage and diaphragm during sleep. J. Appl. Physiol. 43: 600–602, 1977.

5285. Muller, N. L., Francis, P. W., Gurwitz, D., Levison, H., and Bryan, A. C. Mechanism of hemoglobin desaturation during rapid-eye-movement sleep in normal subjects and in patients with cystic fibrosis. Am. Rev. Respir. Dis. 121: 463–469, 1980.

5286. Remmers, J. E., DeGroot, W. J., Sauerland, E. K., and Anch, A. M. Pathogenesis of upper airway occlusion during sleep. J. Appl. Physiol. 44: 931–938, 1978.

5287. Jamal, K., McMahon, G., Edgell, G., and Fleetham, J. A. Cough and arousal responses to inhaled citric acid in sleeping humans (abstract). Am. Rev. Respir. Dis. 127: 237, 1983.

5288. Huxley, E. J., Viroslav, J., Gray, W. R., and Pierce, A. K. Pharyngeal aspiration in normal adults and patients with depressed consciousness. Am. J. Med. 64: 564–568, 1978.

5289. Sullivan, C. E., Zamel, N., Kozar, L. F., Murphy, E., and Phillipson, E. A. Regulation of airway smooth muscle tone in sleeping dogs. Am. Rev. Respir. Dis. 119: 87–99, 1979.

5290. Martin, R. J., Block, A. J., Cohn, M. A., Conway, W. A., Hudgel, D. W., Powles, A. C. P., Sanders, M. H., and Smith, P. L. Indications and standards for cardiopulmonary sleep studies. Sleep 8: 371–379, 1985.

5291. Cohn, M. A., Rao, A. S. V., Broudy, M., Birch, S., Warson, H., Atkins, N., Davis, B., Stott, F. D., and Sackner, M. A. The respiratory inductive plethysmograph: a new non-invasive monitor of respiration. Bull. Eur. Physiopathol. Respir. 18: 643–658, 1982.

5292. Lemen, R., Benson, M., and Jones, J. G. Absolute pressure measurements with hand-dipped and manufactured esophageal balloons. J. Appl. Physiol. 37: 600–603, 1974.

5293. West, P. and Kryger, M. H. Continuous monitoring of respiratory variables during sleep by microcomputer. Methods Inf. Med. 22: 198–203, 1983.

5294. Burwell, C. S., Robin, E. D., Whaley, R. D., and Bickelmann, A. G. Extreme obesity associated with alveolar hypoventilation—a Pickwickian syndrome. Am. J. Med. 21: 811–818, 1956.

5295. Gastaut, H., Tassinari, C. A., and Duron, B. Etude polygraphique des manifestations épisodique (hypnique et respiratoires), diurnes et nocturne, du syndrome de Pickwick. Rev. Neurol. 112: 568–579, 1965.

5296. Jung, R. and Kuhlo, W. Neurophysiological studies of abnormal night sleep and the Pickwickian syndrome in sleep mechanisms. Prog. Brain. Res. 18: 140–160, 1965.

5297. Guilleminault, C., Tilkian, A., and Dement, W. C. The sleep apnea syndromes. Annu. Rev. Med. 27: 465–484, 1976.

5298. Storr, J., Barrell, E., and Lenney, W. Asthma in primary schools. Br. Med. J. 295: 251–252, 1987.

5299. Zorick, F., Roth, T., Kramer, M., and Kless, H. Exacerbation of upper airway sleep apnea by lymphatic lymphoma. Chest 77: 689–690, 1980.

5300. Orr, W. C. and Martin, R. J. Obstructive sleep apnea associated with tonsillar hypertrophy in adults. Arch. Intern. Med. 141: 990–992, 1981.

5301. Mezon, B. J., West, P., Maclean, J. P., and Kryger, M. H. Sleep apnea in acromegaly. Am. J. Med. 69: 615–618, 1980.

5302. Conway, W. A., Bower, C. G., and Barnes, M. E. Hypersomnolence and intermittent upper airway obstruction: occurrence caused by micrognathia. J.A.M.A. 237: 2740–2742, 1977.

5303. Haponik, E. F., Smith, P. L., Bohlman, M. E., Allen, R. P., Goldman, S. M., and Bleecker, E. R. Computerized tomography in obstructive sleep apnea. Correlation of airway size with physiology during sleep and wakefulness. Am. Rev. Respir. Dis. 127: 221–226, 1983.

5304. Rivlin, J., Hoffstein, V., Kalbfleisch, J., McNicholas, W., Zamel, N., and Bryan, A. C. Upper airway morphology in patients with idiopathic obstructive sleep apnea. Am. Rev. Respir. Dis. 129: 355–360, 1984.

5305. Brown, I. G., Bradley, T. D., Phillipson, E. A., Zamel, N., and Hoffstein, V. Pharyngeal compliance in snoring subjects with and without obstructive sleep apnea. Am. Rev. Respir. Dis. 132: 211–215, 1985.

5306. Block, A. J., Faulkner, J. A., Hughes, R. L., Remmers, J. E., and Thach, B. Factors affecting upper airway closure. Chest 86: 114–122, 1984.

5307. Rodenstein, D. O. and Stanescu, D. C. The soft palate and breathing. Am. Rev. Respir. Dis. 134: 311–325, 1986.

5308. Riley, R., Guilleminault, C., Herran, J., and Powell, N. Cephalometric analyses and flow-volume loops in obstructive sleep apnea patients. Sleep 6: 303–311, 1983.

5309. Shelton, R. L. Jr. and Bosma, J. F. Maintenance of the pharyngeal airway. J. Appl. Physiol. 17: 209–214, 1962.

5310. Suratt, P. M., Dee, P., Atkinson, R. L., Armstrong, P., and Wilhoit, S. C. Fluoroscopic and computed tomographic features of the pharyngeal airway in obstructive sleep apnea. Am. Rev. Respir. Dis. 127: 487–492, 1983.

5311. Anch, A. M., Remmers, J. E., Sauerland, E. K., and DeGroot, W. J. Oropharyngeal patency during waking and sleep in the Pickwickian syndrome: electromyographic activity of the tensor veli palatini. Electromyogr. Clin. Neurophysiol. 21: 317–330, 1981.

5312. Weitzman, E., Pollak, C., Borowiecki, B., Burack, B., Shprintzen, R., and Rakoff, S. The hypersomnia-sleep apnea syndrome: site and mechanisms of upper airway obstruction. In: Guilleminault, C. and Dement, W. C. (eds.). Sleep Apnea Syndromes. Alan R. Liss, New York, 1978.

5313. Brouillette, R. T. and Thach, B. T. A neuromuscular mechanism maintaining extrathoracic airway patency. J. Appl. Physiol. 46: 772–779, 1979.

5314. Sauerland, E. K. and Harper, R. M. The human tongue during sleep: electromyographic activity of the genioglossus muscle. Exp. Neurol. 51: 160–170, 1976.

5315. Markowe, H. L. J., Bulpitt, C. J., Shipley, M. J., Rose, G., Crombie, D. L., and Fleming, D. M. Prognosis in adult asthma. Br. Med. J. 295: 949–952, 1987.

5316. Krol, R. C., Knuth, S. I., and Bartlett, D. Jr. Selective reduction of genioglossal muscle activity by alcohol in normal human subjects. Am. Rev. Respir. Dis. 129: 247–250, 1984.

5317. Bonora, M., St. John, W. M., and Bledsoe, T. A. Differential elevation by protriptyline and depression by diazepam of upper airway motor activity. Am. Rev. Respir. Dis. 131: 41–45, 1985.

5318. Patrick, G. B., Strohn, K. P., Rubin, S. B., and Altose, M. D. Upper airway and diaphragm muscle responses to chemical stimulation and loading. J. Appl. Physiol. 53: 1133–1137, 1982.

5319. Weiner, D., Mitra, J., Salamone, J., and Cherniack, N. S. Effect of chemical stimuli on nerves supplying upper airway muscles. J. Appl. Physiol. 52: 530–536, 1982.

5320. Sullivan, C. E. and Issa, F. G. Obstructive sleep apnea. Clin. Chest Med. 6: 633–650, 1985.

5321. Guilleminault, C., Van den Hoed, J., and Mitler, M. M. Clinical overview of the sleep apnea syndrome. In: Guilleminault, C. and Dement, W. C. (eds.). Sleep Apnea Syndromes. Alan R. Liss, New York, 1978.

5322. Strohl, K. P., Saunders, N. A., and Sullivan, C. E. Clinical aspects of sleep apnea syndromes. In: Sullivan, C. and Saunders, N. A. (eds.). Sleep and Breathing, Vol. 14. Lung Biology in Health and Disease. Marcel Dekker, New York, 1984.

5323. Guilleminault, C. and Winkle, R. A review of 50 children with OSAS. Lung 159: 275–287, 1981.

5324. Yoss, R. E. and Daly, D. D. Narcolepsy. Arch. Intern. Med. 106: 168–171, 1960.

5325. Wynne, J. W. Obstruction of the nose and breathing during sleep. Chest 82: 657–658, 1982.

5326. Harmen, E. M., Wynne, J. W., and Block, A. J. The effect of weight loss on sleep-disordered breathing and oxygen desaturation in morbidly obese men. Chest 82: 291–294, 1982.

5327. Guilleminault, C. and Hayes, B. Naloxone, theophylline, bromocriptine, and obstructive sleep apnea. Negative results. Bull. Eur. Physiopathol. Respir. 19: 632–634, 1983.

5328. Brownell, L. G., West, M. P., Sweatman, P., Acres, J. C., and Kryger, M. H. Protriptyline in obstructive sleep apnea: a double blind trial. N. Engl. J. Med. 307: 1037–1042, 1982.

5329. Sullivan, C. E., Issa, F. G., Berthon-Jones, M., and Eves, L. Reversal of obstructive sleep apnea by continuous positive pressure applied through the nares. Lancet i: 862–865, 1981.

5330. Berry, R. B. and Block, A. J. Positive nasal airway pressure eliminates snoring as well as obstructive sleep apnea. Chest 85: 15–20, 1984.

5331. Rapaport, D. M., Garay, S. M., and Goldring, R. M. Nasal CPAP in obstructive sleep apnea: mechanisms of action. Bull. Eur. Physiopathol. Respir. 19: 616–620, 1983.

5332. Strohl, K. P. and Redline, S. Nasal CPAP therapy, upper airway muscle activation, and obstructive sleep apnea. Am. Rev. Respir. Dis. 134: 555–558, 1986.

5333. Cooper, K. R. and Phillips, B. A. Effect of short-term sleep loss on breathing. J. Appl. Physiol. 53: 855–858, 1982.

5334. Berthon-Jones, M. and Sullivan, C. E. Time course of change in ventilatory response to CO_2 with long-term CPAP therapy for obstructive sleep apnea. Am. Rev. Respir. Dis. 135: 144–147, 1987.

5335. Sullivan, C. E., Issa, F. G., Berthon-Jones, M., McCauley, V. B., and Costas, L. J. V. Home treatment of obstructive sleep apnoea with continuous positive airway pressure applied through a nose-mask. Bull. Eur. Physiopathol. Respir. 20: 49–54, 1984.

5336. Guilleminault, C. and Mondini, S. Need for multidiagnostic approaches before considering treatment in obstructive sleep apnea. Bull. Eur. Physiopathol. Respir. 19: 583–589, 1983.

5337. Lowe, A. A., Gionhaku, N., Takeuchi, K., and Fleetham, J. A. Three dimensional CT reconstructions of tongue and airway in adult subjects with obstructive sleep apnea. Am. J. Orthod. 90: 364–384, 1986.

5338. Lowe, A. A., Santamaria, J. D., Fleetham, J. A., and Price, C. Facial morphology and obstructive sleep apnea. Am. J. Orthod. 90: 484–491, 1986.

5339. Bradley, T. D., Brown, I. G., Grossman, R. F., Zamel, N., Martinez, D., Phillipson, E. A., and Hoffstein, V. Pharyngeal size in snorers, non-snorers, and patients with obstructive sleep apnea. N. Engl. J. Med. 315: 1327–1331, 1986.

5340. Fujita, S., Conway, W. A., Sicklesteel, J. M., Wittig, R. M., Zorick, F. J., Roehrs, T. A., and Roth, T. Evaluation of the effectiveness of uvulopalatopharyngoplasty. Laryngoscope 95: 70–74, 1985.

5341. Simmons, F. B., Guilleminault, C., and Silvestri, R. Snoring, and some obstructive sleep apnea can be cured by oropharyngeal surgery. Arch. Otolaryngol. 109: 503–507, 1983.

5342. Guilleminault, C., Hayes, B., Smith, L., and Simmons, F. B. Palatopharyngoplasty and obstructive sleep apnea syndrome. Bull. Eur. Physiopathol. Respir. 19: 595–599, 1983.

5343. Conway, W., Fujita, S., Zorick, F., Sicklesteel, J., Roehrs, T., Wittig, R., and Roth, T. Uvulopalatopharyngoplasty. One year follow-up. Chest 88: 385–387, 1985.

5344. Hyland, R. H., Jones, N. L., Powles, A. C. P., Lenkie, S. C. M., Vanderlinden, R. G., and Epstein, S. W. Primary alveolar hypoventilation treated with nocturnal electrophrenic respiration. Am. Rev. Respir. Dis. 117: 165–172, 1978.

5345. Cirignotta, F. and Lugaresi, E. Some cineradiographic aspects of snoring and obstructive apneas. Sleep 3: 225–226, 1980.

5346. Lugaresi, E., Coccagna, G., Farneti, P., Mantovani, M., and Cirignotta, F. Snoring. Electroencephalogr. Clin. Neurophysiol. 39: 59–64, 1975.

5347. Koskenvuo, M., Partinen, M., Sarna, S., Kaprio, J., Langinvaino, H., and Heikkila, K. Snoring as a risk factor for hypertension and angina pectoris. Lancet i: 893–896, 1985.

5348. Coccagna, G., Mantovani, M., Brignani, F., Parchi, C., and Lugaresi, E. Continuous recording of the pulmonarey and systemic arterial pressure during sleep in syndromes of hypersomnia with periodic breathing. Bull. Physiopathol. Respir. 8: 1159–1172, 1972.

5349. Naeye, R. Pulmonary arterial abnormalities in the sudden infant death syndrome. N. Engl. J. Med. 289: 1167–1170, 1973.

5350. Bruhn, F., Mokrohisky, S., and McIntosh, K. Apnea associated with respiratory syncytial virus infection in young infants. Pediatrics 90: 382–386, 1977.

5351. Hunt, C., McCulloch, K., and Brouillette, R. Diminished hypoxic ventilatory responses in near miss SIDS. J. Appl. Physiol. 50: 1313–1317, 1981.

5352. Moore, G. C., Zwillich, C. W., Battaglia, J. D., Cotton, E. K., and Weill, J. V. Respiratory failure associated with familial depression of ventilatory response to hypoxia and hypercapnia. N. Engl. J. Med. 295: 861–865, 1976.

5353. Schiffman, P., Westlake, R., Santiago, T., and Edelman, N. Ventilatory control in parents of victims of sudden infant death syndrome. N. Engl. J. Med. 302: 486–491, 1980.

5354. Zwillich, C., McCullough, R., Guilleminault, C., Cummiskey, J., and Weil, J. V. Respiratory control in the parents of sudden infant death syndrome victims. Pediatr. Res. 14: 762–764, 1980.

5355. Acres, J. C., Sweatman, P., West, P., Brownell, L., and Kryger, M. H. Breathing during sleep in parents of sudden infant death syndrome victims. Am. Rev. Respir. Dis. 125: 163–166, 1982.

5356. Butler, J. The pulmonary function test: cautious overinterpretation (editorial). Chest 79: 498–500, 1981.

5357. Trask, C. H. and Cree, E. M. Oximeter studies on patients with chronic obstructive emphysema awake and during sleep. N. Engl. J. Med. 266: 639–642, 1962.

5358. Coccagna, G. and Lugaresi, E. Arterial blood gases and pulmonary and systemic arterial pressure during sleep in chronic obstructive pulmonary disease. Sleep 1: 117–124, 1978.

5359. Douglas, N. J., Calverley, P. M. A., Leggett, R. J. E., Brash, H. M., Flenley, D. C., and Brezinova, V. Transient hypoxemia during sleep in chronic bronchitis and emphysema. Lancet i: 1–4, 1979.

5360. Skatrud, J. K., Dempsey, J. A., Iber, C., and Berssenbrugge, A. Correction of CO_2 retention during sleep in patients with chronic obstructive pulmonary disease. Am. Rev. Respir. Dis. 124: 260–268, 1981.

5361. Koo, K. W., Sax, D. S., and Snider, G. L. Arterial blood gases and pH during sleep in chronic obstructive pulmonary disease. Am. J. Med. 58: 663–670, 1975.

5362. Leitch, A. G., Clancy, L. J., Leggett, R. J. E., Tweedale, P., Dawson, P., and Evans, J. I. Arterial blood gas tensions, hydrogen ion and electroencephalogram during sleep in patients with chronic ventilatory failure. Thorax 31: 730–735, 1976.

5363. Mao, Y., Semenciw, R., Morrison, H., MacWilliam, L., Davies, J., and Wigle, D. Increased rates of illness and death from asthma in Canada. Can. Med. Assoc. J. 137: 620–624, 1987.

5364. Abraham, A. S., Cole, R. B., and Bishop, J. M. Reversal of pulmonary hypertension by prolonged oxygen administration to patients with chronic bronchitis. Circ. Res. 23: 147–157, 1968.

5365. Leggett, R. J., Cooke, N. J., Clancy, L., Leitch, A. G., Kirby, B. J., and Flenley, D. C. Long term domiciliary oxygen therapy in cor pulmonale complicating chronic bronchitis and emphysema. Thorax 31: 414–418, 1976.

5366. Flick, M. R. and Block, A. J. Nocturnal vs. diurnal arrhythmias in patients with chronic obstructive pulmonary disease. Chest 75: 8–11, 1979.

5367. Tirlapur, V. E. and Mir, M. A. Nocturnal hypoxemia and associated electrocardiographic changes in patients with chronic obstructive airways disease. N. Engl. J. Med. 306: 125–130, 1982.

5368. Fleetham, J. A., Fera, T., Edgell, G., and Jamal, K. The effect of theophylline therapy on sleep disorders in COPD patients (abstract). Am. Rev. Respir. Dis. 127: 85, 1983.

5369. Turner-Warwick, M. On observing patterns of airflow obstruction in chronic asthma. Br. J. Dis. Chest 71: 73–86, 1977.

5370. Clark, T. J. H. and Hetzel, M. R. Diurnal variation of asthma. Chest 81: 675–680, 1982.

5371. Emergency and Continuous Exposure Guidance Levels for Selected Airborne Contaminants. Vol. 7. Board on Environmental Studies and Toxicology. National Academy Press, Washington, D. C., 1987.

5372. Shapiro, C., Montgomery, I., and Catterall, J. R. Breathing bronchoconstriction and sleep stage in nocturnal asthma (abstract). Thorax 37: 238, 1982.

5373. Catterall, J. R., Douglas, N. J., Calverley, P. M., Brash, H. M., Brezinova, V., Shapiro, C. M., and Flenley, D. C. Irregular breathing and hypoxaemia during sleep in chronic stable asthma. Lancet i: 301–304, 1982.

5374. Barnes, P., Fitzgerald, G., Brown, M., and Dollery, C. Nocturnal asthma and changes in circulating epinephrine, histamine and cortisol. N. Engl. J. Med. 303: 263–267, 1980.

5375. Clark, T. J. H. and Hetzel, M. R. Diurnal variation of asthma. Br. J. Dis. Chest 71: 87–92, 1977.

5376. O'Malley, C. D. and Saunders, J. B. deC. M. Leonardo da Vinci on the Human Body. Henry Schuman, New York, 1952.

5377. Lioy, P. J., Spektor, D., Thurston, G., Citak, K., Lippmann, M., Bock, N., Speizer, F. E., and Hayes, C. The design considerations for ozone and acid aerosol exposure and health investigations: the Fairview Lake summer camp—photochemical smog case study. Environ. Int. 13: 271–283, 1987.

5378. Fowler, W. S. Lung function studies. V. Respiratory dead space in old age and pulmonary emphysema. J. Clin. Invest. 29: 1439–1444, 1950.

5379. Comroe, J. H. Jr. (ed.). Pulmonary function tests. In: Methods in Medical Research, Vol. 2. Year Book Medical Publishers, Chicago, 1950.

5380. Dubois, A. B. New concepts in cardio-pulmonary physiology developed by the use of the body plethysmograph. Third Bowditch Lecture. Physiologist 2: 8–23, 1959.

5381. Mead, J. Volume displacement body plethysmograph for respiratory measurements in human subjects. J. Appl. Physiol. 15: 736–740, 1960.

5382. Yeh, M. P., Adams, T. D., Gardner, R. M., and Yanowitz, F. G. Turbine flowmeter vs Fleisch pneumotachograph: a comparative study for exercise testing. J. Appl. Physiol. 63: 1289–1295, 1987.

5383. Nunn, J. F., Campbell, E. J. M., and Peckett, B. W. Anatomic subdivisions of the volume of respiratory dead space and the effect of the position of the jaw. J. Appl. Physiol. 14: 174–176, 1959.

5384. Agostoni, E. Mechanics of the pleural space. In: Macklem, P. T. and Mead, J. (eds.). Handbook of Physiology, Section 3, Vol. 3, Pt. 2. American Physiological Society, Bethesda, MD, 1986.

5385. Salazar, E. and Knowles, J. M. An analysis of pressure-volume characteristics of the lungs. J. Appl. Physiol. 19: 97–104, 1964.

5386. Hoppin, F. G. Jr., Stithert, J. C. Jr., Greaves, I. A., Lai, Y.-H., and Hildebrandt, J. Lung recoil: elastic and rheological properties. In: Macklem, P. T. and Mead, J. (eds.). Handbook of Physiology, Section 3, Vol. 3, Pt. 1. American Physiological Society, Bethesda, MD, 1986.

5387. Bourbon, J. R. and Rieutort, M. Pulmonary surfactant: biochemistry, physiology and pathology. News Physiol. Sci. 2: 129–132, 1987.

5388. Anthonisen, N. R. Tests of mechanical function. In: Macklem, P. T. and Mead, J. (eds.). Handbook of Physiology, Section 3, Vol. 3, Pt. 2. American Physiological Society, Bethesda, MD, 1986.

5389. Hyatt, R. E. Forced expiration. In: Macklem, P. T. and Mead, J. (eds.). Handbook of Physiology, Section 3, Vol. 3, Pt. 1. American Physiological Society, Bethesda, MD, 1986.

5390. Wilson, T. A., Rodarte, J. R., and Butler, J. P. Wave-speed and viscous flow limitation. In: Macklem, P. T. and Mead, J. (eds.). Handbook of Physiology, Section 3, Vol. 3, Pt. 1. American Physiological Society, Bethesda, MD, 1986.

5391. Whipp, B. J. and Pardy, R. L. Breathing during exercise. In: Macklem, P. T. and Mead, J. (eds.). Handbook of Physiology, Section 3, Vol. 3, Pt. 2. American Physiological Society, Bethesda, MD, 1986.

5392. Milic-Emili, J. Static distribution of lung volumes. In: Macklem, P. T. and Mead, J. (eds.). Handbook of Physiology, Section 3, Vol. 3, Pt. 2. American Physiological Society, Bethesda, MD, 1986.

5393. Laine, G. A., Allen, S. J., Williams, J. P., Katz, J., Gabel,

J. C., and Drake, R. E. A new look at pulmonary oedema. News Physiol. Sci. 1: 150–153, 1986.

5394. Fidone, S. J. and Gonzalez, C. Initiation and control of chemoreceptor activity in the carotid body. In: Cherniack, N. S. and Widdicombe, J. G. (eds.). Handbook of Physiology, Section 3, Vol. 2, Pt. 1. American Physiological Society, Bethesda, MD, 1986.

5395. Fitzgerald, R. S. and Lahiri, S. Reflex responses to chemoreceptor stimulation. In: Cherniack, N. S. and Widdicombe, J. G. (eds.). Handbook of Physiology, Section 3, Vol. 2, Pt. 1. American Physiological Society, Bethesda, MD, 1986.

5396. Widdicombe, J. G. Reflexes from the upper respiratory tract. In: Cherniack, N. S. and Widdicombe, J. G. (eds.). Handbook of Physiology, Section 3, Vol. 2, Pt. 1. American Physiological Society, Bethesda, MD, 1986.

5397. Coleridge, H. M. and Coleridge, J. C. G. Reflexes evoked from tracheobronchial tree and lungs. In: Cherniack, N. S. and Widdicombe, J. G. (eds.). Handbook of Physiology, Section 3, Vol. 2, Pt. 1. American Physiological Society, Bethesda, MD, 1986.

5398. Shannon, R. Reflexes from respiratory muscles and costovertebral joints. In: Cherniack, N. S. and Widdicombe, J. G. (eds.). Handbook of Physiology, Section 3, Vol. 2, Pt. 1. American Physiological Society, Bethesda, MD, 1986.

5399. Von Euler, C. Brain stem mechanisms for generation and control of breathing pattern. In: Cherniack, N. S. and Widdicombe, J. G. (eds.). Handbook of Physiology, Section 3, Vol. 2, Pt. 1. American Physiological Society, Bethesda, MD, 1986.

5400. Siggaard-Anderson, C. The Acid-Base Status of the Blood. Munksgaard, Copenhagen, 1974.

5401. Wasserman, K., Whipp, B. J., and Casaburi, R. Respiratory control during exercise. In: Cherniack, N. S. and Widdicombe, J. G. (eds.). Handbook of Physiology, Section 3, Vol. 2, Pt. 2. American Physiological Society, Bethesda, MD, 1986.

5402. Forster, R. E. II, DuBois, A. B., Briscoe, W. A., and Fisher, A. B. The Lung: Physiological Basis of Pulmonary Function Tests. 3rd ed. Year Book Medical Publishers, Chicago, 1986.

5403. Otis, A. B. An overview of gas exchange. In: Farhi, L. E. and Tenney, S. M. (eds.). Handbook of Physiology, Section 3, Vol. 4. American Physiological Society, Bethesda, MD, 1986.

5404. Forster, R. E. Diffusion of gases across the alveolar membrane. In: Farhi, L. E. and Tenney, S. M. (eds.). Handbook

of Physiology, Section 3, Vol. 4. American Physiological Society, Bethesda, MD, 1986.

5405. Farhi, L. E. Ventilation-perfusion relationships. In: Farhi, L. E. and Tenney, S. M. (eds.). Handbook of Physiology, Section 3, Vol. 4. American Physiological Society, Bethesda, MD, 1986.

5406. West, J. B. Climbing Mount Everest without oxygen. News Physiol. Sci. 1: 23–27, 1986.

5407. Bennett, P. B. and Elliot, D. H. The Physiology and Medicine of Diving. Bailliere Tindall, London, 1975.

5408. Wanner, A. and Cutchavaree, A. Early recognition of upper airway obstruction following smoke inhalation. Am. Rev. Respir. Dis. 108: 1421–1423, 1973.

5409. Pruitt, B. A., Flemma, R. J., DiVicenti, F. C., Foley, F. D., and Mason, A. D. Pulmonary complications in burn patients. J. Thorac. Cardiovasc. Surg. 59: 7–18, 1970.

5410. Whitener, D. R., Whitener, L. M., Robertson, K. J., Baxter, C. R., and Pierce, A. K. Pulmonary function measurements in patients with thermal injury and smoke inhalation. Am. Rev. Respir. Dis. 122: 731–739, 1980.

5411. Haponik, E. F., Munster, A. M., Wise, R. A., Smith, P. L., Meyers, D. A., Britt, E. J., and Bleecker, E. R. Upper airway function in burn patients. Am. Rev. Respir. Dis. 129: 251–257, 1984.

5412. Bonsignore, G., Bellia, V., Ferrara, G., Mirabella, A., Rizzo, A., and Sciarabba, G. Reproducibility of maximum flows in air and He-O$_2$ and of ΔVmax$_{50}$ in the assessment of the site of airflow limitation. Eur. J. Respir. Dis. 61(Suppl. 106): 29–34, 1980.

5413. Bachofen, M. and Weibel, E. R. Basic patterns of tissue repair in human lungs following unspecific injury. Chest 65(Suppl.): 11S–13S, 1974.

5414. Campbell, E. J. M. and Green, J. H. The variations in intraabdominal pressure and the activity of the abdominal muscles during breathing: a study in man. J. Physiol. 122: 282–290, 1953.

5415. Druz, W. S. and Sharp, J. T. Activity of the respiratory muscles in upright and recumbent humans. J. Appl. Physiol. 51: 1552–1561, 1981.

5416. Herbison, G. J., Jaweed, M. M., and Ditunno, J. F. Muscle fiber atrophy after cast immobilization in the rat. Arch. Phys. Med. Rehabil. 59: 301–305, 1978.

5417. Green, M. Respiratory muscle testing. Bull. Eur. Physiopathol. Respir. 20: 433–436, 1984.

5418. Bates, D. V. Disturbance of respiratory function. In: Oswald, N. C. (ed.). Recent Trends in Chronic Bronchitis. Lloyd-Luke Ltd, London, 1958.

INDEX

INDEX

Page numbers followed by t refer to tables.